Pharmacology and Drug Information for Nurses

Pharmacology and Drug Information for Nurses

FOURTH EDITION

The Society of Hospital Pharmacists of Australia

W.B. Saunders
Baillière Tindall

Harcourt Brace & Company
Sydney   Philadelphia   London   Toronto

W. B. Saunders/Baillière Tindall

An imprint of
Harcourt Brace & Company, Australia
30-52 Smidmore Street, Marrickville, NSW 2204

Harcourt Brace & Company
24–28 Oval Road, London NW1 7DX

Harcourt Brace & Company
Orlando, Florida 32887

National Library of Australia Cataloguing-in-Publication Data

Pharmacology and drug information for nurses.

4th ed.
Includes index.
ISBN 0 7295 1414 5.

1. Drugs. 2. Pharmacology. 3. Nursing. I. Society of
Hospital Pharmacists of Australia.

615.1024613

Editor: Roslyn Roberts
Cover and page design: Pamela Horsnell
Proofread by Ronald W. Buck
Index compiled by Glenda Browne
Typeset in Century Old Style by Brad Turner
Printed in Australia by McPherson's Printing Group

Jeffery D. Hughes, BPharm, GradDipPharm,
MPharm
Senior Pharmacist
Sir Charles Gairdner Hospital
Perth, WA

Ann E. James, BPharm(Hons), MSHP
Senior Pharmacist
Drug Information/Clinical Trials
Alfred Hospital
Melbourne, Vic

Judith Kirby, BPharm
Pharmacist in Charge
NSW Poisons Information Centre
The Childrens Hospital
Sydney, NSW

Helen A. Kohlhardt, BSc, DipNutDiet
Dietitian
Royal North Shore Hospital
Sydney, NSW

Deborah L. Lalich, BPharm, GradDipHosp
(Formerly Senior Pharmacist, Sir Charles
Gairdner Hospital, Perth)
Perth, WA

Brian J. Lilley,
Deputy Director of Pharmacy
Royal Children's Hospital
Melbourne, Vic

Kerrie A. Love, BPharm, GradDipHospPharm
Senior Pharmacist
Royal Children's Hospital
Melbourne, Vic

Heather J. Lyall, BPharm,
GradDipHospPharm
Deputy Director of Pharmacy
Geelong Hospital
Geelong, Vic

Anne E. McFarlane, BPharm, DHP, FSHP
Consultant in Pharmacy
(Formerly Assistant Director of Pharmacy
Royal Darwin Hospital
Darwin, NT)
Castlecraig, NSW

Ross D. MacPherson, BPharm, DHP(Syd),
BMed(Hons), PhD, FSHP, MPS
Department of Primary and Emergency Care
Newcastle, NSW

Terry A. Maunsell, BPharm, FSHP, MPS
Director of Pharmacy
Prince Henry Hospital
Sydney, NSW

Richard J. Millard, MBBS, FRCS, FRACS
Associate Professor of Neurology
Department of Urology
Prince Henry and Prince of Wales Hospitals
Sydney, NSW

Kingsley Ng, MSc, BPharm, DipFDA, FAIPM,
MPS
Director of Pharmacy
Westmead and Parramatta Hospitals and
Community Health Services
Sydney, NSW

Marie Thérèse Rosenberg, PhC, FSHP
Pharmacy Consultant
Mater Misericordiae Hospitals
Brisbane, Qld

Margaret P. Shaw, PhC, MPS, MSHP
Senior Pharmacist
Sydney Eye Hospital
Sydney, NSW

Marian M. Townsend, BPharm,
DipHospPharm
Deputy Chief Pharmacist
Wollongong Campus
The Illawarra Regional Hospital
Wollongong, NSW

LIST OF REVIEWERS

Anne Adams
Senior Lecturer, Faculty of Nursing
University of Technology, Sydney
Sydney, NSW

John Alexander
Nurse Educator
Woden Valley Hospital
Canberra, ACT

David Arthur
Head, Department of Community and Mental
Health Nursing
University of Newcastle
Newcastle, NSW

Mavis Comadira
Clinical Nurse Consultant, Accident and
Emergency Department
Royal Children's Hospital
Brisbane, Qld

Julie Corby
Dermatology Centre
Lidcombe Hospital
Sydney, NSW

John Daly
Associate Professor of Nursing
Head, School of Health and Human Services
Faculty of Health Studies
Charles Sturt University
Wagga Wagga, NSW

Patricia Davidson
Clinical Research Coordinator
Cardiovascular Medicine
Prince Henry Hospital
Sydney, NSW

Anne-Marie Dunning
School of Nursing
Royal Brisbane Hospital
Brisbane, Qld

Ken Hambrecht
Coordinator, Nursing Education
Epworth Hospital
Richmond, Vic

Susan Hyde
Clinical Nurse Specialist, Oncology Unit
Sir Charles Gairdner Hospital
Perth, WA

Kirsten James
Clinical Nurse Teacher, Staff Development
Austin Hospital
Melbourne, Vic

Terry Leane
Clinical Nurse Consultant (Infection Control)
Repatriation General Hospital
Adelaide, SA

Desolie Lovegrove
Illawarra Public Health Unit
Kieraville, NSW

Belle Mangen
Cardiac Clinical Nurse Consultant
Royal North Shore Hospital
Sydney, NSW

Jenny Martin
Lecturer, Tasmanian School of Nursing
Launceston, Tas

Julienne Onley
Coordinator, Gerontological Nursing
NSW College of Nursing
Sydney, NSW

Jan Paterson
Clinical Nurse Consultant (Continence)
Repatriation General Hospital
Adelaide, SA

Carmen Pochman
School of Nursing
Royal Brisbane Hospital
Brisbane, Qld

Nita Purcal
Senior Lecturer, Midwifery
University of Western Sydney
Richmond, NSW

Sharon Rowland
Respiratory Nurse
Repatriation General Hospital
Adelaide, SA

Judy Sankey
Lecturer, Tasmanian School of Nursing
Launceston, Tas

Wendy Tomlinson
Clinical Nurse Teacher, Surgical
Austin Hospital
Melbourne, Vic

Heather Vogelzang
Clinical Nurse Consultant, Psychiatry
Repatriation General Hospital
Adelaide, SA

Bronwyn Walkem
Coordinator, Third Year Bachelor of Nursing
Tasmanian School of Nursing
Launceston, Tas

CONTENTS ▆▆▆▆▆▆▆▆▆▆▆▆▆▆▆▆▆▆

LIST OF TABLES

LIST OF FIGURES

PREFACE

In planning for the fourth edition of *Pharmacology and drug information for nurses* it was necessary to take into account the changes that had occurred not only in drug development and the clinical use of drugs but also the changes that had occurred in nurse education. Attention had to be given to ensuring that the information contained in the text satisfied the requirements of the nurse studying in the university environment. The content of the fourth edition has been increased accordingly. Drug monographs have been expanded to include mechanisms of action; pharmacokinetics; detailed information on drug doses; instructions for drug administration; and the precautions to be observed when administering drugs to patients.

The first section of the book has been totally revised with the first two chapters focussing on the basic principles of pharmacology – pharmacodynamics and pharmacokinetics. The original format of utilising disease states as chapter topics has been retained and several new chapters have been added, including liver disease, drugs used in critical care, drug therapy in pregnancy and labour, and a chapter on drug administration which discusses the nurse's responsibilities as part of the medication team. With the extension of the nurse's role in this area, especially with regard to the administration of intravenous doses of drugs, it is important that the nurse is aware of the legal and other issues relating to safe drug administration.

The format of this edition has been radically changed to speed its use as a reference text. New features are: expanded drug and drug group monographs with information listed under standardised headings; chapter numbers and titles on the right margins which function as a thumb index; chapter titles on left hand pages and important chapter sections on right hand pages; learning objectives at the beginning of chapters; test your knowledge questions at the end of chapters with answers provided at the end of the book; and a useful index listing generic names in bold, trade names in italic with cross references to generic names. We trust that nurses will find these changes of benefit.

My thanks go to the team of authors who have contributed to this edition. With the ever increasing demands placed on today's health care professional it is very much to their credit that they have so willingly given of their time and expertise to make this publication possible.

My special acknowledgements go to Ms Virginia Richardson and Mr Chris Alderman for their guidance in the development of this new edition; to the editorial panel, Dr Ross Holland, Ms Ros McKinnon, Ms Treasure McGuire and Dr Greg Peterson, who so ably assisted me with this production; and to my husband Peter for his support throughout the project.

I trust that the information contained in these pages will provide a useful tool for our nursing colleagues in their professional practice.

Margaret Duguid
Editorial Coordinator

General Principles

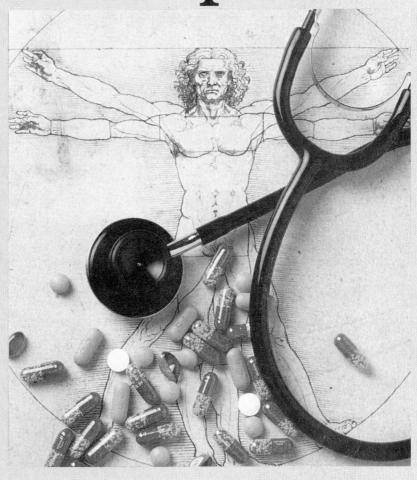

Pharmacodynamics

CHRISTOPHER P. ALDERMAN

O B J E C T I V E S

At the conclusion of this chapter the reader should be able to:

1. Describe the various ways in which drugs act;

2. Outline factors which may influence individual response to drug therapy;

3. Outline factors which may contribute to adverse drug reactions;

4. Describe the basis of interactions between drugs and the management of these interactions; and

5. Identify the patient at risk for drug dependence or withdrawal, list drugs causing dependence and describe the complications of intravenous drug abuse.

PHARMACODYNAMICS

The science of pharmacodynamics is complementary to that of pharmacokinetics and may be described as the study of the way in which drugs produce their various effects within the body. A consideration of pharmacodynamics addresses not only the mechanisms by which a drug produces a therapeutic effect, but also the adverse effects of the drug, the effects of concurrent administration of other drugs, the influence of patient specific factors, such as sex, age and weight, and the effects of long-term drug therapy. Whilst pharmacokinetic influences may account for variations in individual response, differences in drug activity may also result from pharmacodynamic variation. Careful consideration of the known pharmacodynamic characteristics of drugs used in the treatment of the individual patient can be a useful tool in tailoring drug therapy for maximum therapeutic effect with minimum unwanted reactions.

MECHANISMS OF DRUG ACTION

Research has revealed that drugs produce their effects in the body through a variety of complex mechanisms. An understanding of a drug's mechanism of action allows the design of other drug therapy with improved efficacy and can sometimes be used to predict and manage toxicities. In some situations the action of drugs mimics or modifies a normal bodily process which occurs under the influence of endogenous compounds (compounds produced within the body). In other cases, the mechanism of drug action remains unclear, and the knowledge of the effects of the drug within the body is based largely on individual observations and population data.

Some drugs are known to act through a number of possible mechanisms and in some cases beneficial effects and adverse reactions may arise through different pathways and mechanisms. For example, sulfonamides produce a therapeutic antimicrobial effect by interfering with bacterial metabolism, whilst their dermatological adverse effects are thought to be hypersensitivity reactions.

RECEPTORS

With many drugs, effects within the body are caused by a chemical interaction between the drug and a structure within the body referred to as a receptor.

Endogenous compounds, such as hormones and neurotransmitters, have been identified as chemical compounds which interact with, or bind to, receptors and produce a physiological effect. The end effect of this interaction is usually modification of a physiological or biochemical process and an alteration in the rate, extent or nature of the function concerned. For example, when the neurotransmitter acetylcholine binds to its receptors on muscle tissue the muscle fibres contract. The binding of compounds to receptors may also produce a decrease in the rate or extent of a physiological process.

Not uncommonly it is the results of observation of the physiological or biochemical effects of endogenous compounds which are utilised in drug design. In some cases the chemical structure of the drug bears little resemblance to the endogenous compound, in other cases it is identical. For example, by modifying the genetic code of certain bacteria or yeasts it is possible to artificially produce compounds normally found within the body. These methods, sometimes referred to as *genetic engineering techniques* or *recombinant DNA technology*, allow the artificial production of proteins and hormones which are identical in structure and activity to those normally found in the human body. Examples of these types of drug products in use in clinical practice are synthetic human growth hormone, human insulin and erythropoietin.

Drugs which produce similar effects to endogenous compounds are referred to as **agonists**, whilst those which produce an opposite effect are called **antagonists**.

Agonists are compounds which bind to a receptor and produce a physiological effect similar to, but possibly of lesser or greater intensity, the effect observed when the receptor is bound by the naturally occurring hormone or neurotransmitter. On the other hand, when an antagonist binds to a receptor, the effect is usually a decrease in the rate or extent of the physiological function. An antagonist usually works as a receptor blocker. The antagonist binds to the receptor in competition with the normal physiological compound and this competition reduces the intensity, rate or extent of the function of the cell or organ system. When binding to the receptor the antagonist may, but not always, produce an effect in its own right, and this effect can be similar or different to that produced by the natural compound.

Further research has revealed that subclasses of receptors exist and that under certain circumstances a given drug may act as both a receptor agonist and antagonist. For example, opioid drugs such as morphine bind to a variety of receptors which appear to have separate effects. Some produce analgesic effects while others may be responsible for side effects such as sedation, respiratory depression or euphoria. The so-called partial opioid agonists may produce analgesia without causing all the side effects associated with drugs of this type. Naloxone, however, is a pure opioid antagonist and is used to reverse effects of opioids, e.g. respiratory depression.

ENZYME INHIBITORS

Not all drugs act by direct binding to receptor sites. Enzymes are proteins found throughout the body and serve as catalysts for various chemical reactions which occur in the course of the normal functions of organ systems. Enzymes usually facilitate the conversion of one chemical compound to another. In some cases the chemical is converted from an active compound into one with little or no pharmacological activity, whilst in others the conversion results in the production of a chemical with enhanced pharmacological properties.

Enzymatic degradation is the mechanism by which endogenous neurotransmitters are inactivated. Drugs such as the cholinesterase inhibitors (e.g. physostigmine, neostigmine) will prolong and augment the activity of the neurotransmitter acetylcholine producing an effect similar to that caused by a receptor agonist. In the converse situation, drugs may produce a therapeutic effect by inhibiting the conversion of an inactive compound into one with a pharmacological effect. For example, the angiotensin converting enzyme inhibitors such as captopril and enalapril act by preventing the transformation of angiotensin I to angiotensin II, a potent pressor compound which causes increased blood pressure.

The inhibition of enzyme activity may be reversible, that is the administration of a sufficient dose of an antagonist drug will reverse the net pharmacological effect. For example, the administration of atropine, an antagonist of acetylcholine, can reverse the cholinergic effects of anticholinesterase drugs such as neostigmine. On the other hand, enzyme inhibition may be irreversible, that is the body must synthesise new enzyme before the effects of the inhibitor are diminished. For example, some monoamine oxidase inhibitors (MAOIs) produce irreversible inhibition of the enzymes responsible for the degradation of neurotransmitters in the central nervous system thus producing their antidepressant effects. Irreversible inhibition also occurs in other enzyme systems which catalyse the breakdown of vasoactive amines such as tyramine in the gut wall and liver and this is responsible for the important drug–drug and drug–food interactions associated with this type of drug. The body must synthesise new monoamine oxidase enzymes before the effects of the inhibitor are diminished. This process usually takes 14–21 days, the 'washout time' commonly recommended before the commencement of drug therapy which may cause an interaction.

ANTIMETABOLITES

Some drugs act by interfering with the normal biochemical reactions which take place at a subcellular level. Drugs which act as antimetabolites are often very similar in chemical structure to substances utilised by cells in normal biochemical processes. However, subtle differences in structure mean that whilst the cell may use the compound as a substrate in a chemical reaction, the result of that reaction will not be the same as that of the endogenous compound. The biochemical function of the cell or even the rate of cell multiplication or division may subsequently be altered, producing a therapeutic effect. The drawback with many antimetabolite drugs is that their activity is relatively non-selective.

The antimetabolite drugs include a number of the antineoplastic agents, which are absorbed by dividing cells and utilised in the production of nucleic acids. For example, when cytarabine is absorbed into the dividing cell the similarity of the drug to the native nucleotide appears to inhibit the activity of enzymes involved in the synthesis of nucleic acids. Furthermore, a modified derivative of cytarabine may be incorporated into the nucleic acids, producing DNA and RNA which does not function in the same fashion as the normal genetic material.

However, cytarabine is utilised by all cell lines, particularly those which are rapidly dividing. Thus, as well as the rapidly dividing cell lines of a neoplasm, these drugs exert a cytotoxic effect on other cell lines which are rapidly multiplying, e.g. blood, hair and skin cells and cells in the gastrointestinal lining, producing side effects such as anaemia, leucopenia, alopecia and mouth ulcers.

MISCELLANEOUS MECHANISMS

Some drugs are specifically designed to have highly selective activity. For example, many antibiotics are highly toxic to bacterial cells whilst producing no significant effects on the metabolic pathways of the host organism. Penicillins exert a bactericidal effect through inhibition of mucopeptide synthesis in the bacterial cell wall causing the cell wall to break down. Mammalian cells do not have a cell wall (simply a cell membrane) and are not affected by this action of the penicillins.

The concept of administering an externally derived compound normally produced by the body has been used therapeutically for some time. For example, a blood transfusion replaces blood lost due to trauma or surgery. Similarly, immunoglobulins derived from donated blood may be administered in a variety of clinical settings to boost or confer immunity.

As already discussed it is now possible to produce a range of biologically active compounds which are identical to endogenous compounds by using genetic engineering techniques. The use of drugs produced in this fashion has a number of advantages including minimisation of adverse effects, less risk of transmissible disease associated with products of animal or human source, and the opportunity to avoid the lessening of effect associated with the production of antibodies against proteins of foreign origin.

Antigens are used therapeutically in order to provoke an immune response. For example, preparations of attenuated or killed virus or bacteria are used as vaccines, causing the patient to produce an antibody to that organism and conferring immunity against infection with that pathogen.

Specific antibodies may also be administered therapeutically, and with the refinement of biological manufacturing techniques it is now possible to produce antibodies with a highly specific target site. Muromonab-CD3 is a monoclonal antibody directed against a site on the surface of human T cells and is used as an immunosuppressive agent to reduce rejection of transplanted organs.

Table 1.1 summarises the possible mechanisms of drug action.

TABLE 1.1   Possible mechanisms of drug action

Drug	Therapeutic Use(s)	Proposed Mechanism of Action
RECEPTOR AGONISTS		
β_2 Adrenergic agonists (e.g. salbutamol terbutaline, fenoterol)	Asthma, premature labour	Produce effects on smooth muscle tone (e.g. bronchial, uterine) through selective agonism at β_2 adrenoreceptors
RECEPTOR ANTAGONISTS		
α_1 Adrenergic blockers (e.g. prazosin)	Hypertension	Antagonise contraction of smooth muscle in walls of blood vessels caused by stimulation of α_1 adrenoreceptors
β blocking drugs (e.g. atenolol, metoprolol, propranolol)	Angina, hypertension	Block adrenergic stimulation of β adrenergic receptors in the myocardium and vascular smooth muscle
ENZYME INHIBITORS		
Reversible Angiotensin converting enzyme inhibitors (e.g. captopril, enalapril)	Hypertension, heart failure	Prevents conversion of angiotensin I to angiotensin II (a potent pressor amine)
Irreversible Monoamine oxidase inhibitors (e.g. phenelzine)	Depression, post-traumatic stress disorders	Inhibits degradation of biogenic amines (e.g. noradrenaline) in CNS neuronal synapses by various enzymes
ANTIMETABOLITES		
Pyrimidine nucleosides (e.g. cytarabine)	Cancer chemotherapy	Thought to interfere with DNA synthesis through inhibition of DNA polymerase and limited incorporation in nucleic acids
VACCINES		
Hepatitis B vaccine	Prevention of infection with hepatitis B virus	Recombinantly generated hepatitis B surface antigen stimulates host production of protective antibodies

FACTORS INFLUENCING DRUG RESPONSE

Numerous factors play a role in the response of the patient to a given drug treatment regimen. Some of these influences are explainable in terms of their effects on the pharmacokinetics of the drug, although not all variation in individual response is due to differences in the rate or extent of drug absorption, distribution or elimination. Indeed, in the case of two patients with identical drug plasma levels the therapeutic response may differ. In this situation the judgement of the attending clinician, supported by the input of other members of the health care team, is vital in tailoring drug therapy for optimum results.

DISEASE STATE

In some cases the observed response will depend on the disease state being treated. For example, an advanced condition may not respond in the same fashion to the same drugs as the same disease when active intervention has been instituted at an early stage. The benefits of early intervention are clearly demonstrated in the case of many malignancies, the treatment of psychotic illness and depression and the early treatment of HIV infection and its complications.

In other cases the disease state may predispose the patient to drug effects not seen in other patients. For example, immediately after a cerebrovascular accident, the patient is more susceptible to the hypotensive effects of vasodilating drugs such as hydralazine or prazosin, and syncopal episodes may result. Drugs which produce tachycardia or bradycardia should be avoided if possible in the patient who has recently suffered a myocardial infarction, disturbances in heart rate may precipitate potentially serious ventricular arrhythmias.

For reasons presently unknown, patients with human immunodeficiency virus (HIV) infection are more prone to develop adverse skin reactions to sulfonamides used in the treatment of opportunistic infections than are those without HIV infection.

AGE

The influence of age on individual drug response is often profound. Not uncommonly this can be explained in terms of the drug's pharmacokinetic characteristics. For example, the rate of drug elimination may be different in a neonate, pre-pubescent child, young healthy adult or elderly person. For a more detailed discussion of pharmacokinetics in the extremes of age see Chapter 5 Paediatric Therapeutics and Chapter 6 Geriatric Therapeutics.

On the other hand, pharmacokinetic differences do not always explain variations in drug response observed in specific age groups, e.g. *elderly patients* appear to be much more sensitive to the effects of central nervous system drugs. The 5-year survival rate for *children* treated for some forms of haematological malignancies appears to be considerably better than that of adults in whom intervention has been initiated at approximately the same stage of disease progression. *Neonates* respond in a radically different fashion to other age groups when treated with some drug therapies. The response of the *fetus* to drugs is poorly understood and complicated by variability in drug access across the placenta, and because maternal responses to drugs may be altered in both a pharmacokinetic and pharmacodynamic sense during pregnancy. Also, in addition to producing a pharmacological effect in the fetus, a number of drugs are known to interfere with the normal development of the fetus in utero, see

Chapter 7 Drug Safety in Pregnancy and Lactation.

BODY WEIGHT

In some cases, drug dosage is determined on the basis of the patient's weight. Whilst useful as a broad and general guide, this approach has numerous limitations. Adjustments are frequently necessary in obesity, fluid overload, cachexia, limb amputation and so on. In these situations alternative approaches may be based on ideal body weight, predicted lean body mass or body surface areas. These adjustments are particularly important for drugs with a therapeutic dose close to that dose which produces significant toxicity. These drugs are referred to as drugs of *low therapeutic index* and include digoxin, lithium, anticoagulants, aminoglycoside antibiotics, anticonvulsants and theophylline.

PSYCHOLOGICAL FACTORS

The influence of psychological factors on drug response is poorly understood. For example, the treatment of depressive illness in a patient with chronic pain may lead to an increase in the efficacy of analgesic treatments. However, antidepressants may augment the activity of analgesic drugs even when the presence of clinical depression cannot be demonstrated. Similarly, anxiety states may also influence the outcome of drug therapy.

ADVERSE DRUG REACTIONS ████████

The use of drug therapy for therapeutic purposes is almost always associated with some degree of risk for unexpected and potentially harmful effects. These untoward effects are commonly referred to as *side effects* or *adverse drug reactions* (ADRs). The complex and comprehensive screening process applied prior to the release of drugs onto the general market usually means that the adverse effects profile of a drug is often well established before its widespread use. However, the relatively unpredictable nature of these reactions means that adverse reactions to drugs remain a relatively common and important therapeutic problem.

An adverse drug reaction may arise through mechanisms related to the manner in which the drug produces its therapeutic effects. For example, the drug may produce a response of unexpected or excessive intensity — oral hypoglycaemic drugs have been implicated in hypoglycaemic episodes. To some degree, these types of ADRs are the most predictable and may be prevented or managed with the use of close monitoring.

Another example of this type of effect is when the ADR is not an excessive therapeutic response but may be predicted in terms of the drug's pharmacological action. Knowledge of the drug's mechanism of action can be used to predict and manage adverse effects. For example, leucopenia associated with many cytotoxic drugs can be managed by administration of cell colony stimulating factors or appropriate prophylactic antibiotic cover. The likelihood of side effects is increased when two drugs with similar ADR profiles are administered concurrently (e.g. in some combination chemotherapy regimens) and may need to be managed through dose reductions for one or both drugs.

Adverse effects may also arise through pharmacological properties unrelated to the therapeutic actions of the compound. For example, with the potassium sparing diuretic, spironolactone, the oestrogenic effects of the drug are not involved in the production of diuresis but are known to cause gynaecomastia (breast enlargement) in some patients.

In many cases the adverse effects of drug therapy cannot be predicted from the drug's pharmacological properties. These reactions are sometimes called *idiosyncratic adverse effects* and range in nature from relatively minor effects such as skin rash through to serious drug induced illnesses such as blood dyscrasias, hepatitis and anaphylactic reactions. For example, adverse reactions to the commonly used penicillin antibiotics are most commonly manifested as transient skin rashes of relatively minor significance. However, a small proportion of patients treated with these drugs will suffer a life threatening anaphylactic reaction. About one patient in every one hundred thousand treated with penicillin will suffer a fatal allergic reaction and there may be no indication that the patient is sensitive to the drug. Allergic reactions to penicillins demonstrate the necessity for clear documentation of previous adverse drug reactions in the patient's file. Nearly a quarter of patients who die from allergic reactions to penicillins have had a previous adverse reaction to these drugs.

A number of patient-specific factors may predispose the individual to an adverse drug reaction. The disease state being treated may directly contribute to the risk of side effects. Patients undergoing chemotherapy for advanced malignancies are at greater risk for leucopenia if the disease has already infiltrated the bone marrow. The incidence of skin rashes and other adverse drug reactions in patients treated with antibiotics for opportunistic infections resulting from HIV infection is greater than that observed for patients receiving therapy for other reasons. As already mentioned elderly patients appear more sensitive to the central nervous system effects of many commonly used drugs. Genetic variations in drug metabolism also may increase the likelihood of ADRs with some drugs. For example, the incidence of hydrazine induced hepatitis resulting from treatment with drugs such as phenelzine, isoniazid or hydralazine is higher in slow acetylator phenotypes. In some cases, an external influence may precipitate an adverse drug reaction (e.g. myelosuppression resulting from concurrent chemotherapy and radiotherapy or drug induced photosensitivity reactions). The risk of adverse drug reactions increases in proportion with the number of drugs in the treatment regimen. The elderly patient, often treated with multiple drug therapy and suffering from multisystem diseases, is at special risk of adverse drug reactions.

Under some circumstance an adverse effect which is of relatively minor significance can assume greater importance. For example, hypokalaemia resulting from diuretic use will be of greater significance in the patient also treated with digoxin as the cardiac effects of this drug are enhanced when serum potassium levels are low. Many antihypertensive drugs produce postural hypotension. In elderly patients with osteoporosis (which itself may be drug induced) falls caused by postural hypotension may result in fractures which in turn may necessitate extended hospitalisation.

An important consideration when choosing drug treatment regimens is the risk of adverse drug reactions relative to the effects of the untreated disease. The use of a drug with a high risk of relatively serious adverse effects may be justifiable in the context of a life threatening disease such as metastatic carcinoma, but is insupportable as therapy for a minor disease.

Much of the information used in predicting and preventing ADRs is gathered through voluntary reporting systems. In the event of an adverse drug reaction, it is important that the attending clinician or pharmacist (supported by the input of the health care team) provide details of the adverse reaction and the circumstances surrounding it to the appropriate regulatory body. Details of all ADRs which result in death, admission to hospital, prolongation of hospitalisation or significant morbidity must be reported. In addition, reactions which involve newly marketed or investigational drugs or those which result in congenital birth defects should also be reported promptly.

The considerable range and diversity of adverse reactions to drugs precludes an exhaustive discussion here. Readers should refer to specialist texts for detailed information when necessary.

DRUG INTERACTIONS ■■■■■■■■■■■■ **1**■

The use of more than one drug in a given treatment regimen may give rise to alterations in the therapeutic properties or adverse effect profile for one or more of the drugs involved. The phenomenon whereby the effects of one drug are altered by the concurrent administration of another is referred to as a drug interaction.

Drug interactions may be of minor or major significance and arise through a variety of mechanisms. The potential for drug interactions need not prevent combined treatment. In most cases careful planning and consideration of the pharmacological properties of both drugs and the expected effects of combined therapy will allow appropriate compensatory adjustments to the planned treatment regimen. Because of the variation in individual response to drug therapy certain combinations of drugs may be used without ill effects in some patients, whereas in others the same combination may cause a serious adverse reaction.

Drug interactions may occur with a wide range of medications and the nature and extent of the interaction in the individual patient may vary considerably. Drugs most commonly implicated in important interactions tend to be those of low therapeutic index, e.g. anticonvulsants, theophylline, anticoagulants and lithium. For specific information on drug interactions it is important to refer to a drug information centre, clinical pharmacist or appropriate specialist texts.

PHARMACODYNAMIC INTERACTIONS

Pharmacodynamic drug interactions usually arise as a result of pharmacological or physiological effects common to both drugs involved. These effects may be additive or may work in opposition, thus producing either intensification or diminution of therapeutic or adverse effects. For example, when angiotensin converting enzyme (ACE) inhibitors are administered in the treatment of congestive heart failure their hypotensive effects will be additive with those produced by nitrates administered for the prevention of angina. Another example is the additive sedative and respiratory depressant effects observed when two or more drugs with these properties (e.g. opioids, benzodiazepines, barbiturates, phenothiazines) are administered concurrently. Conversely, the diuretic effect of frusemide or the thiazides may be partially antagonised by the concurrent administration of the non-steroidal anti-inflammatory drugs (NSAIDs) as these drugs may cause sodium and water retention. In some cases, the precise mechanism of

pharmacodynamic interaction remains unclear. For example, the combined use of allopurinol and amoxycillin or ampicillin is known to be associated with an increased incidence of skin rash over and above that observed with the use of either drug alone, although these drugs share no immediately obvious pharmacological connection. Examples of some important pharmacodynamic drug interactions are listed in Table 1.2.

PHARMACOKINETIC INTERACTIONS

Drug interactions may also arise from an alteration in the pharmacokinetic properties of one drug caused by another.

Altered Drug Absorption

Before a drug can produce any effect in the body it must reach its site of action. Some drugs are administered directly into the systemic circulation, others must be absorbed after oral administration (see Chapter 2 Pharmacokinetics). Where two or more

TABLE 1.2. Examples of pharmacodynamic drug interactions

Drug	Drug	Interaction and Proposed Mechanism
ACE inhibitors (e.g. captopril, enalapril, lisinopril)	NSAIDs (e.g. naproxen, ibuprofen)	Decreased hypotensive effects of ACE inhibitors related to inhibition of renal prostaglandin synthesis
Ampicillin, Amoxycillin	Allopurinol	Increased incidence of skin rash — mechanism unclear
Benzodiazepines (e.g. diazepam)	Opioids (e.g. morphine)	Additive respiratory depression — both decrease central respiratory drive in the brainstem
Diuretics (e.g. frusemide)	Digoxin	Diuretic induced hypokalaemia enhances the effects of digoxin on the myocardium

drugs are administered at the same time, the oral absorption of one or both agents may be altered by a variety of mechanisms. In some cases the drugs may bind together chemically in the gut and the resulting complex cannot be absorbed completely. For example, tetracycline binds to calcium, magnesium or aluminium ions in antacid preparations and concurrent administration will lead to inadequate absorption of this antibiotic. Another example is cholestyramine, a resin administered in the treatment of elevated blood lipids. This drug may bind to others (e.g. warfarin, digoxin) interfering with their absorption. Cholestyramine also decreases bile acids in the bowel, hence if absorption of a drug (e.g. cyclosporin A) is dependent on the presence of bile acids serum levels may be decreased. Another mechanism by which a drug interaction influencing absorption may arise is when a drug affects the rate of passage of another compound through the gut. The rate at which some drugs (e.g. the antifungal agent griseofulvin) are absorbed is slow, and the concurrent administration of a drug which decreases bowel transit time (e.g. cisapride) may lead to incomplete absorption.

Altered Drug Elimination

HEPATIC ENZYME INDUCTION AND INHIBITION

Important drug interactions may result from the influence of one drug on the elimination of another. In many cases the concurrent administration of a drug may affect the hepatic metabolism of a second drug. The administration of anticonvulsant drugs or the antitubercular drug rifampicin commonly leads to an increase in the rate of hepatic drug metabolism. This effect is referred to as hepatic enzyme induction and, by increasing the rate of metabolic elimination, can lead to decreased plasma levels of the second drug with possible loss of therapeutic effect. This is particularly important when a strong indication exists for effective treatment. For example, the addition of carbamazepine to the regimen of a patient already receiving warfarin as prophylaxis against pulmonary embolism may lead to a loss of anticoagulant efficacy with potentially serious consequences. Another potential hazard is that the dose of the second drug is sometimes increased to compensate

TABLE 1.3 Examples of pharmacokinetic drug interactions

Drug	Drug	Interaction and Proposed Mechanism
Digoxin	Cholestyramine	Digoxin serum levels decreased — decreased oral absorption caused by cholestyramine
Oral anticoagulants (e.g. warfarin)	Rifampicin	Anticoagulant effects decreased — hepatic metabolism of warfarin induced by rifampicin
Theophylline	Erythromycin	Elevation of serum theophylline levels with possible toxicity — hepatic metabolism of theophylline inhibited by erythromycin
Lithium	NSAIDs (e.g. indomethacin)	Elevation of lithium levels — compromised renal excretion (exact mechanism remains unclear)

for the loss of therapeutic effect. If the interacting therapy is later ceased the dose of the second drug must be reduced to previous levels to avoid the administration of a potentially toxic dose.

Conversely, drug interactions may give rise to a decrease in the rate of hepatic metabolism, *hepatic enzyme inhibition*. Plasma levels of the second drug may rise producing unintended toxicity. Cimetidine, quinolone antibiotics and erythromycin are examples of drugs which produce hepatic enzyme inhibition.

MODIFICATION OF RENAL CLEARANCE

Drug interactions may also result from alterations in the renal excretion of a compound. An important example of this type of interaction is the decrease in renal clearance of lithium caused by the addition of diuretic therapy and the increase in serum lithium levels which results. In another example this type of interaction is utilised therapeutically. Probenecid competes with penicillins for tubular secretion in the kidney and is used clinically to increase serum penicillin levels in the treatment of some infections (e.g. osteomyelitis).

Some examples of pharmacokinetic drug interactions are listed in Table 1.3.

DRUG–FOOD INTERACTIONS

In a small number of cases there are demonstrated important interactions between drugs and foods. The monoamine oxidase inhibitors (MAOIs) include phenelzine and tranylcypromine and are irreversible inhibitors of enzymes which play a role in the breakdown of amine compounds. The amino acid tyramine is found in high concentrations in a limited number of foods (e.g. matured cheese, yeast extract spreads) and is a potent pressor amine. If these foods are eaten whilst the patient is being treated with an MAOI there may be a sudden, hazardous increase in blood pressure which in some cases has led to fatal complications such as cerebral haemorrhage. See Chapter 26 Psychiatric Disorders.

DRUG ABUSE AND DEPENDENCE ▮

DRUG ABUSE

The nature and actions of some types of drugs have given rise to their use for purposes other than those for which they are usually prescribed. In some cases the drug is obtained from illicit sources or with fraudulent prescriptions. Drug abuse loosely refers to the use of drugs of any description for purposes other than a legitimate therapeutic indication. The phenomenon of drug abuse is not new. Compounds such as alcohol, cannabis, cocaine and opium have been subject to abuse by various civilisations for hundreds of years.

The abuse of drugs may be recreational in nature, with the compound self-administered for perceived pleasurable effects or deliberate alteration of mood, producing euphoric or depressive effects. This type of drug abuse accounts for a substantial proportion of non-medical drug use, in particular the use of alcohol or tobacco products is common throughout a variety of societies. The widespread use of tobacco and alcohol is undoubtedly costly in terms of morbidity and mortality, as well as in less definable problems such as domestic violence and loss of productivity in the workplace. The occupational health ramifications of drug abuse in the industrial setting have received considerable attention.

The abuse of opioid drugs originated with the use of opium resin for recreational purposes by various civilisations. Today, the most commonly abused opioid drug is heroin, administered by a variety of routes including by injection. Intravenous heroin use carries a significant risk of drug dependence, as well as a multiplicity of medical and psychiatric complications. Doses are poorly standardised and fatal drug overdose with intravenous opioids is not uncommon. Often, heroin powder is adulterated with various contaminants such as lactose or talc, which in themselves may produce serious complications when administered intravenously, particularly on a long-term basis. The intravenous abuse of drugs has always carried the risk of infectious complications through poor injection techniques or contaminated materials. Sharing of needles or syringes between users has now become a major mode of transmission of HIV. Amphetamines are also abused intravenously and are associated with similar hazards.

A variety of other substances are also abused for recreational purposes. Some, such as cannabis or cocaine, are not usually available through legitimate channels. Others are the so-called 'designer drugs' which are synthetic derivatives of opioids or amphetamines with separate and distinct pharmacological profiles to those of the parent drugs. However, many drugs subject to abuse are actually supplied through conventional means.

Benzodiazepines, barbiturates and narcotic analgesics are all subject to abuse and dependence. A number of educational campaigns designed to minimise the abuse of prescription medicines have been aimed at both prescribers and the community in general.

A different type of drug abuse is that which is directed at specific purposes other than recreation. Stimulant drugs are sometimes self-administered to increase or maintain vigilance or relieve fatigue. Another important type of drug abuse is the growing use of drugs to enhance sporting performance or physical stature. Although anabolic steroids are probably the most notorious example of drug abuse in sport, numerous other instances exist. Some boxers and jockeys use diuretics for the purpose of weight loss, whilst some shooters and archers use β blockers for their steadying effect on aim. A number of fatalities have occurred in cyclists after recombinant erythropoietin was used to stimulate red blood cell production. A much more common example is the use of analgesic drugs to enable athletes to compete even when seriously injured.

DRUG DEPENDENCE

A major risk associated with drug abuse is that of drug dependence. The opioids, amphetamines, cocaine, nicotine, alcohol, benzodiazepines and barbiturates are amongst the drugs which are known to be associated with the syndrome of drug dependence. Both physiological and psychological components may contribute to drug dependence, which has also been called drug addiction. The patient with drug dependence will exhibit drug seeking behaviour and, given the expensive nature of some of the drugs involved (particularly illicit drugs), it is not surprising that drug dependence is associated with criminal activity such as theft, prostitution or drug dealing. Although treatment programs can be instituted with success in some instances, drug dependence usually has a poor prognosis with a very high rate of relapse.

Physical Dependence

The physiological changes induced by chronic drug abuse are associated with the process of physical drug dependence and, in the event of sudden cessation of use of this type of drug (e.g. narcotics, cocaine), it is not uncommon for the patient to undergo a *withdrawal reaction*. The features of a withdrawal reaction often include psychological symptoms (e.g. dysphoria, anxiety, agitation). Physical features such as fever, tachycardia, lability of blood pressure and sweating can accompany effects on mental state and, if left untreated, may progress to major autonomic instability or seizures which are difficult to control. Such effects carry a significant risk of mortality. The syndrome of opioid withdrawal is often distinctly different to that observed with other drugs, and may include features such as nausea and vomiting, diarrhoea, yawning, watery eyes and nose and diffuse body pain. It is crucial that patients at risk are closely monitored to prevent progression to serious complications. Medical staff should be promptly contacted if any signs of drug withdrawal are observed, allowing the early institution of management strategies.

Psychological Dependence

It is important to recognise the psychological aspects of drug dependence as distinct from the physiological changes described above. Anxiety, depression and other psychiatric illnesses are common in patients with drug dependence and in many cases it is difficult to differentiate between cause and effect. Cultural and ethnic influences and the patient's medical history may be important in this regard. Drug dependence may originate from the legitimate use of drugs such as analgesics or sedatives during chronic illness.

The importance of community education programs in the prevention of drug abuse and dependence cannot be understated. Tragically, the high price of drug abuse is often extracted from the young, and resources and personnel must be directed at addressing this enormous problem as an issue of the highest priority.

1

PHARMACODYNAMICS

NURSING IMPLICATIONS

ASSESSMENT

An important aspect of nursing assessment of the patient is an appraisal of the current and planned drug therapy for safety and efficacy. Factors to consider include an assessment of the mechanism of action of the drug or drugs and screening for additive or conflicting pharmacodynamic effects.

Through their knowledge of the potential adverse effects of drugs, nurses should screen for preventable side effects and at the same time evaluate the potential for drug interactions. Where relevant, the nursing assessment should also address the potential in the patient for drug abuse, dependence and withdrawal reactions.

EVALUATION

Nursing evaluation involves recognition of the duplication of pharmacological effects and monitoring of biochemical or physiological parameters which are indicators of pharmacodynamic effects.

Another essential facet of nursing evaluation is screening for potential drug interactions and adverse drug reactions and management of these where relevant.

For the patient at risk of a drug withdrawal reaction it is important that rigorous evaluation for signs of withdrawal be instituted. The use of standard observation 'scoring charts' may be helpful.

ADMINISTRATION

For some forms of drug therapy, the correct method of administration in relation to the specific mode of action of the drug is critical to the therapeutic efficacy of the treatment regimen. For example, chemotherapy for most types of malignancy must be administered in the correct chronological sequence in order to elicit optimum response.

Drug–drug or drug–food interactions may also have relevance in the formulation of drug administration regimens and where specific administration instructions are provided, these should be adhered to.

PATIENT EDUCATION

Patients should be aware of the spectrum of pharmacological effects which may be expected with their therapy. When providing patient education relating to the pharmacodynamic effects of drug therapy information should include:

- A plain language explanation of the mode of action of the drug.

- The expected onset of action of the drug and the usual duration of action.

- Any special instructions for drug administration.

- Any adverse effects which could reasonably be expected to arise from treatment.

- Any unusual adverse drug reactions associated with the drug if these are of potentially important clinical consequence.

- Important drug–drug or drug–food interactions.

- Where applicable, the problem of potential drug dependence or withdrawal.

FURTHER READING

Benet, L.Z., Mitchell, J.R., Scheiner, L.B. (1991), 'Pharmacokinetics: the dynamics of drug absorption, distribution and elemination' in Goodman Gilman, A., Rall, T.W., Nies, A.S., Taylor, P. eds. *The pharmacological basis of therapeutics*. 8th edn. Pergamon Press, New York, pp. 3–32.

Dukes, M.N.G. (1992), *Meyler's side effects of drugs*. 12th edn. Elsevier Science Publishers, Amsterdam.

Jaffe, J.H. (1991), 'Drug addiction and drug abuse' in Goodman Gilman, A., Rall, T.W., Nies, A.S., Taylor, P. eds. *The pharmacological basis of therapeutics*. 8th edn. Pergamon Press, New York, pp. 522–73.

Nies, A.S. (1991), 'Principles of therapeutics' in Goodman Gilman, A., Rall, T.W., Nies, A.S., Taylor, P. eds. *The pharmacological basis of therapeutics*. 8th edn. Pergamon Press, New York, pp. 33–48.

Ross, E.M. (1991), 'Pharmacodynamics: mechanisms of drug action and the relationship between drug concentration and effect' in Goodman Gilman, A., Rall, T.W., Nies, A.S., Taylor, P. eds. *The pharmacological basis of therapeutics.* 8th edn. Pergamon Press, New York, pp. 62–83.

Tatro, D.S. (ed.) (1992), *Drug interaction facts.* Facts and Comparisons, St Louis, USA.

Wood, A.J.J., Oates, J.A. (1991), 'Adverse reactions to drugs' in Wilson, J.D., Braunwald, E., Isselbacher, K.J. et al, eds. *Harrison's principles of internal medicine.* 12th edn. McGraw-Hill, New York.

TEST YOUR KNOWLEDGE

1. List three different mechanisms by which drugs may produce pharmacological effects.

2. Describe two examples of the ways in which the pharmacodynamic response produced by a drug may vary in relation to the disease state being treated.

3. Describe two different types of adverse drug reaction.

4. Outline at least one situation in which a relatively minor adverse drug reaction may assume a greater clinical significance.

5. Name three different drugs which may produce hepatic enzyme inhibition.

6. Define the term low therapeutic index.

7. Outline three serious medical complications associated with intravenous drug abuse.

8. Name five drugs or drug groups which may produce drug dependence.

9. Describe the common symptoms of an acute drug withdrawal reaction.

PHARMACODYNAMICS

1

Pharmacokinetics

CHRISTOPHER P. ALDERMAN

O B J E C T I V E S

At the conclusion of this chapter the reader should be able to:

1. Define common pharmacokinetic terms;

2. Outline the fundamental principles governing the movement of drugs into, within, and out of the body;

3. Discuss the potential clinical relevance of factors which influence the pharmacokinetic properties of drugs; and

4. Describe ways in which a knowledge of the pharmacokinetic profiles of drugs can be used to increase the effectiveness of drug therapy while minimising the potential for toxicity.

PHARMACOKINETICS

The characteristics of drug action within the body are partially governed by the fashion in which the compound is dispersed through body systems. The study of the transit of drugs within the body is called pharmacokinetics, literally the movement of drugs. Through an understanding of pharmacokinetics it is possible to approximately predict a number of parameters which are important in formulating drug treatment regimens. When combined with an understanding of the ways in which drugs produce their effects within body systems (pharmacodynamics), the use of pharmacokinetics allows the adjustment and individualisation of drug therapy, permitting optimal efficacy and economy, and minimising predictable toxicities.

In discussions on pharmacokinetics the usual practice is to consider separately the various parameters which characterise the movement of drugs within the body. To gain an overall understanding of the parameters which influence the action of drugs it is first necessary to consider the means by which the drug enters the body, *absorption*, its movements after absorption, *distribution*, and the means by which the drug ultimately leaves the body, *elimination* (which can be further subdivided into drug *metabolism* and *excretion*). A further complication is that the processes of drug absorption, distribution and elimination usually occur at the same time, with the overall movement of drugs reflecting a combination of these separate processes. A schematic representation of the processes involved in pharmacokinetics is shown in Figure 2.1.

A practical application of pharmacokinetics is selection of the optimum route of delivery for a drug, the dose to be administered and the frequency of administration. The pharmacokinetic characteristics of a drug often determine the formulation of the drug product. Numerous factors influence drug elimination, which in turn influences the treatment regimen used. The distribution of the drug within the body will directly influence its elimination.

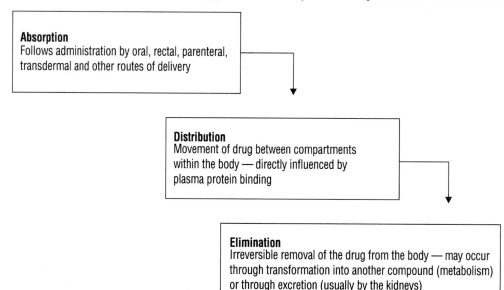

Absorption
Follows administration by oral, rectal, parenteral, transdermal and other routes of delivery

Distribution
Movement of drug between compartments within the body — directly influenced by plasma protein binding

Elimination
Irreversible removal of the drug from the body — may occur through transformation into another compound (metabolism) or through excretion (usually by the kidneys)

FIGURE 2.1 Pharmacokinetics: a schematic representation

DRUG ABSORPTION ████████████████

To produce an effect (either therapeutic or harmful) it is necessary for a drug to enter the body thereby gaining access to its site of action. In most cases the drug enters the systemic circulation and is transported to its site of action by the blood. However, in some situations the site of action can be accessed directly without relying on delivery via the systemic circulation. Examples of drug delivery direct to the site of action include the application of drugs (in creams or ointments) to the skin and the use of bronchodilators via the inhaled route. If systemic absorption occurs in these situations it serves no direct therapeutic purpose and may in fact give rise to side effects. Also, by administering the drug at its site of action side effects are most often minimised and the efficacy of therapy increased.

The process of drug absorption involves the movement of the compound across a membranous structure of some type into the body's internal environment. Drugs can be administered via various routes, but it is necessary to formulate the drug product in a way that allows it to cross the membranous barrier. The nature of some drugs means that the chemical compound is unable to cross the barrier despite optimum formulation. An example of this type of drug is the antibiotic vancomycin, which is not absorbed when administered orally. To achieve a systemic effect in this instance it is necessary to deliver the drug directly into the systemic circulation (i.e. by intravenous injection). In other cases the administration of a drug directly into the systemic circulation is used because the drug is adversely altered during its passage through the gastrointestinal tract (e.g. some proteins or polypeptides are broken down by acid and digestive enzymes in the gut). For example, insulin is destroyed in the gastrointestinal tract and is given parenterally, either by intravenous injection or more commonly by injection into a subcutaneous site from which it is absorbed into the systemic circulation. Delivery directly into the systemic circulation may also enhance effectiveness of the treatment or decrease the time required for its onset of action (e.g. when adrenaline is administered intravenously).

Drug therapy may be administered by a variety of routes. In many cases the preferred route is oral administration because of its convenience, reliability and tolerability. Drugs administered orally usually need to be absorbed into the systemic circulation before producing a therapeutic effect. The exception to this is when the intended site of action is within the lumen of the gastrointestinal tract.

ORAL ADMINISTRATION

Absorption

The process of drug absorption after oral administration, which for most drugs takes place largely within the small intestine, involves several steps. Gastrointestinal disease states such as malabsorption, diarrhoea or 'short bowel syndrome' may impair oral absorption from the gastrointestinal tract. In many cases drugs are administered in solid dose forms and, prior to the process of absorption, must dissolve in the milieu of the gastrointestinal tract. The dissolution of a drug in the fluids in the stomach or bowel is primarily governed by its chemical characteristics, although another important influence is the fashion in which the drug product is formulated (e.g. sustained release or enteric coated formulations). Incomplete dissolution within the gastrointestinal tract may lead to some or all of the administered dose being excreted unchanged in the faeces. In some cases this problem can be overcome by administering a larger dose of drug and accepting that some of the drug will not be absorbed.

A further complication is that for some drugs dissolution is the slowest, or the *rate limiting*, step of absorption, i.e. the rate of transit through the gastrointestinal tract influences the extent of drug absorption. If drug dissolution is particularly slow, factors which lengthen the gastrointestinal transit time will increase drug absorption. These factors may be physiological in nature (e.g. the increase in gastrointestinal transit time observed immediately after myocardial infarction) or may be the result of external influences. Drugs such as morphine and other opioids also have the effect of slowing gastrointestinal transit time and may for this reason influence drug absorption. On the other hand, the oral absorption of drugs which are unstable and broken down in an acidic environment (acid-labile drugs) is decreased by factors which increase stomach emptying time. The presence of food in the stomach delays gastric emptying and may decrease the oral absorption of acid-labile drugs such as flucloxacillin. For this reason drugs such as the acid-labile penicillins should be administered on an empty stomach.

Drug Interactions

Concurrently administered drugs may also influence the absorption of other medications by altering the drug's chemical characteristics. For example, when iron preparations are administered at the same time as tetracycline antibiotics, the two drugs combine forming a non-absorbable complex. Some drugs require an acidic medium for dissolution and oral absorption may be compromised by drugs which inhibit the production of gastric acid. For example, the absorption of the antifungal drug ketoconazole is decreased by the concurrent administration of ranitidine, antacids or other drugs which reduce or neutralise acid in the stomach.

Drug Formulations

The formulation of oral drug products has a significant influence on the characteristics of their absorption from the gastrointestinal tract. A liquid suspension or emulsion of a drug will not yield the intended dose if the preparation is not thoroughly shaken prior to dispensing the dose. The process by which a tablet breaks up and releases its ingredients is called tablet disintegration and different brands of the same drug may produce different effects because of altered tablet disintegration characteristics. Some tablets are coated with a layer which is resistant to acidic environments. *Enteric coated preparations* do not release the drug until reaching the intestine where the ambient pH is higher than that in the stomach. Examples of this type of formulation include enteric coated aspirin and sulfasalazine tablets. This technique also may be used to protect acid-labile drugs from the gastric acid or to protect the gastric mucosa from the irritant effects of some drugs. Occasionally, a pH sensitive coating is used to deliver a drug to a specific point in the lower gastrointestinal tract. *Sustained release preparations* are used to alter the rate of release where an extended action is required, even when the drug is usually rapidly removed from the body (e.g. sustained release theophylline preparations). See Chapter 3 Drug Administration.

Once the drug has been released from the oral dosage form and has dissolved in the gastrointestinal fluids the next step in absorption is the compound crossing the mucosa of the gastrointestinal tract. This usually occurs via a process of *diffusion*, the drug in solution simply moves from an area of relatively high concentration in solution to a second compartment where the concentration is lower. Less commonly, drugs are absorbed by a process of *active transport*, the drug is 'pumped' across a membrane at a faster rate than that achieved by simple diffusion (e.g. lithium). In some cases the chemical modifications to the drug molecule which facilitate its absorption may inactivate the drug pharmacologically. For example, proteins administered orally must be digested by enzymatic action and broken into their constituent amino acids prior to absorption. However, when this occurs the original properties of the compound are lost and the protein loses its usefulness as a drug.

During transit across the gut wall some drugs undergo modifications in chemical structure which alter the properties of the compound. This process, which occurs at other sites within the body, is referred to as *drug metabolism* and in this instance is called *gut-wall metabolism*. The resultant chemical changes which occur mean that some or all of the original drug is lost and that a new compound, a *metabolite*, is formed. Not all orally administered drugs undergo gut-wall metabolism, but in some cases the loss of active compound at this step is so great that the therapeutic efficacy of the drug is significantly diminished. The anti-inflammatory drug sulindac is an exception. It is converted from an inactive precursor form (a *pro-drug*) to the active metabolite during the process of gut-wall metabolism. For further information see Elimination by Metabolism later in this chapter.

First Pass Metabolism

Following transit across the gastrointestinal mucosa the drug must then diffuse across the endothelium of small blood vessels which lie very close to the gastrointestinal lining. These blood vessels form a part of the hepatic portal circulation system and drugs and other compounds (including nutrients) absorbed from the gastrointestinal tract are transported directly to the liver prior to entry into the general systemic circulation. The liver is a major site of drug metabolism and for some drugs a large proportion of the orally administered dose is metabolised before passing into the systemic circulation. In this situation the drug is said to *undergo a significant first pass effect*, and only a relatively small proportion of the drug will reach the target site of action. If this is the case an alternative route of administration is often employed. For example, glyceryl trinitrate, a drug used in the treatment of anginal pain, is subject to a large first pass effect and is usually administered sublingually thus bypassing the hepatic portal circulation.

Other alternative routes sometimes used to circumvent hepatic portal extraction include transdermal and rectal administration. Alternatively, the dose of the drug may be increased when administered orally. For example, although the calcium channel blocker verapamil is well absorbed orally most of the dose is metabolised during the first pass. The oral dose is adjusted to account for this and is much higher than the dose of verapamil administered intravenously.

Enterohepatic Cycling

For certain drugs absorption from the lumen of the gastrointestinal tract may occur after the process of metabolism. This process, enterohepatic cycling, may occur even if the drug was not originally administered via the oral route. After initial absorption the drug undergoes alteration to a metabolite which is then excreted into the gastrointestinal lumen in the bile. The action of bacterial flora in the gut then converts the metabolite back into the parent drug which is subsequently absorbed from the small intestine. Oestrogenic hormones in the oral contraceptive preparations undergo enterohepatic cycling and it is thought that some antibiotics reduce the efficacy of these preparations by interfering with the natural gut flora, resulting in unplanned pregnancy.

Bioavailability

To gain access to the general circulation drugs which are administered orally must overcome significant barriers to absorption. In most cases, not all of the dose administered orally will gain systemic access. The fraction of the drug which is absorbed is usually referred to as the drug's bioavailability. This figure is usually expressed as a decimal fraction or percentage. In the case of a drug with a bioavailability of 0.33 or 33%, two-thirds of the orally administered dose does not reach the systemic circulation. Drugs with very low oral bioavailability are usually not administered by mouth.

ALTERNATIVE ROUTES OF ADMINISTRATION

Whilst many drugs are best administered by the oral route for patient convenience, comfort, safety and economy, for some medications the oral route is impractical or unsuitable. In addition to the intravenous administration of drugs (the medication is injected directly into the systemic circulation) a variety of alternative routes exist for administration. Gaseous anaesthetics such as halothane are rapidly effective when administered by inhalation. The analgesic drug buprenorphine undergoes extensive first pass hepatic metabolism and is administered sublingually. Nitrate antianginal drugs also undergo extensive first pass effects and can be administered sublingually or transdermally (the drug diffuses across the skin through the dermis and into the systemic circulation).

Rectal Administration

In some situations the administration of a drug via the oral route is not practical or possible (e.g. in very young children or patients with an impaired swallowing mechanism) and the rectal route is utilised. The drug is incorporated into a suppository which dissolves or melts at body temperature releasing the drug into the lumen of the rectum. The drug is then absorbed across the mucosa of the rectum where it largely bypasses the hepatic portal circulation. Whilst convenient under some circumstances, rectal administration can be unreliable as the extent of absorption is dependent upon rectal contents and retention of the suppository in the rectum until the absorption process is complete.

Topical Administration

Under some circumstances it is desirable to deliver the drug directly to its site of action. Examples of these modes of administration include the application of drugs, e.g. corticosteroids, to the skin; the use of a drug via the rectal route (when the drug's action is on the mucosa of the rectum itself); the instillation of a drug solution onto the surface of the eye or into the outer ear; and the administration of β agonist bronchodilators, ipratroprium bromide, sodium cromoglycate and corticosteroids by inhalation. Although all of these methods of administration essentially amount to topical drug delivery, specialised dosage forms such as inhalations are discussed in many texts as separate and distinct delivery systems.

Drugs may also be delivered into the systemic circulation using a transdermal delivery system. The drug is formulated so that medication can be released into the circulation through the skin at a known, controlled rate (e.g. glyceryl trinitrate 'patch' systems). In other instances drugs may be absorbed inadvertently through the skin and into the general circulation (e.g. corticosteroids from topical preparations applied to large areas of skin under an occlusive dressing).

Parenteral Administration

When other means of administration are inappropriate or unavailable the drug may be administered by injection (i.e. parenterally). The drug is usually dissolved in an appropriate solvent (commonly water for injection) and is conveyed into the body by way of a needle or cannula. Drugs may be injected directly into the vasculature by intravenous or, rarely, intra-arterial injection. Alternatively, medication can be delivered to a variety of other sites from which there is absorption into the general circulation. Examples of this type of administration include subcutaneous and intramuscular injection.

When the drug is administered intravenously it gains direct access to the systemic circulation. The intensity of effect is sometimes greater when this route of administration is used and the onset of action may be quicker. Care should be taken to ensure that dose forms intended for other parenteral routes (e.g. subcutaneous adrenaline) are not inadvertently administered intravenously. In some cases preparations are formulated specifically for parenteral routes other than intravenous administration (e.g. depot intramuscular injections). Intravenous administration of these formulations will serve no useful purpose and may give rise to dangerous adverse effects such as embolism.

Specific parenteral routes may be used for the delivery of drugs to defined target sites. Opioid analgesics and local anaesthetics are often administered via epidural injection to gain direct access to the sensory neurones in the spinal column. Intraocular injection can be used to deliver a drug into the eye and intrapleural injections are sometimes used to place drugs or chemicals into the pleural cavity. In many cases the aim of these specialised delivery techniques is to localise the effect of the drug, however some absorption of the medication into the systemic circulation does occur. For example, the presence of morphine in peripheral blood can be demonstrated shortly after the epidural administration of this drug.

Under some circumstances systemic access is required but insufficient opportunity or indication exists for the establishment of venous access. (Venous access is associated with a small but significant risk of morbidity and mortality.) In these cases an alternative parenteral route can be used to allow administration of the drug into a site from which general systemic absorption can occur. Subcutaneous injections are placed into the tissue close to the dermal layer of the skin, from here the medication is transported into the vasculature in the subcutaneous tissue.

The intramuscular route of administration is also commonly employed. A drug in solution is injected into a large muscle mass, such as the gluteal or deltoid muscles, and is absorbed into the systemic circulation through the blood vessels supplying the muscle. This route of delivery is generally reliable, but the rate of absorption of the drug may be affected if peripheral perfusion is compromised, e.g. in shock or dehydration. (This also applies for subcutaneous injections.) Another complication is when the administration of a drug into the muscle tissue affects the chemical nature of the drug. For some compounds, e.g. phenytoin and diazepam, the pH of muscle tissue is sufficiently different to that of the injection solution to cause precipitation of the drug product within the muscle. Aside from being particularly painful this also slows absorption from the injection site. In some cases, intramuscular injections are deliberately formulated for slow release from the injection site to achieve sustained action. Examples of these include the depot formulations of some antipsychotic drugs.

DRUG DISTRIBUTION ■■■■■■■■■■■■■■

Following administration and absorption a number of further movements of the drug may occur within the body. Drug distribution refers to the various reversible movements of a drug within the body, usually from one compartment to another. Although drugs may exist in simple solution within the blood or plasma, in many cases the compound is poorly soluble in water and the drug is distributed to sites outside the general circulation.

Drugs produce their therapeutic effects through a variety of mechanisms, in many cases involving the binding of the drug to an appropriate receptor. With some exceptions the receptor is located at a site external to the intravascular space and drug distribution to this site is necessary to elicit drug action. An important principle to remember is that the process of drug distribution to sites outside the blood is reversible. Having been transferred from the general circulation to a site external to the blood the drug will eventually distribute back into the blood from which it will be ultimately removed from the body. An additional complication is that the drug may distribute to several areas within the body at the same time so simultaneous transfer between a number of compartments may occur.

Drug action is usually mediated by binding at a receptor site external to the blood or plasma and it is not normally possible to measure the concentration of drug at its site of action. Instead, the concentration in the blood or plasma is measured and this information is considered in relation to the known pharmacokinetic characteristics of the drug. When a drug is extensively distributed to sites outside the plasma, the plasma concentration may not truly reflect the total amount of drug in the body. The term *volume of distribution* is used to describe that volume which would be consistent with the known amount of drug in the body and the observed concentration in the plasma. For drugs without distribution sites outside the plasma the volume of distribution will be equal to the plasma volume (i.e. about 3 L). When a drug is extensively distributed to sites outside the plasma the volume of distribution (which is a theoretical figure) may be considerably greater than 3 L. An example of the calculations involved in the derivation of a drug's volume of distribution is provided in Figure 2.2.

In some cases the derived volume of distribution can be very large indeed (e.g. the volume of distribution for haloperidol is normally in excess of 500 L). On the other hand, the volume of distribution is never less than the plasma volume.

Another important factor is the rate at which drug distribution occurs. For example, if a drug is rapidly absorbed from the gastrointestinal tract but the process of distribution to the site of action is slow the onset of action for this drug will be slow. The process of drug distribution is in this case the *rate limiting step*. Conversely, if the process of transfer from extravascular sites back into the systemic circulation is slow the removal of the drug from the body will also be slow.

$$\text{Plasma concentration} \quad = \quad \frac{\text{Amount in the body}}{\text{Volume of distribution}}$$

therefore

$$\text{Volume of distribution} \quad = \quad \frac{\text{Amount in the body}}{\text{Plasma concentration}}$$

In the case of a specific patient, an example of the values might be:

Amount of drug in the body (dose administered IV) = 100 mg
Plasma concentration = 5 mg/L

$$\text{Calculated volume of distribution} \quad = \quad \frac{100}{5} \quad = \quad 20 \text{ L}$$

FIGURE 2.2 Calculation of volume of distribution for gentamicin

PLASMA PROTEIN BINDING

Drug distribution is strongly influenced by the propensity of the compound to bind to proteins, in particular those proteins found circulating in the plasma. Such proteins, including albumin, α-1 acid glycoprotein and other specific binding proteins (e.g. corticosteroid binding globulin), are very large molecules which are incapable of diffusing across intact biological membranes. Even when the drug is highly bound to plasma proteins a small proportion remains unbound. The proportion of drug which is not bound to proteins in the plasma is referred to as the *free fraction*. Only unbound drug is able to distribute to sites outside the plasma, but if a drug has a high affinity for sites outside the plasma the small proportion of drug which is unbound tends to distribute to the extravascular site. As the plasma protein binding of drugs is reversible, through the dissociation of the drug from the plasma protein, it is possible for a drug to have a high volume of distribution despite being highly protein bound.

CLINICAL IMPLICATIONS

The properties of a drug's distribution are critical in determining the characteristics of its actions. Drugs act at specific receptor sites and if drug distribution to these sites is slow or limited this will be reflected in the drug's action. Chemical compounds can only be metabolised or excreted out of the body in a free (or unbound) state, thus the properties of the drug's distribution will contribute to determining the duration of the drug's activity. With many drugs the intensity of effect is directly

related to the concentration of the drug at the receptor or in the plasma. In these cases drug distribution will determine the magnitude of pharmacological effect.

The characteristics of drug distribution (including plasma protein binding) may be influenced by a wide variety of factors which will in turn influence the actions of the drug. For example, a number of disease states may directly affect drug distribution within the body. Conditions such as acute viral infections, congestive heart failure or extensive burns may alter the distribution of some drugs into the extravascular compartments. Under some circumstances (e.g. pregnancy, cirrhosis, nephrotic syndrome, malnutrition), the concentrations of plasma proteins may be altered which in turn alters protein binding characteristics. Competition between two drugs for the same protein binding sites may occur, although this type of drug interaction is rarely of clinical significance. When formulating dosage regimens it is important to consider all factors which may affect drug disposition.

DRUG ELIMINATION

Drug elimination is the term which collectively refers to the various ways in which the drug irreversibly leaves the body. The process of drug elimination may be further subdivided into *excretion*, whereby the drug is transported out of the body's internal environment, and *metabolism*, during which the drug is converted into a different chemical entity (this may in turn facilitate excretion of the drug from the body).

Drugs may be eliminated from the body via a number of mechanisms. Whilst very small amounts of drug are sometimes excreted through minor routes of clearance such as perspiration, tears and saliva, these are not major routes of drug elimination. The two major mechanisms by which a drug is eliminated from the body are renal excretion and metabolic elimination (commonly referred to as drug metabolism). However, other routes of elimination may sometimes be important. For example, significant amounts of paraldehyde are eliminated via the lungs in exhaled air, while other drugs are excreted into the bowel and eliminated in the faeces.

DRUG CLEARANCE

Because drugs are distributed to sites external to those from which elimination can occur it is necessary to relate the elimina-

tion from the body to the concentration at the site of elimination. For drug elimination to occur the compound must be presented to the organ system where elimination takes place. Drug clearance is the term used to define drug elimination in relation to the rate of presentation of the drug to the organ system which is the site of elimination. The clearance is measured in units of volume per unit of time. If a drug has a plasma clearance of 3 L per hour, this means that 3 L of plasma are cleared of that drug each hour. If the concentration of the drug in the plasma is 10 mg per L, then the rate of elimination for that drug will be 30 mg per hour. In practical terms factors which influence or alter drug clearance are generally those with the most profound ramifications in clinical practice.

The process of drug clearance by an organ may fall into a number of categories. For some drugs the intrinsic ability of the organ system to clear the drug is very high.

These drugs are said to have a *high extraction ratio*. In this case the rate limiting process in the clearance of the drug is the rate at which the drug is presented to the organ system in which elimination takes place. The clearance of these drugs is sometimes described as *flow dependent*. For example, narcotic analgesics such as pethidine and morphine have high extraction ratios and the rate of clearance is primarily dependent on the rate of liver blood flow (i.e. nearly all drug presented to the liver is cleared during passage through that organ). In this situation clinical circumstances which compromise liver blood flow (e.g. severe congestive cardiac failure) will decrease the rate of hepatic clearance of the drug. Conversely, drugs such as warfarin and diazepam have a *low extraction ratio* and alterations in hepatic blood flow will not have a profound effect on hepatic clearance as the rate limiting process is the intrinsic ability of the liver itself to clear the drug. The intrinsic capacity of the liver for drug metabolism may be altered by external factors including other drug therapy (i.e. drug interactions).

ELIMINATION BY METABOLISM

Most drugs are organic chemicals which may or may not be soluble in water. In order to facilitate drug excretion the process of drug metabolism usually involves the chemical modification of the parent drug, producing a new chemical compound which is more polar in nature and therefore has greater solubility in water. Examples of types of reactions which achieve this effect include oxidative metabolism, or dealkylation of drugs with methyl or ethyl groups.

Drug metabolism takes place at a variety of sites including the kidneys, lungs, muscle tissue, the lining of the gastrointestinal tract and within the circulating blood. However, the major site of drug metabolism is within the liver. Drug metabolism may take place in several steps. For example, a drug may undergo oxidation followed by conversion to a glucuronide metabolite. A further complication is that several types of metabolism may take place in parallel and that different paths of metabolism may compete.

The chemical reactions which take place during drug metabolism usually result in the production of a new compound with less pharmacological activity than the parent compound. In some cases the metabolism of a drug converts it from an inactive form into the active compound. In this case, the parent drug is referred to as a *pro-drug*. Examples include chloral hydrate and sulindac. Another variation is when the drug is converted into another compound with pharmacological activity which may not necessarily reflect that of the parent compound. For example, pethidine is converted into norpethidine which is less effective as an analgesic and may cause convulsions. In this situation the metabolite is referred to as an *active metabolite*. The pharmacological effects of an active metabolite may be useful or, as is the case for norpethidine, harmful.

Hepatic Metabolism

The process of drug metabolism is in most cases mediated through enzyme systems located primarily in the liver. Under certain circumstances the activity of these enzymes may be increased, meaning that the process of drug elimination through metabolism will occur at a faster rate. This phenomenon is referred to as *hepatic enzyme induction*. The clinical consequence of this is that if the rate and extent of drug absorption remains constant and the characteristics of drug distribution do not change (and hepatic metabolism is an important route of elimination for the drug concerned), then the observed plasma level of the drug will normally decrease. Hepatic enzyme induction usually occurs as a result of the influence of a chemical compound from outside the body (an *inducing agent*). For example, cigarette smoking significantly increases the rate of theophylline metabolism, causing decreased theophylline plasma levels. Most commonly the inducing agent is a drug. The induction of hepatic enzymes forms the basis for many of the clinically important drug interactions (see Table 2.1).

Conversely, some drugs and chemicals have the effect of decreasing the rate of hepatic drug metabolism. This process is called hepatic enzyme inhibition and may also give rise to important drug interactions. Provided that drug absorption and distribution are unchanged and that hepatic metabolism is the major route of elimination, enzyme inhibition will cause an increase in plasma drug levels possibly resulting in clinical toxicity. Drugs which can cause enzyme inhibition are also listed in Table 2.1.

TABLE 2.1   Drugs which influence hepatic metabolism

Enzyme inducters	Enzyme inhibitors
Phenytoin	Cimetidine
Carbamazepine	Erythromycin
Barbiturates	Ciprofloxacin
Cigarette smoke	Antifungal drugs
Ethanol	Monoamine oxidase inhibitors

The process of hepatic metabolism cannot be considered in isolation. For example, the influence of hepatic enzyme induction will be more significant for drugs with a low extraction ratio (i.e. the rate of clearance is primarily dependent on the intrinsic capacity of the liver to metabolise the drug, rather than the liver blood flow). Furthermore, if the drug is highly protein bound the rate of clearance will be further compromised. Similarly, hepatic enzyme induction may influence the extent of systemic absorption, which may be decreased because of enzyme induction through an increase in first pass metabolism. In the case of enzyme inhibition the role of other routes of drug elimination (e.g. renal excretion) may become relatively more important and alterations in plasma levels may not necessarily result unless elimination by this route is also compromised.

Renal Excretion

The kidneys are another major site for elimination of drugs from the body. Nearly a quarter of the cardiac output is delivered to the kidneys where filtration of plasma water occurs. If a drug is in solution in the plasma, elimination may be achieved through filtration at the glomerulus in the kidney and the drug excreted into the urine.

The rate at which plasma water is filtered at the functional unit of the kidney (the nephron) is referred to as the glomerular filtration rate. In young, healthy adults this is approximately 100–150 mL per minute. Drugs can also be actively secreted by the renal tubular cells into the urine. In this way the rate of renal clearance of a drug can exceed the glomerular filtration rate. Active secretion is often important when the drug is a weak organic acid, e.g. a penicillin. The uricosuric agent probenecid is also an organic acid and competes with penicillins for secretion in the kidney. Because of this probenecid is used to decrease the rate of renal excretion of penicillins, therefore increasing the plasma levels of these antibiotics. Glucuronide drug metabolites are also actively secreted further facilitating the elimination of drugs from the body.

Another process which occurs in the nephron is reabsorption, the drug or ion diffuses from the filtrate back into the systemic circulation. Although the process of reabsorption is sometimes active, the normal mechanism is one of passive diffusion whereby solute moves from a site of high concentration (the filtrate) to a site of lower concentration (the systemic circulation). Only drugs in the un-ionised state can be reabsorbed. For some drugs altering the urinary pH may result in a higher proportion of the drug in the urine existing in the ionised state, therefore limiting reabsorption and increasing the rate of renal excretion. The overall nature, extent and rate of renal clearance will be a composite of filtration, secretion and reabsorption.

For a drug to be cleared renally it must be transported in solution to the kidney. Drugs which are poorly soluble in water are usually not excreted unchanged by the kidney to any significant extent. These drugs usually undergo conversion to metabolites which are more water soluble. For some drugs a significant proportion of the dose is excreted unchanged in the urine, whilst the remainder is metabolised (the metabolites are excreted in the urine). The sum of the renal and hepatic pathways usually accounts for almost the entire clearance of a drug and for most drugs elimination takes place through both pathways.

The nature of the nephron is such that it allows the filtration of small molecules and ions but will not permit the passage of large molecules into the urine. Plasma proteins are very large molecules and are not usually present in urine (except in certain disease states such as the nephrotic syndrome). When a drug is tightly bound to plasma proteins such as albumin this limits the rate of renal clearance of the drug. For these drugs circumstances which increase the free (unbound) fraction of the drug will lead to an increase in the rate of renal clearance.

For some drugs the major proportion is excreted unchanged in the urine. In these cases a significant decline in renal function will often be accompanied by an increase in drug levels, sometimes resulting in overt toxicity. Drugs for which renal excretion is a major route of elimination include the aminoglycoside antibiotics (e.g. gentamicin, tobramycin), digoxin, lithium and vancomycin. When kidney function is compromised the dose of these drugs or the frequency of their administration should be decreased to avoid accumulation of the drug and possible toxicity. A range of drugs for which excretion of the unchanged compound in the urine is the major route of elimination is given in Table 2.2.

TABLE 2.2   Drugs for which renal excretion is an important pathway of elimination

Antimicrobials	Other drugs
Gentamicin	Digoxin
Tobramycin	Lithium
Amikacin	Disopyramide
Vancomycin	Cisplatin
Amphotericin B	Cimetidine
Flucytosine	Amantadine
Cycloserine	Methotrexate
Acyclovir	

Elimination Half-Life

The rate of clearance of a drug directly determines the rate of decline of the plasma level. The elimination of a drug can be characterised by referring to the time required for the plasma level to decline by a given amount. This is usually achieved by calculating the elimination half-life of the drug. The half-life is that period of time required for the plasma concentration to decrease to 50% of the original value. For example, if the plasma level decreases from 8 mg/L to 4 mg/L after a period of six hours, then the apparent half-life of the drug is said to be six hours. This calculation is based on the assumption that the processes of drug absorption and distribution are complete.

Using the elimination half-life it is possible to make an approximate estimation of the drug's movements within the body. The *steady state concentration* is that blood level when no significant change in the average blood concentration of the drug would be expected, provided the dose of the drug and the rate of elimination are constant. It is known that for most drugs, steady state plasma concentrations are not attained until the drug has been administered for a period of time approximately equal to six times the half-life of the drug. Similarly, the time taken to remove most of the drug from the body after a single dose (or after stopping a maintenance dose) is roughly six times the half-life of the drug. There is a particularly

wide variation in the half-lives of drugs used in clinical practice. The half-lives for a range of commonly used drugs are listed in Table 2.3.

TABLE 2.3 Plasma half-lives for a selection of commonly used drugs*

Drug	Half-life (hours)
Gentamicin	2.5–3.0
Morphine	2–3
Naproxen	14–17
Diazepam	24–48
Warfarin	42
Sodium nitroprusside	0.25
Haloperidol	10–36
Etretinate	2400

*Assumes normal function of major body systems including heart, liver and kidneys.

THERAPEUTIC DRUG MONITORING ■■■

The therapeutic and toxic effects of many drugs are known to be directly related to the concentration of the drug in the plasma or blood. The term therapeutic drug monitoring (TDM) is used to refer to the measurement of drug concentrations (sometimes called drug *levels*) in an attempt to ensure that a good therapeutic response to drug therapy is likely, while at the same time seeking to minimise the toxicities or complications associated with unnecessarily high blood levels.

The use of therapeutic drug monitoring is particularly useful for those drugs with a *low therapeutic index*, that is, where the blood level known to produce therapeutic effects is not greatly different to the level associated with important toxicity. Drugs with a low therapeutic index for which therapeutic drug monitoring is commonly used include gentamicin, theophylline, digoxin, lithium, phenytoin, carbamazepine and amiodarone.

As discussed in earlier sections of this chapter the specific pharmacokinetic profile for a drug in any individual patient may not necessarily be predictable. The dosage schedule which is needed for the safe and effective treatment of one patient may result in a subtherapeutic response or even drug toxicity in another individual. For this reason, therapeutic drug monitoring is used to measure the blood level of the drug and the dosage is adjusted so that the blood level falls within a range known to produce good therapeutic effects without toxicity. This concentration range is often referred to as the *therapeutic range* of the drug.

In most cases the aim of therapeutic drug monitoring is to determine the concentration of the drug in the blood just prior to administration of the next dose. This is called the trough level and is measured to ensure that the level remains in the therapeutic range until the end of the dose interval. If the trough level is greater than the upper limit of the therapeutic range there may be a considerable risk of toxicity, although this depends on the particular drug. Occasionally and especially with some antibiotics, e.g. gentamycin and vancomycin, the aim is to determine the highest concentration of drug in the blood during the dosage interval. This is called the peak level and is determined by measuring the level in blood drawn shortly after administration of the drug.

It is important that the blood for drug level testing is drawn at an appropriate time. As the trough level is determined by measuring the blood level of the drug just prior to the next dose it is sometimes necessary to withhold a scheduled dose until the blood sample has been obtained. The dose can then be administered after the sample has been taken. To allow useful interpretation of the blood level it is important to note details such as the date and time of the last dose, the date and time that the blood sample was taken and the duration of therapy with the drug. Repeat monitoring may be needed to exclude accumulation of the drug to levels which could produce toxic effects.

NURSING IMPLICATIONS

ASSESSMENT

When administered orally drugs must be absorbed across the gastrointestinal mucosa before reaching the systemic circulation. Assessment of the patient should include screening for factors which may alter the rate or extent of oral drug absorption. Such factors include gastrointestinal problems, a variety of acute and chronic illnesses and interacting concurrent drug therapy. Where assessment reveals that the oral route of administration is not practical or effective, alternative routes of administration should be considered. Assessment should also be undertaken to ensure that if parenteral drug therapy is proposed the safest and most effective method of delivery has been selected.

A number of disease states may influence drug distribution producing potentially important effects on pharmacokinetic profiles. The influence of hypoproteinaemia or liver, kidney or heart disease on drug distribution must be considered during the initial assessment of the patient.

During assessment it is crucial that the factors which may potentially influence drug elimination are thoroughly evaluated, as alterations in drug clearance may lead to important complications including drug toxicity or loss of therapeutic effect. Relevant factors include age, body weight, cardiac failure, hepatic or renal impairment or the administration of interacting drugs.

EVALUATION

Given the potentially serious adverse effects which may arise as a result of alterations in the pharmacokinetic profiles of some drugs, continuous nursing evaluation is necessary to allow early intervention when clinical toxicity or lack of therapeutic effect have serious clinical ramifications. Nurses should monitor for signs and symptoms of altered cardiac output and should be familiar with indicators of compromised liver or kidney function.

Variations in the pharmacokinetics of drugs of low therapeutic index (when a small increase in serum concentrations may give rise to important toxicity) will be of particular importance and the patient should be evaluated regularly for signs of clinical toxicity. Some drugs of low therapeutic index in common use include gentamicin, digoxin, lithium, anticoagulants, anticonvulsants and theophylline.

ADMINISTRATION

Nurses should be aware of the principles of pharmacokinetics and apply them during drug administration. The correct method of administration should be adhered to wherever possible to enhance the therapeutic effectiveness of drugs and minimise the incidence of untoward effects.

Particular areas of attention should include: attention to correct timing of administration of oral drugs in relation to food or other drugs; maintenance of the integrity of sustained release or enteric coated oral dose forms (these preparations must be swallowed whole, never crushed or chewed); adequate shaking of liquid oral suspensions or emulsions; and correct use of alternative administration routes when the oral route is ineffective, inconvenient or impractical. Adequate consideration of the appropriate parenteral administration route is also particularly important. In impaired renal function specific dosage schedules may be instituted to avoid accumulation of the drug and subsequent toxicity and it is important to adhere to the planned treatment schedule as closely as possible. The nurse should also be aware of the need for correct timing of doses in relation to blood sampling for therapeutic drug monitoring.

PATIENT EDUCATION

Adequate patient education is especially important when the patient is undergoing therapy with a drug with a low therapeutic index. The patient must be made aware of the signs and symptoms of drug accumulation, and should be aware of the correct actions to take in the event of suspected toxicity. In many instances it is possible to provide patient information in a plain language format which will help to prevent complications associated with drug treatment (e.g. potential drug interactions). Other aspects of patient education may include the provision of advice regarding the actions to take in the event of an omitted dose.

FURTHER READING

Benet, L.Z., Mitchell, J.R., Scheiner, L.B. (1991), 'Pharmacokinetics: The dynamics of drug absorption, distribution and elimination' in Goodman Gilman, A., Rall, T.W., Neis, A.S., Tylor, P. (eds). *The Pharmacological Basis of Therapeutics*. 8th edn. Pergamon, New York, pp. 1–32.
Speight TM (ed) (1989), *Avery's Drug Treatment*. 3rd edn. Adis Press, Auckland.

TEST YOUR KNOWLEDGE

1. Describe two different practical applications for the use of pharmacokinetics in the formulation of individual drug treatment regimens.

2. Outline the ways in which the gastrointestinal transit time may influence the oral absorption of drugs.

3. Define the term significant first pass effect.

4. Calculate the oral bioavailability (as a percentage) for a drug for which 90% of the administered dose is not absorbed after oral administration.

5. Define the term enterohepatic cycling.

6. Calculate the volume of distribution for a drug where the administered IV dose is 150 mg and the observed peak plasma concentration is 3 mg/mL (assume that the process of distribution is complete).

7. What is the term used for that proportion of drug in the plasma which is not bound to plasma proteins. List three clinical situations in which the concentration of proteins in the plasma may change.

8. Define the term pro-drug.

9. List at least four drugs which may cause severe toxicity in patients with altered kidney function.

10. Define the term elimination half-life.

Drug Administration

JULIENNE I. HILDITCH

O B J E C T I V E S

At the conclusion of this chapter the reader should be able to:

1. Describe the responsibilities of the medical officer, the pharmacist and the nurse with respect to drug handling and administration;

2. Discuss the legal requirements relating to the storage and administration of medication;

3. List the various dosage forms in which drugs are available;

4. Describe procedures for drug administration;

5. Describe the rights of the patient with respect to the use of medication; and

6. Discuss patient education about medications.

THE HEALTH CARE TEAM ▬▬▬▬

The prescription, supply, administration and monitoring of drug therapy is primarily the responsibility of three members of the health care team: the medical officer, the pharmacist and the nurse.

The administration of medication is a potentially hazardous form of treatment. It is therefore essential that knowledge and commonsense form the basis of such action. This chapter covers the legal and ethical responsibilities of the nurse as part of the health care team in the administration and storage of drugs, the documentation of drug use and some practical issues related to drug administration.

RESPONSIBILITY OF THE MEDICAL OFFICER

The medical officer is responsible for diagnosis, the prescription of therapy and the monitoring of therapy thereafter.

In the hospital setting medication must be ordered on the appropriate medication chart with due regard to legal requirements, Federal and State department of health regulations and any policy set by the hospital's drug committee, e.g. drug formulary, antibiotic policy.

If there is any doubt in reading or interpreting the prescriber's orders, either by the nurse or the pharmacist, the prescriber must be contacted and clear instructions obtained.

RESPONSIBILITY OF THE PHARMACIST

The pharmacist is legally responsible for the supply and distribution of drugs in accordance with State laws, Federal and State department of health regulations and hospital policies. In addition, the pharmacist is responsible for the manufacture of a variety of specialised products: extemporaneous products (e.g. creams and ointments); paediatric mixtures; intravenous additives; sterile preparations (e.g. total parenteral nutrition solutions); and parenteral doses of cytotoxic drugs.

Many pharmacists work in ward areas where they are responsible for ensuring the supply of medication for each patient, reviewing medication charts to ensure that prescribed drugs and their doses are appropriate and advising on dosage forms, dosage schedules and drug interactions. Educating patients about their medication and how to optimise their treatment is another important role for the pharmacist.

The pharmacist acts as the resource person for drug information and as a consultant to the medical profession, allied health professionals and the nursing staff on all aspects of drug use.

RESPONSIBILITY OF THE NURSE

The nurse is the final link in the chain of supply of drugs to the patient. As the professional responsible for the administration of medication to the patient the nurse must have a thorough knowledge of drug therapy and administration techniques. When medication is being used drug therapy must be incorporated as an integral part of the nursing care plan.

Establishment of a nursing care plan in respect of drug therapy will take into account information obtained by observation and interview of the patient, from relevant family members, from other sources such as patient records, and appropriate professionals (e.g. the community nurse, pharmacist and medical officer). The nursing care plan will need to establish realistic goals for drug therapy. Short-term goals should concentrate on obtaining patient cooperation to gain the maximum benefit from the regimen.

Long-term goals should focus on counselling and patient education to enable self-medication and compliance with therapy. Family members may also require these services to encourage acceptance and understanding of therapy and to enable them to supervise or give home treatment when the patient is incapable of self-medication, or when emergency treatment is necessary.

The patient's physiological and psychosocial state should be assessed with regard to their ability to take medication in the form prescribed. For example, patients who have difficulty swallowing or who are vomiting may require rectal or parenteral medication. Some patients have a particular aversion to certain routes of administration, e.g. injections or rectal administration. Visual, hearing, intellectual or motor impairments that might interfere with the patient's ability to take medications appropriately must also be taken into account.

The nursing care plan should include schedules for drug administration. These should be based on information gained from assessment, knowledge of drug actions, adverse effects, interactions and the prescriber's instructions. Planning should also make allowances for the patient's other activities such as meals and rest periods and other treatments such as physiotherapy. When strict time schedules are essential these should be noted in the nursing care plan.

The nurse is often the professional who is best placed to assess, with patients, their response to therapy. Discrepancies between the goals of care and the results should be critically examined. For example, it may be observed by the nurse or reported by the patient that symptoms are not relieved within an appropriate time. The prescriber must be informed accordingly and a decision made whether to alter the treatment. All this information should be clearly documented in the patient's progess or nursing notes.

LEGAL REQUIREMENTS

The nurse must be aware of, and observe carefully, the laws and regulations relating to drug use. These include State laws, Federal and State department of health requirements, institutional policy, issues relating to professional duty of care, the patient's right to be informed and to refuse treatment.

STATE POISONS ACTS

Each State has a Poisons Act which, with associated regulations, is designed to protect the health and welfare of members of the community. One of the principal concerns of this legislation is to impose some controls on the packaging and labelling, distribution, storage, sale and use of the many potent drugs available. The Poisons Acts provide for the establishment of a Poisons List. All drugs are categorised into a schedule in this Poisons List. For each schedule there are specific rules regulating the use of the drugs listed. All States have now adopted, with a few minor variations, the Standard for the Uniform Scheduling of Drugs and Poisons drawn up by the National Health and Medical Research Council. These schedules are:

Schedule 1
Poisons of plant origin of such danger to health as to warrant their being available only from medical practitioners, pharmacists or veterinary surgeons.

Schedule 2
Poisons for therapeutic use that should be available to the public only from pharmacies or from persons licensed to sell Schedule 2 poisons. Simple analgesics such as aspirin and paracetamol, antacids and mild laxatives are included in this schedule.

Schedule 3
Poisons for therapeutic use that are danger-ous or so liable to abuse as to warrant their availability to the public being restricted to supply by pharmacists or medical, dental or veterinary practitioners. This schedule includes drugs such as glyceryl trinitrate, salbutamol inhalers, some antihistamines and potassium supplements.

Schedule 4
Poisons that should, in the public interest, be restricted to medical, dental or veteri-nary prescription or supply. Also included in this schedule are substances or preparations intended for therapeutic use, the safety or efficacy of which require further evaluation.

Schedule 5
Poisons of a hazardous nature that must be readily available to the public but require caution in handling, storage or use.

Schedule 6
Poisons that must be available to the public but are of a more hazardous or poisonous nature than those classified in schedule 5.

Schedule 7
Poisons which require special precautions in the manufacture, handling, storage or use, or special individual regulations regard-ing labelling or availability.

Schedule 8
Drugs of dependence (e.g. morphine, pethidine). These drugs are also only avail-able on the written prescription of a medical practitioner and have further restrictions to ensure security.

Schedule 9
Poisons which are drugs of abuse, the manufacture, possession, sale or use of which should be prohibited by law.

The schedules of particular importance to nurses are Schedules 4 and 8. The majority of drugs used in the hospital setting belong to these two schedules and nurses must be familiar with the regulations relating to the storage and handling of these drugs. For complete details of all regulations pertaining to the handling and use of drugs nursing staff should make themselves familiar with their own State's Poisons Act and Regulations.

It is illegal for a nurse to 'dispense' any medication. The definition of 'dispensing' in-cludes: packing a drug from a stock bottle into a smaller container; combining two or more containers of medication; transferring drugs from one container to another con-tainer; and re-labelling or over-labelling a container of medication. Apart from the ob-vious danger of a mistake being made in wrongly labelling a medication other prob-lems can occur such as mixing different strengths of medication, different brands of the same drug, different batch numbers and expiry dates. Legally the only person authorised to dispense medication is the pharmacist and, in special circumstances, the medical practitioner.

DRUG STORAGE AND HANDLING ■■■■■■

STORAGE

In the hospital situation the storage of all medication at ward level is the responsibil-ity of the nurse in charge of the ward.

Drugs should be stored at ward level in the same container or carton in which they were issued from the pharmacy. If the label becomes difficult to read the container should be returned to the pharmacy to be re-labelled.

As drugs are toxic substances they must be stored in such a way that patients and the public cannot gain access to them and in compliance with all legal requirements for storage.

Aside from legal considerations two important factors to consider when storing drugs are temperature and expiry dates.

Temperature

Temperature is one of the most critical factors governing the storage of drugs. It is important that the temperature criteria be met if the drug is to have the efficacy and potency stated on the label. Most drugs require storage at room temperatures below 30°C. Some drugs specify that they must be refrigerated, that is, they must be stored at a temperature between 2°C and 8°C. A small number of drugs must be stored frozen, that is, at a temperature below –10°C.

Expiry Dates

Most drugs have an expiry date and if stored correctly will remain useable until the date specified. It is good practice to check the expiry date of all medication before administration. Wastage of drugs can be minimised by stock rotation: replacement stock is always placed at the rear of the shelf ensuring that older stock is used first. Regardless of the expiry date on the container any medication that is discoloured or looks in any way spoiled should not be used. Check with the pharmacy department if any doubt exists.

THE MEDICATION ORDER

Nurses should not administer any medication to any patient unless a valid medication order has been completed by a medical practitioner.

The prescription or medication order must include, in the prescriber's own handwriting, the patient's name and positive identification (e.g. medical record number or patient's address). In some institutions it is acceptable for the name and other identifying particulars to be entered by another person or means (e.g. addressograph label)

as long as the prescriber verifies these particulars with her/his signature. The name and strength of the drug, route of administration, dose and frequency of administration must be specified and the order signed (in full) and dated. An order written by another person is not valid, even if signed by a medical practitioner, except in some specific instances, e.g. emergency telephone orders where hospital policy provides guidelines for acceptable practice. If the order is illegible or there is any doubt as to the prescriber's intention, it must be checked either with senior nursing staff, the pharmacist or the prescriber. Unless the nurse is confident that the order is valid and appropriate she/he has the right and the duty to refuse to administer it.

Nurse Initiated Medication

Individual institutions may approve a list of medications which may be 'nurse initiated' for the treatment of minor conditions which do not warrant assessment by the medical practitioner. Such medication would normally belong to Schedules 2 or 3 of the Poisons List and might include mild analgesics, antacids, laxatives, etc. A written protocol should be available which defines those drugs which may be nurse initiated, the indications for which they are appropriate and any special precautions. Any medication which is nurse initiated should be recorded as specified in the protocol.

RECORD OF ADMINISTRATION

It is general practice for all drug administration to be recorded in the medication record. State laws require that administration of specified drugs of addiction be recorded in a separate drug register. In addition, hospital regulations may require that administration of other substances, such as sedatives and some analgesics, be similarly recorded. The nurse must be aware of, and observe, all regulations.

3

DRUG ADMINISTRATION

The medication should be recorded after it has been given, and the dose, route, time and the initials of the person administering the drug, recorded. If the patient refuses the drug, or if the medication is not administered, the reason should be noted and reported. Administration of a Schedule 8 drug should also be recorded after the drug has been given. It is not acceptable practice to write up in advance that a drug has been given.

ADMINISTRATION

Procedures for drug administration should be designed to ensure that:

'the right patient receives the right drug, in the right dose, by the right route, at the right time.'

THE RIGHT PATIENT

Before medication is given the patient's identity should be checked using the bed-card and identity band, or verbally. Patients should not be asked a closed question such as 'Is your name Mrs Smith?'. A confused or hard of hearing patient may unwittingly answer 'yes' or 'no'. Open ended questions such as 'What is your name?' are safer. If the patient is incapable of a verbal response then some non-verbal response may be acceptable, e.g. nodding. If patients are unable to identify themselves due to unconsciousness or mental incompetence, some other means of identification may be required. These practices vary from institution to institution. Infants should always be identified by their identity bands.

THE RIGHT DRUG

A drug has both a generic name and sometimes numerous trade names. Any order using an unfamiliar trade name should be checked and, if any doubt remains, the pharmacist should be consulted.

Before administering any drug, the label on the container should be checked three times: once when selecting the container; a second time as the container label is checked against the medication order; and a third time as it is returned to storage. An item should never be identified by its container, appearance or normal position in the drug cupboard. If the label on the container is illegible its contents should not be used. It should be returned to the pharmacy. Should the contents be discoloured or non-uniform, again the contents should not be used but returned to the pharmacy.

If the patient expresses doubt or concern about the medication it should be checked again. There is no margin for error in administering drugs.

Nurses must be conversant with the drugs being used by patients in their care, the indication for use, appropriate dosage and adverse reactions which are common or of a serious nature. It is to the nurse that the patient is likely to report signs or symptoms of adverse drug reactions so vigilance in this area is essential.

THE RIGHT DOSE

Before administering any drug the nurse should be confident that the dosage is appropriate. If there is any doubt the nurse should consult the pharmacist or the prescriber before proceeding. If the patient queries the dose it should be checked again. If, after checking with the pharmacist and/or the prescriber, the nurse still has doubts about the dosage, he/she should refrain from administering the drug and inform both the nursing supervisor and the prescriber of this action and the reasons, and document this action.

Particular attention should be paid to decimal points in a dosage and the difference between the symbols for milligrams (mg) and micrograms (μg or sometimes mcg when handwritten).

THE RIGHT ROUTE

Drugs may be administered by a number of different routes. Factors which determine the best route of administration include the patient's general condition, the rapidity of response required, the drug's chemical and physical properties and the site of the desired action. Although the medical officer prescribes the drug and route of administration, the nurse may question such an order when it seems inappropriate, e.g. oral medication for a patient who is vomiting or unable to swallow or the parenteral route for a patient able to tolerate the drug orally. The nurse should also ascertain that a dose form is appropriate to the route of administration.

Drugs may be administered orally, by injection, topically, rectally, vaginally or by inhalation. Specific considerations regarding each route of administration are discussed in the next section.

THE RIGHT TIME

It is important, especially with drugs whose efficacy depends on reaching and/or main-taining adequate blood levels, that drugs are given at the right time. If a drug should be taken before meals to obtain the required blood levels, it should be given about an hour before food. This applies to many of the antibiotics. On the other hand, some drugs must be taken with or after food, either to avoid excessive irritation of the gut (e.g. non-steroidal anti-inflammatory drugs) or to give higher blood levels (e.g. griseofulvin reaches much higher blood levels if given with a fatty meal).

Nurses must also relate their knowledge of the patient's condition to the drug ordered and make a judgement as to the suitability of its administration at any given time, e.g. giving an antihypertensive agent to a patient who is hypotensive, digoxin to a patient with a low apex beat, insulin to a patient with low blood sugar or waking a patient to give a sedative. In this respect nurses need sound knowledge upon which to base such a judgement. It is advisable to check appropriate physical signs before administering such drugs.

Assessment of patient needs is especially important when administering drugs that are to be taken 'when necessary' (pro re nata or prn). For example, careful consideration of the potential causes, physiological and psychological signs and the patient's own assessment are essential to adequately manage pain, a condition for which prn analgesics are frequently ordered.

DOSAGE FORMS ████████████

Drugs are manufactured in a number of different dosage forms. Factors influencing their design include the physical and chemical properties of the drug, the desired pharmacological action, the site of that action, the pharmacokinetic properties, the onset and duration of action required, the route of administration and anticipated adverse reactions.

ORAL DOSAGE FORMS

Oral forms are those taken by mouth. In most cases it is preferable that the patient be given the oral form of a drug as it is usually the most convenient to administer and the least costly dosage form. The disadvantages are the time lag between administration and onset of effect; the necessity for patient co-operation; destruction of some drugs by digestive enzymes or gastric acid; formation of food–drug complexes which make the drug unavailable for absorption; and possible metabolism by the liver before the drug reaches the general circulation. Solid oral dosage forms include tablets, capsules and lozenges.

Tablets

Tablets, which may be moulded or compressed, come in a variety of shapes, sizes, colours and weights. Tablets may contain only the pure drug or be diluted with various inert substances to produce a suitably sized tablet or to aid in the manufacturing process. Some may contain two or more drugs for a combined pharmacological effect. Various tablet forms are available:

- **Plain compressed tablets**

- **Sublingual tablets** — tablets which are dissolved under the tongue, e.g. glyceryl trinitrate tablets (*Anginine*).

- **Buccal tablets** — tablets which are dissolved between the cheek and gum.

- **Sugar coated tablets** — tablets which mask bad odour or taste.

- **Enteric coated tablets** — tablets which are coated to prevent disintegration in the stomach or to preserve the tablet until it reaches the small intestine. This may be necessary to protect the drug from breakdown by the gastric acid in the stomach or to protect the gastric mucosa from damage by the drug (e.g. enteric coated aspirin).

- **Slow or sustained release tablets** — tablets designed to release the drug over a prolonged period either by time selective dissolving of layers or slow release from a matrix. Sustained release dosage forms are being increasingly used to simplify dosage schedules by allowing daily or twice daily dosing (e.g. the theophylline preparations *Nuelin SR*, *Theodur*).

Capsules

A capsule is a drug in powder, pellet or liquid form which has been enclosed in a soluble, cylindrical capsule, usually made of gelatin.

Lozenges

Lozenges are solid doses of medicine that when sucked slowly disintegrate in the mouth. They are used when a local drug action in the mouth or throat is required.

Oral Liquids

There are three main groups of liquid drugs for oral use: solutions, suspensions and emulsions.

- **Solutions** are preparations of one or more drugs dissolved in a solvent, usually water. Various types of solutions are available including:
  Syrups: concentrated solutions of sugar in water into which the medication is dissolved.
  Elixirs: clear, sweetened solutions containing alcohol and water, medication and flavouring.
  Tinctures: alcoholic extracts.

- **Suspensions** are preparations of finely divided powders suspended in a liquid and usually need shaking before use to resuspend the components.

- **Emulsions** are preparations containing either water globules suspended in oil by means of an emulsifying agent or (more usually) fat or oil globules suspended in water (e.g. paraffin emulsion). They require shaking before use.

INJECTABLE DOSAGE FORMS

The term 'parenteral' dosage forms actually refers to all dosage forms other than oral forms. (Parenteral is derived from the Greek language, para meaning beyond and enteron meaning intestine.) Commonly the term is used to describe those dosage forms that are designed to be administered by injection. Injectable drugs usually are presented as either ampoules or vials. Injections are used to insert sterile liquid medicaments into the body. The injection may be:

- **Intravenous (IV):** into the vein.

- **Intramuscular (IM):** into the muscle. Some intramuscular preparations are designed to provide sustained release of the medication over several hours (e.g. procaine penicillin G) or several weeks (e.g. the fluphenazine decanoate preparation *Mod cate*) thereby providing a prolonged effect. Some drugs are not absorbed well by the intramuscular route, e.g. phenytoin is erratically absorbed and can cause tissue damage at the injection site. (See Drug Absorption, Chapter 2 Pharmacokinetics.)

- **Subcutaneous (SC):** into the subcutaneous fat just below the layers of skin.

- Less commonly injections may be **intradermal** — into the skin layers; **epidural** — into the epidural space of the spinal chord; or **intrathecal** — into the subarachnoid space of the spinal chord.

It should be noted that some injectable dosage forms are specific for a particular route of injection and may not be given by other routes. For example, methylprednisolone is available in two formulations, *Solu-Medrol* for intravenous use, and *Depo-Medrol*, a depot preparation for intra-articular or intramuscular administration.

TOPICAL DOSAGE FORMS

Topical forms of drugs are those used externally on the body. They include **creams**, **ointments**, **lotions**, **liniments**, **paints** and **sprays** and may be used locally to lubricate, protect or deliver a drug to a localised area, either the skin or a mucous membrane.

The most common forms in this group are the creams and ointments. Ointments tend to be greasy and therefore emollient and stay on the skin for a long time.

Creams are emulsions of oil in water — non-greasy 'vanishing' creams (e.g. sorbolene cream); or water in oil — greasy (e.g. zinc cream). For further information see Chapter 28 Skin Diseases.

An increasingly important topical dosage form is the **transdermal patch** which allows systemic administration of various drugs via intact skin. They are designed to allow controlled release of the drug which is absorbed continuously through the skin. The patches provide a prolonged systemic effect. Examples are glyceryl trinitrate patches for prevention and treatment of attacks of angina pectoris, hyoscine patches for prevention and treatment of motion sickness and oestrogen patches for hormone replacement.

RECTAL DOSAGE FORMS

Medication may be delivered by the rectal route as suppositories, rectal creams, ointments or foams, or enemas. Rectal administration may be used for local effect, as in constipation or haemorrhoids; to deliver drugs for systemic effect in patients with nausea or vomiting or who are unable to swallow; to decrease gastric irritation (e.g. irritation caused by non-steroidal anti-inflammatory drugs such as indomethacin and naproxen); or in the unconscious patient.

- **Suppositories** are medicated dosage forms designed to melt at body temperature or to dissolve in body fluids. They are designed to deliver medication via the rectal route either for local effect or for systemic absorption.

- **Enemas** are liquid preparations for rectal administration. *Irrigating enemas*, such as soap and water enemas, are usually used to stimulate peristalsis and thus relieve constipation or cleanse the lower bowel in preparation for diagnostic or surgical procedures. *Retention enemas* are designed to be retained within the rectum or colon for a period of time. They are used to treat constipation or to introduce medication (e.g. prednisolone).

Suppositories are considered superior to enemas as a method of delivering drugs as they are easier and more comfortable for the patient to retain.

VAGINAL DOSAGE FORMS

Vaginal preparations include **pessaries**, which are similar to suppositories but are designed for vaginal use, and **vaginal creams and foams**. They are used for the topical application of medication.

INHALATIONS AND RESPIRATORY PREPARATIONS

Various dosage forms have been designed to deliver medication to the respiratory tract to produce both topical and systemic effects.

- **Inhalations** traditionally are given in the form of hot steam to which medications such as eucalyptus oil, menthol or tincture of benzoin compound can be added.

- **Metered dose aerosols** use the power of liquified or compressed gas to expel a dose of medication in the form of a fine powder or mist from the container for inhalation into the lungs.

  An innovation in inhaler therapy is the introduction of *Turbuhaler* inhalers. This inhaler device is breath actuated and thus does not rely on coordination between the inward breath and release of medication.

- **Nebulisers** are mechanical devices driven by compressed air or oxygen which produce a fine aerosol mist of fluid droplets. They are used to deliver medications to the bronchioles.

PROCEDURES FOR DRUG ADMINISTRATION ▮▮▮▮▮▮▮

ORAL ADMINISTRATION

Some general guidelines for giving oral medication are:

- The patient should be sitting upright or in a semi-Fowler's position before administration of any oral medication to facilitate swallowing and minimise the risk of aspiration.

- Water or other fluid should be given with medications (unless contraindicated) to help swallowing.

- If more than one medication has been prescribed the nurse should remain with the patient until all the doses are swallowed.

- Tablets should not be broken unless they are scored, to ensure accurate dosage.

- Capsules should not be opened unless it has been confirmed as appropriate by the pharmacist or prescriber.

- Some tablets and capsules are enteric coated or sustained release formulations and must not be broken, crushed or dissolved. This can be confirmed with the pharmacist. The patient should be advised not to chew these medications. There are increasing numbers of medications available in both plain and sustained release formulations. These dosage forms have quite different absorption characteristics and are not interchangeable (e.g. diltiazem is available as a plain and a sustained release formulation, *Cardizem* and *Cardizem SR*).

- Should a patient vomit shortly after taking an oral medication the vomitus should be checked for signs of undissolved particles and the medical officer notified.

Sublingual and buccal routes of administration are used when a rapid action is desired. These drug forms are specifically designed to be easily absorbed into the blood vessels under the tongue (sublingual) or between the cheek and the gum (buccal). The tablets are completely soluble. Examples are sublingual forms of glyceryl trinitrate and isosorbide dinitrate.

ADMINISTRATION BY INJECTION

The advantages of the parenteral route are: absorption is usually more rapid and predictable than when a drug is given by mouth; some drugs cannot be absorbed by the gastrointestinal tract; and some patients, because they are unconscious, vomiting or unable to swallow, cannot take oral medication. The disadvantages of parenteral therapy include increased cost, discomfort for the conscious patient and a lower level of safety.

Intravenous Administration

Intravenous (IV) doses of drugs are the most critical doses prepared and administered to patients. Penetration of the skin breaches the body's natural defences so strict asepsis must be maintained to avoid infection. Once a drug has been given by the intravenous route it is virtually irretrievable. Adverse reactions to drugs administered intravenously can occur almost immediately. Whenever intravenous therapy is used, emergency equipment and drugs should be readily available. Before giving a drug intravenously the nurse must check:

- The dosage.

- The reconstitution directions (incorrect reconstitution or dilution can render a drug ineffective or at worst dangerous,

e.g. erythromycin must be reconstituted with water for injection, sodium chloride will cause a precipitate to form).

- The method of intravenous administration.

METHODS OF INTRAVENOUS ADMINISTRATION

The recommended method(s) of intravenous administration for each drug are aimed at minimising systemic or local toxicity and maximising therapeutic response. There are three main methods of administering drugs by the intravenous route:

1. Intravenous bolus or push injection.

2. Intermittent infusions using burettes or small volume infusions, e.g. *Minibags*.

3. Large volume infusions.

INTRAVENOUS BOLUS

The advantages of a bolus injection are: an immediate and accurate dosage; the possibility of titrating the dose to the patient's response; and low fluid volume for patients with fluid restriction.

The disadvantages specific to this method include the possibility of serious consequences from a too rapid rate of injection (e.g. phenytoin must be administered at a rate not faster than than 50 mg/minute or hypotension, cardiovascular collapse or central nervous system depression can occur; aminophylline administered too rapidly can cause hypotension, serious arrhythmias and convulsions). Local reactions (e.g. vascular irritation) also can occur and are minimised by diluting known irritant drugs such as ampicillin and erythromycin.

If a drug is to be administered by intravenous bolus the appropriate dilution and rate of injection must be known and strictly followed. For a bolus which needs to be administered over a period longer than five minutes, an intermittent infusion should be considered.

3

DRUG ADMINISTRATION

INTERMITTENT INFUSION

To minimise the problems of vascular irritation and the toxic effects of too rapid injection many drugs are further diluted in a burette or small volume infusion (e.g. a *Minibag*) and infused over a longer period usually 15–60 minutes.

LARGE VOLUME INFUSIONS

Drugs can be added directly to an infusion solution and infused continuously. This practice is fraught with dangers and should only be used when the drug cannot be given any other way.

HAZARDS ASSOCIATED WITH ADDING DRUGS TO INTRAVENOUS FLUID CONTAINERS

BREAKDOWN OF STERILITY

Most intravenous fluids are excellent substrates for the growth of microorganisms and broaching the container of an intravenous fluid may lead to contamination of the fluid with microorganisms. The addition of drugs to infusion flasks or bags should be carried out using aseptic technique, ideally in a laminar flow cabinet in a controlled environment in the pharmacy department. Drugs should be added immediately prior to administration and all solutions should be administered no later than 24 hours after preparation. All solutions containing additives must be appropiately labelled with the drug added, the dose of the drug added, the date and time of the addition, the duration of the intravenous infusion, the signatures of those preparing and checking the solution and the patient's identity.

PARTICULATE CONTAMINATION

Introduction of microscopic particles into an intravenous fluid may lead to microbiological contamination of the fluid, vein damage, thrombophlebitis or thrombus formation. Sources of particles may be airborne dust; skin, hair or lint shed by the operator; particles of glass from ampoules; particles of rubber from intravenous bottles or vials; or organic matter from reconstituted powdered drugs.

DRUG INCOMPATIBILITY

Many factors influence compatibility of drugs with each other and with intravenous fluids. Drug solutions are very sophisticated systems and differences in buffers, pH, preservatives, vehicles, temperature, concentration and even order of mixing can affect compatibility. Incompatibilities may be broadly classified as physical or visual, and chemical. Physical or visual incompatibilities are the result of poor solubility of drugs in solution or of acid–base reactions. They may be typified by the formation of an obvious precipitate, evidence of turbidity or cloudiness, a colour change or evolution of a gas (bubbles). Examples are phenytoin sodium injection which will form a precipate when mixed with solutions of glucose 5%, and diazepam which will precipitate when added to aqueous solutions. However, an incompatibility is not always indicated by an obvious visual change. Chemical incompatibilities involve the irreversible degradation of drugs in solution to form therapeutically inactive or, occasionally, toxic compounds. These incompatibilities may or may not be visually apparent. An example is the degradation of ampicillin sodium when mixed with glucose 5% and stored at room temperature for more than four hours. Many of the degradation reactions are time and temperature dependent.

MULTIPLE ADDITIVES

The dangers of incompatibility are exacerbated when more than one additive is introduced into an intravenous fluid. It is beyond the scope of this chapter to discuss the many known drug–drug and drug–intravenous fluid incompatibilities. There is a variety of texts and references available on this subject. However, some general principles apply.

- Before introducing an additive refer to hospital guidelines, manufacturer's literature or other available references to ensure compatibility. The pharmacy department can provide information and guidance.

- Avoid multiple drug additions to intravenous fluids as they substantially increase the risk of incompatibility.

- After addition of the drug the container should be thoroughly mixed and inspected for particulate matter, precipitation or a change in clarity or colour.

- The only solutions to which additives should be routinely made are glucose 5%, sodium chloride 0.9% and sodium chloride and glucose combinations.

- No drugs should be added to blood, plasma or other blood products, amino acid solutions, lipid preparations, mannitol solutions, dextran and sodium bicarbonate solutions.

ALTERATION OF DRUG AVAILABILITY

An intravenous infusion may be considered to be a sustained release preparation. Depending on the infusion rate it is likely that some drugs may not reach therapeutic blood concentrations if the usual injection dose is added to a large volume of fluid and administered over a prolonged period of time (e.g. many antibiotics). In addition some drugs when added to an infusion container may adsorb onto the glass or plastic of the container and giving set and not reach the patient's circulation and site of action at therapeutic concentrations. For example, with glyceryl trinitrate infusion 40%–80% of the total amount of glyceryl trinitrate in the final diluted solution is absorbed by the PVC tubing of intravenous administration sets currently in general use. Therefore special giving sets must be used.

A drug should be added to an intravenous fluid only when positively indicated and never as a matter of convenience. Many intravenous fluids are now commercially available preloaded with drugs commonly administered in this manner, e.g. potassium, heparin and lignocaine. These should be used wherever possible. When medications are administered by infusion it is usually recommended that an infusion control device be used to control the rate of administration.

Many institutions have specific policies on intravenous administration of drugs, setting out what drugs may be administered by nursing staff and providing protocols for administration. It is a professional responsibility of nurses to become familiar with the policies and procedures of the institution at which they work.

Intramuscular Administration

Absorption of drugs administered by intramuscular injection is similar to that of drugs administered subcutaneously, but is usually more rapid because muscle is more vascularised. Intramuscular injections are more difficult and dangerous to give than subcutaneous injections. If the drug is inadvertently delivered to subcutaneous tissue it is not absorbed quickly and may cause pain and irritation. The possibility of hitting a large nerve or blood vessel should also be kept in mind. The volume of an intramuscular injection is usually less than 3 mL but may be as much as 5 mL.

Subcutaneous Administration

Subcutaneous injections are usually more slowly absorbed than intramuscular injections due to minimal blood flow in subcutaneous fat.

The concept of continuous subcutaneous infusion was introduced to deliver insulin to diabetics. The medication is delivered at a constant rate by syringe pump to the subcutaneous tissue to provide prolonged action. Since its introduction there has been steady development of the technique for patient care in other fields, e.g. systems to deliver morphine for pain control in palliative care.

INHALATIONS, AEROSOLS, NEBULISER SOLUTIONS

The respiratory tract has an enormous area of absorbing epithelium and so is useful for delivering drugs locally to the lungs, e.g. bronchodilators such as salbutamol and

3

DRUG ADMINISTRATION

ipratropium and topical corticosteroids such as beclomethasone. Metered dose aerosols are commonly used to administer these medications. It has been found that up to 50% of asthmatics have inadequate inhaler administration techniques. The nurse has a role to play in reinforcing correct administration technique. The usual procedure for using a metered dose aerosol is to:

- Shake the aerosol.

- Breathe out in a relaxed fashion to the end of a normal breath.

- Place the open end of the mouthpiece between the lips.

- Breathe in slowly through the mouth, at the same time pressing the cannister firmly down into the plastic mouthpiece with the index finger.

- Breathe in slowly and completely. Remove the aerosol from the mouth and hold the breath for 5–10 seconds before breathing out.

- If a second inhalation is necessary wait two minutes before repeating the inhalation.

Various 'spacing' devices are available which reduce deposition of drug in the mouth and help patients when coordination of the inward breath and actuation of the aerosol is a problem. Small volume spacers (e.g. *Misthaler*) allow for a delay of 4–5 seconds between actuation of the aerosol and inhalation of the mist. Large volume spacers of about 750 mL (e.g. *Nebuhaler, Volumatic*) retain the aerosol cloud for 10 seconds or more and may be emptied using several breaths if necessary. Patients who have difficulty with metered dose aerosols may benefit from using these devices.

MEDICATION ERRORS

Strict adherence to the institution's procedures or guidelines for administration of medication should minimise the occurrence of errors. When preparing medications a quiet environment without interruptions is required. Only the nurse who prepares a medication should administer it. However, occasionally a mistake may occur. Medication errors include giving the wrong medication or the wrong dose or administering a medication to the wrong patient. Mistakes in timing of dosages or routes of administration should also be noted. Any medication error should be reported immediately so that appropriate treatment can be initiated if necessary. The patient should be closely monitored. An incident report should be completed. Such reporting will obviously minimise the danger to the patient and documentation of the error may lead to changes in procedures which could help avoid similar mistakes in the future.

RIGHTS OF THE PATIENT

At all times it must be remembered that the patient has rights. These extend to the use of medication. Firstly, the patient has the right to be informed what the medication is for and what beneficial effects might reasonably be expected from its use. The patient also has the right to be informed of adverse reactions that occur commonly with the medication and any potentially serious adverse reactions. In this regard prime responsibility rests with the prescriber, but it is sometimes the pharmacist and often the nurse who performs the counselling function. To be effective, such counselling must be based on knowledge of pharmacology and therapeutics and be tempered with good judgement as to how much information the patient requires.

Secondly, the patient has the right to refuse medication. In the event of a patient so doing, the prescriber should be advised so that alternate treatment may be considered. Obviously there are cases where the patient is incompetent to make such decisions, e.g. the unconscious or mentally disturbed patient, but this does not negate the general principle. Such events should be documented.

PATIENT EDUCATION

Educating the patient, family or other carers should be an essential part of any patient management plan. The patient needs to know what benefits to expect from treatment, what adverse reactions are common and diminish with continued treatment, what adverse reactions are significant and should be referred to a medical practitioner. The correct technique for administration of injections, metered dose aerosols, nebulisers and so on is important to ensure optimum response to therapy. Similarly the timing of medication may be important to maximise the effectiveness of the medication, minimise adverse reactions or aid compliance.

Before teaching a patient about drugs the following factors should be assessed:

- The patient's readiness to learn;

- The patient's ability to receive and use the information effectively;

- The appropriate amount of information to be given to the patient;

- The patient's physical state (e.g. motor and sensory functions);

- Factors likely to interfere with learning (e.g. fatigue, anxiety, fear, pain, social problems); and

- Other people to be included in the program (e.g. family, friends).

Time should be allowed for the education program in the overall nursing plan. Information should be pitched at an appropriate level for the patient, using teaching aids if available. Patients should be encouraged to participate by making some decisions themselves and adequate time for evaluation and feedback should be allocated.

Long-term compliance with a drug regimen may be dependent on successful patient education.

FURTHER READING

Badewitz-Dodd, L.H. (ed) (1993), *MIMS Annual,* MIMS Australia, Sydney.
State Poisons Acts and Regulations.
Trissel, L.A. (1992), *Handbook on Injectable Drugs,* 7th edn, American Society of Hospital Pharmacists, Maryland.

TEST YOUR KNOWLEDGE

1. Describe the responsibilities of the nurse in drug therapy.

2. What is the function of the State Poisons Acts?

3. What schedules of the poisons list are of particular importance to the nurse?

4. Name two drugs which are listed in Schedule 8 of the poisons list.

5. Five factors are involved in ensuring that drug administration procedures are designed correctly. What are these factors?

6. Describe the correct procedure for using a metered dose aerosol.

7. An IV injection of methylprednisolone has been prescribed. Two injectable preparations are available. What are they and which is the appropriate preparation for IV use?

Dose Calculations

JULIENNE I. HILDITCH

O B J E C T I V E S

At the conclusion of this chapter the reader should be able to:

1. Calculate the number of tablets, capsules or volume of liquid required for a specified dose of medication;

2. Calculate flow rates for intravenous infusions;

3. Calculate the administration rate for infusions containing drugs;

4. Calculate a dose based on body weight; and

5. Calculate the quantities required to make up simple solutions, using both percentages and ratios.

CALCULATIONS ▬

Calculations are an integral part of a nurse's daily work. Each medication round requires numerous simple calculations regarding the appropriate number of tablets to be administered, the volume of a mixture to be given, the reconstitution and volume of an injection or the administration rate of an infusion. These calculations are not difficult and with practice can be mastered.

After performing any calculation it is important to look critically at the answer. A calculation that gives an answer that looks implausible probably is and should be reworked. All calculations should be checked with another person.

It cannot be overemphasised how important fluency in these calculations is for safe and effective drug therapy.

ARITHMETIC PRETEST

Students should work through the following exercises. Answers are given at the end of the chapter. If a student is unable to successfully complete this pretest, a review of the appropriate arithmetic principles should be undertaken before proceeding.

Conversion to fractions:

1. $1\frac{3}{7}$ =
2. $2\frac{2}{3}$ =
3. $1\frac{4}{5}$ =
4. $3\frac{1}{6}$ =
5. $4\frac{1}{4}$ =
6. $3\frac{3}{8}$ =

Multiplying fractions:

1. $\frac{1}{4} \times \frac{1}{3}$ =
2. $\frac{3}{5} \times \frac{1}{2}$ =
3. $\frac{1}{6} \times \frac{3}{4}$ =
4. $1\frac{1}{5} \times \frac{5}{7}$ =
5. $\frac{3}{2} \times \frac{4}{6}$ =
6. $\frac{3}{8} \times \frac{2}{7}$ =

Dividing fractions:

1. $\frac{1}{5} \div \frac{1}{6}$ =
2. $\frac{2}{3} \div \frac{4}{6}$ =
3. $\frac{3}{8} \div \frac{1}{5}$ =
4. $\frac{5}{7} \div \frac{3}{4}$ =
5. $1\frac{2}{3} \div 1\frac{2}{3}$ =
6. $1\frac{1}{4} \div \frac{1}{4}$ =

Multiplying decimals:

1. 1.6×3.2 =
2. 2.7×1.75 =
3. 6.0×4.2 =
4. 2.5×1.7 =
5. 16.8×102 =
6. 5.4×30.5 =

Dividing decimals:

1. $16.4 \div 8$ =
2. $3.5 \div 0.7$ =
3. $6.5 \div 1.3$ =
4. $2.12 \div 0.424$ =
5. $7.5 \div 0.3$ =
6. $11.25 \div 3.75$ =

Converting ratios to percentages:

1. 1:2 = %
2. 1:500 = %
3. 1:20 = %
4. 1:2000 = %
5. 1:5000 = %
6. 1:250 = %

Converting percentages to ratios:

1. 1% = :
2. 20% = :
3. 5% = :
4. 0.02% = :
5. 1.5% = :
6. 0.45% = :

INTERNATIONAL SYSTEM OF UNITS ▬

The International System of Units (Système International d'Unités) or SI units are used for all dosage measurements and calculations.

UNITS OF WEIGHT

1 kilogram (kg) = 1000 grams (g)

1 gram = 1000 milligram (mg)

1 milligram = 1000 micrograms (μg)

Only official abbreviations should be used, however, microgram should be written in full to avoid confusion and this policy is used in this book.

UNITS OF VOLUME

1 litre (L) = 1000 millilitres (mL)

Under standard conditions 1 litre of pure water weighs 1 kilogram and 1 millilitre weighs 1 gram. It is important to remember that the gram (g) corresponds in weight to the millilitre (mL) and the kilogram (kg) in weight to the litre (L).

EXPRESSING QUANTITIES AS DECIMALS

Quantities less than one unit are usually written in the next smaller unit. For example, half a gram should be written as 500 mg rather than 0.5 g. If it is necessary to use the larger unit a zero is always placed before the decimal point, e.g. 0.5 g. To write .5 g could lead to confusion if the decimal point is indistinct. If 5 g of a drug were given in error for 0.5 g the mistake could be fatal. Therefore, whole numbers in the smaller unit should be used whenever possible.

CONVERSION BETWEEN UNITS

As 1 gram (g) = 1000 milligrams (mg) to convert grams to milligrams multiply by 1000, e.g.

2 g = (2 × 1000) mg = 2000 mg

2.358 g = (2.358 × 1000) mg = 2358 mg

1.74 g = (1.740 × 1000) mg = 1740 mg

In the last example it was useful to write the 1.74 g as 1.740 g and then multiply by 1000 by moving the decimal place three places to the right.

When converting from milligrams to grams, divide by 1000, e.g.

$$2050\,mg = \frac{2050}{1000}\,g$$
$$= 2.05\,g$$

This corresponds to moving the decimal place three places to the left.

To convert litres to millilitres, multiply by 1000; conversely, to convert millilitres to litres divide by 1000; e.g.

$$1.7\,L = 1.7 \times 1000\,mL$$
$$= 1700\,mL$$

$$960\,mL = \frac{960}{1000}$$
$$= 0.96\,L$$

EXPRESSING PERCENTAGES IN QUANTITATIVE TERMS

Legislation for the labelling of therapeutic goods requires that the strength of a product must be expressed as the amount (usually mg) of active compound per g or mL of product. Previously this strength may have been expressed as a percentage, i.e. parts of active ingredient per 100 parts of product. For example, the strengths of hydrocortisone creams were formerly expressed as percentages such as 0.5%, 1%. The strengths of these creams are now expressed as 5 mg/g and 10 mg/g respectively. This practice mainly affects external preparations such as creams, ointments and eye drops.

Percentage preparations were expressed as weight in weight (w/w), weight in volume (w/v), volume in volume (v/v) and volume in weight (v/w). Thus

1% w/w represented 1 g of a solid dispersed in 100 g of solid product;

1% w/v represented 1 g of a solid dispersed in 100 mL of liquid product;

1% v/v represented 1 mL of a liquid dispersed in 100 mL of liquid product; and

1% v/w represented 1 mL of a liquid dispersed in 100 g of solid product.

When a formula was expressed as a percentage without specifying the units of weight or measure, the convention was that liquids were measured by volume and solids by weight.

As preparations described in percentage terms are still occasionally seen it is necessary to know how to convert from one system to the other.

EXAMPLE: To convert the strength 1% into quantitative terms (mg/g) the following method is used.

Method
The basic units in these types of quantitative expressions are grams for solid preparations and millilitres for liquid preparations.

The expression 1% represents one part per hundred. If the product is a solid (e.g. a cream or ointment) then 1% means 1 g of active ingredient is contained in 100 g of product. To express this in quantitative terms, i.e. in mg/g:

1 g is contained in 100 g

divide each side by 100

$$\frac{1}{100} \text{ g is contained in } \frac{100}{100} \text{ g} = 0.01 \text{ g in 1 g}$$

or remembering the convention about quantities less than 1 g

$$\frac{1}{100} \times 1000 \text{ mg in 1 mg} = 10 \text{ mg/g}$$

If the product is a liquid, e.g. an antiseptic solution or eye drops, then the term 1% means 1 g of active ingredient per 100 mL of product. To express this in quantitative terms, that is mg/mL, the procedure is the same.

MILLIMOLES

In SI units concentration may be expressed either as mass concentration (g/L) or as 'amount of substance' concentration, millimole/L (mmol/L). Millimoles are commonly used to express the quantity of electrolytes in solutions of sodium and potassium.

The term milliequivalent (mEq) has previously been used in a similar context. The use of millimoles is now standard and milliequivalents should not be used. However, as the term milliequivalent may sometimes be seen in older literature it should be noted that millimoles and milliequivalents are not synonymous:

1 mmol = 1 mEq × valency of the ion.

DOSE CALCULATIONS ■

The quantity of a drug given, in terms of numbers of tablets or volume of liquid, may be calculated in a number of ways. Any method of calculation that arrives at the right answer is acceptable, however, only two are presented here:

Method 1, which works from first principles; and

Method 2, which involves the use of a formula.

Regardless of which method is used, it is necessary in all cases to ensure that calculations are performed using the same type of unit throughout, e.g. milligrams, millilitres, percentages, ratio. In many cases a conversion to similar units must be performed before the computation can begin. In addition, it is necessary to specify the type of units to which the answer refers. An answer of six means little, it must specify the units, e.g. six tablets, six litres or whatever the appropriate unit happens to be.

CALCULATIONS FOR SOLID DOSE FORMS

Tablets

EXAMPLE: How many tablets containing 62.5 micrograms of digoxin will be required to give a dose of 0.125 mg?

Method 1

STEP 1
Convert all figures to the same units. As the two doses are in different units, one in micrograms and the other in milligrams, one must be converted to the other, e.g.

$$0.125 \text{ mg} = (0.125 \times 1000) \text{ micrograms}$$
$$= 125 \text{ micrograms}$$

STEP 2
62.5 micrograms = 1 tablet

Divide both sides by 62.5

1.0 microgram $= \dfrac{1}{6.25}$ tablets

Multiply both sides by 125

125 micrograms $= \dfrac{1}{62.5} \times 125$ tablets

$= 2$ tablets

Therefore two tablets of digoxin 62.5 micrograms must be given for a 0.125 mg dose.

Method 2
This method involves application of the following formula:

$$\text{Quantity required} = \frac{\text{dose required}}{\text{dose available}} \times 1 \text{ tablet}$$

STEP 1
As before, convert the dosages to similar units

$$0.125 \text{ mg} = (0.125 \times 1000) \text{ micrograms}$$
$$= 125 \text{ micrograms}$$

STEP 2
Substitute into the formula

$$\frac{\text{dose required}}{\text{dose available}} = \frac{125}{62.5} \times 1 \text{ tablet}$$

$$= 2 \text{ tablets}$$

Therefore 2 tablets of digoxin 62.5 micrograms must be given for a 0.125 mg dose.

Commonsense must always be used to check the answer. For example, it is unusual to administer more than two or three tablets per dose. If a calculation gives an answer that requires the administration of a larger number of tablets it should be checked.

CALCULATIONS FOR LIQUID MEDICATION

Mixtures

CALCULATION OF DOSAGES

EXAMPLE: A dose of 150 mg of amoxycillin is ordered. The suspension available contains 125 mg/5 mL. What volume must be administered.

Method 1

125 mg is contained in 5 mL

1 mg is contained in $\dfrac{5}{125}$ mL

150 mg is contained in $\dfrac{5}{125} \times 150$ mL

= 6 mL

Method 2

Apply the formula:

Volume to be given

$= \dfrac{\text{dose required}}{\text{dose available}} \times \dfrac{\text{volume containing}}{\text{dose available}}$

$= \dfrac{150}{125} \text{ mg} \times 5 \text{ mL}$

= 6 mL

Therefore 6 mL of amoxycillin suspension 125 mg/5 mL must be given for a dose of 150 mg.

After performing any calculation look critically at the answer and ensure that it makes sense. For instance if the dosage form of a drug contains 100 mg in 2 mL and the dosage required is 75 mg the answer must logically be less than 2 mL. Conversely if the dose required is 150 mg the answer must be greater than 2 mL.

Injections

CALCULATION OF DOSAGES

EXAMPLE: A dose of 75 mg of pethidine is ordered. Pethidine is available in ampoules containing 100 mg/2 mL. What volume must be administered?

Method 1

100 mg is contained in 2 mL

Divide both sides by 100

1 mg is contained in $\dfrac{2}{100}$ mL

Multiply by 75

75 mg is contained in $\dfrac{2}{100} \times 75$ mL

= 1.5 mL

Method 2

Apply the formula:

Volume to be given

$= \dfrac{\text{dose required}}{\text{dose available}} \times \dfrac{\text{volume containing}}{\text{dose available}}$

$= \dfrac{75}{100} \text{ mg} \times 2 \text{ mL}$

= 1.5 mL

Therefore 1.5 mL of pethidine injection 100 mg/2 mL will be required for a dose of 75 mg.

CALCULATION OF DOSAGES FOR INJECTIONS THAT REQUIRE RECONSTITUTION

Some injections, mainly antibiotics, are supplied in powder form and have to be reconstituted before use. That is, a diluent must be added to the powder. When the product information specifies exact quantities of diluent to be added and the final strength of the solution the dose is calculated exactly as previously described for liquid medication. Table 4.1 lists some of the commonly used antibiotics with reconstitution details.

TABLE 4.1   Reconstitution details for some commonly used antibiotics

Drug Name	Strength	Diluent*	Volume added (mL)	Final concentration (mg/mL)
Ampicillin	100 mg	WFI	2.0	50
	250 mg	WFI	1.8	125
			2.3	100
	500 mg	WFI	1.7	250
			2.2	200
			4.7	100
	1 g	WFI	1.3	500
			3.3	250
			9.3	100
Cefotaxime	500 mg	WFI	4.8	100
	1 g	WFI	4.6	200
	2 g	WFI	9.0	200
Ceftriaxone	500 mg	WFI	4.85	100
	1 g	WFI	4.7	200
			9.7	100
Ceftazidime	1 g	WFI	3.9	200
Cephalothin	1 g	WFI	3.6	250
			4.6	200
Chloramphenicol	1.2 g	WFI	2.0	400
		or N/S	3.8	250
		or G5%	11.0	100
Erythromycin lactobionate	300 mg	WFI	6.0	50
	1 g	WFI	20.0	50
Flucloxacillin	250 mg	WFI	4.8	50
			2.3	100
			1.8	125
			1.05	200
	500 mg		4.7	100
			3.7	125
			2.2	200
			1.7	250
	1 g		9.3	100
			4.3	200
			3.3	250
			1.3	500
Benzylpenicillin	300 mg	WFI	1.8	150
			1.3	200
			0.8	300
	600 mg		5.6	100
			2.0	250
			0.6	600
Piperacillin	2 g	WFI	8.6	200
	4 g		17.5	200
Ticarcillin	1 g	WFI	4.5	200
	3 g		13.0	200

*WFI = Water for Injection; N/S = Sodium Chloride 0.9% (Normal Saline); G5% = Glucose 5%
Note: Reconstituted solutions may require further dilution before administration.

EXAMPLE: Ampicillin 750 mg IMI is ordered. How many mL from a 1 g vial should be administered?

Reconstitute a 1 g vial with 1.3 mL of water for injection. This gives a solution with a concentration of 500 mg/1 mL (see Table 4.1).

$$1 \text{ mg is contained in } \frac{1}{500} \text{ mL}$$

$$750 \text{ mg is contained in } \frac{1}{500} \times 750$$

$$= 1.5 \text{ mL}$$

Alternatively apply the same formula as that used previously to work out the dose of a liquid preparation.

Occasionally, no final strength is mentioned in the product information. Consider the case of an antibiotic for which a 125 mg dose is required. The antibiotic comes in a vial containing 250 mg to which must be added 2 mL of water for injection. The final volume will be a little over 2 mL because of the space occupied by the powder. The only way to administer a fractional dose is to withdraw and measure the volume of the reconstituted solution and to administer the correct fraction of that volume.

Intravenous Infusions

CALCULATION OF INFUSION RATES FOR ADMINISTRATION SETS

Intravenous administration sets are calibrated to deliver a given number of drops per millilitre of solution. The new international standard for giving sets (macro giving sets) delivers 20 drops/mL. Most sets in Australia now comply with this new standard although there may be some sets still in use which deliver 15 drops/mL. Therefore it is important to know the type of set in use. Paediatric giving sets (micro giving sets) deliver 60 drops/mL.

An intravenous order is usually expressed as a volume to be given over a period of time (e.g. 500 mL over 4 hours) but the rate is estimated by observing the flow in drops per minute. Therefore it is necessary to be able to calculate the conversion from drops per minute to mL per hour and vice versa when using different administration sets.

EXAMPLE 1: What flow rate is required to administer 500 mL of glucose 5% over a period of 4 hours from a set delivering 20 drops per mL?

Method 1

500 mL is to run over 4 hours

$$= \frac{500}{4} \text{ mL to run over 1 hour}$$

$$= 125 \text{ mL to run over 1 hour (60 minutes)}$$

$$= \frac{125}{60} \text{ mL to run over 1 minute}$$

As 1 mL is equal to 20 drops

$$\frac{125}{60} \times 20 \text{ drops will run over 1 minute}$$

$$= 41.67 \text{ drops/minute}$$

The giving set should be set to deliver a flow rate of 42 drops per minute.

Decimal points need not be used as it would be impossible to administer or observe 0.67 of a drop. Adjust the answer to the next whole number.

Method 2

Apply the formula:

Rate (drops/minute)

$$= \frac{\text{volume (mL)} \times \text{number of drops/mL}}{\text{time (hours)} \times 60}$$

$$= 500 \times \frac{20}{4 \times 60}$$

$$= 41.67 \text{ drops/minute}$$

EXAMPLE 2: Calculate the rate of flow required to deliver 75 mL of normal saline per hour using a paediatric or micro giving set.

Method 1

75 mL is to run over 1 hour (60 minutes)

$$= \frac{75}{60} \text{ mL to run over 1 minute}$$

As there are 60 drops per mL

$$\frac{75}{60} \times 60 \text{ drops will run over 1 minute}$$

= 75 drops/minute

Method 2
Apply the formula:

Rate (drops/minute)

$$= \frac{\text{volume (mL)} \times \text{number drops/mL}}{\text{time (hours)} \times 60}$$

$$= 75 \times \frac{60}{1 \times 60}$$

= 75 drops/minute

Therefore to administer normal saline at a rate of 75 mL per hour the flow rate on a paediatric giving set should be set at 75 drops per minute.

It may sometimes be necessary to estimate the time it will take for an intravenous solution to be administered.

EXAMPLE 3: Calculate how long it will take for 1 L of Hartmann's solution to run through at a flow rate of 25 drops per minute using a macro giving set?

Method 1

The flow rate is 25 drops per minute

There are 20 drops/mL

$$= \frac{25}{20} \text{ mL/minute}$$

$$= \frac{25}{20} \times 60 \text{ mL/hour}$$

= 75 mL/hour

Therefore 1000 mL will run through in

$$\frac{1000}{75} = 13.3 \text{ hours}$$

Method 2
Apply the formula:

Time taken (hours)

$$= \text{volume (mL)} \times \frac{\text{drops/mL}}{\text{drops/minute} \times 60}$$

$$= 1000 \times \frac{20}{25 \times 60}$$

= 13.3 hours

Another situation that may arise is the need to administer a given amount of drug over a specified period of time.

EXAMPLE 4: At what rate must a solution containing 1000 mg of lignocaine in 500 mL of solution be given to a patient to administer 3 mg/minute from a set delivering 60 drops per mL?

Method

STEP 1
Calculate how much infusion solution contains 3 mg of lignocaine.

If 1000 mg of lignocaine is contained in 500 mL

1 mg lignocaine is contained in $\frac{500}{1000}$ mL

3 mg lignocaine is contained in $\frac{500}{1000} \times 3$ mL

= 1.5 mL

Thus 1.5 mL each minute will give a dose of lignocaine of 3 mg/minute. This must now be converted to a flow rate.

STEP 2
Convert to a flow rate.

If 1 mL = 60 drops then
1.5 mL = 60 × 1.5 drops
        = 90 drops

Therefore to administer lignocaine at 3 mg/minute from a solution containing 1000 mg/500 mL using an administration set delivering 60 drops/mL, a flow rate of 90 drops/minute must be maintained.

4

DOSE CALCULATIONS

Increasing use is being made of infusion pumps, rate controllers or syringe pumps to achieve precise fluid and dosage control. These require that the infusion rate be set in millilitres of solution per hour (mL/h).

EXAMPLE 5: 10 000 units of heparin in 1000 mL of normal saline is ordered to be given over 8 hours. At what rate should the infusion pump be set (mL/h)?

Method 1
1000 mL is to be given over 8 hours

$$= \frac{1000}{8} \text{ mL given over 1 hour}$$

$$= 125 \text{ mL/hour}$$

Therefore the pump should be set at 125 mL/hour.

Method 2
Apply the formula:

$$\text{Rate (mL/hour)} = \frac{\text{volume (mL)}}{\text{time (hours)}}$$

$$= \frac{1000}{8}$$

$$= 125 \text{ mL/hour}$$

EXAMPLE 6: Heparin 10 000 units is to be given in 30 mL of normal saline over 12 hours using a syringe pump. At what rate should the pump be set?

Method 1
30 mL is to be given over 12 hours

$$= \frac{30}{12} \text{ mL given over 1 hour}$$

$$= 2.5 \text{ mL/hour}$$

Method 2
Apply the formula:

$$\text{Rate (mL/hour)} = \frac{\text{volume (mL)}}{\text{time (hours)}}$$

$$= \frac{30}{12}$$

$$= 2.5 \text{ mL/hour}$$

Therefore the syringe pump should be set at a rate of 2.5 mL/hour.

It is important to know how to do such calculations. However as a matter of convenience a number of tables showing administration rates for intravenous infusions using different administration sets are available. See Tables 4.2 and 4.3.

CALCULATIONS OF DOSES FROM BODY WEIGHT

Occasionally doses may be expressed in terms of dosage per kg of body weight. This requires the nursing staff to weigh the patient and give the appropriate dose based on that weight. This is done simply by multiplying the dose per kg by the weight of the patient (in kg).

EXAMPLE: A dose of 5 mg/kg is to be given to a patient who weighs 70 kg.

Method
Dose required

$$= \text{dose (mg/kg)} \times \text{weight (kg)}$$
$$= 5 \times 70$$
$$= 350 \text{ mg}$$

A variation of this dose may be expressed as: give 1 mg/kg/day in four divided doses. In this instance the total amount to be given per day would be calculated first, then divided into four equal doses and given at six-hourly intervals.

Some infusions are used to administer a drug at a given dose per kg over a specified time.

EXAMPLE: A pethidine infusion prepared by the aseptic addition of 500 mg of pethidine to 500 mL of glucose 5% is to be infused at a rate of 0.3 mg/kg/hour. The infusion is to be controlled by an infusion pump. At what rate should the infusion pump be set to deliver the appropriate amount of pethidine to a 70 kg patient.

TABLE 4.2 Administration rates for intravenous infusions using an adult administration set delivering 20 drops/mL

1 L flask			500 mL flask		
Duration of Infusion (hours)	Drops/min	mL/hour	Duration of Infusion (hours)	Drops/min	mL/hour
24	14	42	24	7	21
18	19	56	18	9	28
16	21	63	16	10	31
12	28	83	12	14	42
10	33	100	10	17	50
8	42	125	8	21	63
6	56	167	6	28	83
4	83	250	4	42	125

TABLE 4.3 Administration rates for intravenous infusions using a paediatric administration set delivering 60 drops/mL

1 L flask			500 mL flask		
Duration of Infusion (hours)	Drops/min	mL/hour	Duration of Infusion (hours)	Drops/min	mL/hour
24	42	42	24	21	21
18	56	56	18	28	28
16	63	63	16	31	31
12	83	83	12	42	42
10	100	100	10	50	50
8	125	125	8	63	63
6	167	167	6	83	83
4	250	250	4	125	125

Method

STEP 1

Dosage required for a 70 kg patient

= 0.3 mg/kg/h
= 0.3 x 70 mg/h
= 21 mg/h

Pethidine infusion contains 500 mg pethidine per 500 mL

= 1 mg pethidine per 1 mL

Therefore 21 mg pethidine is contained in 21 mL of infusion and the dose of 21 mg/hour will be delivered by an infusion run at 21 mL/hour.

A similar calculation is required for a syringe pump.

CALCULATIONS FOR EXTERNAL PREPARATIONS

Antiseptics

Most antiseptic solutions are now supplied diluted to the appropriate concentration for use. However, there may be some instances where a concentrated antiseptic solution has to be diluted before use.

EXAMPLE: A 1:2000 solution of chlorhexidine is required and a 20% solution is available. How much of the 20% solution will be needed to make 1 L of the 1:2000 solution?

Method 1

STEP 1
How much chlorhexidine is in the final solution?

A 1:2000 solution of chlorhexidine contains 1 g of chlorhexidine per 2000 mL, therefore 1000 mL will contain 500 mg of chlorhexidine.

STEP 2
How much chlorhexidine is in the available solution?

The solution available contains 20% chlorhexidine, therefore it contains 20 g of chlorhexidine per 100 mL

STEP 3
To make the final solution we require 500 mg of chlorhexidine:

20 g chlorhexidine is contained in 100 mL

1 g chlorhexidine is contained in $\dfrac{100}{20}$ mL

$= 500$ mg (0.5 g) in $\dfrac{100}{20} \times 0.5$ mL

$= 500$ mg in 2.5 mL of 20% solution

Therefore 2.5 mL of 20% solution diluted with water to 1 L will contain 500 mg chlorhexidine per 1 L which is a 1:2000 solution.

There are numerous ways to do this calculation. A second method involves the application of a formula.

Method 2
Apply the formula:

Amount required

$= \dfrac{\text{strength required}}{\text{strength available}} \times \text{quantity required}$

It is important to remember that when applying a formula all the units must be converted so that they are same type of unit.

STEP 1
As one strength is expressed as a ratio and the other as a percentage one must be converted. It does not matter what units are used as long as they are both the same.
If both strengths are expressed as percentages:

1:2000 = 0.1:200

= 0.05:100

= 0.05%

STEP 2
Substitute into the formula

Amount required

$= \dfrac{0.05}{20} \times 1000$

$= 2.5$ mL

Therefore the amount of 20% chlorhexidine solution required to prepare 1000 mL of 1:2000 solution is 2.5 mL.

ANSWERS TO ARITHMETIC PRETEST

Conversion to fractions:

1. $\frac{10}{7}$
2. $\frac{8}{3}$
3. $\frac{9}{5}$
4. $\frac{19}{6}$
5. $\frac{17}{4}$
6. $\frac{27}{8}$

Multiplying fractions:

1. $\frac{1}{12}$
2. $\frac{3}{10}$
3. $\frac{1}{8}$
4. $\frac{6}{7}$
5. 1
6. $\frac{3}{28}$

Dividing fractions:

1. $1\frac{1}{5}$ 4. $\frac{20}{21}$
2. 1   5. 1
3. $1\frac{7}{8}$ 6. 5

Multiplying decimals:

1. 5.12   4.   4.25
2. 4.725   5. 1713.6
3. 25.2   6.   164.7

Dividing decimals:

1. 2.05   4. 5
2. 5   5. 25
3. 5   6. 3

Converting ratios to percentages:

1. 50%   4. 0.05%
2. 0.2%   5. 0.02%
3. 5%   6. 0.4%

Converting percentages to ratios:

1. 1:100
2. 1:5
3. 1:20
4. 1:5000
5. 15:1000
6. 45:10 000

TEST YOUR KNOWLEDGE

1. Convert the following percentages into quantitative terms: (a) hydrocortisone eye ointment 0.5%; (b) timolol 0.25% eye drops; (c) betamethasone dipropionate cream 0.05%; (d) pilocarpine 6% eye drops.

2. Convert the following quantitative terms into percentages: (a) betamethasone 0.2 mg/g; (b) clotrimazole 10 mg/g.

3. How many frusemide 40 mg tablets must be given for a 10 mg dose?

4. How many digoxin 0.25 mg tablets must be given for a dose of 125 micrograms?

5. How many haloperidol 500 microgram tablets must be given for a 1 mg dose?

6. A dose of 350 mg of potassium chloride has been ordered. A solution containing 1 g in 4 mL is available. What volume must be given?

7. A 100 mg dose of erythromycin has been ordered. Erythromycin suspension containing 125 mg/5 mL is available. How much must be given?

8. From ampoules containing atropine 0.6 mg/mL what volume must be given to give a dose of 900 micrograms?

9. A dose of 160 mg of frusemide is ordered. Each ampoule contains 250 mg/25 mL. How much should you give?

10. Cefotaxime 1.5 g IV is ordered. 2 g vials are available. What volume of reconstituted solution would you administer? (See Table 4.1 for reconstitution details.)

11. What flow rate in drops per minute must be maintained using an administration set delivering 20 drops/mL to give 1 L of normal saline by IV infusion over 12 hours?

12. How many drops per minute must be maintained to administer 50 mL of glucose 10% over 1 hour using a set delivering 60 drops per mL?

13. How long will it take 1 L of Hartmann's solution to run through at 50 drops per minute using a set that delivers 60 drops per mL?

14. How long will 500 mL of glucose 5% take to run through a 20 drop per mL giving set which is set at 40 drops per minute?

15. A patient is ordered 1000 mL of sodium chloride 0.9% containing 20 mmol of potassium to be given over 8 hours using an infusion pump. Calculate at what rate the pump should be set (mL/h)?

16. An infusion of morphine is prepared with 50 mg morphine diluted to 50 mL with normal saline in a 50 mL syringe. A dose of 0.03 mg/kg per hour is ordered. At what rate should the syringe pump be set to deliver this dose for a 60 kg patient?

17. A 70 kg patient is ordered glyceryl trinitrate infusion to commence at a rate of 0.2 microgram/kg/min. The concentration of the prepared infusion pump solution is 100 micrograms/mL. At what rate (mL/h) should the infusion pump be set?.

18. How much sodium hypochlorite concentrate (consider it 100%) is required to make 100 mL of 1:20 solution?

Paediatric Therapeutics

BRIAN J. LILLEY and KERRIE A. LOVE

O B J E C T I V E S

At the conclusion of this chapter the reader should be able to:

1. Discuss factors which should be considered in paediatric drug therapy;

2. Discuss the differences between drug therapy for neonates and older children; and

3. Discuss drugs used particularly in neonates.

GENERAL PRINCIPLES ██████████

Providing drug therapy to infants and children presents a unique set of challenges. There are many physiological differences between children and adults, including variances in vital organ maturity and body composition. These differences greatly influence the actions and effectiveness of drugs. However, pharmacokinetic studies provide little if any information on drug action in infants and children because they are usually performed in adults.

Paediatric pharmacology, therefore, has developed mainly from therapeutic practice and experience in adults and the use of 'scaled down' adult doses. This practice is clinically successful for the majority of drugs which are relatively non-toxic and have a wide margin between therapeutic and toxic doses. Drugs with a narrow therapeutic margin such as the aminoglycoside antibiotics and digoxin, require more sophisticated knowledge and individualised dosage regimens. Doses of such agents are initially based on a mg/kg body weight basis and then modified according to results of serum drug concentration measurements.

Some terms used in this chapter which define stages of human development require definition:

Neonates are babies in the first 4 weeks of life.

Preterm or premature babies are born prior to 37 weeks gestation.

Low birth weight babies weigh less than 2500 g at birth.

Infants are babies from 4 weeks to 2 years of age.

Children are defined as being older than 2 years and less than 12 years of age.

FACTORS INFLUENCING PAEDIATRIC DRUG THERAPY ██████████

Important factors to be considered in paediatric drug therapy are absorption, distribution, metabolism and excretion.

ABSORPTION

Oral Absorption

The gastrointestinal tract, particularly the stomach, undergoes significant changes from birth until around 3 years of age. Before 3 years of age the stomach has low levels of acid and acid labile drugs such as the penicillins show enhanced absorption. On the other hand, this depressed level of acidity may result in reduced absorption of drugs which are weak acids themselves, e.g. phenobarbitone, phenytoin and rifampicin. The incomplete absorption experienced with these anticonvulsants often necessitates their continued parenteral administration.

The delayed gastric emptying seen in neonates and young infants is probably not as important as previously believed. In the first few weeks of life this may be significant but most sick neonates receive their drugs parenterally.

Of considerable importance, particularly to the general public, is the question of drug administration and absorption relative to meals. Current evidence suggests that, with the exception of isoniazid, captopril, rifampicin, phenoxymethylpenicillin and tetracyclines (except doxycycline and minocycline), all medications should be administered with meals to avoid gastrointestinal irritation and to aid compliance.

Topical Absorption

Topical absorption of drugs is enhanced in children and especially in infants. This is a direct result of the relative thinness of the stratum corneum. Absorption may be further enhanced in the presence of burnt or excoriated areas and with occlusive dressings. This has been well documented with the use of corticosteroid creams for eczema and nappy rash in infants, especially when the area treated has been occluded with plastic pants.

Rectal Absorption

Rectal administration may be useful in patients who are vomiting and in infants and young children who are reluctant to take oral medication.

The rectal route is not ideal for all drugs. Drugs with narrow therapeutic margins such as aminophylline should not be administered rectally. Considerable interindividual variation in rectal venous drainage and hence in the extent of drug absorption, can produce toxic drug levels. One drug which is recommended for rectal administration in children is diazepam for the treatment of seizures. Paracetamol can also be safely administered rectally for treatment of pain or fever.

DISTRIBUTION

Numerous factors, including body composition, plasma protein binding and the blood brain barrier influence drug distribution in the various paediatric age groups.

Body Composition

Total body water and fat composition alter significantly during the transition from birth to adult life. Total body water as a percentage of body weight is approximately 80% at birth, 65% at 12 months and 60% for a young adult male.

On the other hand, fat content as a percentage of body weight varies with age, being about 3% in premature infants, 12% in full term neonates, 30% at 1 year of age and about 18% in the average adult.

Therefore, larger mg/kg body weight doses of water soluble drugs need to be given to neonates and infants to achieve plasma concentrations similar to those seen in adults. However, this has to be balanced against diminished hepatic function and renal elimination before arriving at a final dosage recommendation.

Plasma Protein Binding

Drug protein binding is diminished in neonates due to a lower concentration of plasma proteins, particularly albumin, and the lower drug binding capacity of fetal albumin. This may lead to an increase in the fraction of unbound, pharmacologically active drug in the plasma. Moreover, there may be competition between endogenous substances, especially free fatty acids and bilirubin, and drugs for albumin binding sites.

However, when drugs administered to neonates are examined in detail, very few highly protein bound drugs are used. From a practical point of view, highly protein bound drugs such as phenytoin, sulfonamides, salicylates and diazepam should be given with caution in the presence of hyperbilirubinaemia.

In older children, there are a number of disease states which may affect drug protein binding. These conditions include hepatic disease, nephrotic syndrome, chronic renal failure, cardiac failure and malnutrition.

Blood Brain Barrier

The blood brain barrier is a permeability barrier between the circulation and the brain cells bathed in cerebrospinal fluid. The blood brain barrier is functionally incomplete in the neonate and certain substances show increased penetration into the brain. One of the most important factors which determines the rate of transport of drugs across the blood brain barrier is their lipid solubility.

5

PAEDIATRIC THERAPEUTICS

This gives rise to increased brain uptake of barbiturates and morphine in infants.

As meningitis is a relatively common problem in paediatric practice, the extent to which antimicrobial agents penetrate into the cerebrospinal fluid is an important consideration. Although some agents penetrate poorly under normal circumstances, in the presence of meningeal inflammation, penetration may be considerably enhanced so that adequate cerebrospinal fluid concentrations are attained. Drugs in this category include penicillins, cephalosporins, rifampicin and vancomycin. Drugs which penetrate well even in the absence of meningeal inflammation include chloramphenicol and the combination, sulfamethoxazole and trimethoprim.

Although the aminoglycosides continue to be used for meningitis caused by Gram negative organisms, the cerebrospinal fluid concentrations achieved are generally low and inconsistent. Higher concentrations can be obtained by direct intrathecal or intraventricular injections, but controversy exists over the efficacy of such routes of administration. The newer cephalosporins, such as cefotaxime, appear to be more appropriate agents in most cases.

METABOLISM

The various metabolic reactions that occur in the mature liver are not fully developed at birth. Cardiac insufficiency and respiratory distress may also contribute to decreased metabolic activity. Lignocaine, phenobarbitone, phenytoin, diazepam and chloramphenicol show decreased metabolism in the neonate, resulting in increased drug half-lives. Chloramphenicol, if given in usual doses based on body weight, might lead to high concentrations and accumulation of unchanged drug with consequent serious toxicity and circulatory collapse (the grey baby syndrome).

During the first 15 days of life in premature and full term babies decreased metabolism is evident but this is followed by a dramatic increase. Between 1 and 10 years of age hepatic microsomal oxidation is more rapid than in adults. Therefore phenobarbitone, phenytoin and theophylline have shorter half-lives in children than in adults. This more rapid metabolism is almost certainly due to the fact that during childhood the liver is larger relative to body weight than in adult life.

EXCRETION

Renal function is significantly less developed in premature and full term neonates than it is in children and adults. Adult values for glomerular filtration rate are reached after about 3 to 6 months of age, while tubular function does not mature fully until sometime later than this.

Renal function is of particular importance to drug disposition in the neonatal period. Most sick neonates receive antibiotics for suspected or proven infection and most of these agents are water soluble. In general the lower the gestational age of the infant the more prolonged the half-life will be in this period. The rate of elimination increases rapidly during the ensuing weeks so that half-lives similar to those seen in adults are usually achieved by the end of the first month of life.

DRUG USE IN THE NEONATE ■■■■■■

Pharmacological treatment of the neonate is determined by the weight and gestational age of the baby. As previously discussed a preterm baby has poorly developed renal and liver function which will alter metabolism and excretion of some drugs. Thus neonates often require lower, or less frequent, doses of medication.

Advancing technology has greatly improved the outcome for premature babies. The treatment of some neonatal medical conditions is discussed below.

5

PAEDIATRIC THERAPEUTICS

RESPIRATORY CONDITIONS

Respiratory problems are the most common for neonates. Hyaline membrane disease, the major cause of respiratory distress syndrome, is due to a lack of surfactant in the neonatal lung.

Exogenous surfactant can be used prophylactically before the baby's first breath or in the first minutes after birth. Such prophylactic treatment is used only in babies at risk of developing respiratory distress syndrome. Exogenous surfactant can also be administered to rescue babies who develop respiratory distress syndrome in the first 24 hours of life. The optimum treatment regimen has not yet been established.

Up to 90% of neonates weighing under 1000 g will have attacks of apnoea. These attacks are due to underdevelopment of lungs and the respiratory centre in the medulla. Theophylline and aminophylline are thought to have a direct effect on the respiratory centre to stimulate respiration. Neonates tolerate these drugs well and side effects are similar to those experienced by adults.

Neonates are quite sensitive to the respiratory depressant effects of opioids. Opioid analgesics administered to the mother at the time of delivery can cross the placenta. Naloxone is administered to the neonate to reverse the respiratory depression that ensues. Naloxone can be administered by intravenous, intramuscular or subcutaneous injection.

CARDIAC CONDITIONS

Patent ductus arteriosus is another common condition in premature neonates. The ductus arteriosus is a blood vessel connecting the aorta to the pulmonary artery in the fetus. The ductus arteriosus usually closes spontaneously soon after birth but may remain patent in babies born prematurely.

A patent ductus arteriosus may be closed by fluid restriction with or without treatment with frusemide. Indomethacin may be used if the patent ductus arteriosus has not closed within 24 hours. Prostaglandin E (PGE) produced in the wall of the ductus helps to maintain a patent ductus arteriosus. Indomethacin, a prostaglandin synthetase inhibitor, decreases levels of circulating PGE and helps to promote closure. Contraindications include shock, intracranial haemorrhage, high blood urea nitrogen levels, haemorrhagic disease and a low platelet count.

Whilst patent ductus arteriosus can cause problems for the neonate there are some ductus dependent cardiac conditions. In these life threatening cardiac abnormalities a patent ductus arteriosus is necessary to allow some mixing of oxygenated and deoxygenated blood. As already discussed prostaglandins play a role in maintaining a patent ductus arteriosus. PGE is therefore given to maintain a patent ductus arteriosus until corrective surgery can be performed. Prostaglandin E_1 (alprostadil) is available for continuous intravenous infusion. PGE_2 (dinoprostone) is available as dispersible tablets for oral use.

DRUGS USED IN PAEDIATRICS ▐

Theophylline, Aminophylline

TRADE NAMES

Theophylline: *Elixophyllin; Nuelin; Slo-Bid; Theo-Dur.*

MECHANISM OF ACTION

Theophylline causes direct relaxation of the smooth muscle in the respiratory tract and also has a direct effect on the respiratory centre in the medulla to stimulate respiration. The drug acts on the kidney to cause weak diuresis and on the heart to cause increased rate and force of contractions. Aminophylline is a theophylline complex with similar actions and adverse reactions.

PHARMACOKINETICS

Theophylline is well absorbed after oral administration, but rectal absorption is much less reliable. Neonatal absorption of theophylline may be decreased by erratic peristalsis and decreased gastric acidity. Aminophylline can be given intravenously as well as orally. Intramuscular injection of aminophylline is painful and causes sloughing.

Aminophylline and theophylline undergo liver metabolism. Both the parent drug and the metabolites are then excreted by the kidneys. Neonates metabolise theophylline to caffeine, whereas adults convert very little theophylline to the caffeine metabolite.

USES

Theophylline is used as a bronchodilator in asthma. The direct effect on the respiratory centre makes it a drug of choice for neonatal apnoea.

Theophylline is available for oral use as a mixture, tablets and sustained release tablets or sprinkles. Aminophylline is available as a mixture and injection.

Doses of theophylline are titrated to achieve therapeutic serum levels of 40–80 micromol/L for neonatal apnoea and 55–110 micromol/L for the treatment of asthma. The usual starting dose is 5 mg/kg (up to

250 mg) every 6 hours for patients over one year with asthma. The sustained release preparations are usually given 12 hourly: 12 mg/kg/dose for children from 1 to 7 years; 10 mg/kg/dose for 8 to 16 years; and 8 mg/kg/dose (maximum 500 mg) over 16 years of age. For neonatal apnoea, a loading dose of 6 mg/kg (by intravenous injection or orally as a mixture) is given to start and then doses are administered 12 hourly: for babies under 1 week, 2 mg/kg/dose; for babies 1–2 weeks, 3 mg/kg/dose; and for babies over 2 weeks, 4 mg/kg/dose. Aminophylline 10 mg is equivalent to 8 mg of theophylline.

Gastric irritation can be decreased by administration with or after food. Sustained release preparations must not be crushed or chewed. Sustained release capsules may be opened and the beads sprinkled onto soft food. Intravenous aminophylline must be administered slowly to prevent hypotension.

ADVERSE DRUG REACTIONS

Theophylline is a potent drug which is tolerated well by neonates. Adverse effects include gastric irritation; central effects such as irritability and seizures; cardiac effects such as tachycardia; diuresis; and hyperglycaemia.

DRUG INTERACTIONS AND CONTRAINDICATIONS

See Chapter 11 Respiratory Diseases.

Alprostadil, Dinoprostone

TRADE NAMES

Alprostadil: *Prostin VR.*
Dinoprostone: *Prostin E₂.*

MECHANISM OF ACTION

The ductus arteriosus is a blood vessel joining the aorta to the pulmonary artery during fetal life. Prostaglandin E_1 (PGE_1, alprostadil) and prostaglandin E_2 (PGE_2, dinoprostone) are administered to neonates suffering from ductus dependent congenital cardiac abnormalities.

PHARMACOKINETICS

Alprostadil is rapidly metabolised in the lungs. Metabolism is so rapid that alprostadil must be administered as a continuous infusion. Dinoprostone is absorbed when administered orally and is also active when given intravenously. Metabolites of both prostaglandins are excreted in urine.

USES

Alprostadil is administered into a large vein or umbilical artery catheter. It is administered at a rate of 0.1 microgram/minute until an effect is seen. The dose is then decreased to a maintenance dose which may be as low as 0.01 microgram/kg/minute. *Prostin VR* ampoules contain 500 micrograms/mL of alprostadil. *Prostin E2* tablets contain 500 micrograms of dinoprostone. These tablets will disperse in water allowing small doses to be administered orally each hour.

ADVERSE DRUG REACTIONS

Apnoea occurs in up to 12% of neonates treated with alprostadil. Such apnoea is more common in babies less than 2 kg and in the first hour of treatment. Other adverse effects include flushing, bradycardia, hypotension and central nervous system effects such as seizures and temperature elevation. Alprostadil should be avoided in neonates with respiratory distress syndrome or bleeding tendencies. Blood pressure should be monitored during treatment.

DRUG INTERACTIONS

Alprostadil can be used with other drugs such as digoxin, dopamine and diuretics to treat congenital cardiac disease.

PRECAUTIONS AND CONTRAINDICATIONS

Peripheral vasodilation is more common when alprostadil is administered into the umbilical artery.

Long-term administration of alprostadil has been associated with cortical hyperostosis and widening of cranial sutures. These effects are reported to be reversible.

Exogenous Surfactant

TRADE NAMES

Exogenous surfactant: *Exosurf Neonatal.*

MECHANISM OF ACTION

Endogenous surfactant normally lines the lungs, decreasing the surface tension between the alveoli and the air. The presence of endogenous surfactant prevents alveolar collapse during expiration. Exogenous surfactant is administered to neonates at risk of respiratory distress syndrome due to deficiency of endogenous surfactant. Several surfactant preparations have been developed from human amniotic fluid, from animal lung washing or mincing, and synthetically. *Exosurf Neonatal* is a synthetic surfactant.

PHARMACOKINETICS

Exogenous surfactant is administered into the trachea. Little information is available regarding absorption and metabolism, however lung tissue is thought to reutilise exogenous surfactant to synthesise further surfactant.

USES

Exogenous surfactant is used to prevent respiratory distress syndrome (RDS) due to premature birth in the following situations:

- Prophylactic treatment of infants with birth weights greater than 1350 g who are at risk of developing RDS.

- Prophylactic treatment of infants with birth weights greater than 1350 g who have evidence of pulmonary immaturity.

- Rescue treatment of infants who have developed RDS.

Exosurf Neonatal Suspension is reconstituted and administered via a special endotracheal tube without interrupting mechanical ventilation. Administration should only be undertaken by experienced clinicians. The dose is 5 mL/kg/dose. Usually two or three doses are administered at 12 hourly intervals.

ADVERSE DRUG REACTIONS

Exogenous surfactant has relatively few adverse effects. Pulmonary haemorrhage has been reported. Endotracheal tubes may plug with mucus after administration. This may be decreased by suctioning infants prior to administration.

DRUG INTERACTIONS

No drug interactions have been reported at this time.

PRECAUTIONS AND CONTRAINDICATIONS

Infants under 700 g are at an increased risk of pulmonary haemorrhage.

NURSING IMPLICATIONS

The nurse should monitor the heart rate, colour, chest expansion, facial expression, oximeter readings and patency of the endotracheal tube.

Indomethacin

TRADE NAMES

Indomethacin: *Indocid, Arthrexin*.

MECHANISM OF ACTION

Indomethacin is a non-steroidal anti-inflammatory drug (NSAID) which inhibits the synthesis of prostaglandins. Prostaglandins are found in all body tissues so it is not surprising that indomethacin has many actions.

In the kidney, indomethacin decreases levels of vasodilatory prostaglandins leading to sodium and fluid retention. In premature neonates with patent ductus arteriosus decreased PGE allows closure of the ductus and decreases left to right shunting.

PHARMACOKINETICS

In neonates, the bioavailability of oral indomethacin may be as low as 20%. The half-life of indomethacin in neonates is much longer than that in adults. The rate of excretion is directly related to gestational age.

Indomethacin is metabolised in the liver to inactive metabolites, some of which are excreted in the faeces, some in the urine.

USES

In the treatment of patent ductus arteriosus indomethacin can be administered orally or intravenously. Intravenous treatment is considered to be most effective leading to closure in approximately 70% of patients. The first dose is 0.2 mg/kg. Two further doses are given at 8 to 24 hour intervals, the dose depending on the age of the baby. A lower dose of 0.1 mg/kg/day for 6 days has been trialled and shown to have a lower relapse rate.

ADVERSE DRUG REACTIONS

Gastrointestinal side effects are common with indomethacin. Babies are at increased risk of developing necrotising enterocolitis and gastric perforation. Reversible renal failure has been reported in adults with pre-existing renal dysfunction. In neonates urine output decreases after administration of indomethacin but recovers after cessation of treatment. Concomitant administration of frusemide may prevent these renal effects.

Indomethacin reversibly decreases platelet aggregation. There has been an association between indomethacin administration and increased risk of retinopathy of prematurity.

DRUG INTERACTIONS

Aminoglycoside levels require careful monitoring when these drugs are administered to neonates receiving indomethacin. See also Chapter 22 Musculoskeletal Disorders.

PRECAUTIONS AND CONTRAINDICATIONS

Precautions particular to neonates include shock, intracranial haemorrhage and necrotising enterocolitis. See also Chapter 22 Musculoskeletal Disorders.

Naloxone

TRADE NAMES

Naloxone: *Narcan, Narcan Neonatal.*

MECHANISM OF ACTION

Naloxone is a narcotic antagonist which reverses all effects of opiates. Naloxone has no action of its own, acting only when administered after narcotics. It is thought that naloxone competes with opiates for opiate receptor sites.

PHARMACOKINETICS

Naloxone acts rapidly when administered by any parenteral route; subcutaneously, intramuscularly or intravenously. The duration of action is longer after intramuscular administration but is dependent also on the narcotic present.

USES

Naloxone is administered to reverse the respiratory depression, sedation and hypotension caused by narcotics. The neonate may suffer from adverse effects of opiates administered to the mother during labour. Neonates are particularly susceptible to opiate induced respiratory depression. Naloxone is administered to neonates at a dose of 0.01 mg/kg intravenously or 0.07 mg/kg intramuscularly or subcutaneously. The action will last from 1 to 4 hours. The baby must be observed for recurrence of intoxication. Naloxone is available as a 0.4 mg/mL (*Narcan*) and a 0.02 mg/mL injection (*Narcan Neonatal*).

ADVERSE DRUG REACTIONS

Naloxone does not cause adverse effects in its own right. However, the abrupt reversal of opiate effects by naloxone administration can lead to nausea, vomiting and hypertension.

PRECAUTIONS

Naloxone should be administered cautiously to patients who are dependent on opiates including babies of drug dependent women.

Phytomenadione (Vitamin K$_1$)

TRADE NAMES

Phytomenadione: *Konakion*.

MECHANISM OF ACTION

Phytomenadione has the same mechanism of action as naturally occurring vitamin K$_3$ which is necessary for the synthesis of clotting factors in the liver.

PHARMACOKINETICS

Following oral administration of phytomenadione blood coagulation factors increase within 6–12 hours.

Following parenteral administration the increase in clotting factors generally occurs within 1–2 hours. Bleeding is usually controlled within 3–8 hours and a normal prothrombin time may be obtained in 12–14 hours.

USES

Vitamin K is required in the first six weeks of life to prevent a rare but potentially fatal bleeding disorder, haemorrhagic disease of the newborn. For many years phytomenadione was routinely administered intramuscularly to neonates at birth in doses of 0.5–1 mg to prevent this disease. However, recent concern about the association between use of intramuscular phytomenadione and subsequent development of cancer in childhood resulted in a re-evaluation of the use of intramuscular vitamin K.

Many centres now administer vitamin K orally to healthy full term infants in three doses of 1 mg. The first oral dose is given at birth, the second at the time of newborn screening (3–5 days of age) and the third in the fourth week. Infants who are preterm, unwell or unable to absorb oral doses of vitamin K should receive 0.1 mg intramuscularly at birth, followed by further doses (0.1 mg intramuscularly or 1 mg orally) at the time of newborn screening and in the fourth week of life.

ADVERSE DRUG REACTIONS

Phytomenadione is relatively non-toxic. Reactions, which rarely occur, are usually of an allergic nature. Pain, swelling and tenderness at the site of injection have been reported rarely.

5

PAEDIATRIC THERAPEUTICS

Calcium

MECHANISM OF ACTION

Calcium (usually administered as the gluconate) corrects hypocalcaemia which may occur in premature neonates.

USES

Calcium is administered intravenously by diluting calcium gluconate injection to a 2% solution. The diluted solution is administered into a large vein at a rate of 3 mL/kg/hour until normal calcium levels are achieved.

PRECAUTIONS

Rapid infusion can result in decreased blood pressure and bradycardia. Heart rate and blood pressure should be monitored closely during calcium infusion. Calcium salts are incompatible with many other drugs and may precipitate. Compatabilites should be checked carefully before mixing with other infusions.

NURSING IMPLICATIONS

ASSESSMENT

Initial assessment of a child on admission to hospital is extremely important. Weight and height (or length) are used to calculate dosages for medication. It is valuable to know the average weights of children at various ages. When giving doses of medication it is prudent to check the weight on the chart against the child's age. As with adults a history of allergies and adverse drug reactions should be noted.

A child's developmental progress will affect the form of medication chosen and the way in which new medication is introduced. A 2-year old, for example, will often be frightened by a nebuliser pump but is too young for an explanation. A 6-year old may be similarly frightened but may easily comply after a parent has put the mask on and suffered no harm.

Admission to hospital also provides a good opportunity to assess vaccination status. Missed vaccinations can be given whilst the child is in hospital.

ADMINISTRATION

The child's identity must always be certain. Often children cannot or will not identify themselves. The identification band must always be checked immediately before administering medication.

It is essential to check the time of the last dose and the number of doses already given. Nurses have a great responsibility for the safety of young patients. All medications should be locked away.

Dose

As previously discussed most drug doses for children are based on mg/kg body weight calculations. It is, however, important to keep the adult dose of the drug in mind. If the adult dose of a drug is 300 mg it would not usually be appropriate to start a 7-year old on 600 mg, even if this is the dose calculated from mg/kg body weight.

In general, a 7-year old would receive half the adult dose and a 3-year old would receive one-third of the adult dose. These generalisations are a quick check to be used prior to administering medication to children.

Since children grow so quickly, the doses of continuing medication require constant review. Occasionally children are admitted to hospital on suboptimal doses of medication because their increasing size has not been taken into account.

Dosage Calculations

It is good practice to have calculations performed independently by two people. An easy formula for calculating paediatric doses is:

volume of dose required equals

$$\frac{\text{dose required}}{\text{dose available}} \times \text{volume of dose available}$$

For example, a 200 mg dose of penicillin suspension is required. Penicillin mixture is available in two strengths, 125 mg/5 mL and 250 mg/5 mL.

If the 125 mg/5 mL mixture was available:

$$\frac{\text{dose required}}{\text{dose available}} \times \text{volume of dose available}$$

$$= \frac{200 \text{ mg}}{125 \text{ mg}} \times 5 \text{ mL} = 8 \text{ mL}$$

If the 250 mg/5 mL mixture was available:

$$\frac{\text{dose required}}{\text{dose available}} \times \text{volume of dose available}$$

$$= \frac{200 \text{ mg}}{250 \text{ mg}} \times 5 \text{ mL} = 4 \text{ mL}$$

See also Chapter 4 Dose Calculations.

Dosage Form

Oral medications are available in liquid and solid dosage forms. In general children under 6 years require the liquid form, whilst children between 6 and 8 years can usually be persuaded to swallow capsules and tablets.

Mixtures

Suspensions must be shaken well before measuring the dose. Measures should be rinsed with a little water and this should be given to the child as well, to ensure the full dose is administered.

To facilitate the administration of mixtures to infants and children consider the drug's taste, dose form and frequency of administration. The sugar content of mixtures has traditionally been high to improve palatability but this has recently been criticised for increasing the development of dental caries. If the mixture is too pleasant or it is offered to the infant or child as a sweet or lolly, then the possibility of a self-administered overdose increases.

Most mixtures can be diluted but this is not always recommended. If an unpleasant mixture is put into cordial the child then has a larger volume of unpleasant tasting cordial to swallow. In cases of very unpleasant mixture, it is preferable to give the dose and follow this with something pleasant tasting. Cold drinks and ice-cream are good for this because they decrease the taste sensation.

Mixtures should not be added to bottles of infant formula. If the child associates an unpleasant taste with feeds he or she may stop feeding. Further, if the baby drinks only half the bottle then only half of that dose is taken. It is better to give the mixture, diluted with a small amount of fluid if desired, and then give the feed.

When using a medicine dropper or syringe, the medication should be given slowly along the side of the tongue. This prevents children from spitting the mixture out the side of their mouths.

Babies should always be upright and calm when receiving medication. Distressed babies in the prone position can aspirate mixtures, particularly those which have a strong taste.

Tablets

Some manufacturers make tablets especially for children. These tablets are chewable and are usually flavoured. Such chewable tablets are a good introduction to solid dosage forms for children in the 4–8-year age group. Other tablets or capsules may be crushed or opened and mixed with jam, flavoured topping or a small amount of food.

Sometimes it is necessary to halve or quarter tablets. If a tablet is halved, it is good practice to keep the other half for the next dose so that the child has received exactly one tablet over two consecutive doses.

Tablets which are scored are usually easily broken. Shiny, sugar coated tablets are more difficult to break because they slide around when pressure is applied. Sellotape can be used to stick the tablet onto a clean surface. A razor blade or sharp knife can be used to cut the tablet. The pieces of tablet will then peel off the tape.

Not all tablets can be crushed. Some are especially formulated with slow release characteristics or enteric coating to improve their effectiveness. The crushing of such tablets results in the loss of this improved effectiveness and can produce toxicity. For example slow release theophylline tablets (*Nuelin-SR* or *Theo-Dur*) are designed to release their drug over an 8–12-hour period. These tablets may be halved but further crushing will cause the drug to be released over a shorter period of time thereby decreasing the duration of action. More importantly, this may lead to toxic drug levels soon after the dose is taken.

Soluble tablets allow smaller fractions of a tablet to be given. If a tablet is dissolved in a known volume of water a fraction of this can then be administered to even a small baby. It is important to do this only to soluble tablets. Tablets which merely disperse do not give an even solution of drug and are therefore unsuitable for this purpose.

Capsules

Capsules contain powder, beads or liquid. Liquid filled or soft capsules are usually administered whole. Capsules containing powder or beads can be halved or quartered. The capsule can be opened and the powder emptied onto a clean piece of paper. A knife is then used to form a square of powder. The square can then be halved or quartered. A newer dosage form is the bead filled capsule or 'sprinkle'. These capsules are intended to be opened. If the beads are enteric coated they should not be chewed just swallowed. The beads can be sprinkled onto any soft food such as honey or stewed fruit. An alternative is to put them into a small amount of drink. It is then quite easy to suck the beads up through a straw. If the child complains of a bad taste, this indicates that the beads are being chewed.

Drugs Administered by Inhalation

Drugs are often administered to infants and children by a respirator solution delivered by a compressed air nebuliser pump or similar device. Respirator solutions are now available as large multidose bottles or single dose containers (*Nebules* or *Respules*).

At about 4 years of age children can usually manage more portable devices for delivering drugs by inhalation. Salbutamol and beclomethasone are available as powder in capsules, *Rotacaps*. The *Rotacaps* are opened within a *Rotahaler* device and the powder is inhaled. Terbutaline and budesonide *Turbuhalers* are also available. Inhaling through the *Turbuhaler* delivers powder more efficiently to the respiratory system. Spacer devices such as *Volumatics*, *Nebuhalers*, *Misthalers* and *Aerochambers* also decrease the need for accurate coordination. Metered dose aerosols are available but require more coordination for effective use.

Intramuscular Injections

Intramuscular administration is limited as an efficient route of drug administration in infants. The marked changes in relative blood flow to various muscles during development, the relative insufficiency of muscle contractions and the reduced skeletal muscle mass lead to altered and unpredictable absorption from this route in infants.

The pain associated with intramuscular injections is largely due to the volume of the injection. Therefore, the smallest possible amount of fluid should be used to dissolve powder to prepare intramuscular injections.

Those injections presented as reconstitutable powder usually provide information on reconstitution. In the paediatric setting fractions of vials are often required. When this is the case, the actual volume occupied by the powder must be taken into account. Information about powder volumes and reconstitution can be found in product literature. Further information can be obtained from the pharmacy department.

For example, a dose of 125 mg of flucloxacillin is required. Vials containing 500 mg and 1 g are available. If 3.7 mL of water for injection is added to the 500 mg vial the resulting solution contains 500 mg in 4 mL. Thus the powder in the vial occupies 0.3 mL. To obtain the required dose of 125 mg use the formula:

$$\frac{\text{dose required}}{\text{dose available}} \times \text{volume of dose available}$$

$$= \frac{125 \text{ mg}}{500 \text{ mg}} \times 4 \text{ mL} = 1 \text{ mL}$$

See also Chapter 4 Dose Calculations.

Intravenous Injections

The fluid requirements of children dictate special considerations when giving intravenous therapy.

There is a volume of approximately 25 mL in the intravenous tubing between a burette and the patient. Children may be receiving infusions which are running very slowly, as low as 1 mL/hour. If the infusion is running at 5 mL/hour and a drug is added to the burette, it will take 5 hours for the drug to reach the patient. To avoid this problem one might be tempted to increase the rate of the infusion but it is unlikely that the patient will be able to tolerate so much fluid. It is better to administer the drug closer to the patient. If the drug can be given quickly, as a push, the drug could be administered through a three way tap close to the patient. Syringe pumps can also be used to give small volumes of fluid.

PATIENT AND FAMILY EDUCATION

Education of parents and carers should be clear and concise. Nurses along with pharmacists and other health professionals have a responsibility to ensure that parents receive the information necessary for proper treatment at home. The importance of continuing medication at home must be stressed.

5

PAEDIATRIC THERAPEUTICS

FURTHER READING

Robinson, M.J. (1990) *Practical Paediatrics*, 2nd edn, Churchill Livingstone, Melbourne.
Yeh, T.F. (1991) *Neonatal Therapeutics*, 2nd edn, Mosby-Year Book, Sydney.

TEST YOUR KNOWLEDGE

1. Name two factors which affect drug absorption in the neonate.

2. Why does excretion of drugs alter with age?

3. Name two drugs used particularly in neonates.

4. If amoxycillin mixture is available as a 250 mg/5 mL mixture how much is needed for a dose of 350 mg?

5. Name two tablets which should not be crushed or chewed.

Geriatric Therapeutics

DONNA M. DANIELL

O B J E C T I V E S

At the conclusion of this chapter the reader should be able to:

1. Discuss the complex nature of drug therapy and its management in the ageing community;

2. Describe the impact of drugs on an ageing physiology;

3. Identify the different presentations of diseases and medical conditions in the aged;

4. Identify the signs and symptoms of potential adverse drug reactions; and

5. List practical guidelines to assist in optimising drug use in the aged.

THE AGEING POPULATION

'Life is very sweet brother, who would wish to die'

George Burrow 1803–1881.

The Australian population is ageing. This implies that Australia is the type of country that provides a physical and social environment in which a child can be born and have an excellent chance of reaching maturity and surviving into old age.

It is anticipated that the future Australian population will not only have a higher proportion of older people, but the life expectancy of these people will be increased. The percentage of the population over the age of 65 years was 4% in 1901, 10% in 1986 and is expected to reach 12% by the year 2000.

The challenge for medical and allied health professionals is to concentrate efforts into optimising health and to minimise morbidity and mortality in our older age groups. One of the tasks is to ensure the appropriate use of medication and to reduce drug induced illnesses.

Recently, Australian and international studies have drawn attention to high levels of drug use by the aged. Concerns range from the cost of medication to the appropriateness and indeed the safety of current levels of drug usage.

These concerns appear to be justified in light of reports indicating an increased number of drugs being consumed and the higher frequency of adverse drug reactions in this age group. It is not uncommon for an aged person to be prescribed a large number of medications (polypharmacy). A recent survey of a nursing home in Canberra revealed that an average of 7.6 medications, with a range between two and 20 were prescribed per resident. The incidence of drug related hospital admissions of persons over the age of 65 years is estimated to be as high as 25%–30%.

The aged are less physically tolerant of most drugs. They are less capable of metabolising drugs and more susceptible to side effects and interactional effects. As a result they often require a dosage appropriate for geriatric physiology. For the very old, for those that suffer from multiple illness and receive several drugs concurrently rational drug management demands a knowledge of pharmacokinetic and pharmacodynamic changes.

Medications are often not used wisely by the aged. Overdosing, underdosing and erratic dosing intervals can diminish drug action or cause adverse effects. Non-compliance seriously undermines the efficacy of rationally prescribed drugs. When a drug fails to work as hoped, it is too easy to conclude that the patient is a non-responder and either increase the dose or add another drug to the regimen. The inability to manage prescribed medication regimens is a significant factor determining early institutionalised care.

Drug use by the aged person is dominated by the pattern and extent of chronic degenerative diseases established in the middle years of life. It is the prevalence of these diseases that is an essential determinant of the level of drug consumption by the aged patient.

Unfortunately many of the studies reporting high levels of drug utilisation by the aged have concentrated on differences in the use of medication between arbitrarily defined young and old members of a community. This tendency has obscured the important fact that drug use increases progressively throughout the whole period of adult life to finally reach a peak level in the older age group. In effect, high drug use is often the cumulative result of attempts to manage sequential episodes of age related pathology.

It should also be realised that the increase in drug consumption over time is in some ways the result of the increase in effective pharmacological products available on the market. (It is only since the 1940s that effective antibiotic, antihypertensive and psychotropic medications have been available.)

There is a temptation to use 'too little diagnosis and too much drug' in geriatric management. We all too often see the inappropriate use of medication particularly in the treatment of certain conditions. The modification of diet, exercise, physical and emotional environment or other non-drug therapy should be a consideration in the management of conditions such as sleep disturbance, nocturnal agitation, depression, glucose intolerance, postural hypotension, constipation and urinary incontinence.

Fortunately 50%–70% of drug related problems are predictable and preventable through appropriate drug therapy monitoring. It should be remembered that the aged often have low expectations of therapeutic outcomes. There is a tendency among the aged and their professional advisers to attribute the signs and symptoms of disease to mere manifestations of the ageing process.

It is therefore important when attempting to rationalise drug use among the aged not to be led into the error of therapeutic nihilism. The decision to investigate or not to investigate, to treat or not to treat, should seldom be made on the basis of the patient's age.

It is important to individually assess the **risk** and **benefit** of drug therapy in each aged patient. Rules such as 'people over 65 years should not be prescribed more than five drugs' do not have any place in appropriate geriatric care. It is of utmost importance to aim for the highest possible quality of life achievable for a particular patient.

Fundamental to patient management and appropriate drug therapy of the aged is:

- An understanding of the nature of human ageing.

- A basic knowledge of how age related changes modify the presentation of disease.

- An appreciation of how age related changes modify the action and response to drug therapy.

- An understanding of the factors predisposing the aged to adverse drug reactions.

- Access to specific drug information/advice to confirm suspected adverse drug reactions.

- Knowledge of the appropriate management of chronic degenerative disease.

- Multidisciplinary team involvement. This includes the medical practitioner, pharmacist, nurse, occupational therapist, physiotherapist, dietitian and various community services where appropriate.

IMPACT OF AGEING ON RESPONSE TO DRUG THERAPY

PHYSIOLOGICAL CHANGES WITH AGE

The physiological changes that occur with ageing are:

- Alterations in body composition (e.g. a decline in total body size; a decline in total body water; an increase in body fat stores; a decline in lean body mass; and changes in plasma composition).

- A decline in cardiac output and resultant organ blood flow.

- A decline in organ size (e.g. a decline in liver mass and kidney mass).

- Changes in body functioning (e.g. a decline in homeostatic capacity, changes in function of hepatic enzymes, altered tissue responsiveness and reduced glomerular filtration rate).

These changes impact on drug therapy in the aged and have the potential to result in: increased drug plasma concentration; increased duration of drug action; and/or increased drug sensitivity.

6

GERIATRIC THERAPEUTICS

PHARMACOKINETICS

The plasma concentration of a drug is determined by its dose, the time interval between doses, the volume of distribution and its rate of clearance. The plasma concentration of a drug is thus dependant on four factors **absorption**, **distribution**, **metabolism** and **elimination**, all of which may be modified in the ageing process.

The age related changes that affect body composition and renal or hepatic function, alter the pharmacokinetic characteristics of drugs. They may lead to an adverse drug reaction by causing a higher than expected plasma concentration or extended duration of action for a given dose of a drug.

Other age related changes may lead to an adverse drug reaction by increasing the sensitivity of the target organ, i.e. they alter pharmacodynamic characteristics. The expected plasma concentration is not increased.

Absorption

While ageing is associated with a reduction in gastric surface area, reduced blood flow and reduced gastric motility, absorption from the gastrointestinal tract is not significantly affected. The potential interference with drug absorption by food, disease or concurrent medication should be considered.

One drug may physically or chemically impair the absorption of a second drug. For example, antacids, calcium and iron supplements are known to reduce the absorption of many more important drugs such as digoxin and tetracycline antibiotics. Drugs such as metoclopramide and anticholinergics may alter absorption by increasing or decreasing gastric motility.

The timing of a dose in relation to food is an important factor. For example, non-steroidal anti-inflammatory drugs are usually given after food to reduce the risk of gastrointestinal irritation. Penicillins and captopril are usually given on an empty stomach to optimise drug absorption.

Diseases such as neoplasms and diabetes can affect drug absorption.

Distribution

The reduction in total body size can often be masked by obesity, therefore, as age advances body weight becomes a progressively unreliable indicator of metabolic size and less useful for the adjustment of drug dose.

The altered proportion of fat to fluid is significant. In the aged patient water soluble drugs, such as penicillin, ethanol and paracetamol, are distributed into a smaller water compartment than in a younger adult. Therefore for a given dose the plasma concentration of a water soluble drug is likely to be higher in the aged subject.

Similarly, in the aged patient fat soluble drugs, such as anaesthetic agents and diazepam, will be distributed into a relatively larger fat compartment and the plasma concentration is likely to be lower than in the younger person. However, in this case the availability of the drug for clearance will be reduced and consequently the half-life of the drug and therefore its duration of action will be prolonged. For these reasons a reduction in dose is often required.

Drug Binding

The composition of blood serum is known to alter with age. A reduction in albumin concentration and a small increase in $\alpha 1$ acid glycoproteins can impact on drug therapy. Weakly acidic drugs such as phenytoin and warfarin bind to serum albumin, while weakly basic drugs such as propranolol and non-steroidal anti-inflammatory agents bind to α_1 acid glycoproteins. It is probable that under normal circumstances the alterations in concentration of these serum proteins will have little clinical significance. However, when two drugs compete for limited binding sites a clinically significant displacement reaction may occur. Caution is required particularly when administering oral anticoagulants or oral hypoglycaemic agents as both these drug classes are highly protein bound and haemorrhage or hypoglycaemia can result if a second highly protein bound drug is added. Drugs that are highly protein bound are listed in Table 6.1.

TABLE 6.1   Drugs that are highly protein bound

Analgesics (NSAIDs, aspirin)

Anticoagulants (warfarin)

Anticonvulsants (carbamazepine, phenytoin, sodium valproate)

Antidepressants

Antimicrobials (penicillins, nalidixic acid, sulfonamides)

Antihistamines

Antipsychotics

Benzodiazepines

Cardiovascular agents (nifedipine, prazosin, quinidine, verapamil)

Corticosteroids

Diuretics (bumetanide, spironolactone, triamterene)

Oral hypoglycaemic agents

Miscellaneous (bromocriptine, clofibrate, thyroxine, chlormethiazole)

Metabolism

The capacity of the liver, the principle metabolic organ, to metabolise drugs can be reduced with increasing age. The decline in size, blood flow and possible alterations in the hepatic enzyme activity can greatly influence the elimination of a drug and hence increase its duration of action.

Hepatic enzyme activity may be enhanced or inhibited by concurrently administered drugs. The H$_2$ antagonist cimetidine inhibits enzyme action and reduces the metabolism of certain drugs, e.g. benzodiazepines and warfarin. Alcohol and nicotine are known to induce the activity of hepatic enzymes hence potentially enhancing the metabolism of other drugs.

Normally the reduction of hepatic blood flow which occurs in the aged is of no clinical consequence, but when the hepatic capacity is further challenged by congestive heart failure or by hepatic disease the metabolism of drugs is reduced and adverse effects may occur.

Drugs with potentially reduced hepatic clearance are listed in Table 6.2.

While hepatic drug metabolising capacity declines with age routine liver function tests are often normal. A dosage reduction should be made for most drugs which undergo hepatic metabolism. The potential for an adverse drug reaction induced by a drug interaction between two hepatically metabolised drugs should be considered.

Where possible a drug that does not rely on hepatic metabolism should be considered.

TABLE 6.2   Drugs with potentially reduced hepatic clearance in the aged

Alprazolam	Glibenclamide
Amitriptyline	Ibuprofen
Antidepressants	Metoprolol
Antipsychotics	Nitrazepam
Carbamazepine	Pethidine
Chlordiazepoxide	Phenytoin
Chlorpropamide	Propranolol
Diazepam	Theophylline
Flurazepam	Tolbutamide

Elimination

Limitations in renal function are most frequently revealed by the elimination of drugs from the body and the maintenance of sodium, potassium and water balance. It has been estimated that the reduction in kidney function approaches 10% each decade after the age of 40 years. Disease and lifestyle factors can damage kidney function even further.

In contrast to the liver where the decline in drug metabolising capacity is variable and is not reflected in common tests of hepatic function, age changes in renal function are more constant and are reflected in changes in creatinine clearance. It is important to note that the serum creatinine does not adequately reveal this reduction in function and may appear normal even in quite impaired kidney function.

When dehydration or congestive heart failure is present or when drugs such as antihypertensives or non-steroidal anti-inflammatory agents which reduce renal blood flow are given, the filtration rate may further fall. Medications requiring dosage reduction when renal function is reduced are listed in Table 6.3.

PHARMACODYNAMICS

The effect of a drug depends not only on the plasma level but also on the responsiveness of the tissues. The effect of a drug at its site of action may be altered in the aged person.

The aged brain, the bladder's detrusor muscle, the eye and the haemopoietic system appear to be more sensitive to drugs while certain parts of the cardiovascular system appear less sensitive to particular drugs. For example, with the benzodiazepines greater impairment occurs at lower doses than that seen in young people. The haemopoietic system appears to be more sensitive to warfarin and the incidence of bleeding is increased. The β blocking activity of propranolol and the tachycardic response to exercise decreases with

TABLE 6.3 Drugs with potentially reduced renal clearance in the aged

ACE inhibitors	Methyldopa
Allopurinol	Nitrofurantoin
Aminoglycosides	NSAIDs
Acyclovir	Norfloxacin
Cephalosporins	Penicillins
Cimetidine	Quinidine
Ciprofloxacin	Sulfonamides
Digoxin	Tetracyclines
Ethacrynic acid	Thiazide diuretics
Lithium	Triamterene
Metformin	Trimethoprim
Methotrexate	

age, while both angiotensin converting enzyme inhibitors and calcium channel blocking agents have been shown to produce a greater fall in blood pressure in the aged.

Certain drugs limit the capacity of redistribution of blood from areas of low to high metabolic need and to respond adaptively to exercise and postural stress. Hence drugs that may impair blood flow to peripheral tissue, e.g. antihypertensives, antiarrhythmics, negative inotropic drugs and diuretics must be used with extreme caution.

IMPACT OF AGEING ON CLINICAL PRESENTATION OF DISEASE ████████████

The clinical presentation of disease and its subsequent diagnosis is complicated by two factors: multiple diseases and increased physiological vulnerability.

INCREASED PHYSIOLOGICAL VULNERABILITY

Ageing decreases the homeostatic capacity of the individual to respond to both environmental and metabolic stress. This factor has an impact on the maintenance of normal blood pressure, electrolyte and fluid balance, insulin response, body temperature, and postural control.

As age advances this physiological vulnerability becomes a progressively significant factor in determining the clinical presentation of disease.

In the aged person the presentation of a disease is frequently determined by the most vulnerable body system rather than by the usual symptoms of the primary disease. Hence, the manifestation of a disease in the aged is often different from the manifestation of the same disease in a young person. For example, an infection may present with non-specific symptoms such as confusion, breathlessness, impaired balance regulation or urinary incontinence. The diagnosis of pneumonia without fever or pulmonary symptoms, or urinary tract infection without fever, frequency, burning and scalding on micturition, can easily be overlooked.

In the younger individual gripping chest pain with its characteristic radiation is the indication of a heart attack. However, in aged patients this is the presenting symptom in very few cases. Non-specific symptoms such as breathlessness, unexplained heart failure, mental confusion, ataxia or simply increased apathy and lack of motivation may be the only presenting symptoms.

The aged frequently have a generalised diminished perception of pain and temperature, further complicating the diagnosis of several disorders.

SPECIFIC CLASSES OF MEDICATION

Many drugs have consistently been identified as the cause of potentially severe side effects and adverse drug reactions in the aged. Often the expression of the reaction is in a limited range of geriatric syndromes. Table 6.4 lists the drugs associated with the common geriatric syndromes of confusion, depression, postural hypotension, Parkinson's disease, constipation and

6

GERIATRIC THERAPEUTICS

TABLE 6.4 Drugs associated with common geriatric syndromes

	Confusion	Depression	Postural hypotension	Parkinson's disease	Constipation	Urinary incontinence
Anticholinergics	+	+	+		+	+
Anticonvulsants	+	+	+			
Antidepressants	+		+		+	+
Antihypertensives						
β blockers	+	+	+			+
Methyldopa	+	+	+			+
Prazosin	+	+	+			+
Antiparkinsonian agents	+	+	+			
Antipsychotics			+	+	+	+
Benzodiazepines	+	+	+		+	+
Corticosteroids	+	+				
Digoxin	+	+				
Diuretics	+		+		+	+
Hypoglycaemic agents	+		+			
Opioid analgesics	+		+		+	

urinary incontinence. It is notable that five of these syndromes are central nervous system disorders.

The ageing central and autonomic nervous systems are uniquely vulnerable to pharmacological stress and it is this vulnerability that offers a possible explanation of why adverse drug reactions in this age group typically find clinical expression in this restricted range of syndromes.

A drug has the capacity to influence the nervous system adversely by crossing the blood brain barrier (usually due to lipid solubility); by disturbing the system's extracellular environment (electrolytes, glucose, etc); and through its anticholinergic activity. Drugs with anticholinergic activity cause constipation, dry mouth, mydriasis, drowsiness, confusion, palpitations and arrhythmias, and urinary retention (particularly a problem for men with prostatic disorders), see Table 6.5.

Considerable confusion with diagnosis can result if it is overlooked that medication may be the cause of many common conditions presenting in the aged patient. It is wise to approach a patient presenting with one of the common geriatric syndromes with a high degree of suspicion and to investigate potential causes carefully.

TABLE 6.5 Drugs with anticholinergic activity

Antiarrhythmics (disopyramide, mexiletine, quinidine)
Antihistamines (All excluding 'non-sedating' class)
Antiparkinsonian agents (amantadine, benzhexol, benztropine, biperidine)
Antipsychotics
Antispasmodics (atropine, belladonna, dicyclomine, glycopyrrolate, hyoscine, propantheline, orphenadrine)
Tricyclic antidepressants

IMPACT OF AGEING ON ADVERSE DRUG REACTIONS

PREDISPOSING FACTORS

Biological, social and medical factors interact to predispose the aged to adverse drug reactions. The complexity of contributing factors is summarised in Figure 6.1.

Issues such as the cognitive state of the patient, the nature and level of clinical disease and the presence of disability as well as social and economic circumstances interact with the diagnostic and management skills of the doctor to determine the success or otherwise of drug therapy.

Seven factors have been identified as posing particular risks in the community. These factors are age/sex, number of drugs, drug dose/duration, drug type, noncompliance, multiple diseases and poor management practices.

Age and Gender

The physical consequences of ageing impact on drug therapy to increase the risk of adverse drug reactions. The number of reports of adverse drug reactions is higher in females than in males and therefore females are considered to be at greater risk.

Number of Drugs

POLYPHARMACY

The prescription of many drugs (polyprescription) results in polypharmacy. As the number of prescribed drugs rise the likelihood of harmful drug interactions is increased as is the probability of poor patient compliance. It is important to be aware that the aged may have many sources of medications. They may be under the care of several doctors, e.g. consulting one doctor for one complaint and a second doctor for another complaint. They may also obtain medication from several pharmacies. The doctor may be unaware of non-prescription medications purchased over the counter from supermarkets, health food stores and pharmacies. The aged person may be oblivious to the fact that self-diagnosing and treating skin, bowel, respiratory and other ailments may seriously interfere with prescribed medications. It is often difficult for the doctor or pharmacist to detect and intervene at this level. The nurse visiting the patient at home is in an ideal position to observe medication consumption, storage and compliance.

DRUG INTERACTIONS

Drugs that are known to interact can be administered concurrently as long as ade-

quate precautions are taken such as close monitoring of drug therapy and dosage adjustment for any altered response. However, if another agent with similar therapeutic properties and a lesser risk of drug interaction is available, it should be used.

It is therefore advisable to consult the pharmacist on the relevance of a documented drug interaction in view of a particular patient's history and medical condition.

Drug Dose/Duration

Polypharmacy is undoubtedly a highly important factor contributing to adverse drug reactions. However, to concentrate exclusively on this factor ignores the point that the high prevalence of drug reactions among the aged can be traced largely to dose related reactions. It has been estimated that 50%–70% of adverse drug reactions

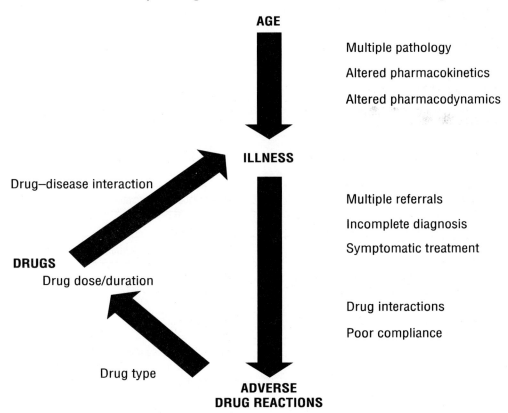

FIGURE 6.1   Factors contributing to adverse drug reactions

result from an extension of the normal pharmacological action of the drug. They are due to altered pharmacodynamic and pharmacokinetic characteristics in the aged who, as a result, are likely to show an increased plasma concentration of the drug for a given dose.

Drug Type

Many drug classes have been identified as causing specific problems in the aged. The risk and benefit in the use of these drugs should be considered carefully with respect to a particular patient's vulnerability. The patient's response and the presentation of an adverse drug reaction should be closely monitored. Drugs which pose particular risks to the aged are listed in Table 6.6.

Non-Compliance

While progressive impairment of cognitive and physiological functions increases the sensitivity of the aged patient to drug therapy, it also increases the probability of errors occurring in the taking of medication.

It is imperative that the patient and carers have a clear understanding of how, why and when a particular drug is to be taken. Aids to compliance such as *Dosettes* and *Webster* packing, timing devices and tailoring the medication regimen to the individual's particular lifestyle should be considered.

Multiple Diseases

CHRONIC DEGENERATIVE DISEASES

Chronic degenerative diseases are those that dominate the ageing process and include

TABLE 6.6 Drugs posing a particular risk to the aged

Drug	Reaction
Aminoglycosides (gentamicin, tobramycin)	Ototoxicity, nephrotoxicity
β blocking drugs	Confusion, respiratory difficulties, aggravation of congestive heart failure
Chlorpropamide	Hypoglycaemia, alcohol intolerance, water retention
Chlorthalidone	Dehydration, incontinence, electrolyte disturbance
Digoxin	Confusion, visual disturbances, loss of appetite
Disopyramide	Urinary retention, constipation
Ethacrynic acid	Deafness
Lithium	Urinary incontinence, dehydration
Metformin	Lactic acidosis
Methyldopa	Drowsiness, depression
Nitrofurantoin	Peripheral neuropathy
Oestrogen	Fluid retention and aggravation of congestive heart failure
Opioid analgesics	Confusion
Tetracycline	Rising blood urea levels

chronic obstructive airways disease, coronary artery disease, chronic neurological diseases and osteoarthritis.

Chronic degenerative diseases have the following characteristics: they are multifactorial rather than single aetiology; the underlying process is universal in its occurrence; the process commences early in life ultimately causing irreversible structural damage to the body systems involved; and individuals differ only in the rate of progress, not the presence or absence of these processes.

The environment plays an important role in the development of chronic degenerative disease and consequently the application of the principles of preventive medicine in the early years of life is critical. Non-drug management such as the modification of diet, exercise and physical and emotional environment should be considered as alternatives for the management of these diseases. For example, heat, exercise, diet changes, simple analgesics, e.g. paracetamol, and joint supports could be considered in the management of arthritis before full non-steroidal anti-inflammatory therapy is commenced.

DRUG–DISEASE INTERACTIONS

As well as contributing to polypharmacy, multiple diseases increase the risk of a drug prescribed for one condition adversely affecting a co-existing disease state, thus causing a significant drug–disease interaction. The disease may be aggravated or the interaction may be expressed as an idiosyncratic reaction, apparently unrelated to the nature of the disease or drug.

The aged, because of their high medication use, are particularly vulnerable to interactions of this nature. For example, in cardiac failure antidepressants may increase the risk of cardiac arrhythmias; β blockers may cause bradycardia and aggravate heart failure; non-steroidal anti-inflammatory agents may cause fluid retention; and verapamil may cause heart block.

Poor Management Practices

Poor management practices contribute significantly to polypharmacy and ultimately to adverse drug reactions. They include incomplete diagnosis, multiple referrals and inappropriate use of medication.

Incomplete diagnosis can result in symptomatic treatment, e.g. insomnia not recognised as induced by antihypertensive therapy being treated with a sedative agent.

Multiple referrals occur when specialist referrals are poorly co-ordinated and the general practitioner loses case control and is unaware of the patient's total number of prescribed medications.

Inappropriate use of medication includes the use of drugs to modify behaviour, e.g. in dementia. The appropriate use of behaviour modifying drugs in a long-term care setting is a complex issue with many factors contributing to the risks and benefits of drug therapy. Although residents' rights, safety and well being are a priority when administering psychotropic drugs, consideration must also be given to the safety of other residents and staff.

These factors increase the likelihood that the aged patient will be exposed to large numbers of medications and develop adverse drug reactions.

DRUG RELATED ILLNESS

Adverse drug reactions or drug related illness can result from a complexity of contributing factors. These factors find expression in one or several of the medication errors summarised below:

- No drug prescribed for appropriate indication

- Patient taking the wrong drug

- Patient taking too little of the right drug

- Patient taking too much of the right drug

- Medical problems resulting from patient not taking the drug for various reasons

6

GERIATRIC THERAPEUTICS

(pharmaceutical, economic, psychological and sociologic)

• Medical problem resulting from an adverse drug reaction

• Medical problem resulting from drug–drug, drug–disease, drug–food interactions

• Age related changes leading to increased drug plasma concentration

• Age related changes leading to increased drug sensitivity

• Patient taking drug for no medically valid reason.

Rational drug management demands knowledge of the pharmacodynamic and pharmacokinetic parameters that may be altered in the aged. In summary, the following general guidelines for drug use in the aged should be considered wherever possible:

1. Drugs that have been consistently implicated in causing adverse drug reactions in the aged should be avoided.

2. A drug with a shorter elimination half-life should be chosen.

3. The dosage of a renally cleared drug should be reduced when reduced renal function is known.

4. The frequency of doses should be reduced (compliance is improved with minimal dosage frequency). A drug should be generally administered once per half-life.

5. The aim should be to achieve the lowest effective dose. Adjustments to dosage should be made slowly allowing full stable blood levels to be achieved before a dosage increment, i.e. 'start low—go slow'.

6. A drug that that is not reliant on hepatic metabolism should be chosen.

7. Goals for drug treatment should be determined.

8. The patient should be monitored carefully for anticipated adverse reactions.

9. A time frame for re-evaluation of efficacy should be determined.

For the very old and those suffering from multiple diseases and receiving several drugs concurrently, appropriate adjustment to type of drug, dosage and frequency must be made.

For healthy older people receiving short-term drug therapy the clinical impact of these changes may be insignificant. However, individual assessment of the patient is still essential.

NURSING IMPLICATIONS

The role of the nurse in the care of the aged is well established. Nurses are often quite closely associated with patients and their carers. Hence they are able to observe drug taking practices in action, monitor drug use, detect medication errors and watch for changes in the health of their patients.

Frequently nurses are solely responsible for initiating medical consultations particularly in long-term care institutions. The nurse is therefore well placed for co-ordinating the effects of other health workers and community groups with the aim of increasing quality of life and maintaining independence.

ASSESSMENT

Information must be recorded on behalf of the patient. The aim is to determine a particular patient's functional capacity and to record baseline parameters so progress can be monitored. In relation to drug therapy, information considered of benefit includes: age, height, weight, fat distribution, food and drug allergies, diet and nutrition; medical history; current medical diagnosis; medication history; liver function, renal function, electrolyte levels and blood screening results; mobility, vision, coordination, hand dexterity; level of independence in activities of daily living, e.g. dressing, feeding, bathing; and cognitive assessment.

EVALUATION

All too frequently instances of polypharmacy, mismanagement of medication and inappropriate prescribing are encountered and it is essential not to become complacent.

It is important to remember that 50%–70% of adverse drug reacations are predictable and preventable. For each patient's medication regimen the following questions should be considered:

Is there more than one drug from a single *drug class*?

Is the *drug dose* appropriate for geriatric physiology?

Is the *dose frequency* regimen likely to be complied with? Is the frequency appropriate for the particular drug's half-life?

Is the *dosage form* appropriate or would another route of administration be better for this patient?

Check the *drug indication* — is the medication still required?

What *adverse drug reactions* are known for this particular agent? Is the patient being monitored for adverse reactions?

Are there any drugs being given that may cause *drug interactions*?

Does the patient have a particular disease that may be affected by one or more of the prescribed drugs, i.e. a *drug–disease interaction*?

It is important to utilise the skills of other team members. If in any doubt always seek further advice to confirm and support your intended actions.

MEDICATION ADMINISTRATION

Individual assessment allows the nurse to determine a particular patient's ability to safely administer their own medication or the level of supervision required. This assessment includes the patient's ability to: read labels (often in very faint, small print); remove tablets from foil packaging; remove tablets from child-proof containers; accurately measure liquid preparations; and divide tablets to obtain the required dose.

In many instances suitable alternatives are available, e.g. a change in dosage form or administration route.

Tablets should not be crushed without discussion with a pharmacist. Crushing may influence the integrity of the dosage form design, hence significantly changing the drug's absorption and kinetics. With recent developments in tablet formulation the reason for this may not always be apparent.

Compliance

As compliance is known to decline with complicated medication regimens, the first step is to review a patient's medication regimen and to simplify it where possible. This can be done through discussion with the patient's doctor and pharmacist. When the medications required (including those purchased without prescription and used irregularly) have been decided:

1. Record all medications.

2. Adjust dosage times to suit the individual's daily routine. Meal times have been found to be suitable reminder

3. Provide the patient with a fully updated medication card which states

   DRUG NAME
   DOSE/FREQUENCY
   DOSAGE TIMES

   and may also include

   GENERIC NAME
   COLOUR
   DRUG PURPOSE
   SPECIAL PRECAUTIONS

   Cards or booklets of a similar format can be provided by pharmacists. The patient should be encouraged to carry a copy of these details with them at all times.

4. Set up patient compliance aids where appropriate.

5. Enlist the aid of carers or family members.

6. **Educate the patient or carers on all aspects of their particular medication needs.**

7. **Encourage the patient to wear medical condition alert jewellery, e.g. a *Medialert* bracelet.**

FURTHER READING

Ames, D. (1991), 'Safe hypnotic use in the elderly', *Current Therapeutics* 32(3) pp. 57–64.

Ames, D. and Tuckwell, V. (1992), 'Psychopharmacology and the aged patient', *Current Therapeutics* 33(5) pp. 13–19.

Cristofalo, V.J. (1990). 'Biological mechanisms of aging: An overview'. In Hazzard, R.E.W., Andres, R., Bierman, E.L. and Blass, J.P. (eds). *Principles of Geriatric Medicine and Gerontology* 2nd edn. McGraw-Hill, New York.

Flynn, P. and McLean, S. (1990), 'Drugs in dementia, Specific and symptomatic treatment', *Current Therapeutics* 32(5) pp. 65–67.

'Geriatric Nursing', *American Journal of Care of the Ageing.* The American Journal of Nurses Company, New York.

Rose, B.S. (1987), 'NSAIDs in the elderly', *Current Therapeutics* 28(5) pp. 17–23.

Russell, B.M. (1986), 'Urinary tract infections in the elderly', *Current Therapeutics* 27(10) pp. 27–41.

Scharf, S. Christophidis, N. (1991), 'Pharmacokinetics and pharmacodynamics in the aged.' *Australian Journal of Hospital Pharmacy* 21(3) pp. 198–202.

Sinnett, P. (1986). *Drug prescribing for the elderly.* The Centre for the Study of Chronic Disease and Disability, Rehabilitation and Aged Care Service, ACT Community and Health Services, Woden Valley Hospital, Canberra.

Speight, T.M. (1981), *Avery's Drug Treatment Principles and Practice of Clinical Pharmacology and Therapeutics.* 3rd edn Adis Press, Sydney.

Tregakis, B.F. and Stevenson, F.H. (1990), 'Pharmacokinetics in old age', *British Medical Bulletin* 46 pp. 9–21.

Ware, G.J., Holford, N.H.C., Davison, J.G. (1991), 'Unit dose calendar packaging and elderly patient compliance', *New Zealand Medical Journal* 104 pp. 495–497.

TEST YOUR KNOWLEDGE

1. List five physiological changes that are known to occur with ageing that may impact on drug therapy. Discuss the three ways that these changes may impact on drug therapy causing an adverse drug reaction.

2. Why is serum creatinine unsuitable as an indicator of renal function in the aged. List five drugs which should be used with care in the aged with known or suspected reduced renal function?

3. Why should the anticoagulant warfarin be administered with care in the aged?

4. Name the three mechanisms by which a drug may cause confusion as an adverse drug reaction.

5. Mrs A is a 71-year old widow who has recently been exhibiting quite unusual behaviour. Her daughter is concerned about her mother's ability to remain independent and wishes to pursue nursing home admission arrangements. She fears the development of a dementing illness. Over the last two to three months Mrs A has become confused, easily fatigued and very irritable. She has developed a disturbing obsessive/compulsive behaviour constantly complaining that her lace window curtains were dirty and required frequent washing. Detailed questioning revealed that she thought they were yellow-green and possibly mouldy. Her prescribed medications are: frusemide 40 mg daily in the morning; digoxin 250 micrograms

daily; paracetamol 500 mg, 1–2 tablets 4-hourly when required; piroxicam 20 mg at night; *Mylanta* suspension, 20 mL when required; and *Coloxyl* 120 mg, 1–2 tablets at night.

(a) Consider how appropriate each drug and drug combination is for this patient. List five drug interactions, drug–disease interactions or administration factors to be considered in the review of Mrs A's medication.

(b) Which drug could be suspected of precipitating the confusion, fatigue and irritability? What other symptom could also be caused by this drug?

(c) What measures could be taken to improve Mrs A's compliance and maintain her independence?

6

GERIATRIC THERAPEUTICS

Drug Safety in Pregnancy and Lactation

RONALD P. BATAGOL

O B J E C T I V E S

At the conclusion of this chapter the reader should be able to:

1. Discuss the risks and benefits of drug use during pregnancy;

2. Describe the Australian Pregnancy Categorisation Scheme;

3. List the drugs contraindicated in pregnancy;

4. Describe the principles involved in drug transfer to the neonate through breast milk; and

5. Discuss how potential problems with drug use during breast feeding can be minimised.

DRUG SAFETY IN PREGNANCY ▆▆▆▆▆

The study of the effects of drugs on the developing fetus began in earnest after the thalidomide episode of the early 1960s. Thalidomide was a drug given to promote sleep and was believed to be reasonably safe for human use at the time. However, throughout the world approximately 8000 women who had received the drug gave birth to infants with a major defect in limb development. Flipper-like structures replaced the normal limb appendages, a condition called phocomelia. This type of defect had not been revealed in the experimental work prior to the release of the drug.

From that time regulating authorities in almost every country in the world set up very stringent standards and methods for toxicological and adverse drug reaction testing. Networks of adverse drug reaction reporting mechanisms were set up to document reported adverse effects.

THE AUSTRALIAN PREGNANCY CATEGORISATION SYSTEM

A recent development has been the adoption by the Australian Drug Evaluation Committee (ADEC) of the Australian Pregnancy Categorisation System which classifies and categorises drugs and drug groups, according to their safety in pregnancy. The system (based on one already operating in Sweden) was implemented during 1989 to assign drugs and drug groups according to the established risk or otherwise to the fetus, arising from their use during pregnancy.

The Australian categorisation consists of five separate categories:

Category A

Drugs which have been taken by a large number of pregnant women and women of childbearing age without any proven increase in the frequency of malformations or other direct or indirect harmful effects on the fetus having been observed.

Category B

Drugs which have been taken by only a limited number of pregnant women and women of childbearing age without an increase in the frequency of malformation or other direct or indirect harmful effects on the fetus having been observed.

As experience of effects of drugs in this category in humans is limited, results of toxicological studies to date (including reproduction studies in animals) are indicated by allocation to one of three subgroups:

Group B1
Studies in animals* have not shown evidence of an increased occurrence of fetal damage.

Group B2
Studies in animals* are inadequate and may be lacking but available data show no evidence of an increased occurrence of fetal damage.

Group B3
Studies in animals* have shown evidence of an increased occurrence of fetal damage, the significance of which is considered uncertain in humans.

Category C

Drugs which, owing to their pharmacological effects, have caused or may be suspected of causing harmful effects on the human fetus or neonate without causing malformations. These effects may be reversible.

Category D

Drugs which have caused, are suspected to have caused or may be expected to cause an

*Animal studies submitted in support of new drug applications must conform to New Drug Form Guidelines.

increased incidence of human fetal malformations or irreversible damage. These drugs may also have adverse pharmacological effects.

Category X

Drugs that have such a high risk of causing permanent damage to the fetus that they should not be used in pregnancy or when there is a possibility of pregnancy.

The Australian categorisation system has provided a useful basis for identifying the relative teratogenic and fetotoxic risks of various drugs and drug groups. Since 1990 drug monographs and product information have included the categorisation rating for each drug. However, frequently there is a need for further clarification and explanation of the risk to benefit ratio in a way that cannot be adequately covered by a risk categorisation system. In such cases an Obstetric Drug Information Centre should be contacted for a more detailed assessment.

DRUG TRANSFER TO THE FETUS

What actually happens when a drug is consumed by a pregnant woman? In almost every case, both the mother and the fetus are affected. Drug transfer occurs normally across the placenta from the maternal arterial blood supply by way of intervillous space into the umbilical vein (Figure 7.1).

For any substance to pass from the maternal blood stream to the fetal blood supply it must traverse what used to be called the 'placental barrier'. In fact, it is transferred through the syncytiotrophoblast, a single layer of multinuclear syncytium with no distinct cell boundaries, and the cytotrophoblast, a single layer of cuboidal cells with distinct cell boundaries (also called the layer of Langerhans). There may be some scattered mesoderm beneath this layer of cells (Figure 7.2).

In common with other semipermeable cell membranes, these two primary layers are composed of phospholipid or lipoprotein and carry a surface charge. There is also a pH difference between maternal blood and fetal blood. Fetal blood is slightly more acidic, about 0.15 pH units lower than maternal blood. Therefore, substances that are fat (lipid) soluble and in their non-ionised form will be transferred more readily. The transfer of drugs that are weak bases will be promoted as they ionise more readily in the more acidic fetal blood and thus produce a higher concentration in the fetal

7

DRUG SAFETY IN PREGNANCY AND LACTATION

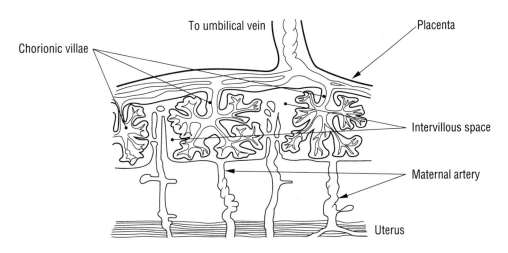

FIGURE 7.1   The placental wall — site of drug transfer

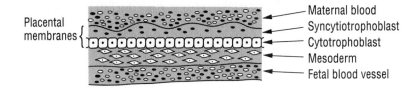

Placental membranes {
Maternal blood
Syncytiotrophoblast
Cytotrophoblast
Mesoderm
Fetal blood vessel

FIGURE 7.2 Cross section of placental tissues showing the placental–fetal membranes

bloodstream at equilibrium than in the maternal bloodstream. This has an important application in the timing of administration of narcotics (e.g. pethidine) for pain relief as these drugs are weak bases. Other drugs that are also rapidly transferred to the fetus include alcohol, barbiturates, anaesthetic agents and phenothiazines. Drugs that are unlikely to pass to the fetus (unless an extremely high concentration exists in the maternal bloodstream) include heparin, which is a large molecule with a strong electronegative charge, and the neuromuscular blocking agents (muscle relaxants), which are highly ionised and have a low fat solubility.

Other factors affecting drug transfer include metabolic and functional changes of the placenta during gestation. The tissue layers between the fetal capillaries and the maternal blood become thinner as pregnancy progresses, decreasing from 25 micrometres (µm) early in gestation to around 2 µm at term. In addition, the capability of the placenta to metabolise drugs increases as term approaches.

While some substances are actively transported across the placenta by enzymatic reaction and pinocytosis, the majority are transferred by passive transport, some by facilitated diffusion when the size and shape of the molecule makes a contribution, but for the most part by simple diffusion from an area of high concentration to an area of low concentration. This means that virtually any drug will pass from mother to fetus if a sufficiently high concentration gradient is produced, unless it is destroyed or altered during passage. For these reasons the term 'placental barrier' misrepresents the situation. The expression placental 'sieve' appears in recent literature and is more in accord with current understanding of placental function.

Nursing staff need to regard seriously questions from pregnant women about their medication and to take the necessary time to educate them by discussing the risk to benefit factors that may be involved.

Why Do Women Need to Take Any Drugs During Pregnancy?

There are times when drug use in pregnancy is essential to treat serious medical conditions. Pregnant women who are diabetic, hypertensive or epileptic require continuous therapy for these conditions. Without such therapy their own health would be at risk and the developing fetus would probably not survive. Given the complexity and range of drugs available it is essential to be able to evaluate one drug against another with respect to hazards from use during pregnancy and to avoid exposing the developing fetus to unnecessary risks for trivial reasons. For example, the risks associated with the casual use of sedatives and tranquillisers without good therapeutic justification. Aside from teratogenic considerations the effects of prolonged or chronic use of medications during pregnancy need to be considered. It is well recognised that some of the earlier benzodiazepines have pharmacologically active metabolites with extremely long half-lives that accumulate in the fetus. The long-term use of diazepam in pregnancy often gives rise to hypotonia and hypothermia in the fetus, with the condition persisting long after birth. This can result in the 'flat baby syndrome' characterised by lethargy and poor sucking reflexes. When treating pregnant or breastfeeding women the evaluation of risk to benefit factors of use of the drug must be considered.

Obstetric Drug Information Centres can provide information about the potential for harm or benefit from the use of a particular drug. The clinical evaluation of such information in relation to the individual patient must then be made by the prescriber in association with the patient who needs to be involved in an informed decision both for the sake of patient compliance and to avoid undesirable legal consequences.

For example, most textbooks advise against the use of sulfamethoxazole–trimethoprim compound during pregnancy, based on the manufacturers' warning about the possible risks from the folate antagonist effect of trimethoprim. However, this drug combination is used extensively in clinical practice to treat infections in the pregnant patient and, in spite of extensive use over a long period of time, no reports of adverse effects of use during pregnancy have appeared in the world literature at the time of writing. Much more pertinent is the often unstated information that sulfamethoxazole–trimethoprim compound should be used near the time of delivery only after very careful evaluation as the long-acting sulfonamide component causes release of bilirubin from protein-binding sites in maternal and fetal plasma. In most instances this will not be clinically significant but certainly may be if the fetus already has abnormally high bilirubin levels because of prematurity or ABO or Rhesus incompatibilities. In this case a further release of bilirubin from the protein binding sites could significantly raise levels and cause kernicterus with the possibility of mental retardation. The important factor is to examine the potential for possible harm to the individual patient, based on a knowledge of the specific drug and the clinical condition of both mother and child.

DRUGS AND TERATOGENICITY IN PERSPECTIVE

Some 3% of newborn infants have an anomaly which is detected at birth. There are many known causes of congenital abnormalities, including maternal metabolic imbalance, infections, chromosomal aberrations, genetic transmission and a variety of other factors, often acting together. Some 6000 chemical agents are known to produce congenital abnormalities in experimental animals, but fewer that 25 are known to cause defects in humans.

To classify a drug as a teratogen, two basic criteria must be fulfilled:

1. the drug must be present during the critical phase of development; and
2. the drug should produce a statistically significant rate of a pattern or cluster of abnormalities in experimental animals.

Some known teratogens are:

Alcohol

Anticonvulsants (particularly phenytoin, sodium valproate, carbamazepine)

Anticoagulants (warfarin, other coumarin derivatives)

Antineoplastic drugs

Antithyroid drugs

Cocaine

Danazol

Diethylstilboestrol

Iodides

Lithium

Penicillamine

Retinoids

Tetracyclines

Thalidomide

7

DRUG SAFETY IN PREGNANCY AND LACTATION

WHICH DRUGS SHOULD BE AVOIDED IN PREGNANCY?

This is not a question that can be answered simply. Many matters are involved, such as the time during pregnancy when the drug is given, the dose of the drug, the medical condition of the mother, and any known allergic and genetic factors from both parents.

As a general rule every effort should be made to totally avoid medications of any kind during the period of organogenesis (the first eight weeks of pregnancy), except when serious medical conditions require urgent treatment and the risk to benefit factors have been carefully evaluated by prescriber and patient. The same special care should be exercised in the period just before delivery when the physiological systems of mother and baby can be modified by drugs such as aspirin, long-acting sulfonamides and the non-steroidal anti-inflammatory medications.

There is still considerable discussion in the world literature about the list of drugs that have been proven to be teratogenic or dysmorphogenic. The Australian Risk Categorisation System gives a good working guide. For more detailed information about a particular drug the reader should refer to specialised publications. Alternatively, an Obstetric Drug Information Centre should be consulted. These centres have access to authenticated and epidemiologically sound data and can advise on the reliability of various reports and studies.

Drugs Contraindicated in Pregnancy

DIETHYLSTILBOESTROL

Diethylstilboestrol (DES), a synthetic oestrogen, was used from the 1940s to the 1960s for treating miscarriage. It was subsequently found to be the cause of a rare form of adenocarcinoma of the vagina in women who were exposed to the drug in utero 15 to 20 years earlier.

WARFARIN, ORAL ANTICOAGULANTS

Warfarin and other oral anticoagulants have been linked to a cluster of congenital malformations when used during pregnancy. Heparin, however, can be used during pregnancy as it is a large molecule with a strong electronegative charge and does not cross the placental wall. For more detailed information on the prophylaxis and treatment of thromboembolism in pregnancy see Chapter 20 Drug Therapy in Pregnancy and Labour.

ISOTRETINOIN, ETRETINATE

The retinoids, isotretinoin and etretinate, are used for severe acne and psoriasis and are well established human teratogens. It is important for women to avoid pregnancy for at least two years after discontinuing etretinate treatment.

TETRACYCLINES

Tetracyclines are known to cause hypoplasia of tooth enamel and discolouration of teeth when used late in pregnancy and should be avoided at any stage of pregnancy. The potential dangers to the fetus from tetracyclines are well documented and among the best known in the general community because of the obvious effect of teeth staining. Tetracyclines are concentrated in chelated form in the enamel and dentine of developing teeth, resulting in irreversible discolouration and enamel hypoplasia. They also cause a reversible inhibition of skeletal growth in premature infants.

Research centres now claim that tetracyclines can be regarded as safe for use during pregnancy for the first 120 days of gestation. From 120 days to 240 days the effect is on the primary or baby teeth, and from 240 days of gestation up to around 10 years of age the effect is on the permanent teeth.

This illustrates the importance of a balanced evaluation of drug choice. Although tetracyclines would never be the drug of first choice during pregnancy, it is a fairly common practice for women in their late teens to have tetracyclines prescribed for acne, often over an extensive period. Should they continue taking such medication well into their pregnancy, unnecessary exposure of the fetus may take place during a critical period.

Although many drug manufacturers have a standard warning for their products regarding safety of use during pregnancy, this warning is not always passed on to the consumer. The greatest dangers to the fetus are posed during the early weeks of organogenesis during the period that pregnancy may not even be suspected, and even when it is, the woman may not be aware that her former daily routine of drug taking could present a threat to her developing child.

COCAINE

Use of cocaine during pregnancy carries the risk of abruptio placentae with fetal death as well as intestinal and limb abnormalities.

ALCOHOL

There is established evidence for what has been called the 'fetal alcohol syndrome', a pattern of facial and cardiovascular defects seen in infants whose mothers were heavy alcohol users during pregnancy. (See section on Self-Administered Drugs.)

DANAZOL

Danazol, used for endometriosis, has an androgenic effect and may cause virilisation in the female fetus. It should not be used during pregnancy.

IODIDES

Iodides may give rise to fetal goitre. (See section on Self-Administered Drugs.)

Drugs Which Must be Used With Caution in Early Pregnancy

The following drugs need to be used with caution in early pregnancy: trimethoprim–sulfamethoxazole, metronidazole, lithium, anticonvulsants and oral hypoglycaemic agents.

TRIMETHOPRIM–SULFAMETHOXAZOLE

The safety of trimethoprim–sulfamethoxazole in pregnancy has already been discussed in a previous section.

METRONIDAZOLE

Metronidazole used to be contraindicated in pregnancy on the basis of questions of mutagenicity in laboratory tests. After 30 years of use it has been established that metronidazole does not exhibit mutagenicity in humans and may be used if it is the drug of choice for a specific infection during pregnancy. (It is listed as B2 in the Australian Risk Categorisation System).

LITHIUM

It has been established that there is a slightly increased incidence of cardiovascular defects in the offspring of women taking lithium during pregnancy. However, the risk versus the benefit needs to be carefully considered in cases where lithium treatment is essential to the health of a woman who is pregnant or wishes to become pregnant.

ANTICONVULSANTS

Anticonvulsants are discussed under epilepsy in Chapter 20 Drug Therapy in Pregnancy and Labour.

ORAL HYPOGLYCAEMIC AGENTS

Oral hypoglycaemic agents exhibit a degree of teratogenicity in animal testing. They are not used during pregnancy as gestational diabetes is managed with insulin. (See Chapter 20, Drug Therapy in Pregnancy and Labour.)

Drugs Which Must be Used With Caution in Late Pregnancy

NARCOTIC DRUGS

This group of drugs is important not only for their therapeutic use but because of the increased non-medical use and abuse amongst young people and, therefore, women of childbearing age.

HEROIN

Heroin (diamorphine) is the 'prototype' drug of the group.

Withdrawal symptoms and respiratory depression are frequently seen in infants of addicts. These infants are often of low birth-weight and prone to infections.

METHADONE

Methadone is frequently used to treat heroin addiction. Methadone withdrawal in an infant may be a potentially more severe problem than heroin withdrawal, with exposed infants exhibiting a higher incidence of seizures as part of their withdrawal syndrome. Also, a 'late withdrawal syndrome' has been reported which may be explained by the pharmacokinetic differences between the two drugs. Such infants require a longer period of time to recover. However, infants of methadone treated women are generally in better condition than those of untreated patients.

The long-term effects of in-utero exposure to narcotics is unknown.

DIAZEPAM

A withdrawal syndrome called the 'floppy infant syndrome' (or 'flat baby syndrome') has been recognised in some infants whose mothers received 10–15 mg of diazepam daily during the last months of pregnancy. The symptoms include tremulousness, hypotonia and hyper-reflexia.

LITHIUM

Lithium induced neonatal toxicity is an established fact. The effects include poor suckling, effects on muscle tone and poor respiratory effort.

ASPIRIN, SALICYLATES

Aspirin and salicylates used late in pregnancy may cause haemorrhage in the newborn infant due to platelet dysfunction and diminished Factor VII activity. Also, it has been suggested that there is an increased risk of kernicterus in the infant. (See section on Self-Administered Drugs.)

INDOMETHACIN

Indomethacin has been associated with neonatal thrombocytopenia when used late in pregnancy.

Self-Administered Drugs

In addition to prescribed medications, many pregnant women regularly consume a variety of self-administered drugs including nicotine, alcohol, iodides and analgesics. It is important for nursing staff, especially midwives, to be aware of the patient's total medication profile so adverse reactions and interactions of drugs can be recognised.

NICOTINE

The effects produced by nicotine as a result of smoking during pregnancy are well recognised and documented. It has been demonstrated that the extent of adverse effects is directly proportional to the number of cigarettes smoked, with resulting symptoms including low birth-weight infants, miscarriage and premature delivery, stillbirth and neonatal death, as well as an increased incidence of bleeding during pregnancy, abruptio placentae, placenta praevia and premature and prolonged rupture of the membranes.

While these physical effects have been well known and documented for more than a decade, many women have reasoned 'If I have a smaller baby, it will mean an easier birth, so I'll keep on smoking'. In fact, a smaller baby is more likely to become stressed during birth, leading to a more complicated delivery.

Smoking has a three-fold effect on the developing fetus. Firstly, nicotine is a vasoconstrictor, thus closing down the size of placental blood vessels. Secondly, smoking increases blood viscosity, thus further restricting blood flow. Finally, the gases produced by smoking, primarily carbon monoxide, replace oxygen in the blood transport of gases to the fetus. The combined effect of these three mechanisms is to greatly diminish oxygen transport to the fetus at the time when oxygen is essential to the rapid cell division needed for brain development. The major effect is therefore neurological, with long-term life potential and prospects for quality of life being affected. Recent follow-up studies have reported post-natal growth deficiency and impaired mental development. Such children score lower on tests for reading ability, vocabulary, perceptual motor skills, IQ, cognitive ability and mathematics. Sound medical evidence continues to accumulate that the threat to fetal well-being is so great that women should be strongly encouraged to stop smoking as soon as pregnancy is recognised or, even better, when the possibility of pregnancy may exist.

ALCOHOL

There is increasing evidence that the greatest concern with the injudicious use of alcohol during pregnancy is the long-term neurological effect, rather than the more immediately obvious physical deformities. The fetal alcohol syndrome originally included symptoms such as growth retardation, specific facial malformations, joint and limb deformities and cardiac defects. The term now also covers neurobehavioural conditions, including: functional disturbances, such as abnormal sleep patterns and unusually high levels of hyperactivity; learning disabilities including mental retardation unresponsive to early or later intervention; inability to concentrate; behavioural problems related to high levels of activity; and speech and language problems. Such information should be communicated to patients to assist them to make an informed decision about any possible intake of alcohol during their pregnancy. Major investigations in Europe indicate that the syndrome may be caused by the chronic ingestion of alcohol, causing a risk factor that may rise as high as 30%. While an occasional social drink appears to cause no problems, pregnant women are well advised to avoid a level of alcohol consumption that could cause long-term hardships for their children or, better still, to avoid alcohol altogether for the duration of their pregnancy.

ASPIRIN

The effect of aspirin on blood coagulation mechanisms is well documented. When pregnant women consume more than 300 mg of aspirin in the week prior to delivery, diminished Factor VII and impaired platelet aggregation have been observed in umbilical cord blood. In addition, by inhibiting prostaglandin synthesis in the mother unnecessarily prolonged labour may result. Also, the inhibition of prostaglandin synthesis in the fetus may cause premature closure of the ductus arteriosus and consequent cardiac failure. To avoid these problems and the potential dangers of maternal and neonatal haemorrhage, mothers should avoid ingestion of aspirin for at least the week before delivery.

Additionally, a number of neonatal centres have reported that aspirin (and similar drugs that inhibit synthesis of prostaglandins such as indomethacin, naproxen and ibuprofen) may be the cause of retained fetal circulation after birth, particularly if they have been taken for any lengthy period during pregnancy. This has been described as persistent primary pulmonary hypertension or increased lung blood pressure, which militates against the transfer to extrauterine circulation. The drug tolazoline (*Priscol*) is used to treat this condition.

IODIDES

Excessive intake of iodides during pregnancy may result in fetal goitre, leading to airway obstruction and interference with brain function because of inadequate thyroid hormone production. Some common cough mixtures contain iodides. While infrequent therapy poses no known problems, long-term ingestion of such medications during pregnancy could be sufficient to cause problems for the neonate.

VITAMINS AND HERBAL PRODUCTS

A number of 'health preparations' such as kelp tablets are rich in iodine content and should be used with caution. They are often taken in large quantities by women who are unaware of the potential dangers of products that are safe in normal doses but can cause untoward effects if taken in high dosage during pregnancy. Also, they may not inform pharmacists or health store personnel that they are pregnant, so appropriate warnings may not have been given. Nursing staff at hospitals and clinics may be able to provide such information for women at their early antenatal appointments. Information of this kind can be of great benefit to the mother and her unborn child. In this era of 'macro' doses of vitamins and minerals and 'health preparations' it is important to advise a balanced approach to self-medication to avoid any possible harmful effects through excess dosage. There has been at least one case report of a baby fatally poisoned in utero by the mother consuming toxic quantities of a herbal tea. Herbal preparations such as comfrey and coltsfoot contain pyrrolizidine alkaloids which may be toxic in large doses. There is an overall absence of standardisation and uniform testing for, and a lack of safety data on the wide range of herbal preparations on the market. Poisonings can occur because of the misidentification of a plant or the unknown or ignored toxicity of a correctly identified plant.

Drugs which should be avoided during pregnancy are listed in Table 7.1.

NURSING IMPLICATIONS

It is important to ensure that pregnant women are aware of the risks arising from inappropriate use of prescribed and self-administered drugs which may have adverse effects in pregnancy. Nurses and other health professionals can assist women to better understand which drugs may cause problems when taken during pregnancy.

TABLE 7.1   Examples of drugs which should be avoided during pregnancy

---

Drugs which must not be used in pregnancy
Diethylstilboestrol
Warfarin, oral anticoagulants
Isotretinoin, etretinate
Tetracyclines
Cocaine
Danazol

Drugs which must be used with caution in early pregnancy
Trimethoprim–sulfamethoxazole
Metronidazole
Lithium
Anticonvulsants
Oral hypoglycaemic agents
Self-administered drugs
  Nicotine
  Iodides
  Alcohol

Drugs which must be used with caution in late pregnancy
Narcotic drugs
  Heroin
  Methadone
Diazepam
Lithium
Aspirin, salicylates
Indomethacin
Self-administered drugs
  Nicotine
  Iodides
  Alcohol
  Vitamins
  Herbal products

DRUG SAFETY IN LACTATION ▊▊▊▊▊

Over the past 30 years there has also been a growing awareness of the need for caution when recommending medication for mothers who are breast feeding. While only a small list of items are totally contraindicated, many others may produce undesirable side effects in the nursing infant. For example, many sedative and tranquillising drugs may be transferred to the baby causing drowsiness and poor feeding habits. This may result in increased anxiety on the part of the mother thus negating the original intent of the maternal therapy. During breast feeding it is important to restrict drug therapy to essential medical indications and to avoid the casual use of medications when realistic alternatives such as patient education, reassurance and attention to physical comfort may be all that are needed.

The same basic principles apply to the transfer of drugs in breast milk as to the transplacental passage of drugs. Breast milk can be viewed as an oil-in-water emulsion containing droplets of fat in an aqueous medium in which lactose, inorganic salts and protein are in solution. Within the breast, this emulsion is separated from the mother's blood by a semipermeable membrane that is lipid in composition and allows a similar exchange to that involved in placental transfer. Water, electrolytes and small water soluble molecules are able to pass through small pores in the membrane, while larger molecules, including most drugs, traverse the lipid membrane by simple passive diffusion from an area of high concentration to one of low concentration.

Additionally, breast milk has a lower (more acid) pH than maternal serum. Hence many drugs, such as those that are weak bases, are more ionised on the milk side of the membrane encouraging a higher concentration of total drug in the milk compared with that in the serum. Drug binding to plasma proteins is a another factor, as most drugs are significantly more strongly bound to plasma proteins than to milk proteins. This means that fat soluble drugs in their non-ionised form will transfer readily into breast milk, especially when the dosage given produces a high maternal serum level of the drug. The nature of the drug, especially molecular size, also will affect the degree of transfer, as will the amount of protein binding of the drug in the mother's bloodstream. It has been demonstrated that 'back diffusion' of drugs can take place from breast milk to maternal plasma as the concentration falls in the mother's bloodstream due to metabolism and excretion of the drug. Therefore timing of infant feeding in relation to the time of the mother taking the medication is another important factor.

This brief summary of the principles involved in drug transfer into breast milk illustrates that it is often difficult to give a simple 'yes' or 'no' answer to an enquiry about whether breast feeding should be stopped when a course of drug therapy is prescribed for the mother. As in the case of drugs used in pregnancy, it is wise to check with an Obstetric Drug Information Centre about the most recent findings on any particular drug and relate this information to the individual patient's medical condition to evaluate the individual risks and benefits. Prescribers who include the mother in the decision making process gain the benefit of optimal patient compliance and minimal parental anxiety.

Publications vary when listing drugs that should be totally avoided while breastfeeding; Table 7.2 lists examples of drugs that are generally contraindicated during lactation.

7

DRUG SAFETY IN PREGNANCY AND LACTATION

TABLE 7.2 Examples of drugs contraindicated in lactation

Drug	Comment
Phenindione (warfarin and heparin are not contraindicated)	Can cause bleeding tendencies in the breast fed infant
Iodides, carbimazole (propylthiouracil may be used)	Suppression of thyroid function and goitre in the infant
Benzodiazepines	'Flat baby syndrome'; lethargy, especially in low birth weight and premature infants
Chloramphenicol	Possible infant blood dyscrasias
Ergot preparations	May cause symptoms of ergotism (vomiting, diarrhoea)
Lithium compounds	Hypotonia, difficulty in feeding, failure to thrive. Proper neonatal hydration and correct maternal serum levels may minimise risk
Oestrogens	Hormonal effects on infant
Radioactive preparations	Feeding may be resumed when milk is no longer radioactive
Sulfonamides	Neonatal jaundice and kernicterus

WAYS TO MINIMISE INFANT DRUG INTAKE FROM BREAST MILK

While drug information, research, reports and experience with the use of a drug may indicate its apparent safety, the necessity of using the drug should still be considered and certain questions asked:

i. Is it really necessary to take this drug? If the condition is self-limiting the therapy may only ameliorate some of the symptoms. Symptoms (such as rash, itch, cough or runny nose) could possibly be endured for a short period for the sake of peace of mind regarding the safety of the child. If treatment is necessary the availability of some safe alternative should be considered.

ii. Is systemic therapy needed? Is it necessary to produce a 'total body' effect by oral or parenteral administration of the drug? Perhaps topical or local therapy may be as effective as systemic therapy without raising any concern about milk transfer of the drug. For a rash, creams or ointments could be used rather than antihistamine tablets, which may cause infant drowsiness, and nasal drops or sprays for a congested or runny nose rather than 'cold tablets' which may produce irritability and sleeplessness in the infant.

If systemic therapy is needed, then the following questions should also be asked to help to evaluate the risk to benefit balance in each case:

i. According to information currently available is the drug regarded as safe therapy in the neonatal period? For example most tables and charts list metronidazole as either contraindicated whilst breast feeding or to be used with caution. In clinical practice the drug is used extensively for mothers in the postpartum period, especially following abdominal surgery, to prevent or treat anaerobic infection. Thirty years of experience with the drug indicates its apparent safety. Also, metronidazole is commonly used in intensive care nurseries to treat necrotising enterocolitis in the neonatal period and in infancy. At the time of writing available knowledge indicates that the only concern is the metallic taste of the drug in the breast milk, which may cause a temporary lack of interest in feeding in some cases.

ii. What is the milk to plasma ratio of the drug? How much of the drug would a breast-fed infant receive per day from six to eight feeds, each of approximately 100 mL? Would this daily ingestion of the particular drug constitute a therapeutic dose for the infant, or is the quantity transferred in the milk too small to be clinically significant? For example, the anticonvulsant drug phenytoin sodium achieves about 25%–50% of plasma concentration in milk. As the therapeutic range for the mother (as confirmed by serum level testing) is 10–20 micrograms per mL, then the content of the drug in the milk would be at the most 5–10 micrograms per mL, or 500–1000 micrograms per 100 mL of milk. Expressed in milligrams, this would be 0.5–1.0 mg per feed, which would be regarded in most instances as clinically insignificant to the infant. It should also be remembered that in the case of epileptic mothers (and mothers being treated for other chronic conditions, e.g. collagen diseases), the neonate would have been exposed to higher levels of the same drug in the intrauterine period than it would be as a consequence of breast feeding. Thus any possible adverse effect should be apparent shortly after birth. This emphasises the importance of paediatricians being made aware of maternal therapy so appropriate neonatal monitoring and assessment can be performed. In turn, liaison can then be made with the mother's obstetrician or physician to discuss any possible or necessary adjustment to maternal drug therapy.

If drug therapy is absolutely necessary infant drug intake can be minimised by:

1. Drugs that can be given as a single daily dose should be taken just before the child's longest sleep period. Feeding can thus be avoided during peak milk levels of the drug.

2. If a drug must be given several times a day the mother should take the drug immediately after nursing. The pharmacokinetics of most drugs ingested by breast feeding women are such that administration of the drug at this time will allow back diffusion to take place and will result in the lowest amount of drug in the milk at the subsequent feeding.

NURSING IMPLICATIONS

Most women are now highly motivated to breast feed their babies. A recent survey in a major Australian maternity hospital showed that over 90% of mothers were breast feeding at the time of discharge. Encouragement and reassurance are therefore most appropriate, as well as expert advice when adjustments have to be made because of the mother's medical condition. Specific information about a particular drug can be obtained from the pharmacy department in the hospital and from Obstetric Drug Information Centres in each state. Avoid uninformed personal opinion that may cause subsequent confusion or concern.

Careful observation of all breast fed infants whose mothers are receiving drug therapy should be routine. Nurses should ensure that both paediatricians and obstetricians are made aware of any adverse effects or any change from normal neonatal functions.

7

DRUG SAFETY IN PREGNANCY AND LACTATION

FURTHER READING

Australian Drug Evaluation Committee. (1992), *Medicines in pregnancy — an Australian categorization of risk*, 2nd edn. AGPS, Canberra.

Batagol, R.P. (1993) *Drugs in pregnancy*, The Royal Women's Hospital, Melbourne.

Batagol, R.P. (1993) *Drugs and breast feeding*. CSL Ltd, Melbourne.

Briggs, G.G., Jaffe, S.J. and Freeman, R.K. (1990), *Drugs in pregnancy and lactation*, 3rd edn. Williams & Wilkins, Baltimore.

Gleicher, N. (1992), *Principles and practice of medical therapy in pregnancy*, 2nd edn. Appleton & Lange, Norwalk.

Llewelyn-Jones, D. (1990) *Fundamentals of obstetrics and gynaecology*, Vol 1, 5th edn. Faber & Faber, London.

Speight, T.M. (1987), *Avery's drug treatment*, 3rd edn. Adis Press, Auckland.

TEST YOUR KNOWLEDGE

1. Describe the mechanisms involved in drug transfer to the fetus. Which drugs will be more likely to accumulate in the fetal bloodstream?

2. List some of the drugs that should be avoided during early pregnancy.

3. List those drugs which are contraindicated whilst breast feeding.

Immunisation

BRIAN J. FEERY

O B J E C T I V E S

At the conclusion of this chapter the reader should be able to:

1. Define the terms vaccine, immunisation, passive immunisation, antigen, antibody, antitoxin, immunoglobulin;

2. Describe the method of active and passive immunisation;

3. Name the vaccines and sera in common use;

4. List the contraindications for vaccination; and

5. List the major side effects of vaccination and their treatment.

GENERAL PRINCIPLES ▮▮▮▮▮▮▮

Immunity in its broadest sense covers all the mechanisms which enable the host to resist the entry, multiplication and harmful effect of pathogenic organisms. Immunity to infection is not an absolute entity. It may be modified by age, nutrition, infection and therapy.

Immunity may be naturally or artificially acquired. Naturally acquired active immunity results from infection. Naturally acquired passive immunity results from the transference across the placenta of maternal antibodies. Artificial active immunity results from immunisation with vaccines and artificial passive immunity results from receiving immunoglobulin or antisera. See Figure 8.1.

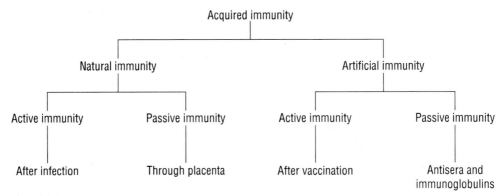

FIGURE 8.1   Classification of acquired immunity

The aim of immunisation is to produce an immune response sufficient to protect an individual against a clinical attack of disease. The purpose of active immunisation is to induce lasting immunity but passive protection may be conferred by giving immunoglobulin or heterologous antisera.

It is possible through immunisation to provide substantial if not complete protection against many infectious diseases. The degree of protection varies from almost absolute long-term protection against toxin mediated diseases such as tetanus and diphtheria to moderate short-term protection against diseases such as typhoid and influenza. With live viral vaccines such as poliomyelitis and measles, mumps and rubella vaccines, protection rates of about 95% are achieved. This protection subsequently may be boosted by subclinical infection.

ACTIVE IMMUNISATION ▮▮▮▮▮▮▮

Active immunisation denotes the induction of immunity including both humoral and cellular immune responses by the administration of vaccines. Active immunisation depends on the existence of adequate immune responses. Such responses may be impaired by neoplastic disease, by immunosuppressive therapy or by infection, such as human immunodeficiency virus (HIV) infection. Nevertheless, the majority of patients with such conditions will respond with an antibody response to inactivated vaccines including inactivated poliomyelitis vaccine. The protective immune response following inactivated vaccines depends on the production of specific antibodies to the infecting organism or to toxins produced by such organisms.

The magnitude and duration of the antibody response depends on the age of the vaccinee, the nature and mass of the antigen in the vaccine, the number of doses given, the interval between doses and the capacity of the individual to produce antibodies.

Once a primary response to the vaccine has been elicited the recipient retains a specific imprint of the stimulus in the form of sensitised cells and will respond rapidly to a subsequent challenge with the same antigen either in the form of a dose of vaccine or an infection by the relevant organism.

The immune response to live attenuated vaccines resembles more closely the response to natural infection in that both protective cellular and humoral responses follow such vaccination. In addition to the systemic antibody and cell mediated responses to infection with attenuated vaccine viruses, local antibody and cell mediated responses are induced when such vaccines are given by the natural route of infection, e.g. after orally administered Sabin poliomyelitis vaccine.

In general, live bacterial and viral vaccines are contraindicated in immunosuppressed individuals. It is recommended however, that infants and children with HIV infection should be given measles, mumps and rubella vaccine but not live poliomyelitis vaccine. The rationale is that the risks of infection are considered to be much greater than the risks of vaccination for measles, mumps and rubella, but live viral poliomyelitis vaccine must not be given to HIV infected patients because of the risk of persistent infection and paralytic poliomyelitis.

INACTIVATED VACCINES

Primary Course

The first injection of a vaccine is the primary or sensitising dose. Microbial antigens from the vaccine induce an immune reaction in the regional lymph glands. This reaction involves phagocytosis and processing by macrophages, stimulation of T and B lymphocytes which undergo blast transformation and proliferation, and finally the production of families of sensitised cells including antibody forming plasma cells and memory cells (see Figure 8.2). This immune response is controlled by cytokines, which are produced by lymphocytes, macrophages and other cells involved in the immune system. Cytokines are mediators or hormones which act specifically on a range

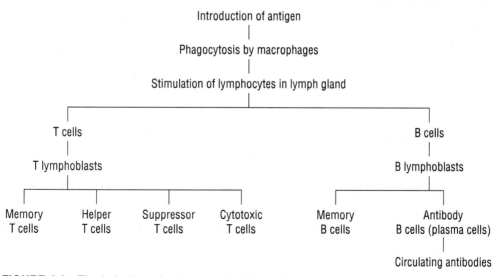

Introduction of antigen
|
Phagocytosis by macrophages
|
Stimulation of lymphocytes in lymph gland

T cells — T lymphoblasts — Memory T cells, Helper T cells, Suppressor T cells, Cytotoxic T cells

B cells — B lymphoblasts — Memory B cells, Antibody B cells (plasma cells) — Circulating antibodies

FIGURE 8.2   The induction of active acquired immunity

8

IMMUNISATION

of cells including granulocytes and lymphocytes and control cellular metabolic activity, chemotaxis, cytotoxicity, immunoglobulin production and the inflammatory response. Cytokines are responsible for the numerous interactions of the T and B cells systems and thus modulate the immune response.

The response to the first injection of vaccine or primary response is different from responses to subsequent doses. With the primary response there is usually a lag period of at least a week before antibody is detectable in the circulation. Antibody titres rise to reach a peak between the second and fourth week. The titre then falls over the ensuing months, eventually becoming undetectable. The duration of the antibody response will, of course, vary from antigen to antigen and will depend also on the height of the initial peak. The height of this peak is related to the size of the initial dose.

Re-exposure to the same antigen weeks, months or even years later evokes a secondary response, which is different from the primary response. There is a marked proliferation in the numbers of sensitised cells with the second and subsequent doses of protein and peptide vaccines. These cells include both memory cells and antibody producing plasma cells. Antibody appears much more rapidly, the titre is much higher and the peak level is reached within 7–14 days. The subsequent decline in antibody is much slower than that observed after primary antigenic stimulation. Adequate immunisation with inactivated vaccines usually involves a primary course of at least two or three doses of vaccine at intervals of at least four weeks, and a booster dose after 6–12 months.

In contrast with the dosage schedule for protein and polypeptide vaccines, immunisation with polysaccharide vaccines (e.g. pneumococcal or meningococcal vaccines) requires only one dose, because such vaccines tend to persist in the tissue and stimulate an ongoing response.

The type of immunoglobulin response depends on the antigens in the vaccine. Protein antigens induce initially an IgM response followed by an IgG immunoglobulin response. Occasionally IgG as well as IgM type responses are observed after polysaccharide vaccines, perhaps because of antigenic determinants on the molecule which cross react with groups on other bacterial antigens. Systemic IgA immunoglobulin responses are observed in the serum but local IgA antibody is not produced when inactivated vaccines are given parenterally.

Booster Doses

Booster doses of inactivated vaccine are necessary at intervals ranging from six months with cholera vaccine to 10 years with tetanus vaccine in order to maintain a satisfactory level of immunity. These doses stimulate a rapid increase in antibody levels which persist in most cases for long periods. Repeating booster doses too frequently does not induce progressively higher levels of immunity, and may be harmful because each successive dose increases the risk of inducing hypersensitivity reactions in the recipient.

Interval Between Doses

Immunisation with vaccines containing protein antigens involves more than one dose to induce an adequate immune response. The recommended minimum interval between doses in the primary immunisation course is four weeks. It has been found that this interval is necessary to achieve an optimum response, but longer intervals between injections do not impair the ultimate response or necessitate the addition of extra doses. It is never necessary to repeat any of the doses of a primary course, even though the recommended interval has been exceeded by months or even years. This is because the initial dose induces an immunological memory response involving T and B cells and this memory enables the individual to respond with a secondary response to subsequent doses.

Adjuvants are sometimes used in vaccines to enhance antibody responses. Thus toxoids (e.g. tetanus toxoid) which have been adsorbed onto mineral carriers such as aluminium hydroxide or phosphate, are more potent antigens than when used alone, and the dose required to produce immunity can be reduced. Vaccines containing adjuvants should be given by deep intramuscular injection because the aluminium may act as an irritant if given superficially.

Combined Vaccines

Combined vaccines have obvious advantages over single vaccines, e.g. fewer injections are required for primary immunisation. Combined vaccines are prepared and tested to ensure there will be no depression of antibody responses due to competition between antigens, e.g. Triple Antigen, which contains diphtheria, tetanus and pertussis vaccine, and M-M-R II vaccine which contains measles, mumps and rubella components.

LIVE VACCINES

The immune response induced by live attenuated vaccines more closely resembles the response induced by natural infection. It involves not only circulating IgM, IgG and IgA antibody responses but also cellular immune responses including T cell responses which are important in combating natural infections. When vaccine is administered by the natural route of infection, e.g. oral Sabin poliomyelitis vaccine, then local IgA antibody and local cellular responses are induced as well as systemic responses. It is usually assumed that these responses will give greater protection than inactivated vaccines but this has not always been demonstrated. Live viral vaccines usually induce long-term immunity after a single dose and may increase the possibility of the eradication of wild-type infection. They may, however, cause clinical manifestations of illness in individuals with immune deficiencies and in a small proportion of normal vaccinees.

Common viral and bacterial vaccines are listed in Tables 8.1 and 8.2 respectively. The recommended schedule for childhood immunisation is shown in Table 8.3.

8

IMMUNISATION

TABLE 8.1 Common viral vaccines

Vaccine	Trade name(s)	Description	Route of administration
Measles, mumps, rubella vaccine	*M-M-R II*	Live attenuated measles, mumps and rubella vaccine	Subcutaneous
Poliomyelitis vaccine	*Polio Sabin (Oral)*	Live attenuated poliomyelitis vaccine	Oral
	Enpovax HDC	Inactivated poliomyelitis virus vaccine	Subcutaneous
Yellow fever vaccine	—	Live attenuated vaccine	Subcutaneous
Hepatitis A vaccine	*Havrix*	Inactivated hepatitis A vaccine	Intramuscular
Hepatitis B vaccine	*H-B-Vax II, Engerix-B*	Adjuvanted inactivated recombinant hepatitis B vaccine	Intramuscular
Influenza vaccine	*Fluvax, Vaxigrip, Influenza Vaccine*	Inactivated influenza split virion vaccine	Subcutaneous
Japanese encephalitis vaccine	—	Inactivated Japanese encephalitis virus vaccine	Subcutaneous
Rabies vaccine	*Imogam, Merieux*	Inactivated rabies virus vaccine	Subcutaneous

TABLE 8.2 Common bacterial vaccines

Vaccine	Trade name(s)	Description	Route of administration
Diphtheria, tetanus, pertussis vaccine	*Triple Antigen (DTP)*	Adsorbed diphtheria and tetanus toxoid and inactivated pertussis vaccine	Intramuscular
Diphtheria, tetanus vaccine	*CDT Vaccine*	Adsorbed diphtheria and tetanus toxoid vaccine	Intramuscular
	ADT Vaccine	Adsorbed dilute diphtheria toxoid and tetanus toxoid vaccine	Intramuscular
Diphtheria vaccine adsorbed	—	Adsorbed diphtheria toxoid	Intramuscular
Diphtheria vaccine adsorbed (diluted for adult use)	—	Adsorbed diphtheria toxoid	Intramuscular
Tetanus vaccine	*Tet-Tox*	Adsorbed tetanus vaccine	Intramuscular
Cholera vaccine	—	Inactivated bacterial vaccine	Subcutaneous
Plague vaccine	—	Inactivated bacterial vaccine	Subcutaneous
Typhoid vaccine	—	Inactivated bacterial vaccine	Subcutaneous
	Typhim Vi	Polysaccharide vaccine	Intramuscular
	Typh-Vax (Oral)	Live attenuated bacterial vaccine	Oral
Haemophilus influenzae vaccine	*Act-HIB, HibTITER, PedvaxHIB, ProHIBiT*	Polysaccharide antigen vaccine	Subcutaneous
Meningococcal vaccine	*Mencevax ACWY*	Polysaccharide antigen vaccine	Subcutaneous
Pneumococcal vaccine	*Pneumovax 23*	Polysaccharide antigen vaccine	Subcutaneous
Tuberculosis vaccine	*Dried BCG Vaccine*	Live attenuated bacterial vaccine	Intradermal
Q fever vaccine	*Q-Vax*	Inactivated vaccine	Subcutaneous

TABLE 8.3 NHMRC standard childhood immunisation schedule (August 1994)

Age	Disease(s)	Vaccine
2 months	Diphtheria, tetanus, pertussis Poliomyelitis *Haemophilus influenzae* type b (Hib) (Schedule 1 or 2***)	*Triple Antigen** (DTP) Sabin vaccine (OPV) Hib vaccine (a or b or c**)
4 months	Diphtheria, tetanus, pertussis Poliomyelitis Hib (Schedule 1 or 2***)	*Triple Antigen* Sabin vaccine Hib vaccine (a or b or c**)
6 months	Diphtheria, tetanus, pertussis Poliomyelitis Hib (Schedule 1 only***)	*Triple antigen* Sabin vaccine Hib vaccine (a or b**)
12 months	Measles, mumps, rubella Hib (Schedule 2 only***)	Measles, mumps, rubella (MMR) Hib vaccine (c**)
18 months	Diphtheria, tetanus, pertussis Hib (Schedule 1 only***)	*Triple Antigen* Hib vaccine (a or b**)
Prior to school entry (4–5 years)	Diphtheria, tetanus, pertussus Poliomyelitis	*Triple Antigen* Sabin vaccine
10–16 years	Measles, mumps, rubella	MMR
15 years or prior to leaving school	Diphtheria, tetanus Poliomyelitis	Adult diphtheria and tetanus (ADT) Sabin vaccine

Contraindications to pertussis component
Triple Antigen should be omitted and CDT used instead for:
(i) infants known to have active or progressive neurological disease including recent convulsions; and
(ii) infants who have had any major reactions following *Triple Antigen*, e.g. fever (40.5°C);
convulsions (uncommon); hypotonic/hyporesponsive episodes (uncommon); shock, anaphylaxis,
thrombocytopenia and encephalopathy (all extremely rare); severe local reactions; and persistent
screaming (more than 3 hours).
These children should be given CDT Vaccine at 2 months, 4 months and 18 months of age.

Hib vaccines
**a = HbOC (*HibTITER*); b = PRP-T (*Act-HIB*); c = PRP-OMP (*PedvaxHIB*).
*** Schedule 1 Hib vaccination applies to the use of HbOC and PRP-T, the selected vaccine is given
at 2, 4, 6 and 18 months. Schedule 2 Hib vaccination refers to the use of PRP-OMP which is
given at 2, 4 and 12 months. A fourth Hib vaccine (PRP-D, *ProHIBiT*) is approved for use as a
single injection for children over 18 months of age. As specific product recommendations vary
always refer to the product information.

8

IMMUNISATION

PASSIVE IMMUNISATION ▮▮▮▮▮▮▮▮▮▮▮

Passive immunisation is used to protect people who are at risk of disease or envenomation and who are known to be or suspected of being susceptible to such challenge. Passive immunisation involves the administration of human antibodies in normal immunoglobulin or heterologous antibodies in antisera or antivenoms.

IMMUNOGLOBULIN

Normal immunoglobulin is prepared by fractionation of serum from large pools of human blood donations and therefore contains the spectrum of antibodies present in the population of blood donors. The fractionation process inactivates human pathogens so the product cannot transmit infection to recipients. It is available as a 16% solution for intramuscular administration and as a 6% solution for intravenous administration.

Immunoglobulin preparations with high antibody levels to specific diseases are available, e.g. hepatitis B immunoglobulin, rabies immunoglobulin, tetanus immunoglobulin, varicella-zoster immunoglobulin, cytomegalovirus immunoglobulin and Rh D immunoglobulin.

The main indication for giving normal immunoglobulin is the management of patients with hypogammaglobulinaemia and agammaglobulinaemia. Other indications include the prevention of viral infections such as hepatitis A, measles, chickenpox, hepatitis B and rabies, and the prevention of sensitisation of the fetus to the Rh D antigen on maternal red blood cells.

When large numbers of immunoglobulin doses are required, the 6% intravenous solution (Intragam) is used.

The duration of the protection afforded by immunoglobulin is related to the half-life of the product and the size of the dose, e.g. in patients with agammaglobulinaemia and hypogammaglobulinaemia it is necessary to give large doses of immunoglobulin once a month. In the prevention of hepatitis A it has been found that a dose of 2 mL will give good protection to adults for 5–6 weeks, but 5 mL is required for protection for 5–6 months.

HETEROLOGOUS ANTISERA

Passive immunisation may also involve the use of heterologous antisera. Heterologous antisera are produced in mammals. The horse is most commonly used since it has a large blood volume and is an efficient producer of antibodies, but cattle, sheep, goats and rabbits have been used. Animals are immunised with vaccines or toxins. After antibody formation has reached an optimum level, serum is collected and fractionated to separate the immunoglobulin fraction. The resulting product is a concentrated solution of the antibody fraction of serum. Antivenoms to snake bite, tick bite and spider bite are made by this method.

Since heterologous antiserum, even after the most careful refinement, contains protein material foreign to humans it may cause allergic reactions of varying severity in sensitive people. These reactions may be severe and sometimes life threatening, e.g. anaphylactic shock or serum sickness reactions.

Antivenoms may be given by the intramuscular route (e.g. red back spider antivenom) or by the intravenous route (e.g. snake antivenoms). Snake antivenom is administered after dilution by slow intravenous infusion. Administration is usually preceded by an appropriate dose of antihistamine and corticosteroid. Adrenaline is used in small doses to control any acute hypersensitivity reactions. Detailed instructions on administration are included in the product information leaflets. Other antivenoms available include box jellyfish, diphtheria, funnel-web, gas gangrene, sea snake, stonefish and tick antivenoms.

PRECAUTIONS

Immunisation is one of the safest and most effective procedures in modern medicine, but there are precautions and contraindications to be observed when giving any dose of vaccine or immunoglobulin. These precautions are listed in the product literature which must be consulted before giving any immunising agent.

In general the precautions can be listed under three headings: the recipient, the immunising agent and administration.

THE RECIPIENT

Age

The recommended age for the administration of specific vaccines results from public health considerations which include the risk of disease at certain ages, the capacity of individuals of certain ages to respond to vaccines and the possibility of adverse reactions. The NHMRC Schedule for childhood immunisation is based on these considerations (see Table 8.3).

Allergy

Most modern vaccines contain negligible quantities of allergenic substances but individuals with a history of acute hypersensitivity or anaphylactic reactions to egg protein must not be given egg based vaccines such as influenza vaccine, typhus vaccine, yellow fever vaccine or Q-fever vaccine.

Measles and mumps vaccines are prepared in cell cultures of chicken embryo cells. It is extremely rare that acute hypersensitivity reactions follow the administration of these vaccines but due precautions must be observed, e.g. egg sensitive infants should be given measles or mumps vaccines or measles–mumps–rubella vaccine only after appropriate skin testing has been completed and when facilities for the treatment of acute hypersensitivity reactions are available.

State of Health

The state of health of persons to be vaccinated should be noted. In general the risks of vaccination are considerably less than the risks of natural infection. In the presence of an acute illness, however, it is usually better to defer vaccination in case complications of the illness are confused with reactions to vaccination.

Inactivated vaccines may be given to patients with chronic illness and immune deficiency conditions and, in general, such patients will respond to such vaccines in a satisfactory manner.

Live bacterial and viral vaccines are contraindicated in immunosuppressed individuals. It is recommended however, that infants and children with HIV infection should be given measles–mumps–rubella vaccine but not live poliomyelitis vaccine. The rationale is that the risks of infection are considered to be much greater than the risks of vaccination for measles, mumps and rubella, but live viral poliomyelitis vaccine must not be given to HIV infected patients because of the risk of persistent infection and paralytic poliomyelitis.

Pregnancy

There is no convincing evidence that vaccination with inactivated vaccines causes any severe complications during pregnancy. However, it would be prudent to avoid giving vaccines which may be accompanied by systemic reactions.

There is no evidence that the live viral vaccines, yellow fever vaccine and poliomyelitis vaccine, cause problems during pregnancy. On grounds of theoretical risk to the fetus, vaccines such as measles–mumps–rubella vaccine are contraindicated, but there is negligible evidence of any risk to the

8

IMMUNISATION

fetus in mothers inadvertently given rubella vaccine in the early weeks of pregnancy.

History of Prior Reactions to a Vaccine

If a patient has suffered a previous reaction to an immunising agent an attempt must be made to determine the cause of the reaction before further doses are given. It may be possible to defer vaccination or give a different vaccine, e.g. combined diphtheria–tetanus vaccine instead of *Triple Antigen*, or to give fractional doses under an antihistamine cover, e.g. tetanus vaccine.

THE IMMUNISING AGENT

Vaccines, immunoglobulins and antisera must be appropriately transported and stored to retain their potency and efficacy. To ensure that the effectiveness of vaccines is maintained, vaccines need to be transported and stored at temperatures between $2°C$ and $8°C$ (see Table 8.4). Each package will have a batch number and expiry date which should be noted before the product is administered. In addition, the product leaflet will contain relevant information about precautions, administration and possible side effects.

TABLE 8.4 Stability of some standard vaccines at different temperatures

Vaccine	Stability at different storage temperatures			
	0–8°C	22–25°C	35–37°C	Above 37°C
Diphtheria and tetanus toxiods	3–7 years	Several months	About 6 weeks	2 weeks at 45°C: loss of potency after a few hours at 60–65°C
Pertussis vaccine	18–24 months, although with continuous slow decrease of potency	Variable: some vaccines stable for 2 weeks	Variable: some vaccines with a 50% loss of potency after one week	About 10% loss of potency per day at 45°C: rapid loss of potency at 50°C
Freeze dried measles vaccine	2 years	Retains satisfactory potency for 1 month	Retains satisfactory potency for at least 1 week	50% loss of potency after 2–3 days at 41°C: 80% loss of potency after 1 day at 54°C
Reconstituted measles vaccine	Unstable: should be used in one working session	Unstable: 50% loss of potency after 1 hour, 70% loss after 3 hours	Very unstable: titre may be below acceptable level after 2–7 hours	Inactivation within 1 hour at temperatures above 37°C
Oral polio vaccine	6–12 months	Unstable: 50% loss of potency after 20 days: some vaccines may retain satisfactory titres for 1–2 weeks	Very unstable: loss of satisfactory titre after 1–3 days	Very unstable at 41°C, 50% loss of potency after one day, complete loss of potency after 1–3 hours at 50°C

Note: Vaccines which are most unstable at room temperature are oral polio vaccine and reconstituted measles vaccine.

Adapted from: World Health Organization (1993), *The immunological basis for immunization. 1. General immunology expanded program on immunization*. World Health Organization, Geneva.

ADMINISTRATION

All immunising agents should be given with appropriate aseptic techniques using separate disposable syringes. The route of administration will be recommended in the product leaflet, e.g. oral, intradermal, subcutaneous, intramuscular or intravenous. Vaccines and antisera should be administered in an area where there is minimal opportunity for local, neural, vascular or tissue injury. Subcutaneous injections are usually administered into the deltoid area. Intradermal injections are generally given on the volar surface of the forearms. The exception to this rule is human diploid cell rabies vaccine where reactions are less severe in the deltoid area. The preferred site for intramuscular injections is in the deltoid muscle of the upper arm in adults and children aged 12 months and over. The anterolateral aspect of the upper thigh should be used for infants less than 12 months of age. The gluteal intramuscular injection is *not* recommended for vaccines. Skin cleansing and sterilisation are carried out in the usual way.

A documented record should be made of the patient's name, date, agent given and batch number, and any adverse reactions to the agent. Unusual adverse reactions should be reported to the manufacturer and to the Adverse Drug Reactions Advisory Committee (ADRAC).

8

IMMUNISATION

ADVERSE REACTIONS ███████████

Adverse reactions to immunisation are generally mild and occur at reasonably low frequency. Severe reactions are uncommon and disabling effects are exceedingly rare.

LOCAL REACTIONS

Local reactions including redness, tenderness and induration at the site of injection occur in about half the recipients of *Triple Antigen* (DTP) vaccine, in less than a third of the recipients of influenza vaccine and infrequently in infants given MMR vaccine. The administration of prophylactic paracetamol 15 mg/kg body weight given at or just before the immunisation and repeated 3–4 hourly thereafter for two to three doses can reduce the incidence of minor side effects and febrile reactions.

SYSTEMIC REACTIONS

Systemic reactions such as fever, malaise and myalgia starting 6–12 hours after administration and persisting for one to two days occur in up to 30%–40% recipients of *Triple Antigen* (DTP) vaccine, but much less frequently (5%–10%) with other vaccines such as influenza vaccine or combined diphtheria and tetanus (CDT) vaccine.

Acute allergic reactions such as acute anaphylaxis are exceedingly rare. Delayed allergic reactions such as local inflammatory reactions or serum sickness reactions may be observed infrequently after tetanus vaccine but more commonly after the administration of antiserum.

TREATMENT OF ADVERSE REACTIONS

Mild local and general reactions may be regarded as an inevitable association with a number of immunisation procedures. In general management can be limited to observation, reassurance or the administration of a mild analgesic such as paracetamol.

Acute hypersensitivity reactions are exceedingly rare. The most appropriate treatment is the administration of adrenaline injection (1:1000) by subcutaneous injection.

The initial dose for adults is 0.5 mL repeated as necessary. The initial dose for infants is from 0.05 mL for infants aged 3–6 months to 0.1 mL for infants aged 12 months. When the symptoms of acute hypersensitivity have been relieved corticosteroids may be given to assist recovery and antihistamines may be useful in the treatment of urticaria or angioedema.

CONTRAINDICATIONS

Immunisation is contraindicated if the patient is suffering from any major illness or allergy; has ever had a fit or an illness of the nervous system; has had a severe reaction to a previous immunisation, such as a temperature over 39°C or persistent screaming or collapse or convulsions; is suffering from a malignant condition such as lymphoma or leukemia; has had any other immunisation in the last month; has had immunoglobulin or a blood transfusion in the last three months; or is under treatment with cortisone or a similar drug.

RULES FOR AVOIDING REACTIONS

1. Use sterile disposable syringes and needles.

2. Always store immunising agents as directed by the manufacturer.

3. Check patient's history for previous reactions or allergies.

4. Select site for injection to avoid blood vessels and other important structures, e.g. use deltoid region of arm or lateral aspect of thigh.

5. After insertion of the needle pull back on plunger (aspirate) to make sure needle is not in a vein.

6. Have adrenaline 1:1000 injection available in case of anaphylaxis.

7. Make sure patient (or parent) knows what agent has been given and give a written record of immunisation.

NURSING IMPLICATIONS

1. The patient's age, state of health and history of allergy or previous reactions to vaccinations should be determined before vaccination is commenced. Whether the patient is pregnant or likely to become pregnant during the course of vaccination should also be determined.

2. Strict attention should be paid to the state of equipment and vaccine before vaccination is commenced. Vaccines must be stored and reconstituted as directed by the manufacturer. Agents should be used at room temperature and not straight from the refrigerator and should be shaken before use to ensure an even dispersal of the contents of the container.

3. Nursing staff should be aware of possible reactions and how to avoid and treat them before vaccination is commenced. Adrenaline (1:1000) should be available for use in case of anaphylaxis and the nurse must be prepared to institute cardiopulmonary resuscitation procedures if necessary.

4. The patient/parent should be informed of the possible side effects and adverse reactions that may occur. For example, with *Triple Antigen* (DTP) most children will have a slight fever and will be irritable within two days after having the injection. More than one half of children develop some soreness and swelling in the area where the injection was given. Paracetamol should be given to relieve a fever and soreness. With MMR, children occasionally will develop a fever with or without a rash 5–10 days after immunisation. Paracetamol can be

given for the fever and children who develop a rash are not infectious to others. With rubella, mild reactions, which include fever, sore throat, enlarged lymph glands, rash and arthritis, may occur one to three weeks after immunisation. Mild discomfort or pain persisting a few days after tetanus injection is common and may also occur 10 days or so after injection. Too frequent administration of tetanus vaccine may provoke hypersensitivity reactions. For severe reactions such as temperatures above 39°C, persist-

ent screaming, convulsions or episodes of limpness and paleness, patients/parents should be advised to consult their local doctor or local casualty department.

5. The patient or, in the case of a child, the parent should be informed of which agent is being administered and advised of the importance of retaining written records of immunisation and of attending for any subsequent doses to complete the course of immunisation or to maintain the state of immunity.

8

IMMUNISATION

FURTHER READING

National Health and Medical Research Council Immunisation Procedures (1994) 5th edn. AGPS, Canberra.

Roitt, I.M. (1991) *Essential Immunology.* 7th edn. Blackwell Scientific, Oxford.

TEST YOUR KNOWLEDGE

1. Define immunity.

2. What is an antigen?

3. What are antibodies?

4. Describe (a) active immunity; (b) passive immunity.

5. Which is the drug of choice for the treatment of anaphylactic shock: adrenaline; an antihistamine; a corticosteroid?

Poisonings and their Treatment

JUDITH KIRBY

O B J E C T I V E S

At the conclusion of this chapter the reader should be able to:

1. List nine groups of substances with potential for causing human poisoning, with examples from each group;

2. Understand the principles of management of poisoning, including initial therapy and exceptions;

3. List 10 specific antidotes and describe their mode of action;

4. List five routes of contact by which poisoning may occur, with examples of substances toxic via these routes and their effects;

5. Understand the concept of 'range of toxicity'; and

6. Understand the role of Poisons Information Centres.

TOXICOLOGY

In the sense of being a study of poisons and their effects on animals (including humans), toxicology predates recorded history. Poisons are mentioned on the Ebers papyrus, written about 1500 BC. They have figured prominently in Roman and Greek histories and through the Middle Ages when, for example, the Borgias illustrated a working knowledge of the dosage and actions of poisons, if rather less interest and knowledge in how to treat their effects.

Paracelsus (1493–1541) could be regarded as the initiator of the modern approach to toxicology. He first took an interest in identifying a particular toxin, the use of experimentation to examine responses to various chemicals in the therapeutic and toxic context and the potential involvement of environmental agents in toxicology. One statement attributed to Paracelsus is still relevant: 'All substances are poisons; there is none which is not a poison. The right dose differentiates a poison and a remedy.'

While intentional homicidal poisonings have decreased as a major section of the study of toxicology, suicide attempts in adults and unintentional, accidental poisonings in young children are still major problems.

In adults, industrial or agricultural accidents are significant causes of poisoning. In all age groups, environmental and work contact with chemicals forms an area of increasing interest.

TOXICITY

TYPES OF CONTACT

The type of contact with potentially poisonous substances is significant and the extent of poisoning will depend on the substance concerned and its chemical properties. Table 9.1 provides some illustrations of possible contacts with some representative toxins.

Water soluble substances, for example, are unlikely to be absorbed through the skin to produce systemic toxicity. However, if they are strongly acidic (e.g. sulfuric acid) or alkaline (e.g. caustic soda) they may react with the skin to cause a chemical burn. Some fat soluble substances (e.g. organophosphates such as parathion and malathion) can be absorbed through the skin to produce systemic toxicity.

A similar situation applies with ingestion, when local irritation, absorption, or both, may occur depending on the chemical nature of the poison. It should be noted that when a potential irritant like caustic soda has been swallowed there may be local burning in the mouth. However, the absence of burning in the mouth cannot be taken as indicative that there will not be serious burns in the oesophagus or stomach. In some cases the substance is swallowed quickly causing severe burns to the oesophagus but no effects in the mouth.

RANGE (RESPONSE AND DOSE)

The relevance of dose to toxicity can be well expressed by an example. Common salt (NaCl) in appropriate quantities is essential to life, with normal serum levels in the range 130–150 mmol/L. Levels of 150–160 mmol/L can result in central nervous system symptoms including convulsions in approximately 10% of patients. Death is a frequent occurrence if levels exceed 185 mmol/L. Two level dessertspoonfuls of sodium chloride (approximately 500 mmol of sodium) would, if retained and absorbed,

TABLE 9.1   Methods of contact with poisons

Type of Contact	Some Possible Effects	Example of Poison
Ingestion	Local effects in gastrointestinal tract Systemic effects	Overdose of medicines, some plants, petroleum distillates, pesticides
Topical — skin	Local irritation	Caustic soda (corrosive alkali)
	Absorption through skin to cause systemic poisoning	Organophosphate pesticide
Topical — eye	Local irritation	Acid and alkali, some plants, e.g. naked lady, arum lily
	Specific effects on eye	Atropine
Inhalation	Irritation in upper and lower respiratory tract	Chlorine gas
	Absorption and systemic poisoning	Carbon monoxide (exhaust fumes)
Injection	Systemic	Overdose of therapeutic drugs
	Local irritation, necrosis	Many cytotoxic drugs

raise the serum sodium level of a two-year-old child by about 50 mmol/L — a potentially lethal dose. Repeatedly, cases have been reported where children have died of salt overdose when it has been administered as an emetic. It should never be used for this purpose in children.

WAYS OF EXPRESSING TOXICITY

Unfortunately no simple relationship exists between the toxic dose of a substance and the therapeutic dose. For some substances the toxic dose is close to the effective therapeutic dose (e.g. cytotoxic drugs, digoxin). For other drugs the therapeutic dose can be increased immensely before a toxic dose is reached (e.g. penicillin).

Therapeutic Index

The therapeutic index is the ratio of the toxic dose to the effective dose. It gives an estimate of the relative safety of a drug in its normal usage. It is estimated as the ratio of LD_{50} (lethal dose in 50% of cases) to ED_{50} (effective dose in 50% of cases). As different effects may require different doses a single drug may have a number of therapeutic indices. In practice a substance is usually referred to as having a 'high' or 'low' therapeutic index.

The term, LD_{50}, is commonly used in toxicology literature. It is the dose which will kill 50% of an experimental population. For example, for the drug imipramine an oral dose of 625 mg/kg given to a group of 100 rats would kill 50 of them. Thus, it is said to have an oral LD_{50} (in rats) of 625 mg/kg. These data are helpful, but there is wide variation among species as shown in Table 9.2.

TABLE 9.2 Species differences in LD$_{50}$ for imipramine

LD$_{50}$ (oral, rats)	=	625 mg/kg
LD$_{50}$ (oral, mouse)	=	448 mg/kg
LD$_{50}$ (oral, dog)	=	100 mg/kg

Cases have been reported of children dying after ingestion of 15–30 mg/kg of imipramine. Hence, while animal data may be helpful, great caution must be exercised in using them to predict effects in humans.

ACUTE AND CHRONIC POISONING ▬

Poisoning may be either acute (a single contact with a toxin) or chronic (repeated contacts with a toxin which can build up over a period of time).

The build-up of toxin or its effect may also be referred to as 'cumulative'. Often the symptoms of a chronic overdose differ from those of an acute overdose. For example, a patient with acute lead poisoning (after ingestion of a soluble lead salt) may present with abdominal pain, vomiting, diarrhoea, metallic taste, black stools, oliguria, collapse or coma. A patient with chronic lead poisoning is more likely to present with a characteristic 'lead line' on the gums and very non-specific symptoms of appetite loss, weight loss, constipation, vomiting, headache, weakness or loss of recently developed skills.

EPIDEMIOLOGY

During 1990 poisoning accounted for 617 deaths in Australia.

In childhood and adult poisonings the most common exposures involve household chemicals and medication. Most deaths and serious intoxications are caused by ingestion of pesticides and medication, paracetamol and benzodiazepines being the drugs used most frequently.

Of those calls handled by Poisons Information Centres in Australia approximately 85% are accidental and 15% intentional exposures.

DETAILS OF AN INDIVIDUAL POISONING

In few cases will there be an accurate history of the quantity of substance swallowed, or even what the substance was. Adults who have attempted to take a suicidal dose of a substance are notorious for giving inaccurate histories of the quantity of substance ingested and may in fact be unconscious at the time of presentation.

The history of childhood poisoning will usually involve the patient (often too young to talk) having been found sitting amidst tablets or liquid spread across the floor. How much has been spilled and how much ingested cannot be accurately estimated. Children in the 'at risk' age group (one to three years) cannot be relied on not to swallow something that tastes unpleasant. They may have ingested much more or much less than the parent thinks has been swallowed. At best, an educated guess can be made based on the maximum that could have been swallowed. In some circumstances blood or urine assays may indicate the drug and quantity absorbed.

MANAGEMENT

In spite of the common association in people's minds between poisons and antidotes, there are very few substances for which an antidote exists.

The management of poisoning in the majority of cases involves two steps and occasionally a third: maintaining vital functions; removing contact between the poison and the patient; and applying specific treatment (if appropriate). Some aspects are summarised in Table 9.3.

TABLE 9.3 Management of poisoning

1. Maintain vital functions
Respiration, cardiovascular function, fluid and electrolyte maintenance, safeguard kidney function

2. Remove contact between poison and patient
If no contraindication, perform gastric lavage (or occasionally induce emesis); wash off skin or eye with water. Remove patient from gaseous poison. Speed excretion: catharsis, diuresis, dialysis. Prevent further absorption by adsorption onto activated charcoal

3. Treat symptomatically, administer antidote if available for specific toxin

Gastric Decontamination

The last few years have seen a change in thought amongst clinical toxicologists on the preferred method of gastric decontamination. In the past, the induction of vomiting, usually using ipecac syrup, was commonly thought to be the most effective way to empty the stomach, especially with paediatric patients. Recent studies have shown that the use of activated charcoal to adsorb the toxin results in lower serum levels than either induction of vomiting or the use of gastric lavage alone.

Activated charcoal uses the process of adsorption which involves using a chemical with a particularly large surface area and hence prevents the toxin from being absorbed into the blood stream. Some drugs adsorbed by activated charcoal are shown in Table 9.4.

It is given as a slurry with water (or sometimes the initial dose is mixed with a cathartic such as sorbitol). This slurry should be a mix of 1 to 8 up to 1 to 10 of activated charcoal to water, although the latter results in large volumes for the patient to swallow. If too concentrated a slurry is used the charcoal can cause a physical obstruction.

The current approach to management of a patient who has recently ingested a toxic amount of substance is to first aspirate the stomach contents and then to administer activated charcoal at a rate of 0.25 g/kg/hour or a single dose of 1 g/kg body weight.

The advantages of this type of approach over the widely used emesis evacuation methods of the past are:

- lower serum levels of absorbed toxin;
- administration of charcoal or oral antidotes not delayed waiting for the cessation of ipecac induced vomiting; and
- no ipecac complications, e.g. lethargy, diarrhoea.

Repeated doses of charcoal have been shown to be useful with some toxins, e.g. theophylline, phenobarbitone and carbamazepine.

TABLE 9.4 Drugs adsorbed by activated charcoal

Analgesics
Aspirin and sodium salicylate
Dextropropoxyphene
Paracetamol
Mefenamic acid

Hypnotics and Sedatives
Barbiturates including barbitone, pentobarbitone, quinalbarbitone
Glutethimide
Benzodiazepines

Tranquillisers and Antidepressants
Chlorpromazine
Imipramine
Nortriptyline

Others
Chloroquine
Chlorpheniramine
Ipecacuanha
Isoniazid
Phenylpropanolamine
Propantheline

POISONINGS AND THEIR TREATMENT 9

Ipecac syrup might still be used in some situations, e.g. serious intoxications occurring in areas remote from medical help and ingestion of sustained release iron tablets by children.

It should also be stated at this point that the induction of vomiting is not without some adverse effects. For example, occasionally patients suffer Mallory-Weiss syndrome (gastric tears) with the dramatic vomiting which ensues and deaths from gastric rupture have been reported. A child who received only 15 mL of ipecac syrup died of this complication in 1987. Up to 13% of patients suffer diarrhoea, lethargy or drowsiness. Therefore, in many patients (especially children) who have ingested doses that are not likely to cause serious toxicity it may be best to manage them conservatively, i.e. with observation and supportive care alone.

In summary, the recommended approach to gastric decontamination in patients with recent, serious intoxications would be to pass a large bore orogastric tube (or a nasogastric tube in some children), with airway protection if indicated, and lavage the stomach, then commence charcoal at 0.25 g/kg/hour.

There are three important situations where gastric emptying and charcoal should NOT be used. They are:

1. Following ingestion of corrosive substances (strong acids or alkalis, caustic soda, drain cleaners, dishwashing machine detergent) as there is the possibility of perforation of the stomach or oesophagus and of further burning when the substance is vomited or aspirated.

2. Following ingestion of petroleum distillates (e.g. petrol, kerosene, mineral turpentine, some polishes and fly sprays) as these may be aspirated into the lungs causing a chemical pneumonitis and they are not adsorbed by charcoal.

3. If the patient is convulsing.

Catharsis

Hastening the passage of gastrointestinal contents by administering a laxative helps remove unabsorbed poison from the body. This needs to be achieved without creating fluid and electrolyte imbalance problems due to the effects of the cathartic.

Commonly used cathartics in the treatment of poisoning are mannitol or sorbitol. Neither are primarily absorbed from the gastrointestinal tract nor adsorbed onto activated charcoal. Common doses are:

Mannitol 20%–25% or Sorbitol 70%
    Children: 1–2 mL/kg orally
    Adults: 100–150 mL orally

The approximate gastric transit time for sorbitol or mannitol is 2–3 hours.

FIRST AID AND NURSING IMPLICATIONS

Management of poisoning necessitates emphasis on first aid and hospitalisation.

First aid measures include the thorough assessment and identification of patient problems. Prompt intervention is imperative. These are, in essence, the 'ABC' of first aid.

FIRST AID

- **A cleared airway, adequate breathing and circulation should be ensured.**

- **The patient should be moved away from any toxic substance.**

- **Any toxic substance should be removed from the patient, e.g. by hosing or washing a substance from the body or removing contaminated clothing.**

- **Convulsions should be managed if they occur.**

- **Any vomitus should be saved if possible.**

- The patient should be transported to hospital as soon as possible and, if known, the following noted and relayed to ambulance personnel or hospital staff: the bottle or container of the substance; the original purpose of the substance; the actual shape or form, colour, odour or texture of the substance; the length of time of exposure to the poison or time since ingestion; and any abnormal signs which have been observed, e.g. fits, twitching, hallucinations or excited behaviour.

ASSESSMENT

- On arrival at hospital any cardiovascular, respiratory or circulatory problems (e.g. cardiac arrhythmias or abnormal respiratory patterns) must be carefully assessed.

- Any particular signs relevant to individual toxic substances should be noted and assessed, e.g. carbon monoxide poisoning often results in a pinkish tinge in the lips and nail beds, arsenic overdose often results in a garlicky smell to the breath.

- Assessment of consciousness level is essential. If possible the toxic substance should be identified to enable the appropriate treatment to be chosen and the correct method of elimination to be implemented.

ELIMINATION OF POISON

Depending on the type of poison or toxic substance and various contraindications, some of the following methods may be appropriate for elimination of the substance.

The most common methods are gastric lavage and emesis (especially in children). Currently the use of adsorbents, e.g. activated charcoal, is thought to be the most effective method of gastric decontamination.

Haemodialysis, charcoal haemoperfusion or peritoneal dialysis may augment these measures but the degree of usefulness depends on the special characteristics of the toxic substance. These measures are used infrequently.

Decontamination by removal of clothing and washing of the skin may be helpful in some gaseous or liquid exposures.

The mainstay of management of the poisoned patient involves supportive care.

ADMINISTRATION

The nurse should understand the procedure for inserting orogastric and nasogastric tubes and be aware of the signs of misplacement or dislodgement, e.g. coughing, respiratory distress. Extreme caution is essential to ensure charcoal does not enter the respiratory system. Charcoal should not be given if there is any doubt about the placement of the tube. The charcoal solution should be given relatively slowly to avoid vomiting and aspiration.

9

POISONINGS AND THEIR TREATMENT

ANTIDOTES

Contrary to popular belief there are few poisons for which there are specific antidotes. However, when the few that do exist are used they may be life saving. Table 9.5 lists the antidotes likely to be encountered.

TABLE 9.5 Antidotes for specific poisons

Antidote	Poison	Notes
Acetylcysteine	Paracetamol	Intravenous. Commence as soon as possible, not later than 10 to 12 hours after ingestion
Atropine	Organophosphate and carbamate insecticides	Large doses needed
Calcium (calcium gluconate, milk)	Fluoride	
Calcium disodium edetate (EDTA)	Lead	
Desferrioxamine	Iron	
Dicobalt edetate	Cyanide	
Digoxin FAB fragments	Digoxin overdose	
Flumazenil	Benzodiazepines	
Dimercaprol	Heavy metals: mercury, arsenic	
Naloxone	Narcotics, dextroproxyphene	
Penicillamine	Copper, lead	
Physostigmine	Anticholinergic drugs	Short duration of action
Pralidoxime (PAM)	Organophosphate insecticides	Do **not** use with carbamates, use early

SPECIFIC AGENTS

Acetylcysteine

TRADE NAMES

Acetylcysteine (*N*-acetylcysteine, NAC): *Parvolex.*

MECHANISM OF ACTION

Acetylcysteine is used as an antidote to paracetamol poisoning. In part the liver toxicity of paracetamol is due to a build up of toxic metabolites of paracetamol. Acetylcysteine is thought to restore glutathione (which conjugates these toxic metabolites or acts as a substrate for these toxic metabolites).

USES

When acetylcysteine is used in the treatment of paracetamol overdose it needs to be given as early as possible after the ingestion, certainly before 10–12 hours have elapsed. For intravenous use, the dose is 150 mg/kg in 200 mL of glucose 5% over 15 minutes followed by 50 mg/kg in 500 mL of glucose 5% infused over four hours followed by 100 mg/kg in 1 L of glucose 5% over 16 hours, i.e. a total of 300 mg/kg in 20 hours. In children the quantity of intravenous fluid used should be modified according to age and weight.

ADVERSE DRUG REACTIONS

Hypersensitivity reactions occur with intravenous administration of acetylcysteine. They are manifested as urticaria, flushing, diaphoresis, pruritus and, rarely, transient hypotension, tachycardia and bronchospasm.

Atropine

MECHANISM OF ACTION

Atropine blocks the action of acetylcholine accumulated at nerve junctions and end plates in the parasympathetic nervous system (mainly affecting 'muscarinic' receptors in smooth muscle, heart and exocrine glands, see Chapter 10 Drugs and the Autonomic Nervous System). It dries up excessive respiratory and other secretions, dilates pupils, causes flushing and reduces bradycardia. Unfortunately it has little effect on muscular weakness including of the respiratory muscles.

PHARMACOKINETICS

When given intravenously atropine is rapidly cleared from the blood and distributed throughout the body. Levels drop quickly within the first 10 minutes and then decrease more gradually. After intravenous administration it crosses the blood brain barrier. It is incompletely metabolised in the liver and excreted in the urine as unchanged drug and metabolites. After intravenous administration, the elimination half-life is between 3.7 and 4.3 hours.

USES

Discussion in this section relates only to the use of atropine for anticholinesterase poisoning. Doses are far in excess of those for other therapeutic uses.

For an adult, this may approximate 4–8 mg intravenously every 10–15 minutes, in children 0.05 mg/kg/dose is given every 2–5 minutes until an atropine-like effect is observed.

For information on adverse drug reactions, precautions and contraindications see Chapter 10 Drugs and the Autonomic Nervous System.

Calcium

Calcium (e.g. calcium gluconate, milk in some mild cases) is used as an antidote to fluoride poisoning. Calcium reacts with the soluble fluoride to form insoluble calcium fluoride and hence prevent absorption from the stomach.

For information on pharmacokinetics, uses, adverse drug reactions, precautions and contraindications see Chapter 32 Drugs Used in Critical Care.

Calcium Disodium Edetate

Calcium disodium edetate (EDTA or calcium disodium versenate) is an effective chelator of extracellular lead, resulting in a 20 to 50-fold increase in urine excretion. It could theoretically be used to bind iron, zinc, manganese, beryllium and copper. It indirectly removes lead from soft tissue, the central nervous system and red blood cells. Lead is bound to the nitrogen and oxygen atoms of EDTA forming a 5-membered heterocyclic ring.

PHARMACOKINETICS

EDTA is poorly absorbed from the gastrointestinal tract after oral administration. It is distributed mainly in the extracellular fluid and does not appear in red blood cells; 5% of the plasma concentration may be found in the cerebrospinal fluid. It is excreted almost entirely unchanged in the urine

9

POISONINGS AND THEIR TREATMENT

within 24 hours. The elimination half-life after intramuscular administration is between 1.4 and 3 hours.

USES

For the treatment of lead poisoning in adults EDTA is given as a 1 g dose intravenously over a period of at least two hours, twice daily for up to five days. Therapy is interrupted for two days and followed by an additional 5-day course of therapy if indicated.

Dosing may be based on body weight. A dose of 50 mg/kg/day is recommended in mild cases and 75 mg/kg/day in more severe cases. It may be given intramuscularly at the same dose level as the intravenous regimen. To avoid the pain associated with the injection it is recommended that the concentrated 20% solution be mixed with procaine prior to the injection. Each 1 mL of concentrate is mixed with 1 mL of 1% procaine to produce a final concentration of 0.5% procaine.

ADVERSE DRUG REACTIONS

EDTA is nephrotoxic and causes renal tubular necrosis. Other side effects include anaemia, hypotension, fatigue, myalgia, headache, joint pain, fever and histamine-like reactions, e.g. sneezing and nasal congestion. Dermatitis has been reported.

PRECAUTIONS AND CONTRAINDICATIONS

EDTA should be used with caution if at all in patients with impaired renal function. It can chelate endogenous metals, including zinc, and may increase their excretion.

Desferrioxamine

TRADE NAMES

Desferrioxamine: *Desferal*.

MECHANISM OF ACTION

Desferrioxamine is a specific chelator of ferric (Fe^3) iron. It combines with the iron to form a water soluble complex which is readily excreted in the urine and the bile.

PHARMACOKINETICS

Desferrioxamine is poorly absorbed from the gastrointestinal tract and therefore is given parenterally. It is metabolised in the liver and excreted by the kidney. It has a half-life of just over one hour.

USES

In the treatment of iron poisoning desferrioxamine is normally given by intravenous infusion at a rate not exceeding 15 mg/kg/hour. Subsequent doses can be reduced when the serum iron level falls below the total iron binding capacity (TIBC). A total dose of 80 mg/kg/24 hours should not be exceeded.

ADVERSE DRUG REACTIONS

Rapid intravenous injection of desferrioxamine may cause flushing and urticaria. There have been some cases of anaphylactic reactions. The most common adverse effects include gastrointestinal disorders, dysuria, fever, hypotension, tachycardia and skin rashes. Cataract formation, visual disturbances and hearing loss have been reported with prolonged treatment.

DRUG INTERACTIONS

Interactions have been reported with ascorbic acid and phenothiazines.

PRECAUTIONS AND CONTRAINDICATIONS

Desferrioxamine is contraindicated in patients with severe renal disease and should be used with caution in patients with impaired renal function.

Dicobalt Edetate

TRADE NAMES

Dicobalt edetate: *Kelocyanor*.

MECHANISM OF ACTION

Cyanide exerts toxicity by inhibiting cellular respiration through blocking the enzyme cytochrome oxidase. Dicobalt edetate is a chelating agent that forms a relatively non-toxic stable ion complex with cyanide.

USES

Dicobalt edetate should only be used in confirmed cyanide poisoning and never as a precautionary measure. In adults, a dose of 600 mg (two 20 mL ampoules) is administered, the contents of one ampoule being given over one minute. In children the dose should be adjusted according to body weight.

ADVERSE DRUG REACTIONS

Dicobalt edetate may cause hypotension, tachycardia and vomiting. Anaphylactic reactions have been occasionally reported.

PRECAUTIONS AND CONTRAINDICATIONS

Dicobalt edetate should not be injected in conditions other than known cyanide poisoning.

Digoxin Fab Fragments

This product is the first of a new group of antidotes — fragments of specific antibodies raised to particular chemical entities — in this case digoxin. Digoxin has a greater affinity for the antibodies than for tissue binding sites and the digoxin antibody complex is then rapidly excreted in the urine.

TRADE NAMES

Digoxin Fab Fragments: *Digibind.*

PHARMACOKINETICS

Digoxin Fab fragments have a small volume of distribution and are eliminated through renal filtration. By comparison, digoxin normally has a very slow excretion rate.

USES

Digoxin Fab fragments are given in digoxin poisoning. The dosage should be calculated in relation to the total digoxin in the body. Each vial containing 40 mg of Fab fragments will complex with 60 micrograms of digoxin.

ADVERSE REACTIONS

Rapid withdrawal of the positive inotropic effects in patients with poor cardiac reserves and hypersensitivity reactions are potential problems. Fab fragments are immunogenic and therefore patients treated more than once may experience an acute hypersensitivity reaction.

Dimercaprol

TRADE NAMES

Dimercaprol (BAL, British antilewisite): *B.A.L.*

MECHANISM OF ACTION

Dimercaprol is a chelating agent that contains ligands that bind heavy metals in preference to the body's sulfydryl groups. The product of the chelate–metal combination is less toxic and more easily excreted from the body than the heavy metals.

PHARMACOKINETICS

After intramuscular injection maximum blood concentrations of dimercaprol may be attained within one hour. Dimercaprol is metabolised and rapidly excreted in the bile and urine.

USES

Dimercaprol is used as an antidote for arsenic, mercury or gold poisoning. It is given as a deep intramuscular injection of 3–5 mg/kg every four hours for the first two days, then twice daily for a week.

ADVERSE DRUG REACTIONS

When doses exceed 5 mg/kg most patients experience vomiting, seizures and even coma within 1–6 hours.

PRECAUTIONS

Dimercaprol should be used with care in patients with hypertension or impaired renal function. It should not be used in patients with impaired hepatic function unless due to arsenic poisoning.

9

POISONINGS AND THEIR TREATMENT

It should not be used in the treatment of cadmium, iron, lead or selenium poisoning as the complexes formed are more toxic than the metals themselves.

Flumazenil

TRADE NAMES

Flumazenil: *Anexate*.

MECHANISM OF ACTION

Flumazenil is a benzodiazepine antagonist which acts competitively at central nervous system benzodiazepine receptors and hence reverses the central sedative effects of benzodiazepine drugs.

PHARMACOKINETICS

After intravenous administration flumazenil is widely distributed in the body and about 50% is bound to plasma proteins. It is rapidly cleared from the plasma by hepatic metabolism. The elimination half-life of the drug is 53 minutes.

USES

It is used to reverse the sedative effects of benzodiazepine drugs. This may be of value in diagnosing and treating benzodiazepine overdosage or reversing benzodiazepine induced anaesthesia.

ADVERSE DRUG REACTIONS

Infrequently reported adverse effects include dizziness, vertigo, anxiety, palpitations, fearfulness, depression, agitation and tearfulness. These may be related to benzodiazepine withdrawal. Seizures may occur if convulsant drugs have been taken or the patient has benzodiazepine withdrawal.

DRUG INTERACTIONS

Interactions with other drugs have not been reported.

PRECAUTIONS AND CONTRAINDICATIONS

Known hypersensitivity to the drug is a contraindication to its use. Consideration should be given to re-sedation of patients, especially those who have taken a long acting benzodiazepine. It should be used cautiously in patients with a known benzodiazepine dependency as acute benzodiazepine withdrawal may be precipitated.

Naloxone

TRADE NAMES

Naloxone: *Narcan*.

MECHANISM OF ACTION

Naloxone is an opioid (narcotic) antagonist. It removes opiate drugs from receptor sites and then binds rapidly to these opiate receptors. It resensitises the respiratory centre to CO_2 which then acts as a respiratory stimulant, resulting in tachypnoea and rapid arousal. Naloxone is considered to be a pure antagonist with no agonist effects.

PHARMACOKINETICS

Onset of effect is within 2–3 minutes of intravenous administration. The duration of effect is short. It acts for about 45–70 minutes and occasionally for up to 4 hours. If administered orally it is rapidly inactivated on the first pass through the liver. When given parenterally it is rapidly distributed to all tissues. The elimination half-life is 30–100 minutes. The half-life in neonates is approximately 2.5–3.5 hours because of their inability to metabolise the drug adequately.

USES

Naloxone is used to reverse central nervous system depression, including respiratory depression, induced by natural or synthetic opioids. For adults an initial dose of 0.4–2 mg should be given intravenously and repeated at intervals of 2–3 minutes. If no response has been observed after 10 mg has been administered, the diagnosis of opioid toxicity should be questioned. The initial dose in children is 0.01 mg/kg body weight intravenously, followed by a second dose of 0.1 mg/kg if there is no clinical improvement. Naloxone can be given by continuous intravenous infusion to avoid repeated doses due to the prolonged effects of opioid analgesics. The addition of 2 mg to 500 mL of normal saline or 5% glucose solution provides a concentrate of 0.004 mg/mL. The rate of administration should be titrated to the patient's response.

ADVERSE DRUG REACTIONS

There have been reports of nausea, vomiting, hypertension, cardiac arrhythmias, pulmonary oedema and seizures. These effects are generally seen in patients given naloxone postoperatively and adverse effects tend not to be a problem with therapeutic doses.

PRECAUTIONS AND CONTRAINDICATIONS

Care should be taken with patients, including newborns of mothers who are or may be physically dependent on opioids, since administration of naloxone may precipitate withdrawal symptoms. Those patients who have received potentially cardiotoxic drugs or who have pre-existing cardiac disease may experience fluctuations in blood pressure, cardiac arrhythmias or pulmonary oedema.

Penicillamine

MECHANISM OF ACTION

Penicillamine is a penicillin degradation product. It is a potent chelator of copper, gold, lead, mercury and zinc and promotes the excretion of metals in the urine.

USES

In the management of lead poisoning the usual oral dose is 1–1.5 g/day for 1–2 months given 2 hours before or 3 hours after meals.

For information on pharmacokinetics, adverse drug reactions, drug interactions, precautions and contraindications see Chapter 22 Musculoskeletal Disorders.

Physostigmine

MECHANISM OF ACTION

Physostigmine is a carbamate cholinesterase inhibitor which allows accumulation of acetylcholine at the neuroreceptor sites. It crosses the blood-brain barrier.

PHARMACOKINETICS

The maximum onset of action occurs within 5 minutes of intravenous injection. Its effect may last less than 1 hour or as long 4 hours. It is rapidly metabolised and has a half-life of 1–2 hours.

USES

It is used to treat poisoning by anticholinergic drugs such as atropine and hyoscine. It should be used cautiously but is indicated if the patient is suffering myoclonic convulsions, severe hallucinations, hypertension or supraventricular arrhythmias. The dose is 2 mg by slow intravenous injection (no faster than 1 mg/minute). A second dose of 1–2 mg may be given in 20 minutes if no reversal has occurred. In children the dose is 0.02 mg/kg every 5 minutes until a response is seen (maximum 0.1 mg/kg) followed by 0.5–2 micrograms/kg/minute.

ADVERSE DRUG REACTIONS

Bradycardia, hypotension, ventricular arrhythmias, seizures, abdominal cramping, vomiting, diarrhoea, hypersalivation, miosis. A cholinergic crisis with respiratory paralysis, bronchospasm and laryngospasm may occur.

DRUG INTERACTIONS

Physostigmine is about 45%–55% protein bound. Quinidine, frusemide, paracetamol, theophylline and verapamil can decrease physostigmine binding and increase the unbound fraction. When used with succinylcholine it may lead to respiratory and cardiovascular collapse.

PRECAUTIONS AND CONTRAINDICATIONS

Atropine should always be available to reverse the toxic effects of physostigmine if necessary. It should not be used in the presence of asthma, gangrene, glaucoma, diabetes, cardiovascular disease, pregnancy, hyperthyroidism, mechanical obstruction of the intestinal or urogenital tract or any vagotonic state. Patients receiving succinylcholine or depolarising neuromuscular blocking agents should not receive physostigmine.

Pralidoxime

MECHANISM OF ACTION

Pralidoxime (PAM) is a cholinesterase re-activator that effectively reverses the phosphorylation of the enzyme caused by organophosphates.

PHARMACOKINETICS

Cholinesterase regenerating activity occurs within one hour but the duration is short and the drug may require re-administration. It has a large volume of distribution and is excreted unchanged in the urine.

USES

Pralidoxime is used together with atropine in the treatment of organophosphate poisoning. A dose of 1–2 g diluted in 100 mL sodium chloride 0.9% is infused intravenously over 30 minutes. This dose may be repeated in one hour if muscle weakness is still present. A maximum dose of 12 g in 24 hours has been suggested. A child would receive an intravenous dose of 20–40 mg/kg.

ADVERSE DRUG REACTIONS

Adverse effects of pralidoxime include tachycardia, dizziness, drowsiness, nausea, headache, hyperventilation, diplopia, laryngospasm and muscle rigidity. Rapid intravenous administration (more than 500 mg/minute) can cause tachycardia, laryngospasm and muscle rigidity.

DRUG INTERACTIONS

Thiamine will reduce the clearance of pralidoxime.

PRECAUTIONS AND CONTRAINDICATIONS

A reduction in dosage may be necessary in patients with impaired renal function. Caution is required when administering pralidoxime to patients with myasthenia gravis. It should not be used to treat carbamate poisoning.

NURSING IMPLICATIONS

The nursing implications for the use of antidotes are shown in Table 9.6.

TABLE 9.6   Nursing implications for the use of antidotes

Antidote	Poison	Nursing Implications
Acetylcysteine	Paracetamol	**Assess:** Time since ingestion; pulmonary and liver function; renal function; blood sugar level. **Administer:** IV, must be given within 12 h of ingestion. IV: 150 mg/kg in 200 mL glucose 5% over 15 min, then 50 mg/kg in 500 mL glucose 5% over 4 h; then 100 mg/kg in 1 L glucose 5% over 16 h; total: 300 mg/kg in 20 h.* **Evaluate:** Therapeutic effect, liver function, paracetamol blood level.

* A specialised paediatric text or Poisons Information Centre should be consulted for paediatric doses.

TABLE 9.6 cont.

Antidote	Poison	Nursing Implications
Atropine	Organophosphate and carbamate insecticides (cholinesterase inhibitors)	**Assess:** Blood pressure, pulse rate, headache, confusion, pulmonary secretions, GIT disturbances, profuse sweating, muscle twitching, convulsions. **Administer:** 4–8 mg IVI (10–15 min to atropinisation) resulting in a rapid pulse (100 beats/minute), dry skin, dilated pupils. Children: 0.05 mg/kg repeated every 2–5 min to atropinisation.* **Evaluate:** Therapeutic effect, which may only be partial.
Calcium disodium edetate (EDTA)	Lead	**Assess:** Renal function and temperature. **Administer:** 1 g IV in 250–500 mL sodium chloride 0.9% or glucose 5% over 2 h, every 12 h for 5 days. Children: 50 mg/kg/24 h by IV infusion for 5 days.* **Evaluate:** For renal toxicity and hyperthermia.
Calcium gluconate	Fluoride	**Assess:** Muscle weakness, seizures. **Administer:** Orally. IV, 10 mL of 10% injection undiluted or diluted with 10 mL sodium chloride 0.9% over 3 min. Repeat every 1–6 hours if needed.* **Evaluate:** Urine output, blood pressure, ECG.
Desferrioxamine	Iron	**Assess:** Blood pressure and pulse rate; pulmonary, GIT, renal and cerebral function; previous allergies. **Administer:** IV injection at a rate not exceeding 15 mg/kg/h, with a total dose of 80 mg/kg in 24 h.* **Evaluate:** Therapeutic effect, allergic reaction, hypotension.
Dicobalt edetate	Cyanide	**Assess:** Blood pressure, metabolic acidosis, cardio-pulmonary function, previous allergies. **Administer:** 300 mg IV over 1 min; additional 300 mg with oxygen and ventilation support.* **Evaluate:** Therapeutic effect, vomiting and anaphylactic reaction.
BAL	Mercury, arsenic, gold	**Assess:** Blood pressure, pulse rate, fits, consciousness. **Administer:** 3–5 mg/kg IM (painful injection) every 4 h for 2 days then reduce over one week. **Evaluate:** Therapeutic effect, adverse effects such as anorexia, restless behaviour, hypertension and tachycardia, fever and epilepsy, and coma.
Flumazenil	Benzodiazepines	**Assess:** Benzodiazepine dependence, other drugs taken by patient. **Administer:** 1 mg/min IV undiluted up to 10 mg. May need maintenance dose 0.5 mg/h diluted in sodium chloride 0.9% for long acting benzodiazepines. **Evaluate:** Return of normal responses of central nervous system.

POISONINGS AND THEIR TREATMENT

TABLE 9.6 cont.

Antidote	Poison	Nursing Implications
Naloxone	Narcotics, dextroproxyphene, pentazocine	**Assess:** Narcotic addiction. **Administer:** IV, IM or SC or by IV infusion. **Evaluate:** Return of normal respiration; onset of withdrawal symptoms in addicted patients.
Penicillamine	Copper, lead, mercury	**Assess:** Blood pressure, pulse rate, blood screening, renal function, previous allergies. **Administer:** Orally. **Evaluate:** Therapeutic effect, hypersensitivity reactions including skin rashes.
Physostigmine	Atropine, hyoscine, propantheline	**Assess:** Coma, epilepsy, hallucinations, blood pressure, cardiac status. **Administer:** IV, 1 mg/min, only for specific indications until anticholinesterase effect reached or symptoms controlled. **Evaluate:** Motor activity, GIT, irritability, pupil changes, hypertension, bradycardia, vomiting, bronchospasm, hypotension.
Pralidoxime	Organophosphate pesticides	**Assess:** Current drug regimen, concurrent use of atropine, blood pressure, conciousness. **Administer:** Within 36 h of ingestion; IV injection over 5–10 min or infusion in glucose 5% at rate not greater than 500 mg/min; adults: 1 g repeated if necessary every 8 h to maximum of 12 g/24 h. Children: 20–50 mg/kg over 30 min, then up to 10 mg/kg/h. **Evaluate:** Therapeutic effect, adverse effects, e.g. weakness, diplopia, headache, nausea, laryngospasm, tachycardia.

THE POISONS INFORMATION CENTRES

Each Australian state has a Poisons Information Centre. These centres have been set up to provide up to date information on poisoning to both the general public and the medical and paramedical professions. Although most are situated in children's hospitals, information pertaining to adult poisonings is readily available from them.

Information can be provided on the extent of a particular problem, ingredients of ingested substances (under certain circumstances) and first aid or more detailed management of poisoning.

The state centres, addresses and telephone numbers are listed below. In any situation where any doubt exists as to the management of a poisoning, the appropriate centre should be contacted for advice.

POISONS INFORMATION CENTRES

Australian Capital Territory
Woden Valley Hospital
Garran ACT
Canberra (06) 285 2852

New South Wales
Children's Hospital
Bridge Road
Camperdown
Sydney (02) 692 6111
NSW callers outside Sydney 008 251 525

Northern Territory
Casuarina Hospital
Darwin
Darwin (089) 22 8842

Queensland
Royal Children's Hospital Brisbane
Herston Road
Herston
Brisbane (07) 253 8233
Qld callers outside Brisbane 008 177 333

South Australia
Adelaide Children's Hospital (Inc)
King William Road
North Adelaide
Adelaide (08) 04 6117
SA callers outside Adelaide 008 182 111

Tasmania
Royal Hobart Hospital
Liverpool Street
Hobart
Hobart (002) 38 8485
Tas callers outside Hobart area 008 001 400

Victoria
Royal Children's Hospital
Flemington Road
Parkville
Melbourne and Vic callers outside
Melbourne area 0055 15678

Western Australia
Princess Margaret Hospital,
Thomas Street
Subiaco
Perth (09) 381 1177
WA callers outside Perth area 008 119 244

9

POISONINGS AND THEIR TREATMENT

FURTHER READING

Albertson, T.E., Derlet, R.W, Foulke, G.E., Minguillon, M.C., Tharratt, S.R. (1989), Superiority of activated charcoal alone compared with ipecac and activated charcoal in the treatment of acute toxic ingestions. *Annals of Emergency Medicine* 18:56–59.

Ellenhorn, M.J, Barceloux, D.G. (1988), *Medical toxicology. Diagnosis and treatment of human poisoning.* Elsevier, New York.

Haddad, L.M, Wincester, J.F. (1988), *Clinical management of poisoning and drug overdose.* Saunders, Philadelphia.

Klaassen, C.D, Amdur, M.O, Doull, J. (1986) *Casarett and Doull's toxicology. The basic science of poisons.* Macmillan, New York.

Knight, K.M., Doucet, H.J. (1987) 'Gastric rupture and death caused by ipecac syrup'. *Southern Medical Journal*, 80:786.

McLuckie, A., Forbes, A.M., Ilett, K.F. (1990) 'Role of repeated doses of oral activated charcoal in the treatment of acute intoxications'. *Anaesthesia and Intensive Care* 18: 375.

Tenenbein, M., Cohen, S., Sitar, D.S. (1987) 'Efficacy of ipecac-induced emesis, orogastric lavage and activated charcoal for acute drug overdose'. *Annals of Emergency Medicine*, 16: 838.

TEST YOUR KNOWLEDGE

1. List nine common groups of substances causing poisoning.

2. (a) List three initial steps in management of a poisoned patient. (b) Note exceptions to generalisations in 2(a).

3. List two substances likely to cause serious delayed poisoning effects.

4. For which of the following would you contact a Poisons Information Centre:

(a) advice on ingredients of a substance swallowed by an infant; (b) advice on how to manage a particular poisoning; (c) advice about a plant poisoning; (d) advice on where to send a redback spider.

5. List four poisons which have antidotes. Name the antidotes.

6. The LD_{50} of a drug 'X' is said to be 700 mg/kg (oral, rats). The potential fatal dose in humans will be: (a) 700 mg/kg; (b) 1 g/kg; (c) 100 mg/kg; (d) cannot tell from data.

7. If a patient presents having ingested 700 mg/kg of drug 'X' referred to in the previous question they should be: (a) observed closely and are likely to have significant toxic effects; (b) sent home at once, 700 mg/kg in rats doesn't mean it will harm humans.

8. You are asked to prepare activated charcoal slurry for administration to a poisoned patient. The ratio of activated charcoal:water you should use is: (a) 1:1 (equal parts); (b) 1:5; (c) 1:8 to 1:10 (within this range); (d) 1:15 to 1:20 (within this range).

Therapeutics

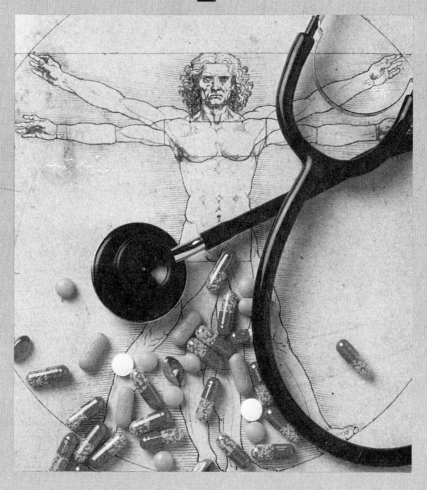

Drugs and the Autonomic Nervous System

ANN E. JAMES

O B J E C T I V E S

At the conclusion of this chapter the reader should be able to:

1. Describe the structure of the nervous system and the role of transmitter substances and receptors;

2. Identify the actions of sympathetic and parasympathetic nerve stimulation on major organs of the body; and

3. Identify and list drugs that influence nervous system function.

THE AUTONOMIC NERVOUS SYSTEM

The following section is intended as a brief review of the physiology of the autonomic nervous system. The autonomic nervous system has been variously described as the vegetative, visceral or involuntary nervous system. Its major function is to regulate the internal environment of the body without conscious control. Specifically, it regulates the heart; the smooth muscle of the respiratory, vascular, gastrointestinal and gentiourinary systems; secretions; and some temperature regulating mechanisms. Despite the name 'involuntary nervous system', there is obvious interaction with the central nervous system. One such example is the effect of fear on heart rate.

STRUCTURE

The autonomic nervous system consists, peripherally, of two sets of fibres: input or afferent fibres, and output or efferent fibres. Integration of the afferent and efferent fibres occurs in the central nervous system. The nerve axons leaving the central nervous system connect with peripheral neurones which in turn innervate the effector cells on the end organ. The cell bodies of these peripheral neurones (where they connect, or synapse, with axons from the central nervous system) occur in clusters known as ganglia.

Afferent Fibres

Information is brought into the autonomic nervous system via sensory afferent fibres, which obtain information from innervated organs, muscles and glands, for processing in the central nervous system.

Efferent Fibres and Central Autonomic Connections

Conversion of input information (received via afferent fibres) into output action occurs via efferent fibres at a number of levels. This ranges from the simple reflex arc in the spinal cord to complex interactions at various levels within the central nervous system and the subsequent outflow via efferent or motor fibres.

THE PERIPHERAL AUTONOMIC NERVOUS SYSTEM

The major divisions of the autonomic nervous system are the sympathetic and parasympathetic nervous systems. When the sympathetic division is stimulated, responses described as the 'fear, fright and flight' are initiated. These responses include dilated pupils, hair standing on end, increased blood flow through the muscles and increase in heart rate. Parasympathetic stimulation generally produces opposing effects to those of the sympathetic division, e.g. constriction of the pupils, increased peristalsis and a slowing of the heart rate.

The Sympathetic Nervous System

The preganglionic sympathetic nerve fibres leave the spinal cord from the thoracic and lumbar sections, synapse in ganglia adjacent to the spinal cord with postganglionic fibres, which then continue on to the innervated muscle or organ.

The Parasympathetic Nervous System

The preganglionic parasympathetic nerve fibres leave the spinal cord from the midbrain, medulla and sacral portions of the central nervous system and synapse in ganglia situated either in, or close to, the innervated organ or muscle. Consequently, the postganglionic parasympathetic nerve fibre is much shorter than the sympathetic postganglionic fibre.

Differences Between Sympathetic and Parasympathetic Nerves

One of the major differences between the sympathetic and parasympathetic systems is the way in which sympathetic fibres spread after reaching their ganglia. There may be up to 20 branches from a single sympathetic nerve fibre after it reaches the ganglia, whereas it is common for there to be only one parasympathetic fibre both before and after the ganglia. This is possible because of the short length of parasympathetic postganglionic fibres, which allow the terminal ganglia to be located either in, or very near, the organs being innervated. Thus a discharge within the sympathetic nervous system will produce a more generalised effect than the more discrete and localised effect of parasympathetic discharge.

TRANSMITTERS

In order to transfer information from the central nervous system to the effector organ, the synapse at the autonomic ganglion and the gap at the junction with the effector organ (neuroeffector junction) must be crossed with the aid of a chemical substance known as a transmitter.

The two main transmitters involved are acetylcholine and noradrenaline. **Acetylcholine** activates all autonomic ganglia, all parasympathetic neuroeffector junctions and some sympathetic neuroeffector junctions. On the other hand, **noradrenaline** activates most sympathetic neuroeffector junctions (see Figure 10.1).

The transmitter, after release from the nerve cell ending, is thought to work on a specific portion of the postjunctional cell called a receptor. After interaction with the receptor, the transmitter is either destroyed by an enzyme (cholinesterase in the case of acetylcholine or monoamine oxidase in the case of noradrenaline) or taken back up into

10

DRUGS AND THE AUTONOMIC NERVOUS SYSTEM

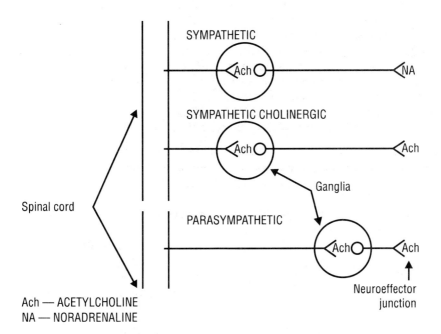

FIGURE 10.1 Location of transmitters

the nerve ending. If this did not occur the receptors would be continually stimulated.

RECEPTORS

Receptors are generally named after the transmitter which activates the receptor. Hence, cholinergic receptors are activated by acetylcholine and noradrenergic receptors by noradrenaline. In the autonomic ganglia, activation of the nerve receptor by the transmitter leads to depolarisation and the continuation of the nerve impulse along the postganglionic nerve fibre. Activation of the receptor at the effector organ may result in contraction or relaxation (usually of smooth muscle) depending on the organ.

An agent used to act on the receptor in a similar way to the transmitter is termed an **agonist**; an agent used to prevent the action of the transmitter at the receptor is termed an **antagonist.**

Cholinergic Receptors

Receptors which respond to acetylcholine or to drugs which mimic the effect of acetylcholine (cholinergics or cholinomimetics) are of two types, nicotinic and muscarinic. **Nicotinic receptors** are mainly involved at ganglia and at skeletal muscle junctions. **Muscarinic receptors** are the main receptors at effector cells. Several subtypes of muscarinic receptors have been identified and these have been termed M_1, M_2 and M_3 receptors. Limited information is available regarding the location of these receptors although, generally, M_1 receptors are found in ganglia and various secretory glands; M_2 receptors are mainly found in the myocardium and may be present in smooth muscle; and M_3 receptors are found in smooth muscle and secretory glands. Drugs which stimulate muscarinic receptors and which mimic the effect of postganglionic parasympathetic nerve stimulation are called parasympathomimetics. Drugs which antagonise the effect of postganglionic parasympathetic nerve stimulation are called parasympatholytics.

Noradrenergic Receptors

Noradrenaline and drugs which mimic the effect of postganglionic sympathetic nerve stimulation are called sympathomimetics. The sites on which these drugs act are called α receptors and β receptors. The classification into α and β receptors is basically determined by the specific physiological activities of sympathomimetic agents. β Receptors are further divided into β_1, β_2 and β_3 receptors. β_1 Receptors are found in the heart and β_2 receptors mainly in the lungs. The difference in the location of β receptors provides an opportunity to selectively stimulate specific types of receptors without stimulating all β receptors throughout the body. This has significant implications for clinical practice. The presence of β_3 receptors has only recently been identified and their function is not yet fully understood.

α Receptors are divided into α_1 and α_2 receptors. α_1 Receptors are located after the nerve junction where they are responsible for the initiation of excitatory responses. It was originally thought that α_2 receptors were located only on the presynaptic nerve terminals. It has now been found that α_2 receptors are also present at postjunctional or non-junctional sites in several tissues. Activation of presynaptic α_2 receptors inhibits the release of transmitters.

ACTIONS OF SYMPATHETIC AND PARASYMPATHETIC NERVE STIMULATION

To gain an understanding of the various actions of drugs, such as sympathomimetics, parasympathomimetics and other drugs which influence the function of the autonomic nervous system, it is necessary to have a basic understanding of the physiological effects produced directly by the autonomic nervous system. In many instances organs are innervated by both parasympathetic and sympathetic nerves, each producing an opposing effect, their activity being orchestrated to effect appropriate organ response. A knowledge of their interrelationship is essential for the understanding of the role of drug intervention in autonomic nervous system function. A summary of effects is shown in Table 10.1

TABLE 10.1 Responses produced by sympathetic and parasympathetic nerve stimulation

Organ innervated	Adrenergic receptor	Adrenergic responses	Cholinergic responses
Heart	β_1	Sinus tachycardia; force of contraction of atria and ventricles is increased	Sinus bradycardia; decreased AV conduction; decreased atrial contractility
Arterioles			
Skin	α_1, α_2	Constriction	Dilation
Skeletal muscle	α	Constriction	Dilation
	β_2	Dilation	
Cerebral	α_1	Constriction (slight)	Dilation
Coronary	α_1, α_2	Constriction	Constriction
	β_2	Dilation	
Renal	α_1, α_2	Constriction	
	β_1, β_2	Dilation	
Pulmonary	α_1	Constriction	Dilation
	β_2	Dilation	
Lungs			
Tracheal and bronchial muscle	β_2	Relaxation	Contraction
Intestine			
Motility and tone	$\alpha_1, \alpha_2, \beta_1, \beta_2$	Decrease	Increase
Sphincters	α_1	Contraction	Relaxation
Secretion	α_2	Inhibition	Stimulation
Stomach			
Motility and tone	$\alpha_1, \alpha_2, \beta_2$	Decrease	Increase
Sphincters	α_1	Contraction	Relaxation
Secretion		Inhibition(?)	Stimulation
Salivary glands	α_1	Sparse, thick secretion	Profuse, watery secretion
	β	Amylase secretion	
Bladder			
Detrusor	β_2	Relaxation	Contraction
Trigone and sphincter	α_1	Contraction	Relaxation
Uterus	α_1, β_2	Variable	Variable
Eye			
Radial muscle, iris	α_1	Contraction (mydriasis)	
Sphincter muscle, iris			Contraction (miosis)
Ciliary muscle	β_2	Relaxation for far vision	Contraction for near vision

Adapted from: Goodman, L. S., Gilman, A. G., Rall, T. W., Nies, A. S., Taylor, P., eds. (1990), *Goodman and Gilman's the pharmacological basis of therapeutics*, 8th edn., Pergamon Press, New York, pp. 89–90.

10

DRUGS AND THE AUTONOMIC NERVOUS SYSTEM

DRUGS ACTING ON THE AUTONOMIC NERVOUS SYSTEM ▮▮▮▮▮▮▮▮

Both the sympathetic and parasympathetic nervous system contain several mechanisms by which drugs can affect normal autonomic nervous system functions. Several of these are common to both systems and include:

- Drugs which mimic the effect of either sympathetic or parasympathetic stimulation, e.g. the sympathomimetics and parasympathomimetics;

- Drugs which interfere with the enzymatic destruction of transmitters, e.g. the monoamine oxidase inhibitors (MAOIs) and anticholinesterases; and

- Drugs which block the receptor to the transmitter, e.g. β blocking drugs, adrenergic neurone blocking drugs, α blocking drugs and anticholinergics.

DRUGS ACTING ON THE PARASYMPATHETIC SYSTEM

Parasympathomimetics: Bethanechol, Carbachol, Pilocarpine

Parasympathomimetics are drugs which mimic the effects of parasympathetic nerve stimulation.

TRADE NAMES

Bethanechol: *Urecholine*; *Urocarb*.
Carbachol: *Isopto Carbachol*.
Pilocarpine: *Pilopt*; *Isopto Carpine*; *P.V. Carpine*.

USES

Clinical indications for the use of these drugs, their usual strength and forms are shown in Table 10.2.

ADVERSE DRUG REACTIONS

The adverse reactions of parasympathomimetics include abdominal discomfort, salivation, flushing of the skin and sweating. Large doses produce more pronounced parasympathetic effects.

PRECAUTIONS AND CONTRAINDICATIONS

Bethanechol is contraindicated in hyperthyroidism, pregnancy, peptic ulcer, bronchial asthma, pronounced bradycardia or hypotension, vasomotor instability, coronary artery disease, epilepsy and Parkinson's disease, following gastrointestinal or bladder surgery, in gastrointestinal or bladder obstruction and spastic gastrointestinal disturbances, and in acute inflammatory lesions of the gastrointestinal tract or peritonitis.

The injectable form of bethanechol is intended for subcutaneous administration only. It should never be given intramuscularly or intravenously as violent symptoms due to severe cholinergic overstimulation will occur.

Anticholinesterase Drugs: Distigmine, Ecothiopate, Edrophonium, Neostigmine, Physostigmine, Pyridostigmine

Anticholinesterase drugs interfere with the enzyme cholinesterase which is responsible for the destruction of acetylcholine.

TRADE NAMES

Distigmine: *Ubretid*.
Ecothiopate iodide: *Phospholine Iodide*.
Edrophonium chloride: *Tensilon*.
Neostigmine: *Prostigmin*.
Pyridostigmine bromide: *Mestinon*.

USES

Clinical indications for the use of these drugs, their usual strength and forms are shown in Table 10.3.

TABLE 10.2   Parasympathomimetics

Drug	Strength and Dose Form	Indication
Bethanechol	10 mg, 25 mg tablets; 5 mg subcutaneous injection	Postoperative urinary retention; postoperative intestinal atony; neurogenic atony of bladder
Carbachol	1.5%, 3% eye drops	Glaucoma
Pilocarpine	0.5% to 6% eye drops	Glaucoma

TABLE 10.3   Anticholinesterases

Drug	Strength and Dose Form	Indication
Distigmine	5 mg tablets; 0.5 mg injection	Atony of urinary tract; postoperative urinary retention; myasthenia gravis
Ecothiopate iodide	0.03%, 0.06%, 0.125%, 0.25% eye drops	Glaucoma
Edrophonium chloride	10 mg injection	Diagnostic agent for myasthenia gravis
Neostigmine	15 mg tablets; 0.5 mg and 2.5 mg injection	Myasthenia gravis; antidote to non-depolarising neuromuscular blocking drugs; postoperative intestinal atony; urinary retention
Physostigmine salicylate	0.5 mg injection	Tricyclic antidepressant overdose
Pyridostigmine bromide	10 mg, 60 mg tablets; 180 mg slow release tablets	Myasthenia gravis; antidote to non-depolarising neuromuscular drugs

10

DRUGS AND THE AUTONOMIC NERVOUS SYSTEM

ADVERSE DRUG REACTIONS

Adverse reactions to anticholinesterase drugs are due to excessive stimulation of cholinergic receptors (both muscarinic and nicotinic) and include vomiting, abdominal pain, diarrhoea, salivation, sweating, lacrimation, miosis, bradycardia, hypotension, dyspnoea, urinary urgency and muscular twitching. These adverse effects can be controlled with atropine.

PRECAUTIONS AND CONTRAINDICATIONS

These drugs should be used with caution in conditions where the potentiation of cholinergic effects is undesirable, e.g. vagotonia, bronchial asthma, heart disease, peptic ulcer, epilepsy and Parkinson's disease.

TABLE 10.4 Parasympatholytics (anticholinergics)

Drug	Strength and Dose Form	Indication
Atropine sulfate	0.1 mg, 0.4 mg, 0.5 mg, 0.6 mg, 1.0 mg, 1.2 mg injection	Preoperative medication; antidote for parasympathomimetics; vagal inhibition; sinus bradycardia; AV block
	0.5%, 1% eye drops; 1% eye ointment	Ophthalmic examination
Benzhexol	2 mg, 5 mg tablets	Parkinson's disease; drug induced extrapyramidal disorders
Benztropine mesylate	0.5 mg, 2 mg tablets; 2 mg injection	Parkinson's disease; drug induced extrapyramidal disorders
Biperiden hydrochloride	2 mg tablet	Parkinson's disease; drug induced extrapyramidal disorders; nocturnal cramps
Cyclopentolate hydrochloride	1% eye drops	Mydriasis; cycloplegia; ophthalmic examination
Dicyclomine hydrochloride	10 mg tablet; 5 mg/5 mL syrup	Gastrointestinal tract spasm
Glycopyrrolate	0.2 mg injection	Preoperative and intraoperative medication
Hyoscine	1.5 mg transdermal patch	Motion sickness
Hyoscine butylbromide	10 mg tablet; 10 mg suppository; 20 mg injection	Renal, biliary and gastrointestinal tract spasm
Hyoscine hydrobromide	400 µg injection	Preoperative medication (usually combined with papaveretum)
	0.3 mg tablet	Motion sickness
Ipratropium bromide	20 µg/puff inhaler; 250 µg/mL nebuliser solution	Asthma
Orphenadrine citrate	100 mg tablet	Muscle spasm
Orphenadrine hydrochloride	50 mg tablet	Parkinson's disease; drug induced extrapyramidal disorders
Propantheline bromide	15 mg tablets	Gastrointestinal tract spasm
Procyclidine hydrochloride	5 mg tablet	Parkinson's disease; drug induced extrapyramidal disorders
Tropicamide	0.5%, 1% eye drops	Mydriasis; cycloplegia; ophthalmic examination

Parasympatholytics: Atropine, Benzhexol, Benztropine, Biperiden, Cyclopentolate, Dicyclomine, Glycopyrrolate, Hyoscine, Ipratropium, Orphenadrine, Propantheline, Procyclidine, Tropicamide

The parasympatholytics (anticholinergics) are drugs which block muscarinic receptors.

TRADE NAMES

Benzhexol: *Artane.*
Benztropine mesylate: *Cogentin.*
Biperiden hydrochloride: *Akineton.*
Cyclopentolate hydrochloride: *Cyclogyl.*
Dicyclomine hydrochloride: *Merbentyl.*
Glycopyrrolate: *Robinul.*
Hyoscine (scopolamine): *Scop.*
Hyoscine butylbromide: *Buscopan.*
Hyoscine hydrobromide: *Kwells.*
Ipratropium bromide: *Atrovent.*
Orphenadrine citrate: *Norflex.*
Orphenadrine hydrochloride: *Disipal.*
Propantheline bromide: *Pro-Banthine.*
Procyclidine hydrochloride: *Kemadrin.*
Tropicamide: *Mydriacyl.*

USES

Clinical indications for the use of these drugs, their usual strength and form are listed in Table 10.4.

ADVERSE DRUG REACTIONS

Adverse reactions to parasympatholytics include drying of salivary secretions, decreased sweating as well as mydriasis, blurred vision, tachycardia, constipation, urinary hesitancy and retention.

PRECAUTIONS AND CONTRAINDICATIONS

Use with caution in patients with severe heart disease and in elderly patients because of the possibility of urinary retention. These drugs must be avoided in patients with glaucoma, obstructive disease of the gastrointestinal tract or intestinal atony.

DRUGS ACTING ON THE SYMPATHETIC SYSTEM

Sympathomimetics: Adrenaline, Dobutamine, Dopamine, Ephedrine, Fenoterol, Isoprenaline, Methoxamine, Noradrenaline, Orciprenaline, Phenylephrine, Ritodrine, Salbutamol, Terbutaline, Tetrahydrazoline, Tramazoline

Sympathomimetics are drugs which mimic the effect of sympathetic nerve stimulation. They vary in their ability to stimulate α, β_1 and β_2 receptors.

TRADE NAMES

Adrenaline hydrochloride: *Epifrin.*
Adrenaline acid tartrate: *Medihaler Epi.*
Dobutamine: *Dobutrex.*
Dopamine: *Intropin.*
Ephedrine hydrochloride: *Fedrine.*
Fenoterol hydrobromide: *Berotec.*
Isoprenaline hydrochloride: *Isuprel.*
Isoprenaline sulfate: *Medihaler Iso.*
Methoxamine hydrochloride: *Vasylox Junior.*
Noradrenaline acid tartrate: *Levophed.*
Orciprenaline sulfate: *Alupent.*
Phenylephrine hydrochloride: *Avil Nasal Spray; Nasalate; Nyal Decongestant Nasal Spray; Neo-Synephrine Ophthalmic; IsoptoFrin; Prefrin; Visopt.*
Ritodrine hydrochloride: *Yutopar.*
Salbutamol: *Respolin; Ventolin.*
Terbutaline: *Bricanyl.*
Tetrahydrazoline hydrochloride: *Visine.*
Tramazoline hydrochloride: *Spray-Tish.*

USES

These drugs show a wide range of receptor specificities, thus providing clinicians with a variety of therapeutic solutions. For example, the drugs adrenaline, isoprenaline and salbutamol may all be used in the treatment of asthma. Adrenaline stimulates α, β_1 and β_2 sympathetic receptors and is therefore regarded as having the least specific action. Isoprenaline is regarded as being more

10

DRUGS AND THE AUTONOMIC NERVOUS SYSTEM

TABLE 10.5 Sympathomimetics

Drug	Receptor Stimulated	Strength and Dose Form	Indications
Methoxamine hydrochloride	α	0.25% nasal drops	Decongestant
Phenylephrine hydrochloride	α	0.25% nasal cream, 0.5% nasal spray	Nasal decongestant
		10% eye drops	Vasoconstriction and pupil dilation in uveitis; wide angle glaucoma
		0.12% eye drops	Minor eye irritation; eye inflammation
Tetrahydrazoline hydrochloride	α	0.05% eye drops	Mild eye irritation
Tramazoline hydrochloride	α	120 µg/puff nasal spray	Nasal decongestant
Adrenaline hydrochloride	α, β	1 in 1000 (1 mg/1 mL) injection, 1 in 10 000 (1 mg/10 mL) injection	Anaphylactic shock; bronchospasm; hypersensitivity reactions; cardiac arrest
		0.004% eye drops	Open angle glaucoma
Adrenaline acid tartrate	α, β	1 in 1000 (1 mg/1 mL) injection	Anaphylactic shock; bronchospasm; hypersensitivity reactions; cardiac arrest
		0.35 mg/puff inhaler	Bronchospasm; asthma; hypersensitivity reactions
Ephedrine hydrochloride	α, β	30 mg, 60 mg tablets	Decongestant; bronchospasm; narcolepsy; catalepsy; hypotension
		1% nose drops	Nasal decongestant
Noradrenaline acid tartrate	α, β	1 in 1000 injection	Hypotension
Dobutamine hydrochloride	β_1	250 mg injection	Heart failure
Dopamine	β_1	40 mg/mL injection; 80 mg/mL and 160 mg/mL syringes	Hypotension; low cardiac output; low urine output (in shock)
Isoprenaline hydrochloride	β_1, β_2	1 in 5000 (0.02 mg/mL) injection	Cardiac arrest; bradyarrhythmias
Isoprenaline sulfate	β_1, β_2	0.1 mg/puff inhaler	Bronchospasm; asthma
Fenoterol hydrobromide	β_2	0.2 mg/puff inhaler; 0.1% respirator solution	Asthma; bronchitis
Orciprenaline sulfate	β_2	0.75 mg/puff inhaler	Asthma; bronchitis

TABLE 10.5 continued

Drug	Receptor Stimulated	Strength and Dose Form	Indications
Ritodrine hydrochloride	β_2	10 mg tablets; 10 mg/mL injection	Prevention of premature labour
Salbutamol	β_2	100 µg/puff inhaler; 0.5% respirator solution; 0.5 mg, 5 mg/5 mL injection; 4 mg tablets; 2 mg/5 mL syrup; 200 µg rotacap; 2.5 mg, 5 mg nebules	Asthma; bronchitis; prevention of premature labour
Terbutaline	β_2	250 µg/puff inhaler; 1% respirator solution; 0.1 mg, 0.5 mg injection; 5 mg tablets; 1.5 mg/5 mL syrup; 0.5 mg/inhalation turbuhaler	Asthma; bronchitis

specific for the treatment of asthma as it stimulates only β_1 and β_2 sympathetic receptors. However, salbutamol has the most specific effect of all three drugs because it predominantly stimulates β_2 sympathetic receptors and is used as the sympathomimetic of choice in asthma.

Clinical indications for these drugs, the receptors they stimulate, their usual strength and dose form are listed in Table 10.5.

ADVERSE DRUG REACTIONS

Adverse reactions associated with sympathomimetic agents differ, depending on receptor specificity. In general they include increased blood pressure and heart rate, palpitations, fear, restlessness and tremor. Increased specificity generally narrows the adverse effect profile, e.g. the most common adverse effect of β_2 sympathomimetics is skeletal muscle tremor.

PRECAUTIONS AND CONTRAINDICATIONS

These drugs should be used with caution in hypertensive or hyperthyroid patients, diabetics, and patients with cardiovascular disease or glaucoma. Existing symptoms in psychoneurotic patients may also be exacerbated.

Monoamine Oxidase Inhibitors: Moclobemide, Phenelzine, Procarbazine, Selegiline, Tranylcypromine

Monoamine oxidase is one of the enzymes partially responsible for the destruction of noradrenaline. Two forms of the enzyme have been identified and have been named monoamine oxidase A and monoamine oxidase B. Most monoamine oxidase inhibitors (MAOIs) are non-specific and irreversibly inhibit both types of monoamine oxidase. Recently, however, agents which selectively inhibit either the A or B form have been identified. For example, the antidepressant moclobemide is a selective, reversible inhibitor of MAO type A while the antiparkinsonian agent selegiline is a selective inhibitor of MAO type B.

TRADE NAMES

Moclobemide: *Aurorix*.
Phenelzine sulfate: *Nardil*.
Procarbazine: *Natulan*.
Selegiline: *Eldepryl*.
Tranylcypromine sulfate: *Parnate*.

10

DRUGS AND THE AUTONOMIC NERVOUS SYSTEM

USES

The MAOIs, the receptor inhibited, strength and dose form and clinical indications for use are shown in Table 10.6.

ADVERSE DRUG REACTIONS

Adverse reactions associated with non-selective MAOIs include hypertensive crisis, orthostatic hypotension, dizziness, palpitations, weakness, dry mouth and drowsiness. Hypertensive crisis is less likely to occur with the selective MAOIs as they cause only minimal potentiation of the pressor response to dietary tyramine (see below).

PRECAUTIONS AND CONTRAINDICATIONS

As these agents inhibit the action of one of the enzymes partially responsible for the destruction of noradrenaline, they can produce potentially serious interactions, on occasion life threatening, when combined with agents which cause either the release of more noradrenaline or the direct stimulation of adrenergic receptors. In particular, concomitant administration of non-selective MAOIs with tricyclic antidepressants, anti-cold preparations (α receptor stimulants) or foods containing tyramine, should be avoided because of the risk of hypertensive crisis. If a hypertensive crisis occurs, phentolamine at a dose of 5–10 mg should be used intravenously and may be repeated if necessary. MAOIs may also suppress anginal pain and should be used with caution in patients with angina or coronary artery disease. They should also be used with caution in patients with Parkinson's disease and hyperthyroidism.

α Blocking Drugs: Phenoxybenzamine, Phentolamine, Prazosin, Tolazoline

These drugs interfere with sympathetic transmission by non-competitively blocking α adrenergic receptors.

TRADE NAMES

Phenoxybenzamine hydrochloride: *Dibenyline*.
Phentolamine mesylate: *Regitine*.
Prazosin hydrochloride: *Minipress*.
Tolazoline hydrochloride: *Priscoline*.

USES

Examples of α blocking drugs, their strength and dose form and indications are shown in Table 10.7.

ADVERSE DRUG REACTIONS

Adverse reactions to α blocking drugs are mainly associated with vasodilation and include flushing, 'goose flesh' and a feeling of chilliness or warmth. Hypotension, dizziness and tachycardia may be experienced.

TABLE 10.6 Monoamine oxidase inhibitors

Drug	Receptor Inhibited	Strength and Dose Form	Indication
Non-selective inhibitors			
Phenelzine sulfate	MAO A, MAO B	15 mg tablet	Depression
Tranylcypromine sulfate	MAO A, MAO B	10 mg tablet	Depression
Procarbazine	MAO A, MAO B	50 mg capsule	Neoplastic disease
Selective inhibitors			
Moclobemide	MAO A	150 mg tablet	Depression
Selegiline	MAO B	5 mg tablet	Parkinson's disease, depression

TABLE 10.7 α Blocking drugs

Drug	Strength and Dose Form	Indication
Phenoxybenzamine hydrochloride	10 mg capsule; 100 mg/2 mL injection	Phaeochromocytoma; urinary retention due to neuropathic bladder; shock unresponsive to conventional therapy; peripheral vascular disease
Phentolamine mesylate	10 mg injection	Phaeochromocytoma; peripheral vascular disease
Prazosin hydrochloride	1 mg, 2 mg, 5 mg tablets	Hypertension; Raynaud's disease; severe refractory congestive heart failure
Tolazoline hydrochloride	100 mg/4 mL injection	Persistant pulmonary hypertension of newborn

10

DRUGS AND THE AUTONOMIC NERVOUS SYSTEM

PRECAUTIONS AND CONTRAINDICATIONS

Overdosage, particularly with intravenous forms of these drugs, may lead to hypotension which should be treated with noradrenaline infusion. Adrenaline should not be used as it may cause a paradoxical fall in blood pressure.

β Blocking Drugs: Alprenolol, Atenolol, Metoprolol, Oxprenolol, Pindolol, Propranolol, Sotalol, Timolol

β adrenergic blocking agents compete with adrenaline and noradrenaline for available β receptor sites. They are prescribed for the management of hypertension, cardiac arrhythmias and angina. β blocking drugs may be divided into drugs which block both β_1 and β_2 receptors and drugs which preferentially block β_1 receptors, that is, cardioselective β blockers.

TRADE NAMES

Alprenolol: *Aptin.*
Atenolol: *Noten; Tenormin.*
Metoprolol: *Betaloc; Lopressor, Minax.*
Oxprenolol: *Corbeton; Trasicor.*
Pindolol: *Barbloc; Visken.*
Propranolol: *Deralin; Inderal.*
Sotalol: *Sotacor.*
Timolol: *Blocadren.*

USES

Clinical indications for the use of both types of β blocking drugs, their strength and dose form are shown in Table 10.8.

For further information on these drugs see Chapter 12 Cardiovascular Diseases.

Adrenergic Neurone Blocking Drugs

These drugs deplete noradrenaline stores from adrenergic nerve endings and block the release of noradrenaline from adrenergic nerve endings. None are currently marketed in Australia.

TABLE 10.8 β Blocking drugs

Drug	Strength and Dose Form	Indication
Non-selective β blocking drugs		
Alprenolol	100 mg tablet	Angina pectoris; hypertension; cardiac arrhythmias
Oxprenolol	20 mg, 40 mg tablets	Angina pectoris; hypertension; cardiac arrhythmias
Pindolol	5 mg, 15 mg tablets	Angina pectoris; hypertension; cardiac arrhythmias
Propranolol	1 mg injection; 10 mg, 40 mg, 160 mg tablets	Angina pectoris; hypertension; cardiac arrhythmias; migraine
Sotalol	160 mg tablet; 80 mg/8 mL injection	Cardiac arrhythmias
Timolol	5 mg tablet	Angina pectoris; hypertension; cardiac arrhythmias
Selective β blocking drugs		
Atenolol	50 mg tablet; 5 mg injection	Angina pectoris; hypertension
Metoprolol	50 mg, 100 mg tablets; 5 mg injection	Angina pectoris; hypertension

FURTHER READING

Goodman, L. S., Gilman, A. G., Rall, T. W., Nies, A. S., Taylor, P., eds. (1990), *Goodman and Gilman's the pharmacological basis of therapeutics*, 8th edn. NY, Pergamon Press.

Guyton, A. C. (1991), *Textbook of medical physiology*, 8th edn. Philadelphia, W.B. Saunders Company, pp. 667–78.

Landsberg, L., Young, J. B. (1991), *Physiology and pharmacology of the autonomic nervous system*, In: Wilson, J. D., Braunwald, E., Isselbacher, K. J. et al, eds. *Harrison's principles of internal medicine*, 12th edn. New York, McGraw-Hill Inc., pp. 380–92.

TEST YOUR KNOWLEDGE

1. Describe briefly: (a) the structure of the autonomic nervous system; (b) the role of cholinergic receptors and which transmitters are present; (c) the role of adrenergic receptors and which transmitters are present.

2. Define the following terms: (a) agonist; (b) antagonist; (c) parasympathomimetic; (d) anticholinergic.

3. What is the response to sympathetic stimulation of the following organs: (a) heart; (b) lungs; (c) uterus?

4. What is the response to parasympathetic stimulation of the following organs: (a) intestine; (b) blood vessels; (c) heart?

5. Give two examples of drugs that have the following actions: (a) parasympathomimetic; (b) anticholinesterase; (c) sympathomimetic; (d) β adrenergic blocker; (e) α adrenergic blocker.

Respiratory Diseases

CHRISTOPHER P. ALDERMAN

O B J E C T I V E S

At the conclusion of this chapter the reader should be able to:

1. Describe the fundamental principles of the drug therapy used in the treatment of asthma, chronic obstructive airways disease and respiratory tract infections;

2. Outline the mechanism of action, clinical pharmacokinetics, dosage and administration, adverse drugs reactions, drug interactions and contraindications to therapy for a range of drugs used in the treatment of respiratory diseases; and

3. List those drugs which may produce serious adverse effects in the respiratory tract in susceptible patients.

GENERAL PRINCIPLES ███████████████

The importance of the lungs as a major organ system is well recognised, and the efficient functioning of the lungs, together with the brain, heart, kidneys and liver, is fundamental to sustaining life. This importance is reflected in the significant consequences of disease in the pulmonary system. Conditions such as asthma, chronic obstructive airways disease (COAD), infections in the lungs or airways, interstitial lung disease or cancers of the respiratory tract are relatively common and cause significant morbidity and mortality despite new sophisticated treatments. However, effective drug therapy is available for many of these conditions and offers both improved prognosis and quality of life for the patient. As with all drug therapy pharmacological treatment in respiratory disease is governed by weighing the potential benefits against the potential hazards of drug therapy.

Many of the drugs used in respiratory therapy are potent agents, sometimes with a low therapeutic index (i.e. the therapeutic dose is close to or the same as that producing significant adverse effects).

As the health professional in contact with the patient at the point of drug administration, the nurse is in the best position to monitor for adverse effects or drug toxicities. Similarly, most of these drugs are administered using complex delivery techniques and the nurse must be familiar with these in order to ensure maximal benefit for the patient. Patient education is an important part of respiratory drug therapy and commonly the patient is treated with a complicated combination of agents capable of producing additive, complementary or, in some cases, toxic effects. In view of these and other considerations it is important that nurses understand and actively participate in the drug treatment of patients with respiratory disease.

BRONCHODILATOR THERAPY ███████████

The basic function of the pulmonary system is to facilitate the exchange of gases into and out of the general systemic circulation. Blood is delivered to the pulmonary circulation directly from the heart. Gas exchange occurs at the functional units of the lung, the alveoli, where oxygen inhaled through the bronchial tree diffuses into the blood, is bound to carrier sites on the haemoglobin in red blood cells and carried to the various tissues around the body. Conversely, it is also at the alveoli that carbon dioxide diffuses out of blood and into the airways where it is transported out of the body in exhaled air.

The bronchioles are flexible tubes composed of a variety of tissues. The walls of the bronchioles contain small muscle fibres. Whilst these smooth muscle fibres are not under voluntary control they are capable of contraction, which leads to a narrowing of the diameter of the tubing. This may impede the passage of air into and out of the airways and is often referred to as bronchoconstriction or bronchospasm which, if severe, may produce a variety of respiratory symptoms or even death.

The smooth muscle tissue found in the bronchioles is under the control of a variety of chemical compounds which act at receptors. The action of these compounds may result in contraction or relaxation of the muscle fibres producing a narrowing or widening of the diameter of the airway tubing. This effect can occur through antagonism at some receptor sites, or through agonism at others (see Chapter 1 Pharmacodynamics).

The bronchodilators are probably the most commonly used drugs in the treatment of disease in the respiratory tract. As the terminology implies, the principal action of these drugs is to produce dilation or widening of the tubing which constitutes the bronchial tree. In bronchoconstriction bronchodilator drugs are used to increase the diameter of the smaller airways which enables the air to move more freely to and from the alveoli.

While these drugs are often a mainstay in the treatment of respiratory diseases they produce their most significant benefit where the underlying condition is chiefly related to bronchospasm. In most cases however, the contraction of the smooth muscle in the bronchial tree is responsible for only a part of the increased resistance to airflow, with other mechanisms such as mucosal oedema or mucous plugging also decreasing the effective diameter of the airways. In these cases it is important that other specific therapy, such as anti-inflammatory drugs or bronchial hygiene measures, also be employed as reliance on symptom relief with bronchodilator treatment may lead to dangerous under-treatment.

Currently available bronchodilator drugs may be subdivided into three broad classes: the $\beta2$ agonists, the anticholinergic drugs and the the xanthine derivatives (theophylline and related drugs), see Table 11.1. A variety of other bronchodilator drugs are currently under development and can be expected to impact significantly on patient care within the foreseeable future.

11

RESPIRATORY DISEASES

TABLE 11.1   Bronchodilator drugs classified according to pharmacological effects

$\beta2$ Agonists

Short acting agents
 Orciprenaline
 Salbutamol
 Terbutaline
 Fenoterol

Long acting agents
 Salmeterol
 Formoterol

Anticholinergic drugs
 Ipratropium bromide

Xanthine derivatives
 Theophylline
 Aminophylline
 Choline theophyllinate

$\beta2$ AGONISTS

Orciprenaline, Salbutamol, Terbutaline, Fenoterol, Formoterol, Salmeterol

The $\beta2$ agonists ($\beta2$ adrenergic receptor agonists) are the most commonly employed bronchodilator agents in clinical use. An-

other term sometimes used for these drugs is $\beta2$ sympathomimetic agents.

TRADE NAMES

Orciprenaline: *Alupent.*
Salbutamol: *Ventolin; Respolin.*
Terbutaline: *Bricanyl.*
Fenoterol: *Berotec.*
Salmeterol: *Serevent.*

MECHANISM OF ACTION

Receptors of various types are found on the smooth muscle fibres in the walls of the bronchioles. Both the sympathetic and parasympathetic nervous systems determine the tone of bronchial smooth muscle. Stimulation of $\beta2$ adrenergic receptors through the sympathomimetic nervous system results in relaxation of bronchial smooth muscle. $\beta1$ receptors are also stimulated (to a lesser extent) by these drugs, and this phenomenon may account for some of the observed side effects of these agents.

Before the introduction of specific $\beta2$ agonists, relatively non-specific agents such as adrenaline were used to provide a means by which bronchodilation could be achieved by adrenergic agonism. Adrenaline still has an important therapeutic application in this area and is often used to treat acute bronchospasm associated with anaphylactic or allergic reactions. The relative selectivity of the β2 agonists is associated with a decreased incidence of the systemic adverse effects seen with previous therapies.

PHARMACOKINETICS

The β2 agonists are administered in a variety of different dosage forms and the pharmacokinetics of these drugs are influenced by the mode of administration.

Drugs such as salbutamol and terbutaline are relatively well absorbed when administered orally and have a rapid onset of action despite undergoing a significant first pass effect. These drugs are also effective when administered by inhalation. When given by this route they produce a much more rapid response (in some patients a therapeutic response is observed within minutes). Systemic absorption is known to occur after administration by inhalation. At least some of this effect is thought to arise through inadvertent swallowing of some of the inhaled dose followed by the standard process of drug absorption from the gastrointestinal tract. The extent of systemic absorption after administration by inhalation is therefore variable and is affected by the inhaler technique of the individual patient.

The plasma half-life of salbutamol ranges from 2–7 hours; but for this drug and for others of this type the duration of effect correlates only poorly with the known pharmacokinetics, particularly when the drug is administered by inhalation.

USES

The β2 agonists are used to produce bronchodilation in a variety of clinical circumstances. The desired therapeutic effect is to reduce the resistance to the passage of air through the bronchial tree, which in turn produces improved gas exchange and relief from symptoms such as chest tightness and breathlessness. These properties mean that the β2 agonists are commonly employed in the treatment of acute and chronic asthma and in the palliative therapy of chronic obstructive airways disease. These drugs may also be used to allow easier access to the

lower airways during diagnostic procedures such as bronchoscopy.

Given the influence of the route of administration on the pharmacokinetics of these drugs the dose administered will depend on the route of delivery chosen. Relatively lower doses are used when the drug is delivered by metered aerosol ('puffer'). For example, each actuation of a salbutamol aerosol dispenses a dose of 100 micrograms. When used as a nebuliser solution a relatively larger amount of salbutamol is used (2.5–5.0 mg), although a significant proportion of the nebulised dose does not reach the airways. These doses may be repeated every four hours or, under exceptional circumstances, more often than this. Salbutamol may also be administered by the oral route, the adult dose is 2–4 mg three to four times daily. Salbutamol injection may be administered by the subcutaneous, intramuscular or intravenous routes. The dose used varies in accordance with the route selected, with smaller doses required for intravenous administration. In all cases, appropriate dosage adjustments should be made for the paediatric patient. Similar principles for dosage and administration apply for other β2 agonist drugs when used as bronchodilators.

ADVERSE DRUG REACTIONS

The side effects of the β2 agonists are principally related to the stimulation of β receptors located in sites external to the bronchial smooth muscle. Cardiovascular effects include tachycardia and occasionally palpitations, although these effects occur more frequently when the recommended maximum dosage rate is exceeded. Tremor is a relatively common dose related reaction and is thought to be related to the action of the drug on skeletal muscle fibres. Central nervous system side effects such as agitation, nervousness, insomnia and others are also associated with drugs of this type. Hypokalaemia may be observed with the β2 agonists and is particularly common when the drugs are administered intravenously.

In some instances a patient may develop an allergic reaction resulting from the contact of nebuliser solution with the skin and mucous membranes. These rare reactions are usually easily recognisable by a rash in the shape of the nebuliser mask.

DRUG INTERACTIONS

The β_2 agonist bronchodilators do not appear to be implicated in serious pharmacokinetic interactions with other drug therapy. In general, these agents may be used safely in combination with other treatments, although it is important to bear in mind the potential for interactions of a pharmacodynamic nature. For example, the increase in heart rate caused by β_2 agonists may be compounded by the concurrent use of other drugs which cause tachycardia. This may be particularly important when a pre-existing medical condition such as ischaemic heart disease places the patient at risk. Similarly, the toxic effects of digoxin on myocardial muscle tissue are increased by hypokalaemia, hence the decrease in the serum potassium caused by β_2 agonists assumes greater importance in some patients.

PRECAUTIONS AND CONTRAINDICATIONS

The place of inhaled β_2 agonists in the treatment of asthma is the subject of ongoing debate in the medical literature. Some work implicates β_2 agonists as a causative factor in relation to increased asthma mortality, although further clarification is required. Explanations for this finding include an increased tendency for self-treatment with β_2 agonists available without prescription, and that this type of therapy is generally directed at the control of symptoms (e.g. breathlessness) rather than control of the underlying disease process with other appropriate therapy (e.g. anti-inflammatory corticosteroid treatment).

Tolerance to the bronchodilator effects of these drugs may occur with prolonged or excessive use. Adequate patient education is required to address this potentially important problem and patients should be urged to seek prompt medical attention if persistent or severe symptoms occur.

ANTICHOLINERGIC DRUGS

Ipratropium

TRADE NAMES

Ipratropium bromide: *Atrovent.*

MECHANISM OF ACTION

Bronchial smooth muscle tone is determined by input from both the sympathetic and parasympathetic nervous systems. Agonism at the cholinergic receptor site produces contraction of the bronchial smooth muscle, resulting in bronchoconstriction. Conversely, cholinergic receptor antagonists, the anticholinergic drugs, produce a relaxation of the bronchial smooth muscle, leading to bronchodilation. Ipratropium bromide is the only example of an anticholinergic bronchodilator drug in clinical use at the time of writing.

PHARMACOKINETICS

Ipratropium is poorly absorbed if administered orally, and is formulated for delivery only by inhalation. Inadvertent swallowing of this drug after administration by aerosol does not produce significant systemic absorption. Furthermore, ipratropium is not absorbed to any significant extent from the lungs after administration by inhalation (estimated systemic absorption after administration of a dose by metered aerosol is approximately 5%), meaning that significant systemic anticholinergic effects are not commonly observed with this agent. Any small amount of ipratropium which is systemically absorbed is cleared by metabolism, with a plasma half-life of approximately 4 hours.

USES

Ipratropium is currently available for administration by inhalation using two different delivery systems. A metered dose aerosol can be used to deliver a standardised dose of 20 micrograms of ipratropium bromide. The advantages of this dosage form include convenience and portability. Alternatively, a solution of ipratropium

11

RESPIRATORY DISEASES

bromide (concentration 0.025%) is available for use in nebulisers and may be preferred where poor inhaler technique or severe symptoms of bronchospasm render the use of the metered dose inhaler impractical.

The bronchodilator effects observed with ipratropium are useful in the treatment of asthma or chronic obstructive airways disease (particularly where there is superimposed bronchoconstriction). Ipratropium is particularly effective in the treatment of asthma in young children, whilst in older patients the β_2 agonists are generally more effective. Ipratropium may be useful as a substitute for those patients in whom the β_2 agonists produce unacceptable side effects, or as a method for enhancing the magnitude or duration of bronchodilation achieved with first-line drugs. Ipratropium solutions may be mixed with β_2 agonist solutions for immediate use in a nebuliser, although the stability of such admixtures cannot be guaranteed. The mixed solution should not be allowed to stand for an extended period of time before use.

The normal recommended dose for adult patients is two puffs of the metered aerosol spray up to four times a day. Alternatively, 1 mL of nebuliser solution may be administered by inhalation up to every six hours (in short-term therapy of severe symptoms the dose may be increased to 2 mL every six hours). For paediatric patients the dosage rate should be modified, with a maximum recommended dose of 1 mL of nebuliser solution administered four times a day.

ADVERSE DRUG REACTIONS

Because of the relatively minor extent of systemic absorption of ipratropium, clinically significant adverse reactions to this drug are comparatively uncommon. However, systemic anticholinergic effects may occasionally be seen, including dry mouth, blurred vision, acute urinary hesitancy or retention, or precipitation of acute angle closure glaucoma. Furthermore, ocular effects may occur through inadvertent topical delivery of the drug to the surface of the eye due to misplacement of the nebuliser mask

or unintentional transfer of the drug to the eye from the hands after mixing solutions. The importance of the uncommon systemic anticholinergic side effects of this drug may be considerably enhanced by the presence of pre-existing medical conditions such as prostatic hypertrophy, ischaemic heart disease or narrow (closed) angle glaucoma.

Although very uncommon, a paradoxical bronchoconstrictor response has been reported to occur in some patients after the administration of ipratropium. The mechanism by which this arises is unclear, particularly as the bronchospasm in these patients cannot always be reproduced with atropine. It has been suggested that the bronchospasm is an allergic reaction to the preservative in the solution or may occur due to an alteration in sputum viscosity.

DRUG INTERACTIONS

As previously mentioned the low systemic absorption of ipratropium limits its potential for important adverse drug reactions or drug interactions. However, the possible potentiation of the effects of other drugs with anticholinergic properties should be considered.

Ipratropium nebuliser solution appears to be compatible when mixed with solutions of β_2 agonist drugs, provided the admixture is used promptly. However, ipratropium solutions should not be mixed with solutions of sodium cromoglycate, as the effectiveness of both drugs will be compromised.

PRECAUTIONS AND CONTRAINDICATIONS

Patients should be screened for possible contraindications to therapy with anticholinergic drugs prior to the introduction of therapy with ipratropium. In particular, narrow angle glaucoma or urinary outflow obstruction may be exacerbated and therapy in patients with these conditions should be introduced with care, if at all. Patients should be reviewed soon after the introduction of ipratropium therapy to exclude a paradoxical worsening of bronchoconstriction related to airway hyper-reactivity.

XANTHINES

Theophylline and Derivatives

Theophylline is a methylxanthine derivative which has been in clinical use for many years. The drug has wide ranging pharmacological effects but is most commonly employed for its therapeutic effects on the tone of bronchial smooth muscle. Derivatives of theophylline such as aminophylline have been synthesised in an attempt to achieve increased water solubility to allow administration by the intravenous route.

TRADE NAMES

Theophylline: *Theo-Dur; Nuelin*; *Austyn.*

MECHANISM OF ACTION

Theophylline is known to inhibit the activity of the enzyme system responsible for the degradation of cyclic adenosine monophosphate (CAMP), and increased concentrations of this compound lead to the relaxation of bronchial smooth muscle. Whilst this effect may account for the bronchodilator effects of these drugs when used in asthma, the full nature of the mechanism by which bronchodilator effects are produced remains unclear. (Phosphodiesterase inhibition can only be consistently demonstrated at serum concentrations greater than those conventionally used in therapy.)

Even less clear is the mechanism by which theophylline produces therapeutic effects in obstructive airways disease. Postulated mechanisms include increased central respiratory drive, enhanced diaphragmatic contractility, and a decrease in fatigue in respiratory accessory muscles.

Further investigations are required to clarify the way in which theophylline produces its effects in both chronic obstructive airways disease and asthma.

PHARMACOKINETICS

The pharmacokinetics of theophylline are complex and have a direct influence on the clinical use of the drug.

Theophylline is well absorbed when administered by the oral route. However, because the elimination of this drug may be rapid in many patients, theophylline is often formulated as slow release tablets (e.g. *Theo-Dur, Nuelin SR*). In this way, despite the relatively rapid elimination of the drug from the blood, the concentration is maintained within the therapeutic range for up to 12 hours. This is more convenient for the patient, often resulting in improved compliance with the prescribed treatment.

Aminophylline may be administered by the intravenous route when a rapid response is needed (e.g. acute bronchospasm) or the patient is unable to tolerate oral intake. When starting treatment with intravenous aminophylline a 'loading dose' is sometimes administered followed by a constant intravenous infusion. It is important that an infusion pump (or at least a burette) is used to prevent 'run-through' accidents with potentially serious consequences. Aminophylline may also be administered by the rectal route and this method is sometimes employed in children. However, the variable and unreliable rate and extent of absorption of drugs administered rectally means that administration by this route should probably be avoided where possible.

Theophylline has a low therapeutic index, with the therapeutic serum concentration relatively close to that level which can produce serious toxicity. For this reason monitoring of theophylline serum concentrations is often used to ensure that the pre-dose theophylline level remains within the therapeutic range, usually 10–20 micrograms per mL. At levels below this range the therapeutic response is likely to be less than ideal, whereas if the level is significantly greater than this range, the likely outcome will be dose related toxicity. It is important for nurses to be familiar with the early signs of theophylline toxicity, such as nausea, vomiting, tachycardia, nervousness and insomnia, as prompt detection of elevated serum levels can prevent serious toxic symptoms such as cardiac rhythm disturbances or convulsions.

The major route of elimination of theophylline from the body is metabolism in the liver. The rate at which hepatic clearance of theophylline takes place depends on a number of important influences, which in turn largely determine the dosage administered. For example, the influence of age on the rate of theophylline clearance may be profound. The half-life may be up to 50 hours in premature infants, decreasing to 1.5–9.5 hours in children older than 6 months. The half-life increases to 3–13 hours in non-smoking adults and may increase further in the elderly. The influence of heart failure, hepatic insufficiency or other acute or chronic illness on theophylline metabolism may be profound. Tobacco smoking or other drug therapy can also affect the drug's metabolism (see Drug Interactions).

USES

Theophylline is used for its bronchodilator properties in the treatment of asthma and also may be useful in enhancing the quality of life in patients with chronic obstructive airways disease.

When administered orally, theophylline is best given immediately after or during a meal to minimise gastric irritation and side effects such as nausea and vomiting. A range of sustained release preparations are available, including controlled release tablets (*Theo-Dur, Nuelin SR*) and slow release pellets (*Nuelin Sprinkles*) suitable for administration (mixed into soft food) to children. The rate of theophylline dosage required will vary in accordance with individual pharmacokinetic parameters and should be adjusted in accordance with tolerance and observed serum concentration. It is important that the patient receive adequate information and education regarding the various forms of theophylline, so that the potential for inadvertent double-dosing can be minimised.

ADVERSE DRUG REACTIONS

Nearly all the side effects of theophylline are dose related and are usually reversed with the withdrawal of therapy or a dose reduction. The incidence of adverse reactions is generally much higher with serum concentrations higher than the recommended range.

Gastrointestinal side effects are probably the most common adverse reactions, and nausea or vomiting, in particular, may be troublesome. Other gastrointestinal side effects of theophylline include gastric reflux, epigastric discomfort and haematemesis. Although there is a component of gastric irritation associated with the oral administration of theophylline (which can be reduced by administration with food), gastrointestinal side effects may occur with theophylline derivatives administered by any route.

Central nervous system side effects such as nervousness, restlessness, irritability and insomnia are also relatively common with theophylline; seizures may occur in theophylline toxicity. The most common cardiovascular side effect is tachycardia and is more frequent in patients in whom the serum concentration is greater than the recommended range.

DRUG INTERACTIONS

Theophylline derivatives exhibit important drug interactions of both pharmacokinetic and pharmacodynamic types. These drugs may, for example, produce additive gastric irritation or an increase in heart rate when used concurrently with other agents with these effects.

The range of pharmacokinetic drug interactions for theophylline has been extensively documented. A variety of drugs, including cimetidine, erythromycin and ciprofloxacin, is known to inhibit the hepatic metabolism of theophylline, reducing the clearance and leading to potential toxicity. On the other hand, the concurrent administration of the anticonvulsant drugs phenytoin or carbamazepine, or the use of the antitubercular drug rifampicin may result in the induction of theophylline metabolism resulting in a subtherapeutic serum concentration. Smoking is also known to induce hepatic metabolism of theophylline and smokers commonly require higher maintenance doses than other patients. A summary of some important drug interactions is provided in Table 11.2.

PRECAUTIONS AND CONTRAINDICATIONS

Caution should be used to prevent the possibility of important interactions with other drug therapy. In the presence of significant cardiac disease the effects of theophylline on the cardiac rate and rhythm may assume greater importance. Patients with serious liver disease are likely to have a slower rate of theophylline metabolism.

Adequate monitoring of the serum concentration of theophylline is essential during extended use and in patients taking potentially interacting drugs or who have

TABLE 11.2   Some important drug interactions for theophylline and its derivatives

Drugs which may *increase* serum theophylline levels

Erythromycin
Ciprofloxacin
Cimetidine
Oral contraceptives

Drugs which may *decrease* serum theophylline levels

Phenobarbitone
Phenytoin
Carbamazepine
Rifampicin

concurrent liver or heart disease, as the effects of theophylline toxicity may result in significant morbidity or mortality.

11

RESPIRATORY DISEASES

ANTI-INFLAMMATORY THERAPY

CORTICOSTEROIDS

The corticosteroid drugs (steroids) are very widely used in a variety of diseases and have multiple pharmacological actions. So widespread is the use of these agents in clinical practice that a saying has been coined which claims that 'no patient ever dies without steroids'. However, in addition to their wide range of useful pharmacological effects, the steroids also cause serious side effects in nearly all major body systems. Thus, although the steroids are often effective therapy, the decision to initiate treatment with these agents should be undertaken only after careful consideration of the potential benefits weighed against the potential for adverse reactions. Furthermore, if a decision is taken to use steroid therapy, the lowest possible effective dose should be employed using the most localised route available for the shortest possible time.

Another important consideration in the planning of steroid therapy regimens is the influence of this drug therapy on endo-

genous production of corticosteroids. When extended treatment with steroids is used the negative feedback mechanism controlling stimulation of the adrenal glands to produce steroid compounds causes downregulation of endogenous corticosteroid production. Abrupt withdrawal of steroids after prolonged therapy may lead to acute adrenal insufficiency. This complication is potentially life threatening and patients should be counselled to ensure that treatment is not discontinued abruptly without medical supervision. As acute illnesses, infections or surgery may alter endogenous steroid production, dose adjustments may be necessary in these situations.

Corticosteroids are used clinically for their potent anti-inflammatory effects mediated through both vascular and cellular pathways, and it is this effect which is most commonly utilised in the treatment of respiratory disease.

Systemic Corticosteroids: Methylprednisolone, Hydrocortisone, Prednisolone, Betamethasone

Steroids are administered systemically in the treatment of asthma and acute exacerbations of chronic obstructive airways and in the management of autoimmune diseases such as interstitial pneumonitis or alveolitis. In some particularly severe cases ongoing maintenance steroid therapy must be administered by the systemic route, usually with an increased incidence of severe adverse effects.

TRADE NAMES

Betamethasone: *Celestone*.
Hydrocortisone sodium succinate: *Solu-Cortef, Efcortelan*.
Prednisone: *Deltasone; Panafcort; Sone*.
Prednisolone: *Deltasolone; Panafcortelone; Solone*.
Methylprednisolone sodium succinate: *Solu-Medrol*.

MECHANISM OF ACTION

In respiratory diseases such as asthma, steroids produce therapeutic benefit through an anti-inflammatory effect thought to be achieved through both cell mediated and vascular mechanisms. The steroids reduce the permeability of blood vessels as well as interfering with cell mediated immunity. Other anti-inflammatory effects are produced by stabilisation of leucocyte lysosymal membranes and the prevention of migration of macrophages into areas of inflammation.

PHARMACOKINETICS

The majority of steroid agents are well absorbed when administered orally, although when the oral route is not practical or when rapid onset of action is required alternative routes may be utilised. Following absorption steroids are in general extensively distributed to sites outside the plasma, although some drugs (e.g. cortisol) are bound to specific carrier plasma proteins.

A number of steroids (e.g. cortisone and prednisone) must undergo metabolic transformation before they become pharmacologically active (i.e. they are pro-drugs). The major route of elimination for the corticosteroids is hepatic metabolism.

USES

The considerable variety of therapeutic applications for the corticosteroid agents is reflected in the range of dosage regimens employed in the treatment of various diseases. Furthermore, the route of steroid administration and the chemical form of the drug (e.g. esters, salts) influence the dose administered.

In many instances, corticosteroid therapy is administered orally in the form of prednisolone or prednisone, with the aim of providing the lowest effective dose given in a way that minimises the influence on the body's own steroid production. This approach is used in the treatment of asthma. The normal practice is to begin therapy at a dose estimated to produce a prompt response, often using a parenteral formulation of hydrocortisone or methylprednisolone. After a short period of stabilisation, the steroid can often be withdrawn completely (provided there is no reason to suspect that suppression of endogenous steroid production has taken place). On the other hand, when therapy has been extended or courses of treatment frequent, a gradual scaled reduction in the dose may be necessary, with the aim of eventually withdrawing corticosteroids or at least achieving the lowest possible maintenance dose. In respiratory disease, inhaled steroid therapy may allow the patient to be weaned off prednisolone and may be commenced before systemic steroids have been withdrawn.

It may sometimes be necessary to administer corticosteroids orally as maintenance therapy, as the inhaled route may not provide adequate control. However, such treatment is associated with a higher incidence of adverse effects and should be reserved for patients with essentially intractable disease. Strategies to minimise this problem of suppression of endogenous production of steroids include administration of the lowest effective dose in the morning and, if possible, on alternate days.

ADVERSE DRUG REACTIONS

Despite their widespread use the corticosteroids are considered by many clinicians to be the drugs most commonly associated with significant adverse reactions. Especially when administered systemically these drugs can produce side effects in nearly every body system. This has become a major factor in discouraging their use in the treatment of relatively simple and uncomplicated diseases.

Metabolic effects are relatively common, although these are usually related to the size of the dose employed and the duration of therapy. Central nervous system effects are not uncommon, and again are related to the dosage schedule employed. Adverse effects which affect the musculoskeletal system may be particularly devastating, and include osteoporosis, avascular bone necrosis and proximal myopathies. Orally administered corticosteroids are thought to account for a significant proportion of drug induced peptic ulcer disease, as well as anaemia arising from a variety of sources. These and other relatively frequent adverse effects contribute to the well earned reputation of the steroids as a causative factor in drug induced illness. A summary of some adverse effects of the corticosteroids is provided in Table 11.3.

The relative severity and frequency of steroid induced adverse drug reactions means that there is a significant role in this area for the practice of preventive medicine. Also, the potential role for a variety of health professionals, including nurses, is significant and may contribute to a significant decrease in the morbidity and mortality associated with the use of these drugs.

DRUG INTERACTIONS

Significant drug interactions related to the corticosteroids are generally limited to those of a pharmacodynamic nature. The salt and fluid retention associated with corticosteroid use may decrease the efficacy of diuretics or other drugs used in the treatment of heart failure or oedematous states. The concurrent administration of steroids and non-steroidal anti-inflammatory drugs (NSAIDs) may result in an increased risk of drug induced peptic ulcer disease. The likelihood of significant gastrointestinal bleeding appears to be increased with concomitant use of steroids and anticoagulants.

11

RESPIRATORY DISEASES

TABLE 11.3 Some adverse drug reactions associated with corticosteroid drugs

System	Adverse Drug Reaction
Central nervous system	Psychosis, mania, depression
Eyes	Cataracts
Gastrointestinal tract	Peptic ulcer disease
Cardiovascular system	Salt and water retention, hypertension, oedema
Musculoskeletal system	Osteoporosis, proximal myopathy, delayed wound healing
Metabolism	Hyperglycaemia, weight gain
Skin	Friability, purpura, hirsutism
Blood	Anaemia, elevated white blood cell count
Immune system	Immunosuppression, increased susceptibility to infection

The immunosuppressive effects of some drugs (e.g. cytotoxic agents) may be enhanced by steroid therapy. Steroids may diminish the immune response to some vaccines.

More rarely a pharmacokinetic interaction may be demonstrated with these agents. In particular, hepatic enzyme inducing drugs such as anticonvulsants or rifampicin may necessitate the use of higher doses of corticosteroids to provide effective anti-inflammatory therapy.

PRECAUTIONS AND CONTRAINDICATIONS

Systemic corticosteroid therapy should be undertaken with care in patients with significant immunosuppression. Close monitoring of blood glucose levels is needed in patients with established diabetes mellitus or glucose intolerance. In patients with a history of peptic ulceration or gastroesophageal reflux systemic corticosteroid treatment should be undertaken with caution, possibly employing prophylactic cover using a drug to reduce the likelihood of peptic ulceration.

Patients should be counselled regarding the possibility of an increased incidence of infections during systemic treatment with steroids and that the signs and symptoms of infection may be masked. Owing to the possibility of suppression of endogenous production of steroids, patients receiving long-term therapy should be provided with specific counselling regarding the possible hazards of sudden or abrupt cessation of therapy. A possible solution to this problem is use of an alert system (e.g. bracelet, pendant or card) carried by the patient to alert medical staff in the event of the need for emergency medical treatment.

Inhaled Corticosteroids: Beclomethasone, Budesonide

The high incidence of important adverse drug reactions associated with systemic administration of steroids, the effectiveness of these agents in the treatment of severe respiratory disease and the sophistication of delivery techniques available for administering drugs to relatively localised sites within the bronchial tree, have all contributed to the common use of inhaled corticosteroid drugs in the treatment of respiratory disease.

TRADE NAMES

Beclomethasone: *Becotide; Becloforte.*
Budesonide: *Pulmicort.*

MECHANISM OF ACTION

The effectiveness of inhaled corticosteroid agents such as beclomethasone or budesonide in the treatment of inflammatory lung disease (i.e. asthma) has now been proven beyond reasonable doubt. This method of delivery appears to result in the systemic absorption of relatively low amounts of the administered dose, and correspondingly suppression of endogenous production of corticosteroids is limited.

PHARMACOKINETICS

A small proportion of the dose of steroids administered by inhalation is absorbed from the lung and gastrointestinal tract into the systemic circulation where the pharmacokinetic profile reflects that of steroids administered by mouth. The systemic absorption of steroids delivered by inhalation appears to be directly related to the total daily dose delivered. However, the lower incidence of systemic adverse effects confirms that the overall amount of drug entering the systemic circulation is low after administration by inhalation. Most systemic absorption occurs through inadvertent swallowing of inhaled doses, and can be minimised through good inhaler technique. The use of inhaled steroids may provide a means by which the dose or duration of systemic steroid treatment may be minimised.

Whilst originally administered by inhalation up to four times a day, it is now acknowledged that corticosteroids such as budesonide and beclomethasone are effective when administered twice daily. In this way patient compliance is enhanced and the regimen of inhaled drugs (often complex for patients with serious respiratory disease) can be simplified considerably.

USES

Inhaled corticosteroids, administered twice daily using a metered dose inhaler delivery system or by nebulisation, now have an established place in the therapy of asthma. The optimal time for administration is after a bronchodilator. This enables maximum penetration of the steroid into the lower part of the bronchial tree. The place of inhaled corticosteroid therapy in the treatment of other lung diseases, such as emphysema and chronic bronchitis, is less well established and requires further investigation.

When administered in equipotent doses, the anti-inflammatory effects of inhaled beclomethasone and budesonide appear to be roughly equivalent. The differences appear to be mainly related to the mode of delivery. Beclomethasone is available as an aerosol delivery system while budesonide is available as an inspiration driven inhaler unit. Claims for superiority in terms of the rate and extent of systemic drug absorption and adverse effects are largely unsubstantiated and patient preference is often the major determinant for the agent selected. Some patients are unable to coordinate the inhaler actuation and inhalation—for these patients an aerosol may be a poor choice. Other patients with severe airways disease may have difficulty in delivering an effective dose using an inspiration driven device—for these an aerosol with an appropriate spacing or chamber device may be preferable. When administered by nebuliser, budesonide must be delivered using specialised apparatus to avoid local irritation. Budesonide nebuliser solution is also light sensitive.

Inhaled corticosteroid products such as beclomethasone are also administered as nasal sprays in the treatment of allergic rhinitis. When employing this form of treatment it is important that the patient understands that, unlike nasal decongestant sprays, no immediate relief is provided by the drug. In fact, many patients complain of an initial transient increase in nasal congestion before any improvement is noted.

ADVERSE DRUG REACTIONS

Although some studies suggest that inhaled steroids administered at high doses over sustained periods may produce systemic adverse effects such as bone demineralisation, evidence at this stage suggests that the adverse effects of inhaled steroids are largely limited to local manifestations.

Hoarseness and pharyngitis are not uncommon with inhaled corticosteroids. Oral infections with *Candida albicans* often occur in patients treated with high dose inhaled steroids. The incidence of this complication may be minimised by the use of warm water gargles after administration. The use of appropriate spacing devices may also reduce the incidence of local oral adverse effects.

DRUG INTERACTIONS

Significant drug interactions with the inhaled corticosteroids appear to be uncommon.

PRECAUTIONS AND CONTRAINDICATIONS

Suppression of adrenal production of endogenous steroids is unlikely when these drugs are administered by inhalation, but cannot be excluded in patients undergoing high dose therapy for extended periods.

PREVENTIVE THERAPY

Sodium Cromoglycate

The principle use for sodium cromoglycate is the preventive treatment of inflammatory disease of the respiratory tract (including the nasopharynx) and the eyes. (Oral preparations are available in some countries for use in applications outside respiratory medicine.)

TRADE NAMES

Sodium cromoglycate (cromolyn sodium): *Intal.*

11

RESPIRATORY DISEASES

MECHANISM OF ACTION

The principal mode of action for sodium cromoglycate appears to be the inhibition of the release of cell substances responsible for mediating the inflammatory process. These substances include histamine and other chemicals which are released from sensitised mast cells following the formation of antigen-antibody complexes. Sodium cromoglycate has no direct anti-inflammatory or bronchodilator effects.

PHARMACOKINETICS

Very little of the administered dose of cromoglycate is absorbed into the systemic circulation, regardless of the method of administration. After oral administration, nearly all of the dose is excreted unchanged in the faeces. The very small amount of drug which does reach the systemic circulation is rapidly eliminated through renal and biliary excretion.

USES

Sodium cromoglycate is administered by inhalation for prophylactic treatment of asthma. The dose is delivered using a nebuliser or metered dose inhaler up to four times a day. The aim of therapy is to stabilise mast cells thus preventing bronchospasm produced by mediator substances such as histamine. Sodium cromoglycate has no bronchodilator properties and should be administered after drugs such as salbutamol have produced their clinical effects. The onset of action may be slow and extended therapy for up to 4–6 weeks may be required before the full extent of response is known.

Sodium cromoglycate may also be administered as a nasal spray for prophylaxis of allergic rhinitis. An ophthalmic preparation is also available and is used for prophylaxis of allergic conjunctivitis.

ADVERSE DRUG REACTIONS

Systemic adverse drug reactions are not commonly associated with inhaled cromoglycate therapy. The most important side effects reported are those related to the local irritant effects of the powder. Transient irritation of the throat and, less commonly, acute bronchospasm have been associated with cromoglycate therapy. For this reason, administration of inhaled sodium cromoglycate is not recommended during acute asthma attacks.

PRECAUTIONS AND CONTRAINDICATIONS

Patients with a history of demonstrated reactions attributable to local irritation secondary to cromoglycate should not be treated with this drug.

ANTI-INFECTIVE THERAPY ▮▮▮▮▮▮

Infections of the respiratory tract are relatively common, and may range in severity from relatively minor problems, such as sinusitis or laryngitis, through to life-threatening pneumonias. Whilst specific issues relating to the use of antibiotic drugs are covered in Chapter 30 Infectious Diseases, a number of aspects specific to the respiratory tract are important for an understanding of the treatment these infections.

The choice of an appropriate antibiotic treatment for use in respiratory tract infection is influenced by a number of factors, including the organism thought to be implicated. In particular, the likely pathogens which need to be considered include *Streptococcus pneumoniae, Haemophilus influenzae* and *Moraxcella catarrhalis*, although others such as *Pseudomonas* and *Staphylococcus* sp. must also be considered, especially in the hospitalised patient. In keeping with this, antibiotics commonly employed for respiratory tract infections include phenoxymethylpenicillin, amoxycillin (with or without clavulanic acid), doxycycline and other tetracyclines, erythromycin and trimethoprim–sulfamethoxazole. Under certain circumstances, infections caused by atypical organisms may necessitate the use of a specific antibiotic (e.g. erythromycin for the treatment of *Legionella* sp. infections).

The site from which the infection is acquired also plays an important role. Infections acquired in the community may demonstrate a different pattern of resistance to those acquired in a hospital ward or intensive care unit. A knowledge of local resistance patterns may be helpful in determining the most appropriate antibiotic for use in these infections. In addition, antibiotic therapy in respiratory tract infections cannot be effective unless the drug gains adequate access to the organism, thus antibiotics must penetrate well into the sputum to be effective.

Patient specific factors also play a role in the selection of therapy. A known allergy to penicillins, cephalosporins, sulfonamides or other agents may necessitate the use of alternative drugs. Likewise, some patients fail to tolerate drug therapy for other reasons, e.g. many patients experience nausea and vomiting when treated with erythromycin. Drug interactions can also be important. For example, when erythromycin or ciprofloxacin are used in patients taking theophylline, the dose of theophylline may need to be reduced. Especially for elderly patients, compliance with prescribed therapy is best when relatively simple drug regimens are used—doxycycline administered once daily after food may produce better compliance than penicillins administered four times daily on an empty stomach.

11

RESPIRATORY DISEASES

EXPECTORANTS, MUCOLYTICS AND COUGH SUPPRESSANTS ▮▮▮▮▮

For many years various pharmacological agents have been used in attempts to alter the nature of the sputum or to enhance the effectiveness with which it could be removed from the respiratory tract. Although these therapies remain popular and are sold in a confusing variety of products available without a prescription, the medical use of expectorants and mucolytics is becoming less common, probably because of the lack of convincing evidence of their effectiveness.

EXPECTORANTS

Expectorants include such products as potassium iodide mixture and senega and ammonia liquid. These preparations were thought to enhance the effectiveness with which the sputum was cleared from the respiratory tract, probably by stimulating the cough mechanism. Very little objective evidence exists for their effectiveness, and it is now thought that the most appropriate means for encouraging the removal of sputum from the respiratory tract are measures such as chest physiotherapy or steam inhalations. Hydration status is also important, as an inadequate fluid intake may lead to the formation of thick, sticky mucus which is difficult to expectorate. Current evidence suggests that drug therapy has little or no role to play in this area.

MUCOLYTICS

Mucolytics are a related group of compounds represented by such agents as bromhexine (*Bisolvon*) and acetylcysteine (*Mucomyst*). The mechanism of action is to render sputum less viscous by disrupting bonds within the mucous, supposedly aiding in the evacuation from the bronchial tree. Although still employed occasionally, clinical trials investigating the effectiveness of these drugs have failed to demonstrate consistent benefits.

COUGH SUPPRESSANTS

Cough suppressants (antitussives) are compounds used to reduce the frequency and severity of cough, and may be particularly useful in the treatment of the dry, unproductive cough. However, under other circumstances their use is not appropriate (e.g. in purulent bronchitis or bronchiectasis). Most cough suppressants are opiates or related drugs, with their activity mediated through the suppression of the cough reflex at a central level. Codeine, morphine, opium and others have been used as cough suppressants although agents with less widespread systemic effects and abuse potential may be preferred. Pholcodine and dextro-methorpan are commonly used for these purposes. In the process of deciding to use a cough suppressant, it is important to evaluate and treat the underlying cause of the cough.

NASAL DECONGESTANTS

Although corticosteroids such as beclomethasone (*Beconase, Aldecin Nasal*) may be administered by nasal inhalation for the treatment of nasal congestion associated with allergic rhinitis, the majority of drugs used as nasal decongestants are sympathomimetic agents which relieve congestion through local vasoconstriction in the nasal mucosa.

Drugs such as xylometazoline (*Otrivin*), tramazoline (*Spray-Tish*) and oxymetazoline (*Drixine*) are delivered by nasal spray, and provide relief from nasal congestion. Repeated or prolonged use of these drugs often results in diminished effectiveness, a phenomenon referred to as tachyphylaxis. Because of this topical decongestants are only indicated for short-term use, 5–7 days, and should not be used more frequently than directed. Patients with hypertension should be treated cautiously with these drugs, as systemic absorption may result in sympathomimetic effects such as tachycardia and increased blood pressure. Patients being treated with a monoamine oxidase inhibitor (MAOI) should not receive treatment with sympathomimetic drugs.

ADVERSE RESPIRATORY EFFECTS OF DRUGS AND ADDITIVES

A wide variety of drugs and additives have been associated with adverse effects manifested in the respiratory system. Although in many cases these reactions are minor, fatal adverse reactions also occur. Some of the drugs known to cause adverse respiratory effects are listed in Table 11.4.

ASPIRIN AND NON-STEROIDAL ANTI-INFLAMMATORY DRUGS

Aspirin is known to produce bronchoconstriction in some patients, and is implicated in exacerbating the symptoms of asthma in others. Acute bronchospasm caused by aspirin may be potentially fatal, and appears to occur more frequently in patients with nasal polyps. Given that a wide variety of products contain aspirin without the labelling necessarily reflecting this, extensive counselling is required for the patient with demonstrated aspirin sensitivity. A written list of aspirin containing products may prove to be a useful counselling aid. Aspirin induced bronchospasm may occur even with very low doses.

Non-steroidal anti-inflammatory drugs (NSAIDs) are related to aspirin and are also known to cause bronchospasm in some pa-

RESPIRATORY DISEASES 11

TABLE 11.4   Some examples of drugs which may cause adverse respiratory effects

Drug Class	Drug
Aspirin, NSAIDs	Aspirin, indomethacin, ibuprofen, diclofenac, piroxicam, tenoxicam, sulindac, naproxen, tiaprofenic acid, ketorolac
β Blockers	Atenolol, propranolol, metoprolol, oxprenolol, pindolol and timolol. Betaxolol and timolol eye drops
Angiotensin converting enzyme (ACE) inhibitors	Captopril, enalapril, perindopril, lisinopril, fosinopril, ramipril
Drugs derived from biological sources	Vaccines, immunoglobulins, antivenoms, asparaginase, antibiotics, monoclonal antibodies
CNS depressants	
Opiates	Morphine, pethidine, methadone, codeine
Benzodiazepines	Diazepam, nitrazepam, midazolam, oxazepam
Others	Barbiturates, antidepressants, chloral hydrate, antipsychotics
Drugs causing idiopathic pulmonary reactions	Amiodarone, bleomycin, methotrexate, penicillamine

tients. Where the existence of aspirin sensitivity can be demonstrated, cross-sensitivity with NSAIDs should be assumed. This effect appears to be class specific, with no one agent implicated to a lesser or greater degree than others. At the time of writing at least one death from acute bronchospasm as a result of the use of a NSAID purchased without a prescription had been reported in Australia.

β ADRENERGIC BLOCKING DRUGS

β Adrenergic blocking drugs (the β blockers) are used in the treatment of hypertension and other cardiovascular diseases as well as topically as eye drops in the treatment of glaucoma. These drugs may cause bronchoconstriction in susceptible patients even when administered only as ophthalmic preparations. Careful patient monitoring is needed at the introduction of β blocker therapy, and the use of appropriate alternative treatments should be considered if there is any doubt. Asthmatic patients should not be treated with systemic β blockers.

ANGIOTENSIN CONVERTING ENZYME INHIBITORS

The angiotensin converting enzyme inhibitors (ACE inhibitors) such as captopril, enalapril, lisinopril, perindopril and others may all cause a variety of adverse respiratory effects. These reactions are thought to arise through an inhibition of enzymes responsible for the breakdown of prostaglandins and kinins in the lung, and may range from cough (probably the most common) through to anaphylaxis. Although usually acute, these reactions may occur some weeks after the introduction of therapy. Cross sensitivity between various agents of this class is known to occur.

BIOLOGICAL PRODUCTS

Drug products derived from human, animal, microbial or plant sources may produce allergic reactions which include important respiratory effects. Examples of these products include human immunoglobulins, monoclonal antibodies, vaccines, antivenom preparations, antibiotics (e.g. penicillins), asparaginase and others. The incidence of serious reactions is so high for some products (e.g. antivenoms) that prophylactic antihistamines and steroids are usually given.

IDIOPATHIC PULMONARY REACTIONS

A variety of drugs may produce idiopathic lung reactions which may be potentially serious. For example, amiodarone, methotrexate, gold salts, penicillamine and others may cause pneumonitis or alveolitis.

CENTRAL NERVOUS SYSTEM DEPRESSANTS

Most drugs with central nervous system depressant effects have the ability to significantly depress central nervous system respiratory drive. Respiratory depression is associated with opiates, benzodiazepines, barbiturates and antidepressants, and may contribute to the cause of death in overdose. For some of these agents respiratory depression can sometimes be reversed by the administration of a specific antagonist drug, e.g. naloxone to reverse opiate effects.

EXCIPIENTS, PRESERVATIVES AND FOOD ADDITIVES

Adverse reactions to additives to food and pharmaceutical products may also be important. Compounds known to be associated with these types of reaction include tartrazine, sodium metabisulfite, mono-sodium glutamate and others. The nature of the reaction may vary from relatively minor problems such as cough, through to life threatening bronchospasm and anaphylaxis.

NURSING IMPLICATIONS

ASSESSMENT

Patients with serious respiratory disease also often suffer from other illnesses which will be important in overall management. The presence of heart disease, diabetes mellitus, peptic ulcer or diseases of other major organ systems should be noted by the nurse during the patient's assessment as they may have a significant influence on the drug therapy used to treat respiratory illness. Conversely, the use of respiratory drug therapy may have a substantial influence on the status of other disease states. Baseline observations of respiratory and cardiovascular parameters, colour, signs of hypoxia and hypercapnia should be documented.

Nurses must know which drugs are to be used on a regular basis for prophylaxis and which are used for an acute attack of bronchoconstriction.

Another important aspect of the nursing assessment of the patient should be an estimation of the patient's ability and motivation to comply with a complex regimen of drug therapy. Issues to consider include inhaler technique and compliance with previously prescribed therapy.

EVALUATION

Strict attention to accurate monitoring and recording of observations is necessary when caring for the patient with respiratory illness as alterations in parameters such as body weight, blood pressure, heart rate, respiratory rate, body temperature and others may provide a means for early detection of deterioration of disease state or drug toxicity. Under other circumstances specialised evaluation may be needed, such as the monitoring of blood sugar levels. Measurement of peak expiratory flow rate or other spirometry is often used to provide information regarding the status of respiratory illness, and repeat measurement after the administration of bronchodilators may provide an indication of the extent of response to this therapy.

ADMINISTRATION

In many cases the processes for the administration of drugs used in the treatment of respiratory illness are complex and often involve specialised delivery techniques. The nurse should be aware of the special requirements for the efficient administration of these drugs. For example, it is necessary to maintain knowledge of the correct use and maintenance of metered dose inhalers and nebulisation equipment.

Sodium cromoglycate, salbutamol and beclomethasone are available in capsules for inhalation via mechanical devices such as a *Spinhaler* or *Rotahaler*. Correct selection of the device specified by the manufacturer for the prescribed substance is important. Patient education on the proper use of the inhaler is particularly important for therapeutic benefit to be obtained.

Several of the β agonists, e.g. salbutamol, are available as nebuliser solutions for use in intermittent-positive-pressure breathing therapy or can be delivered as vapours with gases inhaled through nebulisers. The appropriate dose form must be selected with careful attention paid to the prescription for dose, diluent, gas (air or oxygen) and rate of delivery. The nurse must be familiar with the correct use and adjustment of each type of apparatus.

Mixing different medications in a nebuliser is common practice, but there is some doubt about the chemical compatibility and resulting clinical efficacy of such combinations. It would appear that sodium cromoglycate may be mixed with the

RESPIRATORY DISEASES

11

adrenergic agents and ipratropium, although these mixtures should be used promptly. Current information on mixing these solutions should be sought from the pharmacist.

It is important to follow precisely the instructions for administration of these drugs. For example, sustained release preparations such as *Theo-Dur* and *Nuelin SR* must be swallowed whole, other drugs such as steroids should be given immediately after food to minimise the likelihood of gastrointestinal side effects. Inhaled steroids should be administered 5–10 minutes after bronchodilators and adequate attention must be paid to oral hygiene (i.e. rinsing mouth with water, brushing teeth) after inhaled steroids so that oral complications such as thrush infections can be minimised. Spacer devices may also improve delivery techniques and reduce the incidence of local complications.

Intravenous infusions of aminophylline should not be 'caught up' if running too slowly. Cardiovascular effects may occur with too rapid infusions. An infusion pump or microdrip giving set should be used for maintenance of accurate flow rates. No drugs should be added to aminophylline infusions without first consulting the pharmacist or reliable literature because incompatibilities are extremely common. The dangers of rapid injection cannot be overemphasised, but care must be taken with all routes of administration.

PATIENT EDUCATION

The nurse can play an important role in the education of the patient in respect to respiratory drug treatment. Inhaler technique, equipment maintenance, peak expiratory flow rate monitoring and the correct use of orally administered and inhaled therapy are all areas in which adequate patient education must be undertaken. Nurses can also reinforce the work of pharmacists in educating patients about the nature of respiratory disease, the appropriate use of bronchodilators and self-administration techniques.

The reason for therapeutic failure of aerosol and inhaler treatment can be faulty technique, particularly In the very young and the elderly. Patients must be taught correct techniques and be observed during self-administration to evaluate the effectiveness of teaching. Placebo aerosols and inhalers are available for teaching purposes. Parents must be present when young children are being taught. Patients must be cautioned about over-use and advised of the importance of following recommended doses. They must be able to distinguish between drugs intended for prophylactic use and those intended for the treatment of an acute attack.

As with all drug therapy education the information provided should be in plain language and should be discussed with the other members of the multidisciplinary health care team.

FURTHER READING

Avery, G.S. (1987), 'Respiratory Diseases' *Drug Treatment*. 3rd edn. Adis Press, Sydney, pp. 812–854.

TEST YOUR KNOWLEDGE

1. Define the term bronchodilator and describe how drugs of this type are thought to produce their therapeutic effects.

2. Provide examples of three separate types of bronchodilator drugs and briefly outline the various routes by which they may be administered.

3. Give three examples of drugs which are β_2 agonists and describe the common adverse reactions observed with this class of drugs.

4. Outline the correct chronological order for the administration by inhalation of the following drugs: terbutaline, budesonide and ipratropium bromide.

5. Provide examples of three drugs which may result in theophylline toxicity if administered concurrently with this agent.

6. Describe at least two situations in which the systemic administration of corticosteroid drugs may exert an important influence on the course of other intercurrent disease states.

7. Outline a range of adverse effects which might be expected to occur in patients treated with extended oral corticosteroid therapy.

8. Provide two examples of corticosteroid drugs which can be administered by inhalation.

9. List at least four factors which should be taken into account when selecting antibiotic therapy for the treatment of respiratory tract infections.

10. Provide four examples of drug therapy which can produce adverse drug reactions which affect the respiratory tract.

11

RESPIRATORY DISEASES

Cardiovascular Diseases

TERRY A. MAUNSELL

O B J E C T I V E S

At the conclusion of this chapter the reader should be able to:

1. Name the main drugs used in the treatment of cardiovascular disease;

2. Describe the mechanism of action of these drugs;

3. List the common adverse reactions associated with the use of these drugs; and

4. Discuss the implications for patient care which arise from the use of these drugs.

TREATMENT AND PREVENTION OF ANGINA PECTORIS

Angina pectoris is characterised by paroxysmal discomfort in the anterior chest. The discomfort occurs as a result of insufficient coronary blood flow leading to myocardial hypoxia. The discomfort which varies greatly in severity, is felt most often behind the sternum or across the chest but may radiate down or occur solely in one or both arms or into the jaw, throat, shoulders or back. In addition to discomfort the patient may suffer extreme apprehension. The most commonly associated symptom is dyspnoea.

Factors which predispose a patient to angina include obesity, high serum lipid levels, arrhythmias, hypertension, anaemia and hyperthyroidism. Acute attacks may be triggered by factors which increase myocardial oxygen demand such as exercise, emotional stress or exposure to cold.

In many cases pain relief may be obtained by removing the cause of the attack, e.g. angina of effort may be relieved by rest. In other situations drug therapy may be necessary.

In general treatment is aimed at improving myocardial oxygen sypply and decreasing the myocardial oxygen demand.

NITRATES

Glyceryl Trinitrate, Isosorbide Dinitrate, Isosorbide Mononitrate

The principal action of the nitrates is relaxation of vascular smooth muscle resulting in general vasodilation. Peripheral vascular resistance is decreased via a selective action on the venous capacitance vessels with a resultant venous pooling of blood and decreased venous return to the heart. This decrease in preload is accompanied, to a lesser extent, by a reduction in afterload through vasodilation of the arteriolar vessels.

The result is decreased myocardial oxygen demand. In addition, a redistribution of coronary blood flow may occur resulting in an increase in supply of oxygen to ischaemic areas.

TRADE NAMES

Glyceryl trinitrate: *Anginine*; *Nitradisc*; *Nitrobid*; *Nitrolingual*; *Transiderm Nitro*; *Tridil*.
Isosorbide dinitrate: *Isordil*.
Isosorbide mononitrate: *Imdur*.

PHARMACOKINETICS

Glyceryl trinitrate and isosorbide dinitrate are absorbed from both the oral mucosa and gastrointestinal tract. Isosorbide mononitrate is only absorbed from the gastrointestinal tract.

They undergo extensive metabolism in the liver and are eliminated by the kidneys. Absorption also occurs through the skin from an ointment base or transdermal delivery system.

Onset of action is more rapid following sublingual administration than either oral or topical administration.

USES

Glyceryl trinitrate 600 micrograms and isosorbide dinitrate 5 mg are administered sublingually (under the tongue) to relieve acute attacks of angina. An effect occurs within two to three minutes. If pain relief does not occur the dose may be repeated within a few minutes to a maximum of three tablets in 15 minutes.

Glyceryl trinitrate is also available as a metered dose aerosol. Each dose delivers 400 micrograms of glyceryl trinitrate in the form of spray droplets beneath the tongue.

Initially one dose should be sprayed under the tongue followed by a second spray if pain relief has not occurred within five minutes. No more than two metered doses are recommended.

Glyceryl trinitrate may also be administered as an intravenous infusion for the treatment of angina attacks. The initial dose is 5 micrograms per minute increasing by 5 micrograms per minute every five minutes until a response is obtained or adverse haemodynamic effects occur.

Glyceryl trinitrate may also be used topically for long-term prophylactic treatment of angina. Transdermal patches which release 5 mg or 10 mg of the drug over a 24-hour period are applied to a hairless area of the body at the same time each day. The drug can also be applied in ointment form using an applicator paper to measure the dose, usually 3–5 cm, and then spreading a thin, uniform layer onto a non-hairy skin area every four to six hours.

Isosorbide dinitrate and isosorbide mononitrate tablets administered orally are used for prophylactic treatment of angina. The usual dose of isosorbide dinitrate is 5–20 mg administered one hour before food, three or four times a day.

Isosorbide mononitrate is administered in a single daily dose of 60–120 mg.

ADVERSE DRUG REACTIONS

Nitrates may cause flushing of the face, dizziness, tachycardia and severe headache. Headache is most frequent early in therapy and usually disappears with continued treatment. Overdosage of the intravenous preparation may cause vomiting, severe hypotension, reflex tachycardia and transient headache. Local reactions to the topical preparations may occur. Some patients transferred to the metered dose spray from sublingual tablets may experience a transient increase in side effects.

Tolerance to the nitrates may occur with long-term administration of topical dosage forms. Intermittent therapy, e.g. removal of the patch during the night, can reduce this effect.

Sudden withdrawal of nitrate therapy can lead to rebound angina.

DRUG INTERACTIONS

Alcohol, antihypertensive agents, anticholinergic agents, tricyclic antidepressants or phenothiazines may potentiate the hypotensive effects of the nitrates. Caution should be observed with the concomitant use of pancuronium or morphine with intravenous glyceryl trinitrate.

PRECAUTIONS AND CONTRAINDICATIONS

Nitrates should be used with caution in patients with increased intracranial pressure or low systolic blood pressure and are contraindicated in patients with severe anaemia. Intravenous administration is contraindicated in patients with anaemia, constricted pericarditis, hypotension, increased intracranial pressure and uncorrected hypovolaemia and should be used with caution in patients with impaired renal function.

β BLOCKING DRUGS

Atenolol, Metoprolol, Oxprenolol, Pindolol, Propranolol, Timolol

β Blocking drugs (β blockers) are used in the prevention of angina.

They competitively block the stimulation by sympathetic nerve impulses of β receptor sites at nerve endings within the myocardium ($β_1$ receptors) and vascular smooth muscle ($β_2$ receptors). $β_2$ Receptors are also present in bronchial smooth muscle and in the uterus.

Blockade of cardiac receptors reduces heart rate, myocardial contractility, cardiac output and blood pressure, particularly during exercise. Myocardial oxygen demand is reduced. The reduction in heart rate may also increase coronary blood flow and hence oxygen supply by prolonging the diastolic interval during which coronary flow occurs.

β Blocking drugs differ in their relative affinity for β_1 and β_2 receptors. Propranolol, pindolol, timolol and oxprenolol block β receptors at all sites and are classified as 'non-selective'. Atenolol and metoprolol are more selective for β_1 receptors and are termed 'cardioselective'.

TRADE NAMES

Atenolol: *Tenormin*; *Noten*.
Metoprolol: *Betaloc*; *Lopressor*.
Oxprenolol: *Trasicor*; *Corbeton*.
Pindolol: *Visken*; *Barbloc*.
Propranolol: *Inderal*; *Deralin*.
Timolol: *Blocadren*.

PHARMACOKINETICS

β Blocking drugs are absorbed from the gastrointestinal tract. Propranolol, metoprolol, timolol, oxprenolol and pindolol undergo extensive metabolism in the liver. All are mainly eliminated by the kidney.

USES

β Blocking drugs are administered orally for the prophylactic treatment of angina. The cardioselective β blocking drugs are preferred to the non-selective agents as, in usual doses, they have a greater effect on β_1 receptors and have a reduced incidence of side effects which are mainly due to the effect on β_2 receptors. However, cardioselectivity is relative and dose dependent.

The usual doses of β blocking agents used for prophylactic treatment of angina are listed in Table 12.1.

ADVERSE DRUG REACTIONS

β Blocking drugs are generally well tolerated. Adverse effects include bradycardia, hypotension, nausea, vomiting, diarrhoea, lassitude, impotence, bronchospasm and cold extremities. β Blocking drugs may precipitate heart failure in patients with inadequate cardiac function.

Sudden withdrawal of β blocking drugs can exacerbate angina symptoms or precipitate myocardial infarction in patients with coronary artery disease.

TABLE 12.1   Doses of β blocking drugs for angina prophylaxis

Drug	Dosage
Cardioselective	
Atenolol	50–100 mg once daily
Metoprolol	50–100 mg twice daily
Non-selective	
Oxprenolol	20–40 mg three times daily
Pindolol	2.5–5 mg three times daily
Propranolol	40–80 mg two or three times daily
Timolol	5–10 mg three times daily

DRUG INTERACTIONS

The concomitant use of β blocking drugs and calcium channel blockers with myocardial depressant effects (verapamil, diltiazem) can reduce myocardial contractility and impair AV conduction.

β Blocking drugs can cause a loss of diabetic control in patients treated with insulin or oral hypoglycaemic agents.

β Blocking drugs will potentiate the hypotensive action of antihypertensive agents.

PRECAUTIONS AND CONTRAINDICATIONS

Caution must be exercised in patients undergoing surgery due to the possibility of an interaction between β blocking drugs and anaesthetic agents. Anaesthetic agents which produce myocardial depression, e.g. ether, chloroform or cyclopropane, are contraindicated.

As β blockade may mask the clinical signs of developing or continuing hyperthyroidism, caution should be exercised when β blocking drugs are used in hyperthyroid patients.

As β blockade masks the symptoms of a hypoglycaemic attack (other than sweating) caution should be exercised when β blocking drugs are used in diabetic patients.

The use of β blocking drugs is contraindicated in patients with heart failure, sinus bradycardia, bronchospasm (including asthma) and allergic disorders which suggest a predisposition to bronchospasm. They should be used with caution in patients with peripheral vascular disease.

CALCIUM CHANNEL BLOCKERS

Diltiazem, Nifedipine, Verapamil

Calcium channel blocking drugs act by reducing the slow inward current of calcium ions across the cell membrane in cardiac muscle and in vascular smooth muscle.

This reduction in calcium flow results in decreased myocardial contractility, heart rate and AV conduction. The reduction in contraction of vascular smooth muscle, which causes both coronary and peripheral dilation, is the basis for the drugs' ability to decrease ventricular afterload and cardiac work and to prevent coronary vasospasm.

Calcium channel blockers alleviate symptoms of resting angina by relieving coronary artery spasm thus increasing myocardial oxygen supply. In angina of effort the beneficial effect appears to be due to both reduced myocardial oxygen demand and improved myocardial perfusion.

Clinically important differences among the calcium channel blockers, e.g. their effects on myocardial contractility, cardiac conduction and the peripheral circulation, influence the selection of a particular agent.

TRADE NAMES

Diltiazem: *Cardizem*; *Vasocardol*.
Nifedipine: *Adalat*; *Anpine*.
Verapamil: *Anpec*; *Cordilox*; *Isoptin*.

PHARMACOKINETICS

Diltiazem, nifedipine and verapamil are all absorbed from the gastrointestinal tract. All undergo extensive metabolism in the liver and are eliminated by the kidneys, mainly as metabolites.

USES

Calcium channel blockers are administered orally for the prophylactic treatment of angina.

Nifedipine is the calcium channel blocker of choice in patients with co-existing heart failure because of its greater effect on the peripheral circulation and afterload. The usual dose is one or two 10 mg capsules three to four times a day.

Both verapamil and diltiazem have a negative inotropic effect and should be avoided in patients with heart failure.

The usual dose of diltiazem used for the treatment of angina is 60–90 mg three to four times a day and of verapamil 40–80 mg three to four times a day.

ADVERSE DRUG REACTIONS

Nifedipine produces mild side effects as a result of its vasodilatory action. These include headache, flushing, dizziness, hypotension and leg oedema. Nausea and vomiting are less common.

Adverse reactions to diltiazem include headache, dizziness, hypotension, nausea and rash.

Verapamil is usually well tolerated. More common reactions include constipation, flushing, headache and dizziness.

DRUG INTERACTIONS

Verapamil and diltiazem increase plasma levels of digoxin and cyclosporin. Serum drug levels and the patient's clinical response will need to be monitored. The hypotensive effects of antihypertensive drugs may be potentiated by all calcium channel blockers.

PRECAUTIONS AND CONTRAINDICATIONS

Caution should be observed when β blocking drugs are used in conjunction with verapamil or diltiazem, as congestive cardiac failure, arrhythmias and severe hypotension may occur.

The use of verapamil or diltiazem is contraindicated in patients with sick sinus syndrome, second or third degree AV block or congestive heart failure.

CARDIOVASCULAR DISEASES

12

NURSING IMPLICATIONS

ASSESSMENT

During acute attacks, the typical characteristics of angina pain must be distinguished from other types of chest pain.

The duration of a particular attack should be noted, since myocardial infarction can result from long periods of myocardial ischaemia.

Before prophylactic treatment begins cardiovascular status including heart rate, blood pressure and respiratory status should be documented.

ADMINISTRATION

Sublingual Nitrates

The time taken for the *tablets* to relieve pain should be noted.

Dosage may be repeated in a few minutes, up to a total of three tablets in 15 minutes, if relief is not obtained and the blood pressure is not compromised. The tablets should be administered with the patient in a recumbent position. When administering isosorbide dinitrate the 5 mg sublingual tablet should be selected.

The potency of sublingual nitrates may be affected by heat, moisture and light. The tablets should be stored in tightly closed, light occluding containers and kept in a cool, dry place. Expiry dates should be noted. It is recommended that glyceryl trinitrate tablets are discarded three months after opening the bottle.

With *metered dose aerosols* the dosage may be repeated after five minutes if pain relief has not occurred. No more than two metered doses are recommended. During administration the patient should be in the sitting position.

Oral Nitrates

Isosorbide dinitrate tablets should be given one hour before food. Isosorbide mononitrate tablets should not be crushed or chewed, however they can be halved. They should be given with half a glass of fluid.

Topical Nitrates

Transdermal patches are applied to a hairless area, usually the chest or upper arm, and the site rotated from day to day. If the application has been ordered for less than 24 hours per day, the time it is to be removed should be noted.

The ointment should be measured using the applicator paper provided and applied to the skin in a thin layer. It should not be rubbed in. Care should be taken by nursing staff to avoid contact of the ointment with their skin.

Intravenous Nitrates

Glyceryl trinitrate solution for intravenous use is not for direct intravenous injection. It must be diluted before use with 5% glucose or 0.9% sodium chloride solutions strictly in accordance with manufacturer's instructions. Dilution of intravenous solutions should be made only in glass parenteral solution bottles and polyethylene rather than PVC giving sets used as glyceryl trinitrate is absorbed into PVC. Dosage and flow rates require constant monitoring.

Calcium Channel Blockers

As calcium channel blockers are available in different strengths and dosage forms, care must be taken to select and administer the correct strength and dosage form. As the different dose forms have different absorption profiles, inappropriate substitution of one formulation for another can lead to harmful effects and/or delay in response, e.g. *two nifedipine 10 mg capsules are not equivalent to one 20 mg tablet.*

EVALUATION

Relief of chest pain during an acute attack must be documented together with the time taken to achieve relief and the number of tablets required. The occurrence of adverse effects and their acceptability to the patient should be noted.

Failure of *nitrates* to relieve chest pain may indicate that myocardial infarction is occurring and appropriate action must be taken. Recording of 12-lead ECGs during chest pain and recovery may be used to document the effects of nitrates. Regular monitoring of heart rate and blood pressure is recommended for patients on prophylactic treatment.

Patients receiving β *blocking drugs* should be observed for signs of bronchospasm or cardiac failure.

Patients receiving *nifedipine* may require periodic elevation of feet to relieve ankle oedema.

PATIENT EDUCATION

Patients receiving *nitrates* should be made aware of:

(a) the correct method of sublingual and aerosol administration;

(b) the need to carry sublingual or aerosol preparations at all times;

(c) the correct storage of tablets; and

(d) the correct method of applying topical preparations.

Patients receiving β *blocking drugs* should be made aware of:

(a) the early signs of cardiac failure (e.g. ankle swelling, reduced exercise tolerance) and respiratory problems (e.g. wheezing); and

(b) the need to notify their medical practitioner of these signs and if dizziness and tiredness are causing problems.

Patients receiving the *calcium channel blockers* should be made aware of:

(a) the need to modify diet or take stool softeners if verapamil is being taken.

All patients should be made aware of:

(a) side effects which may occur; and

(b) the problems caused by modifying or stopping treatment without medical advice.

CARDIOVASCULAR DISEASES

12

TREATMENT OF CONGESTIVE CARDIAC FAILURE

In congestive cardiac failure (CCF) a reduction in myocardial contractility is responsible for the inability of the heart to maintain adequate cardiac output when the body is at rest or undergoing normal activity. The major clinical symptoms and signs such as dyspnoea, orthopnoea, fatigue and weakness arise as a consequence of venous congestion and cardiac compensation. Drug therapy is aimed at improving myocardial contractility, reducing oedema and reducing the preload and afterload on the heart.

CARDIAC GLYCOSIDES

Digoxin

Digoxin is a cardiac glycoside. Its principal action is to increase the force of myocardial contraction. This increased force of contraction or positive inotropic action leads to increased cardiac output, decreased heart size, decreased venous pressure and consequent relief of oedema. Digoxin also slows the heart rate (negative chronotropic action) partly mediated by a direct effect on the vagus nerve and partly because of a reflex mediated reduction in rate due to improved cardiac output. In addition digoxin reduces conduction through the AV node which leads to protection of the ventricles from atrial tachyarrhythmias.

TRADE NAMES

Digoxin: *Lanoxin*.

PHARMACOKINETICS

About 75% to 80% of the administered dose is absorbed from tablets. Only small amounts are metabolised in the liver. It is eliminated principally as unchanged drug by the kidneys.

The elimination half-life is prolonged in patients with renal failure necessitating a reduction in dose in these patients. If plasma concentrations of the drug are to be determined, blood samples should be taken at least 6 hours after the daily dose.

USES

Digoxin is used for the treatment of congestive cardiac failure. As the therapeutic index (the margin between the therapeutic dose and the toxic dose) is narrow, the dosage has to be carefully adjusted to the needs of the individual patient. Factors which must be considered include patient's age, lean body mass and renal function.

If rapid digitalisation is required 500 micrograms to 1.5 mg may be given orally as a single dose or in three or four divided doses at intervals of four to six hours. (Digitalisation is the process of bringing a patient's blood concentration of digoxin to a therapeutic level). If there is not a need for rapid digitalisation, a loading dose is omitted and digitalisation is achieved slowly over a week with doses of 125–500 micrograms daily. The usual maintenance dose is 62.5–250 micrograms daily. In urgent cases digoxin can be administered intravenously for rapid digitalisation provided that the patient has not received digoxin during the preceding two weeks. The dose given is 125–250 micrograms at intervals of four to

six hours, to a total dose of 250 micrograms to 1 mg.

ADVERSE DRUG REACTIONS

The incidence of toxic effects is high due to the narrow therapeutic index. These effects include gastrointestinal disturbances such as nausea, vomiting, anorexia and diarrhoea, as well as cardiac symptoms such as sinus bradycardia, ectopic beats, bigeminy and ventricular fibrillation. Fatigue, headache, mental confusion and blurred or coloured vision are other effects which may occur.

Toxicity due to accumulation of digoxin is treated by:

1. withdrawal of the drug;

2. correction of hypokalaemia if present; and

3. use of antiarrhythmic drugs as indicated.

DRUG INTERACTIONS

The plasma levels of digoxin are increased by many other drugs including verapamil, diltiazem, quinidine and amiodarone. The absorption of digoxin can be reduced by the simultaneous administration of antacids or cholestyramine.

PRECAUTIONS AND CONTRAINDICATIONS

Digoxin toxicity may be induced by hypokalaemia, so potassium levels should be closely monitored in patients receiving concomitant diuretic and digoxin therapy. Smaller doses of digoxin hould be given when patients have reduced renal clearance.

The only absolute contraindication to digoxin use is toxicity due to cardiac glycosides.

DIURETICS

The volume of urine produced by the body is controlled by several factors. The most important mechanism involved is related to the amount of sodium reabsorbed through the proximal portion of the renal tubule.

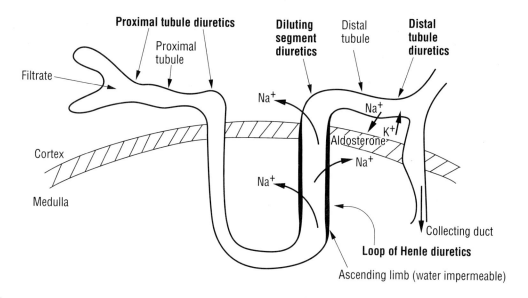

FIGURE 12.1 Diagrammatic representation of the renal tubule showing the main sites of action of various classes of diuretics. (Adapted from: Morgan, T.O. (1978), *Current Therapeutics* 19(1) p. 35.)

Increased reabsorption of sodium leads to increased reabsorption of water, resulting in decreased urine formation. Other important factors are acid–base balance, and the effects of aldosterone and antidiuretic hormone.

Diuretics act within the kidney to increase production of urine, usually by blocking the reabsorption of sodium. This leads to decreased reabsorption of water resulting in increased formation of urine and hence reduction in oedema.

The main sites of action of various classes of diuretics are shown in Figure 12.1.

Frusemide, Bumetanide, Ethacrynic Acid, Metolazone

The diuretics used most frequently to treat the oedema of cardiac failure are frusemide, bumetanide and ethacrynic acid. These act at the loop of Henle, as well as at most proximal sites. They are often referred to as 'loop diuretics'.

Metolazone which acts at both the diluting segment and proximal sites of the renal tubule is often used in conjunction with the loop diuretics when the oedema is refractory to treatment with the loop diuretics alone. Figure 12.1 shows the main sites of diuretic action. For further information on diuretics see section on use of diuretics in hypertension in this chapter.

TRADE NAMES

Frusemide: *Lasix*; *Uremide*; *Urex*.
Bumetanide: *Burinex*.
Ethacrynic acid: *Edecril*.
Metolazone: *Diulo*.

PHARMACOKINETICS

Frusemide, bumetanide and ethacrynic acid are all absorbed from the gastrointestinal tract and undergo metabolism in the liver. They and their metabolites are excreted primarily by the kidney with some biliary excretion also occurring.

Metolazone is absorbed from the gastrointestinal tract but does not undergo any significant metabolism. It is primarily excreted by the kidney with some biliary excretion also occurring.

USES

Loop diuretics are used orally for the treatment of oedema associated with cardiac failure. Frusemide and bumetanide can also be administered parenterally (intravenously or intramuscularly).

Frusemide has a wide therapeutic range (20–400 mg). In most cases 40 mg once daily suffices, however, this dose can be increased if no results are obtained. Daily doses greater than 120 mg are best divided into two or three doses. Once the oedema has begun to respond, the dose is adjusted to individual requirements.

Parenteral administration of frusemide in an initial dose of 20–40 mg is indicated whenever rapid diuretic action is required, when intestinal absorption is impaired or when oral administration is impossible.

Most patients respond to 1 mg of bumetanide administered as a single dose. If the response is not adequate, a second or third dose may be given at four to five hour intervals, up to a maximum of 10 mg in refractory patients. When administered parenterally, an initial dose of 0.5–1 mg is used.

Ethacrynic acid is used orally in doses of 50 mg, once or twice daily.

Metolazone is used in doses of 2.5–5 mg once daily to treat oedema. For maintenance therapy, the daily dose is reduced or administered every two to three days.

ADVERSE DRUG REACTIONS

Nausea, diarrhoea, fluid and electrolyte imbalance and muscle cramps are the most common side effects of diuretic therapy.

Potassium loss with its associated symptoms of weakness and lassitude may be marked. Replacement potassium therapy is commonly required. Increases in serum creatinine and uric acid levels may also occur. Transient deafness can result from loop diuretics, usually following the administration of large doses.

DRUG INTERACTIONS

Concomitant steroid therapy can increase the risk of hypokalaemia. Diuretics will potentiate the hypotensive action of antihypertensive agents. Administration with aminoglycosides may increase the risk of ototoxicity.

PRECAUTIONS AND CONTRAINDICATIONS

A high potassium diet or the addition of potassium supplement therapy is advisable with some diuretic therapy to prevent hypokalaemia, see section on diuretics in hypertension in this chapter.

When administered intravenously, frusemide and bumetanide should be given slowly.

Patients with prostatic hypertrophy must be observed for signs of urinary obstruction particularly after intravenous administration of diuretics. Diuretic therapy is contraindicated in anuric patients.

Spironolactone

The hormone aldosterone causes sodium retention at the distal portion of the renal tubule. Spironolactone is an aldosterone antagonist. It blocks the action of aldosterone causing a loss of sodium, a weak diuretic effect and retention of potassium.

TRADE NAMES

Spironolactone: *Aldactone.*

PHARMACOKINETICS

Spironolactone is absorbed from the gastrointestinal tract and is metabolised extensively by the liver. Spironolactone and its metabolites are excreted primarily by the kidneys with some biliary excretion also occurring.

USES

Spironolactone is used in the management of oedema associated with cardiac failure. It can also be used in combination with other diuretics when oedema is resistant to single therapy.

The dosage normally used is 25–200 mg per day in divided doses.

ADVERSE DRUG REACTIONS

Gastrointestinal symptoms, drowsiness and headache are among the adverse effects. Gynaecomastia may develop and is reversible on discontinuation of therapy.

DRUG INTERACTIONS

When used in conjunction with digoxin, spironolactone has been shown to increase the serum digoxin level.

PRECAUTIONS AND CONTRAINDICATIONS

As spironolactone conserves potassium, potassium supplements should be used with caution. The use of spironolactone is contraindicated in acute renal insufficiency, significant renal impairment and hyperkalaemia.

VASODILATORS

Vasodilators are used as an adjunct in the treatment of congestive cardiac failure. The reduction of afterload by arteriolar dilators causes a reduction in left ventricular end-diastolic pressure and oxygen consumption, while raising stroke volume and cardiac output. The reduction of preload by venodilators relieves pulmonary congestion. The vasodilators used include the angiotensin converting enzyme (ACE) inhibitors, captopril, enalapril and lisinopril, the direct acting vasodilator, hydralazine and the α_1 adrenergic blocking agent, prazosin.

ACE Inhibitors: Captopril, Enalapril, Lisinopril

Angiotensin converting enzyme inhibitors block the production of angiotensin II, a potent vasoconstrictor. By decreasing the production of angiotensin II vascular tone is reduced. In patients with cardiac failure reductions in total peripheral resistance and pulmonary vascular resistance occur and cardiac output is improved without a change in heart rate.

TRADE NAMES

Captopril: *Capoten*.
Enalapril: *Renitec*; *Amprace*.
Lisinopril: *Zestril*; *Prinivil*.

PHARMACOKINETICS

Captopril is rapidly absorbed from the gastrointestinal tract and is extensively metabolised. Captopril and its metabolites are excreted by the kidneys.

Enalapril is rapidly absorbed from the gastrointestinal tract and following absorption is rapidly and extensively metabolised to enalaprilat, the active form of the drug. It is excreted by the kidneys.

Lisinopril is absorbed from the gastrointestinal tract. It does not undergo metabolism and is excreted unchanged by the kidneys.

USES

Captopril, enalapril and lisinopril are administered orally for the treatment of congestive cardiac failure. Treatment is initiated with a low dose with the patient closely supervised to determine the initial effect on blood pressure. The dose is then gradually increased to a maintenance dose according to the patient's response.

The initial dose of captopril is 6.25 mg with a maintenance dose of 25–50 mg three times a day.

The initial dose of enalapril is 2.5 mg with a maintenance dose of 10–20 mg daily in a single or divided dose.

The initial dose of lisinopril is 2.5 mg once daily with a maintenance dose of 5–20 mg per day administered in a single daily dose.

ADVERSE DRUG REACTIONS

Taste disturbances, rash, gastrointestinal disturbances and hypotension are among the adverse effects of ACE inhibitors. Persistant cough occurs in about 5% of patients.

Proteinuria, neutropenia and agranulocytosis have been reported, primarily in patients with pre-existing renal impairment.

DRUG INTERACTIONS

Hypotension is potentiated when antihypertensives and ACE inhibitors are used concurrently. Hyperkalaemia can result if ACE inhibitors and potassium supplements or potassium sparing agents are used together.

PRECAUTIONS AND CONTRAINDICATIONS

ACE inhibitors should be used with caution in patients with renal impairment because of the possibility of neutropenia, agranulocytosis or proteinuria occurring.

They should also be used with caution in patients with sodium depletion, hypovolaemia and those undergoing dialysis as severe hypotension can occur.

Hydralazine

Hydralazine reduces peripheral resistance and blood pressure as a result of a direct vasodilatory effect on vascular smooth muscle. The effect on the arterioles is greater than that on the venous system. Hydralazine markedly decreases systemic vascular resistance and increases cardiac output in patients with congestive cardiac failure.

TRADE NAMES

Hydralazine: *Apresoline*; *Alphapress*.

PHARMACOKINETICS

Hydralazine is rapidly absorbed from the gastrointestinal tract and is extensively metabolised in the gastrointestinal mucosa during absorption and in the liver. Some patients metabolise the drug at a slower rate, they are termed 'slow acetylators'. The drug and metabolites are rapidly excreted by the kidneys.

USES

Hydralazine is used in conjunction with other therapy in the treatment of congestive cardiac failure. The dosage used is initially 50 mg three times a day with adjustment according to individual response and requirement.

ADVERSE DRUG REACTIONS

Headache, flushing and tachycardia are common at commencement of therapy. However, these are usually transient and dose related.

Vomiting, oedema, urticaria and skin rashes have also been reported. A syndrome resembling acute systemic lupus erythematosus (SLE) has occurred in patients receiving doses of more than 200 mg daily for prolonged periods.

DRUG INTERAC IONS

Hypotension may occur when monoamine oxidase inhibitors (MAOIs), tricyclic antidepressants or antihypertensive agents are used concurrently with hydralazine.

PRECAUTIONS AND CONTRAINDICATIONS

Hydralazine should be used with caution in patients who are slow acetylators or have decreased renal function as they are more at risk of developing drug induced SLE.

Prazosin

Prazosin produces both arteriolar and venous dilation as a result of its selective, competitive inhibition of α_1 adrenergic receptors. In patients with congestive cardiac failure prazosin decreases systemic blood pressure, systemic vascular resistance and pulmonary vascular resistance and increases cardiac output.

TRADE NAMES

Prazosin: *Minipress*; *Pressin*.

PHARMACOKINETICS

Prazosin is absorbed from the gastrointestinal tract and is extensively metabolised in the liver. It is primarily eliminated via the bile and faeces.

USES

Prazosin is used in combination with other drugs in the treatment of congestive cardiac failure. Initial doses of 0.5–4 mg daily in divided doses are used and the dosage carefully titrated to maintenance therapy doses of 4–20 mg daily in divided doses.

ADVERSE DRUG REACTIONS

Postural hypotension, palpitations, dizziness and drowsiness are the most commonly reported side effects. Urinary frequency, oedema and diaphoresis can also occur.

DRUG INTERACTIONS

Concomitant use of antihypertensives can result in hypotension.

PRECAUTIONS AND CONTRAINDICATIONS

Caution should be exercised when initiating therapy or when rapidly increasing the dose, as excessive postural hypotension may occur resulting in syncope and loss of consciousness. The first dose should be given either under observation or in the evening when the patient is lying in bed.

NURSING IMPLICATIONS

ASSESSMENT

A baseline of cardiac function including apex rate, peripheral pulse rate, rhythm and quality of the pulse wave, degree of oedema, urine output, weight, electrolyte status and blood pressure should all be assessed before treatment begins.

ADMINISTRATION

Digoxin

Digoxin therapy should be withheld when the heart rate, measured at the apex, is less than 60 beats per minute counted over one full minute. Any change of rate of rhythm should be noted.

Great care should be taken to administer the correct dose for individual patients, given the range of strengths and similarity of names of different preparations. Particular care is essential when giving the drug to children. The drug is best given after food to reduce local gastrointestinal irritation. When administering parenterally,

slow intravenous infusion is the preferred route. It should be given over a period of at least five minutes. Digoxin injection may be added to 5% dextrose, 0.9% sodium chloride or 4% dextrose plus 0.18% sodium chloride infusion fluids.

Diuretics

Diuretics are best given in the early part of the day because of the increase in urine output, time of onset of action and duration of action. If divided doses are prescribed, it is advisable to give the second dose during the early afternoon. They are best given after or with food to minimise gastrointestinal irritation. When administering frusemide or bumetanide intravenously, administration should be over one to two minutes. Intravenous infusion over 30–60 minutes is used for large doses.

ACE Inhibitors

Captopril should be given one hour before food for maximum absorption.

Blood pressure monitoring is essential after the first dose of all vasodilating agents.

EVALUATION

The therapeutic effects of all agents used to treat congestive cardiac failure are decreased respiratory difficulty, peripheral oedema and tiredness and increased pulse volume and urinary output, as well as other signs of improved cardiac function such as mental alertness and exercise tolerance. The patient's appetite should improve and nausea disappear as congestion of the gastrointestinal blood vessels decreases.

Evaluation of digoxin toxicity can be difficult because of the similarity of the features of congestive cardiac failure and digoxin toxicity.

Gastrointestinal disturbances apparent before digoxin therapy may not indicate toxicity, but an initial improvement followed by anorexia, nausea or vomiting, is likely to be drug related. Digoxin serum levels are useful in assessing toxicity. All new rhythm disturbances should be investigated and any visual disturbances noted.

Patients should be observed for signs of dehydration if diuresis is excessive.

PATIENT EDUCATION

Patients treated with *digoxin* should be taught how to count peripheral pulse rates and should be made aware of signs of digoxin toxicity. They should be told of the different strengths of tablets available and of the need to take the correct dose. The distinction between generic and trade names should be made to avoid double dosing by the patient.

Patients treated with *diuretics* should be made aware that increased urine output is the expected and desired effect of diuretics. They should be informed of the time to onset and duration of action of the diuretic to enable them to determine the regimen which best suits their daily routine. The importance of a potassium rich diet and the correct method of taking potassium supplements should be emphasised when applicable.

Patients taking *vasodilators* should be alerted to the possibility of hypotension, e.g. lightheadedness and dizziness, occurring with the use of this therapy.

All patients should be alerted to the side effects which may occur with their medication. The need for compliance with their medication regimen and also of any fluid restriction they may require should be stressed. Patients should be made aware of the early signs of recurring congestive cardiac failure such as ankle swelling and reduced exercise tolerance.

TREATMENT OF HYPERTENSION ████████

Hypertension causes an increased risk of myocardial infarction, heart failure, stroke and renal failure and is associated with reduced life expectancy. Treatment is aimed at modifying the three major systems which determine the level of blood pressure: the blood volume, the cardiac output, and peripheral resistance to blood flow.

The use of non-pharmacological measures to reduce hypertension is worthwhile. Cessation of smoking, weight reduction, regular exercise, reduction of alcohol intake to two to three drinks per day and salt restriction are all positive methods of reducing elevated blood presssure without the use of drugs.

The selection of an appropriate drug may be influenced by many factors including severity of hypertension, age and concomitant diseases. Combinations of antihypertensive agents permit control of blood pressure with lower dosage of individual agents and a subsequent reduction in side effects. This reduction in side effects is important, as many patients have asymptomatic hypertension and adverse drug reactions may result in non-motivated patients discontinuing their therapy.

The mechanisms by which drugs exert an antihypertensive effect are diverse and many drugs are used as first-line treatment.

ACE INHIBITORS

Captopril, Enalpril, Fosinopril, Lisinopril, Ramipril, Perindopril, Quinapril

Angiotensin converting enzyme (ACE) inhibitors are thought to lower blood pressure primarily through suppression of the production of angiotensin II, a potent vasoconstrictor. The arterial and possibly venous dilation which occurs results in a decrease in total peripheral resistance with no change or an increase in heart rate, stroke volume, or cardiac output. The decrease in angiotensin ll production also leads to a reduction in aldosterone secretion. This results in decreased sodium and water retention which may contribute to the hypotensive action.

TRADE NAMES

Captopril: *Capoten.*
Enalapril: *Renitec*; *Amprace.*
Fosinopril: *Monopril.*
Lisinopril: *Zestril*; *Prinivil.*
Ramipril: *Tritace*; *Ramace.*
Perindopril: *Coversyl.*
Quinapril: *Accupril*; *Asig.*

PHARMACOKINETICS

In addition to the ACE inhibitors previously discussed under treatment of congestive cardiac failure, there are several other ACE inhibitors used in the treatment of hypertension.

Fosinopril is slowly absorbed from the gastrointestinal tract and is metabolised in the gastrointestinal mucosa and liver to fosinoprilat, the active form of the drug. It is excreted by the kidneys and in the faeces.

Ramipril is absorbed from the gastrointestinal tract and is metabolised in the liver to ramiprilat, the active form of the drug. It is excreted by the kidneys.

Perindopril is rapidly absorbed from the gastrointestinal tract and is metabolised in the liver, to perindoprilat, the active form of the drug. It is excreted by the kidneys.

Quinapril is absorbed from the gastrointestinal tract and metabolised to quinaprilat, an active metabolite. It is primarily excreted by the kidneys with some faecal excretion occurring.

USES

The dosage of ACE inhibitors used in the treatment of hypertension is usually higher than that used in the treatment of congestive cardiac failure. Treatment is initiated with a low dose and the dose titrated against the blood pressure.

Usual maintenance doses of ACE inhibitors in the treatment of hypertension are listed in Table 12.2.

TABLE 12.2 Maintenance doses of ACE inhibitors in hypertension

Drug	Dosage
Captopril	50 mg twice daily one hour before food
Enalapril	10–40 mg daily in one or two divided doses
Lisinopril	10–20 mg daily in a single dose
Fosinopril	20–40 mg daily in a single dose
Ramipril	5–10 mg daily in a single dose swallowed whole with water during or after meals
Perindopril	4–8 mg daily in a single dose before meals
Quinapril	10–40 mg daily in a single dose before meals

For adverse drug reactions, drug interactions, precautions and contraindications see ACE inhibitors in the section on treatment of congestive cardiac failure in this chapter.

CALCIUM CHANNEL BLOCKERS

Diltiazem, Nifedipine, Verapamil, Amlodipine, Felodipine

Calcium channel blockers inhibit the contractile process of vascular smooth muscle, thereby dilating the systemic arteries. This dilation results in a decrease in total peripheral resistance and a lowering of systemic blood pressure.

TRADE NAMES

Diltiazem: *Cardizem*; *Vasocardol.*
Nifedipine: *Adalat*; *Anpine.*
Verapamil: *Anpec*; *Cordilox*; *Isoptin.*
Felodipine: *Agon*; *Plendil.*
Amlodipine: *Norvasc.*

CARDIOVASCULAR DISEASES

12

TABLE 12.3   Maintenance doses of calcium channel blockers in hypertension

Drug	Dosage
Diltiazem tablets	60–120 mg three times daily
Diltiazem SR capsules	90–120 mg twice daily swallowed whole
Nifedipine tablets	20–40 mg twice daily
Verapamil tablets	80–160 mg two or three times daily
Verapamil SR capsules	160–240 mg once daily swallowed whole
Verapamil SR tablets	240 mg once or twice daily swallowed whole
Felodipine tablets	5–10 mg twice daily
Felodipine ER tablets	10–20 mg once daily, taken whole with water
Amlodipine	2.5–10 mg once daily

USES

The calcium channel blockers diltiazem, nifedipine and verapamil previously discussed in the section on prevention of angina are all used in the treatment of hypertension. However, there are different formulations of the drugs available to treat hypertension and care must be taken to select the correct formulation, as the different dosage forms are not interchangeable.

In addition to these agents amlodipine and felodipine are used in the treatment of hypertension. Both are absorbed from the gastrointestinal tract and are extensively metabolised in the liver. Excretion is mainly by the kidneys with some faecal excretion also occurring.

The usual maintenance doses of calcium channel blockers for the treatment of hypertension are listed in Table 12.3.

For information on pharmacokinetics, adverse drug reactions, precautions and contraindications see the section on calcium channel blockers in the prevention of angina. The adverse effects of felodipine are similar to those of nifedipine.

ADRENERGIC RECEPTOR BLOCKING AGENTS

β Blocking Drugs: Atenolol, Metoprolol, Oxprenolol, Pindolol, Propranolol, Timolol

Although the precise mechanism of the hypotensive action of β blocking drugs has not been determined it is postulated that they reduce blood pressure by blocking peripheral adrenergic receptors (decreasing cardiac output), decreasing sympathetic outflow from the central nervous system, and/or suppressing renin release.

TRADE NAMES

Atenolol: *Noten*; *Tenormin*.
Metoprolol: *Betaloc*; *Lopressor*.
Oxprenolol: *Corbeton*; *Trasicor*.
Pindolol: *Barbloc*; *Visken*.
Propranolol: *Deralin*; *Inderal*.
Timolol: *Blocadren*.

USES

The usual maintenance doses of β blocking agents used in the treatment of hypertension are listed in Table 12.4.

For information on pharmacokinetics, adverse drug reactions, precautions and

TABLE 12.4 Maintenance doses of β blocking drugs in hypertension

Drug	Dosage
Cardioselective	
Atenolol	50–100 mg once daily
Metoprolol	100–450 mg in one or two divided doses
Non-selective	
Oxprenolol	160–320 mg in two or three divided doses
Pindolol	10–30 mg in two or three divided doses
Propranolol	160–480 mg in two or three divided doses
Timolol	20–40 mg in two divided doses

contraindications see section on β blocking drugs in prevention of angina.

α and β Receptor Blocking Agents: Labetalol

Labetalol is a non-selective β blocking drug and a selective α_1 adrenergic blocking agent. It produces a decrease in systemic arterial blood pressure and systemic vascular resistance without a substantial reduction in heart rate or cardiac output.

TRADE NAMES

Labetalol: *Presolol*; *Trandate*.

PHARMACOKINETICS

Labetalol is rapidly absorbed from the gastrointestinal tract and is extensively metabolised in the liver and in the gastrointestinal tract. Labetalol and its metabolites are excreted by the kidneys and in the faeces.

USES

Labetalol is used orally in the treatment of hypertension. The usual maintenance dose is 200–400 mg twice daily.

ADVERSE DRUG REACTIONS

Dizziness, headache, lethargy, eye irritation, skin rashes and tingling of the scalp have been reported. Bronchospasm may occur in susceptible individuals.

PRECAUTIONS AND CONTRAINDICATIONS

The same precautions and contraindications apply as for β blocking drugs.

Post-Synaptic α Blocker: Prazosin

Prazosin blocks α_1 receptors causing vasodilation of both the arteriolar and venous systems, resulting in a reduction in peripheral vascular resistance and blood pressure.

The maintenance dose of prazosin used in the treatment of hypertension is 6–15 mg daily in two or three divided doses.

For further information see section on use of prazosin in the treatment of congestive cardiac failure.

CENTRALLY ACTING DRUGS

Methyldopa

The mechanism of the hypotensive action of methyldopa is a reduction of sympathetic outflow from the central nervous system. A decrease in peripheral resistance occurs.

TRADE NAMES

Methyldopa: *Aldomet*; *Hydopa*.

PHARMACOKINETICS

Methyldopa is partly absorbed from the gastrointestinal tract and is extensively metabolised in the gastrointestinal tract and the liver. It is excreted by the kidneys.

USES

Methyldopa is used orally in the treatment of hypertension. The recommended oral dosage range is 250 mg to 3 g daily in two or three divided doses. An intravenous preparation is also available.

ADVERSE DRUG REACTIONS

Drowsiness occurs during initial treatment and when the dose is increased.

Headache, weakness, nasal stuffiness, impotence, dry mouth and bradycardia are other early reactions. Orthostatic hypotension may occur and is an indication for dosage reduction. Haemolytic anaemia is a rare complication.

DRUG INTERACTIONS

Phenothiazines and tricyclic antidepressants may reduce the hypotensive effects of methyldopa therapy.

PRECAUTIONS AND CONTRAINDICATIONS

Methyldopa should be used with caution in patients with a history of liver disease and is contraindicated in patients with acute hepatic disease.

Acquired haemolytic anaemia has occurred rarely in association with methyldopa therapy. Haemoglobin and/or haematocrit determinations should be performed if clinical symptoms indicate the possibility of anaemia.

Clonidine

Clonidine stimulates α_2 adrenergic receptors in the central nervous system causing inhibition of sympathetic outflow. This reduces both peripheral vascular resistance and cardiac output, resulting in a lowering of blood pressure.

TRADE NAMES

Clonidine: *Catapres.*

PHARMACOKINETICS

Clonidine is well absorbed from the gastrointestinal tract and undergoes metabolism in the liver. Excretion is mainly by the kidneys but significant faecal excretion also occurs.

USES

Clonidine is used both orally and parenterally in the management of hypertension. Oral maintenance doses normally used are 150–300 micrograms two to three times a day.

ADVERSE DRUG REACTIONS

Drowsiness, dry mouth, nausea, vomiting and constipation are the most common adverse effects. Rebound hypertension has been associated with sudden withdrawal of the drug. Patients should be advised not to alter their dosage or run out of tablets.

DRUG INTERACTIONS

Clonidine may potentiate the actions of central nervous system depressants such as alcohol, opiates or other analgesics, sedatives or anaesthetics. Tricyclic antidepressants may decrease the hypotensive effect of clonidine.

PRECAUTIONS AND CONTRAINDICATIONS

Termination of oral therapy should be gradual (over more than seven days) as sudden cessation is associated with rebound hypertension. Clonidine is contraindicated in patients with sick sinus syndrome.

DIRECTLY ACTING VASODILATORS

The mechanism of action of this group of drugs is to produce vasodilation resulting in a drop in blood pressure.

Hydralazine

Hydralazine has a direct vasodilatory effect on vascular smooth muscle; the effect on arterioles is greater than on veins. The decrease in blood pressure is accompanied by an increase in heart rate, cardiac output and stroke volume, probably because of a reflex response to decreased peripheral resistance.

The oral maintenance dosage used for treatment of hypertension is usually 200 mg daily in two divided doses.

Hydralazine is also administered parenterally in the treatment of hypertensive emergency, see Chapter 32 Drugs Used in Critical Care and Chapter 20 Drug Therapy in Pregnancy and Labour.

For information on pharmacokinetics, adverse drug reactions, precautions and contraindications see section on treatment of congestive cardiac failure.

Minoxidil

Minoxidil selectively relaxes arteriolar smooth muscle causing a reduction in peripheral resistance and systemic blood pressure.

TRADE NAMES

Minoxidil: *Loniten*.

PHARMACOKINETICS

Minoxidil is rapidly absorbed from the gastrointestinal tract and is metabolised in the liver. Minoxidil and its metabolites are excreted by the kidneys.

USES

Minoxidil is used as adjunctive therapy in patients with severe hypertension failing to respond to multiple therapy.

The usual maintenance dose is 5–40 mg daily in two or three divided doses.

ADVERSE DRUG REACTIONS

Dermatological reactions including hirsutism (occurring in 50%–70% of patients), pruritus and rashes, and cardiovascular reactions, including pericarditis, pericardial effusions, tachycardia, salt and water retention and ECG changes, are the most common side effects.

DRUG INTERACTIONS

The hypotensive effect is potentiated when minoxidil is administered with other antihypertensive agents.

PRECAUTIONS AND CONTRAINDICATIONS

Patients with renal failure or undergoing dialysis should be closely supervised to prevent exacerbation of renal failure due to the salt and water retention caused by minoxidil.

Minoxidil is contraindicated in phaeochromocytoma.

DIURETICS

Diuretics were formerly used as first-line treatment in mild to moderate hypertension but now tend to be used in combination with other agents.

The doses and onset and duration of action of some common diuretics are listed in Table 12.5.

TABLE 12.5 Dose ranges and onset and duration of action of some common diuretics

Drug	Dosage	Onset of Action	Duration of Action
Amiloride	5–10 mg	2 h	10 h
Bendrofluazide	2.5–10 mg	2 h	12 h
Bumetanide	1–10 mg	30 min	4 h
Chlorothiazide	0.25–1 g	2 h	10 h
Chlorthalidone	25–100 mg	2 h	24 h
Cyclopenthiazide	0.25–1 mg	2 h	12 h
Ethacrynic acid	50–400 mg	20 min	6 h
Frusemide (low dose)	20–80 mg oral	15 min	4 h
	20–100 mg IV	2 min	2 h
Frusemide (high dose)	0.5–2 g oral	15 min	4 h
	0.25–2 g IV	2 min	2 h
Hydrochlorothiazide	25–100 mg	2 h	6 h
Indapamide	2.5–5 mg	2 h	14 h
Methyclothiazide	2.5–10 mg	2 h	12 h
Spironolactone	25–400 mg	24 h	72 h
Triamterene	100–200 mg	2 h	10 h

Thiazide Diuretics: Chlorothiazide, Bendrofluazide, Hydrochlorothiazide, Methyclothiazide, Cyclopenthiazide, Chlorthalidone

Thiazide diuretics inhibit sodium reabsorption at the diluting segment of the ascending limb of the renal tubule (see Figure 12.1). They also have an antihypertensive effect independent of the diuretic effect. This is thought to be due to direct arteriolar dilation. The thiazide diuretics commonly used include chlorothiazide, bendrofluazide, hydrochlorothiazide, methyclothiazide and cyclopenthiazide. Chlorthalidone is a diuretic pharmacologically similar to the thiazides.

TRADE NAMES

Chlorothiazide: *Chlotride.*
Bendrofluazide: *Aprinox.*
Methyclothiazide: *Enduron.*
Cyclopenthiazide: *Navidrex.*
Chlorthalidone: *Hygroton.*
Hydrochlorothiazide: *Dichlotride.*

PHARMACOKINETICS

Thiazides are absorbed from the gastrointestinal tract and are excreted by the kidneys mainly unchanged.

USES

Thiazides are used alone or in combination with other antihypertensives to treat hypertension. The doses used are listed in Table 12.6.

ADVERSE DRUG REACTIONS

Hypokalaemia, increases in plasma uric acid and glucose levels and increases in serum cholesterol and triglyceride levels are adverse effects associated with thiazide therapy. Nausea, vomiting, abdominal cramps and rash can also occur.

DRUG INTERACTIONS

The hyperglycaemic effect of the thiazides may reduce the diabetic control of antidiabetic agents. The use of thiazides in combination with lithium therapy may result in lithium toxicity. The use of concurrent thiazide and corticosteroid therapy will exacerbate potassium depletion.

PRECAUTIONS AND CONTRAINDICATIONS

Thiazides should be used with caution in patients with severe renal disease and are contraindicated in patients with anuria.

Care must be taken to avoid hypokalaemia in patients on digoxin therapy. Thiazides are contraindicated in patients allergic to sulfonamides.

Non-Thiazide Diuretics: Indapamide

The drugs principal site of action is the cortical diluting segment of the distal tubule.

TRADE NAMES

Indapamide: *Dapa-Tabs*; *Natrilix.*

PHARMACOKINETICS

Indapamide is rapidly and completely absorbed from the gastrointestinal tract. It is extensively metabolised in the liver and is excreted mainly as metabolites, primarily by the kidneys with some biliary excretion.

USES

Indapamide is used orally in the treatment of hypertension. The dosage used is 2.5 mg as a single daily dose.

TABLE 12.6 Doses of thiazide diuretics in hypertension

Drug	Dosage
Chlorothiazide	250 mg–1 g once daily
Bendrofluazide	2.5–10 mg once daily
Methyclothiazide	2.5–10 mg once daily
Cyclopenthiazide	0.25–0.5 mg once daily
Chlorthalidone	25–50 mg once daily
Hydrochlorothiazide	25–50 mg once daily

ADVERSE DRUG REACTIONS

Electrolyte changes are the most common side effects. These include hypokalaemia, hyponatraemia and hypochloraemia. Other adverse effects include headache and dizziness.

DRUG INTERACTIONS

No interactions have been reported between indapamide and oral hypoglycaemic agents, anticoagulants, uricosurics and anti-inflammatory agents.

PRECAUTIONS AND CONTRAINDICATIONS

Caution should be used in treating patients with severe hepatic disease. Treatment should be discontinued if increasing azotaemia and oliguria occur in patients with impaired renal function.

Potassium Sparing Diuretics: Amiloride, Triamterene

Amiloride and triamterene act directly on the distal renal tubule to inhibit sodium–potassium ion exchange. As their diuretic effect is weak they are usually used for their potassium sparing effects in combination with other more effective diuretics. Two combination products, hydrochlorothiazide–amiloride, and hydrochlorothiazide–triamterene, are available.

TRADE NAMES

Amiloride: *Kaluril*; *Midamor*.
Triamterene: *Dytac*.
Hydrochlorothiazide–amiloride: *Moduretic*.
Hydrochlorothiazide–triamterene: *Dyazide*.

PHARMACOKINETICS

Amiloride and triamterene are absorbed from the gastrointestinal tract and triamterene is metabolised in the liver. Both amiloride and triamterene are excreted by the kidneys with faecal elimination of amiloride also occurring.

USES

Both amiloride and triamterene are administered orally. The usual doses are amiloride 5 mg once daily and triamterene 100 mg daily.

ADVERSE DRUG REACTIONS

Nausea, abdominal pain, headache and rash are side effects associated with the use of these drugs. Hyperkalaemia can occur especially in renal failure or when potassium supplements are used. Hyponatraemia can also occur.

DRUG INTERACTIONS

The use of these agents with ACE inhibitors can increase the risk of hyperkalaemia. The concurrent use of lithium may result in lithium toxicity.

PRECAUTIONS AND CONTRAINDICATIONS

Amiloride and triamterene should be used with caution in patients with hepatic insufficiency and are contraindicated in patients with renal insufficiency. They should be used with caution in diabetic patients as these patients are more sensitive to changes in serum potassium.

POTASSIUM SUPPLEMENTS

Potassium supplements are added to some diuretic therapies to compensate for the loss of potassium.

Potassium Chloride

TRADE NAMES

Potassium chloride: *Span K*; *Slow K*; *Chlorvescent*; *Kay Ciel*.

PHARMACOKINETICS

Potassium chloride is absorbed from the gastrointestinal tract. Slow release preparations allow for a gradual release of the drug over a large segment of the intestine. It is eliminated by the kidneys.

USES

Potassium chloride is administered orally in the form of slow release tablets (*Span K, Slow K*), effervescent tablets (*Chlorvescent*) or in solution (*Kay Ciel*). The dosage is adjusted according to individual requirements. In cases of severe potassium depletion, the potassium chloride can be administered by intravenous infusion.

ADVERSE REACTIONS

Oral potassium preparations can cause nausea, vomiting, abdominal pain and diarrhoea. Intravenous infusion can cause pain at the site of injection and phlebitis. Rapid intravenous administration can cause serious cardiac arrhythmias and cardiac arrest, see Chapter 14 Drugs Used in Renal Failure.

DRUG INTERACTIONS

The concurrent use of potassium supplements with potassium sparing diuretics or ACE inhibitors can lead to hyperkalaemia. Hypokalaemia will not be reversed by potassium if bicarbonate is given concurrently.

PRECAUTIONS AND CONTRAINDICATIONS

Because of the possibility of potassium chloride causing gastrointestinal irritation it should be used with caution in patients with a history of peptic ulcer. Potassium chloride is contraindicated in patients with marked renal failure.

NURSING IMPLICATIONS

ASSESSMENT

Establishment of the baseline arterial pressure is essential for monitoring the effects of antihypertensive drugs. Because of the many different drugs used to treat high blood pressure, nursing staff must check on the adverse effects of, and precautions to be taken with, each drug. It should be remembered that elderly patients are more likely to suffer from adverse effects.

ADMINISTRATION

Antihypertensive Therapy
Antihypertensive therapy should be initiated with small doses and the dose titrated according to the patient's re-

sponse. Therapy should not be ceased suddenly. The availability of different strengths and dosage forms for many drugs makes selection and administration of the correct dose and form most important as dosage forms are often not interchangeable.

Potassium Supplements
Enteric coated potassium chloride tablets must be swallowed whole, with a glass of water. Effervescent tablets should be dissolved in water or fruit juice, and the liquid dosage form diluted in a glass of water or fruit juice, prior to administration. All dosage forms should be given with or after food.

Intravenous administration of potassium chloride must be by intravenous infusion in a diluted form. The concentration of the solution should not exceed 80 mmol/L and the rate of infusion should not exceed 30 mmol/hour; 5% glucose, 0.9% sodium chloride or glucose plus sodium chloride infusion fluids may be used.

EVALUATION

Evaluation of a patient's response to antihypertensive therapy involves monitoring both arterial pressure and the occurrence of adverse drug reactions.

Arterial presssure must be recorded accurately and under reproducible conditions. The patient should rest for about 10 minutes before the pressure is measured. Recordings taken in the lying, sitting and standing positions will allow for evaluation of postural hypotension. This problem which manifests as dizziness or faintness on rising, can be minimised by instructing the patient to sit and then stand slowly. Depending on the policy of the individual institution it may be necessary to measure the blood pressure before the administration of each dose. Patients should be observed for signs of hypotension. Persistent hypotension should be reported as there may be a need to adjust the dosage of the antihypertensive agent.

Nurses should be alert for the adverse reactions reported for each drug, especially bronchospasm in patients taking β blocking agents. They should also be aware that rebound hypertension may occur if the antihypertensive drugs are withdrawn or the dosage decreased suddenly.

PATIENT EDUCATION

The medical consequences of uncontrolled hypertension, and the need to take medication regularly and to have regular medical checks, should be stressed to the patient. Family support is helpful in establishing a regular dosage regimen which will enhance compliance.

Risk factor modification through cessation of smoking, weight reduction, reduction of alcohol intake, salt restriction and regular exercise, should also be part of the patient's education.

The patient should be made aware of the adverse effects they may encounter. They should be told that therapy should not be stopped suddenly and advised to contact their medical practitioner if the adverse effects are unacceptable as a different drug therapy can be substituted.

Patients should be advised particularly of the hypotension which may occur with the first dose of antihypertensive agents. Patients commencing therapy with methyldopa or clonidine should be told of the drowsiness which can occur on commencement of therapy and advised to take caution when driving and/or operating machinery.

Patients taking minoxidil should be advised to limit their salt intake and of the need to comply with their diuretic regimen, as salt and water retention may diminish the effectiveness of minoxidil therapy.

CARDIOVASCULAR DISEASES

12

TREATMENT OF CARDIAC ARRHYTHMIAS

A cardiac arrhythmia is a disturbance of the normal rhythm of the heart. This condition may be brought about by abnormal SA node rhythm, ectopic foci generating premature beats or pacemaker shifts, circus movements or conduction blocks.

ANTIARRHYTHMIC AGENTS

Antiarryhthmic drugs can be divided into four classes according to their mechanism of action.

Class I drugs *cause sodium channel blockade* and are divided into three groups. Class IA drugs, e.g. quinidine, procainamide and disopyramide, cause moderate phase-O depression, slow conduction and usually prolong repolarisation. Class IB drugs, e.g. lignocaine, mexilitene and phenytoin, cause minimal phase-O depression, slow conduction and usually shorten repolarisation. Class IC

drugs, e.g. flecainide, cause marked phase-O depression, slow conduction and have little effect on repolarisation.

Class II drugs, e.g. propranolol, atenolol and esmolol, *cause β adrenergic blockade* thus inhibiting the effects of the sympathetic nervous system on the heart.

Class III drugs, e.g. amiodarone, bretylium and sotalol, *prolong repolarisation* by widening the entire action potential which increases refractoriness.

Class IV drugs, e.g. verapamil, *cause calcium channel blockade* by antagonising calcium influxes through slow channels during phase 2 of the action potential.

Quinidine

Quinidine, a class IA agent, decreases the excitability of the cardiac muscle and depresses conduction velocity and myocardial contractility.

TRADE NAMES

Quinidine: *Quinidoxin*; *Kinidin Durules*.

PHARMACOKINETICS

Quinidine is absorbed from the gastrointestinal tract and is metabolised in the liver. Quinidine and its metabolites are excreted by the kidneys.

USES

Quinidine is used orally in the treatment of a wide range of atrial and ventricular arrhythmias. The doses normally used are 200–300 mg of conventional tablets (*Quinidoxin*) every four hours or 500–750 mg twice a day of a long acting preparation (*Kinidin Durules*).

ADVERSE DRUG REACTIONS

The incidence of adverse drug effects is high. Diarrhoea, nausea and vomiting are the most common. Tinnitus and dizziness and hypersensitivity reactions including rash, haemolytic anaemia, thrombocytopenia and drug fever, can also occur. Cardiotoxic effects include conduction defects, ventricular tachycardia or flutter and complete AV block.

DRUG INTERACTIONS

Quinidine may increase the effect of oral anticoagulants. Digoxin plasma levels are increased by the concurrent administration of quinidine and digoxin toxicity may result. The dose of digoxin should be halved if quinidine is also being given. Used in high doses quinidine can potentiate the hypotensive effects of antihypertensive agents. Concomitant administration of amiodarone, cimetidine or verapamil will increase serum quinidine concentrations.

PRECAUTIONS AND CONTRAINDICATIONS

Quinidine should be used with caution in patients with digoxin toxicity, congestive cardiac failure or pre-existing hypotension. The use of quinidine is contraindicated in patients with AV block in the absence of a pacemaker, previous or current thrombocytopenia, or a previous hypersensitivity reaction to the drug or related cinchona derivatives.

Procainamide

Procainamide, a class IA agent, has a similar action to that of quinidine, increasing the threshold to electric stimulation in both the atria and the ventricle.

TRADE NAMES

Procainamide: *Pronestyl*; *Procainamide Durules*.

PHARMACOKINETICS

Procainamide is absorbed from the gastrointestinal tract and is metabolised in the liver. N-Acetylprocainamide (NAPA), a metabolite, has significant antiarrhythmic properties. Procainamide and its metabolites are excreted by the kidneys.

USES

Procainamide is most commonly used for ventricular arrhythmias but is also used for atrial arrhythmias. It is usually administered orally, however when oral therapy is not feasible or a rapid therapeutic effect is necessary, parenteral administration is used.

The oral maintenance dose is 3–4.5 g per day in three or four divided doses for long acting tablets (*Procainamide Durules*) or 0.5–1 g every four to six hours for conventional capsules (*Pronestyl*).

If parenteral administration is necessary intramuscular administration is the method of choice as it is less likely to be accompanied by large falls in blood pressure. The intramuscular dose is 0.5–1 g every six hours. Procainamide can also be administered by direct intravenous injection or intravenous infusion. When using the direct intravenous regimen 100 mg is administered every five minutes at a rate not exceeding 50 mg per minute, until the arrhythmia is suppressed or the maximum dosage of 1 g has been administered. To maintain therapeutic levels an infusion may then be started at a rate of 2–6 mg/minute. If the intravenous infusion regimen is used an initial dose of 500–600 mg is infused over 25 to 30 minutes and then changed to a maintenance rate of 2–6 mg/minute.

ADVERSE DRUG REACTIONS

Anorexia, nausea, vomiting, bitter taste and urticaria are among the reported side effects. A syndrome resembling SLE has been reported in patients on long-term procainamide therapy. Cardiovascular effects include conduction defects, ventricular tachycardia and complete AV block. Severe hypotension may occur following rapid intravenous administration.

DRUG INTERACTIONS

Concomitant use of procainamide and cimetidine may result in increased plasma levels of procainamide and NAPA and subsequent cardiotoxicity. Possible additive hypotensive effects may occur if patients receiving antihypertensive agents are given procainamide parenterally or in high doses.

PRECAUTIONS AND CONTRAINDICATIONS

Procainamide should be used with extreme caution in patients with marked disturbance of AV conduction, digoxin toxicity, renal or hepatic disease or congestive cardiac failure. Patients on long-term therapy should have antinuclear antibody (ANA) titres measured at regular intervals. The drug should be discontinued if a rise in titres occurs. It is contraindicated in patients with complete AV block, myasthenia gravis or if the patient has a hypersensitivity to procainamide or related drugs.

Disopyramide

Disopyramide, a class IA agent, has a similar action to quinidine. It appears to be better tolerated than quinidine or procainamide.

TRADE NAMES

Disopyramide: *Norpace*; *Rythmodan*.

PHARMACOKINETICS

Disopyramide is rapidly absorbed from the gastrointestinal tract and undergoes metabolism in the liver. Excretion of disopyramide and its metabolites is mainly by the kidney with some faecal excretion also occurring. Its plasma half-life is prolonged in patients with renal or hepatic disease.

USES

Disopyramide is used for the treatment of both atrial and ventricular arrhythmias. The oral route is the most common but intravenous administration can also be used.

The usual oral dose is 300–800 mg per day in four divided doses. The intravenous dosage can be given either by slow intravenous injection or by an initial intravenous injection followed by an infusion. The regimen for direct intravenous injection is 2 mg/kg given slowly over 10 to 15 minutes with a repeat dose if necessary provided the dose does not exceed 300 mg during the first hour. If the second regimen is used the initial bolus injection is given over 10 to 15 minutes, followed by an infusion of disopyramide at a rate of 0.4 mg/kg/hour up to a maximum of 800 mg per day. When a patient is transferred from intravenous to oral maintenance therapy, 200 mg is given orally immediately on cessation of the infusion or injection, followed by 200 mg every eight hours for 24 hours.

ADVERSE DRUG REACTIONS

The most common adverse reactions are associated with the anticholinergic properties of the drug. They include dry mouth, blurred vision, urinary hesitancy and

CARDIOVASCULAR DISEASES

12

constipation. These effects are usually dose related and may be eliminated by reducing the dose.

DRUG INTERACTIONS

The dosage of warfarin may need to be adjusted when concurrent disopyramide therapy is used.

PRECAUTIONS AND CONTRAINDICTIONS

Disopyramide should be administered with caution and in reduced dosage in patients with renal or hepatic insufficiency. Because of its anticholinergic properties disopyramide should not be used in patients with glaucoma or urinary retention unless adequate over-riding measures are taken.

Disopyramide should not be administered to patients with poorly compensated or uncompensated congestive cardiac failure or hypotension. It is contraindicated in patients with cardiogenic shock or pre-existing second or third degree AV block.

Lignocaine

Lignocaine, a class IB agent, acts by stabilising cell membranes thus reducing the incidence of ectopic beats.

Lignocaine is a local anaesthetic and a class I (membrane stabilising) antiarrhythmic agent which acts by combining with fast sodium channels to inhibit recovery after repolarisation.

TRADE NAMES

Lignocaine: *Xylocaine*; *Xylocard*.

PHARMACOKINETICS

Lignocaine is absorbed from the gastrointestinal tract but it passes into the hepatic portal circulation and only a very small portion reaches the systemic circulation unchanged. The drug has a rapid onset of action following intravenous administration (after an intravenous bolus injection it takes approximately two minutes for lignocaine to reach the central circulation). Its duration of action is 10 to 20 minutes. Lignocaine is extensively metabolised in the liver and the elimination half-life is prolonged in patients with liver disease, myocardial infarction and/or congestive cardiac failure and following continuous intravenous infusion for more than 24 hours.

USES

Lignocaine is mainly used in the treatment of ventricular arrhythmias. Because of the small proportion which reaches the systemic circulation after oral administration the drug is administered either intramuscularly or more commonly, intravenously. The usual intramuscular dose is 4 mg/kg.

When the intravenous route is chosen a bolus dose is given followed by an infusion. The initial bolus dose is 1 mg/kg injected slowly over one to two minutes. The infusion should be commenced within 10 minutes and is administered at a rate of 2–4 mg per minute. In order to maintain therapeutic blood levels in the first few hours of infusion therapy further bolus injections of 50–100 mg may be given at 15–20-minute intervals. No more than 300 mg lignocaine should be administered during a one-hour period. Infusions should be discontinued within 24 hours after the last sign of arrhythmia.

Lignocaine is available in many forms. The 100 mg/5 mL ampoules or 100 mg/10 mL pre-loaded syringes are used for bolus doses and the 1000 mg/10 mL ampoules for preparation of infusions.

ADVERSE DRUG REACTIONS

Adverse effects mainly involve the central nervous system and are dose related. They include drowsiness, dizziness, nervousness, blurred or double vision, tinnitus, and nausea and vomiting. High plasma concentrations of lignocaine may cause cardiovascular side effects including arrhythmias, bradycardia, heart block and hypotension. Local thrombophlebitis may also occur in patients receiving prolonged intravenous infusions.

DRUG INTERACTIONS

The concurrent use of other antiarrhythmic drugs can cause potentiation of cardiac effects and toxicity. The concurrent administration of lignocaine and cimetidine or propranolol may result in increased serum concentrations of lignocaine with resultant toxicity.

PRECAUTIONS AND CONTRAINDICATIONS

Lignocaine infusion should be used with caution in patients with liver disease, congestive cardiac failure, severe respiratory depression, bradycardia, hypovolaemia, shock and those over 70 years of age.

Lignocaine is contraindicated in patients with Stoke-Adams syndrome or severe degrees of SA, AV or intraventricular heart block in the absence of an artificial pacemaker; in the treatment of supraventricular arrhythmias; and in patients with known hypersensitivity to the amide-type local anaesthetics.

Mexiletine

Mexiletine, a class IB agent, acts like lignocaine by stabilising cell membranes thus reducing the incidence of ectopic beats.

TRADE NAMES

Mexiletine: *Mexitil.*

PHARMACOKINETICS

Mexiletine is almost completely absorbed from the gastrointestinal tract. It is extensively metabolised in the liver and with its metabolites is excreted by the kidneys.

USES

Mexiletine is used both orally and parenterally for the management of ventricular arrhythmias. An initial loading dose is desirable to compensate for the rapid phase of tissue distribution. An oral dose of 400 mg followed by 200–250 mg three times daily commencing two hours after the loading dose is the usual regimen. If absorption is delayed, e.g. by acute myocardial infarction or prior administration of an opioid analgesic, intravenous therapy may be desirable. The dosage regimen used is 200–250 mg given at a rate of 25 mg/minute followed by infusion at a rate of 1 mg/minute for one hour, then 0.5

mg/minute. When changing from intravenous to oral maintenance therapy, the oral dose should be commenced on discontinuation of the intravenous infusion.

ADVERSE DRUG REACTIONS

Adverse effects include nausea, vomiting, unpleasant taste, hypotension, bradycardia, drowsiness and confusion. These effects are usually dose related and can often be reversed by reducing the dosage.

DRUG INTERACTIONS

Metoclopramide increases the rate but not the extent of absorption. Concurrent use of phenytoin will result in reduced plasma levels of mexiletine. Drugs which alter the urinary pH may affect the plasma concentration of mexiletine.

PRECAUTIONS AND CONTRAINDICATIONS

Mexiletine should be used with caution in patients with cardiac, renal or hepatic failure, sinus node dysfunction, conduction defects, bradycardia or hypotension.

Phenytoin

The anticonvulsant agent phenytoin also has antiarrhythmic effects. It is classed as a IB agent and depresses automaticity and improves atrioventricular conduction.

TRADE NAMES

Phenytoin: *Dilantin.*

PHARMACOKINETICS

See Chapter 25 Neurological Disorders.

USES

Phenytoin can be used in the treatment of ventricular arrhythmias, particularly those induced by digoxin. The recommended intravenous dosage is 3–5 mg/kg initially by direct intravenous injection which can be repeated if necessary, at a rate not exceeding 50 mg per minute.

Orally, a priming dose of 1 g is given and for maintenance therapy a dose of 100 mg every six hours is recommended.

ADVERSE DRUG REACTIONS

Adverse effects from short-term use include slurred speech, nystagmus, mental confusion and dizziness. Pain, tissue necrosis and inflammation may occur at the site of injection. For adverse reactions with long-term use see Chapter 25 Neurological Disorders.

DRUG INTERACTIONS

Numerous interactions occur when drugs are taken concurrently with phenytoin, see Chapter 25 Neurological Disorders.

PRECAUTIONS AND CONTRAINDICATIONS

Phenytoin should be administered intravenously with extreme caution to patients with respiratory depression, myocardial infarction or congestive cardiac failure. Treatment should be discontinued if a skin rash appears. Intravenous use is contraindicated in patients with sinus bradycardia, SA or AV block or Stoke-Adams syndrome.

Flecainide

Flecainide, a class IC agent, depresses conduction velocity and prolongs the refractory periods.

TRADE NAMES

Flecainide: *Tambocor.*

PHARMACOKINETICS

Flecainide is rapidly and almost completely absorbed from the gastrointestinal tract and is extensively metabolised in the liver. Flecainide and its metabolites are excreted almost completely by the kidneys with a small amount excreted in the faeces.

USES

Flecainide is used for the treatment of ventricular and supraventricular arrhythmias. It is used orally for maintenance treatment with intravenous administration being used for rapid control or short-term prophylaxis of the arrhythmia. The intravenous dose used is 2 mg/kg given over not less than 10 minutes. Oral therapy is commenced with a dosage of 100 mg every 12 hours with dosage increases if necessary until a maximum daily dose of 400 mg is reached.

ADVERSE DRUG REACTIONS

The majority of side effects occur on initiation of therapy and are often alleviated by dosage reduction. The most common adverse effects are dizziness, visual disturbances and headache. The most serious side effect is the arrhythmogenic effect of new or exacerbated ventricular arrhythmia.

DRUG INTERACTIONS

Concurrent administration of flecainide and propranolol can exacerbate effects in patients with impaired left ventricular function.

PRECAUTIONS AND CONTRAINDICATIONS

Flecainide should be used with caution in patients with a history of congestive cardiac failure. It is contraindicated in patients with cardiogenic shock, second or third degree AV block or right bundle branch block, unless a pacemaker is present to sustain rhythm.

β Blocking Drugs

β Blocking drugs decrease conduction velocity through the SA and AV nodes and decrease myocardial automaticity. They are classified as class II agents and are useful in the management of many cardiac arrhythmias but are generally less effective in the management of ventricular arrhythmias. For pharmacokinetics, adverse drug reactions, precautions and contraindications see section on β blocking drugs in prevention of angina in this chapter.

Sotalol

Sotalol, a class III agent, has a major effect of prolonging the atrial and ventricular refractory periods in addition to its non-selective β blocking activity.

TRADE NAMES

Sotalol: *Sotacor*.

PHARMACOKINETICS

Sotalol is well absorbed from the gastrointestinal tract. It is excreted unchanged by the kidneys.

USES

Sotalol is used for the treatment and prevention of cardiac arrhythmias. It is mainly given orally with intravenous administration being used for the management of acute arrhythmias. The recommended oral dose is 160–240 mg daily in two divided doses. The intravenous dose is 0.5–1.5 mg/kg administered over a 10-minute period and repeated at six-hourly intervals if necessary.

For adverse effects, drug interactions, precautions and contraindications see section on β blocking drugs in prevention of angina in this chapter.

Amiodarone

Amiodarone, a class III agent, prolongs the duration of the entire action potential and increases both atrial and ventricular refractory periods.

TRADE NAMES

Amiodarone: *Cordarone X*.

PHARMACOKINETICS

Amiodarone is slowly and variably absorbed from the gastrointestinal tract following oral administration. It is extensively metabolised, probably in the liver and possibly in the intestinal lumen and/or gastrointestinal mucosa. Amiodarone and its metabolites are mainly excreted in the faeces.

USES

Amiodarone is used in the prevention and treatment of serious ventricular and supraventricular arrhythmias. Due to poor absorption and wide interpatient variability in absorption, the initial loading and sub-

sequent maintenance dosage schedules of the drug need to be individually titrated. Both oral and parenteral routes of administration are used. If oral therapy is used, treatment should be commenced with 200 mg three times daily for one week, then reduced to 200 mg twice daily for a one week and then reduced to 200 mg daily, or less if appropriate. The parenteral dose should be given as an intravenous infusion of 5 mg/kg over a period of 20 minutes to 2 hours, followed by repeated infusions up to a total of 15 mg/kg per 24 hours. When transferring from intravenous to oral therapy an overlap of up to two days is recommended.

ADVERSE DRUG REACTIONS

Most of the adverse effects to amiodarone are related to dosage and duration of therapy. They include headache, insomnia, vivid dreams, photosensitivity, skin discolouration, nausea, disturbances of thyroid function and abnormal liver function tests. Microdeposits of iodine in the cornea, which do not affect vision, occur in practically all patients who take amiodarone for longer than six months. Pulmonary fibrosis is a rare but serious side effect.

DRUG INTERACTIONS

Amiodarone interacts with digoxin causing a significant increase in plasma levels of digoxin. Amiodarone also potentiates anticoagulant therapy.

PRECAUTIONS AND CONTRAINDICATIONS

Amiodarone should be used with caution in patients with congestive cardiac failure. It is contraindicated in patients with severe sinus node dysfunction, second or third degree AV block or a history of thyroid dysfunction. Regular liver and thyroid function tests should be performed on all patients receiving long-term treatment with amiodarone.

Verapamil

The calcium channel blocker, verapamil has class IV antiarrhythmic effects. These are primarily due to the increase in the refractory period of the AV node, and a prolongation of conduction time. The rate of conduction within the atria and ventricles is unaffected.

TRADE NAMES

Verapamil: *Isoptin*; *Cordilox*.

USES

Verapamil is used intravenously for the management of supraventricular tachycardias. The usual initial intravenous dose is 5–10 mg given slowly and repeated if necessary after 5 to 10 minutes. For adverse drug reactions, precautions and contraindications see section on calcium channel blockers in prevention of angina in this chapter.

NURSING IMPLICATIONS

ASSESSMENT

Baseline assessment of vital signs and cardiac rhythm are essential. Since antiarrhythmics may be ineffective in patients with hypokalaemia and hypomagnesaemia, potassium and magnesium levels should be normalised prior to their administration. Constant ECG monitoring is essential during infusion of antiarrhythmics. Nurses caring for patients in the initial stages of treatment must be able to read and interpret ECGs and be proficient in cardiopulmonary resuscitation techniques.

As antiarrhythmics are often given intravenously, a history of hypersensitivity is significant. Drug interactions can occur between some antiarrhythmics and digoxin, so an accurate, recent drug history is necessary; families can be of assistance in many cases.

ADMINISTRATION

Closely regulated infusions will often be required so infusion pumps are recommended.

Procainamide injection which is colourless initially, may develop a slight yellow colour in time. This does not indicate a change which would prevent its use, but a solution any darker than light amber or discoloured in any other way should not be used.

Intravenous infusions of *disopyramide* are prepared by adding 200 mg of disopyramide to 500 mL of infusion fluid. Suitable infusion fluids are 0.9% sodium chloride and 5% glucose.

A concentration of 2–4 mg *lignocaine* per ml in 5% glucose or 0.9% sodium chloride infusion solutions is normally used for lignocaine infusions. However, with higher doses, and in cases in which it is desired to limit fluid intake, a higher concentration may be used. Solutions showing discolouration should not be used. Several strengths of lignocaine are available for bolus injection and slow infusion, so care must be taken to select the appropriate strength.

Mexiletine injection should be diluted for infusion by adding 200 mg to 500 mL of 5% glucose or 0.9% sodium chloride solutions.

Phenytoin is normally given by direct intravenous injection at a rate not exceeding 50 mg per minute. The addition of phenytoin solution to an intravenous infusion is not recommended due to its poor solubility and resulting precipitation.

Flecainide can be given by intravenous injection in an emergency situation with continuous cardiac monitoring. A dose of 2 mg/kg up to a maximum of 150 mg can be given over not less than 10 minutes. Flecainide injection for infusion should only be diluted with glucose 5%.

Amiodarone injection should be administered as a dilute solution in 250 mL 5% glucose. It is not compatible with saline. Amiodarone can be absorbed into PVC infusion bags and sets, so it is preferable to prepare the infusion solution in glass bottles.

When administering *sotalol* intravenously, the required dose should be added to 0.9% sodium chloride or 5% glucose, to provide a concentration of sotalol betweem 0.1 mg/mL and 2 mg/mL.

When administering oral antiarrhythmic medications, care must be taken to select the correct dosage form. Long acting preparations must be swallowed whole, not crushed, broken or chewed. Quinidine preparations should be given with food to minimise gastric irritation.

EVALUATION

The effect of antiarrhythmic drugs on cardiac arrhythmias is most accurately evaluated by ECG monitoring. Patients with atrial flutter or fibrillation may have developed atrial thrombi and embolisation may occur when atrial contractions are re-established. They should therefore be observed for signs of life threatening complications of arterial or pulmonary embolism.

Clinical signs of therapeutic action are related to improved cardiac output. Nurses need to be aware of the adverse reactions associated with the use of each drug.

PATIENT EDUCATION

Patients should receive thorough instruction about their dosage regimen and be instructed not to stop or alter their therapy without consulting their medical officer. They should be made aware of adverse effects they may experience and be told of any ways to minimise these, e.g. taking quinidine with food, use of sunblock preparations when taking amiodarone. Families should be directed to cardiopulmonary resuscitation training programs because of the possibility of cardiac emergencies.

TREATMENT OF HYPERLIPIDAEMIA ▰▰

Hyperlipidaemia is a group of disorders characterised by increased concentrations of various plasma lipoproteins. There are several types of lipoproteins involved: chylomicrons, very low density lipoproteins (VLDL), low density lipoproteins (LDL) and high density lipoproteins (HDL). There are six different categories of hyperlipidaemia according to which lipoprotein(s) is (are) in excess. The two main indicators of hyperlipidaemia are the plasma levels of cholesterol and triglycerides. There is a strong familial incidence of hyperlipidaemia.

Hyperlipidaemia greatly increases the risk of atherosclerosis and other heart disease, as well as xanthoma and pancreatitis. Non-drug therapies and other measures are the initial treatments for hyperlipidaemia. These include dietary management (restriction of total and saturated fat and cholesterol intake), weight control, adequate physical activity, restriction of alcohol intake and the management of potentially contributing underlying disease, e.g. diabetes mellitus, hypothyroidism. These measures should be continued when drug therapy is commenced. There are several drugs currently available for the treatment of hyperlipidaemia. The choice of drug depends on the type of hyperlipidaemia to be treated.

BILE ACID SEQUESTRANTS

Cholestyramine, Colestipol

The resins cholestyramine and colestipol are bile acid sequestrants which adsorb bile acids in the intestine, forming a non-absorbable complex that is excreted along with un-

changed resin in the faeces. This results in the partial removal of bile acids from the enterohepatic circulation by preventing their reabsorption. This increased faecal loss of bile acids leads to an increased oxidation of cholesterol to bile acids, a decrease in LDL in plasma and a decrease in serum cholesterol levels. Serum triglyceride levels may increase or remain unchanged.

TRADE NAMES

Cholestyramine: *Questran*.
Colestipol: *Colestid*.

PHARMACOKINETICS

Cholestyramine and colestipol are not absorbed from the gastrointestinal tract.

USES

Cholestyramine and colestipol are used for reduction of elevated serum cholesterol in patients with primary hypercholesterolaemia (elevated LDL). The recommended doses are: cholestyramine 12–16 g per day; and colestipol 15–30 g per day.

Both are taken in two or four divided doses. The powders must be mixed with water or other fluid and taken before food.

ADVERSE DRUG REACTIONS

The most common adverse effects are gastrointestinal and include constipation, nausea, flatulence, abdominal discomfort and vomiting.

DRUG INTERACTIONS

The bile acid sequestrants may delay or reduce the absorption of oral medications given at the same time. Drugs likely to be adversely affected include digoxin, thyroxine and anticoagulants. It is recommended that cholestyramine or colestipol be taken at least one hour before or four hours after other medication.

PRECAUTIONS AND CONTRAINDICATIONS

Bile acid sequestrants may interfere with normal fat absorption and therefore may prevent absorption of the fat soluble vitamins A, D and K, so it may be necessary to administer supplementary vitamins A and D. Serum triglycerides should be measured periodically to ensure that significant changes have not occurred.

HMG-CoA REDUCTASE INHIBITORS

Simvastatin, Pravastatin

The main mechanism of action of simvastatin and pravastatin is the inhibition of HMG-CoA reductase, an enzyme necessary for the synthesis of cholesterol. The production of LDL is reduced and its catabolism increased. The net result is a reduction in total plasma cholesterol, LDL and VLDL. In addition a moderate increase in HDL and decrease in plasma triglyceride occur.

TRADE NAMES

Simvasatin: *Lipex; Zocor*.
Pravastatin: *Pravachol*.

PHARMACOKINETICS

Simvastatin is absorbed from the gastrointestinal tract and undergoes metabolism in the liver to the active form of the drug. It is primarily excreted in the faeces.

Pravastatin is absorbed from the gastrointestinal tract, metabolised in the liver and primarily excreted in the faeces.

USES

Simvastatin and pravastatin are used in the treatment of severe forms of hypercholesterolaemia, i.e. when cholesterol elevation is the primary problem after diet and other treatments have failed. For both drugs dosage is usually commenced at 10 mg per day as a single dose in the evening, with dosage adjustments being made if necessary at four-week intervals to a maximum of 40 mg per day. Patients should be placed on a cholesterol lowering diet before beginning treatment and should continue on this diet during treatment.

ADVERSE DRUG REACTIONS

The most common adverse effects are diarrhoea, nausea, flatulence, rash, headache and myopathy.

DRUG INTERACTIONS

The anticoagulant effect of warfarin is potentiated by simvastatin. Fibric acid derivatives (clofibrate, gemfibrozil), nicotinic acid or immunosuppressants (including cyclosporin) increase the risk of myopathy. Bile acid sequestrants have an additive cholesterol lowering effect.

PRECAUTIONS AND CONTRAINDICATIONS

Liver function tests should be performed before treatment begins and periodically thereafter. HMG-CoA reductase inhibitors should be used with caution in patients with a history of alcohol abuse and/or who have a past history of liver disease. Their use is contraindicated in patients with active liver disease or unexplained persistent elevation of serum transaminases. Because of the risk of myopathy caution should be exercised if the patient reports muscle pain, tenderness or weakness. Their use is contraindicated in patients with myopathy secondary to other lipid lowering agents.

MISCELLANEOUS HYPOLIPIDAEMIC AGENTS

Nicotinic Acid

The precise mechanism by which nicotinic acid decreases serum cholesterol and triglycerides is unknown. However, it does decrease the rate of synthesis of VLDL and LDL by the liver and increase the rate of removal of chylomicron triglycerides from the plasma.

TRADE NAMES

Nicotinic acid: *Tri-B3 SR*; *Nikacid*.

PHARMACOKINETICS

Nicotinic acid is readily absorbed from the gastrointestinal tract and is excreted largely unchanged by the kidneys. No significant metabolism occurs.

USES

Nicotinic acid is used for the treatment of hypercholesterolaemia and hypertriglyceridaemia. To minimise side effects initial treatment should commence with doses of 250 mg twice a day of the long acting preparations increasing the dosage gradually to 1 g or 1.5 g twice daily, or with 250 mg three times daily of standard formulation tablets increasing slowly to 1 g or 1.5 g three times daily. All doses should be taken after food.

ADVERSE DRUG REACTIONS

The most common adverse effects are nausea, vomiting, tachycardia, pruritus and abnormal liver function. Patients taking standard formulation tablets may experience marked flushing.

DRUG INTERACTIONS

Concurrent use of nicotinic acid with antihypertensive agents may have an additive vasodilatory effect and produce postural hypotension. The use of bile acid sequestrants with nicotinic acid will result in additional lowering of serum cholesterol level.

PRECAUTIONS AND CONTRAINDICATIONS

Nicotinic acid should be used with caution in patients with gall bladder disease or a history of jaundice. It is contraindicated in patients with severe hypotension, liver disease or active peptic or duodenal ulcer.

Gemfibrozil

The mechanism of action of gemfibrozil has not been definitely established. It produces a reduction in total cholesterol, LDL, VLDL and triglycerides and an increase in HDL.

TRADE NAMES

Gemfibrozil: *Lopid*.

PHARMACOKINETICS

Gemfibrozil is well absorbed from the gastrointestinal tract and after metabolism in the liver is excreted by the kidneys.

USES

Gemfibrozil is used in the treatment of hypercholesterolaemia and hypertriglyceridaemia. The usual dose is 600 mg twice a day half an hour before meals.

ADVERSE DRUG REACTIONS

Gastrointestinal effects, including diarrhoea, abdominal pain, nausea and flatulence, are the most common adverse effects. Headache and dizziness have also been reported.

DRUG INTERACTIONS

Gemfibrozil may potentiate the effect of oral anticoagulants such as warfarin.

PRECAUTIONS AND CONTRAINDICATIONS

The use of gemfibrozil is contraindicated in patients with pre-existing gallbladder disease and in those with hepatic or severe renal dysfunction.

Probucol

The exact mechanism of action of probucol is unknown. It has however been shown to increase the catabolism of LDL, increase the excretion of bile acids in the faeces and inhibit cholesterol synthesis. The effect on triglycerides is variable and it decreases HDL.

TRADE NAMES

Probucol: *Lurselle.*

PHARMACOKINETICS

Only a small amount of probucol is absorbed from the gastrointestinal tract. The absorbed drug is slowly excreted in the faeces.

USES

Probucol is used for the treatment of primary hypercholesterolaemia. The recommended dose is 500 mg twice daily with meals.

ADVERSE DRUG REACTIONS

The most common adverse effects of probucol are diarrhoea, flatulence, abdominal pain and nausea. Cardiovascular effects such as prolongation of the QT interval and ventricular fibrillation have been reported.

DRUG INTERACTIONS

An additional lowering of serum cholesterol occurs when bile acid sequestrants and probucol are used concurrently.

PRECAUTIONS AND CONTRAINDICATIONS

Probucol is contraindicated in patients with uncontrolled congestive cardiac failure, with evidence of recent or progressive myocardial damage or findings suggestive of ventricular arrhythmias.

Clofibrate

The exact mechanism of action of clofibrate is unclear. It has several antilipidaemic actions such as increasing the rate of metabolism of triglyceride rich lipoproteins and decreasing triglyceride synthesis. These actions result in a net reduction in serum triglyceride and VLDL concentrations.

TRADE NAMES

Clofibrate: *Atromid S.*

PHARMACOKINETICS

Clofibrate is readily absorbed from the gastrointestinal tract. It is rapidly metabolised in the liver to the active form, clofibric acid. Clofibric acid and other metabolites are excreted by the kidneys.

USES

Clofibrate is used for the treatment of Type III hyperlipidaemia (elevated triglyceride and cholesterol levels). The recommended dose is 500 mg three times a day or 1 g twice a day after meals.

ADVERSE DRUG REACTIONS

The most common adverse effects are nausea, diarrhoea, muscle cramping, headaches, rash, dry skin, alopecia and impotence. Myalgia or myositis may occur. Liver function tests may rise.

DRUG INTERACTIONS

Clofibrate will potentiate the activity of oral anticoagulants. Concurrent use with HMG-CoA reductase inhibitors will increase the risk of myopathy.

PRECAUTIONS AND CONTRAINDICATIONS

Clofibrate should be used with caution in

patients with low serum albumin levels, e.g. nephrotic syndrome or impaired renal function, as myalgia or myositis may develop. It should also be used with caution in patients with a history of jaundice or hepatic disease. Clofibrate should not be used in patients with a history of, or existing, gall bladder disease or stones; acute impairment of renal or hepatic function; or primary biliary cirrhosis.

NURSING IMPLICATIONS

ASSESSMENT

Accurate assessment of plasma cholesterol and triglyceride levels must be performed before treatment begins. A fasting blood sample should be used for analysis as plasma levels of cholesterol and triglyceride rise after meals.

ADMINISTRATION

The bile acid sequestrants, cholestyramine and colestipol should not be given in the dry form as accidental inhalation or oesophageal distress can result. They should be mixed with water or fruit juice and left to stand for a few minutes and stirred again to ensure the powder is fully wet. They are best taken before meals.

Other medications should be given one hour before or four hours after the bile acid sequestrants to minimise possible interference with their absorption.

EVALUATION

The progress and effectiveness of therapy is monitored by following the changes in cholesterol and triglyceride levels.

PATIENT EDUCATION

Patients should be advised about the correct time to take their medication and of side effects which may occur. Patients taking cholestyramine or colestipol may need to take a laxative preparation. Patients should be educated about the need for compliance with drug regimens and their compliance regularly assessed. It is important to stress that drug therapy is an adjunct to dietary therapy and other measures such as weight control and physical activity in the treatment of hyperlipidaemia.

CARDIOVASCULAR DISEASES

12

FURTHER READING

American Hospital Formulary Service Drug Information, (1994), American Society of Hospital Pharmacists, Bethesda.

Goodman and Gilman's The Pharmacological Basis of Therapeutics (1985) 7th edn. Macmillan, New York.

Herfindal, E.T., Gourley, D.R., Lloyd Hart, L., eds. (1988), *Clinical Pharmacy and Therapeutics*, 4th edn. Williams Wilkins, Baltimore.

Harrison's Principles of Internal Medicine, 13th edn. (1994) McGraw Hill, New York.

Speight, T. Ed. (1987) *Avery's Drug Treatment*, 3rd edn. Adis Press, Sydney.

Vaughan Williams, E.M. (1975), 'Classification of antidysrhythmic drugs', *Pharm Ther, 1, 115.*

TEST YOUR KNOWLEDGE

1. Define the terms: (a) cardiac arrhythmia; (b) diuretic; (c) congestive cardiac failure.

2. Match the following drugs to the disease state in which they are used.
Drugs: Digoxin, sotalol, clofibrate, isosorbide dinitrate, frusemide.
Disease state: Oedema, angina pectoris, congestive cardiac failure, hyperlipidaemia, cardiac arrhythmias.

3. Match each of the following drugs to the side effect which may result from its use.
Drugs: Nicotinic acid, captopril, verapamil, procainamide, disopyramide.
Side effect: SLE syndrome, urinary retention, cough, flushing, constipation.

4. Assign each of the following drugs to its pharmacological class: Atenolol, chlorothiazide, diltiazem, enalapril, bumetanide, colestipol.

TABLE 12.7 Summary table — drugs used in the treatment of cardiovascular diseases

Drug	Uses	Mechanism of Action	Adverse Effects
Digoxin	Congestive cardiac failure	Increases force of contraction of cardiac muscle, slows heart rate	Gastrointestinal disturbances; cardiac arrhythmias; fatigue; headache; mental confusion; blurred vision
NITRATES Glyceryl trinitrate	Sublingual tablets, aerosol — acute angina. IV infusion — acute angina; control of blood pressure; congestive cardiac failure associated with myocardial infarction. Ointment — angina prophylaxis. Transdermal discs — angina prophylaxis. Sublingual — acute angina.	Dilation of vascular smooth muscle, reduction in myocardial oxygen demand	Flushing; headache; hypotension; tolerance
Isosorbide dinitrate	Oral — angina prophylaxis	As for glyceryl trinitrate	As for glyceryl trinitrate
Isosorbide mononitrate	Oral — angina prophylaxis	As for glyceryl trinitrate	As for glyceryl trinitrate
β BLOCKING AGENTS Non-selective agents: Propranolol Oxprenolol Timolol Pindolol	Prevention of angina, hypertension, arrhythmias	Reduce heart rate, cardiac output, myocardial irritability, extent and force of contraction and myocardial oxygen demand	Bradycardia; hypotension; nausea; vomiting; diarrhoea; lassitude; visual disturbances; nightmares; hallucination; rash; paraesthesias; hypoglycaemia; weight gain; bronchoconstriction, myocardial infarction after abrupt withdrawal
Cardioselective agents: Atenolol Metoprolol	Prevention of angina, hypertension, arrhythmias		
α and β BLOCKING AGENTS Labetalol	Hypertension	Reduces peripheral resistance and blocks reflex tachycardia	As for β blocking agents

12 CARDIOVASCULAR DISEASES

TABLE 12.7 continued.

Drug	Uses	Mechanism of Action	Adverse Effects
POSTSYNAPTIC α BLOCKING AGENTS			
Prazosin	Congestive cardiac failure, hypertension	Blocks postsynaptic α receptors causing vasodilation	First-dose postural hypotension; tachycardia; fluid retention; drowsiness; urinary frequency; diaphoresis
CENTRALLY ACTING DRUGS			
Clonidine	Hypertension	Reduce cardiac output and peripheral resistance	*Clonidine*: drowsiness; dry mouth; constipation; fluid retention; rebound hypertension and arrhythmias on withdrawal.
Methyldopa			*Methyldopa*: weakness; dreams; sedation; impotence; fluid retention; tiredness; depression
CALCIUM CHANNEL BLOCKERS			
Verapamil	Angina, hypertension, arrhythmias	Block entry of calcium ions into cells producing vasodilation and lowering peripheral resistance, reduce heart rate, conductivity and contractility	Constipation (verapamil); headache; flushing; tachycardia; dizziness; oedema; muscle cramps; liver damage; hypotension with first dose (nifedipine); gingival enlargement (rare)
Nifedipine			
Diltiazem			
Felodipine			
Amlodipine			
ACE INHIBITORS			
Captopril	Hypertension, congestive cardiac failure	Inhibit enzyme responsible for conversion of angiotensin I to angiotensin II thereby causing vasodilation	Rash; taste loss; cough; dizziness; headache; gastrointestinal upset; proteinuria; neutropenia; agranulocytosis; hyperkalaemia
Enalapril			
Lisinopril			
Fosinopril	Hypertension		
Perindopril			
Ramipril			
Quinapril			

TABLE 12.7 continued.

Drug	Uses	Mechanism of Action	Adverse Effects
DIRECTLY ACTING VASODILATORS			
Hydralazine	Congestive cardiac failure, hypertension	Direct action on peripheral blood vessels causing vasodilation and reducing peripheral resistance	*Hydralazine:* headache; flushing; tachycardia; vomiting; oedema; rashes; urticaria; SLE.
Minoxidil	Hypertension		*Minoxidil:* pericarditis; pericardial effusion; salt and water retention; oedema; reflex tachycardia; arrhythmia; hypotension; hirsutism; rash; pruritus; dyspnoea; bronchospasm
ANTIARRHYTHMIC AGENTS			
Quinidine	Atrial and ventricular arrhythmias	Depression of myocardial contractility, conduction velocity and excitability	Nausea; vomiting; diarrhoea; rash; haemolytic anaemia; thrombocytopenia; drug fever; potentiates digoxin toxicity
Procainamide	Atrial and ventricular arrhythmias	See quinidine	See quinidine
Disopyramide	Atrial and ventricular arrhythmias	See quinidine	Dry mouth; constipation; urinary hesitancy; blurred vision; dry nose; potentiates digoxin toxicity
Lignocaine	Postinfarction, ventricular arrhythmias	Stabilises cell membrane reducing incidence of ectopic beats	Nausea; vomiting: anorexia; dizziness; tremor; confusion; nervousness; disorientation
Mexiletine	Ventricular arrhythmias	See lignocaine	Uncommon and dose related, hypotension; bradycardia; drowsiness; confusion; nausea; unpleasant taste

12 CARDIOVASCULAR DISEASES

TABLE 12.7 continued.

Drug	Uses	Mechanism of Action	Adverse Effects
Phenytoin	Ventricular arrhythmias	Depresses automaticity, improves conduction	Slurred speech; nystagmus; mental confusion; dizziness
Flecainide	Ventricular and supraventricular arrhythmias	Depression of myocardial conduction, little effect on duration of action potential	Tinnitus; palpitations; dizziness; chest pain; visual disturbances; rash; dyspnoea; headache; nausea
Sotalol Amiodarone	Ventricular and supraventricular arrhythmias	Prolong cardiac action potential and atrial and ventricular refractory periods	*Sotalol:* see β blocking agents. *Amiodarone:* Corneal deposits; photosensitivity; skin discolouration; bradycardia; conduction disturbance; hypotension; hypo or hyperthyroidism; peripheral neuropathy; extrapyramidal effects; vertigo; metallic taste; nightmares
Verapamil	See calcium antagonists		
DIURETICS Thiazides: Bendrofluazide Chlorothiazide Chlorthalidone Cyclopenthiazide Hydrochlorothiazide Methyclothiazide	Hypertension; congestive cardiac disease; oedema	Prevent sodium reabsorption in ascending limb of renal tubule; direct action on blood vessel walls	Gastrointestinal irritation; dehydration; potassium depletion; increased plasma levels uric acid and glucose; rash
Loop diuretics: Frusemide Bumetanide Ethacrynic acid	Hypertension; congestive cardiac disease; oedema	Prevent sodium and water reabsorption in kidney	Elevated serum uric acid; deafness; hypokalaemia; hyperglycaemia

TABLE 12.7 continued.

Drug	Uses	Mechanism of Action	Adverse Effects
Metolazone	Hypertension, congestive cardiac disease; oedema	Inhibit sodium reabsorption at cortical diluting site and in proximal convoluted tubule	See thiazide diuretics
Indapamide	Hypertension	In low dose corrects hypertension, at higher doses only diuretic	Similar to thiazides but without hyperglycaemia
Potassium sparing diuretics: Spironolactone	Oedema; hypertension	Antagonises action of aldosterone at distal portion of renal tubule	Drowsiness; lethargy; gynaecomastia; hyperkalaemia; hyponatraemia
Amiloride Triamterene	Oedema; hypertension	Retains potassium at distal portion of renal tubule while preventing water reabsorption	Hyperkalaemia; hyponatraemia
POTASSIUM SUPPLEMENTS Potassium chloride	Potassium loss caused by diuretics	Replaces potassium	Gastric irritation; potassium overload
HYPOLIPIDAEMIC AGENTS Bile acid sequestrants: Cholestyramine Colestipol	Hypercholesterolaemia	Bind to bile acids in GIT and excreted in the faeces	Constipation, flatulence, unpleasant taste; may delay or reduce absorption of oral medications given at same time; may prevent absorption of fat soluble vitamins A, D and K
HMG-CoA reductase inhibitors: Simvastatin Pravastatin	Hypercholesterolaemia	Inhibit HMG-CoA reductase, an enzyme necessary for cholesterol synthesis	Nausea; diarrhoea; flatulence; rash; headache; myopathy

12 CARDIOVASCULAR DISEASES

TABLE 12.7 continued.

Drug	Uses	Mechanism of Action	Adverse Effects
Nicotinic acid	Hypercholesterolaemia, hypertriglyceridaemia	Decreases hepatic synthesis of VLDL and LDL and removes chylomicron triglycerides from plasma	Flushing; tachycardia; pruritus; vomiting; nausea
Gemfibrozil	Hypercholesterolaemia, hypertriglyceridaemia	Inhibits cholesterol synthesis and increases rate of metabolism of triglycerides	Nausea; flatulence; diarrhoea; abdominal pain; headache; dizziness
Probucol	Hypercholesterolaemia	Increases catabolism of LDL and the faecal excretion of bile acids and inhibits cholesterol synthesis	Diarrhoea; flatulence; nausea; abdominal pain; prolongation of QT interval
Clofibrate	Hypercholesterolaemia, hypertriglyceridaemia	Inhibits cholesterol synthesis, increases metabolism of triglycerides	Diarrhoea; muscle cramps; headaches; rash; impotence; myalgia

Blood Disorders

ANN L. CARTER

O B J E C T I V E S

At the conclusion of this chapter the reader should be able to:

1. Name representative drugs from each pharmacological class discussed;

2. Describe the pharmacological action of the drugs acting on the haematopoietic system and list the disease states in which they are employed;

3. List the common adverse effects of the drugs discussed;

4. Give examples of drugs with a low therapeutic index;

5. Name the antidotes for heparin and warfarin;

6. Name the drugs which have an effect on platelet function; and

7. List the nursing implications of the use of drugs acting on the haematopoietic system.

THE CLOTTING SYSTEM ▐

Platelets, clotting factors and various other substances involved with blood coagulation and clot dissolution act in balance to keep blood flowing through the cardiovascular system but stop it flowing out of the vessel when a break appears in its wall. Ideally, bleeding stops very soon after a cut or abrasion and clots do not form in intact blood vessels.

Clot formation is achieved with the conversion of fibrinogen to fibrin. This conversion is activated by thrombin which is produced by the 'clotting cascade' shown in Figure 13.1. It has two sections, the intrinsic and extrinsic systems. A break in a vessel wall, or presence of a 'foreign' surface, stimulates the 'coagulation cascade'. Once complete, the fibrinolytic system works to break down and lyse the clot which was formed.

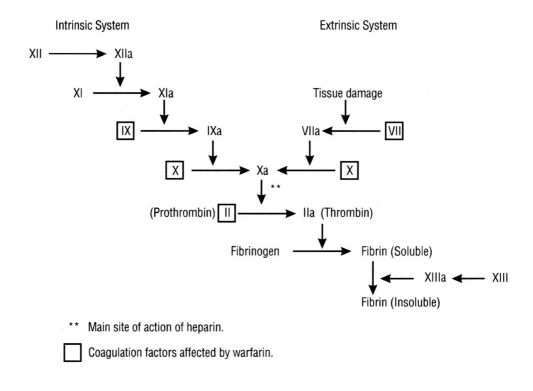

FIGURE 13.1 Intrinsic and extrinsic systems of blood coagulation

The activity of the clotting system can be measured in several ways: whole blood clotting time; activated partial thromboplastin time (APPT), which measures the activity of the intrinsic system; thrombin clotting time; prothrombin and preconvertin test (PTT); the prothrombin index (PI), which measures the extrinsic system; and the International Normalised Ratio (INR). The results of these tests depend on the reagents used and it is very hard to compare results obtained from different laboratories. One exception to this is the INR where results are converted to a common scale.

It is sometimes necessary to suppress the activity of the clotting system. Conditions for which this may be necessary include:

- After implantation of artificial prostheses, e.g. heart valves, because blood has a greater tendency to form clots on 'foreign' surfaces.

- In prophylactic treatment for patients who have developed a deep vein thrombosis (DVT), or pulmonary embolus (PE). This treatment does not alter the clot that has already formed but is aimed at preventing the formation of further clots.

- Following myocardial infarction (MI) as a prophylactic measure to prevent, or limit, further infarction.

A number of different groups of drugs affect the coagulation system in a variety of ways. The modes of action and clinical uses of these agents will be discussed in the following pages. These agents fall into the following groups: antithrombotic drugs (anticoagulants and antiplatelet agents); coagulant drugs; fibrinolytic drugs; drugs used in the treatment of immune thrombocytopenia; drugs affecting haematopoiesis (haematopoietic agents); and iron chelating agents. Lipid lowering agents (hypolipidaemic agents) are discussed in Chapter 12 Cardiovascular Diseases.

ANTITHROMBOTIC DRUGS ▮▮▮▮ 13 ▮

ANTICOAGULANTS

The anticoagulants are used to reduce the body's ability to form clots. These drugs have a low therapeutic index, i.e. the difference between the dose required to produce a therapeutic effect and that which produces a toxic effect is very small.

Patients who are anticoagulated are at risk of bleeding and haemorrhage. Considerable care must be exercised by nursing staff to prevent untoward bleeding in these patients. Patients must be informed of the dangers and taught how to avoid or minimise them.

There are two main groups of anticoagulants in general use: injectable anticoagulants, heparin and heparin-like drugs, and the oral anticoagulants, warfarin and phenindione. Neither group has a direct effect on clots that have already formed. The use of anticoagulant drugs is prophylactic only.

Heparin

Heparin is a large mucopolysaccharide molecule. It is found in small amounts in mast cells. Commercially it is obtained from the intestines or lungs of pigs, cattle and sheep. It is a complex molecule which occurs in different sizes. For this reason, the dose of heparin is not measured in milligrams but in units of anticoagulant activity, i.e. the dose is written as 15 000 units and not 50 mg.

TRADE NAMES

Heparin calcium: *Caprin*; *Calciparine*; *Calcihep*; *Uniparin-Ca*.
Heparin sodium: *Uniparin*.

MECHANISM OF ACTION

Figure 13.1 shows how heparin inteferes with the clotting cascade. It prevents the conversion of prothrombin to thrombin by increasing the activity of antithrombin III (heparin cofactor). Antithrombin III controls the rate of conversion of prothrombin to thrombin. The effect of heparin on coagulation is immediate but lasts only as long as the drug is present in the body.

It is very difficult to measure the blood level of heparin. It is more useful, and easier, to measure the effect it has had on coagulation. This is done by measuring the APPT.

BLOOD DISORDERS

PHARMACOKINETICS

Heparin is a delicate molecule which is destroyed by gastric acid and so it must be administered parenterally. The half-life of heparin is very short, approximately 90 minutes.

USES

In the treatment of DVT or PE the dose of heparin necessary to achieve a given effect varies from patient to patient. The normal range of APPT is 20–30 seconds. Heparin is normally given in a dose which will prolong the APPT to between two and three times that of normal. The APPT should be checked at least once daily while the patient is receiving heparin.

INTRAVENOUS ADMINISTRATION

If heparin is given intermittently (e.g. every 4 hours) as a bolus injection the patient may be over-anticoagulated (and at risk of bleeding) just after the dose and may be under-anticoagulated just before the next dose (and at risk of clotting). For this reason heparin is usually given by constant infusion. It is important that the rate of heparin administration is constant and an infusion pump should be used to control the rate of infusion.

Heparinised saline (50 units in 5 mL) is sometimes used to flush intravenous lines.

SUBCUTANEOUS ADMINISTRATION

Postoperative patients and those on prolonged bed rest have a low, but significant, risk of deep vein thrombosis. Full anticoagulation is not necessary to decrease this risk. Heparin is given to such patients in a dose of 5000 units subcutaneously two to three times daily. Measurement of the APPT is not necessary with this dose level of heparin.

OTHER ROUTES OF ADMINISTRATION

Other routes of heparin administration should be avoided, e.g. intramuscular injection is painful and haematoma formation common.

ADVERSE DRUG REACTIONS

The most serious complication of heparin therapy is bleeding which can occur as haematuria, epistaxis, petecchiae, internal haemorrhage and melaena (often from previously unrecognised gastrointestinal lesions). Care must be taken that the patient has no other cause of reduced clotting ability, e.g. low platelet count, haemophilia, other drugs altering clotting function (e.g. warfarin, aspirin).

DRUG INTERACTIONS

Care must be taken with any other drugs which also affect clotting ability, e.g. aspirin, non-steroidal anti-inflammatory agents, dipyridamole.

It is often necessary to give other parenteral medications to a patient during an infusion of heparin. Drugs must not be mixed in intravenous lines or cannulae unless there is evidence that they are physically compatible in the concentrations and equipment being used. The pharmacy department can provide this information.

PRECAUTIONS AND CONTRAINDICATIONS

Commercial heparin is derived from animals and some patients may experience allergic reactions to it. These reactions may take the form of pruritus or a mild fever. Heparin induced thrombosis thrombocytopenia syndrome (HITTS) is a rare reaction to heparin. It is characterised by a dramatic fall in platelet count and/or a tendency for multiple clot formation. The treatment of HITTS and other causes of low platelet count are discussed later in this chapter.

The heparin molecule is too large to cross the placental barrier. It can, therefore, be used to anticoagulate the mother without fear of directly harming the fetus. Very strict control and monitoring must be maintained as any maternal bleeding will harm both the fetus and mother.

See also Adverse Drug Reactions.

ANTIDOTE

The action of heparin can be antagonised by the use of protamine sulfate. Protamine binds to heparin and the complex of the two molecules is inactive. Protamine sulfate is used in heparin overdose and for rapid reversal of the effects of heparin prior to surgery and at the end of procedures such as cardiac angiography.

Protamine sulfate is given intravenously at a dose of 1 mg for every 100 units of heparin. When calculating the dose to be given it is important to allow for the heparin that has degraded since the last dose was given. Due to the risk of hypotension, bradycardia and dyspnoea from depression of the myocardium, protamine sulfate must be given slowly, i.e. the dose must be administered over at least 10 minutes and not more than 50 mg administered in two hours.

Protamine is not an antidote for the heparinoids and has only a partial effect with low molecular weight heparin (LMWH).

LMWHs and Heparinoids

The low molecular weight heparins (LMWH) (enoxaparin, fraxiparin and tinzaparin), and the heparinoids (danaparoid) are various sized fractions of the heparin molecule. They have been developed to retain the efficacy of heparin therapy while minimising the risk of associated bleeding.

TRADE NAMES

Enoxaparin: *Clexane*.
Fraxiparin: *Fragmin*.
Tinzaparin: *Logiparin*.
Danaparoid: *Orgaron*; *Org 10172*.

MECHANISM OF ACTION

The precise mechanism of action is unclear but it is thought that the LMWHs have greater specificity for inhibition of factor Xa than heparin and cause minimal inhibition of thrombin. Local haemostasis is much less affected compared with heparin therapy. The strength is quoted in antifactor Xa units per mL.

PHARMACOKINETICS

Approximately 90% of a subcutaneous dose is absorbed. The half-life is longer than that of heparin and so these drugs need only be given once or twice daily.

USES

They are administered intravenously or subcutaneously for treatment of acute deep vein thrombosis and thromboprophylaxis after surgery. If therapy is prophylactic, routine monitoring of coagulation status is not required. LMWHs can be tried in patients with heparin allergy but some cross sensitivity has been shown. Danaparoid has been shown to be safe in HITTS.

ADVERSE DRUG REACTIONS

Adverse reactions are similar to those seen with heparin, i.e. bleeding, allergy (urticaria, hypotension, anaphylaxis, fever, pruritus, skin necrosis).

PRECAUTIONS AND CONTRAINDICATIONS

As these compounds have similar effects to heparin the same precautions apply.

Warfarin, Phenindione

Warfarin and phenindione are oral anticoagulants. (Aspirin, dipyridamole and sulfinpyrazone are also used orally to anticoagulate patients but act through inhibition of platelet aggregation and not by an effect on clotting factors. See Antiplatelet Agents.)

TRADE NAMES

Warfarin: *Coumadin*; *Marevan*.
Phenindione: *Dindevan*.

MECHANISM OF ACTION

Warfarin and phenindione are structurally related to vitamin K. They act by inhibiting the formation of the vitamin K dependant clotting factors (II, VII, IX, X) in the intrinsic system (see Figure 13.1). The effect of warfarin and phenindione can be measured by the PI and INR. The APPT does not measure the effect of warfarin

BLOOD DISORDERS

13

and the PI does not measure the effect of heparin.

PHARMACOKINETICS

Warfarin is well absorbed orally and circulates bound to plasma protein. The full effect of warfarin administration is not seen until the clotting factors present before warfarin administration have been removed from the circulation. This takes four to five days. Similarly the effect of warfarin continues after administration has ceased until the body has manufactured new clotting factors.

USES

Warfarin has a low therapeutic index and the dose must be titrated for each patient. When a patient is commenced on warfarin therapy the PI or INR should be measured daily until it is stable. Thereafter it must be measured at regular intervals. Any alteration in diet, the state of health or other drug therapy may alter the effect of warfarin and the dose may have to be adjusted. Patients remain on warfarin therapy as long as the benefits of therapy outweigh the risks involved. This can be for three to six months after a myocardial infarction or for life after heart valve prosthesis placement.

ADVERSE DRUG REACTIONS

As with heparin the main adverse effect is bleeding. Special care is needed if the patient has any other bleeding tendency, e.g. peptic ulceration, wounds. Other reactions are less common and include urticaria, dermatitis, fever, nausea and diarrhoea. Phenindione can cause serious and even fatal sensitivity reactions.

DRUG INTERACTIONS

Many drugs interact with warfarin and these interactions have potentially very serious effects. Each patient should have their medication evaluated before starting warfarin therapy and any new medication should be chosen carefully. These interactions can occur through several mechanisms:

- Potentiation of anticoagulant effect, e.g. with heparin, aspirin;
- Delayed metabolism or excretion, e.g. with cimetidine;
- Increased rate of metabolism, e.g. with phenytoin, thyroxine;
- Displacement from albumin, e.g. with non-steroidal anti-inflammatory drugs;
- Alteration of vitamin K levels, e.g. with change in diet, broad spectrum antibiotics; and
- Alteration in rate of clotting factor synthesis, e.g. with anabolic steroids, oestrogens.

Some examples of drugs which interact with warfarin are listed in Table 13.1.

PRECAUTIONS AND CONTRAINDICATIONS

As it crosses the placenta and can cause fetal malformations and induce fetal haemorrhage, warfarin is contraindicated in pregnancy. It has also been detected in breast milk and should be used with caution in nursing mothers.

TABLE 13.1 Examples of drug interactions with warfarin

Drugs which increase the activity of warfarin
Aspirin, heparin, chloral hydrate, cimetidine, amiodarone, ketoconazole, nalidixic acid, thyroxine, erythromycin, metronidazole, sulfonamides
Drugs which decrease the activity of warfarin
Barbiturates, phenytoin, cholestyramine, rifampicin, sucralfate, griseofulvin, vitamin K
Drugs which have varying effects on warfarin activity
Allopurinol, tricyclic antidepressants, broad spectrum antibiotics, vitamin supplements[*]

[*]These preparations contain varying amounts of vitamin K.

BLOOD DISORDERS

13

ANTIDOTE

The effects of warfarin can be reversed by administration of synthetic vitamin K, phytomenadione (*Konakion*). For several days after administration of vitamin K the patient remains refractory to the effects of warfarin. Vitamin K cannot be used for 'temporary' reversal of oral anticoagulation. If re-anticoagulation is needed after administration of vitamin K, heparin or another type of anticoagulant must be used.

Heparin/Warfarin Changeover

Most patients requiring anticoagulant therapy will be started on heparin as it has an immediate effect. Warfarin therapy is usually started several days before heparin is ceased so the full effect of warfarin is achieved prior to cessation of heparin therapy.

NURSING IMPLICATIONS

ASSESSMENT

Observe the patient for signs of bleeding (e.g. melaena, haematuria, bruising). The possibility of drug interactions should be thoroughly checked when any drug is given to a patient on anticoagulants. Assess the patient and their family for anxiety about the condition or the treatment involved.

ADMINISTRATION

The dose of heparin is often altered by changing the rate of flow of the infusion. Calculation of the dose change and the necessary change in drip rate must be made and checked very carefully.

With subcutaneous administration correct injection technique is important to minimise pain and the possibility of haematoma formation. The site of injection should be rotated.

For drugs with a low therapeutic index it is important that patients receive the same amount of drug at each dose. For example, different brands of tablets may have different bioavailabilities, i.e. the patient may absorb 60% of the drug in brand X tablets but 80% of the drug in brand Y tablets. This difference may be significant and patients must always take the same brand of tablet. Warfarin should always be prescribed by brand name and the patient told to continue taking that brand only. Careful checking must be performed to ensure the correct dose and brand is administered. Some institutions require anticoagulant administration to be checked by two people. A regular time should be established for administration. This makes comparisons of blood levels easier and assists with patient compliance.

Action should be taken to minimise the hazards in the patient's environment and to prevent unnecessary bleeding. Care should be exercised when handling the patient. Pressure caused by either fingers or devices, e.g. blood pressure measuring devices, should be avoided.

Special care should be taken to minimise blood loss from venipuncture sites. Bruising, which can be extensive, painful and unsightly, can occur if this is not done. Intramuscular injections must be avoided whenever possible.

EVALUATION

Evaluation of physiological response to anticoagulants is by frequent clotting tests. Initially these are performed daily until the desired response has been achieved. Several formulae based on the patient's age, weight and renal function have been developed to help determine the appropriate dose. These formulae do not replace the use of clotting tests.

With low dose prophylactic therapy tests of clotting ability may not be required.

When blood is required for coagulation tests it must not be taken from the limb (and especially the line) through which the anticoagulant therapy was administered.

PATIENT EDUCATION

It has been shown that patients are more likely to comply with medication orders if they know why they are being asked to do so. Various companies produce educational booklets on anticoagulation therapy. These should be made available to the patient.

Points that should be discussed with the patient include:

- The reason for anticoagulant therapy and its expected duration;

- The importance of checking for, and reporting, any signs of bleeding (including back pain or headache which may represent internal bleeding);

- The importance of compliance and not to try to 'catch up' missed doses;

- The possibility of drug interactions and the need to inform anyone prescribing other types of medication that they are on anticoagulant therapy, this includes self-medication and non-prescription items;

- The importance of avoiding preparations containing aspirin (see Chapter 22 Musculoskeletal Disorders and Chapter 23 Pain Relief), paracetamol shoud be used if a mild analgesic is needed;

- The need to inform doctors, dentists and other health care providers that anticoagulant therapy is being taken;

- The advisability of wearing or carrying an identification disc in case of medical emergencies or accidents;

- The importance of complying with blood test schedules to avoid over or under dosage, the need for dose changes and how to make up doses from the range of tablet strengths available;

- The importance of adherence to the suggested diet; and

- The contraindication to the use of warfarin during pregnancy.

Patients who are injecting themselves subcutaneously should be instructed to select a suitable abdominal site for injection (the anterolateral abdominal wall is the preferred site, however, if this is not available the thigh is a suitable alternative); to pinch up the skin at the chosen site, swab the top of the fold and insert the needle perpendicularly and completely; to withdraw the plunger slightly to ensure that a blood vessel has not been entered; and then to slowly inject the heparin.

ANTIPLATELET AGENTS

Aspirin, Dipyridamole, Sulfinpyrazone

TRADE NAMES

Aspirin: *Solprin*; *Disprin*; *Cardiprin*; *Cartia*; *Astrix*.
Dipyridamole: *Persantin*.
Sulfinpyrazone: *Anturan*.

MECHANISM OF ACTION

Platelet aggregation is controlled by a delicate balance between the formation of thromboxanes and prostacyclin. The antiplatelet agents, aspirin, dipyridamole and sulfinpyrazone, inhibit the aggregation of platelets by interfering with the formation of the prostaglandins, thromboxane A2 and prostacyclin. In low doses (e.g. 100 mg/day) aspirin inhibits the formation of thromboxane A2 by inhibiting the enzyme prostaglandin cyclo-oxygenase but does not affect prostacyclin formation. In high doses it also affects prostacyclin. Dipyridamole enhances levels of prostacyclin but its exact mechanism of action is not clear. Prostacyclin (epoprostenol) can be used as an alternative to heparin during coronary bypass surgery and renal dialysis, as it limits thrombus formation.

PHARMACOKINETICS

Aspirin, dipyridamole and sulfinpyrazone are absorbed orally. The effect of aspirin is irreversible, i.e. it lasts as long as the life of the platelet. The effect of dipyridamole and sulfinpyrazone only lasts while the drug is present in the blood.

USES

The antiplatelet agents are given either alone or in combination to prevent thrombotic events, e.g. in the prevention of myocardial infarction, the prevention of further myocardial infarction, and in the presence of angina or transient ischaemic attacks (TIA) to prevent stroke.

The dose of aspirin used is 100–150 mg daily. Dipyridamole is given in a dose of 100 mg four times daily.

ADVERSE DRUG REACTIONS

Adverse reactions which occur are nausea; bleeding; hypersensitivity reactions with aspirin; and headache and facial flushing with dipyridamole.

Ticlopidine

TRADE NAMES

Ticlopidine: *Ticlid.*

MECHANISM OF ACTION

Ticlopidine inhibits platelet fibrinogen binding and subsequent platelet–platelet interactions. The effect lasts for the life of the platelet (i.e. it is irreversible). The release of platelet contents is also inhibited.

PHARMACOKINETICS

Ticlopidine has a long (and variable) half-life. It is well absorbed after oral administration and extensively metabolised. The rate

of metabolism is dose and age dependent (e.g. elderly people take longer to clear the same dose from the body).

USES

Ticlopidine tablets are used to decrease the risk of stroke and mortality after transient ischaemic attacks, especially in those intolerant to aspirin.

ADVERSE DRUG REACTIONS

A reversible neutropenia occurred in 2.4% of stroke patients who received the drug in clinical trials. Therefore it is recommended that full blood counts be performed every two weeks for the first three months of therapy.

Other reactions include thrombocytopenia, increased cholesterol levels, diarrhoea, nausea, rash and gastrointestinal pain.

PRECAUTIONS AND CONTRAINDICATIONS

As elderly patients clear the drug more slowly care should be taken with dosage. The safety of ticlopidine when given with other agents affecting coagulation has yet to be established.

NURSING IMPLICATIONS

ASSESSMENT

Platelet function tests need to be performed to assess the effects of anticoagulants. (The effect on coagulation is not measured by clotting tests.) The patient should also be assessed for bleeding tendencies and adverse reactions.

ADMINISTRATION

Aspirin should be taken with food to decrease gastric irritation. Ticlopidine is better absorbed if given with food. Dipyridamole should be given on an empty stomach.

Action should be taken to minimise hazards in the patient's environment and to prevent unnecessary bleeding. Pressure caused by either the fingers or devices such

as blood pressure measuring equipment should be avoided.

PATIENT EDUCATION

The patient should be taught:

- **To check for and report any bleeding or bruising;**
- **That concurrent aspirin administration should be avoided; and**
- **To use paracetamol if a mild analgesic is needed.**

If taking ticlopidine the patient should be informed of the need for, and importance of compliance with, regular blood tests.

Dextrans

Dextrans are low molecular weight polysaccharides. There are two main formulations, dextran 40 and dextran 70 which have molecular weights of 40 000 and 70 000 respectively.

Dextrans decrease platelet adhesiveness and venous stasis and are used in the prophylaxis of venous thrombosis when patients are unable to receive heparin. The other, and main, use of dextran is for plasma volume expansion after shock or trauma.

TRADE NAMES

Dextran 40: *Rheomacrodex.*
Dextran 70: *Macrodex.*
Dextran 1: *Promit.*

PHARMACOKINETICS

Dextrans are not absorbed after oral administration and so must be given intravenously. They are renally excreted and administration should be stopped if signs of renal impairment appear.

USES

For prophylaxis of venous thrombosis a 500 mL dose may be administered intrave-

nously daily for two to three days, then on alternate days for up to two weeks.

ADVERSE DRUG REACTIONS

Severe allergic reactions can occur due to the dextran combining with circulating antibodies. This combination triggers the immune response which varies with the size of the complex. These reactions can occur within a few minutes of starting therapy and include mild to generalised urticaria, pruritus, angioedema, nasal congestion, wheezing, nausea, vomiting, fever, chills, arthralgia, flushing, bronchospasm, hypotension, anaphylactic shock, and respiratory and cardiac arrest.

It is possible to decrease these reactions by giving a very small molecule, dextran 1 just before the dextran 40 or 70 infusion. Dextran 1 must not be combined with the dextran infusion.

PRECAUTIONS AND CONTRAINDICATIONS

Congestive heart failure can be exacerbated by the plasma volume expansion induced by dextran administration.

NURSING IMPLICATIONS

ASSESSMENT

The patient should be monitored for signs of volume expansion and overload, e.g. increased pulse and respiratory rates, wheezing, shortness of breath.

Renal function should be checked before infusions are commenced. If impairment is found therapy may have to be decreased or discontinued. Vital signs should be documented prior to the commencement of the infusion so that a baseline is established.

ADMINISTRATION

As an allergic reaction to dextran may occur soon after administration starts the patient should be observed closely at the commencement of the infusion. If a reaction develops the infusion should be stopped immediately. Resuscitation equipment, adrenaline, steroids and antihistamines should be readily available. If dextran 1 is used it should be given 15 minutes before commencing the dextran 40 or 70 infusion. The two infusions should not be given at the same time.

COAGULANT DRUGS

Bleeding disorders can be caused by an absence of, or deficit in, any one of the factors involved with clot formation, e.g. platelets, clotting factors, the fibrinolytic system. Vascular damage from trauma or surgery can also lead to prolonged or excessive bleeding.

The fibrinolytic system works to break down the fibrin clots once they have been formed. Excess activity of the fibrinolytic system will lead to bleeding. Wherever possible the treatment of these disorders is by correction of the defect, e.g. factor VIII transfusions for haemophiliac patients, platelet transfusions for thrombocytopenia, ascorbic acid for patients with scurvy. When this is not possible several drugs can be used to enhance clot formation or stability.

DRUGS WHICH ENHANCE CLOT FORMATION

Thrombin

Thrombin (*Thrombin, Thrombostat, Thrombinar*) is the substance which activates the conversion of fibrinogen to fibrin and hence enhances clot formation. Thrombin is applied as a solution directly to the bleeding surface. It causes fairly rapid clot formation. It cannnot be used systemically as it causes extensive intravascular clotting which may result in death. It is used by dentists to arrest bleeding after tooth extraction and to stop blood oozing from damaged capillaries and small venules.

Oxidised Cellulose

Oxidised cellulose (*Oxycel*) does not act on the clotting system. On contact with blood it swells and sticks to the surface to form an artificial clot. Care must be taken with its placement to avoid pressure or constriction of surrounding structures when it swells. Once haemostasis has been achieved it should be carefully removed.

DRUGS WHICH ENHANCE CLOT STABILITY

Aminocaproic Acid, Tranexamic Acid, Aprotinin

The agents used to enhance clot stability are aminocaproic acid, tranexamic acid and aprotinin. These drugs prevent a clot which has formed from being broken down by the fibrinolytic system. They do not increase clot formation. Tranexamic acid is said to be ten times as potent as aminocaproic acid.

TRADE NAMES

Aminocaproic acid: *EACA*; *Amicar*.
Tranexamic acid: *Cyclokapron*.
Aprotinin: *Trasylol*.

PHARMACOKINETICS

Tranexamic acid is given orally as tablets. It is rapidly absorbed and is exreted in the urine. Aprotinin and aminocaproic acid must be given parenterally. They are renally excreted.

USES

These drugs are prescribed to decrease bleeding usually from extravascular sites following trauma or surgery, e.g. after

13

BLOOD DISORDERS

prostate and urinary tract surgery. Tranexamic acid may be used to decrease excessive menstrual losses and where the site of gastrointestinal blood loss cannot be identified.

These drugs can be used prophylactically in combination with factor VIII replacement before dental extraction and minor surgery in haemophiliac patients. Aminocaproic acid and tranexamic acid can also be used as antidotes after excessive fibrinolytic agent administration. Aprotinin use is being investigated as a means of reducing blood loss in surgery involving extracorporeal circulation, e.g. heart/lung machines.

ADVERSE DRUG REACTIONS

Adverse reactions to the clotting agents are common. Nausea, diarrhoea, skin rashes, headaches, hypotension and weakness have all been reported. Aprotinin is of bovine origin and allergic reactions, such as urticaria and hypotension, have occurred. Nasal stuffiness has been noted after aminocaproic acid administration. Tranexamic acid is said to have a lower incidence of adverse effects than aminocaproic acid.

PRECAUTIONS AND CONTRAINDICATIONS

These agents are renally excreted so the dose must be decreased if renal impairment is present. Blockage of the urinary tract has occurred in the presence of marked haematuria.

These agents cross the placenta and have been reported to harm the fetus. They should only be used in pregnancy when the benefits outweigh the risks to the fetus. They must be used with care if the patient has any other tendency to clot, e.g. angina, coronary artery disease, transient ischaemic attacks.

NURSING IMPLICATIONS

ASSESSMENT

If these drugs are to be given, renal function should be measured and the dose altered accordingly. Patients are often very worried and anxious about blood loss. Accurate assessment of any blood loss is essential.

ADMINISTRATION

Doses can be high and the patient may find it easier to take a liquid rather than a large number of tablets. If an oral formulation of aminocaproic acid is not available the intravenous form can be substituted in an emergency. The reverse does not apply. Infusions of aminocaproic acid must be given slowly to minimise the risk of bradycardia or cardiac arrhythmias.

EVALUATION

Continuous assessment of blood loss and checking for signs of hypercoagulation is necessary. Renal function should be monitored as renal impairment is an indication for reduction in dose.

FIBRINOLYTIC DRUGS

Fibrinolytic agents are enzymes which can dissolve clots. They convert plasminogen to plasmin which then acts to degrade fibrin, fibrinogen and other proteins involved in clot formation. They are used to dissolve clots which have already formed. They are more effective when given as soon as possible after the clot has formed (preferably within four hours of the onset of pain). They are used for dissolution of thrombi in a number of conditions including pulmonary embolism, deep vein thrombosis and myocardial infarction and to lyse clots in the eye and occluded arteriovenous cannulae.

Although all are effective at recanalising occluded coronary arteries, re-occlusion occurs following acute administration of each agent. The use of aspirin and/or heparin to try and reduce the rate of re-occlusion is currently being studied. The risk of bleeding complications must be carefully assessed.

Streptokinase

TRADE NAMES

Streptokinase: *Kabikinase*; *Streptase*.

USES

Streptokinase is obtained from certain strains of haemolytic streptococci. In coronary artery occlusion it is given as a short infusion over 30–60 minutes. It has a relatively longer half-life than tissue plasminogen activator (tPA). At 24 hours the two drugs produce a similar rate of patency in previously occluded blood vessels. Streptokinase has also been used with some success to unblock central venous catheters and injection ports.

PRECAUTIONS AND CONTRAINDICATIONS

As streptokinase is obtained from bacteria it has a high antigenic potential and the body can produce antibodies to it very quickly. This can lead to severe allergic reactions (including hypotension and anaphylaxis) especially if administration is prolonged or repeated, and tolerance (very high doses may be needed to produce an effect). To avoid these effects it has been recommended that streptokinase not be given again within 5–90 days after the last dose. However, recent information suggests that the drug should not be readministered within 12 months. Pretreatment with antihistamines and/or corticosteroids has also been tried to minimise these reactions.

The antibodies which develop to streptokinase may also develop after streptococcal infection. These antibodies take approximately three months to decline and streptokinase should not be used during this time. Urokinase and tPA do not cause this problem.

Tissue Plasminogen Activator

TRADE NAMES

Tissue plasminogen activator (tPA, alteplase): *Actilyse*.

USES

Tissue plasminogen activator is produced by recombinant DNA technology. It has the same actions as streptokinase but binds more specifically to the fibrin in a clot. It is given as a bolus injection followed by a 3-hour infusion. Maximum patency is obtained at 90 minutes.

Anistreplase (*Emanase*) is another drug in the same family with similar actions.

Urokinase

TRADE NAMES

Urokinase (urinary plasminogen activator): *Ukidin*.

USES

Urokinase has similar properties to streptokinase and is obtained from human urine or tissue culture of kidney cells. It is given as an infusion in pulmonary embolism and limb ischaemia as well as for coronary artery occlusion.

ADVERSE DRUG REACTIONS

Bleeding is the main adverse effect and can occur from any site (e.g. injection site, damaged mucosa, menstruation). Minor haemorrhage has been reported in 5%–10% of patients, serious haemorrhage in 1%–2%. Other reactions include urticaria, itching, flushing, nausea and fever (which may be reduced by giving corticosteroids).

DRUG INTERACTIONS

Heparin, oral anticoagulants and antiplatelet agents may increase the risk of haemorrhage if given with these agents and their concurrent use should be monitored very closely.

Hypotension may occur when morphine is given concurrently.

PRECAUTIONS AND CONTRAINDICATIONS

Contraindications have been classified into absolute and relative.

Absolute contraindications include active bleeding, a history of cardiovascular accident, intracranial or intraspinal surgery or trauma within two months, intracranial neoplasm, arteriovenous malformation, aneurysm and severe uncontrolled hypertension.

Relative contraindications include recent major surgery, organ biopsy, recent obstetric delivery, cardiovascular disease, recent gastrointestinal bleeding, recent trauma, hypertension, bacterial endocarditis, haemostatic defects, severe liver dysfunction, pregnancy, diabetic retinopathy, advanced age, oral anticoagulant therapy, prolonged cardiopulmonary resuscitation.

These relative contraindications should be considered against the situation of each patient and a decision made as to whether the drug should be used.

NURSING IMPLICATIONS

These drugs should only be used in units which have developed protocols for their use and staff are familiar with the drugs, e.g. coronary and intensive care units and emergency departments.

ASSESSMENT

An allergy history should be obtained. Patients must be continually observed for anaphylaxis and other signs of allergy. During therapy puncture sites (such as peripheral and central intravenous catheter sites), wounds, intubation sites and urinary catheters are potential sites for blood loss. These must be kept to a minimum. A tissue perfusion baseline is established for upper and lower extremities. Blood flow may be assessed by a Doppler flowmeter. Colour, temperature, capillary filling and movement should also be checked and blood pressure measured regularly.

ADMINISTRATION

Care must be taken not to shake or unnecessarily agitate the solutions of these drugs. Agitation causes bubbles to form which take a very long time to disperse and may delay treatment.

Unnecessary handling of the patient should be avoided. Intramuscular injections are contraindicated. If invasive procedures must be performed, pressure must be maintained on the site for at least 15 minutes and then a pressure dressing applied. This action is especially important if arterial puncture is used to obtain samples for blood gas analysis. Care of mucous membranes, especially where endotracheal tubes or catheters are used, must be scrupulous.

EVALUATION

Treatment is monitored by frequent clotting tests and by the disappearance of the thrombotic lesion. Anaphylaxis, other signs of allergy and the need for high doses are criteria for discontinuation of therapy. Circulation must be monitored throughout the treatment. Puncture sites, the gastrointestinal tract and the urinary system should be monitored for signs of bleeding until clotting function returns to normal.

DRUGS AFFECTING BLOOD VISCOSITY

Oxpentifylline

Oxpentifylline is a xanthine derivative. It appears to increase the flexibility of erythrocytes and decrease platelet aggregation. It produces a decrease in blood viscosity and an improvement in blood flow in very small vessels.

TRADE NAMES

Oxpentifylline: *Trental*.

PHARMACOKINETICS

It is well absorbed orally and undergoes extensive first pass metabolism in the liver. The half-life increases as the dose increases. It is renally excreted as metabolites.

USES

Oxpentifylline is used in peripheral vascular disease to increase the circulation after stenosis and in intermittent claudication. The effect may take 2–4 weeks to become apparent.

ADVERSE DRUG REACTIONS

Adverse reactions mainly affect the gastrointestinal tract and the central nervous system. Nausea, dyspepsia, vomiting and belching are common but occur less frequently with the sustained release formulation. Dizziness, headache and tremor are also widely noted. Angina and chest pain have been reported.

PRECAUTIONS AND CONTRAINDICATIONS

As it is a xanthine derivative, oxpentifylline is contraindicated in those intolerant to caffeine and theophylline. It may potentiate the effects of antihypertensive agents.

DRUG INTERACTIONS

Bleeding may be more common in patients taking oxpentifylline and anticoagulants. It is recommended that these patients have coagulation tests performed more frequently.

NURSING IMPLICATIONS

ADMINISTRATION

Oxpentifylline is available as slow release tablets. These should be administered with meals to minimise the gastric irritation.

PATIENT EDUCATION

To encourage compliance the patient must be told that it may take some weeks for the effect of therapy to become apparent.

BLOOD DISORDERS

13

DRUGS AFFECTING HAEMATOPOIESIS

Anaemias are due to many different causes, e.g. insufficient production or excessive destruction of cells, excessive loss of cells and deficiencies of the factors needed for haematopoiesis.

Insufficient production of cells may be due to decreased production by bone marrow (e.g. aplastic anaemia) or other diseases which decrease red cell production (e.g. renal failure). For information on anaemia due to renal disease and its treatment with erythropoietin see Chapter 14 Drugs Used in Renal Failure. Treatment involves bone marrow transplant, corticosteroids, anti-T-cell immunoglobulins and colony stimulating factors. Supportive care with blood transfusions and antibiotics is often necessary. Excessive destruction of cells may be due to radiotherapy, chemotherapy or autoimmune disease.

Excessive loss of cells may occur through breakdown or bleeding, e.g. haemolytic anaemia, thalassaemia. As many of these conditions are hereditary it is often not possible to correct the cause of bleeding. Multiple blood transfusions are needed by many of these patients to maintain their haemoglobin level. Desferrioxamine is used to treat the iron overload which can develop from multiple transfusions (see Iron Overload).

Deficiencies of the factors needed for haematopoiesis (iron, folic acid, vitamin B_{12}) may cause iron deficiency anaemia and pernicious anaemia.

Iron

Iron deficiency is the commonest cause of anaemia in Australia. Iron is used in the synthesis of haemoglobin. The total body iron content is 3–5 g of which 60% is present in haemoglobin.

PHARMACOKINETICS

Usually only 10% of dietary iron is absorbed, but absorption is increased in iron deficiency states. Most commercial preparations of iron are the ferrous form as this is more easily absorbed from the gastrointestinal tract. Unabsorbed iron is excreted in the faeces giving them a black colour.

USES

Oral iron therapy will increase the haemoglobin level by 1–2 g/100 mL per week. After the desired level has been reached therapy must be continued for several weeks to allow body stores to be replaced.

Iron can also be given by the intravenous and intramuscular routes. The total dose, based on the haemoglobin level and the patient's weight, is given by intravenous infusion in one or two doses. Parenteral administration of iron is associated with a high incidence of adverse reactions and is only used when the haemoglobin level is very low and immediate treatment is needed, or the patient cannot tolerate oral iron.

ADVERSE DRUG REACTIONS

Several reports of severe adverse reactions, including anaphylaxis, have been reported with parenteral iron preparations. Other reactions include nausea, black and 'tarry' stools (from unabsorbed iron) and constipation with oral preparations.

DRUG INTERACTIONS

Oral iron preparations inactivate some antibiotics (e.g. tetracyclines and quinolones) and absorption of iron may be decreased. Iron preparations and tetracycline antibiotics should be administered at least three hours apart.

PRECAUTIONS AND CONTRAINDICATIONS

Although relatively harmless to adults, iron

preparations are potentially fatal if taken in overdose by children. Such an event should be treated as a medical emergency. Iron preparations should be stored well out of reach of children and in containers with child resistant closures.

NURSING IMPLICATIONS

ADMINISTRATION

The strength of oral preparations of iron can be expressed in two ways, either as the amount of iron in the tablet (e.g. 105 mg iron) or as the amount of ferrous sulfate in the tablet (e.g. 350 mg). Ferrous sulfate tablets 350 mg contain 105 mg iron. It is important to check which form the prescriber has ordered to identify the dose required and the correct amount of iron to give.

Oral administration of iron can cause nausea. Iron is better absorbed if it is administered on an empty stomach but if patients experience nausea it can be given with meals. Liquid preparations of iron can stain the teeth and should be administered through a straw.

Intramuscular injection of iron can be very painful. To avoid staining the skin a 'Z' track injection technique should be used. The dose should be split between the two buttocks.

PATIENT EDUCATION

Patients should be told that their stools will become black and that this is not necessarily a sign of gastrointestinal bleeding. Once the haemoglobin level has returned to normal, patients feel much better and may be tempted to stop therapy. They should be reminded of the need to continue therapy to replace body stores of iron.

Iron Overload

Each unit of whole blood contains approximately 250 mg of iron. People with haemolytic disorders often require multiple transfusions every few weeks. As a result they can very easily become overloaded with iron. The excess iron is deposited in the heart, liver, skin, pancreas and other tissues and produces symptoms of organ damage such as heart failure, diabetes and skin pigmentation. Desferrioxamine (*Desferal*) is a chelating agent which is used to remove excess iron. It is also used in the treatment of acute iron poisoning (see Chapter 9 Poisonings and Their Treatment).

Adverse reactions to desferrioxamine are rare. Pain at the injection site, allergy, skin and cardiac problems have been reported.

NURSING IMPLICATIONS

ASSESSMENT

Organ damage from excessive iron levels should be evaluated and appropriate therapy given.

ADMINISTRATION

Desferrioxamine can be given by intravenous, intramuscular or subcutaneous injection. The dose is titrated to achieve the desired rate of iron excretion. It has a greater effect when given by continuous infusion rather than intermittently. Intravenous administration may be slightly more effective, but is often less convenient than subcutaneous administration. Many patients receive their desferrioxamine as a 10–12-hour subcutaneous infusion overnight. A portable infusion pump or syringe driver is used to regulate the infusion.

EVALUATION

At the start of desferrioxamine treatment the urinary iron excretion should be measured

BLOOD DISORDERS

13

daily. Once stable, it can be measured less frequently but should be measured at least once a fortnight.

PATIENT EDUCATION

If the patient is to administer an infusion at home they must be taught, and be proficient in, all the appropriate techniques, i.e. aseptic technique, drawing up the injections and using the syringe driver or infusion pump. The nurse must be sure the patient fully understands all the procedures involved and how to manage any problems which may arise. The patient should be warned that their urine may develop a reddish discolouration.

Folic Acid, Vitamin B$_{12}$

Both folic acid and vitamin B$_{12}$ are needed for haematopoiesis. The absorption of vitamin B$_{12}$ is dependent on 'intrinsic factor' which is secreted from the parietal cells of the stomach wall. Some people are deficient in intrinsic factor and so cannot absorb adequate amounts of vitamin B$_{12}$. When this deficiency becomes clinically apparent it is known as pernicious anaemia.

TRADE NAMES

Vitamin B$_{12}$ (hydroxycobalamin):
Neo-Cytamen.
Vitamin B$_{12}$ (cyanocobalamin): *Cytamen.*

PHARMACOKINETICS

Both folic acid and vitamin B$_{12}$ are usually well absorbed from the gastrointestinal tract and are available in sufficient quantities in a balanced diet.

Following intramuscular administration hydroxycobalamin is absorbed more slowly and retained in the body longer than cyanocobalamin.

USES

Folic acid is used to treat megaloblastic and macrocytic anaemias caused by folic acid deficiency. Folic acid deficiency is due to

malabsorption, decreased intake or increased needs. It is well absorbed after oral administration even in malabsorption states. The daily requirement is 100–200 micrograms. This requirement may be increased in certain disease states.

When the B$_{12}$ deficiency is not due to a lack of intrinsic factor, vitamin B$_{12}$ replacement can be given orally as cyanocobalamin. If the deficiency is due to a lack of intrinsic factor, replacement therapy must be given parenterally usually by intramuscular injection.

ADVERSE DRUG REACTIONS

Administration of folic acid alone may precipitate a neuropathy in patients who are deficient in vitamin B$_{12}$.

Discomfort at the site of injection is the most common adverse reaction to vitamin B$_{12}$. A few patients will experience llergic reactions. On rare occasions anaphylaxis has been reported after parenteral administration of hydroxycobalamin.

DRUG INTERACTIONS

Folic acid may reduce the anticonvulsant effect of phenytoin by decreasing phenytoin serum levels. The effects of methotrexate may also be reduced if folic acid is given concurrently.

NURSING IMPLICATIONS

ADMINISTRATION

Cyanocobalamin and hydroxycobalamin are the two parenteral forms of vitamin B$_{12}$. The body retains a greater percentage of a dose of hydroxycobalamin and so it can be given less frequently than cyanocobalamin (every three months instead of every month). Treatment regimens are designed to replace body stores (with several weekly intramuscular injections of hydroxycobalamin) and then to replace daily losses (with intramuscular injections every three months).

Care must be taken not to confuse folic acid with folinic acid, see Chapter 31 Cancer Chemotherapy.

PATIENT EDUCATION

Dietary inadequacy is one of the most common reasons for these anaemias. The patient should be referred to a dietitian for information. The nurse should reinforce the need for continued adherence to the recommended diet. The treatment of pernicious anaemia with folic acid and vitamin B$_{12}$ is not curative. It is replacement therapy only. Patients must understand that if they stop therapy the symptoms will reappear. They must be informed that therapy will be long term or for life.

COLONY STIMULATING FACTORS

Colony stimulating factors are glycoproteins which affect the growth of blood cells and many other cells and processes. They are produced by recombinant DNA technology. The recombinant products appear to be biologically equivalent to the naturally occurring colony stimulating factors and the cells produced appear to be functionally identical to those produced normally. Their effects are dose related but there is a large variation in patient response to the same dose.

Many different colony stimulating factors are being developed. Granulocyte colony stimulating factor (G-CSF) and granulocyte macrophage colony stimulating factor (GM-CSF) are already available. Interleukin 3 (IL3) and macrophage colony stimulating factor (M-CSF) are currently being investigated. Erythropoietin (a red cell colony stimulating factor) is discussed in Chapter 14 Drugs Used in Renal Failure.

These agents are also being studied for use in aplastic anaemia, burn injuries, hairy cell leukaemia and AIDS. It is hoped that they will enable larger doses of marrow suppressing drugs to be given (e.g. zidovudine, chemotherapy).

It is important to realise that the colony stimulating factors only ameliorate the marrow suppression and not the other toxicities of these drugs (e.g. neurotoxicity).

The optimum dose, duration and timing of therapy has not yet been established.

GM-CSF: Sargramostim

Sargramostim (granulocyte macrophage colony stimulating factor, GM-CSF) is naturally produced by T-lymphocytes, monocytes, fibroblasts and endothelial cells. It is given intravenously or subcutaneously to accelerate recovery of cell counts after bone marrow transplant and chemotherapy for non-Hodgkins' lymphoma, Hodgkins' disease and acute lymphoblastic leukaemia.

PHARMACOKINETICS

Colony stimulating factors are not orally bioavailable. Given intravenously they have a short half-life (approximately 2.5 hours) and therefore need to be given by infusion. After subcutaneous administration blood levels are maintained for 12–16 hours. The site of elimination is not yet known.

ADVERSE DRUG REACTIONS

At low doses mild constitutional reactions (e.g. fever, headache, myalgias) are common and can usually be controlled with antipyretics and analgesics (e.g. paracetamol). Phlebitis or erythema may occur at the site of administration. At high doses fluid accumulation (peripheral oedema and pleural effusions) have been reported. Dyspnoea has occurred but resolved when the infusion rate was halved.

PRECAUTIONS AND CONTRAINDICATIONS

GM-CSF should not be given to patients with excessive leukaemic or myeloid blast cells as it may worsen their disease.

G-CSF: Filgrastim, Lenograstim

Filgrastim and lenogastrim are preparations of granulocyte colony stimulating factor (G-CSF). Filgrastim (*Neupogen*) is produced naturally by monocytes, fibroblasts and endothelial cells. Lenograstim (*Granocyte*) is recombinant human granulocyte colony stimulating factor (rHuG-CSF) and is produced by recombinant DNA technology. Both stimulate neutrophil production and are used to shorten and lighten the neutropenia associated with chemotherapy, bone marrow transplantation and other chronic neutropenias.

PHARMACOKINETICS

See GM-CSF.

ADVERSE DRUG REACTIONS

Mild constitutional reactions (see GM-CSF) are common. Bone pain and myalgias occur more frequently and fever less often.

NURSING IMPLICATIONS

ASSESSMENT

Patients receiving these drugs have compromised immune systems. It can be difficult to distinguish if fever is due to infection or an adverse drug reaction. In either case appropriate therapy must be instituted promptly.

ADMINISTRATION

GM-CSF and G-CSF can be given by subcutaneous injection or intravenous infusion. If the final concentration of a GM-CSF infusion is less than 10 micrograms/mL albumin needs to be added to the infusion to prevent adsorption of the drug onto the delivery system. Vials should not be shaken vigorously as the solution will froth up and may decrease the amount that can be drawn up in the syringe. Solutions that are cloudy or contain lumps or flakes should not be used.

EVALUATION

The rise of blood cell counts must be followed to confirm the dose and duration of therapy needed.

PATIENT EDUCATION

As patients are immunocompromised they should be educated about the need to avoid infection and appropriate hygiene. Patients who are self-administering subcutaneous injections should be instructed on correct injection technique, to avoid vigorous shaking of the vials, not to use solutions that are cloudy or contain lumps and to store the vials in a refrigerator.

DRUGS USED IN THE TREATMENT OF THROMBOCYTOPENIA

The normal platelet count range is $150–500 \times 10^9$/L. When the number of platelets drops significantly below this level the patient is at risk of both internal and external bleeding.

Bone marrow failure, viral illness and chemotherapy can cause decreases in the platelet count. Some drugs (e.g. gold, quinine, heparin) can also cause acute and profound thrombocytopenia. When the precipitating agent is unknown this reaction is called idiopathic thrombocytopenic purpura.

An antibody to the platelet–drug combination may be demonstrated (e.g. in heparin induced thrombosis/thrombocytopenia syndrome, HITTS). In such cases platelet transfusions are of little benefit as the transfused platelets are rapidly destroyed by the antibody.

Treatment with corticosteroids, intravenous immunoglobulin or splenectomy aims to reduce the immune system's destruction of platelets.

CORTICOSTEROIDS

Methylprednisolone, Prednisolone

Parenteral methylprednisolone and oral prednisolone are given in short high dose courses to depress the immune reaction against platelets. Typically 1 mg/kg/day of prednisolone is given for 5–10 days. At this dose level, use of the drug should be tapered off rather than abruptly stopped.

For information on the adverse reactions, precautions and nursing implications related to corticosteroid therapy see Chapter 19 Endocrine Diseases.

INTRAVENOUS IMMUNOGLOBULIN

Immunoglobulin G

Immunoglobulin G (IgG) is the major immune globulin in serum. It is prepared commercially from pooled blood donations that have been treated to remove contaminants and infectious particles (e.g. hepatitis B virus, HIV).

TRADE NAMES

Immunoglobulin G: *Intragam; Sandoglobulin.*

MECHANISM OF ACTION

Several mechanisms of action have been postulated but agreement has yet to be reached on its mechanism of action in the treatment of idiopathic thrombocytopenic purpura.

PHARMACOKINETICS

The half-life of IgG is difficult to evaluate due to the body's own production but appears to be shorter than that of native IgG (approximately 3 weeks).

USES

The main use of intravenous immunoglobulin is replacement in primary (e.g. aplastic anaemia) and secondary (e.g. AIDS) deficiency states. It is given every few weeks to maintain the immunoglobulin level close to 'normal'. It has also been shown to protect against some bacterial infections in patients with B cell malignancies.

In the treatment of idiopathic thrombocytopenic purpura and HITTS 400 mg/kg/day is given for approximately five days. Higher doses of 1 g/kg/day have been effective in refractory cases. A dose response curve has yet to be determined.

ADVERSE DRUG REACTIONS

Tachycardia, headache, chest tightness, fever, mild hypertension and lumbar pain occur in approximately 2% of patients after infusion. The incidence and severity is related to the rate of infusion. Severe reactions are rare. If a reaction occurs the infusion should be slowed or stopped. It can usually be restarted (slowly) when the reaction has been controlled.

Pre-medication with antihistamines has been tried to reduce the incidence and severity of reactions.

PRECAUTIONS AND CONTRAINDICATIONS

Small amounts of IgA remain in the commercial preparations. Allergic reactions are therefore possible.

BLOOD DISORDERS

13

NURSING IMPLICATIONS

ASSESSMENT

Patients with thrombocytopenia are at extreme risk of haemorrhage. They should be handled gently and their environment made as safe as possible. Invasive procedures must be kept to a minimum. Intramuscular administration of drugs is contraindicated. Blood pressure monitoring should only be performed if deemed necessary. Fever may be due to infection or a reaction to infusion and should be noted and investigated promptly.

ADMINISTRATION

Oral steroids should be given with food to decrease gastric irritation.

Immunoglobulin powders need to be reconstituted gently to avoid foaming. Infusions should be started slowly and the infusion rate increased according to the patient's ability to tolerate the drug.

A close watch for signs of distress or other adverse reactions should be maintained throughout the infusion.

EVALUATION

Some patients do not respond to immunoglobulin therapy and so the platelet count must be monitored to ensure that platelet numbers rise in response to treatment and that the rise is maintained.

PATIENT EDUCATION

The patient should be informed of the precipitating factor of the thrombocytopenia and how to avoid it; how to recognise signs of thrombocytopenia (e.g. bleeding, bruising, petecchiae) and the need to report it; the importance of avoiding knocks and cuts, e.g. by use of an electric razor, and the need for compliance with the steroid regimen and how to taper the dose when stopping therapy.

FURTHER READING

Gilman, A.G., Rall, T.W., Nies, A.S., Taylor, P., eds. (1990), *Goodman and Gilman's the pharmacological basis of therapeutics*. 8th edn Macmillan Press.

Ibister, J.P. (1986) *Clinical haematology: a problem orientated approach*. Williams and Wilkins, Sydney.

Metcalf, D. 'The colony stimulating factors: discovery, development and clinical applications'. *Cancer*, 65, 2185–2195.

Speight, T.M., ed. (1987) *Avery's drug treatment: principles and practice of clinical pharmacology and therapeutics*. 3rd edn Adis Press.

TEST YOUR KNOWLEDGE

1. List two examples of each of the following: (a) anticoagulants; (b) clotting agents; (c) fibrinolytic agents; (d) drugs affecting platelet function; (e) drugs affecting red cell growth.

2. Name the antidote for: (a) heparin; (b) warfarin.

3. Describe the pharmacological actions of: (a) streptokinase; (b) thrombin; (c) low dose aspirin.

4. List the disease states in which the following drugs are used: (a) intravenous immunoglobulin; (b) vitamin B_{12}; (c) warfarin; (d) tranexamic acid; (e) G-CSF.

5. What are the common adverse effects of: (a) oral iron preparations; (b) heparin; (c) GM-CSF.

6. List some of the drugs which interact with: (a) warfarin; (b) iron.

7. List the nursing implications in the use of: (a) dextran; (b) aminocaproic acid; (c) parenteral iron preparations.

TABLE 13.2 Summary table — drugs used in the treatment of blood disorders

DRUG GROUP Drug Name	Uses	Action	Adverse Effects	Nursing Implications
ANTICOAGULANTS				
Heparin Low molecular weight heparin Heparinoids Warfarin	DVT, PE, after MI, prosthesis implantation.	Prevents conversion of prothrombin to thrombin.	Bleeding, local irritation, mild pyrexia.	**Assess:** For bleeding tendencies (i.e. liver disease, recent surgery, GI conditions, wounds, other drugs affecting coagulation); probability of compliance; potential drug interactions; anxiety about condition; laboratory tests. **Administer:** Check all labels carefully for correct route of administration; do not massage injection site; use infusion pumps for continuous IV therapy. **Evaluate:** For any signs of bleeding (e.g. urine, stools); hypersensitivity; ADRs; drug interactions. **Educate:** Importance of compliance with drugs/laboratory tests, common food–drug interactions; to assess for bleeding; protect from trauma; sources of information.
Phenindione	DVT, PE, after MI, prosthesis implantation.	Inhibits synthesis of clotting factors II, VII, IX, X.	Bleeding, drug interactions.	
ANTIPLATELET AGENTS				
Aspirin Dipyridamole Sulfinpyrazone	Before and after MI, stroke prevention.	Inhibit platelet aggregation.	Nausea, bleeding, headache, facial flushing.	
Ticlopidine	Stroke prevention.	Inhibits platelet aggregation.	Neutropenia, GI intolerance.	
Dextran 40, 70	DVT, PE.	Decrease platelet adhesiveness, and venous stasis.	Mild to severe allergy, volume overload, bleeding.	

13 BLOOD DISORDERS

TABLE 13.2 continued

DRUG GROUP Drug Name	Uses	Action	Adverse Effects	Nursing Implications
COAGULANT DRUGS Thrombin	Arrests oozing from small blood vessels.	Activates conversion of fibrinogen to fibrin.	Excess clot formation.	**Assess:** For anxiety; blood loss; renal function; pregnancy. **Administer:** Give IV infusions slowly. **Evaluate:** Blood loss, hypercoagulation, renal impairment, ADRs.
Oxidised cellulose	Arrests small vessel bleeding.	Forms artificial clot.	Pressure or stricture of surrounding structures.	
Aminocaproic acid Tranexamic acid Aprotinin	Arrest internal bleeding after trauma or surgery.	Inhibit normal mechanism of clot breakdown.	Hypotension, nausea, diarrhoea, rash, pruritus, cardiac arrhythmias, allergy, nasal stuffiness.	
FIBRINOLYTIC AGENTS Streptokinase Tissue plasminogen activator (tPA) Urokinase	Dissolve formed clots. PE, coronary artery occlusion.	Activate conversion of plasminogen to plasmin.	Allergic reactions; anaphylaxis, antibody development; haemorrhage.	**Assess:** Allergy history, blood loss, other causes of bleeding, potential drug interactions, time since clot formation. **Administer:** According to protocol, minimal handling of patient, no IM injections, apply 15 minutes pressure at any site of invasive procedure. **Evaluate:** Clotting tests; allergy; anaphylaxis.
BLOOD VISCOSITY AGENTS Oxpentifylline	Intermittent claudication.	Increased flexibility of erythrocytes.	Nausea, vomiting, headache, dizziness, tremor.	**Administer:** Take with food. **Educate:** Delay before effect apparent.

TABLE 13.2 continued

DRUG GROUP Drug Name	Uses	Action	Adverse Effects	Nursing Implications
HAEMATOPOIETIC AGENTS				
Iron	Iron deficiency.	Haemoglobin formation.	Nausea, constipation, black/tarry stools.	**Assess**: Diet, GI bleeding. **Administer**: Liquid iron through straw; 'Z' track technique for IM injection. **Evaluate**: Blood count; recurrent GI bleeding; ADRs. **Educate**: Need for long-term therapy and compliance; to check for signs of bleeding; dark stools with oral iron; dietary modification; protect children from iron overdose.
Folic acid	Folic acid deficiency.	Required for red blood cell synthesis.	Rare.	
Vitamin B$_{12}$ (cyancobalamin, hydroxycobalamin)	Vitamin B$_{12}$ deficiency, pernicious anaemia.	Required for red blood cell synthesis.	Rare; discomfort at injection site; allergy after parenteral administration.	
GM-CSF G-CSF	Shorten and lighten neutropenia associated with chemotherapy, bone marrow transplantation; chronic neutropenia.	Stimulate target cell growth.	Fever, myalgia, bone pain, fluid overload.	**Assess:** Need for supportive therapy. **Administer:** IV or SC as appropriate. **Evaluate:** Rise in cell counts. **Educate:** Need for hygiene; report signs of infection.

13 BLOOD DISORDERS

TABLE 13.2 continued

DRUG GROUP Drug Name	Uses	Action	Adverse Effects	Nursing Implications
IRON CHELATING AGENTS				
Desferrioxamine	Iron overload.	Binds iron which is then renally excreted.	Pain at injection site, allergy (rare).	**Assess:** Urinary iron excretion; other organ damage. **Administer:** IV or SC infusion. **Educate:** Need for compliance; aseptic technique; drawing up injection; operating infusion pump; possible red discolouration of urine.
AGENTS USED IN THROMBOCYTOPENIA				
Methylprednisolone, prednisolone	Increase platelet count.	Immunosuppressant.	Nausea, immunosuppression.	**Assess:** Bleeding tendency; need for supportive therapy. **Administer:** Give steroids with food, IgG infusion to be reconstituted gently, started slowly and increased as patient can tolerate. **Evaluate:** Rise in platelet count. **Educate:** Risk factors for recurrence; to avoid cuts, scratches, etc; report signs of thrombocytopenia; compliance with steroid regimen.
Intravenous Immunoglobulin	Increase platelet count.	Interference with immune reaction to antibody.	Hypotension.	

Drugs Used in Renal Failure

KINGSLEY NG

O B J E C T I V E S

At the conclusion of this chapter the reader should be able to:

1. Describe the basic concepts of drug management in problems associated with renal failure, with particular reference to renal osteodystrophy, hyperkalaemia, renal hypertension and anaemia;

2. List the uses of drugs and their main side effects;

3. Name three commonly used immunosuppressive agents and list their main side effects; and

4. Describe the effect of renal failure and dialysis on the excretion of drugs.

RENAL FAILURE

The kidney is responsible for the elimination of many products of metabolism such as urea, uric acid and creatinine. It also controls the excretion of electrolytes and water and thus regulates the internal environment of the body. If the kidney fails breakdown products of dietary constituents will accumulate in the blood and water and electrolyte balance can no longer be maintained. Depending on the degree of kidney damage and provided that some renal function remains, the accumulation of metabolic products can be limited by a careful choice of diet. This usually involves protein and salt restriction. However, when a kidney has lost most (90%–95%) if not all of its function, control by diet is no longer possible. In order to maintain life the diseased kidney must be replaced with a functional one (i.e. transplantation) or have its functions performed by means of artificial or mechanical devices. The technique employed for the latter process is dialysis.

The outlook for patients with end-stage renal disease has been improved substantially over the past three decades by the development of dialysis and renal transplantation. These two techniques enable thousands of individuals with irreversible renal failure to lead a normal or near normal life. However, it is not uncommon to encounter problems associated with renal failure in spite of dialysis therapy. Some of these problems include vitamin deficiency, renal osteodystrophy, hyperkalaemia, hypertension, acidosis and anaemia.

There are also problems associated with transplantation, such as rejection and the side effects of immunosuppressive therapy. This chapter looks at some of the pharmacological agents which are employed to prevent or manage these problems. A brief discussion on the principles of dialysis is also included.

PRINCIPLES OF DIALYSIS

The principles of dialysis are relatively simple. If a patient's blood is placed on one side of a semipermeable membrane and a solution of known composition on the other, substances which the membrane is permeable to will move from the area of high concentration to the area of low concentration. Thus if the blood levels of substances such as urea and uric acid are high and these substances are absent from the dialysis solution, they will pass from the blood to the dialysis solution. Similarly if the blood potassium is low, and the potassium concentration in the dialysis solution is in the normal range, potassium will pass from the dialysis solution into the blood. Based on this principle, any abnormal electrolyte levels in patients with renal failure may be corrected by using a dialysis solution which contains the most important electrolytes in concentrations which are normal for healthy individuals. As waste products such as urea, uric acid and creatinine are absent from dialysis solutions they can be removed from the patient's blood by dialysis. Dialysis can be used to remove fluid from overhydrated patients. This is done by adding substances such as glucose to the dialysis solution until it is hypertonic with respect to blood or by creating a hydrostatic pressure gradient between blood and the dialysate. Due to the difference in hydrostatic or osmotic pressure, water will move from the patient to the solution.

Not only waste products are removed by dialysis. Essential body constituents such as the water soluble vitamins are also removed by the process. A number of drugs and poisons may be removed from the blood by dialysis and this technique has been used to treat certain types of drug intoxication (or toxicity) and poisoning. Dialysis can be performed either in the patient's peritoneal cavity (peritoneal dialysis), using the peritoneum as the semipermeable membrane, or outside the patient's body (haemodialysis), using an artificial kidney machine with a

dialysis membrane of cellulose or similar material.

DRUG TREATMENT OF PREDIALYSIS PROBLEMS

HYPERTENSION

Control of blood pressure is an important aspect in the management of all forms of renal diseases. If hypertension is left untreated, deterioration of renal function is inevitable and can also lead to other vascular complications. In some patients hypertension can be relieved by fluid restriction, dialysis and salt restriction. Renal hypertension due to stenosis of the renal artery may be surgically cured in selected patients.

The medical treatment of renal hypertension does not differ in principle from other forms of hypertension. The antihypertensives commonly employed include β blocking drugs and calcium channel blocking agents, vasodilators and angiotensin converting enzyme (ACE) inhibitors. For further information on these agents see Chapter 12 Cardiovascular Diseases.

It should be noted that ACE inhibitors should be used with caution in renal impairment as they cause retention of potassium and have been shown to cause a decline in renal function. Diuretics, which are frequently included in antihypertensive regimens in patients without renal failure, are of limited value in the presence of renal insufficiency. Potassium sparing diuretics such as spironolactone and amiloride may cause fatal hyperkalaemia when given to patients with renal failure and are therefore contraindicated.

HYPERKALAEMIA

As urinary potassium excretion is reduced in oliguric renal failure, potassium retention and hyperkalaemia often become a problem. The treatment of hyperkalaemia is a matter of urgency as it can cause life threatening cardiac arrhythmias and arrest. Such patients require cardiac monitoring and emergency treatment.

Glucose and Insulin

Usually 50 mL of 50% glucose together with 10–12 units of neutral insulin is given intravenously. When glucose enters the cells under the influence of insulin it carries potassium with it. The onset of the effect is rapid, but potassium will leave the cells if the glucose infusion is not kept up.

Some physicians advocate the use of glucose alone in non-diabetic patients since these patients can produce their own insulin quite rapidly in response to infused glucose and the use of glucose and insulin is associated with significant hypoglycaemia.

Sodium Bicarbonate

Administration of sodium bicarbonate is another measure by which serum potassium can be rapidly lowered. It is administered as an intravenous infusion of 500 mL isotonic sodium bicarbonate. The bicarbonate induces potassium ions to enter the cells and thus reduces plasma potassium. The effect is rapid but temporary, buying time for other measures, such as dialysis, to be instituted.

Salbutamol

Salbutamol (*Ventolin, Respolin*), given either intravenously or in large doses via a nebuliser is as effective as intravenous glucose and insulin in treating hyperkalaemia in patients with renal failure. It acts by stimulating the β2 adrenergic receptors. This leads to activation of the Na–K adenosine triphosphatase pump and movement of potassium into cells.

Despite inducing an increase in heart rate and blood glucose levels, salbutamol is reported to be well tolerated and lacks serious side effects.

The reported effective intravenous dose is 0.5 mg, diluted in 100 mL of 5% glucose and administered over a 15-minute period. A dose of 15–20 mg, diluted in normal saline and administered via a nebuliser, is also reported to be effective. For further information on salbutamol see Chapter 11 Respiratory Diseases.

Calcium

Hyperkalaemia can lead to cardiac arrhythmia and subsequent death. The arrhythmia can be reversed or prevented by the administration of calcium, usually in the form of an intravenous infusion of calcium gluconate or calcium chloride. Calcium has no effect on the serum potassium concentration. For further information see Chapter 32 Drugs Used in Critical Care.

Polystyrene Resins: Sodium Polystyrene Sulfonate

TRADE NAMES
Sodium polystyrene sulfonate: *Resonium A.*

MECHANISM OF ACTION
Sodium polystyrene sulfonate is a cation exchange resin which releases sodium and hydrogen ions in exchange for potassium ions, the bound potassium ions are then excreted in the faeces.

USES
Sodium polystyrene sulfonate is used in the treatment of hyperkalaemia. However, its onset of action is not rapid (hours to days) and its effectiveness depends on the amount of potassium to be removed. For rapid correction of severe hyperkalaemia, immediate administration of faster acting

agents, such as intravenous glucose and insulin, is necessary as a temporary measure to lower serum potassium while other longer term potassium lowering therapy is prepared.

The usual adult dose is 15 g up to four times a day. A suggested dose for children is up to 1 g per kg body weight daily in divided doses.

It is given orally in a little water or may be made up into a paste with some sweetened vehicle. It may also be mixed with a diet appropriate for a patient in renal failure. *It should not be given in fruit juices which have a high potassium content as this may reduce the exchange capacity of the resin.*

When oral administration is difficult, sodium polystyrenc sulfonate may be administered rectally in a suspension of 30–50 g resin in 100 mL of an aqueous vehicle such as sorbitol solution, given as a retention enema once or twice daily. Children may be given similar rectal doses to those suggested by mouth, however, care is needed as excessive dose or inadequate dilution can cause impaction of the resin.

ADVERSE DRUG REACTIONS

Gastric irritation, anorexia, constipation, nausea, vomiting and occasionally diarrhoea may occur. Large doses in elderly patients may cause faecal impaction. Constipation can be minimised by concomitant use of non-magnesium containing laxatives.

DRUG INTERACTIONS

It should not be administered concomitantly with digoxin, antacids containing aluminium or magnesium, or fruit juices.

PRECAUTIONS AND CONTRAINDICATIONS

Patients can develop serious hypokalaemia from sodium polystyrene therapy and frequent determination of serum potassium levels is necessary. Symptoms of hypokalaemia should also be watched for and the decision to cease treatment assessed individually as serum potassium levels may not always reflect intracellular deficiency. Hypokalaemia can enhance the effects of cardiac glycosides and sodium polystyrene sulfonate should be used with caution in patients receiving digoxin.

Administration of sodium polystyrene sulfonate can result in sodium overload. It should be used with caution in patients who cannot tolerate even a small increase in sodium load, e.g. patients with severe congestive heart failure, severe hypertension or marked oedema.

Sodium polystyrene sulfonate is not totally specific for potassium in its action, and small amounts of other cations such as magnesium and calcium can be lost during treatment. Thus patients receiving the resin should be monitored for electrolyte disturbances.

Cation donating antacids, phosphate binders or laxatives such as magnesium hydroxide or calcium carbonate may reduce the potassium lowering effect of sodium polystyrene sulfonate. Metabolic alkalosis has also been reported in patients with renal disease after the concomitant oral administration of these agents.

Calcium Polystyrene Sulfonate

TRADE NAMES

Calcium polystyrene sulfonate: *Calcium Resonium*.

MECHANISM OF ACTION

Calcium polystyrene sulfonate is a cation exchange resin which releases calcium ions in exchange for potassium and other cations.

USES

It is used in a similar way to sodium polystyrene sulfonate in the treatment of hyperkalaemia and is preferred in patients who cannot tolerate any increase in sodium load.

ADVERSE DRUG REACTIONS, PRECAUTIONS AND CONTRAINDICATIONS

See sodium polystyrene sulfonate.

Although sodium loading is not a problem, calcium overloading and hypercalcaemia may occur. Patients should be monitored for electrolyte disturbances particularly hypokalaemia and hypercalcaemia. *It should not be used in patients presenting with renal failure together with hypercalcaemia.*

Dialysis is the most effective means for the treatment of hyperkalaemia but often takes time to arrange. These measures may be used if severe hyperkalaemia is present until dialysis can be instituted.

ACIDOSIS

Sodium Bicarbonate, Calcium Carbonate

The metabolic acidosis of renal failure may be corrected by oral administration of sodium bicarbonate (*Sodibic*), the dose required varying from patient to patient. For chronic acidosis, 30–60 mmol (i.e. 3–6 capsules) per day is generally required. Calcium carbonate in adequate doses has also been shown to be effective in reducing acidosis and may be used when sodium is contraindicated.

DRUGS IN RENAL FAILURE

14

DRUG TREATMENT OF DIALYSIS PROBLEMS

VITAMIN DEFICIENCY

Vitamin Supplements

In the past, vitamin supplements (in the form of B complex with C tablets) were usually given to uraemic and dialysis patients as their vitamin intake can be limited by the dietary restrictions placed on them and significant amount of the soluble vitamins B, C and folic acid are lost during dialysis. However, with modern dialysis techniques and more flexible diets, vitamin deficiency is not a common problem. Some centres tend not to give 'prophylactic' vitamin therapy but to use specific treatment when vitamin deficiency is detected.

Supplementation with fat soluble vitamins such as vitamins A and D which are not removed by dialysis is unnecessary and risky. On prolonged ingestion, particularly with high doses, they tend to accumulate in the body and cause hypervitaminosis. In the case of vitamin D some patients may already be taking some form of this vitamin for the management of renal osteodystrophy (see next section). Additional amounts of this vitamin in these patients is undesirable and potentially dangerous. Similarly, vitamin preparations containing minerals or trace elements, such as magnesium, should be avoided because of the possibility of toxicity from these components.

RENAL OSTEODYSTROPHY

The term, renal osteodystrophy, refers to any bone disease occurring in a patient with renal disease. In these patients the progressive loss of functional renal tissue causes a defect in the ability to convert vitamin D into the active form, 1,25-dihydroxycholecalciferol ($1,25\text{-}(OH)_2D3$). This deficiency of $1,25\text{-}(OH)_2D3$ causes a decrease in absorption of calcium from the intestine and contributes to the development of hypocalcaemia. Hyperphosphataemia, which occurs as a result of decreased phosphate excretion during loss of renal function, also contributes to a decrease in the synthesis of $1,25\text{-}(OH)_2D3$ via inhibition of the renal enzyme responsible for the conversion of vitamin D from its precursor to the active form. Phosphate elevation can also reduce calcium concentration by complexation. Low serum calcium levels stimulate the parathyroid glands to secrete parathyroid hormone, which stimulates osteoclast activity leading to bone destruction and the release of calcium into the circulation. Elevated parathyroid hormone

levels or secondary hyperthyroidism is a major characteristic of renal failure. Bone demineralisation is, however, only one major aspect of renal osteodystrophy, other factors such as erratic bone formation are also involved.

Longstanding renal osteodystrophy can lead to morbidity and mortality and is not easily amenable to treatment. The most effective approach is to initiate early preventive measures. Such measures include supplementation of the deficient hormone $1,25\text{-}(OH)_2D3$ (calcitriol), and maintenance of normal serum phosphorus and calcium through dietary control and use of phosphate binders.

Calcitriol

TRADE NAMES

Calcitriol: *Rocaltrol*.

MECHANISM OF ACTION

The major known action of calcitriol is stimulation of intestinal absorption of calcium. Recent evidence suggests that it also has a direct suppressive effect on the synthesis and release of parathyroid hormone.

PHARMACOKINETICS

Calcitriol is rapidly absorbed from the intestine after oral administration. It has been shown that peak serum concentrations are reached within 3–6 hours following oral single doses of 0.25–1 microgram. The half-life of calcitriol ranges from 3–6 hours and the duration of pharmacological activity of a single dose is about 3–5 days.

USES

Calcitriol is used for the treatment of hypocalcaemia in patients with uraemic osteodystrophy, hypoparathyroidism and vitamin D resistant rickets.

It is available as 0.25 microgram capsule. The optimal daily dose must be carefully determined for each patient. The recommended initial dose for the treatment of uraemic osteodystrophy is 0.25 microgram once a day. The dosage may be increased by

0.25 microgram per day at two to four week intervals if a satisfactory response in biochemical parameters and clinical manifestations of the disease state is not observed. During the dosage titration period, calcium levels should be closely monitored (levels should be measured at least twice weekly).

Hypercalcaemia is a common side effect of daily calcitriol treatment. 'Pulse therapy', with high doses given twice a week at the end of dialysis, has been shown to be effective in reducing parathyroid hormone secretion with less hypercalcaemia.

ADVERSE DRUG REACTIONS

Since calcitriol is the active form of vitamin D, adverse effects are, in general, similar to those experienced with excessive vitamin D intake. Most common reactions include hypercalcaemia, drowsiness, weakness and constipation.

DRUG INTERACTIONS

Cholestyramine has been reported to reduce intestinal absorption of fat soluble vitamins and may reduce the absorption of calcitriol.

Calcitriol should be used with caution in patients receiving digoxin, because hypercalcaemia in such patients may precipitate cardiac arrhythmias. It should also be used with caution in patients taking thiazide diuretics as concomitant use may precipitate hypercalcaemia.

PRECAUTIONS AND CONTRAINDICATIONS

The use of calcitriol in renal patients must be carefully supervised and frequent biochemical monitoring is essential. Excessive dosage can result in hypercalcaemia and metastatic calcification of soft tissue.

Since calcitriol is the most potent form of vitamin D, other vitamin D or vitamin D containing compounds must be withheld during treatment to avoid the development of hypervitaminosis D.

As high serum phosphate levels are found in patients with renal failure, a rise in serum calcium (due to an increase in intestinal calcium absorption subsequent to calcitriol administration) tends to produce deposition of calcium phosphate in soft tissue. Further, calcitriol itself may also increase plasma phosphate levels. Thus, if treatment with calcitriol is indicated the serum phosphate must be controlled with phosphate binders before starting therapy (see next section). Small doses must be used and any increase in dose should be gradual and monitored.

Calcitriol is contraindicated in hypercalcaemia, vitamin D toxicity, pregnancy and breast feeding.

Phosphate Binders: Aluminium Hydroxide, Calcium Carbonate

As mentioned previously, high serum phosphate levels are found in patients with renal failure. An increase in serum calcium levels can produce deposition of calcium phosphate in soft tissues if the serum phosphate level is not adequately controlled. Phosphate binders such as aluminium hydroxide or calcium carbonate are used to reduce serum phosphate concentration. They are given with meals with the aim of binding dietary phosphate in the bowel and preventing its absorption.

USES

The sole use or concurrent use of non-aluminium based binders such as calcium carbonate is preferred to minimise aluminium absorption and resultant toxicity. Calcium carbonate can also serve as a calcium supplement and reduce metabolic acidosis. However, it is not as effective as aluminium hydroxide in decreasing phosphate levels and may increase the risk of hypercalcaemia and extraosseous calcifications, especially when used with calcitriol.

There are a number of aluminium hydroxide and calcium carbonate preparations available (see Table 14.1). To facilitate stabilisation it is desirable to use the same preparation throughout the treatment.

DRUGS IN RENAL FAILURE

14

TABLE 14.1 Phosphate binders available in Australia

Proprietary Name	Dosage Form	Composition
Alugel	Suspension	Aluminium hydroxide 320 mg/5 mL
Alu-Tab	Tablet	Aluminium hydroxide 600 mg
Amphogel	Suspension	Aluminium hydroxide 321 mg/5 mL
Cal-Sup	Flavoured tablet	Calcium carbonate 1250 mg
Caltrate	Tablet	Calcium carbonate 1500 mg
Calcimax	Chewable tablet	Calcium carbonate 750 mg
Aludrox	Suspension	Aluminium hydroxide 306 mg–magnesium hydroxide 97.5 mg/5 mL
Mylanta II	Suspension	Aluminium hydroxide gel 400 mg–magnesium hydroxide 400 mg/5 mL

The use of magnesium salts as phosphate binders is somewhat controversial. It has been reported that magnesium carbonate is effective but magnesium oxide and trisilicate are ineffective. Also, magnesium salts may have deleterious effects on bone mineralisation and the central nervous system.

Other phosphate binders have been introduced recently but further studies are required to establish their safety and efficacy.

ADVERSE DRUG REACTIONS

Patients with renal failure can accumulate significant amounts of aluminium from ingestion of aluminium based phosphate binders or exposure to aluminium in the water supply. It is now evident that excessive exposure to aluminium in patients with renal failure may cause dementia, severe osteomalacia and microcytic anaemia.

Both aluminium hydroxide and calcium carbonate can cause constipation.

DRUG INTERACTIONS

Aluminium hydroxide can interfere with the absorption of other drugs and should be taken at least two hours apart from other drugs.

ANAEMIA

Anaemia is almost universal among patients with chronic renal failure. The mechanisms underlying the anaemia are complex. These involve blood loss associated with haemodialysis and blood testing, bleeding, shortening of red cell survival, dietary restriction and inadequate secretion of erythropoietin (the hormone responsible for the production of red blood cells). Inadequate secretion of erythropoietin is the major cause of uraemic anaemia.

Iron

Iron supplements may be required to prevent or correct iron deficiency resulting from blood loss, bleeding or dietary restriction. Iron is available in different salts and in different forms. The common salts used are ferrous sulfate and ferrous gluconate. Various iron preparations are available in the form of capsules, tablets, controlled release tablets and syrup. Iron can cause constipation and turn faeces black. It can also cause gastric discomfort and vomiting in some patients. For further information on iron preparations see Chapter 13 Blood Disorders.

Erythropoietin

Erythropoietin is an endogenous glycoprotein produced primarily by the kidney. It is the major regulator of erythropoiesis, the process which results in the production of red blood cells.

Erythropoiesis is regulated by a feedback mechanism in the kidney which senses and responds to the oxygen level in the blood. When the level is low, erythropoietin secreting cells in the kidney increase their release of the hormone which stimulates precursor cells in the bone marrow resulting in an increased production of erythrocytes.

In chronic renal failure, the kidneys progressively lose their functions including the secretion of erythropoietin. Erythropoietin deficiency is considered to be the major cause of uraemic anaemia and replacement therapy with the hormone is a logical approach to treating the problem.

Recombinant human erythropoietin (r-HuEPO) is manufactured by genetic engineering (DNA recombinant) technology. It is identical to natural erythropoietin.

The efficacy of recombinant human erythropoietin in correcting anaemia of end-stage renal disease has been demonstrated in several clinical studies. Its use has eliminated the need for repeated blood transfusions which can have undesirable consequences including transmission of infectious disease, iron overload, haemolytic reactions and induction of cytotoxic antibodies that can affect the success of subsequent organ transplants.

TRADE NAMES

Erythropoietin: *Eprex*.

PHARMACOKINETICS

Recombinant human erythropoietin is broken down in the gastrointestinal tract and must be given parenterally, either intravenously or subcutaneously.

It has been shown that peak serum concentrations of recombinant human erythropoietin are reached immediately after intravenous injection. Its mean half-life after intravenous administration ranges from 4.0–6.1 hours in normal volunteers and 6.5–9.3 hours in patients with chronic renal failure. The half-life in dialysis patients is about 25 hours after subcutaneous administration. The major routes of elimination are thought to be predominantly non-renal.

USES

Recombinant human erythropoietin is currently approved in Australia for the treatment of symptomatic or transfusion dependent anaemia associated with chronic renal failure.

The recommended starting dose is 50 units/kg body weight three times a week, administered as an intravenous injection over 1–2 minutes or by subcutaneous injection. It may be necessary to titrate the dose at monthly intervals to adjust the rate of increase in haemoglobin. The total maintenance dose can be given as one or two injections per week when a stable haemoglobin level is reached.

ADVERSE DRUG REACTIONS

The most serious adverse effect observed is development or exacerbation of hypertension, infrequently leading to encephalopathy and seizures. Seizures have also been observed in patients receiving erythropoietin who were not hypertensive, especially during the first three months of treatment.

Clotting of arteriovenous fistulas and shunts has occurred in some patients, and higher doses of heparin may be needed for adequate anticoagulation during haemodialysis.

Other reported adverse reactions include hyperkalaemia, flu-like symptoms, headache, bone pain, chills and skin reactions.

DRUG INTERACTIONS

There are no known clinically significant drug interactions but the effect of recombinant human erythropoietin may be potentiated by co-administration of a haematin agent, e.g. ferrous sulfate when iron deficiency is present.

DRUGS IN RENAL FAILURE

14

PRECAUTIONS AND CONTRAINDICATIONS

Recombinant human erythropoietin should be used with caution in patients with pre-existing hypertension, ischaemic vascular disease, a history of seizures, porphyria, gout or suspected allergy to any component of the product.

The need for contraception in women of child-bearing age should be evaluated as it is not known whether recombinant human erythropoietin crosses the human placenta or whether it can cause fetal harm when administered during pregnancy. Animal studies have shown that it has different effects on the fetus in different species and at different dose levels.

The drug is contraindicated in patients with uncontrolled hypertension, a known sensitivity to human albumin or a known sensitivity to products derived from mammalian cells. It should also be avoided in patients with a high risk of thrombosis and in aluminium toxicity.

DRUG TREATMENT OF TRANSPLANTATION PROBLEMS

REJECTION AND IMMUNOSUPPRESSIVE AGENTS

Kidney transplantation is the treatment of choice for many patients with end-stage renal failure. It allows them to have a near normal lifestyle. However, there is one major disadvantage and this is the need for continuous medication to suppress the immune system which would normally destroy the transplanted kidney (rejection).

Tissues from a transplanted kidney present as foreign antigenic cells and provoke an immune response in the recipient. If unchecked the response will lead to destruction of the transplanted kidney. Such an immune response is a complex process and involves cell populations of the immune system and chemicals secreted by these cells. The process mainly involves T cell subsets and chemicals known as cytokines, particularly interleukins 1 and 2 (IL-1 and IL-2). B-cells and other effector cell types are also involved. To enable the transplant to be accepted or tolerated it is necessary to suppress the recipient's immune response.

With recent advances in immunosuppressive therapy there has been a significant improvement in the success of renal transplantation and a reduction in patient morbidity and mortality.

The availability of an increasing number of immunosuppressive agents has led to the development of various combination immunosuppressive regimens. These combinations have been used in an attempt to increase efficacy and decrease adverse reactions. The agents act at different levels of the recipient's immune response and when used together their effects are additive and the side effects of individual agents minimised through the use of smaller doses.

Corticosteroids

The corticosteroids are an important class of immunosuppressive agents. Despite the introduction of a number of new agents they remain the mainstay of immunosuppressive therapy and are used in most transplant recipients.

The immunosuppressive effects of the corticosteroids are complex and not fully elucidated. The proposed mechanism of action is inhibition of lymphocyte production, especially T cells, and suppression of the inflammatory response.

The two corticosteroids most commonly used are prednisolone for oral use and methylprednisolone for intravenous administration. The dosage employed depends on a number of factors, including whether the drugs are being used for prophylaxis or treatment.

ADVERSE DRUG REACTIONS

The adverse effects of steroids are numerous and well documented (see Chapter 19 Endocrine Diseases).

Many side effects, such as cushingoid appearance, psychiatric disturbance and myopathy, are uncommon if the dose used does not exceed 30 mg per day. On the other hand, complications such as the thin skin syndrome, osteoporosis and cataracts, are related to long-term use even if the dose is relatively low.

PRECAUTIONS AND CONTRAINDICATIONS

See Chapter 19 Endocrine Diseases.

To avoid problems of sudden withdrawal an intravenous form of corticosteroid should be administered to patients who are 'nil by mouth' or have difficulties in taking the drug orally. The dose of corticosteroid should be increased during times of stress.

Azathioprine

TRADE NAMES

Azathioprine: *Imuran; Thioprine.*

MECHANISM OF ACTION

The exact mode of action of azathioprine is yet to be elucidated. The metabolic product, 6-mercaptopurine, is responsible for the majority of its immunosuppressive effects. 6-Mercaptopurine inhibits purine synthesis thereby blocking the production of DNA. This inhibits cell replication, effectively reducing the lymphocytes, particularly T cells, and other cell populations.

PHARMACOKINETICS

Azathioprine is well absorbed from the gastrointestinal tract when given by mouth. After oral or intravenous administration it is rapidly and extensively metabolised to 6-mercaptopurine by enzymes in the liver and other tissues. 6-Mercaptopurine is fur-

ther converted to a number of derivatives. Small amounts of unchanged azathioprine and 6-mercaptopurine are excreted in the urine.

USES

Azathioprine in combination with corticosteroids and/or other immunosuppressive agents is used to facilitate the survival of organ transplants.

It is also used either alone, or more commonly, in combination with corticosteroids in a wide variety of conditions which are considered to be autoimmune in character. These include rheumatoid arthritis, systemic lupus erythromatosus and some severe skin disorders. Its use with a corticosteroid may allow a lower dose of both drugs to be used thus reducing side effects.

ADVERSE DRUG REACTIONS

The major side effect of azathioprine is dose related and reversible bone marrow depression leading to leucopenia. Other side effects include megaloblastic anaemia, alopecia, nausea and hepatotoxicity. When hepatotoxicity occurs the usual practice is to substitute azathioprine with another cytotoxic drug such as cyclophosphamide or chlorambucil. These drugs have similar effects to azathioprine.

DRUG INTERACTIONS

Allopurinol inhibits the metabolism of azathioprine and only one quarter of the usual dose of azathioprine should be given if these two drugs are administered together. As plasma azathioprine levels cannot be measured satisfactorily, a decrease in white blood cell count is the only clue to excessive dosage.

PRECAUTIONS AND CONTRAINDICATIONS

Azathioprine injection should be prepared according to the guidelines for safe handling of cytotoxic drugs. If it is necessary to halve uncoated tablets similar precautions to those recommended for handling azathioprine injection should be followed. Film tablets should not be divided. There is no risk in handling film coated tablets provided the coating is intact.

Patients receiving azathioprine should have regular full blood counts.

The drug is contraindicated in patients known to be hypersensitive to azathioprine. Hypersensitivity to 6-mercaptopurine should be considered as a probable hypersensitivity to azathioprine. Therapy should not be initiated in patients known to be pregnant.

Antithymocyte Globulin

MECHANISM OF ACTION

Antithymocyte globulin (ATG) is produced by immunising animals (usually horses or rabbits) with thymocytes and then harvesting the animal's plasma to obtain the desired antibodies. It acts by coating T lymphocytes (T cells). The antibody coated T cells are then lysed by the complement system and/or removed by the reticuloendothelial system in the liver or spleen. By eliminating the T cells the immune response is attenuated.

USES

ATG is used in combination with other immunosuppressants in the treatment of acute allograft rejection. ATG is for intravenous use only.

The solution should be inspected visually for particulate matter and discolouration. It should be diluted in sodium chloride 0.9% solution before intravenous infusion. The addition of ATG to glucose or highly acidic solutions is not recommended. It should be administered over at least 4 hours.

ADVERSE DRUG REACTIONS

Some of the common side effects include fever, chills, leucopenia, thrombocytopenia and dermatological reactions such as rash and pruritus. Although anaphylactic reaction has been reported the incidence is considered to be low.

The major disadvantages of this type of preparation are the likelihood that low levels of antibodies against other formed elements of the blood are present, and batch to batch variation in potency. With the advent of reagents like monoclonal antibody, which is more specific in action and uniform in potency, the role of ATG in immunosuppressive therapy is being re-appraised.

PRECAUTIONS AND CONTRAINDICATIONS

Patients should be skin tested prior to administration, however, allergic reactions can occur after a negative skin test. ATG is contraindicated in patients who have had a severe systemic reaction to the drug. Patients should be monitored for signs of leucopenia, thrombocytopenia and infection.

Muromonab-CD3

Muromonab-CD3 (murine monoclonal antibody) is an immunoglobulin produced by a monoclonal antibody technique in mice.

TRADE NAMES

Muromonab-CD3: *Orthoclone OKT3.*

MECHANISM OF ACTION

Muromonab-CD3 binds the CD3 molecule on the surface of mature human T cells and blocks their immunological function. Once binding takes place the antibody-coated T cells are removed by the reticuloendothelial system. Removal of functioning T cells after administration of muromonab-CD3 is rapid (within minutes).

USES

Muromonab-CD3 is used to reverse acute rejection epidodes. The recommended dose for the treatment of acute renal allograft rejection is 5 mg/day for 10–14 days. It should only be administered intravenously.

Because the preparation is a mouse antibody most patients develop antibodies after treatment. Thus treatment beyond two weeks or retreatment of second and subsequent rejections may not be effective and safe. The initial antibody formation can be reduced by continuing azathioprine during the course of monoclonal antibody.

The injection should be inspected for particulate matter and discolouration prior to administration. However, because it is a protein solution it may develop a few fine translucent particles which do not affect its potency.

The solution should be drawn into a syringe through a low protein binding 0.22 micron filter. The filter is then discarded and a needle attached for intravenous bolus injection. The injection should be administered in less than one minute.

ADVERSE DRUG REACTIONS

Muromonab-CD3 has a number of initial side effects. Over 70% of patients receiving the antibody develop a high fever. Other first-dose adverse effects include chills, headaches, rigors, hypotension or hypertension. The release of chemical mediators from destroyed T cells is thought to be responsible for these first dose effects.

Severe pulmonary oedema and subsequent death has occurred in patients treated with a greater than 3% weight gain in the week prior to treatment. In each case the weight gain was due to fluid overload.

Other side effects include nausea and vomiting, tremor, chest pains, dyspnoea, wheezing, diarrhoea, aseptic meningitis and seizures. Patients may also have a higher rate of infection, especially viral.

PRECAUTIONS AND CONTRAINDICATIONS

To minimise the severity of these first dose effects, the manufacturer recommends that a 1 mg/kg dose of intravenous methylprednisolone sodium succinate be given prior to the first muromonab-CD3 dose and 100 mg of intravenous hydrocortisone sodium succinate 30 minutes after administration of the antibody. Paracetamol and antihistamines can also be administered with muromonab-CD3 to reduce early reactions.

The first dose adverse reactions may occur 0.5–6 hours after administration. Therefore, the first dose should be administered in hospital and the patient should be closely monitored for 4–6 hours. The dose should not be given in the late evening as problems may occur overnight.

It is important to evaluate patients for fluid overload by chest X-ray and weight gain before treatment with muromonab-CD3 is initiated. Weight should be brought to a value less than or equal to 3% above the minimum weight in the week before the first dose is administered.

Muromonab-CD3 is contraindicated in patients who are hypersensitive to the drug.

Cyclosporin

Cyclosporin represents a major advance in immunosuppressive therapy. It was originally developed as an antifungal agent. Although it was known to possess mild antifungal activity, its marked immunological properties were only discovered during routine screening. Its immunosuppressive efficacy in renal transplantation has now been well demonstrated. The major advantage of cyclosporin is that it does not depress haematopoiesis and has no effect on the function of phagocytic cells.

TRADE NAMES

Cyclosporin: *Sandimmun.*

MECHANISM OF ACTION

The principal effect of cyclosporin is to inhibit the secretion of interleukin 2 and other cytokines from T cells, resulting in prevention of proliferation and differentiation of lymphocytes aggressive to the graft such as cytotoxic T cells and antibody producing cells.

PHARMACOKINETICS

The absorption of cyclosporin from the gastrointestinal tract is incomplete and very variable. It is highly bound to tissues and proteins, including erythrocytes, leucocytes and lipoproteins. Cyclosporin is extensively metabolised by the liver, with more than 15 metabolites currently identified. The rate of metabolism may be decreased in liver disease and in older patients.

DRUGS IN RENAL FAILURE

14

USES

An oral solution and capsules are available for oral administration. Both dosage forms are bioequivalent.

For patients who cannot take the drug orally a concentrate for intravenous infusion is available. The concentrate should be diluted in sterile sodium chloride 0.9% or glucose 5% in glass containers and infused over approximately 2–6 hours.

ADVERSE DRUG REACTIONS

Ironically, the principal adverse effect of cyclosporin is nephrotoxicity. It can occur as an acute reaction in the first days or weeks after transplantation or as chronic toxicity manifested as a slow deterioration of renal function usually after the first year of transplantation. Although nephrotoxicity is more likely to be associated with high serum levels of cyclosporin it can occur with levels within the normal therapeutic range.

Other side effects include hypertension, hyperkaelaemia, hepatotoxicity, gum hypertrophy, hirsutism, gastrointestinal disturbances and central nervous system effects such as headache, seizures and confusion.

DRUG INTERACTIONS

A number of drugs are known to either increase or decrease the blood levels of cyclosporin by inhibition or induction of those liver enzymes involved in the metabolism of cyclosporin. Thus, whenever possible, co-administration of such drugs should be avoided. There are also drugs which can enhance the nephrotoxicity of cyclosporin.

Drugs which are known to increase blood levels of cyclosporin are: danazol, diltiazem, doxycycline, erythromycin, ketoconazole, methylprednisolone (high dose), nicardipine and verapamil.

Drugs which are known to decrease blood levels of cyclosporin are: carbamazepine, isoniazid, phenobarbitone, phenytoin, rifampicin and trimethoprim–sulfamethoxazole injection.

Drugs which are known to enhance the nephrotoxicity of cyclosporin are: aminoglycosides, amphotericin B, ciprofloxacin, colchicine, melphalan, trimethoprim and trimethropim–sulfamethoxazole.

PRECAUTIONS AND CONTRAINDICATIONS

As hyperkalaemia can occur with cyclosporin treatment, patients receiving cyclosporin should avoid high dietary potassium intake and not be given potassium containing medication or potassium sparing diuretics.

Blood tests should be performed regularly to monitor for signs of nephrotoxicity and hepatotoxicity.

The concentrate for intravenous infusion contains polyoxyethylated castor oil (*Cremophor EL*) which has been reported to cause anaphylactoid reactions. Thus, patients receiving intravenous cyclosporin should be observed continuously for at least the first 30 minutes following commencement of infusion and at frequent intervals thereafter.

COMPLICATIONS OF IMMUNOTHERAPY

In addition to the adverse reactions specific to particular agents there are complications which are common to all immunosuppressive agents and immunotherapy in general. These include:

- A higher incidence of cancer, particularly non-Hodgkin's lymphoma and carcinoma of the skin, lip and urogenital tract;

- Increased susceptibility to bacterial infection;

- Increased susceptibility to opportunistic infections, e.g. cytomegalovirus, herpes and fungal infections and *Pneumocystis carinii*.

Prophylaxis against some of these infections is prescribed for transplant patients in some centres.

DRUG ADMINISTRATION IN RENAL FAILURE

Apart from the drugs which are used to treat their basic condition, patients with renal failure also receive a wide variety of pharmacological agents for intercurrent illnesses. Drugs which are mainly excreted in active form by the kidneys (i.e. as unchanged drug or pharmacologically active metabolites) may accumulate in the presence of renal insufficiency resulting in adverse reactions or toxicity. If toxic effects are to be avoided, modification of dosage regimens and careful monitoring is required. This is particularly important with drugs with a low therapeutic ratio, e.g. digoxin and gentamicin. Dosage modification should take into consideration changes in renal function and dialysis. The latter may lower therapeutic concentrations of drugs by causing their removal from the blood into the dialysate but in no case will the rate of removal exceed that performed by normally functioning kidneys.

Dosage regimens are usually modified by administering either normal doses at extended intervals or a reduced dose at normal intervals. Some drugs requiring dosage adjustment are listed in Table 14.2.

For drugs which are highly dialysable, the dose just preceding dialysis and doses scheduled during dialysis are usually omitted and a supplementary dose is given after dialysis. The factors affecting the removal of drugs during dialysis are molecular size, protein binding in plasma and distribution between the plasma and other body fluid compartments. As a generalisation, drugs which are mostly eliminated by the kidneys will undergo significant decreases in concentration during dialysis. For drugs with small molecular weight, losses are less significant with peritoneal dialysis than with haemodialysis because of the lesser efficiency of the peritoneal method.

TABLE 14.2 Some drugs requiring dosage adjustment in renal failure

Allopurinol
Amikacin
Amphotericin B
Cefotaxime
Cefoxitin
Ceftazidime
Cimetidine
Digoxin
Flucytosine
Gentamicin
Magnesium containing antacids
Methotrexate
Netilmicin
Potassium salts
Procainamide
Tobramycin
Trimethoprim–sulfamethoxazole
Vancomycin

NURSING IMPLICATIONS

Vitamin Supplements

Ensure patient awareness of: (a) the importance of taking the specific vitamin preparation prescribed and of avoiding the use of additional non-prescribed preparations; (b) the need for biochemical monitoring during calcitriol therapy; and (c) the importance of taking phosphate binding preparations when prescribed with calcitriol.

Phosphate Binders: Aluminium Hydroxide, Calcium Carbonate

Educate the patient on the need to use the specific preparation prescribed. The drugs should be administered with meals. Other drugs taken concurrently should be given at least two hours before or after aluminium hydroxide which interferes with the absorption of many drugs. Watch particularly for constipation. Dietary restrictions may preclude an increase in fibre or fluid content.

Polystyrene Resins

These drugs should not be administered concomitantly with digoxin, antacids, phosphate binders, laxatives containing aluminium or magnesium or fruit juice. Polystyrene resins cause constipation which may be difficult to treat in view of dietary and drug restrictions.

Antihypertensives

See Chapter 12 Cardiovascular Diseases

Erythropoietin

If the patient is known to have poorly controlled hypertension, previous thrombotic episodes or poorly functioning arteriovenous fistulae alert the medical officer before administration. If the drug is given by the intravenous route, it should be given over 1–2 minutes. Monitor vital signs routinely during and for 30 minutes after the first injection. Blood pressure should be monitored at each dialysis. Transfusion requirements should also be monitored and should be ceased when erythropoietin is commenced.

Corticosteroids

See Chapter 19 Endocrine Disorders.

Azathioprine

Observe patient for signs of bone marrow depression. Protect patient from infection. If stomatitis occurs use appropriate measures such as mouth washes and a soft diet. Observe for biochemical and/or clinical evidence of liver damage.

Educate patients on the reason for immunosuppressive therapy and the necessity to continue therapy as prescribed. When administering azathioprine injection follow the guidelines for safe handling of cytotoxic drugs.

Antithymocyte Globulin

Store ampoules of ATG under refrigeration. Patients should be skin tested for a specific batch to ensure no reaction. During and following administration observe for unwanted effects, including signs of impending anaphylaxis. Have emergency drugs (e.g. adrenaline, corticosteroids) readily available. Observe patient for signs of infection. Inspect the injection solution for particulate matter and discolouration prior to administration.

Monoclonal Antibody

The patient's vital signs and body weight should be closely monitored before treatment. If the weight is greater than 3% of the patient's normal weight, alert the attending medical officer.

Ensure that all premedications, including prophylactic doses of methylprednisolone, hydrocortisone and paracetamol, are given and resuscitation facilities are available before the first dose is administered. Monitor the patient closely for 4–6 hours. The medical officer should be contacted as a matter of urgency if the patient develops signs, or complains, of dyspnoea. Observe for signs of infection.

Inspect the injection solution for particulate matter and discolouration prior to administration. The solution should be drawn into the syringe through a 0.22 micron filter. Inject over less than one minute.

Cyclosporin

Although blood levels may be useful in patient management to minimise side effects and rejection episodes, they are not always reliable and patients must be closely observed for signs of adverse reactions.

Cyclosporin has an oily taste. To mask the taste, the oral solution should be diluted with milk or chocolate milk immediately before administration. For administration of intravenous infusions, glass containers and non-PVC infusion sets should be used.

Educate patients to take cyclosporin doses at the same time each day. Patients taking the oral solution should be instructed to carefully measure the dose using the pipette provided then place the solution in a glass (not plastic) container and mix with milk or chocolate milk. The mixture should be mixed well and swallowed immediately. The glass should then be rinsed with additional milk and the contents swallowed. The pipette should be wiped with a dry tissue, it should not be rinsed with water.

General Concepts

As patients with renal diseases or receiving immunosuppressive drugs are susceptible to infections, strict aseptic technique should be employed for procedures such as changing of dressings and handling intravenous lines. Such patients should not be nursed near patients with respiratory, gastrointestinal, wound or skin infections. Dosage intervals for the administration of drugs to patients with renal failure should be strictly adhered to.

FURTHER READING

Koda-Kimble, M.A., Young, L.Y. (eds) (1992) *Applied therapeutics — the clinical use of drugs*, 5th edn, Applied Therapeutics Inc., Vancouver Washington, pp. 23-1–28-21.
Speight, T.M. (ed.) (1987) *Avery's drug treatment* 3rd edn ADIS Press, pp. 855–909
Wilson, J.D., Braunwald, E., Isselbacker, K.J., et al (eds) (1991) *Harrison's principles of internal medicine* 12th edn, vol 2, McGraw-Hill, pp. 1131–1212.

TEST YOUR KNOWLEDGE

1. Name one drug which is commonly used to treat hypocalcaemia in patients with renal osteodystrophy.

2. What are the indications for use of aluminium hydroxide and/or calcium carbonate, and what is their main side effect?

3. Name two drugs which may be used to treat hyperkalaemia.

4. Are diuretics of any value in the treatment of hypertension in patients with renal failure?

5. Should potassium sparing diuretics be administered to patients with renal failure?

6. What is the most common adverse reaction of erythropoietin. List two other reported adverse reactions.

7. Name three commonly used immunosuppressive agents and list their main side effects.

8. Name two drugs which require modification of dosage regimen when administered to patients with renal failure.

DRUGS IN RENAL FAILURE

14

Drugs Used in Bladder Dysfunction

RICHARD J. MILLARD

O B J E C T I V E S

At the conclusion of this chapter the reader should be able to:

1. Discuss the use of drugs in promoting urinary continence;

2. Describe the place of drugs in promoting bladder emptying;

3. List the types of drugs that can cause urinary retention; and

4. List the common adverse drug reactions to drugs used in the treatment of bladder dysfunction.

BLADDER AND URETHRAL FUNCTION

The bladder has two functions. Firstly, it should store urine at low pressure and without voluntary effort or discomfort. Secondly, when appropriate, it should void to completion under voluntary control (i.e. micturition). The normal bladder fills to about 500 mL capacity every 4–5 hours and voids at about 20–30 mL/second, emptying in less than 30 seconds. This cycle of events requires complex control mechanisms coordinated in the brain stem and is under higher centre control.

The normal bladder and urethra act together to store urine and maintain urinary continence. Continence is preserved when the bladder neck remains closed and when the pressure within the urethra (the urethral closure pressure) exceeds the pressure within the bladder (the intravesical pressure). The intravesical pressure is due partly to the intra-abdominal pressure and partly to the detrusor pressure derived from contraction or tonus in the bladder smooth muscle (the detrusor muscle). See Figure 15.1.

The urethral closure pressure is derived from elastic tissues in the urethral wall and from the muscles of the urethral sphincter mechanism. This sphincter mechanism is made up of both involuntary smooth muscle and voluntary striated (skeletal) muscle surrounding the urethra, augmented and supported by the striated muscles of the pelvic floor. Both smooth and striated components contribute equally to the resting urethral closure pressure and maintain this during bladder filling.

The bladder neck is usually water tight and only opens when the bladder contracts to empty. When it is closed and competent it is a major bulwark against urinary incontinence. However, if the bladder neck is incompetent (e.g. after prostatectomy, bladder neck incision or sometimes multiple childbirth) or if it has been opened by a bladder contraction,

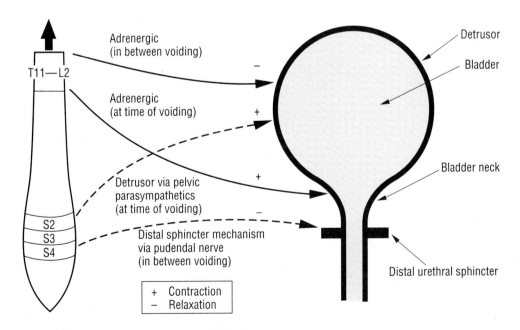

FIGURE 15.1 Neurological control of bladder emptying

continence may still be maintained by the urethral sphincter mechanism. If both the bladder neck and the urethral sphincter mechanism are incompetent or weak, stress incontinence may occur with coughing, sneezing or lifting.

During filling the bladder pressure remains low and the detrusor does not contract until micturition starts. This low pressure occurs because the bladder wall is extremely stretchable and because the bladder is prevented from contracting by inhibitory neural mechanisms. Even under the provocations of bladder fullness, change of posture or exercise, the intravesical pressure remains low due to this central inhibition and micturition can be delayed until it is convenient. The bladder only contracts when voiding is voluntarily initiated at an appropriate time and place. After emptying the bladder does not contract again until the next time that voiding is started. This cycle of events describes normal stable bladder function.

Some people cannot inhibit micturition, and unstable bladder contractions may then occur inappropriately during filling or in response to provocation such as exercise, posture change or the sound of running water. These unstable contractions occur involuntarily and give rise to an urgent and very strong desire to urinate. Urge incontinence is said to occur if the patient loses control before a toilet can be found or a bedpan brought. This type of bladder dysfunction is a common cause of incontinence in the elderly and in patients in whom incontinence is secondary to neurological diseases such as multiple sclerosis, Parkinson's disease, cerebrovascular accident, dementia or spinal injury.

During the act of micturition the first event to occur is relaxation of the sphincter mechanism. This is followed by a coordinated contraction of the detrusor muscle which starts within a few seconds. The detrusor contraction opens the bladder neck and generates sufficient pressure to overcome the remaining outlet resistance and causes urine to flow out. The pressure is sustained until the bladder is empty. The detrusor then relaxes and the urethral closure pressure is restored. Efficient voiding thus requires both an adequate detrusor contraction and synchronous sphincteric relaxation, this is coordinated in the micturition centre in the brain stem.

Indeed, the entire bladder cycle is a constant balance between the intravesical pressure and the forces acting upon the urethra. When the bladder pressure exceeds the urethral closure pressure, urine flows through the urethra causing micturition (if this occurs intentionally) or incontinence (when the event occurs involuntarily).

15

TYPES AND CAUSES OF INCONTINENCE

Stress Incontinence

Stress incontinence is the involuntary loss of urine when the pressure in the bladder exceeds the urethral closure pressure in the absence of a detrusor contraction.

Leakage occurs coincident with sudden rises in intra-abdominal pressure such as coughing, sneezing or straining. It implies incompetence of both the bladder neck and the distal sphincter mechanism.

Urge Incontinence

Urge incontinence is the involuntary loss of urine associated with a strong desire to void. There are two types: sensory and motor.

Sensory urge incontinence is due to discomfort during filling, thus limiting the effective bladder capacity (e.g. discomfort due to bladder inflammation or infection). Motor urge incontinence is due to involuntary detrusor contractions from an unstable bladder. Unstable bladder function may occur idiopathically or may result from bladder outlet obstruction (e.g. prostatic enlargement or bladder neck obstruction), neuropathy or, rarely, with severe intravesical irritation caused by catheters or calculi.

Overflow Incontinence

Overflow incontinence occurs if the intravesical pressure exceeds the urethral closure pressure when the bladder is over full or distended but is not contracting, i.e. in chronic retention. This may be secondary to obstruction or detrusor failure or both.

Bedwetting

Bedwetting is due to an unstable bladder combined with a deep sleep pattern such that when the bladder contracts to empty the sufferer is not awoken.

TABLE 15.1   Drugs which can cause or aggravate incontinence

Agent	Mechanism of Action	Type of Incontinence
Antihypertensive agents Phenoxybenzamine Prazosin Terazosin* Doxazosin* Indoramin* Labetolol	Sphincter relaxation	Stress incontinence
Bladder relaxants Anticholinergic agents Tricyclic antidepressants	Promote incomplete emptying	Overflow incontinence
Bladder stimulants Cholinergic agents Caffeine	Enhance detrusor excitability	Urge incontinence
Sedatives Antihistamines Antidepressants Antipsychotic agents Antianxiety agents Hypnotics	Cloud consciousness (less awareness of bladder sensation)	Urge incontinence
Non-steroidal anti-inflammatory drugs Tiaprofenic acid Naproxen Diflunisal Ibuprofen Sulindac	Transient haemorrhagic cystitis	Sensory urge incontinence
Miscellaneous Alcohol	Lowers central inhibition	Urge incontinence/enuresis
Loop diuretics	Increase bladder filling rate	Urge incontinence
Lithium	Polydipsia	Urge incontinence

*Not available in Australia

Continuous Incontinence

Continuous incontinence is the loss of urine usually in association with an abnormal urinary opening such as a fistula or ectopia of the bladder or ureter.

Drug Induced Incontinence

A variety of pharmacological agents may cause urinary incontinence. Drug therapy should be considered during assessment of incontinent patients. Clearly any drug which reduces urethral resistance may induce or aggravate stress incontinence, especially in the elderly. α Blockers (e.g. prazosin, doxazocin, phenoxybenzamine, terazosin) can cause such problems. Labetolol may also have the same side effect. Other antihypertensive agents, e.g. methyldopa, are thought by some researchers to aggravate incontinence.

Alcohol, loop diuretics and cholinergic agents may aggravate the unstable bladder and thus promote urge incontinence. In contrast, tricyclic antidepressants (but not tetracyclic antidepressants), anticholinergic and antiparkinsonian agents may cause varying degrees of chronic retention and overflow incontinence may result.

In the elderly any agent which clouds consciousness or sedates the patient, either intentionally or unintentionally, may promote urinary incontinence. The ability to recognise not only the desire to pass urine but the appropriate place in which to pass it and to be able to get there in good time are integral to achieving continence in the elderly or demented patient. Hence, in these patients, antidepressants, psychotropic agents, antihistamines, major and minor tranquillisers and sedatives may all promote incontinence.

Consideration of drugs as a possible cause of incontinence is essential to proper patient assessment (see Table 15.1). Dosage modification or elimination can sometimes restore continence without further investigation or treatment.

DRUGS USED TO PROMOTE URINARY CONTINENCE ■

To promote urinary continence it is necessary to achieve either a reduction of intravesical pressures (by suppressing bladder instability) or an increase in urethral closure pressure, or both. The key to successful management of urinary incontinence is the accurate diagnosis of its cause. A careful history and examination are required to detect incontinence due to fistulae or ureteric ectopia requiring definitive surgery. Bladder distension or pelvic floor weakness should be easily detected and a neurological assessment is essential especially in the elderly or those who also have faecal control problems.

Urine culture is essential to detect infection and intravenous urography or cystoscopy may be indicated. A time and volume chart of voiding pattern and incontinent episodes is extremely helpful for an objective assessment since the patient's impressions may be an unreliable guide to causation. Video-urodynamic assessment is definitive, accurately detecting unstable contractions, sphincter weakness, the presence and cause of residual urine or voiding difficulties. Once the cause of the incontinence has been delineated a rational approach to therapy can be formulated.

REDUCTION OF INTRAVESICAL PRESSURE

Reduction of intravesical pressure is indicated when frequency, nocturia, urgency and urge incontinence are due to an unstable or uninhibited neuropathic bladder (e.g. in multiple sclerosis, Parkinson's disease, spina bifida or following a cerebrovascular accident).

DRUGS USED IN BLADDER DYSFUNCTION

15

In such patients bladder relaxants reduce the frequency and strength of the unstable contractions by reducing bladder contractility. This results in symptomatic improvement through an increase in effective bladder capacity and both urinary frequency and nocturia are diminished. Urgency is also diminished giving the patient more time to get to the toilet or commode. Bladder relaxants do not help when the frequency and sensory urgency are the result of intravesical inflammation or infection and these possibilities should always be excluded and treated appropriately.

Patients with high pressure bladders (e.g. autonomous neuropathic bladder resulting from lesions of the pelvic nerve, cauda equina or sacral spinal cord) and in whom the bladder will not empty, can be managed by intermittent catheterisation combined with bladder relaxants to improve the functional capacity and bladder compliance. Compliance is the term used to describe the 'stretchability' of the bladder wall. Low compliance means the wall is stiff and less stretchable resulting in high pressures within the bladder at the end of filling. In this situation drug therapy assists in maintaining urinary continence between catheterisations, sometimes reducing the frequency of catheterisation. Because the bladder pressure is reduced, back pressure on the kidneys is minimised reducing the likelihood of nephropathy. Patients who are being managed with an indwelling catheter may develop detrusor contractions secondary to mucosal irritation. These contractions give rise to bladder spasms which can be painful and cause leakage around the catheter. This type of problem is commonly seen in patients with neuropathic bladder problems, in children and adults who have catheters after bladder surgery and in geriatric patients who frequently pull at their catheters. Such patients benefit from bladder relaxants.

Anticholinergic Agents: Atropine, Hyoscine, Hyoscyamine, Belladonna Alkaloids, Propantheline, Penthienate, Emepromium, Oxybutynin

The detrusor muscle is innervated by postganglionic, parasympathetic nerves and is therefore cholinergic with muscarinic receptors. Anticholinergic agents tend to relax the detrusor and lower the intravesical pressure. They also impair the ability of the bladder to empty and are thus contraindicated in patients with any degree of obstruction to the bladder outlet.

TRADE NAMES

Hyoscine, hyoscyamine: *Donnatabs; Donnatal LA.*
Belladonna alkaloids: *Atrobel.*
Propantheline: *Pro-Banthine.*
Penthienate: *Monodral.*
Emepromium: *Cetiprin.*
Oxybutynin: *Ditropan.*

USES

Atropine is the classic anticholinergic agent but its use is limited by its cardioaccelerator and mydriatic effects. This agent will not completely paralyse the bladder even at high doses suggesting that detrusor muscle contractility is not wholly mediated by muscarinic receptors. Research indicates that β adrenergic receptors in the dome of the bladder may have a role in bladder contractility. In addition non-adrenergic, non-cholinergic nerves may play a role in bladder tonus or neuromuscular transmission. Stimulation of these receptors causes some detrusor responses. Nevertheless, anticholinergic agents remain the mainstay of drugs used to reduce detrusor tonus or contractility.

Hyoscine and hyoscyamine containing preparations have been used and belladonna alkaloids with anticholinergic properties may be tried. Propantheline is used worldwide but some of the more recent synthetic agents appear to be more effective.

Penthienate, emepromium and oxybutynin have been found to be as, or more, effective than propantheline in clinical trials.

Penthienate is a particularly effective anticholinergic agent for use in treating the unstable bladder and urge incontinence in the elderly. Patients with uninhibited (hyper-reflexic) neuropathic bladder dysfunction, such as occurs in multiple sclerosis or after a cerebrovascular accident, may be extremely sensitive to this agent and may require only low dosage to obtain therapeutic benefit. Emepromium careegenate is not available in Australia but is used in Europe.

Oxybutynin is a newer agent combining anticholinergic, analgesic and direct smooth muscle relaxant properties. It is demonstrably superior to the other anticholinergic agents for reducing bladder pressure and enhancing effective bladder capacity. It has replaced many of the other agents in the treatment of incontinence. By contrast, dicyclomine, whilst having some relaxant effect on the bladder and colonic smooth muscle, is disappointing in its effect on urinary symptoms.

Irrespective of which anticholinergic agent is used all are best absorbed when taken on an empty stomach.

ADVERSE DRUG REACTIONS

Dryness of the mouth caused by anticholinergic agents is universal. This side effect limits the tolerable dosage that can be administered and is a reliable guide to the effective absorption of, or compliance with, the medication. Difficulty in reading small print (due to paralysis of accommodation and dilation of the pupil) only occurs at high dosage. Constipation and tachycardia may also occur.

PRECAUTIONS AND CONTRAINDICATIONS

In the elderly and in patients with neuropathy the bladder may be very sensitive to these agents and urinary retention may occur. The patient who responds initially and then relapses into incontinence shortly afterwards should be suspected of developing chronic retention with overflow. The bladder should be checked for residual urine by catheterisation. Dosage reduction is indicated. Alternatively, management by intermittent self-catheterisation may be employed to establish continence.

These agents are contraindicated in the presence of bladder outlet obstruction such as prostatic enlargement and strictures because they may precipitate acute retention of urine. They should be given with caution to patients with glaucoma or myasthenia gravis.

Tricyclic Antidepressants: Imipramine

The tricyclic antidepressants have a role in the management of urological problems due to their weak anticholinergic and ganglion blocking properties. Traditionally they have been used in the treatment of enuretic children. Such children have unstable bladder contractions during the night which fail to wake them. The tricyclic antidepressants attack both elements of the problem. They promote a lowering of detrusor pressures and excitability and an upward shift in the sleep pattern, making it more likely that the child will wake in the night rather than wetting the bed.

In addition to its anticholinergic action imipramine (*Melipramine, Tofranil*) also inhibits reuptake of noradrenaline from postganglionic synapses. This leads to an enhancement of adrenergic effects and augments bladder relaxation by an inhibitory action on the dome of the bladder. It also promotes closure of the male bladder neck and the smooth muscle component of distal urethral resistance.

Other tricyclic agents have no particular advantage over imipramine in the treatment of urinary disorders. The main place of these agents is in the treatment of persistent nocturnal enuresis. In adults they may be used in combination with the anticholinergic agents (when these alone give incomplete urinary control) or as an alternative medication when anticholinergic agents are not tolerated. The sedative action experienced initially by some patients becomes less troublesome with time. Dry mouth, blurring of vision and constipation are generally less

DRUGS USED IN BLADDER DYSFUNCTION

15

marked than with anticholinergic agents. For further information on tricyclic antidepressants see Chapter 26 Psychiatric Disorders.

Smooth Muscle Relaxants: Flavoxate

Flavoxate has a direct smooth muscle relaxant effect of unknown mechanism. It has been promoted as having beneficial effects on the unstable bladder. However, the patient often must take unacceptably large numbers of tablets each day to obtain any noticeable benefit.

β Sympathomimetics: Salbutamol

β Adrenergic sympathomimetics such as salbutamol (*Ventolin*) have mild detrusor relaxant effects. When used alone they are ineffective but they have been used to augment anticholinergic agents. With the advent of newer and more potent anticholinergic agents they are rarely used.

Calcium Channel Blockers: Terodiline, Nifedipine, Flunarizine

This class of therapeutic substances should, on theoretical grounds, be effective in combating the effects of detrusor instability. In practice only terodiline (*Mictrol*) has any useful effect on the unstable bladder in reducing frequency, nocturia, urgency and incontinence. This is only partly due to the calcium channel blocking properties of terodiline which also has quite marked additive anticholinergic properties. Trials have shown terodiline to be at least as effective as oxybutynin in the treatment of urge incontinence. However, it has recently been withdrawn from the market due to a low incidence of fatal cardiac arrhythmia.

Nifedipine (*Adalat*) has minimal anticholinergic properties being solely a calcium channel blocker. Although it has been shown to have an effect on the contractility of detrusor muscle strips in vitro. Its effects on the unstable bladder in clinical trials are disappointing and consequently it has little place in the treatment of incontinence.

Flunarizine has only a limited effect on the unstable bladder in trials to date. Urgency may be reduced but frequency is not affected. Clearly work in this area is in its infancy and this class of drugs may find an important place in the treatment of bladder disorders in the future.

For information on adverse drug reactions, drug interactions, precautions and contraindications for calcium channel blockers see Chapter 12 Cardiovascular Diseases.

Other Agents and Techniques

Prostaglandins have been shown to have a number of effects on the detrusor muscle and have a potentially important role in non-adrenergic non-cholinergic neurotransmission in the bladder. Prostaglandin synthetase inhibitors (non-steroidal anti-inflammatory drugs) reduce the available prostaglandins in the bladder wall and thus may reduce bladder contractility. Flurbiprofen has been tried in the treatment of the unstable bladder with little clinical benefit, however some symptomatic benefit has been reported with indomethacin. Unfortunately, side effects are prominent with most prostaglandin inhibitors and limit their long-term usefulness.

The reduction of intravesical pressure obtained with any of these agents may be disappointing unless high doses are employed. Therapeutic response rates for the various agents range from 30% to 60%, compared with 30% for placebo. The failure of one anticholinergic agent does not preclude success with another agent and it is always worth changing drugs and doses, or trying combinations, to achieve a response. Tachyphylaxis is common with all the drug groups.

Bladder retraining and biofeedback techniques offer a highly successful (75%) alternative to pharmaceutical manipulation for the treatment of motivated patients with unstable bladder problems. When this fails surgery may also be unsuccessful. Nerve block techniques using transvesical phenol injections into the inferior vesical plexuses on each side achieve 65% success rates when bladder training and anticholinergic agents are unsuccessful. After such a procedure the bladder may become hypersensitive to the effects of anticholinergic agents, demonstrating denervation supersensitivity. For the refractory unstable bladder, bladder transection or 'clam' ileocystoplasty may need to be considered.

NURSING IMPLICATIONS

ASSESSMENT

Drugs can only help patients to control their bladders by giving them warning of impending micturition and more time in which to get to the toilet. They are not a substitute for motivation or effort. The patient's willingness and ability to cooperate with treatment need realistic assessment. Factors which may decrease motivation should be identified and rectified, whilst ways of increasing motivation and patient compliance are instituted. The expectation of a positive outcome can act as a motivator to patients, relatives and therapists.

When mobility problems are prominent, as in elderly patients with arthritis or those who are bedridden, the call for assistance needs to be answered promptly. Timed toileting or regular potting may still be required in order to maintain continence but needs to be tailored to the requirements of each individual. Bladder relaxants in such patients can improve the bladder capacity and reduce the number of times that the patient needs to be toileted.

In the elderly or in patients with neuropathic bladder dysfunction, these agents can cause urinary retention especially if there is any degree of bladder outlet obstruction. The nurse should be alert to this possibility and should be prepared to check a residual urine if suspicion is aroused by recurrent urinary infections, overflow incontinence, enuresis, double voiding or abdominal distension whilst patients are taking these medications.

Leakage around an indwelling catheter which is not blocked is due to bladder spasms and can be alleviated by anticholinergic agents and by reducing bladder irritation. Such bladder irritation is caused by catheter traction, urinary infection and large catheter balloons (5 mL balloons on 18F catheters are ideal). Informed nursing management of the chronic indwelling catheter can eliminate leakage around a catheter and reduce the need for pharmacological intervention.

ADMINISTRATION

If a patient with a urinary catheter requires anticholinergic agents because of bladder spasms or leakage around the catheter, administration of the drug must be stopped when the catheter is removed so that normal micturition can be re-established.

EVALUATION

The patient's response to bladder relaxants should be improved continence or decreased leakage around a catheter. Dry mouth can be distressing to patients, especially the elderly. They should be advised to drink and to suck on low sugar lemon flavoured sweets or gum to promote salivation.

PATIENT EDUCATION

Patients need to be informed of the limitations of drug treatment and that their cooperation and conscious contribution to a treatment regimen is important to attaining bladder control. Realistic expectations for treatment outcome should be set and conveyed to the patient. Direction to alternative methods of treatment will be necessary if drug therapy is unsatisfactory. Patients taking imipramine need reassurance that its sedative effects will diminish with time. All patients need to be warned about the possibility of urinary retention occurring and should be advised to seek medical advice if acute retention occurs.

DRUGS USED IN BLADDER DYSFUNCTION

15

STORAGE

Penthienate should be stored in a refrigerator.

DRUGS USED FOR SENSORY URGENCY/FREQUENCY

In clinical practice it is common to encounter patients who have symptoms which suggest detrusor instability but in whom no instability can be detected on urodynamic testing. Many report sensory discomfort or pain on bladder filling suggestive of intravesical inflammation. Urinary infection must be excluded and cystoscopic examination of the bladder is necessary.

A variety of chronic non-bacterial 'cystitis' conditions may be responsible and some are amenable to cystoscopic treatment. Interstitial cystitis is one such condition. It is characterised by an idiopathic chronic relapsing pancystitis which predominantly affects women. The bladder wall contains many histamine secreting mast cells as well as a variety of other chronic inflammatory cells such as lymphocytes. A spectrum of less severe 'mast cell cystoses' exists, all of which can present with similar clinical symptoms.

Symptomatic improvement may follow bladder hydrodistension but relief is invariably transient. In severe cases a course of bladder washouts (usually six) with either oxychlorosene (*Chlorpactin*) or dimethyl sulfoxide (DMSO) can be beneficial. The mode of action of both preparations is unknown. Oxychlorosene is an antibacterial agent with mild detergent properties. The 0.4% solution must be freshly prepared just prior to instillation into the bladder under anaesthesia. Nascent chlorine is liberated within the bladder but whether this is responsible for the therapeutic effect is unknown. Dimethyl sulfoxide has multiple pharmacological actions being a membrane penetrant, anti-inflammatory, local analgesic, bacteriostatic, diuretic, cholinesterase inhibitor, collagen solvent and vasodilator. Several groups have reported 75% response rates in patients with interstitial cystitis when DMSO in a 50% solution was instilled into the bladder without the need for anaesthesia.

An alternative pharmacological approach is based on an attempt to suppress the effect of the mast cells. Antihistamines in combination with non-steroidal anti-inflammatory drugs (indomethacin or naproxen) have been used with anecdotal reports of success.

For patients with no obvious inflammatory lesion on cystoscopy reassurance combined with bladder training techniques can bring relief from frequency and urgency in 90% of cases, presumably through a desensitisation process. Urinary alkalinisation using sodium citrate/bicarbonate preparations (*Ural, Citravescent, Sodibic, Citralka*) may be helpful in patients in whom the symptoms wax and wane. Urethral discomfort may be diminished but frequency and urgency do not always respond. Infection must be excluded by urine culture.

Pentosanpolysulfate is a polysaccharide which, when taken orally or instilled intravesically, can replace the strongly hydrophilic glycosaminoglycan layer which normally lines the bladder epithelium. Deficiencies in the glycosaminoglycan layer have been found in patients who have recurrent urinary tract infections, recurrent stone disease and interstitial cystitis. Glycosaminoglycans prevent bacterial adherence to the bladder mucosa, inhibit crystal formation in the urine and waterproof the bladder lining. They are useful in reducing the incidence of recurrent urinary infections and may be helpful in the treatment of some of the non-bacterial chronic cystitis conditions. There are reports of its beneficial use in interstitial cystitis and in radiation cystitis.

15

ENHANCEMENT OF URETHRAL RESISTANCE

Stress incontinence is the result of incompetence of both the usually watertight bladder neck mechanism (the chief continence mechanism after detrusor stability) and the distal sphincter mechanism. With an incompetent bladder neck continence is still possible if the distal urethral sphincter mechanism is competent. When the distal mechanism and the bladder neck are incompetent, stress incontinence occurs with coughing, sneezing or any sudden rise in intra-abdominal pressure. The competence of the distal mechanism relates to the effective urethral closure pressure which depends on both the elastic and muscular properties of the urethra.

The elastic component of urethral resistance or closure pressure is not amenable to direct pharmacological stimulation although oestrogens may enhance both the urethral elasticity and muscle tone in the postmenopausal female.

The distal urethral mechanism is partly α adrenergic smooth muscle and partly cholinergic striated muscle. Both types of muscle contribute equally to the maintenance of the urethral closure pressure. Thus it is possible to enhance urethral competence by stimulation of either the smooth or striated component of the sphincter mechanism. Both α adrenergic sympathomimetics and cholinergic agents can achieve this but, since the latter also cause an increase in intravesical pressure (nullifying any therapeutic effect on the urethral resistance), only the α receptor stimulators are clinically useful for augmentation of urethral resistance.

The conservative treatment of stress incontinence involves weight reduction and pelvic floor exercises. In the treatment of uncomplicated stress incontinence in women pelvic floor exercise programs augmented by either drugs or electrostimulation of the muscles, achieve 70% success rates even in patients who have had pre- viously unsuccessful surgery. When these measures fail, urodynamic assessment is indicated with a view to surgical intervention.

Drugs are only used as an adjunct to an exercise program or in the treatment of incontinence when surgery is contraindicated or has been unsuccessful. Incontinence due to sphincter weakness or damage after prostatectomy and neuropathic sphincteric weakness (e.g. due to spina bifida) may respond to pharmacological stimulation.

α Adrenergic Sympathomimetics: Ephedrine, Pseudoephedrine, Phenylpropanolamine

α Adrenergic agents increase urethral closure pressure and urethral resistance. They act on the smooth muscle component of the urethral sphincter mechanism, causing contraction. In the male, part of the bladder neck mechanism is α adrenergic smooth muscle and this is also stimulated.

Ephedrine and pseudoephedrine (*Sudafed*) can be helpful, particularly in patients with minor degrees of stress incontinence. Unfortunately many patients cannot tolerate them due to their unpleasant central effects such as nervousness, irritability or insomnia, or to the tachycardia and cardiac dysrhythmias which are sometimes induced.

Phenylpropanolamine is tolerated better and causes fewer central and cardiac effects. Several cases of hypertensive reactions have been reported but seem to be either idiosyncratic reactions or reactions which occurred when another adrenergic agent was taken concurrently. Unfortunately, this preparation is not widely available except in combination with antihistamines in various cold remedies (e.g. *Sinutabs*, *Dimetapp*). In this form the drowsiness caused by the antihistamine makes long-term therapy unacceptable to most patients.

Midodrine is a long acting α adrenergic agent which is both well tolerated and therapeutically effective in patients with stress incontinence.

These agents have the capacity to cause urinary retention in patients with mild degrees of bladder outlet obstruction or detrusor failure. This can be significant when an elderly male requires a decongestant for upper respiratory tract disease, as nearly all the oral preparations contain sufficient amounts of sympathomimetics to cause an increase in urethral resistance leading to acute retention. A topical nasal decongestant is a wiser choice in such patients.

Oestrogens

In the postmenopausal or oestrogen deficient woman, a course of oestrogen therapy over a three-month period may improve urethral competence. This is partly a direct action on the periurethral smooth muscle or elastic tissues and partly because oestrogens sensitise the smooth muscle to circulating catecholamines. Any low dose preparation may be used. If long term use is contemplated the agents used should be selected using the same criteria which apply to hormone replacement therapy (see Chapter 19 Endocrine Diseases). The use of topically applied oestrogen creams (e.g. dienoestrol cream) is helpful in treating concomitant senile (atrophic) vaginitis, but probably does little to improve urethral closure pressures in patients with stress incontinence.

Other Agents

Mazindol (*Sanorex*) is an appetite suppressant with properties similar to dexamphetamine but without the addictive and other side effects. Trials have shown that this agent can improve urethral closure pressure and help 63% of patients with stress incontinence. Some centres have used imipramine for the same purpose. The rationale behind this is that one of the side effects of tricyclic antidepressants is their ability to block the reuptake of noradrenaline into adrenergic nerve endings. This has the effect of sensitising the receptors to circulating catecholamines, thus hav-

ing an adrenergic stimulating effect. This is devious pharmacology and cannot be recommended unless there is another reason for subjecting the patient to the other effects of imipramine.

The drugs used to promote continence are listed in Table 15.2.

TABLE 15.2 Drugs used to promote continence

Bladder Relaxants
Anticholinergic Agents   Atropine   Hyoscine   Propantheline   Penthienate   Dicyclomine   Emepromium*   Oxybutynin
Tricyclic Antidepressants   Imipramine   Amitriptyline
β *Adrenergic Agents*   Salbutamol
Calcium Channel Blockers   Terodiline**
Miscellaneous   Flavoxate*

Urethral Stimulants
α *Adrenergic agents*   Ephedrine   Pseudoephedrine   Phenylpropanolamine   Midodrine*
Oestrogens
Miscellaneous   Mazindol

*Not available in Australia.
**Withdrawn from market.

DRUGS USED TO PROMOTE BLADDER EMPTYING

Inadequate bladder emptying may be due to bladder outlet obstruction, detrusor failure or a combination of both. Ultimately, residual urine occurring in any clinical situation results from a failure of detrusor force. That is, the detrusor fails either to sustain sufficient pressure to completely empty the bladder or it fails to generate sufficient pressure to overcome outlet resistance. Detrusor failure of this kind may be neurogenic, myogenic, psychogenic or pharmacological in origin (see Table 15.3).

TABLE 15.3 Causes of detrusor contractile dysfunction

Neurogenic causes
Autonomous bladder
Sacral/infrasacral spinal cord lesion
Cauda equina lesion
Autonomic neuropathy
Metabolic (diabetes, uraemia, porphyria, hypothyroidism)
Infectious (Guillain-Barre syndrome)
Toxic (alcoholism, heavy metals)
Collagen disease (SLE, polyarteritis)
Carcinomatous
Pelvic surgery
Abdominoperineal excision of rectum
Low anterior resection
Cordoma
Wertheim hysterectomy
Pelvic radiotherapy
Pelvic/sacral fractures
Decompensated neuropathic bladder
Recovery phase after acute spinal cord injury
Myogenic causes
Congenital megacystitis
Overstretch
Acute retention
Chronic retention
Radiation induced
Outlet obstruction
Psychogenic causes
Bashfulness
Pain
Postoperative
Hysterical retention
Pharmacogenic causes
Anticholinergic agents
Ganglion blockers
Tricyclic antidepressants
Anaesthetics (general, epidural, spinal)
Opioids

Some bladders are unable to contract and are called acontractile or areflexic. In the **acontractile bladder** there are no coordinated expulsive contractions of the detrusor and the bladder is therefore unable to empty. Some acontractile bladders can generate some pressure due to abnormal tonus in the bladder wall (hypertonic or low compliance bladder). The degree of tonus is related to the bladder volume such that intravesical pressure rises with bladder filling. If the pressure is high enough the bladder neck may be pulled open and incomplete evacuation of urine can sometimes be achieved by abdominal straining. This is a dangerous situation in which to leave a patient, risking both recurrent infections and renal failure.

The **atonic bladder** which has no tonus in its wall and is unable to contract is very rare. Most doctors are really referring to an acontractile bladder when they talk about an 'atonic bladder'. Pharmacological attempts to stimulate the truly atonic bladder are futile. This type of detrusor contractile dysfunction is best managed by intermittent self-catheterisation or a permanent indwelling urethral or suprapubic catheter.

Other contractile dysfunctions may respond to pharmacological treatment either by bladder stimulation or by reduction of urethral resistance, or both. It must always be remembered that the bladder that cannot contract (acontractile or atonic) will not be stimulated to do so by pharmacological agents. Only a bladder which is able to contract can be stimulated to do better by drugs.

ENHANCEMENT OF DETRUSOR FUNCTION

Bladder function can be enhanced by cholinergic agents which stimulate the post-ganglionic muscarinic nerve ending on the detrusor muscle. Acetylcholine, the classical agent and natural neurotransmitter, is too rapidly degraded and too generalised in effect to be useful and synthetic cholinergic agents are therefore used.

The main indication for the use of bladder stimulation is non-obstructive urinary retention or impaired voiding efficiency. However, when this is due to drugs which depress detrusor function these agents should be discontinued. Outflow obstruction is a contraindication to detrusor stimulation and must be excluded. Postoperative and psychogenic retention may respond to cholinergic agents by injection. Effective voiding function may be restored by bladder stimulation in patients in whom there are ineffective or inadequate detrusor contractions secondary to overstretch of the bladder wall (e.g. after prostatectomy for chronic retention) or secondary to neuropathy.

Bethanechol is widely used to stimulate the neuropathic bladder either in the recovery phase after spinal injury or when incomplete emptying becomes a problem later in management. Stimulation of the autonomous (acontractile) neuropathic bladder associated with cauda equina, conus or pelvic nerve lesions has been used to improve tonus in order to facilitate emptying by straining. If the 'leak point pressure' at which urine escapes from the urethra is above 40 cm water, upper tract damage and renal failure can occur. Particularly in neuropathic bladders concurrent lowering of outlet resistance by drugs or surgery may be required to achieve satisfactory bladder emptying and prevent renal damage. Management by intermittent self-catheterisation is generally preferable. Bladder pressures may need to be lowered by anticholinergic agents to facilitate storage.

Cholinergic Agents: Carbachol, Bethanechol, Distigmine

Carbachol is a choline ester with parasympathomimetic properties. It stimulates the neuromuscular junction of the bladder and bowel. It is cheap and has been widely used in patients with postoperative retention. Some patients do not tolerate it because of the intestinal colic or diarrhoea which it can induce. This intestinal stimulatory effect makes its use in patients who have had a recent intestinal anastamosis somewhat hazardous.

Bethanechol (*Urecholine, Urocarb*) is similar in action to carbachol but seems to have more effect on the urinary bladder and less effect on the bowel. It is generally better tolerated and is useful when long-term therapy is being considered. Large oral doses may be required to achieve the same effect as small injected doses.

Distigmine (*Ubretid*) is a long acting anticholinesterase. It is similar to carbachol and has pronounced detrusor stimulating effect especially when given by injection. It is particularly useful in getting the bladder started again after postoperative retention in the absence of obstruction. Oral distigmine has no advantages over oral bethanechol but is vastly more expensive.

ADVERSE DRUG REACTIONS

The other cholinergic effects of these agents may be troublesome. Stimulation of gastrointestinal muscle and secretions may cause diarrhoea or aggravate peptic ulceration. Sweating, miosis and bradycardia can occur.

PRECAUTIONS AND CONTRAINDICATIONS

These drugs are contraindicated in pregnancy and in patients with asthma or cardiac disease. Retention due to bladder outlet obstruction is an absolute contraindication to the use of these agents.

For further information on cholinergic agents see Chapter 10 Drugs and the Autonomic Nervous System.

REDUCTION OF OUTLET RESISTANCE

Bladder outlet resistance can be reduced by drugs which act on either the smooth muscle or striated muscle components of the distal sphincter mechanism. α Adrenergic blockers relax the smooth muscle component while striated muscle relaxants act on the voluntary striated component.

Bladder outlet obstruction due to urethral strictures, valves or prostatic enlargement requires surgical correction and does not respond to drug therapy. Early or mild degrees of benign prostatic obstruction may be temporarily improved by relaxation of the bladder neck musculature or the smooth muscle within the prostatic gland by α adrenergic blocking drugs. These agents have also been effective for short periods when patients were unfit for, or unwilling to undergo, prostatic surgery. Obstructions such as those which occur at the bladder neck and distal sphincter mechanism are muscular in origin, dynamic in nature. While they are amenable to pharmacological relief, this is seldom of a permanent nature.

The normal bladder neck is actively pulled open by contraction of the detrusor muscle and remains open until the bladder relaxes again. In some men there is a dyssynergia of the bladder neck such that when the detrusor contracts the neck tightens causing obstruction. These men present between 30 and 50 years of age with symptoms of prostatitis or 'prostatism'. Definitive treatment for the condition consists of bladder neck incision, but this carries a risk of retrograde ejaculation and infertility. When fertility is important to the patient the bladder neck can be reversibly relaxed by α adrenergic blockade and the effect monitored by urinary flowmetry.

The normal distal sphincter mechanism relaxes synchronously with a voiding detrusor contraction to facilitate emptying. This normal coordination of the bladder and sphincter during micturition is disturbed as a result of spinal injuries above the sacral segments of the spinal cord and this results in a condition known as detrusor sphincter dyssynergia. In this condition there is a failure of the normal synchronous relaxation of the sphincter during voiding. Instead the sphincter contracts during voiding and may produce complete, partial or intermittent obstruction to the bladder outlet. About 80% of people with spinal injuries have this type of problem which, if not adequately treated, can cause progressive renal damage. Treatment is surgical endoscopic sphincterotomy to remove the obstruction and to enable the bladder to be managed by intermittent suprapubic percussion (to stimulate bladder contraction) and necessitates the use of a condom urinary collecting device. This is impractical for females in whom the condition is better managed by intermittent self-catheterisation or a permanent suprapubic catheter using an anticholinergic agent to suppress unwanted detrusor contractions from the neuropathic bladder. This approach is winning more support amongst male spinal injury patients, providing they have sufficient hand function to be able to self-catheterise.

When the degree of obstruction caused by the dyssynergic sphincter is only mild or intermittent, or when surgery is impracticable or hazardous, a therapeutic trial of drug treatment may be indicated. In such cases the therapeutic attack may be directed towards relaxation of either the smooth muscle or striated muscle components of the sphincter mechanisms. In patients with spastic paraparesis or quadraparesis drugs which relax the striated muscle would be expected to be more effective than smooth muscle relaxants, although both have been employed with clinical success.

In patients with an acontractile bladder, such as the autonomous bladder of cauda equina, conus medullaris or pelvic nerve lesions, reduction of outlet resistance can be employed to enable the patient to empty the bladder by straining. However management by intermittent self-catheterisation is to be

15 ■

DRUGS USED IN BLADDER DYSFUNCTION

preferred. If drug therapy is elected a fine balance needs to be struck between sufficient reduction of outlet resistance to facilitate emptying and reduction to the point of incontinence. Since the pelvic floor striated musculature is generally flaccid in such nerve lesions the use of α adrenergic blockade is the preferred method of lowering outlet resistance in such cases.

α Adrenergic Blockers: Phenoxybenzamine, Prazosin, Indoramin, Alfuzosin, Doxazocin, Terazosin

Phenoxybenzamine (*Dibenyline*), a long acting, cumulative α blocking drug. Phenoxybenzamine acts at two sites on the bladder outlet, relaxing smooth muscle of the male bladder neck and the smooth muscle component of the distal sphincter mechanism of both sexes. It can take up to 10 days to reach its full effect if given in low doses but has the potential to reduce the resting urethral closure pressure by 40%.

Prazosin (*Minipress, Pressin*) is a selective postsynaptic α_1 receptor blocker with similar effects on the bladder outlet. Trials suggest that it may be more effective in lowering bladder outlet resistance and cause less tachycardia than phenoxybenzamine. Prazosin is also used as an antihypertensive agent because of its action in reducing peripheral vascular resistance.

Indoramin and alfuzosin are similar α_1 selective blocking drugs with proven effect in lowering outlet resistance in patients with prostatic obstruction. Doxazocin is a long acting α blocker which has yet to find a place in urological management but can reduce urethral resistance. Terazosin is similar but is of proven efficacy in reducing bladder outlet resistance.

Postural hypotension can be a problem with higher doses of α blocking drugs and requires dosage reduction. Stepwise dosage introduction is recommended especially with prazosin which can have a profound first-dose hypotensive action. Failure of

ejaculation is common due to bladder neck relaxation allowing retrograde ejaculation back into the bladder. There is also a failure of seminal emission from the terminal vas deferens, which is also under α adrenergic sympathetic control. Prazosin can induce or aggravate urinary incontinence in elderly females especially when their control is already tenuous. Nasal congestion, miosis and reflex tachycardia can occur.

These drugs are contraindicated in congestive cardiac failure.

For further information on α blocking drugs see Chapter 12 Cardiovascular Diseases.

Other Agents

5-α Reductase inhibitors, e.g. finasteride, are undergoing trials in the relief of bladder outlet obstruction due to benign prostatic enlargement. Some shrinkage in prostatic size has been documented, however, after two years of use, symptomatic improvement but little objective relief of outflow obstruction has been demonstrated. They may find a place in the treatment of early symptoms of prostatism before significant obstruction develops.

Striated Muscle Relaxants: Baclofen, Diazepam, Dantrolene, Methocarbamol, Orphenadrine

The striated muscle component of the distal sphincter mechanism has cholinergic (nicotinic) somatic innervation. In attempting to facilitate bladder emptying by pharmacological reduction of outlet resistance, the anticholinergic agent selected should not also reduce detrusor contractility. They should not cause respiratory depression, total paralysis or hypotonia.

Baclofen (*Lioresal, Clofen*) is an ideal agent as it affects both periurethral striated muscle and can alleviate skeletal muscle spasms of spinal origin. A derivative of γ aminobutyric acid (GABA), it produces presynaptic inhibition affecting both polysynaptic and monosynaptic transmission. It also diminishes reflex contractions by reducing γ efferent activity from the muscle spindles. Generalised hypotonia and drowsiness may be caused and step wise introduction of the drug is necessary. It can mildly inhibit the detrusor at high doses. It may be the drug of choice for the treatment of detrusor sphincter dyssynergia in spinal patients in whom it can be combined with an α blocker. It is relatively contraindicated in psychotic or epileptic patients.

Diazepam (*Antenex, Ducene, Valium*) is a muscle relaxant, but its central tranquillising effect may make it unacceptable to the patient. It is useful in cases where there is a functional sphincteric outlet obstruction associated with anxiety. In such cases the central effects of the drug may be more therapeutic than its peripheral effect.

Dantrolene sodium (*Dantrium*) reduces skeletal muscle contractility by an inhibitory effect on excitation–contraction coupling beyond the neuromuscular junction, possibly by blocking the release of activator from the sarcoplasmic reticulum. It affects predominantly fast twitch fibres but also affects slow twitch fibres. Its effects are generalised. Profound muscular hypotonia, respiratory depression, hepatocellular damage and drowsiness can occur and limit its usefulness. Dosage titration is necessary, especially when a degree of muscular tonicity is required by the patient for independent locomotion. Its long term use cannot be recommended when the only indication is bladder dysfunction.

Methocarbamol (*Robaxin*) reduces skeletal muscle spasm through a central effect on spinal internuncial neurones. It is claimed not to affect normal muscle tone and to be non-toxic. Its effectiveness in detrusor sphincter dyssynergia is unknown.

Orphenadrine (*Disipal*) has a parasympatholytic action useful in the treatment of muscular rigidity associated with Parkinson's disease or drug induced extrapyramidal muscular dyskinesia. Its use in bladder outlet obstruction is limited by its tendency to reduce detrusor contractility and therefore it is not recommended.

The drugs used to promote bladder emptying are listed in Table 15.4.

TABLE 15.4 Drugs used to promote bladder emptying

Bladder Stimulants

Cholinergic Agents
  Carbachol
  Bethanechol
  Distigmine

Urethral Relaxants

α *Adrenergic Blockers*
  Phenoxybenzamine
  Prazosin
  Indoramin
  Alfuzosin*
  Doxazocin*
  Terazosin*

Striated Muscle Relaxants
  Baclofen
  Diazepam
  Dantrolene

*Not available in Australia

NURSING IMPLICATIONS

Postoperative urinary retention can often be avoided by good nursing management. Getting male patients to stand to void, ensuring privacy in which to do so and administering adequate postoperative analgesia will prevent many problems. Cholinergic agents should not be used in patients who are pregnant, have bronchospasm, cardiac disease or urinary obstruction. Adrenergic blockers should not be used when congestive heart failure is evident.

During trials of micturition using bladder stimulants patients require careful monitoring. Overstretch of the bladder due to prolonged and unsuccessful trials should be avoided.

DRUGS USED IN BLADDER DYSFUNCTION

15

In spinal injury patients cholinergic agents can aggravate detrusor sphincter dyssynergia and result in life threatening autonomic dysreflexia, with headache, sweating and profound hypertension. This is a medical emergency requiring immediate catheterisation to empty the bladder — delay can be fatal due to cerebral haemorrhage.

The occurrence of intestinal colic or diarrhoea may make cholinergic therapy unacceptable to patients. Cardiovascular and respiratory effects should be evaluated. Arterial blood pressure response to the use of adrenergic blockers should be monitored.

WARNING

None of the agents mentioned in this chapter can be recommended for use in the treatment of functional disorders of the bladder associated with pregnancy. Since these disorders run a self-limiting course, an expectant policy is best adopted after careful exclusion of an infective cause.

FURTHER READING

Pearson, B.D., Droessler, D. (1988), 'Continence through nursing care'. *Geriatric Nursing*, 9(6), pp. 347–349.

Shepherd, A.M., Blannin, J.P., Feneley, R.C. (1982), 'Changing attitudes in the management of urinary incontinence: The need for specialist nurses'. *British Medical Journal* (*Clinical Research*), 284(6316), pp. 645–646.

US Department of Health and Human Services. (1992), *Urinary incontinence in adults—clinical practice guideline*. AHCPR Pub. No. 92-0038, Rockville, MD.

Wein, A.J. (1990), 'Pharmacological treatment of incontinence: National Institutes of Health consensus development conference on urinary incontinence in adults, Bethesda, MD, USA, 1988'. *Journal of the American Geriatrics Society*, 38(3), 317–325.

TEST YOUR KNOWLEDGE

1. List: (a) the types of drugs which can be used to relax the bladder; (b) the indications for the use of such agents; (c) what precautions need to be taken?

2. How may the detrusor be stimulated? Under what circumstances are such agents (a) indicated, (b) dangerous, (c) unhelpful?

3. What types of drugs can cause urinary retention?

4. List: (a) the drugs which can be used to lower bladder outlet resistance; (b) their indications; (c) their side effects.

Liver Diseases

DEBORAH L. LALICH

O B J E C T I V E S

At the conclusion of this chapter the reader should be able to:

1. Name the main drugs and doses used in the treatment of hepatic diseases and list important adverse effects;

2. List the nursing implications associated with the treatment of viral hepatitis and alcoholic liver disease; and

3. Give examples of drugs known to have adverse effects on the liver.

THE LIVER ▀▀▀▀▀▀▀▀▀▀▀▀▀▀▀▀▀▀▀▀▀

The liver is the largest gland in the body and is associated with many complex functions. These include the formation of bile, control of carbohydrate metabolism, detoxification of drugs and manufacture of plasma proteins. Diseases of the liver, therefore, have wide reaching consequences and in general are broadly divided into acute or chronic. Acute liver disease (liver failure) may be induced by viral hepatitis, drug toxicity and end-stage alcoholic liver disease. Chronic liver disease may result from chronic viral hepatitis, alcohol abuse or drugs.

This chapter discusses the pharmacological treatment of those conditions confined to the liver. For information on cancer of the liver see Chapter 31 Cancer Chemotherapy.

USE OF DRUGS IN LIVER DISEASE ▀▀▀▀▀▀▀

Hepatic elimination of drugs depends on hepatic blood flow, intrinsic hepatocellular enzyme activity and plasma protein binding. A change in these parameters may affect drug metabolism. The biochemical tests used to assess liver function (AST, bilirubin, etc) are of limited value in predicting the liver's ability to metabolise drugs. At present there are no tests capable of predicting this. In general, chronic liver disease affects drug metabolism more than acute disease.

Hepatic blood flow may be reduced by shock or cardiac failure which reduces the elimination of drugs whose clearances are flow dependent (e.g. lignocaine). Drugs taken orally which undergo high 'first pass' metabolism should have their dose reduced in conditions with reduced hepatic blood flow such as chronic liver disease or the presence of a portosystemic shunt. The drug will have more time to be absorbed into systemic circulation before arriving at the liver where it is inactivated. As a result, the therapeutic effect may be greater. Examples of such drugs are propranolol, metoprolol, nifedipine and verapamil—a reduced first pass effect may produce a more marked reduction in blood pressure.

Drugs which undergo low hepatic clearance (low first pass metabolism) and are independent of hepatic blood flow include phenytoin and sodium valproate. With these drugs the degree of plasma protein binding is important. In liver disease, the production of albumin may be reduced and it is to this protein that many drugs bind. As it is only unbound drug which exerts a therapeutic effect and is metabolised, a reduction in protein binding may result in toxicity. This is particularly important for drugs which are highly protein bound, i.e. more than 90% (e.g. phenytoin). There are no general rules for dose adjustment for these drugs as there are many factors involved. The patient should have blood levels monitored where possible and be closely observed for signs of toxicity.

HEPATITIS ▀▀▀▀▀▀▀▀▀▀▀▀▀▀▀▀▀▀▀▀▀

Hepatitis is defined as 'inflammation of the liver'. The cause of the inflammation may be viral infection, drugs or other toxins (e.g. alcohol). The disease may be further defined as acute or chronic. A carrier state also exists and occurs in 5%–10% of patients who develop acute hepatitis B. Some carriers may be asymptomatic while others develop chronic liver diseases such as chronic active hepatitis and cirrhosis. Non-viral hepatitis frequently responds to withdrawal of the causative agent. Many treatment modalities have been used for viral hepatitis, including corticosteroids, immunosuppressants, interferons and liver transplants, all with limited success.

ACUTE VIRAL HEPATITIS

In recent years advancing technology has enabled the causes of viral hepatitis to be further differentiated and now there are five proposed groups as shown in Table 16.1.

Epstein-Barr virus and cytomegalovirus may also cause acute viral hepatitis.

Symptoms for all types of viral hepatitis are similar and may be divided into three groups: prodromal symptoms, clinical jaundice and the recovery phase (see Table 16.2). Complete recovery may take one to two months for hepatitis A and E and three to four months for hepatitis B and C.

TABLE 16.1 Classification of viral hepatitis

Hepatitis Virus Type	Previously Known As	Route of Transmission	Incubation Period	Complications
A (HAV)	Infectious hepatitis, yellow jaundice	Faeco–oral	2–6 weeks	Usually none; prolonged jaundice is rare
B (HBV)	Serum hepatitis	Intravenous, sexual contact, vertical (mother to infant)	4–6 weeks	Chronic liver disease, carrier state (5%–10%)*, extra-hepatic symptoms, serum sickness, polyarteritis
C (HCV)	Parenteral non A-non B hepatitis	Intravenous, sexual contact, blood transfusion, vertical	1 week–6 months	Chronic hepatitis (20%), chronic liver disease, cirrhosis, ?hepatocellular carcinoma
D (HDV)**	Delta hepatitis	Intravenous, sexual contact, vertical		Increased morbidity and mortality as it usually affects those with existing liver disease
E (HEV)	Enteral non A-non B hepatitis	Faeco–oral	2–8 weeks	Fatal in 1%–2% cases in normal population, up to 10% during pregnancy

*HBV carrier state may be associated with long-term effects including chronic persistent hepatitis, chronic active hepatitis, cirrhosis and hepatocellular carcinoma.
**HDV is dependent upon HBV to replicate; therefore it either co-exists with acute HBV or may supra-infect chronic HBV.

16 LIVER DISEASES

TABLE 16.2 Symptoms of hepatitis infections

Stage	Symptoms*
1. Prodromal phase	May precede jaundice by 1–2 weeks; anorexia, nausea, vomiting, fatigue, malaise, arthralgias, myalgias, headache, photophobia, pharyngitis, cough and coryza; dark urine and clay coloured stools precede jaundice by 1–5 days; increased levels of aspartate aminotransferase (AST) and alanine aminotransferase (ALT).
2. Clinical jaundice	Mild weight loss; distaste for alcohol and cigarettes common; enlarged and tender liver with right upper quadrant pain; pruritus; increased levels of bilirubin
3. Recovery phase	Lasts 2–12 weeks; liver may remain enlarged; abnormal biochemistry

*Some patients with very mild symptoms may have subclinical attacks which pass undetected.

Treatment for all forms of acute hepatitis is largely supportive. Patients should be encouraged to rest and to eat a high calorie diet and avoid fatty foods. As many patients may have increased nausea late in the day, they should be encouraged to have a higher proportion of their diet in the mornings. If the patient is unable to maintain adequate oral intake, then intravenous feeding may be necessary. If the patient experiences severe pruritus, cholestyramine (*Questran*) may be used to reduce bile levels. The usual dose is one sachet three or four times daily mixed with juice or water. Antihistamines such as terfenadine (*Teldane*), astemizole (*Hismanal*) and hydroxyzine (*Atarax*) may be used if cholestyramine is not successful, however, they may precipitate hepatic coma. Drugs which are metabolised by the liver or known to be toxic to the liver should be avoided, e.g. non-steroidal anti-inflammatory drugs, alcohol, oral contraceptive pills. The use of sedatives should also be avoided.

NURSING IMPLICATIONS

Advice should be sought from infection control personnel in each hospital to determine what precautions should be taken when nursing these patients. In general, gloves should be worn when handling body fluids and blood and infectious waste disposed of according to hospital policy. Particular attention should be paid to handwashing after attending to each patient. Each hospital should have a policy for staff vaccination. As there is no specific treatment for acute viral hepatitis, prophylaxis is very important to reduce the spread of the disease.

NEEDLESTICK INJURIES

The nurse should be aware of the hospital policy in relation to needlestick injuries while nursing patients infected with hepatitis viruses. It is important to receive hepatitis B immunoglobulin as soon as possible and to complete the course of hepatitis B vaccine if necessary. Appropriate documentation and follow-up should be implemented according to hospital protocol.

PROPHYLAXIS

Hepatitis A Vaccine

Vaccination against hepatitis A is recommended for travellers to countries with a high incidence of the disease, e.g. South East Asia. Immunoglobulin (human) should be used when contact has been made with a proven case of hepatitis A.

TRADE NAMES

Hepatitis A vaccine: *Havrix*.

USES

Vaccination should take place 6–8 weeks prior to travelling into a high risk area. An initial intramuscular dose of 1 mL is followed by a second dose 2–4 weeks later. This should provide protection for up to one year. Longer protection may be provided by a third dose given 6–12 months after the initial dose. The vaccine should be stored in a refrigerator.

ADVERSE DRUG REACTIONS

The most common adverse effects are local reactions at the injection site, e.g. soreness, mild redness, slight swelling or hardness. These effects are usually mild and transient.

Immunoglobulin (Human)

Immunoglobulin (human) is prepared from the pooled plasma of blood donors and contains IgG (more than 95%), IgM, IgA and other plasma proteins. It also contains anti-hepatitis A virus antibodies.

USES

To provide immunity, immunoglobulin may be used up to two weeks following exposure to persons with hepatitis A. The recommended dose is 0.03–0.06 mL/kg by intramuscular injection.

Immunoglobulin may also be used to provide passive immunity against measles and rubella and in immunodeficiency states. Intravenous forms (*Intragam*, *Sandoglobulin*) are also available, but are generally not used for this purpose.

ADVERSE DRUG REACTIONS

The main adverse effects are pain at the injection site and muscle stiffness which may persist for several hours or days. Repeat injections may cause sensitisation with subsequent allergic reactions.

Hepatitis B Vaccine

A specific vaccine and immunoglobulin are available for hepatitis B virus. The vaccine is used to immunise individuals who are likely to be exposed to hepatitis B virus (e.g. health care workers). The immunoglobulin is reserved for use following exposure to the virus.

TRADE NAMES

Hepatitis B vaccine: *H-B-Vax II*; *Engerix B*.

Each brand is available in several strengths to accommodate the variation in doses required for infants, children and adults. The brands are not directly interchangeable and care should be taken to ensure that the correct brand and dose is administered.

Both are inactivated vaccines derived from hepatitis B virus surface antigen (HBsAg) and produced by recombinant DNA technology. Following a course of three injections, most people develop protective antibodies against hepatitis B virus which provide immunity for up to five years. The vaccine is not effective in preventing hepatitis B if given after exposure but may be given with hepatitis B immunoglobulin if the individual has not previously been vaccinated.

USES

Hepatitis B vaccine is administered as a course of three intramuscular injections into the deltoid muscle for adults or anterolateral thigh for infants and children. Subcutaneous injection may be used if the patient is unable to have intramuscular injections. (It should not be given intravenously or intradermally.) The vaccine is a suspension of HBsAg and should be shaken before use. The injection should be stored in the refrigerator (2–8°C).

LIVER DISEASES

16

TABLE 16.3 Doses for hepatitis B vaccines

Group	Engerix B		H-B-Vax II	
	Strength	**Dose**	**Strength**	**Dose**
Birth to 10 years	Paediatric 10 µg/0.5 mL	0.5 mL (10µg)	Paediatric 5 µg/0.5 mL	0.25 ml (2.5 µg)
11–19 years	Adult 20 µg/1.0 mL	1.0 mL (20 µg)	Paediatric 5 µg/0.5 mL	0.5 mL (5 µg)
Adults	Adult 20 µg/0.1 mL	1.0 mL (20 µg)	Adult 10 µg/1.0 mL	1.0 mL (10 µg)
Dialysis and immunocompromised patients	Adult 20 µg/1 mL	2.0 mL* (40 µg)	Adult dialysis 40 µg/1.0 mL	1.0 mL (40 µg)

*Two 1.0 mL doses should be given at different sites

The recommended doses are outlined in Table 16.3 and should be given at the selected start date, then one month and six months later. Immunocompromised patients often require larger doses to develop immunity. The appropriate interval for booster doses has yet to be determined. It has been suggested that a booster dose be given if the anti-HBs level falls below 10 IU/L.

ADVERSE DRUG REACTIONS

The vaccine is generally well tolerated. The most common reactions are pain and redness at the injection site with occasional swelling and warmth. Low grade fever may occur during the following 48 hours.

PRECAUTIONS AND CONTRAINDICATIONS

As there is a possibility of anaphylactic reactions, an emergency trolley should be on hand.

Hepatitis B Immunoglobulin (Human)

MECHANISM OF ACTION

Hepatitis B immunoglobulin (HBIg) is prepared from human plasma containing high levels of antibodies to HBsAg and reduces the risk of developing hepatitis B infection.

USES

The National Blood Transfusion Committee (NBTC) has made a list of recommendations for the use of HBIg. Briefly, these include staff exposed to significant risk of infection from patients or specimens; any person accidentally inoculated with material or blood known to be HBsAg positive; regular sex partners of individuals with acute hepatitis B; and infants born to HBsAg carrier mothers or mothers who develop acute infection during the third trimester. HBIg is only available in limited supplies and therefore may only be obtained from the Red Cross Blood Transfusion Service for those patients who fulfil the NBTC criteria.

HBIg is given by intramuscular injection at a dose of 0.06 mL/kg (up to 5 mL for adults and 0.5 mL for infants). The dose should be given as soon as possible after exposure, preferably within three days. It will not be effective if given after seven days. Hepatitis B vaccine is frequently given at the same time and should be administered at a separate site.

The injection is available in two strengths, 100 IU and 400 IU, and should be stored in the refrigerator.

ADVERSE DRUG REACTIONS

Adverse effects are uncommon. The main effects are local tenderness and stiffness at the site of injection and occasionally mild fever, malaise and urticaria.

CHRONIC HEPATITIS

Chronic hepatitis is defined as the presence of an inflammatory liver disease in a patient for more than six months. Three categories have been identified: chronic active hepatitis, chronic persistent hepatitis and chronic lobular hepatitis. The last two categories are generally asymptomatic and benign and are not treated.

Chronic active hepatitis may be caused by infection with hepatitis B virus, hepatitis C virus, autoimmune disease or drugs such as methyldopa or isoniazid. Patients with chronic active hepatitis may be asymptomatic or present with liver inflammation, fibrosis or hepatic necrosis which may ultimately progress to hepatic failure, cirrhosis, hepatic cancer and death. Treatment depends on the cause of the hepatitis.

If the cause is not viral, corticosteroid therapy is the treatment of choice. Prednisolone or prednisone is given at a dose of 20–40 mg daily for four weeks and then tapered off gradually over two to three months to 10–20 mg daily. This dose is maintained for at least 24 months as abrupt withdrawal may lead to relapse. Azathioprine (at a dose of 50–100 mg daily) may be added as a 'steroid sparing' agent to allow a reduction in the steroid dose without relapse occurring. The combination prevents or reduces the occurrence of some of the major adverse effects associated with prolonged steroid therapy.

Corticosteroid therapy is of little benefit for chronic active hepatitis of viral origin. Interferon alfa is currently the only drug which will modify the course of chronic hepatitis B or C.

Interferon Alfa

TRADE NAMES

Interferon alfa-2a: *Roferon-A.*
Interferon alfa-2b: *Intron A.*

MECHANISM OF ACTION

The antiviral mechanism of interferon alfa is not completely understood, however two major actions have been established. Interferon stops virus replication and also stimulates the immune system to produce antibodies and killer 'T' cells. Interferons occur naturally in the body as part of its defence mechanism. They are now commercially produced using recombinant DNA technology.

PHARMACOKINETICS

Interferon alfa may only be given parenterally as it is degraded by enzymes in the gastrointestinal tract. It is well absorbed following intramuscular or subcutaneous injection. It is mainly metabolised in the kidney and the metabolites are excreted in the urine. Dosage adjustment is only necessary in severe renal failure.

USES

Interferon alfa has been used in the treatment of chronic hepatitis B and C. Studies have shown cessation of viral replication in approximately 40% of patients. In general treatment is reserved for patients who are hepatitis Be antigen-positive and have had chronic active hepatitis B for at least six months or patients who have had the diagnosis confirmed by liver biopsy.

The recommended dose is 4.5–5.0 million IU by subcutaneous injection three times each week for six months. If there is no response after two months the dose may be increased to 9 million IU three times each week for a further six months. Patients with proven hepatitis C are given 3 million IU by subcutaneous injection three times each week for six months.

ADVERSE DRUG REACTIONS

Most patients develop 'flu-like' symptoms characterised by fever, chills, tachycardia,

16 LIVER DISEASES

malaise, myalgia and headache. These are usually relieved by paracetamol or aspirin and subside as treatment is continued. Symptoms associated with long-term use may include fatigue, weakness, peripheral and central nervous system disturbances (e.g. confusion, depression), blood abnormalities (reduced white blood cells and platelets), hair loss, rash and cardiovascular problems (hypotension, arrhythmias). The frequency of these effects appears to be dose related. In some patients a hepatitis-like illness may develop during the treatment. This is thought to point to a good prognosis and the patient should be reassured that it does not represent relapse.

DRUG INTERACTIONS

Interferon alfa inhibits the cytochrome-P450 enzyme system in the liver and therefore may inhibit the metabolism of other drugs.

Reduced metabolism and subsequent increased toxicity has been observed with theophylline and phenobarbitone.

NURSING IMPLICATIONS

PATIENT EDUCATION

Patients should be advised of the high likelihood that a flu-like illness may develop in the first few weeks of treatment with interferon. Paracetamol should be offered with each dose of interferon to help reduce this problem. Patients should be shown how to self-administer their injections. Information booklets which may be given to patients are produced by the drug companies.

CIRRHOSIS

Cirrhosis may be defined as a diffuse increase in the fibrous connective tissue of the liver producing a nodular or glandular texture. The onset of the disease is insidious and may not be detected until disease is advanced and liver function has been compromised. The complications of cirrhosis are many—portal hypertension, ascites, bleeding varices, anaemia and hepatic encephalopathy—and may have serious consequences. The management of these complications is a combination of diet, bed rest and medication.

PORTAL HYPERTENSION

Portal hypertension occurs as a result of increased resistance to blood flow through a diseased liver. The pressure rises throughout the gastrointestinal tract vessels and the spleen. As a result the blood flow is diverted to small collateral vessels through the oesophagus, abdominal wall and between the spleen and left renal vein.

Complications of portal hypertension include oesophageal and abdominal varices which may rupture, splenomegaly and ascites.

Treatment is aimed at reducing the blood flow through the portal system either surgically (splenectomy, portacaval shunts, e.g.

Le Veen) or with drug therapy. Propranolol has been used with some success in doses of 40–180 mg daily, usually in divided doses (see Chapter 12 Cardiovascular Diseases).

ASCITES

Ascites develops as a result of portal hypertension, low concentrations of plasma albumin and enhanced sodium retention by the kidneys. The amount of fluid accumulated in the peritoneal cavity varies from a few litres to more than 20 litres. This causes considerable abdominal distension and umbilical herniation.

The aim of treatment is to produce slow diuresis of approximately 1 L per day representing a daily weight loss of 0.5–1 kg. This may be achieved with a combination of bed rest, salt restriction of 500 mg to 2 g daily, adequate protein intake and diuretics. Drugs which promote sodium retention (e.g. non-steroidal anti-inflammatory drugs) or contain significant amounts of sodium (e.g. antacids, effervescent preparations) should be avoided.

Spironolactone

Spironolactone is the cornerstone of diuretic therapy in the treatment of ascites. It is used in higher doses than required for treating hypertension and requires three to five days to achieve maximal response.

TRADE NAMES

Spironolactone: *Aldactone*.

USES

Spironolactone is used to treat conditions associated with increased levels of aldosterone, i.e. primary and secondary hyperaldosteronism. These include oedema and ascites associated with congestive heart failure, cirrhosis and the nephrotic syndrome.

In the treatment of cirrhosis, if the urinary sodium:potassium ratio is greater than one, the starting dose is 100 mg daily. If the ratio is less than one the dose is 200–400 mg daily usually given as divided doses. If therapy with spironolactone alone is not effective other more potent diuretics such as frusemide may be added.

For information on mechanism of action, pharmacokinetics, adverse drug reactions, precautions and contraindications see Chapter 12 Cardiovascular Diseases.

OESOPHAGEAL AND GASTRIC VARICES

Portal hypertension causes engorgement of capillaries in the gastrointestinal tract. This may lead to the development of varices, most commonly in the stomach and oesophagus. Rupture of these varices is a medical emergency as about one-third of patients admitted with bleeding oesophageal varices die during initial hospitalisation. Bleeding may occur in 30% of patients with cirrhosis and recurrent bleeding is common.

Following initial resuscitation with plasma expanders (*Haemaccel*) or blood, treatment is divided into two stages: control of active bleeding and prevention of recurrent bleeding.

Control of active bleeding requires the use of vasoconstricting agents (e.g. vasopressin), octreotide, balloon tamponade and sclerosing agents. Balloon tamponade requires the insertion of a tube with an inflatable balloon into the oesophagus. The balloon is inflated close to the point of bleeding and may be left in place for several hours. This procedure has associated problems including a mortality rate of up to 8%.

Injection of the varice with a sclerosing agent such as ethanolamine is often effective in controlling the acute episode and may delay re-bleeding of the varice. Some studies have observed that if re-bleeding does occur, it may be worse than the original episode. Propranolol has been shown to have similar efficacy to sclerotherapy in some trials. Propranolol reduces portal pressure by lowering cardiac output and by splanchnic vasoconstriction.

The incidence of re-bleeding varices is quite high and methods of **prevention of recurrent bleeding** have varying success. At present, surgical ablation of the varice or installation of a portal systemic shunt to reduce portal pressure are the only methods with proven success. There is some evidence that propranolol can reduce the risk of both initial bleeding and re-bleeding. H_2 antagonists (e.g. cimetidine, ranitidine) are often used to reduce bleeding from gastric erosions.

Vasopressin

TRADE NAMES

Vasopressin: *Pitressin*.

MECHANISM OF ACTION

Pitressin is an aqueous solution of synthetic vasopressin with both antidiuretic activity and the ability to enhance smooth muscle contraction in the gastrointestinal tract and produce generalised vasoconstriction.

USES

Vasopressin is used to treat bleeding oesophageal varices; in the management of diabetes insipidus; to prevent or treat postoperative abdominal distention; and to remove gas shadows in abdominal radiography.

In the treatment of bleeding varices, vasopressin is given by intravenous infusion at a rate of 0.4 units per minute which may be increased to up to 0.9 units per minute. The infusion may be prepared in normal saline or glucose 5%. The success rate varies from 9% to 71% and therapy has been associated with significant adverse effects. Some studies have shown that combining a vasodilator (e.g. glyceryl trinitrate) with vasopressin reduces the cardiovascular complications associated with vasopressin therapy without altering its effectiveness in reducing portal pressure. The glyceryl trinitrate may be given sublingually, by patch or by intravenous infusion.

ADVERSE DRUG REACTIONS

The most significant adverse effects include myocardial infarction and left ventricular failure. It is therefore recommended that cardiac monitoring is undertaken when vasopressin infusion is used. The cardiac effects are less pronounced when vasopressin is given by other routes. Localised reactions may occur at the site of injection. Other effects include tremor, sweating, vertigo, 'pounding' in the head and bronchial constriction.

Octreotide

Octreotide (*Sandostatin*), a synthetic analogue of somatostatin, has been shown to reduce splanchnic and hepatic blood flow. In clinical trials it has been found to be as effective as vasopressin without producing severe cardiac effects. The usual dose is 25–50 micrograms/hour by intravenous infusion. Additional bolus doses of 50–100 micrograms may also be used.

HEPATIC ENCEPHALOPATHY

The cause of hepatic encephalopathy is not known. Increased blood levels of ammonia and aromatic amino acids have been associated with its development. Cirrhotic patients break down urea in the gut at a greater rate producing higher levels of ammonia. Lactulose decreases the rate of urea breakdown and facilitates removal of ammonia from the colon. Neomycin has been used in conjunction with lactulose to inhibit colonic bacteria and reduce the formation of ammonia. Oral metronidazole has also been used and is probably as effective as neomycin.

It has been suggested that aromatic amino acids may act as, or stimulate the production of, false neurotransmitters in the central nervous system and therefore cause encephalopathy. To reduce the levels of aromatic amino acids, protein intake should be restricted to 20 g per day. Special protein sources with high levels of other amino acids are thought to be beneficial.

Lactulose

Lactulose is a slightly yellow clear syrup containing lactulose, galactose, lactose and epilactose.

TRADE NAMES

Lactulose: *Duphalac.*

MECHANISM OF ACTION

As a laxative, lactulose is metabolised by bacteria in the colon to acetic, lactic and formic acids and carbon dioxide. This increases osmotic pressure in the colon and increases the water content of the stools. As a result, soft bulky stools are produced which promote peristalsis and subsequent bowel evacuation.

Lactulose inhibits the bacteria which break down urea and therefore the production of ammonia is reduced. As lactulose decreases the colonic pH, the ammonia in the colon is prevented from being reabsorbed and is excreted in the stools as ammonium ions.

PHARMACOKINETICS

Lactulose is poorly absorbed from the gastrointestinal tract and reaches the colon largely unchanged, where bacteria convert it to the active compounds. It is mainly excreted in the faeces.

USES

Lactulose is used in the treatment of hepatic encephalopathy and may be given orally or as an enema. The usual oral dose is 30–45 mL three or four times a day and is adjusted to produce two or three soft stools daily. Improvement in the patient's condition may take 24 hours to occur and if a rapid effect is required, doses initially may be given every hour.

Lactulose may be given at a maintenance dose of 15–30 mL daily to prevent recurrent episodes.

ADVERSE DRUG REACTIONS

Transient flatulence and abdominal cramping occur in about 20% of patients. Less commonly, nausea, vomiting, anorexia and increased thirst may occur.

DRUG INTERACTIONS

Theoretically, concurrent neomycin therapy may inhibit the colonic bacteria required to break down lactulose and prevent the reduction in colonic pH. However, this does not appear to be a problem in practice and the two drugs are frequently prescribed together.

Lactulose should be avoided in patients taking mesalazine as the effectiveness of the latter may be reduced.

PRECAUTIONS AND CONTRAINDICATIONS

Lactulose contains galactose and lactose and therefore should not be given to those patients who require a galactose and/or a lactose free diet. It should be used with caution in diabetics as blood glucose levels may be elevated with prolonged use.

Neomycin Sulfate

Neomycin is an aminoglycoside antibiotic available for oral use. The injection is no longer used because of unacceptable nephrotoxicity and ototoxicity.

MECHANISM OF ACTION

Neomycin inhibits the colonic bacteria and therefore reduces the production of ammonia.

PHARMACOKINETICS

It is poorly absorbed from the gastrointestinal tract and is excreted in the faeces. Its toxicity may be increased in the presence of intestinal obstruction because of the prolonged opportunity for systemic absorption.

USES

Neomycin is most frequently used to sterilise the bowel prior to surgery. In the treatment of acute hepatic encephalopathy, 1 g four times a day is the usual dose. A maintenance dose of 1 g twice daily may then be used.

ADVERSE DRUG REACTIONS

Prolonged oral therapy may result in overgrowth of organisms not sensitive to neomycin, e.g. *Candida* sp. Neomycin may cause ototoxicity and nephrotoxicity, although with oral administration the incidence is very low.

DRUG INTERACTIONS

Neomycin may decrease the absorption of digoxin and reduce serum levels of phenoxymethylpenicillin when given orally. Neomycin may also potentiate the effect of warfarin.

PRECAUTIONS AND CONTRAINDICATIONS

Neomycin should be used with caution in patients with impaired hearing or reduced renal function.

LIVER DISEASES

16

NUTRITION

Patients with alcohol induced cirrhosis must avoid alcohol intake. Abstinence alone may produce improvement. This, in conjunction with a nutritious diet, avoids the need for dietary supplementation. However should hypoprothrombinaemia develop, vitamin K supplementation may be required. Prolonged alcohol intake combined with inadequate diet may cause thiamine (vitamin B₁) deficiency. This may be corrected with intramuscular or oral administration of thiamine.

Vitamin K

Vitamin K is essential for the formation of certain clotting factors. Lack of vitamin K increases the tendency to haemorrhage.

TRADE NAMES

Vitamin K (phytomenadione): *Konakion*.

USES

Vitamin K may be used to treat or prevent haemorrhage associated with low prothrombin levels. Its main indications are as an antidote to oral anticoagulant therapy; neonatal haemorrhage and to replenish low levels of vitamin K as a result of disease, e.g. cirrhosis.

It is available as an injection (for intravenous or intramuscular use) and tablets. The dose is dependent on the indication. In cirrhosis the usual dose is 10 mg daily given as one tablet that should be chewed or sucked then swallowed.

ADVERSE DRUG REACTIONS

The oral dose form is well tolerated with no significant adverse effects. The injection may produce severe and sometimes fatal reactions when given intravenously. It should be diluted and administered slowly. When given by intramuscular injection, pain, redness and swelling occasionally develop at the site of the injection.

NURSING IMPLICATIONS

PATIENT EDUCATION

Patients should be encouraged to abstain from alcohol to prevent further liver damage and enable some recovery. The importance of a healthy diet should be emphasised as should any fluid or salt restrictions.

It is important to avoid night-time sedation (e.g. temazepam, nitrazepam) in patients with advanced liver disease as these drugs may precipitate hepatic encephalopathy and make the patient's neurological status difficult to assess.

LIVER TRANSPLANTATION

Liver transplant candidates are generally those patients who suffer from severe, irreversible liver disease who have not responded to traditional medical and surgical treatment. Transplantation would be considered when the liver failure is caused by non-alcoholic cirrhosis, primary biliary cirrhosis, sclerosing cholangitis, hepatic vein thrombosis and in some cases hepatobiliary cancer. In alcoholic cirrhosis a period of abstinence from alcohol (at least six months) is usually required.

Postoperatively, liver transplant patients may be prone to fluid overload and frequently develop jaundice. As with other types of transplants, immunosuppressive therapy is essential and therefore patients are susceptible to bacterial, fungal and viral infections.

IMMUNOSUPPRESSIVE THERAPY

Immunosuppressive therapy is the same as that for patients with kidney transplants, see Chapter 14 Drugs Used in Renal Failure.

Cyclosporin

Postoperatively, the absorption of oral cyclosporin may be reduced due to external bile drainage. As a result, the bioavailability will be reduced and higher doses may be needed. When the drain is removed absorption will improve and the dose may be reduced. During this period the blood levels of cyclosporin should be monitored frequently.

Cyclosporin is usually commenced the day before the transplant and may be given intravenously for the first 24–48 hours. The intravenous dose is 2–5 mg/kg daily as a single dose diluted in 100 mL of normal saline or glucose 5%. The oral dose is about three times the intravenous dose because of low bioavailability. The initial oral dose is approximately 15 mg/kg (14–18 mg/kg) given as one or two doses daily. This may be reduced to a maintenance dose of 5–10 mg/kg/day after a few weeks.

Adverse effects tend to be dose related and therefore it is recommended that blood levels are maintained between 50 nanograms/mL and 400 nanograms/mL.

For further information on cyclosporin see Chapter 14 Drugs Used in Renal Failure.

DRUG KINETICS IN LIVER TRANSPLANTATION

Transplant recipients undergo an unusual change from failing liver function to normal liver function. As a result, there may be an alteration in drug absorption, distribution and metabolism. Limited studies have shown that after liver transplants the absorption of lipid soluble compounds, such as cyclosporin and vitamins A and E, is considerably improved.

For further information including nursing implications see Chapter 14 Drugs Used in Renal Failure.

PARASITIC LIVER DISEASE

AMOEBIASIS

The major cause of amoebiasis (hepatic abscess) is the protozoa *Entamoeba histolytica*. The cystic form is released from the bowel and infection results when the cyst is ingested and transforms into the active trophozoite. An abscess may develop in the affected tissue, e.g. liver, lung, brain. Treatment is aimed at eradicating the parasite with specific antiamoebic therapy. The recommended treatment in order of preference is listed in Table 16.4.

Diloxanide Furoate

Diloxanide is a directly acting amoebicide which acts principally in the bowel.

TRADE NAMES

Diloxanide furoate: *Furamide*.

PHARMACOKINETICS

Diloxanide furoate is well absorbed from the gut and is metabolised by the liver. Approximately 10% of the dose is not absorbed and it is this component which is active throughout the gastrointestinal tract and excreted in the faeces. It is not active in the liver.

USES

Diloxanide furoate is used primarily in the treatment of intestinal amoebiasis. It is used in combination with metronidazole in hepatic infestations to treat any extrahepatic pools of amoeba. It is available as 500 mg tablets. The usual dose is 500 mg three

LIVER DISEASES

16

TABLE 16.4 Drug treatment of hepatic abscess

Drug	Adult Dose	Paediatric Dose
Metronidazole* followed by diloxanide furoate	600–800 mg tds for 5–10 days	35–50 mg/kg per day in three doses for 5–10 days
	500 mg tds for 10 days	20 mg/kg per day in three doses for 10 days
Tinidazole*	2 g daily for 3–5 days or 600 mg twice daily for 10 days	50 mg/kg per day (maximum 2 g) for 3–5 days

*For further information on metronidazole and tinidazole see Chapter 30 Infectious Diseases.

times a day for 10 days in adults and 20 mg/kg/day in divided doses for 10 days in children.

ADVERSE DRUG REACTIONS

Flatulence or an urticarial rash may occur.

LIVER FLUKES

There are two types of liver flukes that infect the human biliary tract. They are *Clonorchis sinensis* (Chinese liver fluke) and *Fasciola hepatica* (sheep liver fluke). Presenting symptoms range from mild abdominal discomfort and anorexia to severe right upper quadrant pain resembling biliary abscess or pancreatitis. Treatment for both types is with praziquantel.

Praziquantel

TRADE NAMES

Praziquantel: *Biltricide*.

MECHANISM OF ACTION

Praziquantel appears to directly kill susceptible trematodes (flukes, flatworms). It also causes paralysis of the worms which allows them to be dislodged and carried by nor-

mal blood flow to the liver, where them may be removed by host tissue reactions (e.g. phagocytosis).

PHARMACOKINETICS

It is rapidly absorbed and undergoes extensive metabolism by the liver. It is mainly excreted via the kidneys.

USES

In addition to the treatment of liver flukes, praziquantel is also used for *Schistosoma* sp. (blood fluke) infections. It is available as 600 mg tablets which are scored in four segments, each containing 150 mg to facilitate accurate dosing. The dose is 20 mg/kg three times a day for one day for both adults and children. The tablets should be swallowed without chewing, preferably after meals.

ADVERSE DRUG REACTIONS

These are usually mild and transient and include abdominal pain, nausea, vomiting, headache, dizziness, slight drowsiness, pruritus and elevated temperature.

DRUG INDUCED LIVER DISEASE ▮▮▮

Adverse effects of drugs on the liver represent only a small proportion of liver disease. Less than 5% of patients admitted to hospital with jaundice have drug related problems. However, of those presenting with fulminant hepatic failure or hepatic necrosis, 20%–30% are drug induced (e.g. paracetamol overdose).

Drug effects on the liver may be broadly divided into two groups: predictable (intrinsic) and unpredictable (idiosyncratic). The effect may be acute or chronic.

Predictable reactions are usually associated with a toxic dose-response relationship and occur frequently. Idiosyncratic reactions are not related to a specific blood concentration and tend to occur less frequently.

It appears that the risk of liver damage from drugs increases with advancing age (over 70 years), probably as a result of decreased liver blood flow.

Generally, the prognosis for drug induced liver damage is good if the offending drug is withdrawn. However, the type of liver damage is important. If the damage is cytotoxic, then progression to hepatic failure and death may occur. If the damage is more cholestatic, then the prognosis is much better.

Further classification of hepatotoxicity is outlined in Table 16.5.

Many drugs have been associated with adverse effects on the liver. They are too numerous to mention in this chapter. Comprehensive lists are available and the reader is referred to textbooks on adverse drug reactions. Some of the well recognised causes of drug induced hepatic damage are outlined briefly in Table 16.6.

LIVER DISEASES

16

PARACETAMOL OVERDOSE

Paracetamol is metabolised by the liver via conjugation with glutathione to non-toxic metabolites. When excessive amounts of paracetamol are ingested, the liver's stores of glutathione are rapidly depleted resulting in the production of a toxic intermediate metabolite. This then binds irreversibly to liver cells producing cell death and if untreated, hepatic necrosis.

For details on the treatment of paracetamol overdose see Chapter 9 Poisonings and Their Treatment.

TABLE 16.5 Classification of hepatotoxicity

Classification	Effect
Predictable (intrinsic)	
Direct hepatotoxins	Necrosis*, steatosis**
Indirect hepatotoxins	
Cytotoxic	Steatosis and/or necrosis
Cholestasis***	Bile casts blocking bile ducts
Unpredictable (idiosyncratic)	
Hypersensitivity	Cytotoxic or cholestatic
Metabolic abnormality	Cytotoxic or cholestatic

*Necrosis is associated with hepatocellular jaundice and a viral hepatitis-like syndrome. Serum transferases are elevated 10–200 times normal, while alkaline phosphatase is rarely more than three times normal. The fatality rate is between 10% and 50%, usually from fulminant hepatic failure.

**Steatosis is fatty degeneration of the liver with deposition of fat in the hepatocytes. It is associated with mild jaundice and moderate increases in serum transferases.

***Cholestasis is associated with jaundice and pruritis. There are moderate increases in transferases and alkaline phosphatase is increased greater than three fold. The fatality rate is less than 1%.

TABLE 16.6 Drug induced liver damage

Type of Damage	Description	Drugs
Centrilobular necrosis (metabolite related hepatotoxicity)	Often predictable, results from production of toxic metabolites	Paracetamol
	Idiosyncratic, mild to severe hepatic failure	Halothane
Steatonecrosis	Predictable. Accumulation of fat within hepatocytes may cause cells to rupture and become necrotic; reversible if drug withdrawn early	Alcohol, valproic acid
Phospholipidosis	Accumulation of phospholipids in hepatocytes	Amiodarone
Toxic hepatitis	Resembles acute viral hepatitis with eosinophilia and fever	Halothane, methyldopa, nitrofurantoin, isoniazid, aspirin (high dose), ketoconazole
Liver vascular damage	Veno-occlusive disease (phlebitis of central veins in liver causing cirrhosis)	Azathioprine, herbal teas with comfrey
	Peliosis hepatitis (large blood-filled lacunae in the liver which may rupture causing peritoneal haemorrhage)	Testosterone, oestrogens, tamoxifen, azathioprine, danazol
Cirrhosis	Usually develops following a necrotic or cholestatic lesion	Methotrexate (may be decreased by adding leucovorin), vitamin A (high dose)
Chronic active hepatitis		Methyldopa, nitrofurantoin, isoniazid, dantrolene, sulfonamides, paracetamol, chlorpromazine, halothane
Hypersensitivity reactions (may occur as hepatocellular, cholestatic or mixed hepatocellular/cholestatic damage)	Hepatocellular damage associated with fever, rash, arthritis, haemolytic anaemia, liver granulomas	Trimethoprim–sulfamethoxazole, penicillin, flucloxacillin
	Rash, pruritus, abdominal pain and liver granulomas	Erythromycin
	Canalicular cholestasis (mild to moderate increase in bilirubin)	Allopurinol, oestrogens (long term)
	Hepatocellular cholestasis	Chlorpromazine

WILSON'S DISEASE ▮▮▮▮▮▮▮▮▮▮

Wilson's disease is a metabolic disorder causing reduced biliary copper excretion with subsequent copper accumulation in the liver, brain, cornea, red blood cells and kidneys. The symptoms range from asymptomatic (carriers) to symptoms of significant neurological impairment such as ataxia and dysarthria or liver impairment resembling cirrhosis and chronic hepatitis.

The mainstay of therapy is D-penicillamine, however 10% of patients may not tolerate the drug and alternative therapies such as zinc sulfate and chelating agents have been tried.

D-Penicillamine

TRADE NAMES

D-Penicillamine: *D-Penamine*.

MECHANISM OF ACTION

D-penicillamine acts as a chelating agent for heavy metals such as copper and lead which are then excreted from the body.

USES

D-penicillamine is indicated for the manage- ment of Wilson's disease and for the treatment of other heavy metal poisoning such as lead, mercury and gold.

In Wilson's disease, a daily dose of 1500–3000 mg daily is recommended, with a starting dose of 500 mg three times a day. Although increased levels of copper in the urine may be detected almost immediately, symptomatic improvement may be slow.

For information on adverse drug reactions, drug interactions and contraindications see Chapter 22 Musculoskeletal Disorders.

LIVER DISEASES

16

FURTHER READING

Gastrointestinal Drug Guidelines Sub-Committee, Victorian Drug Usage Advisory Committee. (1994), 'Gastrointestinal drug guidelines', Victorian Medical Postgraduate Foundation Inc., Melbourne.

Lau, J.Y.N., Alexander, G.J.M., Alberti, A. (1991), 'Viral hepatitis'. *Gut Supplement*, pp. S47–S62.

Overman, J.A., et al. (1989), 'Role of the nurse in the multidisciplinary team approach to care of liver transplant patients'. *Mayo Clinic Proceedings*, 64, pp. 690–698.

Ptachcinski, R.J., Venkataramanan, R., Burckart, G.J. (1989),' Drug therapy in transplantation' in DiPiro, J.T., Talbert, R.L., Hayes, P.E., Yee, G.C., Posey, L.M., eds, *Pharmacotherapy A pathophysiologic approach*. Elsevier, New York, pp. 75–85.

Thompson, A.D., Bird, G.L.A., Saunders, J.B. (1991), 'Alcoholic liver disease'. *Gut Supplement*, pp. S97–S103.

TEST YOUR KNOWLEDGE

1. What is the most commonly expected adverse effect on commencing interferon treatment and how can it be managed?

2. What is the treatment of choice for hepatitis A infection?

3. (a) Into which muscle should hepatitis B vaccine be given for adults? (b) At what interval should the doses be given?

4. What is the theory behind the use of lactulose in hepatic encephalopathy?

5. What dose of spironolactone is used to treat ascites?

Gastrointestinal Disorders

DAVID G. COSH

O B J E C T I V E S

At the conclusion of this chapter the reader should be able to:

1. Describe the fundamental principles of the drug therapy used in the treatment of acid pepsin disease, inflammatory bowel disease, intestinal motility and associated disorders; and

2. Describe the mechanism of action, clinical use, methods of administration, dosage, adverse drug reactions, drug interactions and contraindications to therapy for drugs used in the treatment of disorders of the alimentary system.

GENERAL PRINCIPLES ▮▮▮▮▮▮▮▮▮▮

The gastrointestinal tract is intimately involved with the absorption of water, electrolytes and nutrients and the elimination of waste. It controls the movement and digestion of food and, importantly, the absorption of drugs. The gastrointestinal tract is subjected to a variety of primary disease states and it can be adversely affected by unrelated disorders affecting other body systems. Technological advances have provided clinicians and scientists with an array of diagnostic equipment and tests which have added significantly to the precision of the diagnosis of many gastrointestinal abnormalities.

Many drugs affect gastrointestinal function. In some circumstances these effects are exploited in the treatment of disease, while in others the effects are undesirable and limit the effectiveness of the particular agent. A large number of drugs from many different classes are used to treat gastrointestinal disorders. Many are used to treat other conditions and the adverse effect profile of the drugs used ranges from relatively innocuous to life threatening. With a few exceptions the majority of the drugs referred to in this chapter have been in clinical use for considerable periods of time and their adverse effect and drug interaction profiles are well documented. The majority of adverse effects seen are predictable and based on their known mechanisms of action.

In many instances patients will be taking medications for long periods of time. Adequate patient education is mandatory to ensure that patients have realistic expectations of the benefits and know of the likely adverse effects of therapy.

ACID PEPSIN DISEASE ▮▮▮▮▮▮▮▮▮▮

PEPTIC ULCER

The term peptic ulcer is used to collectively describe ulcers occurring in either the stomach (gastric ulcer) or duodenum (duodenal ulcer). Under normal physiological conditions there is a balance in favour of protection between factors which promote a healthy gastric mucosa and those which have the potential to cause damage. It is accepted that when inflammation or ulceration occur the balance between these factors has altered.

Smoking, stress and genetic factors have been implicated in the aetiology of peptic ulcer. Whether these factors lead to an alteration in the production of acid and pepsin or whether they impair mucosal defence in their own right is not clear.

Certain medications can damage gastric and duodenal mucosa which is then rendered more susceptible to attack by endogenous acid and pepsin. The drugs most commonly implicated are the non-steroidal anti-inflammatory drugs (NSAIDs) of which aspirin is the prototype. These drugs are used to treat inflammatory arthritic conditions and exert their anti-inflammatory effect by inhibiting prostaglandins. Two prostaglandins (PGI_2 and PGE_2) are involved in maintaining the integrity of the gastric mucosa and their inhibition by NSAIDs is a postulated mechanism for the ulcerogenic effect of these agents. The potential for mucosal damage is to an extent independent of the route of administration, although the salicylates do exert a direct irritant effect. For this reason rectal or parenteral administration of an NSAID does not necessarily prevent adverse gastrointestinal effects. It is now clear that the overall incidence of NSAID induced ulcer disease is not so much an indication of unacceptable risk associated with the use of these agents in the individual patient, but rather is a result of the extremely widespread use of NSAIDs throughout the community.

The organism *Helicobacter pylori* has long been associated with inflammation in both the stomach and duodenum. Duodenal ulcer associated with *H. pylori* colonisation is a recognised entity and is the reason for the use of combination therapy aimed at eradicating this organism from inflamed mucosa.

Zollinger-Ellison syndrome is characterised by gastric hypersecretion and peptic ulceration. This condition is usually associated with a gastrin producing tumour in either the pancreas or another site in the upper gastrointestinal tract. Because of the significantly increased acid output no other aetiological stimulus for peptic ulcer formation is required in patients who have this condition.

GASTROESOPHAGEAL REFLUX DISEASE

The role of the lower oesophageal sphincter is to prevent the retrograde flow of stomach contents into the oesophagus (reflux). When reflux does occur to the extent that symptoms warrant medical attention the condition is referred to as gastroesophageal reflux disease or simply 'reflux'. The spectrum of symptoms varies from occasional heartburn and discomfort which can be readily relieved by antacids to severe oesophageal ulceration which, if left untreated, can result in stricture and an increased risk of oesophageal malignancy. Many of the drugs used to treat peptic ulcer are also used in the treatment of reflux. In considering these drugs in more detail their application in the treatment of both peptic ulcer and reflux will be discussed.

There are a number of agents which are very effective at healing peptic ulcers and many are also used to treat reflux, although their overall success rate in the latter condition is lower. The natural history of both peptic ulcer and reflux is such that when therapy is withdrawn after healing has been effected, relapse is common. The same range of drugs used to heal these disorders is also used to prevent relapse.

ANTACIDS

Aluminium Hydroxide, Magnesium Hydroxide

TRADE NAMES

Aluminium–magnesium combination products: *Almacarb*; *Aludrox*; *Dijene*; *Gastrogel*; *Gaviscon*; *Mucaine*; *Mylanta*.

MECHANISM OF ACTION

Antacids exert their effect by neutralising hydrochloric acid present in the stomach. The most common agents used today are alkaline salts of magnesium and aluminium used either alone or in combination. Sodium bicarbonate is rarely used because it is short acting and systemically absorbed which can lead to metabolic alkalosis. In addition, the sodium load provided by sodium bicarbonate is contraindicated in patients on low sodium diets. Calcium salts have also lost appeal, not because of their lack of efficacy but, in the case of calcium carbonate, its propensity to cause acid rebound when ceased. In the past excessive use of calcium antacids and milk based drinks for ulcer patients led to the 'milk-alkali' syndrome characterised by hypercalcaemia and alkalosis.

USES

When given on an empty stomach antacids will pass through the stomach quickly thereby minimising the time available for neutralising acid. The presence of food in the stomach elevates stomach pH to approximately 5. It is therefore advisable to recommend that antacids be given one hour after food so that the antacid will be retained in the stomach by the presence of food, and then again three hours after food so that the neutralising effect will be maintained as the effect of food begins to wane. If taken in sufficient doses antacids will heal peptic ulcers and can be used to maintain remission. Suspensions are more effective than tablets but less convenient. No doubt the inconvenience of liquid preparations is one of the reasons that antacids are often taken in less than optimal quantities. Antacids can be used together with other agents, e.g. H2 receptor antagonists and omeprazole, when healing or symptom control proves difficult. When aiming to heal a peptic ulcer a dose of 30 mL of a combination antacid containing both 2400 mg of aluminium and magnesium hydroxide given one and three hours after meals and at bedtime is required. Lower doses will provide inadequate acid suppression. For reflux 10–15 mL of the same combination taken every two hours is often required to alleviate symptoms and promote healing. *Gaviscon*, a combination antacid containing magnesium trisilicate, aluminium hydroxide and sodium bicarbonate, also contains alginic acid which is derived from seaweed. Alginic acid forms a viscous gel when it comes in contact with acid. The gel is claimed to sit like a raft on the surface of the stomach contents thereby impeding reflux.

ADVERSE DRUG REACTIONS

Magnesium salts can cause diarrhoea whereas aluminium salts tend to constipate. This fact provides the rationale for combining alkaline salts of both metals in the one suspension in an attempt to minimise bowel disturbances.

DRUG INTERACTIONS

Antacids can interact with other drugs forming insoluble complexes which then minimise or prevent absorption of the drug. Some examples of drugs that form complexes are iron, tetracycline and etidronate. As a general rule most potential interactions can be avoided by separating the ingestion of antacids and other drugs by a two hour interval.

NURSING IMPLICATIONS

ASSESSMENT

The patient should be assessed for changes in bowel habit and their medication orders reviewed for drugs whose absorption may be affected by antacids.

ADMINISTRATION

Mixtures should be shaken well before pouring the dose. Patients should be instructed to chew or suck tablets because if they are swallowed whole there is a risk of intestinal obstruction. Antacids are usually given after meals and at bedtime or more frequently if required.

EVALUATION

The patient should be evaluated for relief of discomfort. If diarrhoea or constipation occur the prescriber should be contacted as a change in the type of antacid may be necessary.

PATIENT EDUCATION

Patients should be warned not to take aspirin unless advised to do so by their doctor.

ANTICHOLINERGIC AGENTS

Atropine is the prototype naturally occurring anticholinergic agent exerting its effect by inhibiting the muscarinic effect of acetylcholine. Belladonna is another naturally occurring alkaloid with anticholinergic properties which was widely used to treat gastric disorders prior to the introduction of synthetic derivatives.

Propantheline, Glycopyrrolate, Dicyclomine

TRADE NAMES

Propantheline: *Pro-Banthine*.
Glycopyrrolate: *Robinul*.
Dicyclomine: *Merbentyl*.

MECHANISM OF ACTION

By inhibiting the action of acetylcholine at effector sites within the parasympathetic nervous system effecting the gastrointestinal tract, muscarinic antagonists reduce gastric motility and acid output. Agents in use include propantheline, glycopyrrolate and dicyclomine. They are now primarily used to control spasm in conditions such as irritable bowel syndrome and infantile colic.

USES

The usual dose of propantheline is 15 mg three times a day before meals and up to 30 mg at bedtime.

ADVERSE DRUG REACTIONS

All anticholinergic agents produce classical atropine-like side effects (dry mouth, blurred vision, urinary retention and constipation) as well as a variety of central nervous system effects including drowsiness, restlessness and irritability (the last two effects are more commonly seen in overdose). Because of widespread effects outside the gastrointestinal tract their use in the treatment of peptic ulcer and motility disorders has declined, although hyoscine is still used to prevent motion sickness.

DRUG INTERACTIONS

Administration in combination with other drugs possessing anticholinergic properties, e.g. the tricyclic antidepressants, will lead to an increased incidence of adverse effects.

PRECAUTIONS AND CONTRAINDICATIONS

Because these drugs cause drowsiness and blurred vision patients should be advised to exercise caution when driving or operating machinery. Patients with prostatic hypertrophy may experience worsening urinary hesitation or retention.

NURSING IMPLICATIONS

ASSESSMENT

The patient's current drug profile should be assessed for use of other atropine-like drugs such as antihistamines or tricyclic antidepressants.

EVALUATION

The nurse should evaluate the patient for signs of the desired response to the drug and observe for adverse effects. Initially the patient may experience a dry mouth. This can be alleviated by giving extra fluids or sweets to suck. The nurse should be alert for reports from the patient of urinary hesitancy or retention. Restlessness or confusion are signs of toxicity and may indicate a need for the dose to be reduced. Bowel function should be monitored as constipation may occur.

PATIENT EDUCATION

Patients should be reassured that side effects such as dry mouth and blurred vision may occur and are predictable side effects of these drugs. They should also be advised that if blurred vision and drowsiness occur, driving a car or operating machinery would be dangerous.

GASTROINTESTINAL DISORDERS

17

H₂ RECEPTOR ANTAGONISTS

Cimetidine, Ranitidine, Famotidine, Nizatidine

TRADE NAMES

Cimetidine: *Tagamet.*
Ranitidine: *Zantac.*
Famotidine: *Pepcidine.*
Nizatidine: *Tazac.*

MECHANISM OF ACTION

Parietal cells located in the gastric mucosa secrete hydrochloric acid in response to a number of stimulae which activate receptors on the cell's basolateral membrane. Two of these receptors, those that are activated by acetylcholine and those activated by histamine, have been targeted by drugs in an effort to block the stimulus for acid secretion and thereby create a more favourable environment for healing of inflamed or ulcerated mucosa. The end result of blocking acid release via inhibiting acetylcholine release in the gut is to also block acetylcholine elsewhere, giving rise to atropine-like side effects. Greater therapeutic success and patient acceptance has been obtained with drugs which block the effect of histamine on H₂ receptors on the parietal cells, thus the name H₂ receptor antagonists.

Four agents are currently available for therapeutic use: cimetidine, ranitidine, famotidine and nizatidine. These drugs reduce both the volume of gastric secretion and its hydrogen ion content. In standard doses they reduce 24 hour gastric acidity by about 60%. A single night time dose can be as effective as twice daily dosing (e.g. 300 mg ranitidine at night versus 150 mg twice a day).

All four drugs can be used to heal peptic ulcers and, in patients where ongoing therapy is indicated, to prevent relapse. Since the introduction of cimetidine in the 1970s the H₂ receptor antagonists have replaced antacids as the first-line agents in the treatment of peptic ulcers. The convenience of once-a-day dosing coupled with their good safety record has contributed to their widespread use. The fear that prolonged use in patients requiring continual therapy might increase the risk of gastric cancer has not been clinically demonstrated.

PHARMACOKINETICS

Cimetidine, ranitidine, famotidine and nizatidine are absorbed rapidly after oral administration. Each is subjected to a degree of first pass metabolism in the liver and a significant amount of each drug is excreted in the urine unchanged. For patients unable to take oral medications, parenteral forms of cimetidine, ranitidine and famotidine are available.

USES

Dose and duration of therapy vary depending on the acid pepsin disorder being treated and whether the aim is resolution of an acute disorder or the prevention of relapse. Dosage regimens for the treatment of peptic ulcer are listed in Table 17.1. Administration via the oral route is effective and parenteral administration is usually reserved for patients who cannot swallow.

ADVERSE DRUG REACTIONS

The risk to benefit ratio of these agents is very favourable. They are effective in the majority of clinical situations in which they are used and are responsible for few serious adverse effects. All have been reported to cause altered bowel habits, nausea, headache and skin rash. Full dose treatment with all four drugs in elderly patients with renal impairment has been linked with confusional states. It is a standard recommendation that in these patients, especially when the drugs are administered parenterally, the dose be reduced. Cimetidine can cause gynaecomastia and impotence due to its ability to enhance the secretion of prolactin and bind to androgen receptors.

DRUG INTERACTIONS

Cimetidine can affect the metabolism of other drugs which depend on the liver's cytochrome P-450 system for their metabolism

TABLE 17.1 Dosage regimens for H_2 receptor antagonists in the treatment of peptic ulcer

Drug	Acute Treatment	Maintenance	Maximum*
Cimetidine	400 mg twice a day or 200 mg three times a day and 400 mg at night or 800 mg at night	400 mg at night	2 g a day
Ranitidine	150 mg twice a day or 300 mg at night	150 mg at night	900 mg a day
Famotidine	40 mg at night	20 mg at night	480 mg a day
Nizatidine	150 mg twice a day or 300 mg at night	150 mg at night	No data

*Maximum doses reserved for hypersecretory states, e.g. Zollinger-Ellison syndrome

and clearance. In practice this can be clinically relevant when cimetidine is co-prescribed with drugs which are metabolised by the liver and have a narrow therapeutic index, e.g. warfarin, theophylline and phenytoin. Careful monitoring of prothrombin time ratio (with warfarin) and plasma levels of theophylline and phenytoin is recommended when these agents are first co-prescribed with cimetidine.

Ranitidine, famotidine and nizatidine have no appreciable effect on drug metabolism.

PRECAUTIONS AND CONTRAINDICATIONS

Dosage adjustments are required in patients with significant renal impairment.

PROSTAGLANDIN ANALOGUES

Misoprostol

TRADE NAMES

Misoprostol: *Cytotec.*

MECHANISM OF ACTION

Misoprostol is an analogue of prostaglandin E_1 (PGE_1). The rationale for its use in treating acid pepsin disease is based on the natural existence of prostaglandins in gastric mucosa and the fact that inhibition of gastric prostaglandins by NSAIDs predisposes patients to peptic ulcer. Misoprostol has demonstrated similar efficacy to the H_2 receptor antagonists in healing peptic ulcers. It is cytoprotective but at the doses used in clinical practice (200 micrograms four times a day) it has acid suppressive properties equivalent to that provided by the H_2 receptor antagonists. Misoprostol appears to be less effective in treating reflux than the H_2 receptor antagonists, but has been shown to minimise the risk of gastric ulceration in patients with dyspeptic symptoms who require NSAIDs.

PHARMACOKINETICS

Misoprostol is rapidly absorbed following an oral dose. Dose reduction in the presence of renal impairment is not required.

USES

The standard dose for both duodenal and gastric ulcer is 200 micrograms four times a day or 800 micrograms twice daily. The drug is also used in doses of 200 micrograms four hourly to prevent stress ulcers in intensive care patients.

ADVERSE DRUG REACTIONS

Abdominal pain and diarrhoea are common dose related adverse effects of misoprostol. However, these effects are often self-limiting when therapy is continued. Gynaecological effects such as menstrual disorders and dysmenorrhoea have been reported in women taking misoprostol and the drug is a potential abortifacient.

PRECAUTIONS AND CONTRAINDICATIONS

Its use in pregnant women, and women of childbearing age without adequate contraception, is contraindicated.

OTHER AGENTS

Sucralfate

TRADE NAMES

Sucralfate: *Carafate*; *SCF*; *Ulcyte*.

MECHANISM OF ACTION

Sucralfate is an aluminium salt of a sulfated sugar. It does not neutralise acid or reduce acid output. In an acid environment it forms a viscous paste which preferentially attaches to inflamed and necrotic tissue in the oesophagus, duodenum and stomach. It therefore exerts a cytoprotective effect by physically protecting damaged mucosa from further exposure to acid. In addition sucralfate binds pepsin thus reducing the activity of this proteolytic enzyme. Other mechanisms such as increased mucosal blood flow and increased local production of prostaglandins have been shown to contribute to its efficacy in healing peptic ulcers. Its efficacy is equivalent to that of the H$_2$ receptor antagonists and misoprostol. Sucralfate, if continued after healing has taken place, will prevent relapse and there is some evidence, awaiting confirmation in larger studies, that the quality of healing obtained with sucralfate is better than that obtained with other

agents. This results in a lower rate of relapse when the drug is discontinued. Sucralfate has shown promise in the treatment of reflux. However, a practical problem with its use in this condition is actually getting the sucralfate to stay in the oesophagus.

USES

The standard dose for the treatment of peptic ulcer is 1 g three times a day one hour before food and at bedtime. In maintenance regimens this dose is reduced to 1 g twice daily.

ADVERSE DRUG REACTIONS

Sucralfate is chemically inert and absorption is insignificant. Each gram of sucralfate contains 190 mg of aluminium and with continued use in patients with severely impaired renal function the possibility of accumulation of aluminium leading to toxicity exists. Avoidance of long-term use in susceptible patients will obviate this risk. Constipation is the most common side effect, occurring in 2%–3% of patients.

DRUG INTERACTIONS

Because sucralfate requires an acid environment in which to exert its therapeutic effect two hours should be allowed between the administration of sucralfate and antacids. H$_2$ receptor antagonists have been used together with sucralfate in the treatment of acid pepsin disease with marginally superior results to those obtained with either drug alone, although the clinical relevance is doubtful. As with antacids, administration of an H$_2$ receptor antagonist and sucralfate should be separated by at least two hours.

Omeprazole

TRADE NAMES

Omeprazole: *Losec*.

MECHANISM OF ACTION

Omeprazole is the first agent of its class available in Australia. It acts by inhibiting the gastric enzyme H$^+$,K$^+$-ATPase proton pump in the parietal cell, reducing the number of hydrogen ions available to combine with chloride ions to form hydrochloric acid. Omeprazole blocks acid release independent of stimulus, resulting in greater inhibition of acid release and the achievement of faster ulcer healing rates than is possible with other antisecretory drugs. When ulcers prove resistant to healing or symptoms remain poorly controlled despite maximal therapy with other drugs, omeprazole may be the drug of choice. Omeprazole has also proven to be very useful in the treatment of severe reflux disease, a condition often poorly controlled with other drugs.

PHARMACOKINETICS

Omeprazole is rapidly effective when given orally and no dosage reduction is required in patients with renal impairment or hepatic insufficiency. Omeprazole is degraded in the presence of acid and for this reason the drug is enclosed within small enteric coated pellets inside gelatin capsules. Contact with gastric acid is avoided and the pellets disintegrate in the small intestine where absorption takes place. The timing of omeprazole administration in relation to food is unimportant.

USES

Omeprazole is given once a day in doses of 20–40 mg although higher doses have been used without ill effect.

ADVERSE DRUG REACTIONS

Omeprazole is well tolerated. However, safety associated with long-term use has yet to be established.

DRUG INTERACTIONS

Omeprazole is metabolised in the liver via the cytochrome P-450 system, and has been shown to interact with diazepam, phenytoin and warfarin. These effects may not be clinically significant but close monitoring of the central nervous system effects of diazepam, plasma levels of phenytoin and the prothrombin time ratio when giving warfarin is recommended when the drugs are first given together.

BISMUTH AND TRIPLE THERAPY

Bismuth Subcitrate

TRADE NAMES

Bismuth subcitrate: *Denol*.

MECHANISM OF ACTION

Bismuth subcitrate has been used for many years in the treatment of peptic ulcer. It has no effect on acid release but, like sucralfate, bismuth subcitrate, in the presence of acid, forms a precipitate on the ulcer surface in both stomach and duodenum therefore affording protection against further attack by acid and pepsin. Bismuth also has a bactericidal effect against *H. pylori* the organism which has been implicated in the pathogenesis of duodenal ulcer. There is now expanding interest in the eradication of this organism as a means of healing duodenal ulcer and preventing relapse.

Triple Therapy

The combination of bismuth with amoxycillin (or a tetracycline in penicillin allergic patients) and either metronidazole or tinidazole is far more effective at reducing the numbers of *H. pylori* in the gut than bismuth alone. It is usual to reserve this form of treatment for duodenal ulcers which have proven to be resistant to other pharmacological measures because of the risk of antibiotic resistance and pseudomembranous colitis.

USES

Bismuth subcitrate is given in doses of 120 mg four times a day half an hour before meals and at bedtime along with amoxycillin (or tetracycline) and metronidazole or tinidazole in conventional doses.

ADVERSE DRUG REACTIONS

A small amount of bismuth is absorbed while most is excreted in the faeces. Bismuth accumulation leading to toxicity in the renally impaired patient on long-term therapy can occur. Blackening of the stools due to

GASTROINTESTINAL DISORDERS

17

the formation of bismuth sulfide in the colon occurs and a black discolouration of the mouth is also common.

DRUG INTERACTIONS

Bismuth subcitrate can combine with milk and antacids so a two hour interval should separate the consumption of these two substances. Similarly bismuth will bind tetracycline antibiotics in the gut leading to reduced antibiotic efficacy.

NURSING IMPLICATIONS

ASSESSMENT

Before administering cimetidine the patient's drug profile should be checked for interacting drugs.

ADMINISTRATION

H_2 Antagonists
Antacid should not be given one hour before or after oral H_2 antagonists.

Intravenous injections should be given slowly. Cimetidine should be diluted with 100 mL of fluid and given over 20 minutes.

Sucralfate
If antacids or H_2 receptor antagonists are co-prescribed with sucralfate, administration should be two hours apart.

Bismuth Subcitrate
Antacids and milk should be avoided during treatment with bismuth subcitrate.

EDUCATION

Patients should be educated to avoid taking antacids with bismuth subcitrate and to take antacids at least one hour before and after H_2 antagonists and sucralfate.

Explain to patients taking bismuth subcitrate that their stools may be darker than usual. Patients should be instructed to chew the tablets before swallowing and that the tablets should be taken half an hour before meals and at bedtime.

PROKINETIC AGENTS

By definition prokinetic agents are drugs that restore, normalise and facilitate motility in the gastrointestinal tract. The role of antacids and antisecretory therapy in the treatment of gastroesophageal reflux disease has been discussed. An additional therapeutic choice in this condition, which may provide additional benefit when added to the treatments already described, is the use of a drug which accelerates gastric transit time in both the stomach and oesophagus. Accelerated transit time minimises contact time between gastric contents and oesophageal mucosa and speeds up the transit of gastric contents from the stomach to the small intestine thereby reducing the likelihood of reflux occurring. Currently used prokinetic agents increase the tone of the lower oesophageal sphincter which further reduces the incidence of reflux.

Metoclopramide

Aside from its role in treating reflux, metoclopramide (*Maxolon*) is widely used in the treatment of nausea and vomiting, especially that associated with the postoperative period and chemotherapy. Its ability to accelerate gastric transit minimises nausea associated with the presence of food in the stomach and it also acts centrally via inhibition of dopamine effects at the chemoreceptor trigger zone. (See section on antiemetics and antinauseants.)

PHARMACOKINETICS

Metoclopramide is rapidly and completely absorbed after oral administration and readily crosses the blood brain barrier accounting for its central nervous system side effects. When given orally it exerts its effect within 30–60 minutes. The half-life of the drug is normally 4–6 hours but is significantly extended in patients with renal failure.

USES

In young adults the normal dose is 5–10 mg three times a day, with the higher dose being used for adults. Dosage should be reduced in patients with significant renal or hepatic impairment. Higher doses (1–2 mg/kg body weight) are used to prevent the nausea and vomiting associated with emetogenic chemotherapy regimens.

ADVERSE DRUG REACTIONS

The central dopamine antagonist effect of metoclopramide is responsible for side effects such as drowsiness, hyperprolactinaemia and extrapyramidal effects seen more commonly in the young and in certain chemotherapy regimens where high doses (1–2 mg/kg) are employed. Transient agitation and restlessness are more common than true dystonic reactions. The movement disorders seen with metoclopramide are similar to those seen with the phenothiazine antipsychotic drugs (e.g. chlorpromazine, thioridazine) and are mediated in the same manner by inhibition of dopamine receptors.

Domperidone

Domperidone (*Motilium*) has similar actions to metoclopramide but because it crosses the blood-brain barrier to only a limited extent it very rarely causes extrapyramidal side effects. However, like metoclopramide, it can cause symptoms related to hyperpro-

lactinaemia (e.g. breast enlargement, galactorrhoea and menstrual irregularities) and occasional abdominal cramping and dry mouth.

Domperidone is rapidly absorbed following oral administration and although clearance is decreased in patients with severe renal impairment, dosage reduction is not usually required when used for a brief illness. However, when the drug is required for long periods of time in patients with significant renal impairment, the dose should be reduced from the normal 10 mg three to four times a day before food to 10 mg once or twice daily.

Cisapride

Cisapride (*Prepulsid*) is the most recently available prokinetic agent and unlike metoclopramide and domperidone it does not have antidopaminergic properties but exerts its effect by increasing the release of the neurotransmitter acetylcholine from postganglionic nerve endings of the myenteric plexus. Cisapride has been termed a 'pan-prokinetic' agent because it increases propulsive motor activity throughout the entire gastrointestinal tract. Cisapride does not exert a central antiemetic action like metoclopramide but when nausea and vomiting are a function of delayed gastric emptying then cisapride is useful. Experience with cisapride suggests that it, like metoclopramide, can be used in many cases in which gastric motility needs to be increased.

Cisapride is rapidly and completely absorbed when given orally. Diarrhoea and abdominal cramping can occur secondary to its prokinetic effect. The dose range usually employed in adults is 5–10 mg three to four times a day with the lower dose used in patients with hepatic or renal impairment.

GASTROINTESTINAL DISORDERS

17

BLOATING AND FLATULENCE ▐█████████

Excess gas in the gastrointestinal tract (usually hydrogen or carbon dioxide) is associated with irritable bowel syndrome, carbohydrate malabsorption, pancreatic insufficency, a diet high in indigestible carbohydrate and coeliac disease. Colic in infants is caused by swallowing of air (aerophagia) with resultant abdominal distension. Simethicone is an agent which lowers surface tension resulting in the coalescence of small bubbles of gas into smaller numbers of larger bubbles which are easier to expel. Proprietary products containing simethicone include *De-Gas*, *Infacol Wind Drops* and *Infacol C Colic Syrup* which also contains the anticholinergic preparation dicyclomine. Peppermint oil (*Mintec*) contains menthol and acts locally in the gastrointestinal tract to relieve flatulence and colic. Capsules are enteric coated to delay release of the contents until the capsule has passed through the stomach and proximal small intestine. The usual dose is one capsule three times a day half an hour before food.

PANCREATIC INSUFFICIENCY ▐███████

Preparations of pancreatic enzymes (*Pancrease, Pancrex, Viokase*) are indicated in conditions where there is a symptomatic reduction in normal pancreatic function, e.g. cystic fibrosis, chronic pancreatitis and after pancreatectomy and gastrointestinal bypass surgery. These preparations are prepared from hog pancreas and contain the enzymes lipase, amylase and protease, which are responsible for the digestion of fat, carbohydrate and protein respectively. Choice of agent and dosage varies depending on the condition, its severity and the patient's diet. They are taken with meals in a dose determined by the severity of the condition with smaller doses accompanying snacks. They must be used with caution in patients allergic to pork. Irritation of the mouth and anus can occur especially when given in high doses to the very young.

NURSING IMPLICATIONS

The patient's faeces should be monitored for signs of steatorrhoea which may indicate non-compliance or ineffective dosage levels. Patients should also be monitored for signs of hypersensitivity.

Patients should be advised not to chew or crush the spheres from the capsule preparations of pancrelipase and encouraged to maintain full compliance with dosage schedules as some preparations are unpleasant to take.

ANTIEMETICS AND ANTINAUSEANTS ▐██

Vomiting is a complex mechanism involving pathways both within and outside the central nervous system. The area postrema lying on the floor of the fourth ventricle and referred to as the chemoreceptor trigger zone, responds to signals from emetogenic drugs, e.g. cisplatin, opioid analgesics, by sending signals to the vomiting centre located in the reticular formation of the medulla. The chemoreceptor zone is outside the blood brain barrier so that it can be acted upon by agents which are unable to cross the barrier.

Agents used to treat nausea and vomiting include antihistamines, dopamine antagonists (phenothiazines, butyrophenones, metoclopramide, domperidone) muscarinic antagonists and the 5HT₃ antagonists.

ANTIHISTAMINES

The antihistamines, also referred to as H_1 receptor antagonists, bind to H_1 receptors in the central nervous system. Meclozine (*Ancolan*), pheniramine (*Avil*) and promethazine (*Phenergan*) are used to prevent motion sickness and the nausea and vomiting associated with vertigo and Meniere's disease. Sedation is the most common side effect seen with these agents and patients need to be cautioned against driving and operating machinery. The antihistamines are well absorbed from the gastrointestinal tract with peak plasma levels achieved in 2–3 hours. For further information see Chapter 29 Antihistamines.

DOPAMINE ANTAGONISTS

The phenothiazines, prochlorperazine (*Stemetil*), thiethylperazine (*Torecan*), chlorpromazine (*Largactil*); the butyrophenones, haloperidol (*Serenace*), droperidol (*Droleptan*); and the prokinetic agents, metoclopramide (*Maxolon*) and domperidone (*Motilium*), all exert their antiemetic effect via central dopamine blockade. All can produce extrapyramidal side effects such as dystonias and muscle rigidity, while the phenothiazines produce anticholinergic side effects. Haloperidol and droperidol should only be used in vomiting resistant to other agents.

The role of metoclopramide and domperidone in treating gastroesophageal reflux via their ability to reduce gastric transit time and increase lower oesophageal sphincter tone has already been discussed. Accelerated gastric transit will reduce nausea and vomiting associated with the presence of food in the stomach. Both agents act centrally at the level of the chemoreceptor trigger zone. Metoclopramide crosses the blood brain barrier more readily than domperidone and for this reason extrapyramidal side effects are more likely with metoclopramide, especially when high doses are used, e.g. in chemotherapy regimens.

ANTICHOLINERGIC AGENTS

Hyoscine patches (*Scop*) provide prolonged cover (approximately 72 hours) but their use can be associated with atropine-like side effects.

5HT₃ ANTAGONISTS

Ondansetron is the first of a new class of antiemetic drugs available in Australia that exert their effect by the selective inhibition of a subtype serotonin receptor (5HT₃). Serotinin is a neurotransmitter found in neurones of both the central and peripheral nervous systems and in the gastrointestinal tract. Ondansetron exerts its antiemetic effect by blocking the stimulatory effect of serotonin on 5HT₃ receptors in both the central nervous system and the gut.

Other members of this drug class, e.g. granisetron and tropisetron, are not yet available in Australia.

Ondansetron

Ondansetron is principally used to antagonise the emetogenic effects of chemotherapy and abdominal radiotherapy. Recently its uses have been extended to include postoperative nausea and vomiting.

TRADE NAMES

Ondansetron: *Zofran*.

PHARMACOKINETICS

Ondansetron can be given orally or intravenously. Oral bioavailability is approximately

GASTROINTESTINAL DISORDERS

17

TABLE 17.2 Dosage regimens for some antinauseants and antiemetics

Drug	Dosage
Antihistamines	
Meclozine	25–50 mg twice a day
Pheniramine	25–50 mg 2–3 times a day
Promethazine	25–50 mg before travelling
Dopamine antagonists	
Prochlorperazine	5–10 mg 2–3 times a day (12.5 mg IM or 25 mg rectally if oral administration not feasible)
Metoclopramide	10 mg three times a day (oral or parenteral)
Domperidone	10 mg 3–4 times a day
Anticholinergics	
Hyoscine patches	Apply to skin behind ear 5–6 hours before travelling (effect can last up to 72 hours)
5HT$_3$ antagonist	
Ondansetron	8 mg 2–3 times a day (oral or parenteral)

60% and peak levels are obtained between 1 and 2 hours after administration. The half-life may be prolonged in the elderly and in patients with severe liver impairment.

USES

For acute nausea and vomiting following emetogenic chemotherapy and radiotherapy the usual adult dose is 8 mg 12-hourly, the first oral dose being given two hours prior to chemotherapy or radiotherapy. If the intravenous route is used then the first dose can be given immediately before the emetogenic stimulus. For patients receiving highly emetogenic therapy (e.g. cisplatin) a daily dose of 32 mg may be necessary. While ondansetron is highly effective in the acute phase of nausea and vomiting its comparative advantage over other agents (e.g. metoclopramide) for delayed nausea and emesis is not well established.

For postoperative nausea and vomiting the adult dose is 4 mg by slow intravenous injection at the time of anaesthetic induction. For established postoperative nausea and vomiting 4 mg is given intravenously, increasing to 8 mg if necessary.

ADVERSE DRUG REACTIONS

Major adverse effects are uncommon. Those most commonly reported include headache and a sensation of flushing or warmth in the head or epigastrum. Doses of more than 8 mg should be given by slow intravenous infusion over at least 15 minutes, since rapid intravenous administration has been associated with a higher incidence of transient visual disturbances.

Table 17.2 lists some common dosage regimens for the antinauseant and antiemetic agents. However these doses are provided as a guide only as doses outside these ranges are used in certain circumstances.

NURSING IMPLICATIONS

ASSESSMENT

Before the administration of an antiemetic the patient's history should be assessed in relation to the type of drug to be used (see Table 17.2).

ADMINISTRATION

Metoclopramide should always be given 15–30 minutes before meals.

Avoid spilling injectable phenothiazines on the skin.

EVALUATION

Response to the drug should be monitored and the patient observed for possible adverse effects. Dystonic reactions should be watched for and reported if they occur, e.g. oculogyric crisis has occurred after a single dose of phenothiazine. If antichol nergic side effects occur offer appropiate explanation to the patient.

PATIENT EDUCATION

Patients should be advised that drowsiness, blurred vision and dry mouth may occur and warned that increased sedation and hypotension may occur if other central nervous depressant drugs (e.g. alcohol, sedatives, opioid analgesics) are used concurrently with antihistamines or phenothiazines and if affected driving a car or operating machinery could be dangerous.

INFLAMMATORY BOWEL DISEASE ▬▬

The term inflammatory bowel disease is used to describe two conditions, ulcerative colitis and Crohn's disease, neither of which is curable. There are other forms of colitis amenable to drug treatment (e.g. microscopic and collagenous colitis) but these are usually managed with the same range of agents used to treat either of the two principal disorders.

The aetiology of both the major inflammatory bowel diseases remains unclear. Five possibilities are commonly quoted: food intolerance, microbiological factors, inflammatory mediators, increased permeability of intestinal mucosa leading to penetration by bacteria or inflammatory cells, and immune mechanisms. The drug therapies used to treat acute exacerbations and maintain patients in remission are usually a mix of different pharmacological agents.

CORTICOSTEROIDS

Corticosteroids are potentially life saving drugs in acute exacerbations of inflammatory bowel disease. They are given intravenously in doses of the order of 100–200 mg of hydrocortisone four times a day. Maintenance oral prednisolone can be given when required in the lowest possible dose to maintain remission once an acute exacerbation has resolved. Both prednisolone and hydrocortisone may also be administered rectally. For further information on the corticosteroids see Chapter 19 Endocrine Diseases.

5-AMINOSALICYLIC ACID DERIVATIVES

Sulfasalazine, Olsalazine, Mesalazine

TRADE NAMES

Sulfasalazine: *Salazopyrin.*
Olsalazine: *Dipentum.*
Mesalazine: *Mesasal.*

MECHANISM OF ACTION

There are currently three oral 5-aminosalicylic acid (5-ASA) preparations available in Australia. Sulfasalazine is the oldest having been developed by a Scandinavian physician in the late 1930s.

GASTROINTESTINAL DISORDERS

17

Sulfasalazine is composed of two drugs, sulfapyridine and 5-ASA, chemically joined. The major portion of a dose of sulfasalazine passes through the stomach and proximal small bowel intact with some minor absorption taking place in the jejunum (both 5-ASA and sulfapyridine if given separately will be absorbed in the proximal small bowel). When the intact drug reaches the terminal small bowel and colon, bacteria act to release the two parent compounds. Sulfapyridine is absorbed and 5-ASA remains in the bowel where it exerts a local anti-inflammatory effect. Formerly sulfapyridine was thought to have no therapeutic effect, simply acting as a carrier for 5-ASA enabling it to reach its site of action. However, the majority of the adverse effects associated with sulfasalazine, of which gastrointestinal intolerance is the most common, have now been attributed to sulfapyridine.

The two newer preparations, olsalazine and mesalazine are 5-ASA preparations without sulfapyridine. Olsalazine consists of two 5-ASA molecules again joined together by a bond which is split by colonic bacteria. Mesalazine consists of beads of 5-ASA coated with a pH dependent acrylic resin. As the beads reach the terminal small bowel and colon the pH rises to 6 at which point the resin coating dissolves releasing 5-ASA.

It is no longer accepted that sulfasalazine itself or sulfapyridine have no therapeutic effect in inflammatory bowel disease. Sulfapyridine has been shown to be responsible for the immunomodulatory effect of sulfasalazine in patients with rheumatoid arthritis, so it is conceivable that it also has a similar effect in inflammatory bowel disease. Until the exact mechanism of these agents is established all that can be said is that the newer 5-ASA derivatives are potentially useful alternative agents for those patients unable to tolerate sulfasalazine. All three can be used in the treatment of remissions of both ulcerative colitis and Crohn's disease, but are more effective in maintaining remission in ulcerative colitis than in Crohn's disease.

USES

Sulfasalazine is usually given in doses of the order of 4 g a day, although higher doses can be used if required and tolerated. Olsalazine is given after meals in doses of 1 g daily for patients in remission and up to 2–3 g a day during an acute exacerbation of disease.

Mesalazine is given half an hour before meals in doses ranging from 250 mg three times a day to prevent relapse of both ulcerative colitis and Crohn's disease. For acute attacks the dose can be increased to a recommended maximum of 1.5 g a day.

ADVERSE DRUG REACTIONS

Sulfasalazine has a range of adverse effects many of which can be attributed to the sulfapyridine component. These include gastrointestinal intolerance, skin rashes, photosensitivity, exfoliative dermatitis, blood dyscrasias, reversible azospermia, renal toxicity, central nervous system effects and hepatotoxicity. The newer compounds are not without side effects although many patients who manifest an adverse reaction to sulfasalazine can be successfully managed with either olsalazine or mesalazine.

DRUG INTERACTIONS

Caution should be exercised when co-administering sulfasalazine with oral anticoagulants, high dose methotrexate and the sulfonylurea oral hypoglycaemics. Sulfasalazine can displace these drugs from plasma protein binding sites thus increasing their therapeutic effect and potential for toxicity.

PRECAUTIONS AND CONTRAINDICATIONS

Significant release of 5-ASA can saturate the bowel's ability to acetylate 5-ASA resulting in the absorption of nephrotoxic unacetylated 5-ASA. This adverse effect has been reported with mesalazine and it is therefore recommended that renal function be monitored in patients receiving mesalazine. The drug should be avoided in patients with pre-existing renal impairment.

For information on the use of *Salazopyrin* in rheumatoid arthritis see Chapter 22 Musculoskeletal Disorders.

IMMUNOSUPPRESSIVE AGENTS

Azathioprine

Azathioprine (*Imuran*) is a potent immunosuppressive agent used to minimise the risk of rejection in organ transplant programs and in the treatment of immune mediated conditions (e.g. rheumatoid arthritis). It has been used in ulcerative colitis refractory to other agents but is more commonly used in Crohn's disease, both in the active phase and to maintain remission. Azathioprine in this setting can reduce the requirement for corticosteroids and is therefore termed 'steroid sparing'. Doses used are normally in the range 1–2 mg/kg body weight per day.

For further information on azathioprine see Chapter 14 Drugs Used in Renal Failure.

OTHER AGENTS

Metronidazole

Metronidazole, like azathioprine, is more commonly used in Crohn's disease than ulcerative colitis. Again, it is prescribed for acute episodes especially in patients with perineal manifestations, e.g. rectovaginal fistulae and abscesses.

While usually well tolerated the most common adverse effects of metronidazole are related to gastric intolerance. Peripheral neuropathy is seen with metronidazole especially when given in high doses for long periods of time. However, there are circumstances when long-term use of metronidazole is justified, e.g. patients who cannot tolerate 5-ASA derivatives or do not respond to these drugs.

For further information on metronidazole see Chapter 30 Infectious Diseases.

ENEMAS

Prednisolone enemas (*Predsol*) and hydrocortisone rectal foam (*Colifoam*) have been available for a number of years. A range of newer steroids (budesonide, tixocortol) and 5-ASA preparations have been formulated in enema preparations and are undergoing evaluation. The success of an enema depends on the susceptibility of the disease to the active ingredient and the anatomic site of the disease. At best an enema will reach the splenic flexure of the colon so that diseased bowel proximal to this site will not be accessed by an enema. This is more likely to be the case in Crohn's disease rather than ulcerative colitis when disease is normally localised in the colon and rectum.

ANTIPERISTALTIC AGENTS

Drugs such as loperamide (*Imodium*), codeine, diphenoxylate (*Lomotil*) are not recommended during acute flare-ups of inflammatory bowel disease because of the risk of bowel obstruction in small bowel Crohn's disease and toxic megacolon in both ulcerative colitis and Crohn's disease. They are useful for the patient at home to prevent urgency and diarrhoea and thereby reduce some of the stress associated with living with inflammatory bowel disease.

BILE SALT BINDERS

The resins cholestyramine (*Questran*) and colestipol (*Colestid*) will bind with bile salts. This can be useful in Crohn's disease involving the terminal ileum which has either been resected, or because of disease, is unable to efficiently reabsorb bile salts. For further information on bile salt binders see Chapter 12 Cardiovascular Diseases.

GASTROINTESTINAL DISORDERS

17

IRRITABLE BOWEL SYNDROME ▉▉▉▉▉▉

This disease is more common in women than men and the spectrum of abnormal bowel habit ranges from constipation to diarrhoea.

Irritable bowel syndrome usually begins relatively early in life, is an entity essentially found in the waking state and is not usually associated with severe weight loss and anorexia. The aetiology is unclear but, as a group, patients with irritable bowel syndrome tend to be more anxious or depressed than the normal population.

Treatment must first concentrate on the exclusion of other disorders especially malignancy which is often a concern to the patient with an irritable bowel. Lifestyle changes may be helpful and an increase in dietary fibre can improve symptoms in a significant number of patients. Mebeverine (*Colofac*) is an antispasmodic drug which reduces colonic contractility. It acts by blocking the entry of sodium and calcium ions into colonic smooth muscle cells and is normally given in a dose of 135 mg three times a day.

DIARRHOEAL DISEASE ▉▉▉▉▉▉

The treatment of diarrhoea can be divided into three phases: symptomatic, supportive and specific. Symptomatic treatment refers to treating the symptoms, supportive therapy is aimed at replacing lost water and electrolytes, while specific treatment depends on a diagnosis having been made.

Symptomatic treatment involves the use of kaolin mixtures and antiperistaltic agents such as codeine, loperamide and diphenoxylate. In many instances the diarrhoea will spontaneously resolve without a cause having been found. For diarrhoea that does not resolve ongoing medical attention will be required, especially in the very young and the frail elderly, in an effort to try and ascertain a treatable cause. Hospitalisation may be necessary to provide supportive treatment in cases of severe electrolyte and fluid depletion and to carry out relevant diagnostic procedures.

The differential diagnoses of diarrhoea are many and include:

- Dietary factors
- Infection
- Inflammatory bowel disease
- Drugs
- Endocrine disease (e.g. diabetes, hyperthyroidism)
- Diverticular disease
- Irritable bowel syndrome
- Lactose intolerance
- Laxative abuse

Drug treatment for diarrhoea is only applicable in certain instances. In some situations diarrhoea may be drug induced and removal of the drug may lead to a return to normal bowel habits.

INFECTION

The majority of cases of acute infectious diarrhoea are mild and self-limiting. Viral causes are the most common while bacteria usually cause more severe illness. Even where a bacterial pathogen has been isolated antibiotics are not always necessary because of the self-limiting nature of many acute episodes of diarrhoea. *Campylobacter jejunum* is probably the most common cause of diarrhoea in Australia and is susceptible to the quinolone antibiotics, norfloxacin (*Noroxin*) and ciprofloxacin (*Ciproxin*). Diarrhoea due to enterotoxigenic *Escherischia coli* (ETEC) and *Shigella* sp. is also treated with the quinolone antibiotics.

Giardia lamblia is the commonest protozoal parasite of the gut in Australia. Transmission is via the faecal-oral route and symptoms, which include diarrhoea, usually begin about 10 days after ingestion of the organism. In adults, either metronidazole 400 mg three times a day for three days or tinidazole 2 g as a single dose which can be repeated in seven days, are effective.

ADSORBENTS

Kaolin

Kaolin adsorbs toxins and improves the bulk and consistency of faeces. It is administered as a suspension alone, in combination with aluminium hydroxide (*Kaomagma*), with pectin which absorbs water forming a gel thereby increasing the bulk of colonic contents (*Kaomagma with Pectin*) and with antiperistaltic agents, e.g. opium or codeine. Adult dosage regimens are of the order of 15–20 mL three times a day.

ANTIPERISTALTIC AGENTS

The opioids (e.g. codeine, morphine) have traditionally been used to inhibit gastric motility and peristalsis. Codeine can be administered orally as a tablet (30 mg) or in combination with agents such as kaolin.

Two synthetic agents, diphenoxylate and loperamide, both of which are chemically related to the synthetic opioid pethidine are widely used to treat diarrhoea. The restrictions which apply to the storage, prescribing and dispensing of the opioids do not apply to these agents.

Diphenoxylate

Diphenoxylate is available in combination with atropine as the proprietary preparation *Lomotil*. It exerts an inhibitory effect on the gastrointestinal tract similar to all opioid agents. Atropine is included in a small dose (0.025 mg per tablet) to discourage abuse.

PHARMACOKINETICS

Diphenoxylate is well absorbed from the gastrointestinal tract and exerts its effect within one hour. The duration of effect is 3–4 hours.

USES

The adult dose of *Lomotil* is two tablets 3–4 times a day reducing to a lower maintenance dose once control of diarrhoea has been gained.

ADVERSE DRUG REACTIONS

Lomotil can cause central nervous system side effects such as malaise, lethargy, confusion, sedation and drowsiness. Its unwanted effects on the gastrointestinal tract can include nausea, vomiting, abdominal distension and discomfort. Overdosage may be accompanied by atropine-like side effects. In the event of an overdose causing opioid side effects these can be reversed by the opioid antagonist naloxone.

PRECAUTIONS AND CONTRAINDICATIONS

Extreme caution should be exercised in using *Lomotil* for patients with advanced liver and/or renal disease. The use of antiperistaltic agents in patients with active inflammatory bowel disease may lead to obstruction and toxic megacolon. These agents should not be used in patients when bowel obstruction or perforation is suspected.

GASTROINTESTINAL DISORDERS

17

Loperamide

Loperamide (*Imodium*) like diphenoxy-late is chemically related to pethidine. It has the same mechanism of action, adverse effects (without the atropine related effects associated with excessive doses of *Lomotil*), and precautions and indications as diphenoxylate.

The adult dose is 4 mg (it is available as 2 mg capsules) followed by 2 mg after each loose bowel action until symptom control has been achieved. Onset of action is usually within 1–3 hours.

NURSING IMPLICATIONS

ASSESSMENT

The patient's fluid and electrolyte status should be assessed and the number, frequency and consistency of all bowel actions documented.

ADMINISTRATION

Adsorbents such as kaolin preparations may be given frequently, e.g. after each bowel action. Antimotility drugs have a structured dosage schedule and excessive dosage must be avoided. When bacterial or viral infection of the bowel is suspected the use of antimotility drugs should be avoided for 24–48 hours so that transit of the infecting organism is not delayed.

EVALUATION

The patient should be observed for a reduction in number of stools and consistency and for atropine-like side effects with antimotility drugs such as *Lomotil*. In severe cases a stool chart and fluid balance chart should be kept.

PATIENT EDUCATION

When patients are taking these drugs at home they should be instructed on the correct dosage regimen and advised against taking excessive doses if the drugs appear not to be working.

ANTIBIOTIC ASSOCIATED DIARRHOEA

Antibiotics can cause diarrhoea because of their inhibition of colonic bacteria involved in metabolising dietary sugars. Unmetabolised sugars can then exert an osmotic effect drawing fluid into the bowel and causing diarrhoea. Another mechanism, and one that is amenable to specific treatment, is diarrhoea caused by a toxin produced by the Gram positive bacillus *Clostridium difficile*. This organism is resistant to many antibiotics and has been shown to proliferate when colonic flora is suppressed during antibiotic administration. This may be too simplistic an explanation as the disease can occur in the absence of antibiotic therapy. However, the fact remains that the condition does occur in patients who have received courses of antibiotic therapy irrespective of the route of administration. It is also important to note that the diarrhoea can present days to weeks after antibiotic exposure. The spectrum of disease varies from a mild diarrhoea to fulminant life threatening colitis. The term pseudomembranous colitis is used when characteristic plaques, easily visible and distinguishable by sigmoidoscopy, are present. Antibiotic associated diarrhoea is best diagnosed by demonstrating the presence of the cytotoxin in the stool.

Treatment

Three antibiotics can be used to treat this disorder: vancomycin (*Vancocin*) which must be given orally in doses of 125–250 mg four times a day; metronidazole 400 mg three times a day; or bacitracin at a dose of 25 000 units four times a day. Treatment should be continued for 7–10 days. Bacitracin is not available in a ready to use dosage form but is obtainable as a powder which can then be made into capsules or prepared as a solution for oral administration. Irrespective of which drug is chosen, relapses do occur and these can be treated with another course of the same antibiotic or an alternative from among the three discussed. The anion exchange resins, cholestyramine and colestipol, can be used to bind the toxin and can be used concurrently with these antibiotics. However, the possibility of the resin binding the antibiotic exists and for this reason dosing should be separated by at least two hours.

CONSTIPATION

The prevalence of constipation increases with age and may be due to a specific disorder (e.g. endocrine disorders such as hypothyroidism and hypercalcaemia), a diet low in fibre, inactivity, poor dentition, inadequate fluid intake, drugs or long-term abuse of stimulant laxatives. Constipation is primarily a colonic problem and any definition of the disorder revolves around reduced stool frequency when compared with the patient's normal bowel habit and the passage of hard stools often accompanied by straining and pain. Faecal impaction, common in the elderly, may paradoxically present as incontinence and diarrhoea when liquid stools are able to pass around the mass of hard faeces. Constipation is a chronic problem in patients with neurological problems, e.g. stroke, multiple sclerosis and motor neurone disease.

The successful treatment of constipation need not always include the use of laxatives. Dietary advice is often pivotal in resolving constipation. An adequate intake of fibre and fluid is important in preventing and treating constipation, a fact which requires reinforcing in a society where the fibre content of the average diet has steadily dropped since the refining of foods began during the industrial revolution.

Certain drugs are known to cause constipation. The opiates are well recognised causes of constipation and this fact is a therapeutic advantage when weak opiates such as codeine, diphenoxylate and loperamide are used to treat diarrhoea (see Antiperistaltic Agents). All drugs which exert an anticholinergic effect, e.g. atropine and derivatives, and benztropine and the tricyclic antidepressants, have the potential to constipate. The aluminium containing antacids, sucralfate and the calcium channel blockers can also cause constipation.

LAXATIVES

It is accepted practice to divide agents used to treat constipation into the following groups. While accepting this division it is worth remembering that the majority act in the same way, i.e. by altering intestinal fluid and electrolyte transport in the colon. Dosage of the majority of agents tends to be variable, based on a need to establish a desirable frequency of bowel actions in the individual patient (see Table 17.3).

Bulk Forming Agents (Fibre)

Ispaghula (*Metamucil, Fybogel*), sterculia (*Normacol*), methylcellulose and bran are effective agents in treating constipation. They increase stool bulk and decrease colonic transport time resulting in the passage of soft, bulky stools. These agents take several days to exert their full effect and care must be taken to ensure that fibre is taken with adequate fluid, i.e. a full glass of water, to minimise the risk of oesophageal and bowel obstruction.

GASTROINTESTINAL DISORDERS

17

TABLE 17.3 Dosage and administration of some agents used to treat constipation

Agent	Dosage and Administration (Adults)
Bulk forming agents (fibre)	
Ispaghula	One rounded teaspoonful in a glass of fluid one to three times a day
Sterculia	1–2 heaped teaspoonfuls once or twice a day with fluid
Stimulants	
Bisacodyl 5 mg	5–10 mg at night
Senna	
Tablets	2–4 tablets at night
Granules	1–2 teaspoonfuls chewed or mixed with hot or cold milk at night
Osmotic agents	
Magnesium sulfate (epsom salts)	1–3 teaspoonfuls in a glass of water daily
Lactulose	15–30 mL daily
Sorbitol 70%	20 mL three times daily
Lubricants	
Liquid paraffin	7.5–15 mL at night
Stool softeners	
Docusate sodium 120 mg	1–2 tablets at night
Docusate sodium with senna	1–2 tablets at night

Stimulants

These drugs stimulate peristalsis by irritating the intestinal mucosa. Two agents commonly used are senna (*Senokot*) and bisacodyl (*Durolax*). They work in 8–12 hours and are therefore suitable to be given at night with the expectation of a result the next morning. Prolonged use of stimulant laxatives places patients at risk of entering a vicious cycle of colonic atony leading to constipation and an increasing dependence on the agents which contributed to the problem in the first place.

Osmotic Agents

Salts of magnesium (sulfate, hydroxide and carbonate) and phosphates (usually given as an enema, e.g. *Travad Enema Solution* containing phosphate salts of sodium), draw fluid into the bowel by osmosis. They are used in various bowel preparation regimens.

Lactulose (*Duphalac*), a synthetic derivative of lactose, also exerts an osmotic effect and although expensive is effective. Lactulose is also used in the treatment of hepatic encephalopathy in patients with cirrhosis of the liver. Onset of action is of the order of one to three days.

Sorbitol is a naturally occurring polyhydric alcohol which is widely used as a sweetening agent in sugar free pharmaceuticals. Sorbitol 70% (*Sorbilax*) is commercially available and is a less costly alternative to lactulose for the treatment of constipation. Like lactulose, sorbitol is not absorbed from the gastrointestinal tract and exerts its laxative action via an osmotic effect.

Lubricants

Liquid paraffin is the most common lubricant agent used either alone or emulsified in an oil-in-water emulsion (*Agarol*) to make it more palatable. Like the stimulants, onset of action is of the order of eight hours. Long-term use of liquid paraffin is associated with diminished absorption of fat soluble vitamins and in the debilitated patient aspiration can cause a lipid pneumonitis.

Hyperosmotic Agents

Glycerin is a hygroscopic agent which attracts water. It is used in suppository form and, like the other osmotic agents discussed, draws fluid into the colon.

Colonic Lavage Solutions

These are iso-osmotic electrolyte solutions containing polyethylene glycol (*Glycoprep*, *Golytely*). They are normally given in volumes of 3–4 L over four hours prior to bowel examination. Insignificant absorption of electrolytes takes place so that in the cardiac compromised patient a significant sodium load is avoided. They can be used to manage constipation which has not been effectively treated with other agents.

Stool Softeners

Docusate sodium (dioctyl sodium sulfosuccinate) is a wetting agent which lubricates the stool and increases its permeability to water. It is available as *Coloxyl* tablets (50 mg and 120 mg), drops for paediatric use, suppositories, an enema concentrate and in combination with senna (*Coloxyl with Senna*).

NURSING IMPLICATIONS

ASSESSMENT

Before the administration of a laxative the nurse should ensure the patient is not suffering from intestinal obstruction or a perforated bowel. All laxatives are contraindicated in these conditions. Patients who are receiving anticoagulant therapy and those who are debilitated should not be given lubricant laxatives as decreased vitamin absorption can occur with these preparations.

ADMINISTRATION

Administration should be timed so that the agent's onset and peak of action occurs at a convenient time and not during the night. Bulk laxatives should be given with a large glass of water as they require a high fluid intake to be effective.

EVALUATION

The patient should be evaluated for relief of constipation and appropiate records made. If the patient remains constipated after the administration of bulk laxatives the fluid intake should be checked and a further assessment made for signs of intestinal obstruction. The patient should be observed for signs of dehydration and electrolyte imbalance especially when saline laxatives have been used or if the patient is very ill or debilitated.

PATIENT EDUCATION

The nurse has an important role as an educator of both patients and the general public regarding how to maintain normal bowel function. Some people have 'bowel phobia' and become habitual users of laxatives which may lead to the 'lazy bowel' syndrome. A high fibre diet, plenty of fluids and regular exercise all contribute to maintenance of normal bowel function.

GASTROINTESTINAL DISORDERS

17

Nurses should be continually alert to prevent the development of constipation in their patients. Prevention or treatment must be carried out to avoid the problem of severe faecal impaction.

HAEMORRHOIDS

Haemorrhoids represent the most common rectal disorder in the community. They consist of venous swelling associated with increased hydrostatic pressure in the portal venous system, often a result of straining. Treatment ranges from Sitz baths, the use of a variety of creams, ointments and suppositories containing various combinations of local anaesthetics, steroids, vasoconstrictors and zinc oxide for its anti-inflammatory effect (*Rectinol, Proctosedyl, Xyloproct*), to definitive surgery. Stool softeners (*Coloxyl*) and fibre (*Metamucil*) are indicated to promote the formation of a softer stool which can be passed without straining.

ANTIHELMINTICS

Antihelmintics are used to treat worm (helminth) infections in humans. Roundworm and threadworm infestations are the two most commonly seen in Australia. The dose of each agent discussed is determined by body weight, while the most common side effects are related to gastric intolerance.

Pyrantel embonate (*Combantrin*) is a single dose agent used to eradicate threadworm, roundworm and hookworm. It is a neuromuscular blocking agent which acts to paralyse worms.

Thiabendazole (*Mintezol*) is indicated in the treatment of threadworm and guinea worm infestations and both cutaneous and visceral larva migrans. It is indicated for the relief of symptoms and fever associated with trichinosis.

Niclosamide (*Yomesan*) is used to treat tapeworm infestations in humans. Patients should be advised to avoid alcohol during treatment.

DISORDERS OF THE MOUTH AND THROAT

Debilitated patients are prone to a variety of disorders of the mouth and pharynx which are potentially extremely painful and can compromise nutritional status in patients who are already malnourished. Good palliative care demands that meticulous attention be given to oral hygiene.

TREATMENT

Certain drugs can predispose patients to oral disorders. For example, inhaled corticosteroids increase the incidence of oral *Candida albicans* infections (thrush). Topical nystatin (*Nilstat*) remains the treatment of choice for oral candidiasis and it is usually given as 1 mL (100 000 units) four times a day. Miconazole in a gel form (*Daktarin*) is another effective agent which can be used in place of nystatin. Povidone-iodine is available as a gargle (*Betadine Sore Throat Gargle*) providing the broad bactericidal and fungicidal action of iodine. Anticholinergic agents and tricyclic antidepressants, which have anticholinergic side effects, reduce saliva output and give rise to a dry mouth (xerostomia) and an increased incidence of infection. Artificial saliva preparations are available (*Saliva Substitute, Saliva Orthana Spray*), however their use is not a substitute for regular mouth toilets. Hydrogen peroxide (6%) solution or *Amosan* sachets containing sodium perborate, which releases hydrogen peroxide when dissolved in water, is an effective agent for cleaning the mouth as part of an oral hygiene routine. Hydrogen peroxide is bactericidal against anaerobic bacteria and because of the effervescence accompanying the release of oxygen it assists in the mechanical removal of adherent debris.

Antiseptic lozenges, topical applications and mouthwashes with and without local anaesthetics (*Cepacol, Bonjela, Cepacaine, Codral*) are useful agents for providing symptom relief but again they should not be used as substitutes for adequate oral hygiene.

The local application of hydrocortisone (*Corlan pellets*) is used in treating apthous ulcers resistant to other treatment modalities, e.g. choline salicylate (*Bonjela*).

Local anaesthetic gels (*Xylocaine Viscous*) produce profound local anaesthesia, but the accompanying loss of sensation can be unpleasant and these preparations are more commonly used to alleviate pain during oral procedures.

Benzydamine (*Diflam*) is a topical NSAID and is available in both solution and lozenge form for the treatment of sore mouth. To avoid side effects associated with the systemic absorption of NSAIDs, the solution should be expectorated after rinsing the mouth.

NURSING IMPLICATIONS

ASSESSMENT

Patients should be assessed for hypersensitivy to the active ingredient. The preparation should be administered as prescribed. The patient should be evaluated for effectiveness of the preparation and any adverse reactions. If appropriate the patient should be instructed to retain the substance in the mouth for a while before swallowing.

Patients using *preparations containing local anaesthetics* should be observed for local adverse effects and advised to avoid hot liquids and hot or abrasive food until the local anaesthetic effect wears off.

Some *antifungal preparations* are suspensions of insoluble powders, the container should be shaken well immediately before administering the dose. The patient should be instructed that when the suspension is applied to the lesion it should be retained in the mouth for some time before swallowing to ensure maximum local effect and to avoid rinsing the mouth, eating or drinking for some time after administration.

GASTROINTESTINAL DISORDERS

17

NURSING IMPLICATIONS– GASTROINTESTINAL DISORDERS

ASSESSMENT

The impact of drugs used to treat gastrointestinal disease on concomitant illnesses and other drugs the patient may be taking must always be taken into consideration. While the patient is in hospital an assessment of their ability to understand and comply with chosen therapy should be undertaken.

EVALUATION

Aside from the normal clinical observations carried out on all patients there are some specific observations which are important for patients with gastrointestinal disorders. A bowel chart on which details such as stool frequency, volume, consistency, colour, smell and presence or otherwise of blood can be recorded is an extremely important aid in arriving at a cause for an altered bowel habit. Accurate recording of body weight is essential where steps have been put in place to improve a patient's nutritional status.

ADMINISTRATION

Patients who are ill and malnourished may not be able to correct their deficit by normal feeding methods and therefore will require tube feeding (nasogastric or gastrostomy) or parenteral nutrition. Fine bore nasogastric tubes and, to a lesser extent, gastrostomy tubes can be readily blocked by solid medications if tablets are not crushed into a fine powder prior to dissolution or the preparation of a suspension. It is imperative to check with the pharmacy department whether or not crushing a tablet or emptying out the contents of a capsule to prepare a solution or suspension will alter the bioavailability of the drug.

PATIENT EDUCATION

Patients should not leave hospital without a clear understanding of the medications they are required to take, any alternative names, what they are for, how long they are to take them, warning signs of serious adverse effects and what their responsibility is in terms of ongoing monitoring (e.g. blood tests, stool examination).

FURTHER READING

Friedman, G. (1989) 'Irritable bowel syndrome: 1. A practical approach'. *American Journal of Gastroenterology*, 84, pp. 863–867.

Katelaris, P., Barr, G. (1990) 'Acute infectious diarrhoea in adults'. *Current Therapeutics*, Dec, pp. 26–34.

McCallum, R.W. (1991) 'Cisapride: A new class of prokinetic agent'. *American Journal of Gastroenterology*, 86, pp. 135–149.

Peppercorn, M.A. (1990) 'Advances in drug therapy for inflammatory bowel disease'. *Annals of Internal Medicine*, 112, pp. 50–60.

Soll A.H., Weinstein, W.M., Kurata J., McCarthy D. (1991) 'Nonsteroidal anti-inflammatory drugs and peptic ulcer disease'. *Annals of Internal Medicine*, 114, pp. 307–319.

Weir, D.G. (1988) 'Peptic ulceration'. *British Medical Journal*, 296, pp. 195–200.

Wynne, H.A., Edwards, C. (1992) 'Laxatives'. *Pharmaceutical Journal*, Jan 4, pp. 17–19.

TEST YOUR KNOWLEDGE

1. Name three drugs from different chemical classes which can be used to heal peptic ulcers.

2. By which route should vancomycin be given when used to treat *Clostridium difficile* associated diarrhoea?

3. Name two drugs, the clearance of which can be reduced by the concomitant administration of cimetidine.

4. What ongoing monitoring should be instituted for patients taking sulfasalazine or azathioprine?

5. Metoclopramide, domperidone and cisapride are all referred to as prokinetic agents. Explain the meaning of the term prokinetic.

6. Describe the mechanism whereby non-steroidal anti-inflammatory drugs damage gastric mucosa.

7. Which of the three currently available 5-aminosalicylic acid derivatives used to treat inflammatory bowel disease should not be given to patients sensitive to sulfonamide drugs?

8. What effect does the administration of metronidazole to patients taking warfarin have on their anticoagulation status?

9. Do tricyclic antidepressants cause diarrhoea or constipation?

10. Describe the mechanism of action of omeprazole. Does it suppress acid output to a greater or lesser extent than that achieved with the H_2 receptor antagonists?

GASTROINTESTINAL DISORDERS

17

TABLE 17.4 Summary table — drug treatment of gastrointestinal disorders

DISORDER/DRUG GROUP Drug Name	Use	Action	Adverse Reactions	Nursing Implications
ACID PEPSIN DISEASE ANTACIDS Aluminium hydroxide Magnesium hydroxide Magnesium carbonate Magnesium trisilicate Calcium carbonate	Peptic ulcers, gastroesophageal reflux	Neutralise gastric acid providing symptom relief, promote healing	*Aluminium salts*: constipation *Magnesium salts*: diarrhoea Antacids can interfere with absorption of some other drugs	**Assess:** Bowel habit; concurrent use of drugs absorption of which may be affected by antacids **Administer**: Variable, most effective if given one and three hours after meals
ANTICHOLINERGIC AGENTS Belladonna compounds Dicyclomine Glycopyrrolate Propantheline	Peptic ulcers, irritable bowel syndrome, colic	Inhibit effect of acetylcholine in GIT thereby reducing gastric motility and acid output	Dry mouth, blurred vision, dilated pupils, tachycardia, constipation, urinary hesitancy, dizziness, mental confusion, see Chapter 10. Incidence increased if patient taking other drugs with anticholinergic effects, e.g. tricyclic antidepressants, antihistamines	**Assess:** For adverse reactions **Administer:** As prescribed, usually up to 1 h before meals and at bedtime (e.g. propantheline)
H₂ RECEPTOR ANTAGONISTS Cimetidine Ranitidine Famotidine Nizatidine	Peptic ulcers, gastroesophageal reflux	Antagonise action of histamine on H₂ receptors in parietal cells, thereby reducing gastric acid output	Altered bowel habit, GI intolerance, headache, skin rash. Hormonal effects and potential drug interactions with cimetidine. Confusion in elderly when given in full doses in renal impairment	**Administer:** As prescribed **Educate:** Patients must be aware of need to complete prescribed course despite possible absence of symptoms

TABLE 17.4 continued

DISORDER/DRUG GROUP Drug Name	Use	Action	Adverse Reactions	Nursing Implications
PROSTAGLANDIN ANALOGUES Misoprostol	Peptic ulcers	Inhibits gastric acid secretion and protects mucosal lining of stomach	Diarrhoea. Potential abortifacient	**Administer**: 100–200 μg 4 times/day **Evaluate**: Bowel habits
OTHER AGENTS Sucralfate	Peptic ulcers	Combines with protein at ulcer site to form protective layer, blocks back diffusion of gastric acid, inhibits action of pepsin and bile	Constipation	**Administer**: As prescribed, usually 4 times/day but can be given twice daily. If antacids or H2 receptor antagonists co-prescribed, administration should be 2 h apart **Evaluate**: Bowel habits
Omeprazole	Peptic ulcers, gastroesophageal reflux	Blocks hydrogen ion release from gastric parietal cell	Usually well tolerated	**Administer**: As prescribed, usually once a day in morning
BISMUTH AND TRIPLE THERAPY Bismuth Subcitrate	Peptic ulcers	Combines with proteins at ulcer site to form protective layer. Used either alone or in combination with other agents (amoxycillin, metronidazale) to eradicate *Helicobacter pylori*	Blackening of stools, discolouration of mouth	**Administer**: As prescribed half an hour before meals. Separate antacids or milk by 2 h

17 GASTROINTESTINAL DISORDERS

TABLE 17.4 continued

DISORDER/DRUG GROUP Drug Name	Use	Action	Adverse Reactions	Nursing Implications
PROKINETIC AGENTS Metoclopramide	Nausea, vomiting, gastroparesis, reflex oesophagitis	Enhances GIT motility and gastric emptying. Acts centrally via inhibition of dopamine effects on chemoreceptor trigger zone	Dystonia, drowsiness	**Assess:** For concurrent use of phenothiazines **Administer:** 10 mg 8-hourly; oral, IM or IV as ordered usually 15–30 min before meals. Larger doses used in chemotherapy regimens **Evaluate:** For signs of extrapyramidal side effects, drowsiness **Educate:** To take 15–30 min before meals
Domperidone	Nausea, vomiting, gastroparesis, reflex oesophagitis	Depresses vomiting mechanisms; enhances GIT motility and gastric emptying	Abdominal cramps, dry mouth	**Administer:** 10 mg 3–4 times/day 15–30 min before meals
Cisapride	Motility disorders	Increases gastric motility via increased release of acetylcholine locally	Diarrhoea	**Administer:** As prescribed before meals

TABLE 17.4 continued

DISORDER/DRUG GROUP Drug Name	Use	Action	Adverse Reactions	Nursing Implications
ANTIEMETICS AND ANTINAUSEANTS ANTIHISTAMINES Meclozine Promethazine Pheniramine	Nausea, vomiting	Act on CNS vomiting centre	Sedation, dizziness, anticholinergic effects; see Chapter 29 *Note:* some antihistamines belong in phenothiazine group	**Administer**: As prescribed **Evaluate**: For drowsiness; anticholinergic side effects; hypotension (especially after IV injection) **Educate**: Warn that drowsiness and dry mouth may occur; advise of potential dangers when driving and operating machinery and of potentiation of sedative effect by other drugs
PHENOTHIAZINES Prochlorperazine Perphenazine Thiethylperazine Chlorpromazine	Nausea, vomiting.	Act on chemoreceptor trigger zone	Extrapyramidal effects, sedation; see Chapter 26	**Administer**: As prescribed **Evaluate**: For signs of extrapyramidal side effects and hypotension (especially after injected doses), signs of skin irritation at injection sites, body temperature **Educate**: advise use of sunscreening agent if necessary, to avoid concurrent use of other CNS depressants, that sedating effect could make driving a car or operating machinery dangerous

17   GASTROINTESTINAL DISORDERS

TABLE 17.4 continued

DISORDER/DRUG GROUP Drug Name	Use	Action	Adverse Reactions	Nursing Implications
ANTICHOLINERGIC AGENTS Hyoscine Dicyclomine	Nausea, vomiting	Act on CNS vomiting centre and central cholinergic pathways	Dry mouth, blurred vision, urinary retention, constipation; see Chapter 10	As for anticholinergic drugs—see Chapter 10
INFLAMMATORY BOWEL DISEASE 5-ASA DERIVATIVES Sulfasalazine Olsalazine Mesalazine	Inflammatory bowel disease	Sulfasalazine breaks down in gut to sulfapyridine and a salicylate. Olsalazine and mesalazine release 5-ASA (salicylate) only	*Sulfasalazine.* Nausea, vomiting, anorexia, rash, Stevens-Johnson syndrome, giddiness, headache, blood dyscrasias, drug fever, azospermia *Olsalazine.* Diarrhoea	**Assess:** For previous hypersensitivity to sulfonamides and salicylates, pregnancy, lactation, with sulfasalazine **Administer:** As prescribed **Evaluate:** For drug effectiveness, adverse effects **Educate:** Correct method of administration; that urine colour might turn orange with sulfasalazine, importance of adequate fluid intake and to recognise indications of adverse effects
ANTIDIARRHOEAL DRUGS ADSORBENTS Kaolin Aluminium hydroxide Attapulgite	Diarrhoea	Adsorb toxins	Constipation	

TABLE 17.4 continued

DISORDER/DRUG GROUP Drug Name	Use	Action	Adverse Reactions	Nursing Implications
ANTIPERISTALTIC AGENTS Codeine phosphate Diphenoxylate Loperamide	Diarrhoea	Inhibit gastric motility and peristalsis	Overdose: nausea, vomiting, constipation, respiratory depression, drowsiness	**Administer:** Adsorbents—frequently as required and after each bowel action until diarrhoea ceases; antimotility drugs—as prescribed **Evaluate:** Response to drug; record stool chart; observe for atropine-like effects with diphenoxylate **Educate:** Correct dosage regimen and advise patients taking opium derivatives and antimotility drugs such as diphenoxylate to avoid excessive dosage

17 GASTROINTESTINAL DISORDERS

TABLE 17.4 continued

DISORDER/DRUG GROUP Drug Name	Use	Action	Adverse Reactions	Nursing Implications
LAXATIVES SALINE LAXATIVES Magnesium sulfate Sodium sulfate Sodium phosphate Potassium phosphate Sodium citrate	Constipation, preoperative bowel evacuation	Attract water, soften faeces, increase bulk	Diarrhoea, electrolyte imbalance	**Assess:** For presence of nausea, vomiting, abdominal pain, possibility of intestinal obstruction or bowel perforation as all laxatives are contraindicated in these situations; assess hydration and electrolyte status; sodium restriction (saline laxatives), anticoagulant therapy (lubricant laxatives) **Administer:** So that onset and peak of action occur at convenient time and not during night; give bulk laxatives with large glass of water; avoid giving bisacodyl tablets with antacids as this could cause premature dissolution of enteric coating, leading to nausea and vomiting **Evaluate:** For required effect and record appropriately; for signs of electrolyte imbalance (especially saline laxatives) **Educate:** About normal bowel function and how to prevent constipation with correct diet, fluids and exercise; that continual use of drugs to relieve constipation can lead to 'lazy bowel syndrome'; advise approximate time laxative effect of the drug will occur; advise to seek medical advice if constipation remains a problem or if laxative is not effective

TABLE 17.4 continued

DISORDER/DRUG GROUP Drug Name	Use	Action	Adverse Reactions	Nursing Implications
BULK LAXATIVES Methylcellulose Bassorin Ispaghula Psyllium Sterculia Bran	Constipation, faecal incontinence	Absorb water increasing stool bulk and causing reflex peristalsis	Diarrhoea, intestinal obstruction	**Assess:** See saline laxatives **Administer:** As prescribed. Agents should be taken with plenty of fluid to minimise risk of obstruction. Takes several days to exert full effect **Evaluate:** For required effect and record appropriately; for signs of intestinal obstruction **Educate:** See saline laxatives
STIMULANT LAXATIVES Senna Cascara Castor oil Bisacodyl	Constipation	Irritation of intestinal mucosa, stimulation of peristalsis	Nausea, diarrhoea, cramping, habituation	**Assess:** See saline laxatives **Administer:** Effect usually occurs within 8–12 hours **Evaluate:** For required effect and record appropriately **Educate:** See saline laxatives
LUBRICANTS AND HYPEROSMOTIC AGENTS Liquid paraffin Glycerin	Constipation	Lubricate intestinal wall, soften faeces	Cramps, diarrhoea, interfere with absorption of fat soluble vitamins and other drugs, anal leakage of oil, lipid pneumonia, habituation	**Assess:** See saline laxatives **Administer:** Effect usually occurs in 8–12 h **Evaluate:** For required effect and record appropriately **Educate:** See saline laxatives
SURFACE ACTIVE LAXATIVES Docusate sodium	Constipation	Detergent-like effect on faecal mass allowing penetration of water and fats thus softening faeces		**Assess:** See saline laxatives **Evaluate:** For required effect and record appropriately **Educate:** See saline laxatives

17 GASTROINTESTINAL DISORDERS

TABLE 17.4 continued

DISORDER/DRUG GROUP Drug Name	Use	Action	Adverse Reactions	Nursing Implications
OTHER AGENTS Lactulose	Constipation, hepatic encephalopathy	Lactulose is broken down in colon into organic acids which cause mild irritation and promote peristalsis		**Assess:** See saline laxatives **Administer:** In hepatic encephalopathy dose to obtain 2–3 reasonably formed bowel motions a day **Evaluate:** For required effect and record appropriately **Educate:** See saline laxatives
ANTHELMINTICS Pyrantel	Threadworm, roundworm, hookworm	Neuromuscular blocking agents in worms	GI side effects	**Assess:** Ability of patient to understand hygiene principles to prevent re-infection; presence of constipation; age and weight **Administer:** As prescribed; therapeutic dose usually calculated according to body weight; give laxative if indicated **Evaluate:** Record if and when bowel action occurs; note presence of helminths; observe for side effects **Educate:** Principles of hygiene to prevent re-infection; correct dosage and date to take follow-up dose; to avoid alcohol with niclosamide
Thiabendazole	Threadworm			
Niclosamide	Tapeworm			

Fluid and Electrolyte Disorders

MARIAN M. TOWNSEND

O B J E C T I V E S

At the conclusion of this chapter the reader should be able to:

1. List the principles involved in the maintenance of body fluid, electrolyte and pH balance;

2. Describe the principles involved in the replacement of deficits by intravenous therapy;

3. Understand the effects of surgical intervention and disease processes on fluid, electrolyte and pH balance; and

4. Assess the response to intravenous therapy and describe adverse effects due to any component of therapy.

BODY WATER

Water is the most abundant constituent of the human body. It represents approximately 50% of the total body weight. However, this varies with age, weight and gender. It can be up to 85% of the total body weight of a premature infant, 75% of an infant born at term, 50% of a 40-year old female and 60% of a 40-year old male. This is because fat is essentially water free and infants have a much lower proportion of adipose tissue in their body make up than adults, with females having a higher proportion than males.

The total body water is distributed in the body in various fluid spaces or compartments. The two major compartments are the intracellular fluid compartment (inside cells) and the extracellular fluid compartment. The extracellular fluid is subdivided into the intravascular component (plasma), interstitial fluid (fluid in the spaces between cells) and lymph. In normal adults approximately 55% of the total body water is intracellular and 35% is extracellular. The remaining water is located in connective tissue, bone and the transcellular compartment comprising the gastrointestinal tract, tracheobronchial tree, various glands, the cerebrospinal fluid and the aqueous humour of the eye. The distribution of total body water is shown in Table 18.1.

TABLE 18.1 Distribution of total body water in adults

Body Water	%	%
Intracellular		55
Extracellular		35
Plasma	7.5	
Interstitial	27.5	
Bone		7.5
Transcellular		2.5
Total		100

FLUID BALANCE

Fluid balance is maintained by altering the intake and excretion of water. Intake is normally controlled by thirst, while excretion is controlled by the renal action of antidiuretic hormone (ADH). ADH is secreted by the posterior pituitary gland and acts on the distal tubules of nephrons to increase water reabsorption. In health, a plasma osmolality of approximately 280 mOsm/kg suppresses plasma ADH to levels low enough to permit maximum urinary dilution. However, when the extracellular fluid volume is reduced and the osmolality of the extracellular fluid is increased, the output of ADH is increased via stimulation of baroreceptors in the left atrium and osmoreceptors in the hypothalamus. The secretion of ADH increases water reabsorption by the kidney which increases the volume of the extracellular fluid and results in a decrease in the extracellular fluid osmolality. In the conscious healthy person thirst also initiates water repletion. As the extracellular fluid is primarily dependent on extracellular sodium (see Electrolytes), sodium regulation is also very important in fluid balance. A contraction of the extracellular fluid impacts directly on cardiovascular function, decreasing cardiac output and arterial blood pressure. A decreased arterial renal pressure reduces the glomerular filtration rate and results in the activation of the renin angiotensin system stimulating the production of aldosterone by the adrenal cortex. This increases sodium reabsorption by the kidneys and increases the extracellular volume.

The normal 70 kg adult at rest in a temperate climate requires approximately 2400 mL of fluid per day to compensate for normal urinary excretion (1500 mL), faecal loss (200 mL) and insensible losses through respiration (500 mL) and sweating (500 mL). Endogenous water is produced from catabolism (300 mL).

CHANGES IN FLUID VOLUME

Volume depletion

Fluid and electrolyte losses which have occurred more slowly are less debilitating than sudden losses. The history will tell how long the patient has been ill and the recent oral and intraveneous intake. Any abnormal losses, e.g. from vomiting, diarrhoea, polyuria, bleeding, sweating, nasogastric suction or enterocutaneous fistulae, can be estimated. A large blood loss from haemorrhage requires replacement by a blood transfusion. Plasma loss (from burns or ascites) necessitates the administration of a plasma protein solution. However, as an initial emergency measure, the infusion of 0.9% sodium chloride in water helps restore intravascular volume depletion, to give haemodynamic stability and the induction of diuresis.

Signs and symptoms depend on the loss and the rapidity with which it has occurred. Extracellular fluid loss may be present without cardiac signs unless associated with intravascular volume depletion.

The examination of the patient primarily involves evaluation of the cardiovascular system. Appropriate assessment may vary from measurement of vital signs to measurement of central venous pressure, pulmonary wedge pressure and cardiac output by invasive monitoring techniques in the more complex case. In compensated intravascular volume depletion, the heart rate is elevated but blood pressure is maintained within a normal range. When the capacity of the haemodynamic compensatory mechanisms are exceeded, signs suggestive of inadequate perfusion will be present, e.g. a low systolic blood pressure, a low mean blood pressure and a low cardiac output.

Monitoring of urine output is also important in the initial evaluation of the extracellular fluid deficit and the assessment of therapy, particularly in the absence of invasive monitoring data such as central venous pressure. A urine output of less than 0.5–1 mL per kg per hour suggests inadequate perfusion.

Further examination will reveal if the eyes are sunken, if the mucosa appears dry and if the tissue is turgid. If so, the interstitial space has also been reduced and must be replenished appropriately. Intracellular fluid is usually not depleted without initial losses from the other compartments.

Measurement of serum electrolytes helps to calculate needs, based on maintenance requirements and apparent deficits or excesses. Knowledge of the relationship between the serum level and the total amount of the electrolyte in the body is necessary to calculate total body deficit or excess. In acute haemorrhage, a blood sample is also needed for typing and crossmatching and a haemoglobin and haemotcrit estimation should also be done.

Volume Excess

Excessive fluid volume may be caused by overload with oral or intravenous fluids or may be due to diseases such as congestive cardiac failure, renal failure or the syndrome of inappropriate antidiuretic hormone. The patient's blood pressure, body weight and central venous pressure will be raised and the fluid balance will be positive.

Pulmonary and/or peripheral oedema may occur. A biochemical analysis reveals a diluted serum with a low concentration of sodium and chloride, and the treatment is fluid and sodium restriction.

ELECTROLYTES

The water of the body contains electrolytes. An electrolyte is a charged particle in solution. Electrolytes which have a positive charge are cations and those with a negative charge are anions.

FLUID AND ELECTROLYTES

18

The electrolyte content of the various compartments differ significantly. Sodium (Na^+), chloride (Cl^-) and bicarbonate (HCO_3^-) are the main electrolytes of the extracellular compartment and potassium (K^+), magnesium (Mg^{2+}) and phosphate ions (PO_4^{2-}) are the main electrolytes of the intracellular compartment, see Table 18.2.

These differences in electrolyte composition are maintained by an active Na^+-K^+-ATPase transport system on the cellular membrane.

TABLE 18.2   Major electrolytes

Electrolyte	Major function (regulation)	Distribution	Normal serum level (mmol/L)	Normal IV requirement (mmol/kg/day)
Sodium (Na^+)	Osmotic pressure and water balance of extracellular fluid; conductivity/excitability of nerves and muscles	50% in extracellular fluid; 45% in bone	135–145	1–2
Potassium (K^+)	Osmotic pressure and water balance of intracellular fluid; acid–base balance; nerve and muscle excitability; enzyme systems	95% in intracellular fluid	3.4–4.8	1–1.5
Calcium (Ca^{2+})	Mineralisation of bone, teeth; neuromuscular transmission; muscular contraction; blood clotting, fibrinolysis	99% in bone; 0.1% in extracellular fluid	2.15–2.55	0.1–0.15
Magnesium (Mg^{2+})	Neuromuscular excitability; co-factor for many enzyme systems	55% in bone; 44% in soft tissues; 1% in extracellular fluid	0.75–1	0.1–0.2
Phosphate (PO_4^{2-})	Mineralisation of bone; buffer system; acid–base balance; high energy bonds	85% in bones; 15% in soft tissues	0.6–1.25	0.5–0.7
Chloride (Cl^-)	Osmotic pressure of ECF; acid–base balance; cell membrane electrical potential; gastrointestinal secretions	Extracellular fluid	93–103	1.3–1.9

OSMOLALITY

Some chemical compounds in solution do not have an electrical charge, they are non-electrolytes, e.g. urea, glucose. They contribute to osmotic pressure, however, as this is dependent on the number of particles in solution not the size or charge of the particle. Osmolality is the measure of the number of osmotically active particles in 1 kg of solution.

The osmotic pressure is identical in all compartments, water moving freely between compartments to maintain this pressure. The major determinants of osmotic pressure in the extracellular fluid are sodium and chloride, and the major determinant in the intracellular fluid is potassium.

A solution is isotonic if it has the same osmolality as plasma (275–295 mOsm/per kg). It is hypotonic if it has an osmolality less than that of plasma and hypertonic if it has an osmolality greater than that of plasma.

Intravenous Solutions

There is a wide variety of intravenous solutions available commercially. These solutions are sterile and free from pyrogens. They differ in tonicity (osmolality), electrolyte content and energy value. They may be colloid or crystalloid solutions. The composition of some commonly used intravenous fluids is shown in Table 18.3.

TABLE 18.3 Composition of some commonly used intravenous fluids

Solution	Type	Tonicity	Na (mmol/L)	K (mmol/L)	Cl (mmol/L)	Other (/L)	Energy (kJ/L)
0.9% NaCl in water	Crystalloid	Isotonic	150	—	150	—	
0.45% NaCl in water	Crystalloid	Hypotonic	75	—	75		
3% NaCl in water	Crystalloid	Hypertonic	500	—	500		
5% Glucose in water	Crystalloid	Isotonic	—	—	—		783
4% Glucose + 0.18% NaCl + 30 mmol KCl in water	Crystalloid	Isotonic	30	30	60		630
Hartmann's	Crystalloid	Isotonic	131	5	112	Lactate 29 mmol Ca 2 mmol	
Haemaccel	Colloid	Isotonic	145	5	145	Polygeline 35 g Ca 12.5 mmol	
6% Dextran 70 in 0.9% NaCl	Colloid	Isotonic	150		150	Dextran 60 g	

FLUID AND ELECTROLYTES

18

Crystalloid Solutions

Crystalloid solutions contain electrolytes or glucose or both. The administration of 5% glucose in water delivers water to all body compartments (i.e. the intracellular fluid and extracellular fluid) proportionately. This is because insulin stimulates the intracellular uptake and metabolism of glucose, so there is no contribution of osmotically active particles. The water moves freely between compartments to maintain an iso-osmotic state and the osmolality of all fluid compartments decreases. The administration of glucose in water solutions represents the administration of free water. In contrast, the intravenous administration of 0.9% sodium chloride in water increases the extracellular, but not the intracellular, fluid compartment. The sodium and chloride are confined to the extracellular fluid by an active transport system. As the solution is isotonic there is no net movement of water from the extracellular fluid to the intracellular compartment. It is the preferred crystalloid solution when an increase in intravascular volume is required.

Colloid Solutions

Colloid solutions (or plasma volume expanders) contain large particles which are osmotically active and which stay in the intravascular space, thus increasing the intravascular volume. They may also contain electrolytes or glucose. They have a tonicity similar to that of plasma.

Albumin solutions are prepared from pooled plasma and are sterilised by heating. They do not require typing or cross matching. They contain sufficient sodium chloride to make them isotonic. They are very expensive and their shelf life at 25°C is 1 year and 5 years at 2–8°C.

Albumin solution 5% is indicated in hypovolaemia due to haemorrhage or plasma loss, e.g. in burns, crush injuries and peritonitis, and is particularly valuable when there is associated hypoproteinaemia. It is also used as a replacement fluid during plasma exchange.

Albumin solution 20% contains relatively less sodium and is used instead of the 5% solution when salt and water overloading is a problem.

Patients must be monitored carefully to avoid circulatory overload. Albumin solutions may cause flushing, urticaria and fever.

Dextrans are polysaccharides which are produced by the action of bacteria on sucrose. The long chains of glucose units formed are of two average molecular weights, dextran 70 with a molecular weight of 70 000 and dextran 40 with a molecular weight of 40 000. Dextran 70 is available as a 6% solution in 0.9% sodium chloride or 5% glucose and dextran 40 as a 10% solution in 0.9% sodium chloride or 5% glucose. The solutions do not require refrigeration.

Dextran 70 solution (*Macrodex*) is used in hypovolaemic shock and the prophylaxis of thromboembolism. It has an intravascular half-life of 6 hours. It exerts a colloid osmotic pressure greater than that of plasma. Dextran 40 solution (*Rheomacrodex*) produces a greater expansion of blood volume than dextran 70 solution but the effect is shorter as its half-life is 2 hours.

Administration of additional electrolytes is necessary to replenish the extravascular space. Dextrans alter normal platelet function and tend to prevent platelet aggregation as well as facilitating fibrinolysis by plasmin, thus the bleeding time is prolonged. Their administration also interferes with cross matching procedures. Both dextrans may cause allergic and, rarely, anaphylactoid reactions. Dextran 40 solutions may cause acute renal failure.

Haemaccel is a 3.5% solution of gelatin produced by hydrolysis of animal collagen. It is not as expensive as albumin solutions and is stable at room temperature for 3 years. It is less efficient as a volume expander than dextran 70 because it has a shorter intravascular half-life and is iso-osmotic with plasma. The plasma volume is increased only by the volume infused.

An advantage of *Haemaccel* over dextran solutions is its lower tendency to produce haemorrhagic complications. However, allergic reactions (ranging from skin rashes and pyrexia to anaphylaxis) are more common although the incidence is low. It contains sodium and a large amount of calcium and should not be infused in the same administration set as blood.

FLUID REPLACEMENT

The administration of intravenous fluids and electrolytes is necessary when oral intake is not possible or inadequate due to surgery, trauma, burns, fever, vomiting, diarrhoea, gastric suction or enterocutaneous fistulae. The situation may also be complicated by disease, e.g. congestive cardiac failure, renal failure or diabetes mellitus.

It is necessary to estimate both fluid and electrolyte requirements and the extent of any deficit or abnormal losses to enable appropriate therapy to be administered. The history, an examination of the patient and determination of the serum electrolytes are needed. It is also fundamental to make an ongoing assessment of the patient's fluid balance status.

Replacement Therapy

In cases of short-term or minor dehydration, the combination of solutions selected for replacement therapy need not be identical in composition with the estimated losses because of the body's homeostatic mechanisms. For example, an otherwise well patient who is nil by mouth for less than 24 hours after a simple uncomplicated procedure could receive 1 L of Hartmann's solution over 10 hours followed by 1 L of 4% glucose and 0.18% sodium chloride in water plus 30 mmol potassium chloride over 10 hours. If the patient is then able to drink adequately intravenous therapy could be discontinued.

However, if dehydration and electrolyte loss are significant, e.g. after major surgery, the regimen of replacement fluid is selected to closely resemble the estimated needs. A patient who has large nasogastric losses will require this fluid to be replaced plus the chloride, sodium and potassium it contains, as well as maintenance fluid and electrolytes. Serial serum electrolytes will need to be measured and the fluid balance continually assessed.

Maintenance Therapy

Maintenance therapy provides the normal requirements of the patient, i.e. fluid, electrolytes and glucose, to minimise protein breakdown. A combination of the crystalloid solutions listed in Table 18.3 is commonly used to achieve this.

ELECTROLYTE IMBALANCES

Sodium Deficit (Hyponatraemia)

Hyponatraemia results from a loss of sodium without a corresponding loss of water or an increased water load without an increased sodium load. It may be caused by gastrointestinal losses (vomiting or gastric suction), excessive sweating, excessive use of diuretics, adrenal insufficiency or water intoxication due to excessive infusions of glucose in water.

It causes extracellular hypotonicity and cellular overhydration resulting in weakness, lethargy, confusion, delirium and convulsions. The ensuing hypovolaemia may lead to circulatory failure. The serum sodium and chloride are low. Treatment is by removal or treatment of the cause, e.g. discontinuation of the diuretic or glucose infusion, and replacement of sodium and chloride, usually with 0.9% sodium chloride in water.

Sodium Excess (Hypernatraemia)

Hypernatraemia results from an excessive intake of sodium, a decrease in sodium output, increased water output or decreased water intake. For example, it may be caused by repeated administration of sodium chloride containing infusions, excessive diarrhoea or inadequate water intake.

It causes extracellular hypertonicity and cellular contraction with thirst, dry mucous membranes, muscle rigidity, hyper-reactive reflexes and central nervous system depression. Convulsions and coma may follow. The serum sodium and chloride levels are high. Treatment is by removal of the cause, if possible, and the administration of intravenous fluids containing low amounts of sodium.

Potassium Deficit (Hypokalaemia)

Hypokalaemia will occur if there is an inadequate intake or excessive loss of potassium. It may be caused by the use of potassium losing diuretics, glucocorticosteroids, amphotericin or excessive losses from the gastrointestinal tract (e.g. due to diarrhoea or vomiting).

It leads to muscle weakness, paralytic ileus, cardiac conduction defects, cardiac arrhythmias, metabolic alkalosis and confusion. The serum potassium and chloride are low and bicarbonate elevated. The ECG may be abnormal. Treatment is by removal of the cause, if possible, and the intravenous administration of potassium chloride. Potassium injections must be well diluted and administered slowly at a maximum rate of 10–20 mmol per hour.

Solutions containing up to 40 mmol/L can be infused into a peripheral line without causing localised pain. If higher concentrations are required, because of the need to restrict fluids, a central vein should be used.

When preparing infusions, bags or bottles must be shaken well and inverted several times after adding the potassium to ensure thorough mixing.

Phlebitis and pain on injection may occur. Rapid intravenous administration may result in hyperkalaemia manifesting as muscle weakness, paralysis, hypotension, cardiac arrhythmias, heart block or cardiac arrest.

Extravasation should be avoided. Potassium must never be given by bolus injection or injected undiluted.

Potassium Excess (Hyperkalaemia)

Hyperkalaemia results from excessive intake or inadequate excretion or release of potassium from damaged cells. For example, it may be caused by excessive administration of potassium, renal failure, metabolic acidosis, crush injuries, the use of angiotensin converting enzyme inhibitors or potassium sparing diuretics, or adrenal insufficiency.

It leads to muscular weakness, diarrhoea, paraesthesia, cardiac conduction defects, bradycardia, cardiac arrhythmias, ventricular fibrillation and cardiac arrest. The serum potassium is high and there are ECG abnormalities. Treatment is by removal of the cause if possible, the discontinuation of potassium intake, the administration of oral or rectal sodium polystyrene sulfonate (*Resonium A*), a cation exchange resin, or the administration of intravenous insulin and glucose. Haemodialysis may be necessary. See Chapter 14 Drugs Used in Renal Failure.

Calcium Deficit (Hypocalcaemia)

Hypocalcaemia may result from inadequate intake of calcium, vitamin D deficiency, metabolic abnormalities such as hypoparathyroidism, acute pancreatitis, magnesium depletion, hyperphosphataemia, renal failure or excessive infusions of citrated blood.

It causes paraesthesia, muscle cramps, tetany, convulsions, cardiac conduction abnormalities and, in the long term, rickets and osteomalacia. The serum calcium is low (correction of the reading is necessary if the serum albumin is also low) and there are ECG abnormalities. Treatment is to correct the cause, if possible, and the administration of a phosphate binding agent or vitamin D, or replacement with intravenous calcium gluconate or calcium chloride given as a bolus injection. For further information see Chapter 32 Drugs Used in Critical Care.

Calcium Excess (Hypercalcaemia)

Hypercalcaemia can result from malignancies, hyperparathyroidism or excessive vitamin D or calcium intake. It causes nausea, vomiting, polyuria, confusion, coma and cardiac arrhythmias. The serum calcium level is high and abnormalities are seen on the ECG. Treatment is by control of the underlying disease, the discontinuation of calcium intake, the administration of 0.9% sodium choloride in water with the diuretic frusemide, or the infusion of disodium pamidronate.

Magnesium Deficit (Hypomagnesaemia)

Hypomagnesaemia results from decreased or inadequate magnesium intake, loss from the gastrointestinal tract, diuretics, acute pancreatitis or chronic alcoholism. It causes neuromuscular excitability with cramps and tetany, central nervous system irritability with confusion and convulsions, and tachycardia. The serum magnesium is low. Treatment is the administration of intravenous magnesium sulfate by bolus injection or infusion. For further information see Chapter 20 Drug Therapy in Pregnancy and Labour.

Magnesium Excess (Hypermagnesaemia)

Hypermagnesaemia is caused by excessive intake, e.g. magnesium containing medication, inadequate excretion, e.g. in renal failure, uncontrolled diabetes mellitus, hypothyroidism or metabolic acidosis. It impairs neuromuscular function, reduces cardiac contraction and can lead to stupor, coma and depression of the respiratory centre. The serum magnesium is high and there may be ECG abnormalities. Treatment is by removal of the cause and intravenous administration of calcium gluconate or calcium chloride. Haemodialysis may be necessary.

Phosphate Deficit (Hypophosphataemia)

Hypophosphataemia results from primary hyperparathyroidism, vitamin D deficiency, metabolic alkalosis, renal tubular defects, glucose based parenteral nutrition, low phosphate intake or chronic alcoholism. It causes impaired cellular energy stores, paraesthesia, weakness, haematologial abnormalities, reduced renal tubular bicarbonate reabsorption, rickets and osteomalacia. The serum phosphate is low. Treatment is by the intravenous infusion of phosphate as the sodium or potassium salt.

Parenteral administration can cause hypocalcaemic tetany, hypotension, oedema and acute renal failure. Excessive administration may cause hyperphosphataemia.

Extravasation should be avoided. Phosphate must never be given by bolus injection or injected undiluted.

Phosphate Excess (Hyperphosphataemia)

Causes of hyperphosphataemia include hypoparathyroidism, vitamin D excess, renal failure, metabolic acidosis or excessive intake. It influences calcium homeostasis with the development of ectopic calcification, secondary hyperparathyroidism and renal osteodystrophy. The serum phosphate level is high. Treatment is of the cause, reducing phosphate intake or the administration of phosphate binding agents. See Chapter 14 Drugs Used in Renal Failure.

Chloride Deficit (Hypochloraemia)

Hypochloraemia may result from a low sodium chloride intake, excessive diuretic therapy, excessive gastric losses, sweating without adequate water intake, potassium depletion or metabolic alkalosis. The serum chloride and potassium are low and the bicarbonate high. Treatment is by the administration of chloride as both the sodium and potassium salt.

FLUID AND ELECTROLYTES

18

Chloride Excess (Hyperchloraemia)

Hyperchloraemia may result from excessive chloride intake, dehydration or hyperchloraemic acidosis. The serum chloride is high. It is treated by a reduction in the administration of chloride.

ACID–BASE IMBALANCE

pH is a measure of acidity. For survival, the acidity of body fluids must be maintained between the very narrow range of 7.35–7.45. A pH of less than 7.35 implies acidosis and above 7.45 alkalosis.

The body has renal and respiratory homeostatic mechanisms and buffer systems (which limit changes in pH) to maintain a pH in the normal range while coping with the constant production of acid (hydrogen ion, H^+). When an imbalance occurs it is either metabolic or respiratory, depending on the cause.

Metabolic Acidosis

Metabolic acidosis may be due to renal disease, ketoacidosis, lactic acidosis, severe vomiting or diarrhoea, and overload with intravenous sodium chloride solutions. It causes fatigue, confusion and coma. Hyperventilation, shock, and vascular collapse can occur. The pH is less than 7.35, the serum bicarbonate is reduced and potassium is high. The pCO_2 is reduced. The treatment depends on the cause and is directed towards the underlying condition. Chronic renal failure and renal tubular acidosis may necessitate intravenous bicarbonate, acute renal failure requires dialysis, and diabetic ketoacidosis requires insulin and intravenous infusions of sodium and potassium chloride.

Metabolic Alkalosis

Metabolic alkalosis is due to chloride depletion from vomiting, gastrointestinal suction or diuretic therapy, severe potassium depletion, excess alkali intake or excess adrenocorticotrophic hormone. It causes apathy, confusion, shallow respiration, irregular pulse, cardiac dilation or decompensation, and muscle tetany and convulsions. The serum bicarbonate level is elevated, potassium and chloride are low and the pH is greater than 7.45. The pCO_2 is elevated. There may be ECG abnormalities. The treatment again depends on the cause of the alkalosis. It is usual to administer intravenous sodium chloride and potassium chloride in water. If severe it may be necessary to use arginine hydrochloride or hydrochloric acid infusions.

Respiratory Acidosis

Respiratory acidosis is due to respiratory dysfunction which leads to inadequate excretion of carbon dioxide by the lungs. This may result from pneumonia, emphysema, bronchiectasis, pulmonary oedema or neuromuscular disorders involving the muscles used in respiration. It causes respiratory distress, tachycardia, cyanosis, weakness and coma. The pCO_2 is elevated and serum chloride is low. The pH is less than 7.35 and the serum bicarbonate is high. Treatment is directed at the cause with the objective of improving respiratory function, e.g. use of antibiotics if pneumonia is the cause or diuretics if pulmonary oedema is the problem. Respiration may have to be assisted.

Respiratory Alkalosis

Respiratory alkalosis is due to an increase in the rate and depth of respiration leading to an excessive loss of carbon dioxide. This may result from anxiety, hysteria, salicylate intoxication, encephalitis, trauma, high altitude or mechanical ventilation. It causes light headedness, paraesthesia, tetany, convulsions and coma. The pH is greater than 7.45, the pCO_2 is low and there is a compensatory decrease in serum bicarbonate. Treatment is directed towards the cause or rebreathing into a bag.

NURSING IMPLICATIONS

ASSESSMENT

The clinical features of specific fluid and electrolyte disturbances and potential causes of disturbance (e.g. vomiting, wound drainage) must be documented so that the patient's response to therapy can be calculated. Patients undergoing surgery should be assessed before surgery to establish a baseline of physiological parameters. Assessment should include weight, cardiovascular and respiratory parameters, temperature and neurological status. The condition of the skin, mucous membranes and tissue turgor are useful guides to hydration.

Nurses must be familiar with local policy on the management of intravenous therapy with regard to: medication orders and documentation of administration; addition of medications to infusions; checking of solutions to be administered; selection and changing of giving sets; management of cannulation sites; and nursing observation and records.

ADMINISTRATION

Cannulae must be secure, but the site should be able to be inspected easily. If an arm vein or hand vein is to be cannulated, the patient will be less restricted if the non-dominant side is chosen. Safety and patient comfort are appropriate criteria in the selection of a method for dressing the cannula site and securing tubing.

Flow rates must be maintained according to the medication order, so frequent and regular checking is essential. Giving sets delivering small or large drops, with or without burettes, should be selected according to the patient's needs and local policy. Giving sets with burettes (delivering small drops) enable good control of flow rate and reduce the potential for over-infusion. Infusion pumps are used where even greater control is needed. Nurses must be familiar with the operation and limitations of pump devices. The cannulation site must be inspected frequently, since pumps can deliver fluid into tissues if cannulae dislodge. The appropriate giving set must be selected for use with the pump. However, no giving set or pump makes skilled nursing management unnecessary. A 'timing tape', attached to the container and showing the expected fluid level at regular intervals, is a useful aid to monitoring flow over long periods.

As a general rule, infusions that are running well behind schedule should not be 'caught up' quickly, because of the dangers of fluid overload. Solutions containing potassium should never be infused faster than the prescribed rate. Discrepancies between the prescribed regimen and the actual delivery over a period of hours must be reported to the prescriber, so that the schedule can be adjusted if necessary.

Adjustments to flow rates may be necessary if medications are added to burettes intermittently. These medications must be delivered at the rate prescribed for them, and the primary infusion adjusted after delivery of the medication. Great care should be taken with labelling, and avoiding too rapid infusion and extravasation of drugs.

Flow may be reduced or stopped by a change in limb position, restrictive clothing, the cannula tip being occluded by the vessel wall, or by the cannula piercing the vessel wall allowing fluid to leak into the tissues. Thrombus formation at the tip of the cannula or in the lumen can occlude flow. Thrombus may be aspirated from the cannula, using aseptic technique, but must *never* be irrigated into the vein, because of the danger of embolus. Air bubbles must always be removed from the giving set for the same reason.

If doubt exists about the position or patency of the cannula, the fluid container can be momentarily lowered below the level of the cannula. Backflow of blood into the tubing indicates that the cannula is properly positioned.

FLUID AND ELECTROLYTES

18

When arterial pressures are recorded with a sphygmomanometer, the cuff should not be applied to the cannulated limb if possible. The vein will be temporarily occluded as the cuff is inflated to systolic pressure, flow will be interrupted and the cannula may become dislodged and need to be replaced.

Accurate fluid balance records must be maintained during intravenous therapy. The record usually acts as both an intake and output record, and the documentation of the administration of prescribed substances. If the medication order is written on the fluid balance record this must then be treated and filed as a legal document. Daily weight records are a reliable adjunct to the fluid balance chart.

EVALUATION

The patient's response to intravenous therapy is evaluated by his/her clinical state and by monitoring blood chemistry and haematological parameters. Cardiovascular and respiratory signs should be observed regularly. The urine output and specific gravity should be monitored with regard to the patient's original condition and the volume and nature of the fluid infused. Changes in thirst, the condition of the mucous membranes and skin turgor should be evaluated against the initial assessment.

A rise in temperature, even with no other signs of infection, may indicate catheter sepsis. Pyrogenic reactions can occur if the infusion fluid is contaminated with bacterial endotoxins. Symptoms usually occur within 30 to 60 minutes of commencing the infusion and include a sudden rise in temperature, headache, malaise, nausea and rigors. The medical officer must be notified, the infusion stopped and the cannula removed. Infusion fluids and cannulae may be sent for microbiological examination. Pyrogenic symptoms may be treated by administration of an antipyretic drug, e.g. aspirin.

The cannula site must be inspected regularly, so that the appropriate action can be taken if tissue infiltration or thrombophlebitis occur. Local infiltration is signified by a sluggish flow rate, pain and swelling around the vein. Hypertonic, acidic or basic solutions and some medication can cause tissue necrosis. Thrombophlebitis and inflammation around the cannula site result from chemical, mechanical or microbiological irritation to the vein. The signs are pain, redness and swelling. The infusion should be discontinued and the cannula resited if either of these problems occurs.

Cardiovascular and respiratory status must be evaluated for signs of circulatory overload or air embolus. Circulatory overload results from infusion of excessive volumes of fluid. Symptoms are elevated venous pressure (and sometimes arterial pressure), venous distention, dyspnoea and production of frothy sputum, indicating pulmonary oedema. The medical officer must be notified, and the infusion slowed down to a rate sufficient only to maintain patency of the cannula. The cannula should not be removed, since intravenous drug treatment might be necessary.

Air embolus results from air being infused through the giving set and a large bubble or bubbles lodging in the pulmonary circulation. Symptoms are dyspnoea, cyanosis, hypotension, tachycardia and loss of consciousness. The infusion must be stopped. Oxygen should be administered with the patient lying on the left side with the head down. The vital signs should be recorded and the medical officer notified immediately.

PATIENT EDUCATION

The reasons for the intravenous therapy, its expected duration and the limitations it will impose on movement and activities should be explained to patients. They should know to report any pain at the cannula site or breathlessness. If the initial disturbance was caused by a fluid or dietary intake problem, advice about avoiding the problem in the future should be given.

FURTHER READING

Oh, T.E. (ed) (1990) *Intensive care manual*, 3rd edn. Butterworths, Sydney.

Phillips, G.D. and Odgers, C.L. (1986) *Parenteral and enteral nutrition, a practical guide*, 3rd edn. Churchill Livingston.

Vickers, M.D., Morgan, M., Spencer, P.S.J. (1991) *Drugs in anaesthetic practice*, 7th edn. Butterworth-Heinemann.

Young, L.Y., Koda-Kimble, M.A. (eds) (1992) *Applied therapeutics — the clinical use of drugs*, 5th edn. Applied Therapeutics Inc, Vancouver, Wa, pp. 635–674.

TEST YOUR KNOWLEDGE

1. The water content of a 70-kg 25-year old male is approximately: (a) 7 L; (b) 28 L; (c) 42 L; (d) 63 L.

2. The most abundant electrolytes of the extracellular space are: (a) sodium and chloride; (b) sodium and potassium; (c) sodium and calcium; (d) chloride and potassium.

3. The most abundant electrolyte of the intracellular space is: (a) sodium; (b) potassium; (c) calcium; (d) phosphate.

4. An isotonic solution has: (a) the same osmolality as plasma; (b) the same concentration of potassium as plasma; (c) the same concentration of sodium as plasma; (d) an osmolality of approximately 290 mosmol per kg.

5. The electrolyte sodium is: (a) a cation; (b) primarily involved with regulation of the water balance of the intracellular fluid; (c) primarily involved with bone formation; (d) primarily involved with blood clotting.

6. A patient who is volume depleted may have: (a) increased pulse, decreased urine output and thirst; (b) increased pulse, normal urine output and hypertension; (c) decreased pulse, normal urine output and hypertension; (d) decreased pulse, decreased urine output and hypertension.

7. The following solutions are all crystalloids: (a) 0.9% NaCl in water, Hartmann's solution, 5% albumin; (b) 0.9% NaCl in water, Hartmann's solution, *Haemaccel*; (c) fresh frozen plasma, dextran 40 in 0.9% NaCl, 5% glucose; (d) 0.9% NaCl in water, 0.9% NaCl + 30 mmol KCl in water, Hartmann's solution.

8. A 70-kg 40-year old healthy male has had an uncomplicated hiatus hernia repair. A suitable IV regimen for use in the 24-hour nil by mouth period after operation might be: (a) 1 L Hartmann's over 24 hours; (b) 3 L 5% glucose, each litre over 8 hours; (c) 1 L Hartmann's over 8 hours, 1 L 0.9% NaCl + 30 mmol KCl over 8 hours, 1 L 5% glucose + 30 mmol KCl over 8 hours; (d) 500 mL dextran 40 in 0.9% NaCl over 1 hour, then 1 L 0.9% NaCl and 10 mmol KCl over 23 hours.

9. A 50-kg 70-year old female with chronic renal failure and congestive cardiac failure has had an uncomplicated hysterectomy. A suitable IV regimen for use in the 24-hour nil by mouth period after operation might be: (a) 1 L Hartmann's over 6 hours, then 3 L 5% glucose each litre over 6 hours; (b) 1 L 4% glucose + 0.18% NaCl with 60 mmol KCl over 24 hours; (c) 1 L Hartmann's over 12 hours then 1 L 5% glucose over 12 hours; (d) 500 mL 0.9% NaCl + 60 mmol KCl over 24 hours.

10. Part of the treatment of metabolic alkalosis might include: (a) infusion of 500 mL 8.4% sodium bicarbonate over 1 hour; (b) infusion of 1 L 0.9% NaCl + KCl over 8 hours; (c) rebreathing into a bag; (d) infusion of 30 mL neutral insulin in 1 L 5% glucose over 24 hours.

FLUID AND ELECTROLYTES

18

Endocrine Diseases

DAVID B. CUNNINGHAM

O B J E C T I V E S

At the conclusion of this chapter the reader should be able to:

1. List the drugs used in the treatment of the major endocrine disorders;

2. Understand the mechanism of action of these drugs;

3. List the adverse effects associated with the use of these drugs; and

4. Describe the implications for patient care which arise from the use of these drugs.

DRUGS AND THE ENDOCRINE SYSTEM ▅▅▅▅▅▅▅▅▅

The endocrine system consists of a number of ductless glands which release hormones, protein or steroid, directly into the blood. These hormones travel in the circulation to distant sites of action where they affect processes of homeostasis, metabolism, reproduction and response to stress. Endocrine diseases such as diabetes mellitus, thyrotoxicosis and Addisons disease are related to either an oversupply or deficiency of these hormones. Drugs used in the treatment of endocrine disorders act in one of five ways:

1. replacement of hormones;

2. stimulation of hormone production;

3. stimulation of hormone release;

4. blockage of hormone production; or

5. blockage of hormone action.

The synthesis of endocrine hormones and their chemical alteration has lead to the production of powerful therapeutic agents such as the corticosteroids which are used in many non-endocrine disorders.

HYPOTHALAMIC AND PITUITARY HORMONES ▅▅▅▅▅▅▅▅▅

The hormones of the hypothalamus act on the pituitary to cause the release of pituitary hormones which have diverse effects on endocrine and non-endocrine organs of the body. Analogues of hypothalamic and pituitary hormones have been developed and are used in the diagnosis and treatment of many endocrine and non-endocrine diseases.

HYPOTHALAMIC HORMONES AND ANALOGUES

Gonadorelin (gonadotropin releasing hormone, GnRH) is used in the assessment of pituitary function and the treatment of amenorrhoea and infertility. Goserelin is an analogue of gonadorelin and has been used in the treatment of metastatic prostate cancer.

Protirelin (thyrotropin releasing hormone, TRH) is used in the differential diagnosis of thyroid disorders.

POSTERIOR PITUITARY HORMONES AND ANALOGUES

Vasopressin (antidiuretic hormone, ADH) is used in the treatment of diabetes insipidus, haemophilia and bleeding oesophageal varices. Desmopressin (DDAVP) is an analogue of ADH which has to a large degree replaced the use of vasopressin in the treatment of diabetes insipidus. The advantages of desmopressin are a longer half-life in plasma and the absence of vasoconstrictor effects. It is given parenterally after pituitary surgery and in unconscious patients. Maintenance therapy is by nasal instillation.

Chlorthalidone, chlorpropamide and carbamazepine have also been used in the treatment of diabetes insipidus.

Demeclocycline *(Ledermycin)*, a tetracycline antibiotic, is used in the treatment of the syndrome of inappropriate secretion of antidiuretic hormone (SIADH). The drug reverses the hyponatraemia seen in this disorder probably by antagonising the action of the hormone on the renal tubule. Treatment is usually started with 900–1200 mg per day in divided doses and then reduced to a maintenance dose of 600–900 mg per day.

Oxytocin is another posterior pituitary hormone and is used in obstetric practice. For further information on oxytocin see Chapter 20, Drug Therapy in Pregnancy and Labour.

Vasopressin

TRADE NAMES

Vasopressin: *Pitressin.*

MECHANISM OF ACTION

The main action of vasopressin is a direct antidiuretic effect on the kidney. Water is reabsorbed by the kidney tubules and the urine is concentrated. Vasopressin also causes contraction of smooth muscle in blood vessels and other organs, in particular the gastrointestinal tract, bladder and gall bladder. Vasopressin causes the release of factor VIII from blood vessels.

PHARMACOKINETICS

Vasopressin is rapidly inactivated by peptidases in various tissues. The liver and the kidney are both important in the clearance of vasopressin from the circulation. Vasopressin is ineffective if given orally.

USES

When used in the treatment of diabetes insipidus vasopressin is given by intramuscular or subcutaneous injection or intranasally. The dose by injection is 5–10 units two to three times daily. This dose must be adjusted to maintain an adequate diuresis. Intranasal dosing is tailored to the patient's response.

Vasopressin is given by intravenous infusion or intra-arterial infusion in the treatment of bleeding oesophageal varices. Vasopressin is used as an aid in abdominal X-ray and to prevent and treat postoperative abdominal distention.

Vasopressin is available as a solution for injection containing 20 units in 1 mL.

ADVERSE DRUG REACTIONS

Anaphylaxis and other allergic reactions may occur after administration of vasopressin. Other adverse effects associated with the use of vasopressin are related to its effect on the vasculature and smooth muscle of the gastrointestinal tract and include pallor, nausea, desire to defaecate, abdominal cramps, increased blood pressure, angina and myocardial ischaemia.

PRECAUTIONS AND CONTRAINDICATIONS

Careful attention to water intake and adequate diuresis is important in patients treated with vasopressin to avoid water intoxication and hyponatraemia.

Vasopressin should be used with caution in patients with cardiac disease because it may cause vasoconstriction and water retention. The antidiuretic effect of vasopressin may also cause problems in patients with chronic nephritis, asthma, epilepsy and migraine.

Desmopressin

MECHANISM OF ACTION

Desmopressin is an analogue of vasopressin and has similar actions. It has a more potent antidiuretic action but markedly less effect on blood pressure.

PHARMACOKINETICS

Desmopressin is ineffective if given orally. After parenteral dosing, bioavailability is approximately 100%. Since bioavailability after intranasal dosing is approximately 10% intranasal doses are normally 10 times greater than parenteral doses.

ENDOCRINE DISEASES

19

USES

In the treatment of diabetes insipidus desmopressin is used by nasal instillation at a dose of 10–40 micrograms or by intravenous or intramuscular injection at a dose of 1–4 micrograms per day. It is usually given in two doses a day but some patients may be controlled with a single daily dose. The dose should be individualised after assessment of patient response.

Desmopressin is available as a 100 micrograms/mL solution for nasal instillation and in 4 micrograms/mL ampoules for parenteral use.

Desmopressin is also used in the diagnosis of disorders of renal concentrating capacity.

In the prophylaxis and treatment of bleeding associated with von Willebrand's disease, haemophilia A and certain platelet disorders, desmopressin may be given by intravenous infusion.

For intranasal administration the dose is loaded into a plastic tube marked to allow measurement of the dose. One end of the tube is placed in the nose and one in the mouth and the dose blown into the nostril.

Doses for intravenous or intramuscular injection should be measured using an insulin syringe.

ADVERSE DRUG REACTIONS

Desmopressin is generally well tolerated and there are few adverse reactions at normal doses used in the treatment of diabetes insipidus. The reactions reported are similar to those seen with vasopressin but the incidence is lower. When large doses are given, e.g. in the treatment of bleeding disorders, desmopressin may cause a decrease in blood pressure.

DRUG INTERACTIONS

Glibenclamide has been reported to reduce the effect of desmopressin in diabetes insipidus.

Chlorpropamide and clofibrate may potentiate the effects of desmopressin.

PRECAUTIONS AND CONTRAINDICATIONS

Careful attention to water intake and adequate diuresis is important in patients treated with desmopressin to avoid water intoxication and hyponatraemia.

Desmopressin should be used with caution in patients with cardiac disease because it may cause water retention. The antidiuretic effect may also cause problems in patients with chronic nephritis, asthma, epilepsy and migraine.

NURSING IMPLICATIONS

Patients should be carefully assessed and educated if they are to self-administer desmopressin. They should be cautioned to avoid excess fluid intake and monitor fluid balance.

ANTERIOR PITUITARY HORMONES AND ANALOGUES

Corticotropin (ACTH) and its analogue tetracosactrin are used in the diagnosis of disorders of the hypothalamic-pituitary-adrenal (HPA) axis. Long acting depot preparations have been used as an alternative to corticosteroid therapy in conditions such as Crohn's disease and rheumatoid arthritis. Some investigators report advantages over corticosteroids such as reduced HPA axis suppression and less growth retardation in children. However, accurate dosing is difficult since the effect depends on the level of response of the patient's adrenal glands.

Human growth hormone (HGH) has been used as replacement therapy in children of short stature who lack the hormone. This product has now been replaced by somatropin, a synthetic human growth hormone produced by recombinant DNA technology, as a result of concern over the transmission of slow viral diseases from products derived from human tissue.

Bromocriptine and octreotide are used in the treatment of acromegaly, a condition of excess growth hormone.

Human follicle stimulating hormone (FSH) is used in combination with human chorionic gonadotropin (HCG) in the treatment of infertility in patients with proven hypopituitarism, see Chapter 21 Contraception and Infertility.

Thyrotropin (thyroid stimulating hormone, TSH) is used in the differential diagnosis of hypothyroidism.

Corticotropin, Tetracosactrin

TRADE NAMES

Corticotropin: *Acthargel.*
Tetracosactrin: *Synacthen; Synacthen Depot.*

MECHANISM OF ACTION

Corticotropin acts by causing the release of corticosteroids from the adrenal glands. Its action is therefore indirect and relies on the presence of an adequate adrenal reserve. Because of this indirect mode of action the effect is less easily controlled than that with corticosteroid therapy. The supposed advantage of corticotropin over corticosteroid therapy is that less adrenal suppression may result.

Tetracosactrin is an analogue of corticotropin and is used in the treatment of corticosteroid responsive conditions and the diagnosis of disorders of the HPA axis.

PHARMACOKINETICS

Both drugs are destroyed by enzymes in the gastrointestinal tract. They are rapidly absorbed following intramuscular injection.

Corticotropin is available as an intramuscular injection in gel form to retard release into the circulation and prolong action. Tetracosactrin is available as a solution for injection (*Synacthen*) and as a long acting depot form (*Synacthen Depot*).

USES

Tetracosactrin as a solution for injection is

given at a dose of 250 micrograms in the diagnosis of adrenal insufficiency.

Corticotropin gel and tetracosactrin depot injection are used in the treatment of corticosteroid responsive conditions such as gout and rheumatoid arthritis. An initial dose of 40–80 units of corticotropin gel or 1 mg of tetracosactrin depot is given by intramuscular injection and then the dose is individualised according to response.

For information on adverse drug reactions, drug interactions and precautions and contraindications see the section on corticosteroids.

Growth Hormones and Analogues

TRADE NAMES

Somatrem: *Somatonorm.*
Somatropin: *Humatrope; Norditropin.*

MECHANISM OF ACTION

Growth hormone of human origin and synthetic growth hormone products stimulate growth and have complex effects on the metabolism of nitrogen, carbohydrates and lipids.

PHARMACOKINETICS

Growth hormone and its synthetic analogues are given by intramuscular or subcutaneous injection. The action of these agents is not directly related to their persistence in plasma.

USES

Human growth hormone has now largely been replaced by the synthetic products somatrem (methionyl human growth hormone) and somatropin (biosynthetic human growth hormone).

These products are used in the treatment of growth failure due to growth hormone deficiency in children. Dosing is complex and related to response which must be carefully monitored.

ADVERSE DRUG REACTIONS

Development of antibodies has been reported and may interfere with treatment.

ENDOCRINE DISEASES

19

Local reactions such as lipoatrophy may occur with prolonged subcutaneous use. Glucose intolerance may occur and require alteration to therapy in diabetic patients.

PRECAUTIONS AND CONTRAINDICATIONS

Treatment with growth hormone products should only be initiated in patients with open epiphyses. Use of these products in patients with other pituitary hormone deficiency states requires caution. Diabetes mellitus will require careful management in patients being treated with growth hormone products.

Octreotide

TRADE NAMES

Octreotide: *Sandostatin*.

MECHANISM OF ACTION

Octreotide is a synthetic analogue of somatostatin. Somatostatin is a naturally occurring hormone which inhibits the release of growth hormone by the pituitary. Somatostatin also has an affect on the release of insulin and glucagon and on gastrointestinal function and motility.

PHARMACOKINETICS

Octreotide is poorly absorbed after oral administration and is usually given by subcutaneous injection or intravenous injection. Peak plasma levels are lower after subcutaneous administration compared to intravenous administration but bioavailability is similar.

The kidney is the most important organ involved in the elimination of octreotide and clearance is significantly reduced in renal failure.

USES

Octreotide is used for the treatment of acromegaly and relief of symptoms associated with gastroenteropancreatic tumours. Its use in gastrointestinal fistulae and oesophageal varices is under investigation.

Octreotide is available as a solution for injection in ampoules containing 0.05 mg, 0.1 mg and 0.5 mg octreotide. The most common method of administration is subcutaneous injection.

In the treatment of acromegaly octreotide is administered in an initial dose of 0.05–0.1 mg every 8–12 hours. Therapy is monitored using growth hormone levels and clinical response and the dose can be increased to a maximun of 0.5 mg every 8 hours if necessary.

ADVERSE DRUG REACTIONS

Octreotide is usually well tolerated. The most commonly reported side effects are related to the gastrointestinal tract and include nausea, vomiting, diarrhoea, abdominal pain and discomfort. Dizziness, headache, fatigue and weakness have also been reported by some patients. Octreotide administration has been associated with the development of gallstones.

Subcutaneous injection may be accompanied by pain at the injection site. Sites of injection should be rotated.

DRUG INTERACTIONS

Insulin doses may need to be reduced in diabetic patients receiving octreotide.

PRECAUTIONS AND CONTRAINDICATIONS

Patients receiving octreotide should be monitored for the development of gallstones, changes in visual fields which may indicate pituitary tumour expansion, and loss of control of diabetes.

Bromocriptine

TRADE NAMES

Bromocriptine: *Parlodel*.

MECHANISM OF ACTION

The major action of bromocriptine is inhibition of the release of prolactin from the anterior pituitary gland. It also suppresses growth hormone levels in some patients with acromegaly and activates dopamine receptors, i.e. it is a dopamine agonist.

PHARMACOKINETICS

Bromocriptine is well absorbed after oral administration and widely distributed to all tissues. Metabolism by the liver is the major route of elimination.

USES

Bromocriptine is used in the treatment of acromegaly. Approximately 50% of treated patients will show a reduction in growth hormone levels and severity of symptoms. It is also used in the suppression of physiological lactation and the treatment of hyperprolactinaemia and Parkinson's disease.

Bromocriptine is available as 2.5 mg tablets and 5 mg and 10 mg capsules.

In the treatment of acromegaly bromocriptine is given in a starting dose of 1.25 mg at night which is then increased slowly over a period of weeks to 10 mg a day. The daily dose may be increased to a maximum of 60 mg and should be divided into four daily doses.

For information on the use of bromocriptine in Parkinsons disease see Chapter 25 Neurological Disorders.

ADVERSE DRUG REACTIONS

Commonly ocurring side effects include nausea, dizziness, drowsiness and headache. These side effects may reduce with continued therapy. Bromocriptine may cause postural hypotension and reversible pallor of the fingers and toes.

In high doses dry mouth, leg cramps, pleural effusions and retroperitoneal fibrosis have been reported as have various neuropsychiatric side effects such as confusion, psychomotor excitation, hallucinations and dyskinesias. Gastric haemorrhage has been reported in patients being treated for acromegaly.

PRECAUTIONS AND CONTRAINDICATIONS

Bromocriptine should be introduced slowly and patients warned of the likelihood of postural hypotension and drowsiness which may interfere with their ability to drive and operate machinery.

Patients should be monitored for the development of gastrointestinal bleeding, retroperitoneal fibrosis and pulmonary effusion. Female patients being treated with bromocriptine should have regular gynaecological assessments. Diabetic patients receiving bromocriptine should be carefully monitored.

Bromocriptine is contraindicated in pregnancy and breast feeding.

THYROID HORMONES AND ANTITHYROID DRUGS

The thyroid gland is responsible for maintaining the optimal level of metabolism for normal physiological function. Thyroxine (T_4) and triiodothyronine (T_3) are the two principal hormones secreted by the thyroid gland. Secretion of these hormones is regulated by thyroid stimulating hormone (TSH) released from the anterior pituitary in response to changes in the internal and external environment. Release of TSH is regulated by neural input from the hypothalamus and negative feedback on the pituitary of circulating thyroid hormones.

Hypothyroidism occurs when there is a low level of thyroid hormones and causes a slowing of metabolic rate, intolerance to cold, weight gain and mental and physical slowing.

Hyperthyroidism or thyrotoxicosis occurs when there is a high level of thyroid hormone and causes weight loss, nervousness, tachycardia, tremor and intolerance to heat.

DRUG TREATMENT OF HYPOTHYROIDISM

The drug treatment of hypothyroidism consists of replacement with synthetic thyroid hormones or natural hormone extracts of animal origin. Synthetic hormones have largely replaced natural hormone preparations because of problems with standardisation of

ENDOCRINE DISEASES

19

potency with products derived from animal thyroid tissue.

Thyroxine

TRADE NAMES

Thyroxine: *Oroxine*.

MECHANISM OF ACTION

Thyroxine is converted in the body to triiodothyronine the active form of the hormone. The major effect of thyroxine is to increase the metabolic rate.

PHARMACOKINETICS

Once daily dosing is possible due to the long half-life of thyroxine but doses need to be individualised because of erratic absorption from the gastrointestinal tract.

USES

Synthetic thyroxine is the preferred agent for replacement therapy in hypothyroidism. Administration of thyroxine should start with small doses and be gradually increased until thyroid function tests are normal and symptoms of hypothyroidism have disappeared. Normal replacement doses usually range from 50–200 micrograms per day. If thyroxine doses are increased too quickly then the patient may suffer from the same symptoms seen in thyrotoxicosis.

ADVERSE DRUG REACTIONS

Adverse effects of thyroid hormone therapy are the same as those seen in patients suffering from hyperthyroidism. Symptoms of over medication may include anginal pain, arrhythmias, sweating, diarrhoea, weight loss and tremor.

DRUG INTERACTIONS

Because of its affect on metabolic rate thyroxine may alter the effect of other drugs given concurrently. The action of anticoagulants may be enhanced by thyroxine administration and diabetic patients may require additional insulin when treated with the drug.

PRECAUTIONS AND CONTRAINDICATIONS

Thyroxine should be used with caution in the elderly and those with cardiac disease or adrenal insufficiency.

Triiodothyronine

TRADE NAMES

Triiodothyronine (liothyronine): *Tertroxin*.

MECHANISM OF ACTION

Synthetic triiodothyronine is also known as liothyronine. It is the active form of thyroid hormone found in the body and is more potent than thyroxine.

PHARMACOKINETICS

Triiodothyronine is more rapidly and completely absorbed than thyroxine but has a shorter half-life.

USES

Triiodothyronine 20 micrograms is equivalent to 60–100 micrograms of thyroxine. Because it is available in a parenteral form and has a more rapid onset of action it is the agent of choice in severe hypothyroid states and where oral therapy is not possible.

For information on adverse drug reactions, drug interactions, precautions and contraindications see thyroxine.

NURSING IMPLICATIONS

ASSESSMENT

The patient's vital signs should be checked and related to their current thyroid status. Temperature, blood pressure, pulse rate and respiration rate are all good indicators of thyroid status. History taking should include attention to recent weight change, appetite, bowel activity, agitation or lethargy and response to environmental temperature. Note should be taken of any intercurrent medical conditions or drug

therapy which may be affected by thyroid hormone administration. Particular attention should be paid to diseases such as diabetes and angina and patients who are taking anticoagulants.

EVALUATION

The vital signs and factors noted during assessment should be monitored during treatment with thyroid hormone products. Through close attention to these factors the adverse effects related to overdose with thyroid hormones may be avoided. Weight, bowel activity, appetite and mental status are all important in monitoring the effectiveness of therapy. Regular biochemical testing of thyroid function is basic to normalisation of thyroid hormone levels. Hypothyroid patients may be particularly sensitive to sedative/hypnotic drugs and they should be used with caution in these patients. Response to drug therapy for other non-thyroid conditions may alter as thyroid hormone levels normalise and dosage adjustments may be necessary.

PATIENT EDUCATION

Drug treatment for hypothyroidism is life long and patients should understand the importance of compliance. It should be stressed that they should not cease taking their medication or alter the dose without consulting a doctor. Patients should be able to recognise the symptoms associated with hypo- and hyperthyroidism and know to contact their doctor if they experience these symptoms.

ANTITHYROID DRUGS

The treatment of hyperthyroidism has three main components, surgical removal of part of the thyroid gland, partial destruction of the thyroid gland by the administration of radioactive iodine and the administration of antithyroid drugs. Patients may require therapy with thyroxine after ablative techniques, e.g. surgery or radioactive iodine. The two major drugs used in the medical treatment of hyperthyroidism are carbimazole and propylthiouracil.

Carbimazole

TRADE NAMES

Carbimazole: *Neomercazole*.

MECHANISM OF ACTION

The major mechanism of action of carbimazole is to prevent the incorporation of iodine into the thyroid hormones.

PHARMACOKINETICS

Carbimazole is rapidly absorbed from the gastrointestinal tract and metabolised to methimazole, the active form of the drug. Methimazole has a short half-life in plasma but the biological effects persist for a longer time. Methimazole crosses the placenta and is present in breast milk.

USES

Carbimazole is used before thyroid surgery to reduce the activity of the thyroid, for prolonged periods to produce remission in Grave's disease and in the treatment of decompensated thyrotoxicosis or thyroid storm. Therapy is started with a high dose (30–60 mg per day in three divided doses) which is continued until the patient is euthyroid, this may take 2–4 months. Therapy is then continued at a lower dose (5–15 mg per day) for 12 to 24 months and the patient is given thyroxine if they become hypothyroid. If the patient experiences a relapse after treatment is ceased ablative therapy may be necessary.

ADVERSE DRUG REACTIONS

Side effects associated with the administration of carbimazole include headache, nausea, rashes, arthralgias, hypoprothrombinaemia, agranulocytosis and jaundice. The most important of these adverse effects is agranulocytosis which has been reported to occur in 0.1%–1% of patients. Onset is sudden and

ENDOCRINE DISEASES

19

may be heralded by sore throat, fevers and mouth ulcers. Agranulocytosis is most common in the first three months of treatment. Drug administration should be stopped immediately. Withdrawal of treatment usually leads to a gradual increase in white blood count. There is cross sensitivity between carbimazole and propylthiouracil and patients who develop agranulocytosis on antithyroid drug treatment will probably require surgery or radioactive iodine.

DRUG INTERACTIONS

Myelosuppressive effects may be additive with those of other drugs.

PRECAUTIONS AND CONTRAINDICATIONS

Carbimazole should be used with caution in pregnancy and breast feeding.

Propylthiouracil

MECHANISM OF ACTION

The major mechanism of action of propylthiouracil is prevention of incorporation of iodine into the thyroid hormones. Propylthiouracil also inhibits the peripheral conversion of T_4 to the biologically active T_3.

PHARMACOKINETICS

Propylthiouracil is rapidly absorbed from the gastrointestinal tract and widely distributed in the body. The drug has a short half-life in plasma but the biological effects persist for a longer time. Propylthiouracil crosses the placenta and is present in breast milk.

USES

Propylthiouracil is used before thyroid surgery to reduce the activity of the thyroid, for prolonged periods to produce remission in Grave's disease and in the treatment of decompensated thyrotoxicosis or thyroid storm. Therapy is started with a high dose (300–450 mg daily in three divided doses) which is continued until the patient is euthyroid, this may take 2–4 months. Therapy is then continued at a lower dose (50–100 mg per day) for 12 to 24 months and the patient is given thyroxine if they become hypothyroid. If the patient experiences a relapse after treatment is ceased ablative therapy may be necessary.

ADVERSE DRUG REACTIONS

See carbimazole.

DRUG INTERACTIONS

Propylthiouracil should be used with caution with heparin and warfarin. Myelosuppressive effects may be additive with those of other drugs.

PRECAUTIONS AND CONTRAINDICATIONS

Propylthiouracil should be used with caution in pregnancy and breast feeding.

Iodine and Potassium Iodide

As part of the preparation for thyroid surgery iodine may be given either as Lugol's solution or as potassium iodide tablets. Large doses of iodine given to patients with hyperthyroidism reduce the friability and vascularity of the thyroid and make surgery easier. This therapy also reduces the likelihood of the release of large amounts of hormone from the gland during surgery causing acute thyrotoxicosis.

Radioactive Iodine

Radioactive iodine, ^{131}I, emits beta rays and has a half-life of about 8 days. When administered to hyperthyroid patients the radioactive iodine is taken up by the thyroid gland where the beta rays destroy thyroid cells resulting in decreased production of thyroid hormones. Radioactive iodine is used in patients who are not candidates for surgery, where medical therapy or compliance is a problem or who relapse after surgery.

NURSING IMPLICATIONS

ASSESSMENT

The patients vital signs should be checked and related to their current thyroid status. Temperature, blood pressure, pulse rate and respiration rate are all good indicators of thyroid status. When taking the history particular attention should be paid to recent weight loss, bowel activity, mood and response to environmental temperature. Note should be taken of co-existing medical conditions and drug therapy which may need to be altered when the patient's thyroid status is altered by treatment.

EVALUATION

The vital signs and factors noted during assessment should be monitored during treatment with antithyroid drugs. Response to treatment can be gauged by close attention to these factors and regular testing of thyroid function. A watch should be kept for the appearance of signs and symptoms of hypothyroidism which may require treatment with thyroxine. Relief from some of the symptoms of hyperthyroidism, e.g. tachycardia, may be obtained by administering the β blocking drug propranolol. Response to drug therapy for non-thyroid conditions may alter as the patient's thyroid status returns to normal and dosage adjustment may be necessary. The patient should be observed for the development of adverse effects with particular attention paid to signs of agranulocytosis, e.g. sore throat, fever, mouth ulcers.

PATIENT EDUCATION

Successful therapy with antithyroid drugs depends on patient compliance and the importance of not discontinuing medication should be stressed to the patient. The patient should be familiar with the symptoms of hypo- and hyperthyroidism and know to consult a doctor if any of these symptoms occur.

The patient should understand the importance of regular medical checks while they are taking antithyroid drugs and be told to report any side effects, particularly those which may indicate the onset of agranulocytosis, to the doctor responsible for their treatment.

OTHER THYROID HORMONES

Calcitonin

The thyroid gland also secretes calcitonin which has important effects on bone turnover and serum calcium levels. Calcitonin lowers serum calcium levels probably by reducing resorption of bone. It is given by subcutaneous injection and has been used in the treatment of Paget's disease, hyperparathyroidism and hypercalcaemia. Calcitonin products are classified according to animal source, i.e. porcine or salmon. Synthetic human calcitonin is also available.

TRADE NAMES

Porcine calcitonin: *Calcitare.*
Salcatonin (salmon calcitonin): *Calsynar; Miacalcic.*
Human calcitonin: *Cibacalcin.*

MECHANISM OF ACTION

Calcitonin inhibits the resorption of bone and therefore acts to lower serum calcium levels.

PHARMACOKINETICS

Calcitonin is inactive when given orally. It is metabolised by the kidney.

The onset of action of salmon calcitonin after intramuscular or subcutaneous injection occurs after 15 minutes, the effect is maximal in four hours and lasts for 8–24 hours. Human calcitonin has a shorter duration of action than salmon calcitonin.

USES

Calcitonin is used in the treatment of Paget's disease and hypercalcaemia. It is administered by intramuscular or subcutaneous injection.

ENDOCRINE DISEASES

19

PORCINE CALCITONIN

In Paget's disease the normal dose ranges from 80 units three times a week to 160 units daily. Response to therapy may not be seen for several months after treatment has commenced. Continued use of porcine calcitonin may result in the production of neutralising antibodies which lead to a decrease in effect. Transfer to salmon calcitonin may restore the effectiveness of treatment. In hypercalcaemia a dose of 4 units/kg is used. If larger doses are necessary salmon calcitonin should be used.

SALMON CALCITONIN

Salmon calcitonin is less antigenic than porcine calcitonin and may be effective in patients who develop resistance to porcine calcitonin. Salmon calcitonin 50 units is equivalent to porcine calcitonin 80 units.

In Paget's disease the normal dose ranges from 50 units three times a week to 100 units daily. As with porcine calcitonin the response to therapy may not be seen for several months after therapy has commenced. Although salmon calcitonin is less antigenic than porcine calcitonin continued use may lead to antibody production and decreased effect. Transfer to synthetic human calcitonin may restore the effectiveness of treatment.

In hypercalcaemia the recommended dose is 4 units/kg body weight every 12 hours increasing to a maximum of 8 units/kg body weight every 6 hours.

HUMAN CALCITONIN

Patients who have developed resistance to other forms of calcitonin may respond to treatment with human calcitonin.

In Paget's disease the normal dose ranges from 0.5 mg three times a week to 0.5 mg daily. The response to therapy may not be seen for several months after therapy has commenced. Antibody production has not been a problem with human calcitonin.

ADVERSE DRUG REACTIONS

Side effects of calcitonin therapy include nausea, vomiting, flushing, tingling of the hands and an unpleasant taste. Inflammatory reactions may occur at the injection site. Hypersensitivity reactions may occur. Human calcitonin is associated with less development of resistance and allergic reactions.

PRECAUTIONS AND CONTRAINDICATIONS

Hypersensitivity reactions may occur with the administration of calcitonin. Skin testing should be considered before initiating therapy and appropriate resuscitation measures should be available.

DRUGS USED IN THE TREATMENT OF DIABETES MELLITUS

The best way to understand diabetes is to consider it as a disease where the basic defect is an absolute or relative lack of insulin. Treatment consists of dietary measures and drug therapy aimed at maintaining normal blood glucose levels and avoiding the short-term and long-term complications of the disease. Diabetic patients are usually classified as insulin dependent or non-insulin dependent.

Patients with insulin dependent diabetes mellitus (IDDM; type 1) have an absolute lack of insulin. They usually present early in life and require insulin therapy for survival. The effect of a lack of insulin on the body's ability to utilise and store glucose, its main source of energy, leads to the signs and symptoms of diabetes. Insulin was first extracted from the pancreas and its therapeutic effect demonstrated in 1922. Since then insulin administration has developed as a cornerstone in the therapy of diabetes.

Patients with non-insulin dependent diabetes mellitus (NIDDM; type 2) have a relative lack of insulin and may be controlled with dietary measures and oral hypoglycaemic drugs.

Patients with non-insulin dependent diabetes may require insulin injections at some stage in their disease.

Hypoglycaemia is a major complication of therapy for diabetes. Initially oral glucose in the form of sugar or glucose sweets may be given but in the unconscious patient intravenous administration of glucose may be necessary. Glucagon, a hormone produced by the alpha cells of the islets of Langerhans, may be used as an alternative to glucose administration in the unconscious patient.

Many drugs administered for the treatment of conditions other than diabetes have the capacity to affect blood glucose levels in the diabetic patient.

Insulin

MECHANISM OF ACTION

Insulin is a polypeptide hormone secreted by the beta cells of the pancreas. It plays a major role in the body's regulation of carbohydrate, fat and protein metabolism.

PHARMACOKINETICS

Insulin is inactivated by gastrointestinal enzymes if taken orally and is usually given by injection. Absorption is affected by a number of factors including the site of injection, route of administration and type of insulin.

The duration of action of insulin is extended by the addition of zinc and protamine. These preparations are classified on the basis of the length of action after subcutaneous administration as short, intermediate, or long acting (see Table 19.1). Biphasic insulin preparations are also available. These are fixed ratio mixtures of short and intermediate acting insulin.

USES

Insulin is used routinely in the management of IDDM. It is also used in NIDDM at times of stress, e.g. surgery, infection or when the diabetes is not adequately controlled by diet.

Many animal species utilise insulin in the same way as humans. Insulin prepared from animal sources differs chemically from human insulin but is effective in the treatment of diabetes. Insulins from cows (bovine insulin) and from pigs (porcine insulin) were used to treat patients for the first 50 years of insulin therapy.

Recently synthetic human insulin has been manufactured using recombinant DNA technology and semisynthetic human insulin has been manufactured by enzymatically altering porcine insulin. An equivalent preparation of human insulin usually has a more rapid onset and shorter duration of action than animal insulin. Human insulin is now used routinely to treat the majority of diabetic patients who require insulin therapy. Initially it was used to treat newly diagnosed diabetics but eventually most other patients stabilised on insulin of animal origin were transferred to human insulin. Bovine insulin is still available and is used for the treatment of patients who require a once daily regimen or who cannot tolerate human insulin.

The most common method of insulin administration is by subcutaneous injection. The injection is usually administered into the thigh, buttocks, abdomen or upper arm. Injection into a limb may result in increased absorption if the limb is strenuously exercised.

Multiple dose injection devices which deliver a metered dose of neutral insulin have been developed. These devices which resemble a fountain pen and contain a replaceable insulin cartridge may be of use in patients who require multiple injections each day or in patients who are unable to measure insulin accurately.

Insulin has been given by continuous subcutaneous infusion using a portable pump capable of delivering a continuous basal rate of insulin and bolus doses at mealtimes.

Nasal administration of insulin has also been tried. Absorption is low and unreliable when insulin is given intranasally but it may have a place in controlling hyperglycaemia associated with meals.

ENDOCRINE DISEASES

19

TABLE 19.1   Insulin preparations

Preparation	Type	Source	Trade name	Onset (hours)	Peak (hours)	Duration (hours)
Regular insulin	Short acting	Bovine	*Insulin 2*	0.5	4	6–8
Neutral insulin	Short acting	Human	*Actrapid HM, Humulin R*	0.5	2–4	6–8
		Bovine	*Hypurin Neutral*			
Isophane insulin	Intermediate acting	Human	*Protophane, Humulin NPH*	2	4–12	24
		Bovine	*Hypurin Isophane*			
Insulin zinc suspension (lente)	Intermediate acting	Human	*Monotard HM, Humulin L*	3	7–15	24
		Bovine	*Lente MC*			
Insulin zinc suspension (ultralente)	Long acting	Human	*Ultratard HM, Humulin UL*	4–6	10–30	36
		Bovine	*Ultralente MC*			
Protamine zinc insulin	Long acting	Bovine		4–8	16–20	24–36
Neutral insulin 15% + isophane insulin 85%	Biphasic	Human	*Mixtard 15/85*	0.5	2–9	24
Neutral insulin 30% + isophane insulin 70%	Biphasic	Human	*Mixtard 30/70, Humulin 30/70*	0.5	4–8	24
Neutral insulin 50% + isophane 50%	Biphasic	Human	*Mixtard 50/50*	0.5	4–8	24

Insulin doses are measured in units of activity and the most commonly used strength is 100 units/mL. Most insulin preparations are suspensions and must be gently shaken before drawing up the dose. When more than one insulin preparation has to be given at the same time the insulin preparations may be mixed in the syringe and one injection given. Insulin should be injected immediately after mixing.

Insulin should be stored under refrigeration at a temperature of 2–8°C but not fro-zen. Insulin preparations are stable for several months at room temperature and the vial of insulin currently in use may be left at room temperature as long as it is kept in a cool place.

The perfect insulin regimen would exactly mimic the normal physiologic secretion of insulin by the pancreas. In the practical situation this perfect insulin regimen cannot be achieved. Insulin regimens must be designed for the individual patient to maintain blood glucose close to normal levels without involving too many injections each day. The time profile of action of a certain insulin is different in each patient and figures quoted for onset, peak and duration of action can only be taken as a guide when devising an insulin regimen for an individual patient.

A number of factors such as illness, infection and exercise may alter the insulin requirement and patients may need to alter their insulin doses in response to the results of blood or urine testing in these circumstances.

One of the most common regimens is a combination of short acting and intermediate acting insulins, i.e. neutral insulin and isophane insulin or insulin zinc suspension (lente), given twice daily. Usually the morning dose is larger than the evening dose. Adjustment of the short acting and intermediate acting components will allow good blood glucose control in a large number of patients. Once a patient's insulin requirements have been calculated it may be possible to transfer them to one of the biphasic preparations, e.g. *Mixtard*, removing the need for the patient to mix the insulins in the syringe. This may be particularly useful in patients who have difficulty measuring and mixing insulin accurately.

Neutral insulin is used intravenously in the treatment of diabetic ketoacidosis and hyperosmolar non-ketotic coma. An intravenous injection of 10–20 units of insulin is given and then an infusion of insulin in sodium chloride 0.9% is commenced.

ADVERSE DRUG REACTIONS

The most serious adverse effect of insulin administration is hypoglycaemia. Usually hypoglycaemia occurs because the insulin dose is too high or because a meal is missed after an insulin injection. The symptoms of hypoglycaemia include giddiness, tremor, palpitations and loss of consciousness which may progress to coma.

Local reactions to insulin injection include lipoatrophy, lipohypertrophy and erythema, pain, swelling and itching at the site of the injection. These local reactions are less common with human insulin. Systemic allergic reactions to insulin and the development of insulin resistance because of the formation of insulin antibodies can occur, these reactions are also less common with the use of human insulins.

DRUG INTERACTIONS

Many drugs used for the treatment of conditions other than diabetes may affect blood glucose control in the diabetic patient. This may lead to a loss of diabetic control or symptomatic hypoglycaemia. Diabetic patients should be monitored closely whenever drug therapy is changed.

Diabetic patients should be warned that β blocking drugs and clonidine may mask the normal symptoms of hypoglycaemia.

Drugs which may increase blood glucose levels when used in combination with insulin include adrenaline, nifedipine, oral contraceptives, corticosteroids, chlorpromazine, thiazide diuretics and thyroid hormones.

Drugs which may decrease blood glucose levels when used in combination with insulin include anabolic steroids, ethanol, fenfluramine, monoamine oxidase inhibitors and salicylates.

ORAL HYPOGLYCAEMIC AGENTS

The majority of oral hypoglycaemics are sulfonylureas. Sulfonylureas currently available for the treatment of diabetes include chlorpropamide, glibenclamide, gliclazide, glipizide, tolazamide and tolbutamide. Metformin is a biguanide oral hypoglycaemic.

TRADE NAMES

Chlorpropamide: *Diabinese.*
Glibenclamide: *Daonil; Euglucon; Glimel.*
Gliclazide: *Diamicron.*
Glipizide: *Minidiab.*
Tolbutamide: *Rastinon.*
Metformin: *Diabex; Diaformin; Glucophage.*

MECHANISM OF ACTION

Sulfonylureas act mainly by increasing release

ENDOCRINE DISEASES

19

TABLE 19.2   Pharmacokinetics of oral hypoglycaemic agents

Drug	Duration of action (hours)	Route of elimination
Sulfonylureas		
Chlorpropamide	>24	Renal, hepatic
Glibenclamide	10–15	Hepatic
Gliclazide	12–15	Renal, hepatic
Glipizide	24	Hepatic
Tolbutamide	5–8	Hepatic
Biguanides		
Metformin	6	Renal

of insulin from the pancreas. The action of the sulfonylureas in lowering blood glucose is also thought to involve extra-pancreatic or peripheral mechanisms but these are not fully understood. There is little difference in effectiveness between the sulfonylureas when given at equipotent doses.

The mechanism of action of metformin is not fully understood but it is thought to involve changes in the absorption of glucose from the gastrointestinal tract, inhibition of gluconeogenesis and increased peripheral utilisation of glucose.

PHARMACOKINETICS

All oral hypoglycaemics are well absorbed from the gastrointestinal tract. The significant pharmacokinetic differences between the oral hypoglycaemics are duration of action and route of elimination from the body (see Table 19.2). These properties influence drug selection in patients with renal or hepatic dysfunction and the number of times the drug must be given each day.

USES

In NIDDM patients who have failed to respond to exercise and diet, therapy with an oral hypoglycaemic drug should be started at a low dose and blood sugar levels monitored. The dose can be increased every two to three weeks until control of blood sugar levels is attained.

The sulfonylureas are the most commonly used oral agents in the treatment of diabetes. Metformin is most commonly used in patients who do not respond satifactorily to therapy with sulfonylureas and dietary measures. It is also useful in overweight patients where it tends to cause a decrease in body weight rather than the increase often associated with sulfonylurea therapy.

Details of dose forms, dose schedules and maximum daily dosages are shown in Table 19.3.

ADVERSE DRUG REACTIONS

Adverse effects of sulfonylurea administration are usually mild and infrequent. Reported adverse effects include gastrointestinal upset, headache, rashes, fever, dermatitis, jaundice, photosensitivity and blood dyscrasias. Sulfonylureas may cause weight gain and therefore should be avoided if possible in obese patients. Chlorpropamide has been reported to cause facial flushing and nausea when taken with alcohol.

The most serious side effect associated with the use of sulfonylureas is hypoglycaemia. The risk of hypoglycaemia is greatest in the elderly and patients with renal or hepatic dysfunction who may accumulate high levels of drug or active metabolites in plasma. Caution is required in the use of these drugs in these patient groups. Short acting drugs should be used. In renal failure drugs with an elimination route that is primarily hepatic should be used.

TABLE 19.3 Dose forms, dose schedules and maximum daily dosages for oral hypoglycaemic agents

Drug	Dose form	Dose schedule	Maximum Daily Dosage
Chlorpropamide	250 mg tablet	100–500 mg/day as a single dose	500 mg/day
Glibenclamide	5 mg tablet	2.5–15.0 mg/day as a single dose	20 mg/day in divided doses
Gliclazide	80 mg tablet	40–80 mg/day as a single dose	160 mg/day as a single dose, may be increased to 320 mg/day in divided doses
Glipizide	5 mg tablet	2.5–15 mg/day as a single dose	40 mg/day in divided doses
Metformin	0.5 g tablet	0.5–1.0 g 1–3 times daily	3 g/day
Tolbutamide	0.5 g	1 g twice daily	3 g/day

Metformin has been reported to cause nausea, vomiting and diarrhoea. Lactic acidosis has been associated with the use of biguanides especially in patients with renal failure. The use of metformin in renal failure should be avoided if possible.

DRUG INTERACTIONS

Many drugs used for the treatment of conditions other than diabetes may affect blood glucose control in the diabetic patient. This may lead to a loss of diabetic control or symptomatic hypoglycaemia. Diabetic patients should be monitored closely whenever drug therapy is changed.

Diabetic patients should be warned that β blocking drugs and clonidine may mask the normal symptoms of hypoglycaemia.

Drugs which may increase blood glucose levels when used in combination with oral hypoglycaemic agents include acetazolamide, adrenaline, nifedipine, oral contraceptives, corticosteroids, chlorpromazine, rifampicin, thiazides and thyroid hormones.

Drugs which may decrease blood glucose levels when used in combination with oral hypoglycaemics include allopurinol, anabolic steroids, chloramphenicol, ethanol, fenfluramine, monoamine oxidase inhibitors, phenylbutazone, probenecid, salicylates and sulfonamides.

PRECAUTIONS AND CONTRAINDICATIONS

Patients being treated with sulfonylureas should be fully educated about diabetes and understand the importance of diet and exercise in the control of their disease. Patients should monitor their blood glucose levels regularly and know when to seek help from their doctor.

Patients should be advised not to drink alcohol while being treated with sulfonylureas as serious hypoglycaemia may result from the combination.

Sulfonylureas should not be used as sole therapy in patients with IDDM or in the treatment of diabetes complicated by ketoacidosis, diabetic coma, major or severe infection or severe trauma. Insulin therapy should be instituted in these situations.

In pregnant diabetic patients oral hypoglycaemic therapy should be replaced with insulin, see Chapter 20 Drug Therapy in Pregnancy and Labour.

ENDOCRINE DISEASES

19

DRUGS USED FOR HYPOGLYCAEMIA

Glucagon

MECHANISM OF ACTION

Glucagon increases blood glucose levels by mobilising hepatic glycogen stores, causing glycogen to be converted to glucose.

PHARMACOKINETICS

Glucagon in plasma is inactivated rapidly in the liver, kidneys and other tissues.

USES

Glucagon is given by subcutaneous, intramuscular or intravenous injection for the treatment of hypoglycaemia in diabetic patients. Glucagon is given in a dose of 1 unit by the easiest route, usually subcutaneous injection, in an unconscious patient when the administration of intravenous glucose is not possible.

ADVERSE DRUG REACTIONS

Glucagon is usually well tolerated. The most common adverse reactions are nausea and vomiting. Rarely hypersensitivity reactions may occur.

PRECAUTIONS AND CONTRAINDICATIONS

Glucagon is only for emergency use in unconscious patients. Diabetic patients and caregivers should understand the importance of proper control of diabetes and management of hypoglycaemia. Patients experiencing hypoglycaemia should always notify their doctor.

Glucagon may not be effective in patients with chronic hypoglycaemia, adrenal insufficiency and starvation because of insufficient hepatic glycogen stores.

It should be used with caution in patients with phaeochromocytoma.

NURSING IMPLICATIONS

ASSESSMENT

In assessing the drug management of diabetic patients the following questions should be asked:

Is the blood glucose control acceptable?

What method is being used to monitor blood glucose levels?

Are they using this method correctly?

What drugs are currently being used to control the blood glucose?

Are these drugs being used correctly?

What other drugs are they taking?

What drugs have been used in the past and is there a history of reactions to any of these drugs?

Is the patient experiencing any adverse reactions to current drug therapy?

Answering these question involves testing blood and urine glucose levels, assessment of the physical condition of the patient and taking a thorough medication history.

EVALUATION

All patients receiving hypoglycaemic agents should have their blood and urine glucose levels monitored while in hospital. Diabetic patients using insulin should have their administration technique and monitoring skill assessed during their stay in hospital. Re-education may be necessary if inadequate technique or monitoring is observed.

Clinical signs and symptoms of hypoglycaemia should be carefully evaluated. Patients being treated with β blocking drugs may not experience the usual warning signs of incipient hypoglycaemia and require special attention.

MANAGEMENT

Management of hypoglycaemia consists of the administration of oral glucose in conscious patients. If the patient is unconscious then glucose 50% injection is given intravenously in a dose of 10–25 mL. If no venous access is available glucagon 1 unit should be administered subcutaneously. Patients should be observed for the development of any other adverse reaction to the hypoglycaemic agent being used.

A protocol should be established for the administration of insulin by intravenous infusion in cases of ketoacidosis and non-ketotic diabetic coma.

PATIENT EDUCATION

Proper education of the diabetic patient is the basis of effective control of the disease.

Most centres who deal with a large population of diabetic patients have a formal diabetic education program. All diabetic patients should attend this program when therapy is commenced, after major changes in their therapy or if they are having problems with blood glucose control.

The education of the diabetic patient should include education of family and close friends where possible. The diabetic patient should understand the disease and the management methods being employed. They should be confident in their ability to administer their therapy and monitor their blood glucose levels. The diabetic patient should be able to recognise the warning signs of hypoglycaemia and know what to do if hypoglycaemia occurs. They should understand the effect of illness, infection, diet and physical activity on their blood glucose control and know when to seek medical advice regarding their diabetes. Regular medical checks are important.

ENDOCRINE DISEASES

19

SEX HORMONES AND RELATED AGENTS

The sex hormones are steroid hormones produced in the body in response to the gonadotropins, follicle stimulating hormone (FSH) and lutienising hormone (LH), released by the anterior pituitary gland. The sex hormones may be divided into three groups: the oestrogens, the progestogens and the androgens.

The female sex hormones, natural oestrogens and progesterone, are responsible for the development of female secondary sexual characteristics and the maintenance of the menstrual cycle. For information on the use of oestrogens and progesterones as oral contraceptives see Chapter 21 Contraception and Infertility. Antioestrogens are drugs which oppose the action of oestrogen. They are used in the treatment of oestrogen sensitive tumours and female infertility due to secondary amenorrhoea.

Testosterone is the naturally occurring androgen produced by the testes in the human male. Androgens are also produced in small amounts by the ovaries and adrenal cortex. The androgenic properties of testosterone are responsible for the development of secondary sexual characteristics and the maintenance of fertility in the male. Testosterone is also an anabolic substance. Cyproterone acetate is classified as an antiandrogen. It inhibits the action of testosterone and is used in the treatment of disorders associated with symptoms of androgen excess.

FEMALE SEX HORMONES

Oestrogens

TRADE NAMES

Conjugated oestrogens: *Premarin*.
Ethinyloestradiol: *Estigyn*.
Oestradiol: *Estraderm*; *Primogyn Depot*.
Oestriol: *Ovestin*.
Piperazine oestrone sulfate: *Ogen*.

MECHANISM OF ACTION

Oestrogenic compounds act on oestrogen receptors in sensitive tissues such as the female genital organs, breast, pituitary and hypothalamus. Oestrogens regulate the female menstrual cycle and maintain female secondary sexual characteristics.

PHARMACOKINETICS

The naturally occurring oestrogens are not active when given orally. Agents used for oral treatment are conjugated natural oestrogens, synthetic derivatives of natural oestrogens and non-steroidal oestrogenic compounds. Oily solutions or aqueous crystalline suspensions of oestrogens are given intramuscularly to achieve a prolonged effect. Oestrogens are well absorbed from the skin and mucous membranes.

Oestrogens are metabolised in the liver into more water soluble compounds which are then excreted by the kidneys.

USES

Natural oestrogenic steroids and synthetic steroidal and non-steroidal agents with oestrogenic properties are used in the treatment of certain neoplastic conditions, e.g. cancer of the prostate, and a number of gynaecological conditions.

The menopause can be seen as a hormonal deficiency syndrome and oestrogens are of use in relieving associated symptoms. Hot flushes, atrophic vaginitis and osteoporosis respond to small doses of oral oestrogens. Oestrogen therapy may be given cyclically or continuously but these agents should not be administered for extended periods unless accompanied by a small dose of progesterone. Unopposed oestrogen therapy may be associated with an increased risk of endometrial cancer. Symptoms associated with vaginitis or vulvitis may be treated with topical preparations. Oestrogen therapy may also be administered by implant or transdermal patch.

Oestrogens are used in the treatment of dysfunctional uterine bleeding and primary dysmenorrhoea. In the treatment of these disorders they are given cyclically in combination with progestogens.

Oestrogens are used to induce the development of secondary sexual characteristics and relieve the symptoms of oestrogen deficiency in patients with primary hypogonadism or ovarian failure but should be used in combination with a progestogen.

Dose forms, indications and dosage schedules are listed in Table 19.4.

ADVERSE DRUG REACTIONS

Sodium and water retention, weight gain, headache, nausea and vomiting, thrombosis, changes in liver function, jaundice, rashes, breast enlargement and tenderness, chloasma, withdrawal bleeding, endometrial carcinoma.

DRUG INTERACTIONS

Drugs which induce the hepatic microsomal enzyme system such as rifampicin, barbiturates, phenytoin and carbamazepine may cause increased metabolism of oestrogens.

Oestrogens may decrease the effect of oral anticoagulants such as warfarin.

PRECAUTIONS AND CONTRAINDICATIONS

Oestrogens should be used with caution in patients who have conditions which may be aggravated by retention of sodium and water and a history of jaundice, diabetes or thyroid disease.

Oestrogens should not be used during pregnancy or lactation, in patients who are at risk from thromboembolic disorders, have a history of liver disease or have oestrogen sensitive tumours.

Long-term therapy with oestrogens in women with a uterus should always be

TABLE 19.4 Dose forms, indications and dosage schedules for oestrogen preparations

Drug	Dose Form	Indication	Dosage Schedule
Conjugated equine oestrogens	Tablets 0.3 mg, 0.625 mg, 1.25 mg Vial 25 mg/5 mL	HRT Female hypogonadism Dysfunctional uterine bleeding	0.3–1.25 mg/day 2.5–7.5 mg/day 25 mg IMI or IVI, repeat if necessary
Ethinyloestradiol	Tablets 0.01 mg, 0.02 mg, 0.05 mg	HRT Amenorrhoea	0.01–0.05 mg twice a day, maintenance 0.01 mg 1–2 times daily Cyclical, up to 0.15 mg/day
Oestradiol	Implants 20 mg, 50 mg, 100 mg Transdermal patches: 2 mg, 4 mg, 8 mg	Oestrogen deficiency syndromes HRT	20–100 mg every 4–8 months One patch applied to skin every 3–4 days
Oestradiol valerate	Ampoules 10 mg/mL	Dysfunctional uterine bleeding; oestrogen deficiency syndromes	IMI according to indication
Piperazine oestrone sulfate	Tablets 0.625 mg, 1.25 mg, 2.5 mg	HRT Female hypogonadism	0.625–5.0 mg/day 1.25–7.5 mg/day

HRT = Hormone replacement therapy

accompanied by a progesterone to reduce the risk of endometrial carcinoma.

Progestogens

TRADE NAMES

Allyloestranol: *Gestanin.*
Dydrogesterone: *Duphaston.*
Hydroxyprogesterone hexanoate: *Proluton Depot.*
Medroxyprogesterone acetate: *Depo-Provera; Provera.*
Norethisterone: *Primolut.*
Progesterone: *Proluton.*

MECHANISM OF ACTION

Progestogens cause changes in the structure and function of breast and endometrial tissue, including induction of secretory changes in the endometrium, relaxation of uterine smooth muscle, production of withdrawal bleeding in the presence of oestrogen and stimulation of mammary alveolar tissue growth.

Synthetic progestogens may also have some oestrogenic and androgenic effects.

PHARMACOKINETICS

Progesterone is ineffective when given orally because of extensive first pass metabolism by the liver. It is given as an oily intramuscular injection. Synthetic analogues of progesterone which are orally active have been developed.

USES

Progestogens are used in the treatment of amenorrhoea, severe dysmenorrhoea and menorrhagia. A progestogen such as norethisterone is given during part of the menstrual cycle. Combination therapy with an oestrogen may be used.

Endometriosis is treated with progestogens either continuously or cyclically in combination with oestrogen therapy.

Premenstrual tension may respond to treatment with a progestogen such as

19

ENDOCRINE DISEASES

TABLE 19.5 Dose forms, indications and dosage schedules for progestogens

Drug	Dose Form	Indications	Dosage Schedule
Allyloestranol	Tablets 5 mg	Threatened or habitual abortion	10–15 mg/day
Dydrogesterone	Tablets 10 mg	Dysfunctional uterine bleeding, threatened or habitual abortion, amenorrhoea	10–40 mg/day
Hydroxyprogesterone hexanoate	Ampoules 250 mg	Habitual abortion	IMI 250–500 mg/week
Medroxyprogesterone acetate	Ampoules 50 mg/mL, 150 mg/mL	Endometriosis	Oral 10 mg 3 times a day IMI 150 mg every 2–4 weeks
	Tablets 2.5 mg, 5 mg, 10 mg	Amenorrhoea, dysfunctional uterine bleeding	Cyclical, with or without oestrogen, 2.5–20 mg/day
Norethisterone	Tablets 5 mg	Endometriosis, menorrhagia, dysmenorrhoea	Cyclical 5–15 mg according to indication
Progesterone	Ampoules 25 mg/mL	Diagnosis of amenorrhoea	1 mL IMI/day for 2 doses

norethisterone either alone or in combination with an oestrogen.

Progestogens are used in the palliative treatment of some cancers, see Chapter 31 Cancer Chemotherapy.

Dose forms, indications and dosage schedules are listed in Table 19.5.

ADVERSE DRUG REACTIONS

Adverse effects include changes in menstrual flow, breakthrough bleeding, breast tenderness, acne, nausea and vomiting, weight gain, allergic reactions, chloasma, cholestatic jaundice, changes in libido.

PRECAUTIONS AND CONTRAINDICATIONS

Progestogens should be used with caution in patients with diabetes, hypertension, liver disease, cardiac disease and renal disease.

Progestogen therapy is contraindicated in patients with a history of thromboembolic disorders, missed or incomplete abortion or undiagnosed vaginal bleeding.

MALE SEX HORMONES AND RELATED AGENTS

Androgens and Anabolic Steroids

TRADE NAMES

Ethyloestrenol: *Orabolin.*
Fluoxymesterone: *Halotestin.*
Mesterolone: *Proviron.*
Methenolone acetate: *Primabolin; Primabolin Depot.*
Nandrolone decanoate: *Deca-Durabolin.*
Oxymetholone: *Adroyd; Anapolin 50.*
Testosterone enanthate: *Primoteston Depot.*
Testosterone undecanoate: *Andriol.*

MECHANISM OF ACTION

Testosterone is the naturally occurring androgen produced by the testes in the human male. The androgenic properties of testosterone are responsible for the development of secondary sexual characteristics and the maintenance of fertility in the male.

Testosterone is also an anabolic substance. Administration of anabolic agents increases the synthesis and decreases the breakdown of protein leading to an increase in skeletal and muscle mass. Anabolic agents also cause retention of sodium, water, potassium, calcium and phosphate. They are also thought to stimulate the production of erythrocytes. A number of agents have been developed which are anabolic but not as androgenic as testosterone. These are called anabolic steroids.

PHARMACOKINETICS

Testosterone is not active orally and has only a small effect if injected due to rapid metabolism and excretion. Various esters of testosterone and synthetic analogues of testosterone have been developed for oral and parenteral use.

Most androgens are metabolised by the liver into more water soluble compounds which are then excreted by the kidneys.

USES

Androgens are used as replacement therapy in patients who are testosterone deficient due to castration or hypogonadism. Therapy with androgens results in the development and maintenance of male secondary sexual characteristics.

Testosterone cypionate, testosterone enanthate, testosterone propionate and testosterone isocaproate are all esters of testosterone which have been used for replacement therapy. Intramuscular injection of depot preparations is the preferred method of administration. Oral preparations such as methyltestosterone and mesterolone are also used.

The anabolic steroids have been used in the treatment of a wide range of disorders including osteoporosis, catabolic states and anaemia. There is little evidence of long-term positive effect in most of these disorders and the risk of androgenic side effects should be considered when they are prescribed.

Anabolic steroids are of benefit in occasional patients suffering from aplastic anaemia

and in the palliative treatment of breast cancer. Anabolic steroids in clinical use include nandrolone, oxymetholone and oxandrolone.

The dose forms, indications and dosage schedules for the androgens and anabolic steroids are listed in Table 19.6.

ADVERSE DRUG REACTIONS

The adverse effects of these drugs are related to their androgenic and anabolic effects. In females all androgens may cause deepening of the voice, growth of facial hair, acne and menstrual irregularities.

Methyltestosterone has been associated with cholestatic jaundice and all these agents will cause salt and water retention. Androgens can cause low sperm counts and infertility if used in high doses in males.

DRUG INTERACTIONS

Androgens may potentiate the effects of oral anticoagulants such as warfarin. Close monitoring and dose adjustment may be necessary in patients taking oral anticoagulants when commencing or discontinuing therapy with androgens.

Androgens may lower blood glucose concentrations and changes in antidiabetic therapy may be necessary in diabetic patients commencing or discontinuing therapy with androgens.

PRECAUTIONS AND CONTRAINDICATIONS

Androgens should be used with caution in patients with diabetes, cardiac disease, renal disease, hypertension and hepatic dysfunction.

Female patients receiving anabolic agents should be monitored for signs of virilisation such as deepening of the voice and menstrual irregularities.

Male patients receiving androgens should be monitored for the development of priapism, excessive sexual stimulation or prostatic hypertrophy.

Androgens are contraindicated in male breast cancer and cancer of the prostate.

ENDOCRINE DISEASES

19

TABLE 19.6 Dose forms, indications and dosage schedules for androgens and anabolic steroids

Drug	Dose form	Indications	Dosage schedule
Androgens			
Fluoxymesterone	Tablets 5 mg	Androgen deficiency Anaemias	2.5–10 mg/day 20–50 mg/day
Mesterolone	Tablets 25 mg	Androgen deficiency	25 mg 3–4 times a day, reduce for maintenance
Methyltesterone	Tablets 5 mg, 25 mg, 50 mg	Androgen deficiency	10–25 mg 3 times a week
Oxymetholone	Tablets 50 mg, 100 mg	Androgen deficiency, anaemias	100–300 mg/day
Testosterone	Implants 100 mg, 200 mg	Androgen deficiency	100–600 mg every 3–6 months
Testosterone enanthate	Ampoules 250 mg/mL	Androgen deficiency	IMI 250 mg every 2–3 weeks, increase interval for maintenance
Testosterone undecanoate	Capsules 40 mg	Androgen deficiency	120–160 mg/day, reduce for maintenance
Anabolic steroids			
Ethyloestrenol	Tablets 2 mg	Growth disorders in boys	0.1 mg/kg/day to maximum 4 mg/day
Methenolone acetate	Tablets 5 mg Ampoules 100 mg/mL	Osteoporosis, breast cancer	Oral 10–20 mg/day IMI 100 mg every 2–4 weeks

ANTIANDROGENIC STEROIDS

Cyproterone Acetate

TRADE NAMES

Cyproterone acetate: *Androcur.*

MECHANISM OF ACTION

Cyproterone acetate blocks the action of androgens at androgen receptors.

PHARMACOKINETICS

Cyproterone acetate is poorly absorbed from the gastrointestinal tract. It is excreted as metabolites in the urine and bile.

USES

Cyproterone acetate is used in the treatment of hypersexuality and sexual deviation in the male. It is given in a dose of 50 mg twice daily after food. Cyproterone acetate has also been used in the treatment of hirsutism and androgenisation in the female and inoperable prostatic carcinoma.

In androgenisation the initial dose is 100 mg daily from days 5–14 of the menstrual cycle, combined with oestrogen therapy. The dose for prostatic carcinoma is 100 mg 1–3 times daily.

ADVERSE DRUG REACTIONS

Adverse effects include fatigue, gynaeco-mastia, infertility in the male, weight changes and changes in hair pattern.

PRECAUTIONS AND CONTRAINDICATIONS

Cyproterone may impair the ability to drive or operate machinery.

Full blood counts, blood glucose levels, liver function tests and adrenocortical function should be monitored regularly. Particular care should be taken in patients suffering from diabetes or adrenocortical insufficiency.

Cyproterone acetate is contraindicated in patients with hepatic disease, malignant or wasting diseases, severe depression, a history of thromboembolic disease and in young male patients in whom physical and sexual maturation is not complete.

NURSING IMPLICATIONS

ASSESSMENT

Assessment of the patient about to be commenced on therapy with sex hormones should include a thorough review of the patient's physical condition and an understanding of the disorder being treated, the agent chosen for therapy and the signs and symptoms which will be used to monitor therapy. Particular attention should be paid to the patient's baseline renal and hepatic function as some of these agents may cause retention of sodium and water and affect hepatic function. The presence of hypertension or cardiovascular disease which may be aggravated by sodium and water retention should be noted.

EVALUATION

Regular medical checks are important for all patients receiving sex hormone therapy. During replacement therapy with sex hormones the patient should be evaluated for normalisation of secondary sexual characteristics. Children being treated with androgens should have their growth rate checked to detect any adverse effect of therapy. Cosmetic measures may assist women who are troubled by the masculinising effect of androgen therapy. Salt and water retention should be monitored by serial weight measurements, blood pressure readings and checks for oedema. Retention of salt and water may respond to diuretic therapy.

PATIENT EDUCATION

The patient should understand the nature of their disease and the drugs being used to treat them. They should be aware of the benefits of treatment and how to recognise the adverse effects which should be reported to their doctor. The patient should understand that replacement therapy is lifetime therapy and that compliance is important if the benefits of therapy are to be maintained.

When patients are commenced on cyproterone therapy they should be warned not to drive or operate machinery if they feel drowsy.

ENDOCRINE DISEASES

19

ADRENAL HORMONES AND ANTIADRENAL AGENTS

The adrenal cortex is an important endocrine gland which secretes two principal hormones: hydrocortisone (cortisol) and aldosterone. The actions of these two corticosteroid hormones are usually classified as glucocorticoid and mineralocorticoid. Glucocorticoid activity mainly affects processes of metabolism while mineralocorticoid activity affects fluid and electrolyte balance. Hydrocortisone is a glucocorticoid with weak mineralocorticoid properties. Aldosterone is a mineralocorticoid.

The basic nature of the systems affected by corticosteroid hormones make it obvious that disorders of adrenal gland function or the administration of pharmacological doses of drugs with corticosteroid activity will have major effects on the function of the human body.

Glucocorticoids affect **carbohydrate and protein metabolism** by promoting the production of glucose from glycogen stores in the liver and opposing the action of insulin, leading to a rise in blood sugar levels. These effects may lead to muscle wasting and osteoporosis.

The administration of corticosteroids or overproduction of natural hormones affect **lipid metabolism** by causing movement of fat stores from peripheral depots to central depots leading to truncal obesity and fat deposition on the face and upper back.

Corticosteroids may cause considerable retention of water and electrolytes thus affecting **electrolyte and water balance**.

Corticosteroid administration may affect the **central nervous system** leading to psychiatric symptoms such as euphoria, depression, apathy and in some cases frank psychosis.

Administration of corticosteroids may cause lysis of **lymphoid tissue** and a decrease in circulating lymphocytes.

Corticosteroids reduce the **inflammatory response** leading to a reduction in the normal signs of inflammation. Systemic or local corticosteroids will cause a reduction in redness, swelling, tenderness and the formation of granulation tissue at a site of injury.

Suppression of the normal **immune response** by corticosteroids may be a desirable effect in the treatment of certain diseases but may also lead to an increased susceptibility to infection.

CORTICOSTEROIDS

Betamethasone, Cortisone, Dexamethasone, Fludrocortisone, Hydrocortisone, Methylprednisolone, Prednisolone, Prednisone, Triamcinolone

TRADE NAMES

Betamethasone: *Celestone.*
Cortisone: *Cortate.*
Dexamethasone: *Dexmethsone; Decadron; Oradexon.*
Fludrocortisone: *Florinef.*
Hydrocortisone: *Hysone.*
Methylprednisolone: *Solu-Medrol.*
Prednisolone: *Panafcortelone; Solone.*
Prednisone: *Deltasone; Panafcort; Sone.*
Triamcinolone: *Kenacort-A.*

MECHANISM OF ACTION

Corticosteroid drugs have been developed which mimic the actions of hydrocortisone and aldosterone. These drugs have varying degrees of the mineralocorticoid and glucocorticoid actions of the naturally occurring hormones.

Mineralocorticoid activity is desirable in the treatment of conditions such as Addison's disease while drugs with high glucocorticoid potency are used in conditions where anti-inflammatory and anti-allergic actions are required. The potency of various corticosteroids is shown in Table 19.7.

PHARMACOKINETICS

Most corticosteroids are well absorbed when given orally. Significant absorption may also occur when these drugs are applied to the skin, conjunctiva or injected into the joint space.

Corticosteroids circulate bound to plasma proteins. At low serum levels most of the circulating drug is bound to corticosteroid binding globulin but at higher serum levels large amounts may be bound to albumin.

TABLE 19.7   Properties of corticosteroids

Drug	Estimated potencies*	
	Glucocorticoid	Mineralocorticoid
Glucocorticoids		
Hydrocortisone	1	1
Cortisone	0.8	0.8
Prednisolone	4	0.25
Prednisone	4	0.25
Methylprednisolone	5	Insignificant
Triamcinolone	5	Insignificant
Dexamethasone	25	Insignificant
Betamethasone	25–30	Insignificant
Mineralocorticoids		
Fludrocortisone	10	300

*Relative potency compared with hydrocortisone

The biological activity of corticosteroids is not directly related to their level in plasma. Hydrocortisone and fludrocortisone have a duration of action of 8–12 hours. Prednisone, prednisolone and methylprednisolone all have a duration of action between 12 and 36 hours. Dexamethasone, betamethasone and triamcinolone have a duration of action between 36 and 72 hours.

The major site of metabolism of corticosteroids is the liver. A small amount of metabolism takes place in the kidney and other tissues. Inactive metabolites are excreted through the kidney.

USES

Corticosteroids should not be used unless the benefits from therapy outweigh the risk of possible adverse effects. When used as suppressive therapy the lowest dose which will produce the desired effect should be used for the shortest possible time.

Once the diagnosis has been established and a dose decided on, the signs and symptoms which will be used to monitor response should be selected and steroid therapy commenced.

Short-term, high dose glucocorticoid therapy is used to suppress disease activity in a wide range of disorders and can be life saving in conditions such as inflammatory bowel disease, status asthmaticus and anaphylaxis.

Severely ill patients will require parenteral therapy. The most commonly used corticosteroid for this purpose is hydrocortisone in doses of 100–200 mg every six hours. Once the condition is under control the patient is transferred to the equivalent dose of an oral corticosteroid. Prednisone (or prednisolone) is most commonly used for this purpose. The dose of the oral corticosteroid is then reduced slowly to a maintenance level or ceased. Reducing the dose too quickly or ceasing the drug prematurely may lead to either a relapse of the condition or acute adrenal insufficiency.

Corticosteroids are used to treat congenital or acquired adrenal insufficiency. The aim of treatment is to simulate the natural daily production of adrenocorticosteroids. The dose should be individualised for the patient but a typical regimen would be hydrocortisone 25 mg in the morning and 12.5 mg at night. Mineralocorticoid replacement with fludrocortisone is not necessary when the adrenal insufficiency is secondary, e.g. pituitary failure or after administration of synthetic corticosteroids, however in primary adrenal failure fludrocortisone 0.05–0.2 mg in the morning is given to maintain normal fluid and electrolyte

ENDOCRINE DISEASES

19

status. In periods of stress the demand for glucocorticoid activity increases and the replacement dose will have to be increased. Failure to adequately increase doses in periods of increased stress, e.g. infection or trauma, may lead to the development of acute adrenal insufficiency, a life threatening condition requiring hospitalisation and parenteral therapy with hydrocortisone.

Glucocorticoids, in particular dexamethasone, are used parenterally in the treatment of raised intracranial pressure. In the treatment of neoplastic disease prednisone is used in chemotherapy regimens and dexamethasone is used as part of the multicomponent regimens for the treatment of chemotherapy associated nausea and vomiting.

Corticosteroids may be used long term in the treatment of diseases such as chronic hepatitis, systemic lupus erythematosus, severe asthma, Crohn's disease and ulcerative colitis.

Local application of corticosteroids is preferred when possible as it is associated with a lower incidence of side effects than systemic therapy. It is important to remember however that significant absorption may occur after local application of corticosteroids.

Betamethasone and budesonide are used by inhalation in the treatment of asthma, see Chapter 11 Respiratory Diseases.

Beclomethasone, dexamethasone and flunisolide are used for symptomatic relief in inflammatory and allergic nasal conditions, see Chapter 11.

Corticosteroids such as hydrocortisone, dexamethasone, fluorometholone, prednisolone and medrysone are used to control inflammation in the eye, see Chapter 27 Eye Disorders. Topical corticosteroids are applied to the ear canal for symptomatic relief in inflammatory conditions.

Rectal preparations and enemas of corticosteroids such as hydrocortisone and prednisolone are used to control symptoms in proctitis and colitis, see Chapter 17 Gastrointestinal Disorders.

ADVERSE DRUG REACTIONS

Administration of corticosteroids may lead to the development of adverse effects which can be understood as exaggerations of the normal physiological functions of the natural hormones. In general the use of short courses of high dose steroids is not accompanied by significant adverse effects, however, long-term use of supraphysiological doses of corticosteroids requires careful management to avoid adverse effects.

Mineralocorticoid effects may lead to sodium and water retention, oedema, hypokalaemia, muscle weakness and exacerbation of heart failure. These effects are most marked with fludrocortisone but are also significant with hydrocortisone and cortisone.

Glucocorticoid effects may lead to hyperglycaemia, osteoporosis, glaucoma, peptic ulceration, mood changes, psychosis, increased susceptibility to infection, atrophy of the skin, steroid dermatitis and the development of a moon face and buffalo hump due to changes in the disposition of adipose tissue.

Long-term high dose corticosteroid therapy may lead to suppression of the hypothalamic-pituitary-adrenal axis which can last for 9–12 months after withdrawal. Abrupt withdrawal may cause a steroid withdrawal syndrome. Corticosteroid withdrawal syndrome may also occur after protracted low dose therapy. Symptoms of the corticosteroid withdrawal syndrome include myalgias, arthralgias and fatigue. Withdrawal of corticosteroid therapy or transfer from systemic to local therapy should be slow and the patient observed carefully for signs of disease recurrence or adrenal insufficiency. The safe rate of reduction varies from individual to individual and from disease state to disease state. There are a number of regimens used for withdrawal but in general a reduction of 2.5–5 mg of prednisone (or equivalent) every 3–7 days is safe. However, the rate of reduction may have to be even lower in some patients.

Hypersensitivity reactions ranging from anaphylaxis to local irritation may accompany either systemic or local use of corticosteroid preparations.

DRUG INTERACTIONS

Corticosteroids may decrease serum salicylate levels. Care should be taken when introducing corticosteroid therapy in a patient receiving salicylates. Doses of the salicylate may have to be increased on introduction of corticosteroid therapy and decreased if steroid therapy is withdrawn.

Corticosteroids may reduce the response to vaccines. If possible vaccination should be delayed until corticosteroid therapy has finished. If this is not possible extra doses of vaccine may be necessary and serological testing to confirm response is necessary.

The metabolism of corticosteroids may be induced by drugs such as rifampicin, phenobarbitone and phenytoin.

PRECAUTIONS AND CONTRAINDICATIONS

Corticosteroids may alter the effectiveness of a large number of other drugs. When corticosteroids are introduced or discontinued consideration should be given to the effect on other disease states being treated. Particular caution is necessary due to the effect of corticosteroids on blood sugar levels, fluids and electrolytes, intraocular pressure, psychiatric state, muscle weakness and the immune response.

Corticosteroids may exacerbate the side effects of other drugs. Particular caution is necessary when they are combined with agents such as non-steroidal anti-inflammatory drugs when there may be an increased risk of peptic ulceration. The potassium wasting effects of diuretics such as frusemide and the thiazides may be made worse by therapy with corticosteroids.

Corticosteroids should be used with care in any patient with a known or suspected infectious disease as their effect on the immune response may lead to an exacerbation of the infection which can be masked by decreased signs of inflammation. In the presence of infection adequate anti-infective therapy must always accompany therapy with corticosteroids.

Corticosteroids should never be withdrawn abruptly as this may lead to adrenal insufficiency or steroid withdrawal syndrome.

Corticosteroids should be used with care in children as these drugs may interfere with normal growth. Administration of corticosteroids at high doses during pregnancy may affect the development of the fetus. Corticosteroids may be excreted in breast milk and should therefore be avoided during breastfeeding.

NURSING IMPLICATIONS

ASSESSMENT

Assessment of the patient on steroid therapy is vitally important if the nurse is to be able to take an active part in the management of the patient's condition. During the normal nursing assessment of vital signs particular attention should be given to those signs which may be useful in evaluating the response to treatment or adverse effects such as salt and water retention, hyperglycaemia and psychiatric changes. The nurse should understand the indication for steroid therapy, the signs and symptoms which will be used to monitor the patient's progress and any co-existing medical conditions, e.g. hypertension or diabetes, which may be adversely affected by corticosteroid administration.

EVALUATION

Regular monitoring of the patient should allow the nurse to recognise changes related to steroid therapy. This evaluation will help in management decisions aimed at effective therapy without unacceptable adverse effects.

Any clinical signs of hyperglycaemia such as increased urinary output or increasing thirst are important. Testing of blood or urine glucose levels may confirm steroid induced diabetes.

Oral steroids may cause gastric irrita-

ENDOCRINE DISEASES

19

tion and exacerbate any existing gastritis or peptic ulcer disease. Any signs of gastrointestinal upset or bleeding should be reported.

Careful attention to any signs of infection is important as these signs may be suppressed in steroid treated patients.

Any changes in the psychiatric state of the patient are important as they may be related to steroid administration.

Complaints of musculoskeletal pain should be evaluated as they may relate to steroid induced myalgia or fractures due to osteoporosis.

Salt and water retention is a common adverse effect of steroid therapy and should be monitored by recording the patient's weight and blood pressure and observing for signs of oedema formation.

MANAGEMENT

Dietary restriction or the administration of hypoglycaemic agents may be necessary in steroid induced diabetes. Salt restriction may be necessary to counter the mineralocorticoid effects of steroids. Hypertension may require drug therapy.

Patients with steroid induced osteoporosis may be prone to fractures and should be moved with care.

Gastrointestinal effects may be minimised by the administration of steroids with meals. Concurrent administration of drugs known to cause gastritis and gastrointestinal bleeding should be avoided.

Care must be taken to avoid infection as the patient is more susceptible to infection and signs of infection may be suppressed. Steroid therapy with high doses or for extended periods should never be stopped abruptly. During withdrawal from long-term corticosteroid therapy the patient should be observed for any signs of reactivation of disease and symptoms of withdrawal.

PATIENT EDUCATION

It is vital that the patient understands the importance of steroid treatment and the serious consequences of suddenly ceasing treatment without medical supervision. This advice applies equally to patients on replacement or suppressive therapy. The patient should be advised to to wear an identification tag and inform their dentist, pharmacist or any other doctor who may treat them that they are taking steroids.

Patients should have regular medical checks and be told about the side effects of steroids but it is important not to frighten them into non-compliance. They should be told to report any symptoms such as increased thirst, weakness, bruising, infections and dyspepsia to the doctor who is treating them.

ANTIADRENAL AGENTS

The antiadrenal agents aminoglutethimide, metyrapone and mitotane are used to treat overproduction of adrenocorticosteroids. When this overproduction is due to a tumour, surgical removal of the tumour is the best treatment but therapy with antiadrenal drugs can be used to control the condition in patients who refuse or are unsuitable for surgery. Drug therapy has also been used to stabilise patients before surgical removal of the tumour. Metyrapone is used in the differential diagnosis of disorders of the pituitary-adrenal axis.

Aminoglutethimide

TRADE NAMES

Aminoglutethimide: *Cytadren*.

MECHANISM OF ACTION

Aminoglutethimide inhibits the synthesis of aldosterone and hydrocortisone from cholesterol.

PHARMACOKINETICS

Aminoglutethimide has good oral absorption; 12%–20% of the drug is excreted as unchanged drug in the urine.

USES

Aminoglutethimide is used to decrease hypersecretion of adrenocorticosteroids caused by tumours of the adrenal cortex and also ectopic corticotropin producing tumours. Aminoglutethimide is also used in combination with metyrapone in the treatment of Cushing's syndrome resulting from pituitary tumours which produce excess corticotropin.

Aminoglutethimide is given orally as 250 mg tablets. The initial dose is 250 mg every 6 hours which is then increased to a maximum of 2 g a day if tolerated.

Hydrocortisone, at a dose of 40 mg a day, is given with aminoglutethimide to suppress pituitary production of corticotropin. Mineralocorticoid supplementation with fludrocortisone may be necessary.

Aminoglutethimide is also used in the treatment of metastatic breast cancer, see Chapter 31 Cancer Chemotherapy.

ADVERSE DRUG REACTIONS

The most frequent side effects of aminoglutethimide are lethargy, drowsiness, vertigo and transient rash. Lethargy and drowsiness occur in 50% of patients but ceases within 2–6 weeks of continued therapy in most patients. However, symptoms may persist in 10% of patients. Transient vertigo may occur initially in 20% of patients but resolves over a period of weeks. Transient rash, occasionally associated with fever, occurs in up to 33% of patients. Bone marrow depression, hypothyroidism and virilisation of female patients have also been associated with the administration of aminoglutethimide.

DRUG INTERACTIONS

Aminoglutethimide increases the rate of metabolism of dexamethasone. The drug decreases the effects of warfarin, theophylline and oral hypoglycaemic agents and the dose of these drugs may need to be increased.

PRECAUTIONS AND CONTRAINDICATIONS

Patients receiving aminoglutethimide should be observed for signs of hypoadrenalism especially during periods of stress. Thyroid function, electrolyte status and haematological indicators should be monitored. The need for corticosteroid replacement therapy should be assessed.

Aminoglutethimide may affect the ability to drive or operate machinery.

Safety in pregnancy and breast feeding has not been established. Use of the drug should be avoided in these patients.

Mitotane

MECHANISM OF ACTION

Mitotane is a cytotoxic agent which selectively attacks adrenocortical cells. Mitotane also inhibits adrenocortical function.

PHARMACOKINETICS

Mitotane is absorbed from the gastrointestinal tract and is given orally. The drug has a long half-life and is distributed in body fat so plasma levels do not plateau until around 8 weeks of continuous therapy. Inhibition of adrenal function begins after 2–4 weeks of continuous therapy and does not appear to be directly related to plasma levels. Mitotane is mainly eliminated by liver metabolism and metabolites are excreted in the urine and bile.

USES

Mitotane is used in the treatment of inoperable adrenocortical carcinoma and Cushing's syndrome. Mitotane is given orally as 500 mg tablets.

In the treatment of adrenocortical carcinoma mitotane is given at a dose of 9–10 g daily in three to four divided doses. Patients are started at lower doses and gradually increased to the maximum tolerated.

In the treatment of Cushing's syndrome doses have ranged from 1–12 g a day. Mitotane can cause adrenal insufficiency and patients will probably require corticosteroid replacement therapy.

ADVERSE DRUG REACTIONS

Side effects of mitotane commonly reported include anorexia, nausea and vomiting, diarrhoea, lethargy, somnolence, dizziness and skin rash.

ENDOCRINE DISEASES

19

DRUG INTERACTIONS

Mitotane may have additive effects with central nervous system depressants. Mitotane may increase the metabolism of drugs such as phenytoin, barbiturates and warfarin. Spironolactone may inhibit the effect of mitotane.

PRECAUTIONS AND CONTRAINDICATIONS

Patients given mitotane are at risk of adrenal insufficiency and corticosteroid therapy is usually necessary. Patients should be hospitalised during the initial stages of mitotane therapy because of the high rate of side effects.

Patients should be warned that mitotane may make them drowsy and impair their ability to operate machinery or drive motor vehicles.

Metyrapone

TRADE NAMES

Metyrapone: *Metopirone.*

MECHANISM OF ACTION

Metyrapone inhibits the synthesis of adrenocorticosteroid hormones in the adrenal cortex. This block is overcome in patients with a normally functioning pituitary by an increase in secretion of corticotropin.

PHARMACOKINETICS

Oral absorption of metyrapone is variable and incomplete. Metyrapone is metabolised by the liver and kidneys. Metabolism may be delayed in patients with liver disease.

USES

The main uses of metyrapone is in the assessment of hypothalamic-pituitary function in disorders of adrenal function.

Metyrapone is given orally as 250 mg capsules. For two days urine collections are taken for determination of baseline urinary steroids. Mitotane is given at a dose of 750 mg every 4 hours for six doses and then another urine collection is taken to estimate the effect of the drug on urinary steroid excretion.

ADVERSE DRUG REACTIONS

Side effects of metyrapone include nausea, dizziness, abdominal discomfort, vertigo, headache and sedation. Bone marrow depression and low blood pressure have been reported with the administration of metyrapone.

DRUG INTERACTIONS

Phenytoin, oestrogens, progestogens, phenothiazines, methysergide, phenobarbitone, amitriptyline, chlordiazepoxide and corticosteroids have all been reported to interfere with the results of testing with metyrapone.

PRECAUTIONS AND CONTRAINDICATIONS

Patients receiving metyrapone are at risk of developing adrenal insufficiency. It should not be used in patients with adrenocortical insufficiency.

The safety of metyrapone use during pregnancy or in breast feeding women has not been proven and its use should be avoided if possible.

NURSING IMPLICATIONS

ADMINISTRATION

Tolerability to central nervous system side effects of aminoglutethimide can be improved by starting with small doses and increasing the dose gradually.

When metyrapone is being used as a diagnostic test it is important that the dose is given at the time charted.

When corticosteroid therapy is ordered as replacement therapy it is important to ensure that it is given every day.

EVALUATION

All these drugs suppress adrenal cortical function and patients should be monitored for signs of adrenal insufficiency.

Patients receiving aminoglutethimide should be observed for signs of hypothyroidism and have their blood pressure monitored as the drug can cause hypotension.

PATIENT EDUCATION

Patients receiving aminoglutethimide should be advised of the course of action to take if hypotension occurs. They should also be warned of the risk of drowsiness with aminoglutethimide and mitotane, particularly in the initial stages of therapy. They should be advised not to drive a motor vehicle or operate dangerous machinery if they feel drowsy.

The importance of taking these medications and associated corticosteroid replacement therapy in accordance with the prescribed dose should be stressed.

FURTHER READING

DiPiro, J. (ed) (1993), *Pharmacotherapy: a pathophysiolocal approach*, 2nd edn, Appleton & Lange, Norwalk, USA.
Koda-Kimble, M.A., and Young L. (eds), *Applied therapeutics — the clinical use of drugs*, 5th edn, Applied Therapeutics Inc., Vancouver, USA.
McEvoy, G. (ed) (1994), *AHFS 94 Drug information*, American Society of Hospital Pharmacists, Bethesda, USA.
Reynolds, J. (ed) (1993), *Martindale the extra pharmacopoeia*, 30th edn, The Pharmaceutical Press, London, UK.

ENDOCRINE DISEASES

19

TEST YOUR KNOWLEDGE

1. Which of the following drugs are used in the treatment of acromegaly: octreotide, somatrem, norethisterone, bromocriptine, desmopressin?

2. Tetracosactrin is an analogue of which of the following hormones: oestrogen, testosterone, corticotropin, triiodothyronine, glucagon?

3. Which of the following statements are true: (a) Thyroxine is the active thyroid hormone in the body. (b) Intolerance to cold is a symptom of thyroxine overdose. (c) Propylthiouracil is used in the treatment of myxoedema coma. (d) Triiodothyronine can be given parenterally. (e) Thyroxine administration may enhance the action of warfarin.

4. Which of the following drugs are sulfonylurea oral hypoglycaemics: tolbutamide, oestriol, glipizide, metformin, glucagon?

5. Which of the following statements is true: (a) Insulin is effective if given by mouth. (b) Insulin should be stored under refrigeration. (c) Metformin is given by subcutaneous injection. (d) Metformin is used to treat type 2 diabetes. (e) Glibenclamide is a biguanide oral hypoglycaemic.

6. Which of the following drugs are used in the treatment of androgen deficiency: methyltestosterone, medroxyprogesterone acetate, bromocriptine, cyproterone acetate, mesterolone?

7. Sodium and water retention is a side effect of which of the following drugs: oestriol, fludrocortisone: mesterolone, insulin, chlorpropamide?

8. Which of the following drugs are corticosteroids: hydrocortisone, aminoglutethimide, oxymetholone, betamethasone, prednisolone?

9. Which of the following are adverse effects of corticosteroid therapy: (a) Salt and water retention. (b) Hypoglycaemia. (c) Intolerance to heat. (d) Muscle weakness. (e) Skin atrophy.

10. Which of the following drugs are used in the treatment of hyperadrenalism: aminoglutethimide, oestradiol, carbimazole, mitotane, mefenamic acid?

Drug Therapy in Pregnancy and Labour

RONALD P. BATAGOL

O B J E C T I V E S

At the conclusion of this chapter the reader should be able to:

1. List the drugs frequently prescribed during pregnancy;

2. Discuss the drugs commonly used to treat medical conditions such as pre-eclampsia, eclampsia and thromboembolism in pregnancy;

3. Discuss the drug therapy of pre-existing conditions such as epilepsy, diabetes and asthma during pregnancy;

4. List the drugs commonly used during labour and at delivery; and

5. Discuss the drugs used for problems occurring during labour and at the time of delivery.

ADVANCE PLANNING

Health promotion and disease prevention are emerging as the fields of medicine that can have the greatest impact for positive patient benefits for the future. In no other area is the potential greater than during pregnancy as the entire basis for quality of life for each individual is determined at this time. Cost benefits too, are obvious, as the expense of maintaining a premature neonate in an intensive care nursery for several weeks is an enormous part of the health care budget for any hospital. If a number of premature deliveries can be prevented — and often the cause is drug related — then the savings per annum could be quite substantial.

Planning for an optimum pregnancy should be the goal of both the mother-to-be and her partner. Ideally, careful avoidance of all drugs should begin well before conception, along with a program of balanced nutrition and exercise. Couples should therefore be encouraged to plan for pregnancy and be aware that disease prevention and health promotion apply particularly in pregnancy and the neonatal period, as positive planning and appropriate therapy can have a profound impact upon the future life prospects of their child.

However, women with pre-existing medical conditions such as asthma, diabetes, epilepsy and hypertension, require continuation of treatment to ensure survival of, and optimum medical care for, both the mother and the developing infant. In these cases it is important to be able to evaluate and select the drug which is effective but has the least likelihood of causing teratogenic or fetotoxic effects. With some drugs it may be necessary to transfer from a preferred form of treatment for the period of the pregnancy and/or while breast feeding. For example, angiotensin converting enzyme (ACE) inhibitors such as captopril and enalapril should be avoided during pregnancy because of their association with several fetal and neonatal complications.

This chapter deals with the treatment of a range of medical conditions during pregnancy and the management of labour, preterm labour and pre-eclampsia.

NORMAL PREGNANCY

IRON THERAPY

Iron therapy is by far the most common form of medication prescribed for the pregnant woman. During a normal pregnancy the serum iron concentration falls during the second and third trimesters in women who do not take iron supplements. As iron exacerbates the possibility of nausea and vomiting in many patients it is common practice to start oral therapy early in the second trimester when any condition of nausea has disappeared. However, women with multiple pregnancies, a documented history of iron deficiency, or low serum ferritin levels early in pregnancy, may require prophylactic iron therapy at an earlier stage.

Iron is best absorbed orally if taken on an empty stomach, however this increases the risk of side effects, including gastric irritation, nausea, vomiting, diarrhoea and constipation, depending on individual response and the type of iron preparation. It is now considered best to take oral iron preparations immediately after food and in particular after the type of food that will maximise its absorption. For example, meals that include meat and green leafy vegetables that contain folic acid (one of the B group vitamins) and ascorbic acid (vitamin C), will aid the absorption of iron. On the other hand, calcium decreases iron absorption and, as most people have milk (containing calcium) with their cereal at breakfast time, it is best to avoid taking iron supplements at that time. Furthermore, if morning sickness persists into the second trimester, it is wise to avoid any iron intake as it may only add to the problem. For all these reasons, the consensus is that oral iron therapy should be taken after the main meal of the day, that is, after the meal which is most likely to include meat and green vegetables, as well as cauliflower, broccoli, potatoes and other high roughage foods.

This rationale supports the recommendation for once daily dosage preparations such as the ferrous sulfate/folic acid slow release preparations (*Fefol, FGF*). Ferrous gluconate preparations (*Fergon*) should also be taken after meals (usually three times a day).

ANTINAUSEANT THERAPY

Another drug therapy frequently prescribed during pregnancy is medication for the treatment of vomiting of pregnancy, 'morning sickness', or its more severe form, hyperemesis gravidarum.

There has been a great deal of professional and public debate about recommendations for this condition since the withdrawal by the manufacturer of the combination product *Debendox*, or *Bendectin* as it was called in the USA. (See Chapter 7 Drug Safety in Pregnancy and Lactation.)

If medications are prescribed expectant mothers are concerned and anxious for the welfare of their babies, while health professionals fear their efforts to alleviate a distressing and potentially harmful condition may result in litigation. However, reviews of the world literature consistently point out that there is no medical or scientific case against the use of time proven antinauseants, including *Debendox*.

Hyperemesis gravidarum itself, when left untreated, poses a possible threat to the fetus because of ketosis, dehydration and malnutrition, leading to the likelihood of growth retardation.

The answer to this problem is to treat a patient only as far as clinically necessary for the individual person. That is, only what is appropriate to gain control of the condition and to avoid any adverse consequences of severe vomiting should be recommended. The treatment used should then be carefully documented in the patient's records, showing it was necessary to proceed to a certain point in a spectrum of treatment for the sake of the woman and her baby. Any suspected adverse effects of any particular therapy should be explained to the woman who should be involved in the final decision about taking any medication. Such agreement should also be documented in the patient's records. While individual prescribers have their own preferences, the following list is a reasonable consensus of opinion from a number of research centres.

Treatment of Nausea

1. Recommend 'dry toast or biscuits'. This will not help many women but for the small percentage who respond it is all that is needed.

2. Suggest an effervescent glucose-saline drink, such as *Dexsal* or *Efferdex*. This will help only a further small percentage of women by 'breaking the bubble' and helping them to feel more comfortable.

3. Next, pyridoxine hydrochloride (vitamin B_6) can be tried. It should be given in a dose high enough to produce definite benefits (50–100 mg twice daily). However, megadoses of pyridoxine should be avoided as there is evidence that doses in excess of 1000 mg daily can cause peripheral neuropathy.

4. If pyridoxine alone is not sufficient to gain control of the condition, meclozine (*Ancolan*) 25 mg tablets can be added,

taken with each morning and evening dose of pyridoxine. Meclozine now has a 25-year 'safety record' and evidence based on the world literature indicates it can be used with safety during pregnancy, especially in such low dosage.

5. If control has not been achieved at this point, it may be necessary for the woman to be admitted to hospital because of the risks of ketosis and dehydration. Crystalloid intravenous solutions, to which is added metoclopramide (*Maxolon*) or prochlorperazine (*Stemetil*) depending on prescriber preference, can be administered to maintain normovolaemia. Another drug which may be used is promethazine (*Phenergan*), also regarded as having a reasonable safety record when used during pregnancy.

6. For a remaining small percentage of women the vomiting may be of psychotic origin. In this case it will be necessary to use drugs such as chlorpromazine (*Largactil*) or haloperidol (*Serenace*). In the extreme situation the cause may be a state of relative adrenal insufficiency. Some of these patients have been given corticosteroids with a rapid response and no recurrence of problems.

In summary, treatment should proceed along the possible spectrum of treatment only as far as necessary to gain control of symptoms for the individual woman and to minimise any possible harm to the fetus, either from the adverse effects of the un-treated condition or from the unnecessary use of medications when a simpler form of therapy would have been sufficient.

ANALGESIC THERAPY

Currently available evidence points to the use of paracetamol (or a combination of paracetamol and codeine) in normal doses, as the drug of choice during pregnancy. The term 'normal doses' should be emphasised as paracetamol in high doses is toxic to the liver and long-term effects of high dosage on the developing fetal liver are yet to be determined. Paracetamol–codeine combinations (*Panadeine, Dymadon Co*) may cause constipation in some women because of the codeine content, but the concurrent use of a mild laxative to gain the benefit of improved pain relief may be regarded as a desirable compromise.

Aspirin still remains the drug of choice for some acute viral illnesses and inflammatory conditions, but should be viewed with caution and prescribed by specialists who are familiar with possible adverse effects if used during pregnancy. Recent reports suggest that there may be an application for low dose aspirin in improving placental blood flow and in the treatment of pre-eclampsia, but again, such therapy should be prescribed only by obstetricians and physicians who specialise in the treatment of medical complications of pregnancy. Women should be cautioned against the use of aspirin as 'self-prescribed' medication while pregnant, especially on a long-term basis (see Chapter 7 Drug Safety in Pregnancy and Lactation).

MEDICAL CONDITIONS ARISING DURING PREGNANCY

PRE-ECLAMPSIA

Hypertension in pregnancy, or pre-eclampsia, occurs in 3% to 8% of all pregnancies, with a slightly higher rate in the primagravida. It is generally accepted that the risk is two to three times greater in diabetics. Women with underlying renal disease are also at a particular risk of developing hypertension and proteinuria during pregnancy.

Pre-eclampsia is marked by a generalised vasoconstriction, which becomes increasingly obvious with increasing severity of the disease and is also associated with coagulation changes. Vasoactive substances, including thromboxane A_2, are released during platelet aggregation and occlusive thrombotic lesions may develop within the renal and uteroplacental circulation. The causes of pre-eclampsia are unknown. Amongst the theories advanced are immunological causes and aberrations in prostaglandin metabolism.

Signs and Symptoms

Pre-eclampsia usually occurs after 20 weeks gestation. It is diagnosed by increased blood pressure accompanied by proteinuria, oedema, or both.

The increase in blood pressure for a diagnosis of pre-eclampsia should be an increase in systolic blood pressure of 30 mmHg or greater or an increase in diastolic blood pressure of 15 mmHg or greater, from measurements obtained prior to 20 weeks of gestation.

Proteinuria is defined as the excretion of at least 0.3 g of protein in a 24-hour specimen of urine.

Oedema is diagnosed by clinically evident swelling, but fluid retention may also be manifested as a rapid increase of weight without evident swelling.

There is also a variant of pre-eclampsia, called the HELLP syndrome (haemolysis, elevated liver enzymes, low platelet count). There may be mimimal elevation of blood pressure and only minimal renal dysfunction, but these patients exhibit severe liver disease with markedly elevated transaminase levels and increased bilirubin levels, severe coagulation changes, platelet counts often below 40 000 and blood test results consistent with microangiopathic haemolytic anaemia. HELLP is a life-threatening medical emergency. Treatment consists of supportive care. The survival rate is high with the metabolic abnormalities improving two days to one week after delivery.

Prevention

Whilst it is not possible to categorically state that pre-eclampsia can be prevented, various measures have been advocated to try to reduce the incidence. These include:

- Restriction of weight gain to 0.5 kg per week in the second half of pregnancy;

- Appropriate dietary advice including limitation of intake of excessively salty foods;

- Regular attendance for antenatal examination including blood pressure examination; and urinalysis for protein.

Other preventive measures, including a high caloric, low protein diet and nutritional supplementation with calcium, magnesium, zinc, fish oil and evening primrose oil, have been advocated. The efficacy of these measures has **not** been substantiated in the literature.

Low-dose heparin has also been widely used in women at risk of developing pre-eclampsia, although its effectiveness has not been proven.

Recently, it has been advocated that the use of low-dose aspirin (60–100 mg per day) may

DRUG THERAPY IN PREGNANCY AND LABOUR

20

prevent pre-eclampsia by suppressing the production of thromboxane A$_2$ by platelets. There are several multicentre studies substantiating these claims and there does not appear to be any notable fetal or maternal side effects. However, because the numbers of patients in whom low-dose aspirin has been used is not great enough to evaluate the likelihood of rare haemorrhagic complications, it is only advocated for women who are at increased risk of developing pre-eclampsia. Its use may also be a contraindication to epidural anaesthesia. Low-dose aspirin is usually discontinued about one week before the due date or planned delivery.

Early detection of pre-eclampsia is obviously desirable and there is currently a great deal of research work being carried out to identify early 'markers' of the likelihood of pre-eclampsia developing. Progression of pre-eclampsia to eclampsia with fitting and coma is a life threatening complication of pregnancy. Eclampsia was a much more frequent occurrence in the past but, in recent years, with the increase in the level of pregnancy monitoring in most countries and close attention to the signs of pre-eclampsia, the incidence of eclampsia has diminished dramatically.

Treatment of Hypertension

Some authorities suggest that bed rest and sedation are as effective as antihypertensive drugs, but there are no conclusive results from clinical trials.

The role of antihypertensive drugs in the treatment of hypertension of pregnancy is summarised below. Since the drugs listed are also used for the treatment of hypertension more detailed information is given in Chapter 12 Cardiovascular Diseases.

Methyldopa

TRADE NAMES

Methyldopa: *Aldomet*.

USES

Methyldopa at a dose range of 0.5–4 g daily, has been the most extensively used agent. Its safety and efficacy have been confirmed in many trials and use over several years. Methyldopa acts on the central nervous system, inhibiting central sympathetic discharge. Follow-up studies of children born of mothers who took methyldopa during pregnancy have identified normal physical and mental development at 10 years of age.

ADVERSE DRUG REACTIONS

Sedation is a side effect of methyldopa. Nasal stuffiness and dry mouth may also be seen in some patients. A positive Coombs test and occasionally haemolytic anaemia may occur. Nevertheless, methyldopa is regarded by many as the drug of choice for hypertension of pregnancy.

β Blocking Agents: Atenolol, Metoprolol, Oxprenolol

TRADE NAMES

Atenolol: *Tenormin*; *Noten*.
Metoprolol: *Betaloc*; *Lopressor*.
Oxprenolol: *Trasicor*; *Corbeton*.

USES

Whilst there have been reports of neonatal hypoglycaemia, bradycardia, respiratory difficulties and fetal intrauterine growth retardation when these drugs have been used, evidence is accumulating that they may be safely used for hypertension of pregnancy. However, some authorities still caution against long-term use.

The β blocking agents atenolol, metoprolol and oxprenolol have been widely used as antihypertensive agents in pregnancy. Some advantages are their gradual onset of action, lack of postural hypotension and the fact that blood pressure is reduced to normal not hypotensive levels.

The dosage ranges for these drugs when used for gestational hypertension are:

Atenolol: 50–200 mg per day.
Metoprolol: 50–200 mg per day.
Oxprenolol: 40–480 mg per day.

ADVERSE DRUG REACTIONS

The non-selective β blocking agents ox-prenolol, propranolol and pindolol are more likely to induce uterine contractions than the selective β blocking agents. For further information on β blocking agents see Chapter 12 Cardiovascular Diseases.

Combined α and β Blocking Agents: Labetalol

TRADE NAMES

Labetalol: *Trandate*; *Presolol*.

USES

Labetalol, a combined α and β blocking agent, is the drug most favoured within the group because it decreases peripheral resistance without changing cardiac output or producing tachycardia.

As there have been some studies which have shown a lower birthweight in the infants of women treated with atenolol compared with alternative treatments including labetalol, labetalol is usually the preferred option.

The dosage range is 200–2000 mg per day.

ADVERSE DRUG REACTIONS

Patients taking labetalol may experience postural hypotension, myalgia or scalp tingling. For further information see Chapter 12 Cardiovascular Diseases.

α Blocking Agents: Prazosin

TRADE NAMES

Prazosin: *Minipress*.

USES

Prazosin is a vascular α adrenergic antagonist. It causes a reduction in mean arterial pressure and peripheral vascular resistance with occasional tachycardia. Experience with its use in pregnancy is limited, but it appears to be safe and generally effective.

The dosage range is 3–30 mg per day.

ADVERSE DRUG REACTIONS

The major side effects of prazosin are related to postural hypotension, including the well-known 'first dose reaction', headache, lassitude and nausea. The first dose effect may be dangerous in the pregnant woman as the lowering of maternal blood pressure may be a potential cause of fetal hypoxia. For further information see Chapter 12 Cardiovascular Diseases.

Antihypertensive Agents Which Should be Avoided

DIURETICS

Diuretics should probably be avoided in the treatment of pregnancy hypertension because of their tendency to cause plasma volume contraction. Pre-eclampsia is associated with a reduction in plasma volume and it is known that fetal outcome is worse in women with chronic hypertension who do not have expanded plasma volume.

ANGIOTENSIN CONVERTING ENZYME INHIBITORS

Captopril (*Capoten*) and enalapril (*Renitec*) are two drugs of this class which are widely used for the treatment of hypertension. These agents should not be used in pregnancy as they have been associated with several fetal and neonatal complications, including hypotension, growth retardation, oligohydramnios, oliguria, renal failure, malformations, stillbirth and neonatal death.

NURSING IMPLICATIONS

For information on assessment, administration, evaluation and patient education for the various drugs used for pre-eclampsia and pregnancy hypertension see Chapter 12 Cardiovascular Diseases and Chapter 25 Neurological Disorders.

DRUG THERAPY IN PREGNANCY AND LABOUR

20

ECLAMPSIA

Management of Hypertensive Crisis

Hypertensive crisis is usually managed in an intensive care unit. Therapy required is parenteral drug and fluid administration to enable adequate blood pressure control, volume expansion with stable plasma protein solution (SPPS), to restore central venous pressure and establish and maintain urine output, continual fetal monitoring by non-stress cardiotocogram and treatment and prophylaxis of convulsions of eclampsia with magnesium sulfate.

The drugs used in the management of hypertensive crisis and the prophylaxis of eclampsia are discussed briefly below. For details on dosages and nursing implications for these drugs see Chapter 12 Cardiovascular Diseases.

Hydralazine

TRADE NAMES

Hydralazine: *Alphapress*; *Apresoline*.

USES

Hydralazine is regarded as a very effective agent for use in hypertensive crises for rapid control of blood pressure.

When used orally the dosage range is 50–300 mg daily. It has low bioavailability and a variable rate of metabolism in the liver.

When used by the parenteral route hydralazine is given initially as a 5–10 mg bolus injection over 5–10 minutes via the peripheral intravenous line, and then by continuous infusion commencing at 5 mg per hour. The rate of infusion should be adjusted according to response and to avoid large drops in blood pressure.

ADVERSE DRUG REACTIONS

Flushing and severe pounding headaches may be experienced with use of hydralazine.

Diazoxide

TRADE NAMES

Diazoxide: *Hyperstat*.

USES

Diazoxide is a potent and rapidly acting vasodilator administered by intravenous injection. When the drug was initially marketed it was recommended that it be given as a 300 mg bolus injection. However, it was subsequently shown that this dose could produce excessive hypotension with resultant cardiovascular and cerebral damage, as well as fetal hypoxia. These complications can be avoided by giving the drug in graded dosage increments.

The dosage is 30 mg every 5 minutes by intravenous bolus injection or 10 mg/minute by infusion. The maximum dosage is usually 150 mg.

Calcium Antagonists: Nifedipine

TRADE NAMES

Nifedipine: *Adalat*; *Anpine*.

USES

The use of nifedipine either orally or sublingually for hypertensive crises is well documented. It has also been used as a uterine muscle relaxant. Nifedipine causes a drop in peripheral vascular resistance and an increase in heart rate and cardiac output.

An oral or sublingual dosage of 10–20 mg reduces blood pressure after 5–10 minutes, with a maximum effect after 20 minutes. For further information on calcium antagonists see Chapter 12 Cardiovascular Diseases.

Magnesium Sulfate

USES

Magnesium sulfate is given intravenously for prevention or treatment of convulsions associated with eclampsia. It acts on both the central and peripheral nervous systems. Peripherally, it exerts a curare-like action on the neuromuscular junction and decreases acetylcholine release. Contraction of vascular smooth muscle is reduced by competition with calcium ions. Vasodilation results with a reduction in blood pressure but without a decrease in uteroplacental blood flow.

A loading dose of 4 g (8 mL of a 50% solution) is given over 15 minutes in 100 mL of glucose 5%. The infusion is continued at 2–3 g (4–6 mL) per hour, preferably given by syringe pump through the peripheral intravenous line, until at least 24 hours after delivery.

ADVERSE DRUG REACTIONS

The patient may experience hot flushing on commencement of treatment. Signs of magnesium toxicity include sweating, hypotension, depression of reflexes and depression of cardiac function. To avoid overdosage magnesium serum levels should be monitored 6-hourly and maintained at 1.7–3.5 mmol/L. However, the dose should be reduced if the knee jerks are abolished, the respiratory rate falls below 10 per minute or magnesium levels greater than 3.5 mmol per L are obtained. Other appropriate monitoring, e.g. coagulation profile, should be carried out as indicated by the clinical condition of the patient.

Magnesium sulfate is a tocolytic agent and increased doses of oxytocin may be required to counter this effect. Also, intra-partum computed tomographic tracings may show variability. Scalp pH determination may be required to differentiate this effect from hypoxia.

Phenytoin Sodium

Phenytoin sodium is also used in the management of convulsions associated with hypertensive crises. It is usually given intravenously as a loading dose of 15 mg/kg, followed by a maintenance dose of 200 mg twice a day. The administration rate of phenytoin must not exceed 50 mg/minute. To reduce burning sensation or irritation on injection the line may be flushed with normal saline.

Sodium Phenobarbitone

Although barbiturates are no longer used as sedatives a single dose of 200 mg of sodium phenobarbitone is still widely used in eclampsia. It is given at the commencement of anticonvulsant therapy.

NURSING IMPLICATIONS

As a general principle, the management of severe pre-eclampsia and hypertensive crisis involves consultation between all members of the patient care management team, high dependency nursing, appropriate eclampsia prophylaxis, blood pressure control, volume expansion and close fetal monitoring by non-stress cardiotocogram. Volume expansion with SPPS may be required to restore central venous pressure and to establish and maintain urine output. Fluid overload must be avoided. Maintenance fluids (glucose/saline) should be limited to 2 L per day, given via a peripheral intravenous line. Once the patient is stabilised, arrangements are usually made for delivery to take place. The central venous pressure line should not be used for magnesium sulfate infusion because of marked side effects with bolus doses. Adequate urine output is essential when using magnesium sulfate infusion. The dose of magnesium sulfate should be reduced or the drug discontinued in the presence of oliguria. It is important to keep either calcium chloride or calcium gluconate on hand for use as an antidote for magnesium toxicity. For further information see Chapter 12 Cardiovascular Diseases and Chapter 25 Neurological Disorders.

THROMBOPHLEBITIS

Superficial thrombophlebitis is the most common thrombotic disorder of pregnancy and occurs with increased frequency in women with varicose veins.

THROMBOEMBOLISM AND DEEP VEIN THROMBOSIS

Development of thromboembolism is associated with fetal and maternal mortality and morbidity. Indeed, it has been estimated that in Australia between 1979 and 1984 pulmonary thromboembolism equalled hypertensive complications as the most frequent cause of death in pregnancy. The pregnant woman is at an increased risk of developing thromboembolic disorders because of a decrease in venous return from the lower limbs, an increase in concentration of clotting factors and the trauma associated with delivery.

Heparin

Prophylaxis with heparin is usually recommended for pregnant women at high risk of developing a deep vein thrombosis and for women with a history of thrombotic or coagulation disorders. The dosage used is usually in the range 5000–7500 units, given subcutaneously 8 or 12-hourly.

For treatment, initial therapy is with intravenous heparin for 2–5 days followed by 5000–10 000 units given subcutaneously 8 or 12-hourly throughout pregnancy.

PRECAUTIONS AND CONTRAINDICATIONS

Heparin induced thrombocytopenia and bone demineralisation may occur.

Bone demineralisation resulting in osteoporosis is a rare complication but of concern. It is believed to be dose related and studies have demonstrated that heparin treatment at high dosage levels affects the serum concentration of one of the vitamin D metabolites. It has also been suggested that low calcium levels may predispose the pregnant woman to the development of heparin induced osteoporosis at a lower dosage than would occur under normal circumstances.

Close monitoring of bleeding time parameters and observation for potential side effects is necessary.

For further information on adverse effects and precautions see Chapter 13 Blood Disorders.

Warfarin

Warfarin crosses the placenta and may cause birth defects, e.g. various facial defects, and inhibit normal bone development in the fetus. Use during the second and third trimesters of pregnancy warfarin has been associated with various central nervous system and eye defects in the fetus and an increased risk of fetal haemorrhage.

Although the exact rate of deformities has not been firmly established, it is probable that 10%–15% of infants exposed to warfarin in utero have some type of abnormality. Approximately 4% show the classic features of warfarin embryopathy — nasal hypoplasia, stippled epiphyses and growth retardation. Use of warfarin late in pregnancy has been associated with fetal, placental and neonatal haemorrhage, which may be the result of the pharmacological effects of the drug. It has also been suggested that the frequency of stillbirth and spontaneous abortion is increased in women exposed to warfarin during pregnancy.

The only situation in which warfarin is likely to be used during pregnancy is in the management of patients with prosthetic heart valves when heparin has not been proved to be of value. There are two possible approaches for these patients. Heparin may be administered by subcutaneous injection 12-hourly throughout pregnancy, in doses adjusted to keep the mid-interval APPT at 1.5 times the control, or alternatively, heparin may be used until the 13th week, then warfarin until the middle of the third trimester, then heparin until term.

If warfarin is used during pregnancy, appropriate patient counselling with a full discussion of the risks and benefits must be carried out, so that an informed decision can be made by the patient.

For information on the use of warfarin as an anticoagulant see Chapter 13 Blood Disorders.

NURSING IMPLICATIONS

For information on assessment, administration, evaluation and patient education see Chapter 13 Blood Disorders.

EPILEPSY

In some women with epilepsy who become pregnant there is an improvement in seizures, whilst in others the condition remains stable or deteriorates.

Theoretically, there are several physiological alterations in pregnancy which may affect the seizure threshold. Plasma levels of progesterone and oestrogen increase and may be factors. In addition progesterone mediated hyperventilation may occur. In some women increased seizure frequency may be a result of plasma volume increases, impaired gastrointestinal absorption of anticonvulsant medication and decreased protein binding and increased hepatic metabolism of medication. Within 4–6 weeks of delivery these physiological changes are reversed. Thus, there is the danger of postpartum anticonvulsant overdosage and potential toxicity if therapy is not reassessed.

Risks and Benefits of Anticonvulsant Use

Over the years there has been a great deal of confusion in the general community regarding the safety of anticonvulsant use during pregnancy.

Congenital malformations in the babies of epileptic women, both treated and untreated, occur at an increased rate compared with the rate in the general population. The rate is generally considered greatest amongst treated epileptics and is around two to three times the rate in the non-epileptic population, or about 6% of live-born births. Cardiac, facial and limb deformities are the malformations most commonly seen. With valproic acid there is an additional 1% risk of spina bifida.

Uncontrolled fitting poses risks of acidosis and hypoxia in the fetus increasing the risk of physical defects, trauma, cerebral palsy and mental retardation. Therefore, the woman requires appropriate counselling on the risks and benefits. If she decides to continue her pregnancy, appropriate drug treatment is given, with close monitoring of the epilepsy and drug therapy throughout the pregnancy.

Recommendations

Anticonvulsant drugs interfere with folate metabolism and folate supplementation is usually recommended in women who are pregnant or contemplating pregnancy (usually 0.5 mg daily). Also, infants of women taking phenytoin, primidone or phenobarbitone during pregnancy are at an increased risk of coagulopathy and intraventricular haemorrhage from vitamin K deficiency. The use of oral vitamin K 20 mg daily for two weeks prior to expected delivery, or 10 mg by intramuscular injection four hours before delivery, will prevent these complications. For further information see Chapter 25 Neurological Disorders.

Whilst no drug is completely safe, if treatment is required to control seizures the lowest effective dose should be given with close monitoring. Generally, the risk of seizures outweighs the risk of teratogenesis. In cases where the patient has been seizure free for some time medication may be withdrawn under strict medical supervision.

DRUG THERAPY IN PREGNANCY AND LABOUR

20

NURSING IMPLICATIONS

The ability of the body to handle antiepileptic drugs is altered during pregnancy. The binding of phenytoin to serum proteins is reduced in the last trimester, increased hydroxylation in the liver occurs, renal clearance may increase and absorption of the drug from the bowel may be reduced. Metabolism of carbamazepine, primidone and phenobarbitone is also altered in pregnancy.

EVALUATION

Because of the individualised nature of the effects of pregnancy on seizure threshold and frequency, it is important that the blood levels of the drugs used are monitored on a regular basis (usually monthly) and the dosage adjusted when necessary. After delivery drug levels should be measured on a fortnightly basis.

PATIENT EDUCATION

Pre-conceptual counselling of these patients is very important. The patient should be advised that the risk of having a baby with a malformation is two to three times greater than the general risk of malformation and that the actual chance of having a normal child is in excess of 90%.

During pregnancy the frequency of seizures has been found to increase in about 45% of patients, remain the same in about 50% and decrease in about 5%. The patient must be counselled on the importance of taking her medication, as prescribed, throughout the pregnancy.

DIABETES

Before the advent of insulin treatment the mortality rate in those few diabetic women who became pregnant was 30% and in the fetus, 50%. Although gestational diabetes was recognised in the early 1900s, it is only over the last 15 years or so that there has been a systematic approach to this disease entity, resulting in a decrease in the fetal mortality rate to 2%–5% for diabetes and a much lower rate for gestational diabetes.

In the insulin dependent patient, insulin requirements change throughout the course of the pregnancy. The first trimester is often marked by increased insulin sensitivity and a tendency to hypoglycaemia. Between 22 and 32 weeks it is usual for insulin requirements to rise, often to as much as twice the dose required before pregnancy or even more in some individuals.

When diabetes is poorly regulated the fetus is subject to meal related hyperglycaemia and stimulation of fetal islet cells which results in hyperinsulinaemia. This, in turn, leads to macrosomia (or 'large for gestational age' infants). In addition, hyperinsulinaemia may inhibit lung maturation leading to a deficiency of surfactant production and an increased incidence of respiratory distress syndrome. Overall, there is a higher incidence of pre-eclampsia and polyhydramnios and an increased rate of caesarean section in diabetic pregnancies compared with the general population. Congenital abnormalities in the infants of diabetic women occur at approximately three times the rate of that of the general population (incidence, 8%–9%).

It is now well established that perinatal mortality and neonatal morbidity are lowest when blood sugar levels are monitored frequently and kept as low as possible. Usually accepted upper limits of normal for pregnant women are 5.5 mmol/L in the fasting state and 7.8 mmol/L post-prandially (around two hours after a meal).

Since the discovery in 1978 that there is a correlation between elevated glycosated haemoglobin levels and fetal malformations, this marker is closely monitored throughout pregnancy.

There is increasing and compelling evidence to suggest that there is a link between early glycaemic control and congenital malformations. Therefore, it is important that women should be counselled before they become pregnant so that good control may be maintained throughout the period of organogenesis (the first 8–10 weeks).

Dietary Management

Dietary management is centred around glucose level monitoring and a meal plan which limits hyperglycaemia and minimises hypoglycaemia. Insulin is used when indicated, oral hypoglycaemic agents are never used. Glucose levels should be monitored continuously. Nutritionally balanced meals and snacks, high in complex carbohydrate and fibre should be arranged to minimise glycaemic episodes and provide a continuing energy source for mother and fetus. Appropriate exercise should be encouraged throughout the pregnancy.

In gestational diabetes insulin is used if blood glucose levels exceed 7 mmol/L.

Insulin

Because exposure to insulin derived from animal sources, especially beef insulin, may lead to the development of anti-insulin antibodies, human insulin is the only insulin used for treatment.

The choice of insulin type and regimen will vary and is dependent on the blood glucose levels. In type 1 diabetes mellitus an intensive insulin regimen, such as a multi-dose regimen using short acting insulin before meals and medium acting insulin at bedtime, provides flexibility and usually improved control. If, before pregnancy, good control was maintained using a more conventional regimen then this is not changed.

In gestational diabetes requiring insulin, twice daily premixed human insulin (e.g. *Mixtard*) or mixed human insulins (e.g. neutral insulin—*Actrapid*; isophane insulin—*Protophane*) are often used. However, because hypoglycaemic episodes are often meal related, short acting insulin given before each meal provides excellent control.

Pen injectors offer a useful method of insulin delivery. The usual considerations concerning insulin administration and storage, and adverse effects, are discussed in Chapter 19 Endocrine Diseases.

Management During Labour and Delivery

When possible the patient does not eat breakfast on the morning of delivery. A reduced dose of insulin, about half the dose, is usually given. An infusion of 150–300 mL of glucose 5% is given to provide calories and prevent ketonuria in labour. In spontaneous labour when the patient may have eaten prior to admission additional insulin may not be required. If the insulin level becomes too high, glucose may be required. Frequent monitoring of blood glucose levels is carried out. Delivery is usually induced with early resort to caesarean section if signs of fetal distress or other complications occur.

If an insulin drip is given it should be stopped at delivery, as insulin requirements rapidly decrease in the postpartum period. Women with gestational diabetes rarely require insulin after delivery, whilst those with non-gestational diabetes will require progressive adjustments to re-establish stabilisation, along with appropriate dietary management.

NURSING IMPLICATIONS

PATIENT EDUCATION

The importance of frequently monitoring blood glucose levels and maintaining good control throughout the pregnancy needs to be emphasised to the patient.

For further information see Chapter 19 Endocrine Diseases.

ASTHMA

It has been estimated that around 4% of pregnant women are affected by asthma during pregnancy. Obviously, prevention and treatment of asthma during pregnancy is aimed at preventing maternal deaths, respiratory failure, status asthmaticus and debilitating wheezing, in addition to ensuring that fetal growth and maturation are not affected. Uncontrolled episodes of asthma have been associated with maternal and perinatal mortality. It has been found that the pregnancy outcome for women with steroid-dependant asthma is almost as favourable as that for the general population, provided the asthma has been effectively controlled during pregnancy.

The prevention and treatment of asthma during pregnancy is similar to that for the non-pregnant patient.

Prevention

Prevention of asthma in pregnant patients with inhaled beclomethasone dipropionate (*Aldecin, Becotide*) is usually effective. Use of inhaled beclomethasone reduces the potential for adverse long-term effects which may result in long-term oral steroid use. Inhaled beclomethasone is regarded as safe for use in pregnancy. Use of inhaled sodium cromoglycate (*Intal*) as a prophylactic agent is also regarded as safe in pregnancy.

Treatment

Drugs used for the treatment of asthma include the β_2 agonists salbutamol (*Ventolin, Respolin*) and terbutaline (*Bricanyl*). All these drugs are listed as Category A in the Australian Medicines in Pregnancy classification and may be regarded as safe for use during pregnancy (see Chapter 7 Drug Safety in Pregnancy and Lactation). Although the β_2 agonist drugs have been given by injection to inhibit labour, there is little or no effect on the uterus when they are used by inhalation.

A short-term course of oral steroids, such as prednisolone 20–50 mg daily for 4–7 days, may be used with safety. In women who have been taking steroids regularly during pregnancy, hydrocortisone is used intramuscularly or intravenously at a dose of around 100 mg every 8 hours for 24 hours during labour. This ensures that adequate exogenous steroid is provided for the physiological stress of labour.

Theophylline preparations are also widely used for their bronchodilator effects. Theophylline and its derivatives do, however, possess a central nervous system stimulant effect. It is well established that theophylline used late in pregnancy can cause symptoms of irritability and jitteriness and even tachycardia in the neonate, especially in low birthweight or premature infants.

The presence of asthma may affect obstetric management. β Blocking agents (atenolol, metoprolol) and labetalol are frequently used for the treatment of gestational hypertension. Although drugs such as labetalol and metoprolol are relatively cardioselective, there is still a residual potential for exacerbation of asthma.

Prostaglandins may also exacerbate asthma. When used to initiate labour dinoprostone vaginal gel is much less likely to be a problem than dinoprost injection. However, it is sensible to have a bronchodilator inhaler on hand when any of the prostaglandins are used. See Chapter 11 Respiratory Diseases for further information on the drugs used in the treatment of asthma.

LABOUR AND DELIVERY

SUPPRESSION OF PRETERM LABOUR

The incidence of premature deliveries is about 8% of all births, yet prematurity accounts for approximately 75% of the perinatal mortality rate. In other words, less than one-twelfth of all births accounts for three-quarters of the deaths associated with childbirth.

Suppression of labour can be achieved with the use of tocolytic drugs and the discovery of these medications has been welcomed by all those involved in obstetrics. The aim of using tocolytic therapy is to delay labour for at least 48 hours, so that steroids can be given to enhance fetal lung maturity.

The following drugs are examples of medications that have been used to inhibit labour although there is some controversy about the indications for their use (e.g. in the management of pregnant women with ruptured membranes and preterm labour).

Magnesium Sulfate

Magnesium sulfate inhibits uterine contractions and is widely used in the treatment of pre-eclampsia and eclampsia. While the magnesium ion causes paralysis of skeletal muscle it has a relaxant effect on smooth muscle by a direct effect on the muscle cell.

It is a relatively safe drug but its role in the suppression of labour has been overshadowed by the more common use of the β_2 sympathomimetic agents such as salbutamol and ritodrine.

Before tocolytic therapy is given both fetal and maternal wellbeing must be assessed. A cardiotocogram is performed to rule out fetal stress. Any maternal contraindications, such as heart disease, to tocolytic drugs need to be assessed.

β_2 Sympathomimetic Agents: Ritodrine, Salbutamol

The β receptors are subdivided into β_1 and β_2 receptors with stimulation of β_1 receptors resulting in increased heart rate and output while β_2 activation causes vasodilation and relaxation of smooth muscle in the uterus and bronchial tree. While further clarification is needed it has been shown that β_1 receptors are dominant in the heart, small intestine and fat cells, while β_2 receptors are dominant in the smooth muscle of the uterus, blood vessels, diaphragm and bronchioli. These basic principles explain the

use of salbutamol and terbutaline as bronchodilators in the treatment of asthma and uterine relaxants in obstetrics and the reverse role of the β blocking agents in the treatment of hypertension.

Ritodrine

Because of its β_2 sympathomimetic activity ritodrine is a potent inhibitor of uterine contractions.

TRADE NAMES

Ritodrine: *Yutopar*.

USES

Ritodrine is used as an intravenous infusion and also orally. When given by infusion the dosage is 50–350 micrograms/minute depending on the cardiovascular response. One recommended regimen is an initial infusion rate of 50 micrograms/minute, increasing by 50 micrograms every 10 minutes until adequate uterine relaxation occurs with a maximum infusion rate of 350 micrograms/minute. If disturbing palpitations or a maternal heart rate in excess of 135 beats/minute are observed the infusion rate is reduced by similar steps until an acceptable heart rate is obtained. When appropriate, the patient can be transferred to oral therapy. The dosage is 10 mg four times a day, or more if necessary.

Salbutamol

Salbutamol is a β_2 agonist in common use in Australian hospitals.

TRADE NAMES

Salbutamol: *Ventolin Obstetric Injection*.

USES

Ventolin Obstetric Injection is a special presentation of salbutamol for obstetric use. It is available as ampoules containing 5 mg in 5 mL as distinct from *Ventolin* ampoules containing 0.5 mg of salbutamol in 1 mL for use in the treatment of asthma. To produce uterine relaxation a suitable solution for infusion

DRUG THERAPY IN PREGNANCY AND LABOUR

20

can be prepared by diluting the contents of an ampoule of *Ventolin Obstetric Injection* in 500 mL of sodium chloride 0.9%, glucose injection or glucose/sodium chloride injection. (The contents of the ampoule should never be injected undiluted by any route.) A dosage regimen of 10–50 micrograms/minute can then be administered with careful monitoring of maternal cardiovascular effects. When a maternal heart rate in excess of 140 beats/minute occurs the dose rate should be reduced or administration of the drug discontinued. When appropriate control has been established some patients may be effectively maintained on oral salbutamol therapy. The recommended initial dose is 8 mg every six hours with suitable adjustments made as necessary. Oral salbutamol may not, however, give the serum levels required.

ADVERSE DRUG REACTIONS

Adverse drug reactions include hand tremor, tachycardia, hypotension, anxiety, headaches and flushing, dizziness, nausea and vomiting. A more severe complication reported recently is pulmonary oedema.

PRECAUTIONS AND CONTRAINDICATIONS

β_2 agonists are contraindicated in hyperthyroidism, diabetes, fetal acidosis (pH 7.1–7.2), active uterine bleeding, maternal cardiac disease and hypersensitivity to this group of drugs. Great care should be exercised when administering these drugs to patients with hypertension and cardiac abnormalities.

Terbutaline (*Bricanyl*) and fenoterol (*Berotec*) are recent additions to this group of medications and have also been used to inhibit labour.

Miscellaneous Agents

Other agents that have been suggested for tocolytic purposes include diazoxide (*Hyperstat*) and hydralazine (*Apresoline*). Both are well known for their roles in the treatment of hypertension. It has been observed that when used in this capacity in late pregnancy women in labour sometimes experienced inhibition of uterine contractions. Various mechanisms of action have been suggested but, since these effects have not been consistently demonstrated, neither drug is commonly recommended for this purpose. Similar observations have been made when general anaesthetic agents are administered to women in labour, particularly the gaseous inhalation type such as halothane (*Fluothane*). A practical application of this has been the use of halothane to assist the manual removal of retained placenta in the third stage of labour. Nifedipine has also been used as a uterine muscle relaxant for the control of premature labour.

There is also substantial evidence that prostaglandins are of critical importance in the initiation and maintenance of human labour. Suppression of endogenous prostaglandin synthesis is the basis for using indomethacin to inhibit pre-term labour occurring at less than 34 weeks. Effects on the fetus, such as those on the ductus arteriosus, renal blood flow and platelets, have been shown to be temporary with rapid reversal on withdrawal of therapy. Dosage used is usually 100 mg rectally as a loading dose, followed by 25 mg orally every 4 hours for 24 hours (or 100 mg rectally every 12 hours for 24 hours). If pre-term labour recurs, a second 24-hour course may be initiated.

NURSING IMPLICATIONS

1. **Close monitoring of infusion strength and rate of administration is necessary.**

2. **Careful monitoring of maternal pulse rate, fluid balance and blood pressure is essential, because these drugs are associated with a number of side effects such as maternal tachycardia and shortness of breath, chest pain and myocardial ischaemia, as shown on electrocardiogram.**

3. Careful observation of the fetal heart rate and the status of the fetus is recommended.

4. Administration should to be stopped if the maternal pulse rate exceeds 140 beats/minute or the woman has tremors or palpitations.

RESPIRATORY DISTRESS SYNDROME

Corticosteroids

An adjunct to the use of tocolytic agents has been the discovery that administration of corticosteroids to a mother with threatened premature delivery may result in early maturation of the fetal lungs and avoidance of the respiratory distress syndrome (hyaline membrane disease), see Chapter 5 Paediatric Therapeutics. In the normal pregnancy the surfactant that promotes respiration is present from about 36 weeks of gestation and is indicated by a lecithin to sphingomyelin ratio (L:S ratio) of 2:1 or greater. It is understood that administration of corticosteroids activates choline phosphotransferase which catalyses the conversion of choline to lecithin.

USES

While dexamethasone is recommended by some centres the preferred regimen is the administration of betamethasone (*Celestone Chronodose*) given as two injections of 12 mg 12 hours apart. This should produce pulmonary maturity within 24 hours and subsequently safe delivery within 48 hours. Discussion in the world literature suggest that the technique is of value up to 34 weeks gestation. Before 26 weeks the fetal lungs are too immature to respond to steroid therapy and after 34 weeks steroids are probably unnecessary unless low surfactant levels are revealed on amniocentesis.

PRECAUTIONS AND CONTRAINDICATIONS

Corticosteroid therapy is usually not employed when infection is present, in severe hypertensive conditions when delivery is planned within 48 hours or when the L:S ratio is found to be good. It has been claimed that in diabetic mothers fetal stress may also contribute to early pulmonary maturity and that medications, e.g. labetalol, used to treat maternal hypertension may also have this effect.

NORMAL LABOUR AND DELIVERY

A normal human pregnancy lasts approximately 40 weeks when delivery of the infant and the placenta are brought about by strong rhythmical contractions of the uterus. This process ordinarily takes place automatically under the influence of endogenous oxytocin and prostaglandins.

For controlled induction of labour, synthetic oxytocin may be administered. At the completion of labour, oxytocic drugs are used routinely. These drugs include synthetic oxytocin available in ampoules containing 2 IU in 2 mL, 5 IU in 1 mL and 10 IU in 1 mL and as a nasal spray; ergometrine maleate available in ampoules containing 0.25 mg and 0.5 mg in 1 mL; and a combination preparation for intramuscular use available in ampoules containing synthetic oxytocin 5 IU and ergometrine maleate 0.5 mg in 1 mL.

Oxytocin

Oxytocin stimulates the rhythmical contractions of the uterus. The postpartum use of oxytocics causes the uterus to become firm and active which reduces the incidence and extent of postpartum haemorrhage. In lactation, oxytocin stimulates milk let-down.

TRADE NAMES

Oxytocin: *Syntocinon*; *Syntocinon Nasal Spray*.

20 DRUG THERAPY IN PREGNANCY AND LABOUR

USES

Oxytocin is used for induction of labour, stimulation of inadequate uterine effort, management of the third stage of labour and for disorders of lactation.

When oxytocin is used for induction or stimulation of labour it is given by a well controlled intravenous infusion in sodium chloride 0.9% or Hartmanns solution. Uterine contractions occur almost immediately and subside within one hour following intravenous administration of oxytocin.

For the management of the third stage of labour an intramuscular injection is given at the birth of the anterior shoulder. Intramuscular injection produces uterine response within three to five minutes, which persists for two to three hours.

The nasal spray containing 40 IU/mL in 5 mL is used for disorders of lactation to improve the milk 'let-down' reflex.

ADVERSE DRUG REACTIONS

Oxytocin has been known to cause serious reactions when given in large or excessive doses, including violent uterine contractions with rupture of the uterus; soft tissue damage; fetal bradycardia and arrhythmias; severe hypertension and subarachnoid haemorrhage; water retention and intoxication with convulsions, coma and death; allergic reactions; and nausea and vomiting.

PRECAUTIONS AND CONTRAINDICATIONS

Oxytocin is contraindicated in severe pre-eclampsia, hypertonic uterine inertia, abnormal fetal posture, placenta praevia, fetal distress or mechanical obstruction of delivery.

Ergometrine

TRADE NAMES

Ergometrine–oxytocin: *Syntometrine.*

USES

Ergometrine maleate is used for the production of rhythmic contractions which increase in both frequency and force and for the treatment of postpartum haemorrhage.

Ergometrine initiates uterine contractions within two to five minutes after intramuscular injection and virtually immediately after intravenous administration. Contractions persist for three hours or more after intramuscular use and for 45 minutes after intravenous use. Because of the severity of contractions produced by ergometrine when given by the intravenous route it is seldom used this way except when needed to control severe postpartum haemorrhage.

The combination product oxytocin–ergometrine is given by intramuscular injection routinely with the birth of the anterior shoulder except in women with elevated blood pressure when the diastolic reading is more than 90 mmHg. In such cases an intramuscular injection of oxytocin alone is used.

ADVERSE DRUG REACTIONS

Ergometrine maleate may cause nausea and vomiting, an occasional increase in blood pressure and peripheral vascular constriction and gangrene.

PRECAUTIONS AND CONTRAINDICATIONS

Oxytocics should be used with caution in patients with pre-eclampsia.

Prostaglandins

The most recent additions to the list of drugs that promote uterine contractions are the prostaglandins. The term refers to a group of compounds that are produced by the action of the enzyme prostaglandin synthetase on the precursor substance arachidonic acid. While many prostaglandins are known only three are commonly used in practice, dinoprostone the E_2 analogue (PGE_2), gemeprost the E_1 analogue (PGE_1) and dinoprost the $F_{2\alpha}$ analogue ($PGF_{2\alpha}$).

TRADE NAMES

Dinoprostone: *Prostin E2 Vaginal Gel.*
Dinoprost: *Prostin F2 Alpha.*
Gemeprost: *Cervagem.*

USES

The mechanism of action of the prostaglandins has yet to be defined although inhibition of the formation of cyclic adenosine monophosphate or an effect on calcium release have been suggested.

Dinoprostone vaginal gel is used to initiate uterine contractions for induction of labour. The initial dose is 1 mg followed by 2 mg if required. The advantages of dinoprostone gel are that early amniotomy is not required and many consider that the effect produced is gentler, more natural and less invasive than oxytocin.

Dinoprost is available as a 5 mg/mL solution in 1 mL and 8 mL ampoules. It can be administered by the extra-amniotic or intra-amniotic route. It is used for therapeutic termination of pregnancy and to initiate uterine contractions to expel the contents of the uterus when intrauterine fetal death has occurred. In clinical trials dinoprost has also been used topically as a gel to 'ripen' the cervix.

Gemeprost is used to ripen the cervix prior to first trimester or mid-trimester termination. It cannot be used for induction of labour as fetal distress from hypertonicity may occur.

ADVERSE DRUG REACTIONS

Prostaglandins have been reported to cause cardiac arrhythmias and sudden cardiovascular collapse. They should be used with caution in patients with asthma. As mentioned, the risks of untoward effects are greatly diminished with the use of dinoprostone gel.

Miscellaneous Drugs

Phenothiazines, such as chlorpromazine (*Largactil*), and prochlorperazine (*Stemetil, Compazine*) are used as adjuncts to pain relief in labour as well as for sedation and treatment of nausea. Promethazine (*Phenergan*) can be employed similarly, with the added benefit of its antihistaminic effect for therapy of itch and rash, a frequent adverse effect of narcotic epidural anaesthesia.

Metoclopramide (*Maxolon, Primperan*) is used as an antiemetic and, more recently, to assist in the promotion of lactation because of its effect of elevating serum prolactin levels.

Lignocaine (*Xylocaine*) is used for local anaesthesia prior to episiotomy. Lignocaine, bupivacaine (*Marcain*) and mepivacaine (*Carbocaine*) are used for epidural anaesthesia.

Narcotics, especially pethidine, are used for pain relief during labour and following caesarean section. Less severe pain, particularly pain following delivery, is commonly treated with paracetamol (*Panadol*), or paracetamol and codeine (*Panadeine, Dymadon Co*).

Laxatives are administered for postpartum constipation. Agents such as docusate sodium (*Coloxyl*) and docusate sodium with senna (*Coloxyl and Senna*) may be used, the former to soften faeces and the latter to soften faeces and promote peristalsis. Senna (*Senokot*), emulsion of paraffin and phenolphthalein (*Agarol*) and plantago and senna granules (*Agiolax*) may also be used.

Antibiotics are given for postpartum and post-caesarean infection and for the treatment of mastitis.

NURSING IMPLICATIONS

Various regimens are used for oxytocin infusion for induction or augmentation of labour, so nursing staff need to become thoroughly familiar with the procedure used in their particular hospital.

EVALUATION

Close patient observation is essential with attention paid to the length and strength of contractions, the interval between contractions, the fetal heart rate and the possibility of water intoxication, in addition to routine obstetric observations. When a patient receives more than 3.5 L of infused fluid in 24 hours the risks of water intoxication increase.

DRUG THERAPY IN PREGNANCY AND LABOUR

20

During administration of oxytocics:

1. The fetal heart rate should be monitored;

2. The duration and amplitude of contractions should be constantly supervised;

3. The drip rate must be closely monitored and the fluid balance accurately recorded;

4. As ergometrine has a tendency to cause peripheral vascular constriction from which gangrene may result patients must be checked for symptoms such as the feet becoming cold, numb or even purple; and

5. Care must be taken not to mix up the oxytocic injections with any injection intended for the infant, e.g. vitamin K injection.

FURTHER READING

Australian Drug Evaluation Committee. (1992) *Medicines in pregnancy — an Australian categorization of risk*, 2nd edn, AGPS, Canberra.

Batagol, R.P. (1993) *Drugs in pregnancy*. The Royal Women's Hospital, Melbourne.

Batagol, R.P. (1993) *Drugs and breast feeding*. CSL Ltd, Parkville.

Briggs, G.G., Jaffe, S.J., Freeman, R.K. (1990) *Drugs in pregnancy and lactation*, 3rd edn. Williams and Wilkins, Baltimore.

Gleicher, N. (1992) *Principles and practice of medical therapy in pregnancy,* 2nd. edn. Appleton & Lange, Norwalk.

Llewelyn-Jones, D. (1990) *Fundamentals of obstetrics and gynaecology*, Vol 1, 5th edn. Faber & Faber, London.

Speight, T.M. (1987) *Avery's drug treatment*, 3rd edn. Adis Press, Auckland.

TEST YOUR KNOWLEDGE

1. List the drugs used prophylactically to prevent pre-eclampsia.

2. What drugs should be avoided in the treatment of pre-eclamptic hypertension?

3. What are the two important side effects of continuous heparin therapy during pregnancy.

4. What are the vitamin preparations that may be used during pregnancy in women taking antiepileptic drugs.

5. Why is human insulin usually chosen for use in pregnant diabetic women who require insulin?

6. Which drugs when used for treatment of pregnancy associated conditions may interfere with control of asthma?

7. Discuss the use of drugs in premature labour at 30 weeks gestation.

8. Which drugs can be used to induce uterine contractions in normal labour?

9. What other drugs are commonly used at the time of delivery, and for what indications?

Contraception and Infertility

RONALD P. BATAGOL

O B J E C T I V E S

At the conclusion of this chapter the reader should be able to:

1. List the main female hormones and outline their role in the ovarian cycle;

2. Describe the use of synthetic hormones as contraceptives;

3. Discuss the side effects of oestrogens and progestagens and apply this information to determine the choice of oral contraceptives for particular patients; and

4. Name the main causes of infertility and briefly outline the hormones used in its treatment.

THE FEMALE SEX HORMONES

The female gonads (ovaries) maintain ova, maintain nutrition and maturity of the female reproductive organs, and sensitise the mucous membrane of the uterus so that it responds to the contact of the developing ovum and assists in implantation.

Two pituitary hormones directly affect the ovaries: **follicle stimulating hormone (FSH)** which, as its name implies, stimulates follicular growth in the ovary as well as controlling the production of oestrogen; and **luteinising hormone (LH)** which, together with FSH, controls ovulation by causing the release of the ovum from the ripened follicle.

Prolactin, also found in the pituitary, is responsible for the secretion of milk. Lactation occurs when the fully developed breast is released from the inhibitory influence which oestrogen and progesterone exert during pregnancy upon the action of prolactin. With the rapid decline of oestrogen and progesterone levels that follow delivery, prolactin from the pituitary gland is able to exert its full effect upon the mammary tissue, and milk production commences.

The two principal female sex hormones are **oestrogen** and **progesterone**. Oestrogen is produced throughout the entire menstrual cycle and is responsible for the regrowth of the lining of the uterus after each menstruation (the proliferative phase). Oestrogen is necessary to stimulate the endometrium just prior to its conversion to a secretory state. Progesterone is produced from the ruptured egg follicle (the corpus luteum) after ovulation, and is therefore present only in the latter half of the menstrual cycle. It is responsible for maintaining pregnancy and is mainly involved in the secretory phase of the menstrual cycle.

Drugs affecting fertility fall into two categories: those which stimulate ovarian activity and those which suppress it. Whereas most drugs are foreign to the body, hormones (used to a large extent in the first category and entirely in the second) are natural secretions of the endocrine glands which exert effects on specific tissues. However, a number of compounds which have pronounced hormonal activity have been synthesised. Mestranol and ethinyloestradiol are synthetic oestrogens, and norethisterone and levonorgestrel are synthetic progestagens.

CONTRACEPTION — OVARIAN SUPPRESSION

Progesterone injection was used in the 1930s as a means to suppress ovulation. However, the era of oral contraception did not begin until 1951 in the USA after Pincus had carried out research on progestagens.

ORAL CONTRACEPTIVES

Oral contraceptives, unlike most other drugs, are prescribed for healthy women and are taken for long periods so that the chance of toxic manifestations is increased. Either oestrogen or progestagen taken orally can be used to inhibit ovulation. Barrier methods of contraception, including both chemical and mechanical means, do not stop ovulation. Their usage is aimed at preventing fertilisation of the ripened eggs.

The natural oestrogen, oestradiol, is not sufficiently active orally, so synthetic ethinyloestradiol is used. However, the menstrual bleeding pattern produced by oestrogen alone is irregular, often prolonged, and unpredictable. For this reason, a progestagen is administered with oestrogen for part of the second half of the cycle. This usually produces a predictable and satisfactory menstrual pattern.

The Combined Pill

The most commonly prescribed type of oral contraceptive is the combined pill. Early types of the combined pill used a combination of various forms of oestrogens and progestagens. For example, *Anovlar*, the first pill released in Australia (1961) contained a combination of ethinyloestradiol 50 micrograms and norethisterone acetate 4 mg. Further development led to improved oral progestagens such as levonorgestrel, which permitted lower dosage of both hormones, e.g. *Microgynon 30* and *Nordette*, released in 1975, contained ethinyloestradiol 30 micrograms and levonorgestrel 150 micrograms. The latest development in progestagens, desogestrel, has less androgenic side effects. It is combined with ethinyloestradiol in the preparation *Marvelon*.

More recent developments sought to imitate the changing hormonal levels of a normal cycle, leading to the biphasic concept (*Biphasil* and *Sequilar* — 1979) and the current triphasic or three-step concept (*Triquilar* and *Triphasil* — 1981; and the most recent addition — *Synphasic*). The triphasic concept was designed 'by women, for women' and aimed to imitate the changing levels of oestrogen and progestagen during the monthly cycle. However, none of the triphasic pills available in Australia at the time of writing completely achieves this aim as progesterone levels are higher and oestrogen levels are lower than those occurring during the natural cycle.

The combined pill is available either as a 21-day pack containing active medication which is taken from the fifth day of the cycle for 21 days, or a 28-day pack containing 7 inert ('sugar' pills) and 21 active pills. The 28-day pack is started on the first day of bleeding, commencing with the inert pills, and continued with a pill taken each day without any break. In this case, again only 21 active pills are taken monthly, but the 28-day pack assists the woman in setting up and maintaining a daily routine, without having to remember when to recommence taking the pills each month.

The Progestagen-Only Pill (Mini-pill)

Small doses of a progestagen, such as levonorgestrel 30 micrograms or norethisterone 350 micrograms, find special application in the immediate postpartum period for lactating mothers and also have been used to minimise the adverse side effects of oestrogen, such as thrombosis.

The compositions and trade names of the fixed, biphasic, triphasic and progestagen-only pills currently available are listed in Table 21.1.

MECHANISM OF ACTION

How then does the 'pill' work? In brief, by preventing ovulation coupled with other possible actions.

While a number of mechanisms can be involved, the major contraceptive effect of the combined pill is to suppress the cyclical activities of the pituitary gland and the ovaries. Combined administration of oestrogen and progestagen imitates the corpus luteum phase of pregnancy, and hormone levels produced (by negative feedback) cause the hypothalamus and the pituitary to remain in a 'resting' state. As a consequence insufficient FSH is released to cause the ripening of the follicles in the ovaries, no LH surges are produced and release of an ovum (ovulation) does not occur.

Other mechanisms include thickening of the cervical mucus making sperm penetration more difficult while thickening of the endometrium is prevented making nidation less likely.

The method of action of the mini-pill (progestagen only) is less clearly defined. It is believed that whilst a mother is fully breastfeeding, the small continuous dose of pro-

CONTRACEPTION AND INFERTILITY

21

TABLE 21.1   Oral contraceptives

Trade name	Oestrogen content (μg)		Progestogen content (μg)			
	Ethinyl-oestradiol	Mestranol	Levonorgestrel	Norethisterone	Ethynodiol diacetate	Desogestrel
Combined Pills						
Fixed preparations						
Marvelon	30					150
Microgynon 30	30		150			
Nordette	30		150			
Brevinor	35			500		
Brevinor-1	35			1000		
Microgynon 50	50		125			
Nordette 50	50		125			
Nordiol	50		250			
Ovulen 0.5/50	50				500	
Ovulen 1/50	50				1000	
Ortho-novum 1/50		50		1000		
Norinyl-1		50		1000		
Biphasic Preparations						
Biphasil	50		50 (11 tabs)			
	50		125 (10 tabs)			
Sequilar	50		50 (11 tabs)			
	50		125 (10 tabs)			
Triphasic Preparations						
Triphasil	30		50 (6 tabs)			
	40		75 (5 tabs)			
	30		125 (10 tabs)			
Triquilar	30		50 (6 tabs)			
	40		75 (5 tabs)			
	30		125 (10 tabs)			
Synphasic	35			500 (7 tabs)		
	35			1000 (9 tabs)		
	35			500 (5 tabs)		
Progestogen-Only Pills						
Microlut			30			
Microval			30			
Micronor				350		
Noriday				350		

Adapted from Badewitz-Dodd, L.H. ed. (1993) *MIMS Annual*, MIMS Australia, Sydney.

gestagen is usually sufficient to augment the postpartum levels of hormones to prevent ovulation from occurring.

When used as an alternative to the combined pill for the non-postpartum woman, thickening of the cervical mucus is thought to be the major antifertility effect of the progestagen-only pill as ovulation will occur in a significant number of these women (40%–60%) and in some, fertilisation will take place. Another effect of the small dose of progestagen is to change the lining of the uterus (the endometrium) making it unreceptive to the fertilised ovum and thus preventing implantation and any further growth of the developing cell mass.

Although it has a failure rate of about 2%, the absence of oestrogenic, progestagenic or androgenic side effects means that the mini-pill is ideal for breast-feeding women. As the mini-pill does not provide cycle control, irregular bleeding is the most common side effect. Whilst not usually a problem for the breast-feeding woman, it may be a source of anxiety for the menstruating woman. Irregular bleeding usually either settles or resolves over weeks or months during long-term use.

ADVERSE DRUG REACTIONS

Most of the side effects caused by oral contraceptives are reversible.

ADVERSE EFFECTS OF OESTROGENS

Nausea

Nausea is maximal on commencing oestrogen and improves as tolerance develops. If nausea continues beyond the third cycle of therapy, a change to a less oestrogenic, more progestagenic formulation may be considered.

Reduction of Lactation

Reduction of lactation will occur thus oestrogen should not be used for fertility control during lactation.

Water And Salt Retention

Water and salt retention may occur as oestrogen increases the osmotic pressure of the tissues. Patients may have difficulty in wearing contact lenses due to tissues holding more fluid. Diuretics, however, are rarely needed. A change to a less oestrogenic preparation may be considered, to counteract cyclical weight gain.

Leg Cramps

Leg cramps may occur especially at night.

Leucorrhoea

Leucorrhoea may occur as oestrogen stimulates the cervical glands to increased activity.

Migraine and Headaches

A principal reason for migraine is the fluid retention caused by the pill. Another reason for migraine and headaches is the withdrawal of oestrogen at the completion of a course of tablets. Those women who experience these symptoms during the pill-free week may be treated with a low dose of ethinyloestradiol. This type of menstrual migraine is not specific to women on the pill.

Hypertension

Hypertension when it occurs is frequently observed in women with a family history of hypertension and in those who develop pregnancy induced hypertension. A small proportion of women (around 5%) may develop hypertension with prolonged use. In some of these women the hypertension may be a coincidence. However, in most the hypertension will resolve after ceasing oral contraceptive use. Occasionally, malignant hypertension may occur. Frequent monitoring of blood pressure is required for all women taking oral contraceptives.

Venous Thromboembolism

Venous thromboembolism is potentially the most important side effect of oral contraceptive use. When oral contraceptive formulations contained much higher oestrogen levels, there was concern about the increased risks of morbidity and mortality due to pulmonary embolism, since the risk is proportional to the oestrogen content. The risks have been minimised with the

21

CONTRACEPTION AND INFERTILITY

low oestrogen content of modern oral contraceptive formulations.

Other Effects

Slight breast development and deposition of fat on the thighs are stimulated by oestrogen.

ADVERSE EFFECTS OF PROGESTOGENS

Weight Gain

All types of progestagens facilitate fat deposition but nortestosterones, e.g. levonorgestrol, also stimulate appetite. This is of particular importance in women who develop diminished glucose tolerance. Progestagens also decrease physical activity. To counteract acyclical weight gain a product with a lower progestagen content may be used.

Breakthrough Bleeding

Breakthrough bleeding often occurs and the menstrual flow is reduced. This effect probably accounts for around 20% of discontinuation of oral contraceptives by women. Bleeding occurring early in the cycle is caused by lack of oestrogenic stimulation, whilst that occurring after the middle of the cycle indicates a progestagen deficiency.

A short course of oestrogen from days 1–7 may be given to counteract persistent breakthrough bleeding. Alternatively, a change to a formulation with a higher oestrogenic content or a change to a triphasic formulation (which has a higher progestagen content after day 7) may be used.

Acne

Acne is related to the type of progestagen and is more common with nortestosterone progestagens. Low progestagenic, predominantly oestrogenic pills, such as *Biphasil*, *Sequilar* or *Ovulen-0.5/50* or preparations containing the progestagen desogestrel, e.g. *Marvelon*, should be used.

Other Effects

Progestagens in high doses can cause breast discomfort, headaches, migraine, premenstrual tension, depression, chronic fatigue, irritability and diminished glucose tolerance. Patients may also develop alopecia, gingivitis, loss of libido, hirsutism, jaundice and chloasma. After ruling out psychological causes, e.g. depression, a decrease in progestagen or an increase in oestrogen may be considered. Pyridoxine may also be of benefit (25–50 mg per day) for some depressed patients. Obviously, other causes of depression need to be ruled out. If the headaches are vascular in nature (throbbing, intense pain, nausea and other central nervous system symptoms) oral contraceptives may aggravate the symptoms and should be stopped. Women who have focal migraines or 'crescendo' migraines should not take oral contraceptives.

Oral contraceptives predispose to monilial infections and treatment with antifungal preparations such as nystatin gives little relief unless the amount of progestagen is reduced at the same time.

Choice of Oral Contraceptive

From this discussion, it is obvious there is not just one 'pill'. However, from the range of formulations available, a suitable choice should be possible after clinical assessment of the woman. Factors to be considered include age, length of menses, length of cycle, breast size, fat and hair distribution, history of acne, lactation and any history of thrombosis or smoking. For lactating mothers, the progestagen-only pill is recommended, especially the levonorgestrel type (e.g. *Microlut*, *Microval*) to minimise any possible effects from oestrogen metabolites during the infant's first year of life.

A typical 'check-list' to determine the most appropriate form of oral contraception for the individual woman would be:

- Does the woman need hormonal contraception? Would her needs be served better by 'barrier' methods of contraception, e.g. condom or diaphragm?

- What is the general condition of the patient? What is her medical and surgical history?

- What is revealed by a complete physical examination? Blood pressure? Body mass? Cardiovascular problems? Clotting difficulties? Pelvis and uterus? Fibroids? Migraine attacks?

- Does the woman have any moral or religious objections to the use of the pill?

When these factors have been considered and there are no reasons for not using the pill, the logical starting point is a low-dose balanced pill, e.g. the triphasic formulations, *Triquilar* and *Triphasil*. Breakthrough bleeding is common with triphasic pills. If the woman has a history of acne or hirsutism, a more oestrogenic preparation, e.g. *Biphasil*, *Brevinor* or *Sequilar*, may be appropriate. If irregular bleeding is a problem, then a balanced low-dose oestrogen formulation, e.g. *Microgynon-30*, *Nordette* or *Ovulen*, may be appropriate, as minimal endometrial buildup occurs.

If the woman has indications of oestrogen intolerance, then the progestagen-only pill would be a possible option. This group includes smokers over 35 years, hypertensive patients and patients with a history of thrombosis.

When contraception is necessary it is medically safe to prescibe oral contraceptives to young adolescents. The pill does not interfere with maturation of the hypothalamic-pituitary-ovarian axis and does not increase the incidence of amenorrhoea, oligomenorrhoea or infertility in later life.

Pill Failure

The combined pill has the distinction of being the most reliable known method of contraception. However, during the past decade numerous reports of 'pill failure' have appeared in the medical literature, raising a measure of concern about the need for special precautions for some patients and the possibility of contraindications when other medications are prescribed concurrently with the pill.

After selection of the most appropriate formulation of the pill for the individual woman, the most obvious reason for pill failure is non-compliance. Breakthrough ovulation can occur if daily doses of the combined pill are forgotten, or if the progestagen-only pill is taken more than three hours after the appropriate time each day. Also, any medical condition causing 'gut hurry', when the dose of hormones is not fully absorbed, can contribute to an increased incidence of unplanned pregnancy.

To understand the possible or potential causes of pill failure it is necessary to understand the process of enterohepatic cycling (see Chapter 2 Pharmacokinetics). This process results in the recirculation of the pill hormones at levels that are sufficient to suppress ovulation. While both oestrogens and progestagens are involved it is accepted that enterohepatic cycling of the oestrogen component is of greater significance.

When the pill is ingested the hormones are absorbed by the body in the upper part of the small intestine and then transported by the portal circulation to the liver where they are: (i) metabolised by hydroxylation in the mixed function oxidase system (the cytochrome P450 pathway); and then (ii) conjugated, that is, transformed into an inactive, more water soluble form (glucuronides and sulfates). From the liver these conjugated steroids are transferred in the bile to the small intestine. Under normal circumstances hydrolysis by enzymes from gut bacteria causes a release of the free, active form of the drug which can then be reabsorbed and returned to the cycle rather than being excreted in the conjugated form in the urine and faeces.

This recycling of the pill hormones has become more important as the doses of hormones in the combined pill have been progressively reduced in recent years. The triphasic pill, now the most frequently prescribed form of oral contraceptive, has only about one-fortieth of the steroid content of the pill formulations that were common when the pill was first introduced in the early 1960s.

With this knowledge of enterohepatic recycling it can be seen that there are at least

CONTRACEPTION AND INFERTILITY

21

three possible ways in which it is theoretically possible for pill failure to occur. These are gut hurry, concurrent administration of other drugs and reduction in gut bacteria.

If the contents of the upper bowel containing the pill hormones do not remain in the absorption area long enough because of **gut hurry**, then insufficient hormones will be absorbed initially to produce appropriate serum levels to prevent ovulation. Thus, during episodes of vomiting or diarrhoea, whether caused by food intolerance or medications, additional contraceptive cover for that particular cycle is usually required. Purgatives and magnesium containing antacids are usually mentioned as items to be used with caution by women taking the pill.

Concurrent administration of other drugs which compete for absorption and metabolism through the same pathway reduce the amount of hormones available for enterohepatic cycling. In most cases it appears that induction of hepatic microsomal enzymes and the consequent increased rates of metabolism are the cause of lowered circulating oestrogen levels.

Drugs in common use which have been implicated as causing such metabolic interactions include: anticonvulsant agents (e.g. phenytoin sodium, carbamazepine, barbiturates, primidone); antituberculous drugs (particularly rifampicin which, because of its potent induction of hepatic microsomal enzymes, should be viewed as one of the few drugs that should be totally contraindicated for concurrent administration with the pill); and antifungal agents (e.g. griseofulvin) which should be used with appropriate caution by women using hormonal contraception. A number of other drugs could be added to this list.

The main point to consider is that if the concurrent administration of any other drug with the pill causes any change from the previously 'normal' condition while taking oral contraceptives, the woman should be referred to her prescriber to assess the need for a possible change in the choice of pill. Breakthrough bleeding is a major indication that a drug interaction may have oc-

curred and women should be advised to use additional contraceptive cover, e.g. barrier methods, for the remaining part of that cycle.

Reduction in gut bacteria has been demonstrated with administration of antibiotics (e.g. broad spectrum penicillins, tetracyclines). The antibiotics can reduce the number of bacteria in the gut and affect absorption of the pill. While some controversy surrounds the explanation of possible causes, it is possible that the killing of such bacteria reduces the enzymes available for hydrolysis of the conjugated forms of the steroid back to the 'free' form, thus causing loss of steroid by excretion and a lowering of the levels of circulating hormones. However, this is not believed to be a major cause of pill failure.

This process can also operate in reverse, that is, when ceasing the concurrent administration of another medication with the pill. For example, the regular ingestion of large doses of vitamin C (ascorbic acid) causes a considerable increase in the level of circulation of oestrogen, effectively turning a low-dose pill into a higher-dose pill with a corresponding increase in oestrogenic side effects. More importantly, however, if the consumption of vitamin C is suddenly ceased, then a dramatic fall in oestrogen levels can occur often with breakthrough bleeding and the possibility of ovulation. Doses of 1 g of vitamin C daily have been reported to cause this effect when the dose is ceased or even taken intermittently. Women who insist on taking regular vitamin therapy should be advised to limit vitamin C intake to 250–300 mg daily while using hormonal contraception.

This discussion outlines the theoretical or potential possibility for pill failure. Indeed it has been suggested that the failure rate of oral contraceptives due to drug interactions is about 0.2–1 per 100 woman years, and that non-ingestion or non-absorption are probably the most important reasons for pill failure.

A knowledge of these interactions as possible causes of pill failure is also important in understanding the need for dosage adjustment of drugs used to treat a number of important medical conditions. Such conditions and therapies include epilepsy, diabetes, hypertension, depressive illnesses and collagen diseases and anticoagulant drugs. Because of competition in the same pathway for metabolism and excretion, re-evaluation of therapy or a dosage adjustment may be required. In some cases it may be wise to recommend another form of contraception. However, patients taking antiepileptic medications will usually obtain satisfactory contraceptive control by using a 50 microgram oestrogen pill. A pill-free period of four, rather than seven days, has also been suggested.

Effects of Missed Pills

There is a great deal of misunderstanding and confusion about what advice should be given to women who miss a dose of oral contraceptive during a cycle. It needs to be emphasised that missing a pill in the middle of a cycle is not as risky as missing a pill at the beginning or the end of a cycle. This is because during the pill-free week ovarian follicles ripen and therefore any increase in the pill-free time may allow ovulation to occur.

It is recommended that if the missed pills are the last of the active pills, the woman should immediately start taking the active pills of the next month's pack and omit the placebo pills of the current cycle. If the pills are missed at the beginning of the cycle other methods of contraception should be used during that cycle. The low dose of levonorgestrel at the beginning of the triphasic pill cycle may make it less reliable if pills are omitted. Furthermore, the 30 micrograms and 40 micrograms sequence of ethinyloestradiol in the triphasic pill is below the 50 micrograms ovulation inhibiting dose.

For women taking low-dose combined pills, contraceptive effectiveness cannot be guaranteed if the pill is taken more than six hours after the due time. For 50 microgram pills the leeway is 12 hours.

With progestagen-only preparations there is some evidence to suggest that only about three days are required to inhibit sperm penetration of cervical mucus and for contraceptive effectiveness to be restored, after a pill is missed. Generally speaking, however, it is assumed that there is an overall need to take progestagen-only pills within three hours of the due time each day.

A simple approach which will safeguard women whichever pills they miss is the 7-day rule: after a missed pill or pills take extra precautions for seven days plus; if the seven days happen to go beyond the end of the current packet start taking the active pills of a new packet with no break. An acceptable alternative is the 14-day rule: after a missed pill or pills take extra precautions for the next 14 days irrespective of bleeding. The latter approach has the obvious advantage that there is no need to explain the difference between active and placebo pills.

The 'Morning After' Pill

The use of high-dose hormone treatment within 72 hours of intercourse to reduce the risk of pregnancy (post-coital conception), is around 95% successful. Whilst various hormones have been used for this purpose, including high doses of pure oestrogens, the currently accepted method (the YUZPE method) is to give two *Nordiol* tablets (ethinyloestradiol 50 micrograms plus levonorgestrel 250 micrograms) followed by a further dose of two tablets in 12 hours. Frequently, antinauseant tablets such as metoclopramide (*Maxolon*) are given half an hour before each dose. The morning after pill must be used within 72 hours of intercourse taking place.

When oestrogen containing preparations are strongly contraindicated but unprotected intercourse has occurred, various progesterone-only preparations have been used, e.g. a regimen of norethisterone 0.35 mg, five tablets daily for five days. The failure rate of progesterone-only methods is higher than with combination regimens and

21

CONTRACEPTION AND INFERTILITY

there is a significant incidence of menstrual disturbances. It is important that patients are informed of the risk of failure, that adequate follow-up must be instituted and that no further unprotected intercourse should occur prior to the next period. Frequent intercourse may be to blame for the apparent failure rate.

Withdrawal bleeding is not a completely reliable indicator that pregnancy has not occurred and it is advisable to perform a pregnancy test at follow-up.

OTHER HORMONAL METHODS OF CONTRACEPTION

Progesterone Injection

Medroxyprogesterone acetate (*Depo-Provera*), a potent inhibitor of the gonadotrophins, can be given intramuscularly. Slowly absorbed, it results in prolonged activity, 150 mg given at three-month intervals producing a reliable method of contraception.

When the patient has a special need for effective contraception and other methods are contraindicated or have failed, *Depo-Provera* is the best choice.

NURSING IMPLICATIONS

ASSESSMENT

Assessment of the woman should include measurement of blood pressure, pulse rate and weight; a full medical history (especially for cerebrovascular disease, hepatic disease, oestrogen dependent tumours, fluid retention and hypertension); and assessment of current health, smoking habits, the possibility of pregnancy or existence of lactation and any current medications.

ADMINISTRATION

The combined pill is self-administered and taken on a cyclical basis. The nurse should stress the importance of taking the pill at the same time each day during the cycle to maintain ovarian suppression.

The progestogen-only pill is taken daily for as long as contraception is desired regardless of menstruation. The nurse should stress that the pill must be taken at the same time every day as it is not as effective as the combined pill. If a delay of more than three hours occurs in taking it, an additional means of contraception is recommended until menstrual bleeding occurs.

EVALUATION

Evaluation is important and should include consideration of adverse effects, e.g. nausea, chloasma (which responds to reduction in sun exposure) and headache (which may respond to simple analgesics). The incidence of migraine, which may necessitate a change in the type of oral contraceptive, should be noted. Weight gain may be helped by reduction in salt and calorie intake. Oedema and hypertension should be constantly watched for. If they occur a change in the method of contraception may be necessary. Women who wear contact lenses may experience difficulty and may need to wear glasses. Breakthrough bleeding, mood changes, monilial infection and acne also should be watched for.

The use of concurrent medication should be evaluated because rifampicin, phenytoin sodium, a variety of antibiotics (including ampicillin) and barbiturates have been implicated in reducing the effectiveness of oral contraceptives (see above). Haematological and endocrine tests may be affected by oral contraceptive therapy.

If diarrhoea and vomiting occur the woman should regard herself as inadequately protected and use additional contraception for the remainder of the cycle.

PATIENT EDUCATION

Education should include the need for regular health checks at least annually. This is essential for women taking the pill on a long-term basis. These checks can be performed by the local doctor or family planning clinic. Women who suffer adverse effects should be encouraged to report their symptoms to their doctor or clinic staff, as a review of their method of contraception may be necessary.

DRUG TREATMENT OF INFERTILITY — OVARIAN ACTIVATION

Infertility can be treated with drugs only when hormone abnormality is the cause. Causes of sterility also include hypothyroidism, tubal blockage and severe mental strain. This chapter deals only with the drug treatments used for hormone abnormalities.

OESTROGENS AND PROGESTAGENS

Ethinyloestradiol, Oestradiol Valerate, Oestrone Piperazine Sulfate

TRADE NAMES

Ethinyloestradiol: *Estigyn*; *Primogyn C.*
Oestradiol valerate: *Progynova.*
Oestrone piperazine sulfate: *Ogen.*

USES

Low hormone levels are frequently the cause of infertility, and therefore oestrogen and/or progesterone replacement therapy is all that is required.

In its naturally occurring form oestradiol is not sufficiently active by oral administration so a synthetic form, ethinyloestradiol, is used for the treatment of sterility caused by low oestrogen levels, e.g. genital underdevelopment. It is slowly metabolised and then excreted in the urine. Orally active forms of oestradiol, such as oestradiol valerate and oestrone piperazine sulfate, also may be used.

Impaired fertility due to failure of nidation may be treated with progesterone replacement therapy. Recently, progesterone pessaries have been used. Progesterone pessaries are, however, not generally available.

ADVERSE DRUG REACTIONS

Side effects of ethinyloestradiol are gastrointestinal disturbances, nausea, vomiting, headache, dizziness, breast tenderness and sodium and water retention.

PRECAUTIONS AND CONTRAINDICATIONS

The use of oestrogens is contraindicated in pregnancy, jaundice and patients with a previous history of blood clotting or impaired liver function.

ANTIOESTROGENS

Clomiphene

TRADE NAMES

Clomiphene: *Clomid.*

MECHANISM OF ACTION

Clomiphene has been described as an antioestrogen or a weak or impeded oestrogen. It competes for hypothalamus and pituitary receptor sites and replaces endogenous oestrogen with weak or impeded oestrogen. This interferes with the feedback mechanism causing an outpouring of gonadotrophic hormones FSH and LH with resultant increased prospects of ovulation. It enlarges

CONTRACEPTION AND INFERTILITY

21

the ovary (a reversible side effect) and ovulation can be obtained in a high proportion of patients with amenorrhoea.

PHARMACOKINETICS

Clomiphene citrate is readily absorbed from the gastrointestinal tract following oral administration. It has a half-life of about five days and appears to be metabolised in the liver. The drug and/or its metabolites are excreted principally in the faeces via biliary elimination.

USES

Clomiphene is indicated when the reason for infertility is failure of nidation.

Depending on the prescriber, clomiphene is usually administered on days 1 to 5, 2 to 6, 3 to 7 or 5 to 9 of the cycle. The dosage for clomiphene is between 25 mg (half a tablet) and 200 mg (4 tablets) daily for five days. Higher doses of clomiphene are sometimes used if ovulation has not occurred with the recommended doses, and the personal experience of the physician has shown it to be efficacious. Patients with hyperandrogenism and clomiphene resistance can also be given dexamethasone 0.25 mg or 0.5 mg at night.

ADVERSE DRUG REACTIONS

Just as lower levels of oestrogen at the menopause cause hot flushes, depression, insomnia and weight gain, so menopausal side effects are often produced by clomiphene since oestrogen levels are lowered. High doses produce ovarian cysts and visual blurring. The incidence of multiple pregnancy is increased.

PRECAUTIONS AND CONTRAINDICATIONS

Clomiphene is contraindicated in patients with liver disease, ovarian cysts and endometrial carcinoma.

DOPAMINERGIC RECEPTOR STIMULANTS

Bromocriptine

TRADE NAMES

Bromocriptine: *Parlodel.*

MECHANISM OF ACTION

Bromocriptine is a peptide ergot alkaloid which does not have the vasoconstricting effect of other ergot compounds. It is described as a dopaminergic receptor stimulant, as it mimics the action of dopamine which suppresses secretion of prolactin by the anterior pituitary. Bromocriptine also acts at the hypothalamic level by stimulating dopaminergic receptor sites in the hypothalamus, as well as either enhancing the release of gonadotrophic hormones (LH and FSH) or restoring the sensitivity of the ovary to gonadotropic stimulation. As elevated prolactin levels cause amenorrhoea and galactorrhoea, treatment with bromocriptine returns pituitary production of prolactin to normal, gonadal sensitivity to gonadotrophins promptly returns and normal ovulation occurs. It can also hasten the return to ovulation following childbirth, so patients who have bromocriptine prescribed for the suppression of lactation should be advised of the need for appropriate contraceptive measures.

PHARMACOKINETICS

Approximately 28% of an oral dose of the drug is absorbed from the gastrointestinal tract following oral administration, however, because of a substantial first-pass effect, only 6% of the dose reaches systemic circulation unchanged. With a fixed dosage there are large variations in plasma concentrations between individuals.

Following oral administration of a single 1.25–5.0 mg dose of bromocriptine, serum prolactin decreases within two hours, is maximally decreased at eight hours, and is still decreased at 24 hours. The maximum obtainable reduction of serum prolactin in hyperprolactinemic patients usually occurs within the first four weeks of bromocriptine therapy.

USES

Bromocriptine is the recommended form of treatment if elevated prolactin levels (caused by pituitary tumour or other pituitary disorders) are the underlying cause of infertility.

The dosage for infertility is one tablet (2.5 mg) twice daily, increasing to three times a day depending on the response shown by serum prolactin level estimations. Bromocriptine should be taken with food to minimise the possibility of gastrointestinal side effects such as nausea and vomiting.

For further information see Chapter 25 Neurological Disorders.

DRUGS FOR ENDOMETRIOSIS

Danazol

Danazol is currently used when endometriosis is the primary cause of infertility. It is a synthetic derivative of ethisterone.

TRADE NAMES

Danazol: *Danocrine*.

MECHANISM OF ACTION

Oral administration of danazol results in reduced plasma levels of the pituitary gonadotrophins, LH and FSH, with suppression of ovulation and menses. It is devoid of progestational and oestrogenic effects, but possesses androgenic activity and associated anabolic properties.

PHARMACOKINETICS

Danazol is absorbed from the gastrointestinal tract and metabolised in the liver.

USES

Danazol is indicated for the treatment of visually proven (e.g. by laparoscopy) endometriosis if surgery has been unsuccessful or is contraindicated, and the required endpoint of treatment is pregnancy. It is also used to treat various endocrine and gynaecological disorders where the control of pituitary gonadotrophins would be expected to have a beneficial effect.

The recommended dosage is 200–800 mg daily in two to four divided doses. Initial treatment is usually one capsule (200 mg) four times daily, although it may be possible to maintain improvement with a reduced dosage once a satisfactory response has been obtained. Treatment should continue for three to six months, but may be extended to nine months if necessary.

ADVERSE DRUG REACTIONS

A large proportion of patients (up to 75%) experience side effects when using danazol. A diuretic is sometimes co-administered for fluid retention. Anabolic side effects include weight gain, but as danazol causes a decrease in sex hormone binding globulin, and this in turn causes an increase in free testosterone (the active form), androgenic side effects are more common. These include deepening of voice (singers should be advised of this), hirsutism, acne and decrease in breast size.

PRECAUTIONS AND CONTRAINDICATIONS

Danazol should not be given during pregnancy or lactation, and to exclude the possibility of pregnancy, treatment should start during menstruation.

GONADOTROPHINS

Gonadotrophins, given parenterally, are also used to treat infertility. A number of specific types are available.

Human Chorionic Gonadotrophin (HCG)

TRADE NAMES

Human chorionic gonadotrophin: *Profasi*; *Pregnyl*; *APL*.

CONTRACEPTION AND INFERTILITY

21

MECHANISM OF ACTION

Human chorionic gonadotrophin (HCG) is a gonadotrophin with predominently luteinising properties. It is produced by the placenta and is obtained from the urine of pregnant women. The action of HCG is virtually identical to that of pituitary LH. HCG stimulates the corpus luteum of the ovary in the pregnant woman to continue production of oestrogen and progestogen, thereby preventing loss of the pregnancy through shedding of the endometrium as would normally occur at the end of that particular cycle.

PHARMACOKINETICS

Because of its polypeptide nature HCG is destroyed in the gastrointestinal tract and, therefore, must be administered parenterally. Following intramuscular administration, an increase in serum HCG concentrations may be observed within two hours. Peak HCG concentrations occur within about six hours and persist for about 36 hours. Serum HCG concentrations begin to decline at 48 hours and approach baseline (undetectable) levels after 72 hours.

USES

Exogenous HCG is used for male infertility due to hypogonadotrophic hypogonadism including eunuchoidism, female anovulatory sterility, ovulation induction in in-vitro fertilisation (IVF) programs and corpus luteum inadequacy.

In women it is given to induce ovulation after follicular development has been stimulated with FSH or menotrophin in the treatment of infertility due to absent or low concentrations of gonadotrophins. Duration of therapy varies but the total dose is in the region of 10 000 units given by intramuscular injection.

In males it has been used in the treatment of cryptorchidism in doses of 500–4000 units three times weekly by intramuscular injection. It has also been used for hypogonadotrophic hypogonadism due to pituitary deficiency and in the treatment of delayed puberty and oligospermia.

Menotrophin

TRADE NAMES

Menotrophin (human menopausal gonadotrophin, HMG): *Pergonal; Humegon.*

MECHANISM OF ACTION

Menotrophin is a purified preparation of gonadotrophin, prepared from the urine of postmenopausal women, and contains both FSH and LH activity. When administered for nine to 12 days menotrophin produces ovarian follicular growth in women who do not have primary ovarian failure. Treatment with menotrophin in most instances results only in follicular growth and maturation. In order to effect ovulation, HCG must be given following the administration of menotrophin when clinical assessment of the patient indicates that sufficient follicular maturation has occurred.

PHARMACOKINETICS

Because of its polypeptide nature menotrophin is destroyed in the gastrointestinal tract and, therefore, must be administered parenterally. Following intramuscular administration of a single dose of menotrophin approximately 8% of the dose is excreted unchanged in the urine.

USES

As indicated above menotrophin followed by chorionic gonadotrophin is used in the treatment of anovulatory infertility due to insufficient gonadotrophins. Menotrophin is administered to induce follicular maturation and endometrial proliferation and is followed by treatment with HCG to stimulate ovulation and corpus luteum formation.

Menotrophin may be given daily by intramuscular injection to provide a dose of 75 units of FSH with 75 units of LH until an adequate response (judged on the basis of daily oestrogen determinations) is achieved, followed after one or two days by HCG. A course of menotrophin should not exceed 12 days. Alternatively, three doses may be given on alternate days followed by HCG one week after the first dose.

Menotrophin is also used in conjunction with HCG to stimulate spermatogenesis in men with hypogonadotrophic hypogonadism in doses of 75 units or 150 units of FSH with 75 units or 150 units of LH three times weekly.

Urofollitrophin

TRADE NAMES

Urofollitrophin (urinary follicle stimulating hormone): *Metrodin.*

MECHANISM OF ACTION

Urofollitrophin is prepared by chromatographic removal of LH from menotrophins which have been purified from postmenopausal urine, and therefore possesses FSH activity but not LH activity.

USES

Urofollitrophin and HCG given in a sequential manner are indicated for the induction of ovulation in the anovulatory infertile patient when the cause of anovulation is a hormonal imbalance. This imbalance is usually an inappropriate ratio of endogenous FSH and LH levels in patients in whom primary ovarian failure has been excluded. Inappropriate levels of LH and FSH in patients with amenorrhoea or other anovulatory states is sometimes known as polycystic ovarian disease. This is characterised by a raised LH and low to normal FSH level.

ADVERSE DRUG REACTIONS

A possible serious complication of human gonadotrophin therapy is the hyperstimulation syndrome. Symptoms range from mild reactions such as lower abdominal pain and swelling, nausea, vomiting and diarrhoea, to more severe complications, including ascites, pleural effusions, haemoconcentration, increased viscosity and coagulation time, and thrombosis. While this potential exists, it should be stressed that such hyperstimulation is usually not a problem, provided that careful monitoring is undertaken as outlined by manufacturers. This usually involves hormone serum level assays.

IN-VITRO FERTILISATION (IVF)

As mentioned earlier this discussion does not include the operative procedures or methods of investigation used to assist patients with physical causes of infertility. However, the hormone therapy used during the IVF procedure is outlined below.

1. While it is preferred that the patient ovulate naturally, if necessary superovulation can be induced with clomiphene administered on days 1–5 of the cycle.

2. On day 6, menotrophin is administered, usually 100 units or more. Dosage is tailored for the individual patient, as determined by measurement of plasma hormone levels.

3. By approximately day 12 the patient will ovulate, depending on the length of the normal cycle. If not, ovulation is 'triggered' by administration of HCG, usually in a dose of around 3000 units. About 10% of IVF patients need this additional step.

4. A further 32–34 hours later, the obstetrician will perform a laparoscopy to aspirate the follicles as the LH surge will usually cause ovulation about 36 hours after the administration of HCG. Hormone level assays can be used to detect this. Often four or five ova are gathered by this procedure. The ova are then fertilised and returned to the uterus, thereby bypassing the problem of a blocked fallopian tube or similar physical abnormality.

GONADOTROPHIN RELEASING HORMONE (GnRH) ANALOGUES

The GnRH analogues are members of a new group of drugs that appear to have great potential for the future. Many research centres claim that GnRH analogues

CONTRACEPTION AND INFERTILITY

21

could prove to be one of the major advances in gynaecology for many years. They are derivatives of the natural hormone GnRH a decapeptide hormone, which, after synthesis and release by the hypothalamus, is transported to the anterior pituitary, where its primary role is to stimulate the secretion of the gonadotrophic hormones FSH and LH. As discussed earlier, these hormones are involved in the cyclical maturing of ovarian follicles and release of an ovum, with relative ratios often being more important than absolute serum levels of either.

There are two possible groups of GnRH analogues under investigation, GnRH antagonists and GnRH agonists, although it is interesting that the agonists (which bind to and stimulate pituitary GnRH receptors) have the potential for both types of action depending on the method of administration. If given in a pulsatile form of administration every one to two hours, thus mimicking the hypothalamic delivery of the hormone, increased synthesis and secretion of FSH and LH will result. If administration is by continuous infusion, however, with no time for the receptors to regenerate between the usual 'pulse' stimulation, the pituitary cells are not able to respond to further stimulation of endogenous GnRH or exogenous agonist therapy and consequently synthesis and secretion of FSH and LH stops. This results in substantially depressed plasma levels of FSH, LH and ovarian steroids, thus producing a reversible state of 'medical castration' or 'pseudomenopause'.

Consequently, these analogues have the prospect of finding application in a wide range of medical conditions, including: endometriosis, leiomyomata (fibroids), polycystic ovarian disease, induction of ovulation, menstrual disturbances (e.g. menorrhagia, dysmenorrhoea and premenstrual syndrome), contraception, hirsutism and in the treatment of hormone sensitive tumours in both men and women. Two of the early forms of GnRH analogues are nafarelin (*Synarel*), with a claimed potency two hundred times that of naturally occurring GnRH, and buserelin, which is understood to be one hundred times more potent than GnRH. Further research and clinical trials will disclose the potential of these new therapeutic agents.

NURSING IMPLICATIONS

ASSESSMENT

Assessment should include consideration of the physical health of both partners, psychosocial aspects and the outcome of any previous attempts to induce ovulation with drugs. The response of the couple to success or failure of fertility treatment also should be assessed. When ovarian activating drugs are to be prescribed for whatever reason the woman must be assessed for the presence of pregnancy and/or lactation, a familial history of gynaecological malignancy and a history of drug reaction and hypersensitivity.

ADMINISTRATION

Administration of HCG should be by intramuscular injection. Clomiphene should not be given to patients with liver disease, ovarian cysts or endometrial carcinoma. Danazol should not be given during pregnancy or lactation. Treatment with danazol should commence during menstruation, and diuretics may need to be given concomitantly.

EVALUATION

Evaluation is essential, and the following should be taken into account: observe for adverse effects, especially sodium and water retention with ethinyloestradiol; signs of ovarian enlargement or cysts and visual blurring with clomiphene; with danazol, the patient should be assessed for signs of oedema, acne and hirsutism.

PATIENT EDUCATION

Patient education is important, and patients should be informed of possible adverse effects of ovarian activators. Important aspects of education include timing of coitus in relation to courses of treatment and informing the couple of the increased incidence of multiple births following treatment with drugs such as clomiphene. Instruction should be given about basal-temperature monitoring and collection of urine for determination of oestrogen levels.

Nurses should be understanding and supportive of the infertile couple while they undergo numerous clinic visits, tests, examinations and questions related to their sexuality. Often it is necessary to reinforce medical counselling and give additional explanations on temperature taking (for ovulation) and the administration of medications.

Nurses, through their experience of working with infertile couples should also be alert to couples' wishes for alternatives (e.g. IVF, adoption) to pharmacological treatment especially if there are continued adverse drug reactions.

FURTHER READING

Filshie M., Guillebaud J., eds. (1989) *Contraception: science and practice*. Butterworths, London.

Guillebaud J. (1990) 'Current recommendations for oral contraception'. *Current Therapeutics* (Nov) pp 87–89.

Healy, D.L., Kovacs, G.T. (1990) 'Contraception'. *Current Therapeutics* (Feb) pp. 11–17.

Lumbers, E.R. (1987) 'Drug effects on reproductive physiology — mechanisms of action'. *Australian Prescriber*, Vol. 10, No. 1, p.4.

McLennan, A.H. (1986) 'Optimum use of oral contraceptives'. *Current Therapeutics*. (Sep) pp 37–48.

Normal, R.J., de Medeiros, S.G. (1991) 'Treatment of female infertility'. *Current Therapeutics*. (Nov) pp 41–48.

Rabone, D. (1990) 'Postcoital contraception. Coping with the morning after'. *Current Therapeutics*. (Jan) pp 45–49.

Shearman, R. (1987) 'Drug effects on reproductive physiology — clinical applications'. *Australian Prescriber*, Vol. 10, No. 1, p.7.

Szarewski, A., Guillebaud, J. (1991) 'Contraception. Current state of the art'. *British Medical Journal* 302 pp. 1224–1226.

Weisberg, E. (1992) 'Triphasics—Have they fulfilled their promise?' *Current Therapeutics* (Jan). pp 11–16.

TEST YOUR KNOWLEDGE

1. List the main female hormones and describe the role of these hormones in the normal ovarian cycle.

2. What types of contraceptive 'pill' are available, and what factors would determine the type of pill chosen for a particular patient?

3. Which of the following are adverse effects of oestrogen? Acne, depression, weight gain, leucorrhoea, hypertension, water retention, migraine, leg cramps, thrombosis, breakthrough bleeding.

4. What are some of the possible causes of 'pill failure'?

5. List the main drug treatments available for female infertility?

CONTRACEPTION AND INFERTILITY

21

Musculoskeletal Disorders

JENNIFER L. BENZIE

O B J E C T I V E S

At the conclusion of this chapter the reader should be able to:

1. Identify the drugs used in the treatment of musculoskeletal disorders;

2. Discuss the mode of action of these drugs and the disease states for which they are used;

3. List the common adverse reactions to drugs used in the treatment of musculoskeletal disorders; and

4. Write brief notes describing the nursing implications related to the drugs mentioned.

DRUGS USED IN ARTHRITIS, RHEUMATOID ARTHRITIS AND RELATED DISORDERS

There are two main classes of agents used in the treatment of arthritis, rheumatoid arthritis and related disorders; the non-steroidal anti-inflammatory drugs and the disease modifying agents.

NON-STEROIDAL ANTI-INFLAMMATORY DRUGS

The non-steroidal anti-inflammatory drugs (NSAIDs) are used for the symptomatic relief of pain and inflammation in a wide range of musculoskeletal conditions such as arthritis, rheumatoid arthritis, ankylosing spondylitis and osteoarthritis. They exert their effect by inhibiting the synthesis of prostaglandins, known mediators of inflammation. The number of NSAIDs on the market has increased rapidly in the past decade. All these drugs have anti-inflammatory, analgesic and antipyretic properties. The NSAIDs share common adverse drug reactions to a greater or lesser extent. These adverse reactions include gastrointestinal upset, peptic ulceration and inhibition of platelet aggregation. All NSAIDs possess the potential for masking the signs and symptoms of infection. They may also cause fluid retention.

Aspirin and Salicylates

The anti-inflammatory effect of aspirin (acetylsalicylic acid) is attained in the plasma salicylate concentration range of 150–300 mg/L, and this is usually achieved with doses of 2.6–6.0 g of aspirin per day.

TRADE NAMES

Aspirin: *ASA* (*Arthritis Strength Aspirin*); *Aspro*; *Bufferin*; *Disprin*; *Ecotrin*; *Solprin*.

MECHANISM OF ACTION

Pain relief is effected by both a central and peripheral action. Aspirin and the salicylates inhibit the synthesis of prostaglandins in inflamed tissues and so prevent sensitisation of pain receptors to substances that appear to mediate the pain response.

PHARMACOKINETICS

Absorption is rapid, partly from the stomach and mostly from the upper small intestine with appreciable plasma concentrations being attained within 30 minutes. After absorption, aspirin is rapidly distributed throughout the body tissues. It readily crosses the placenta.

Aspirin is partially hydrolysed during absorption to salicylate in the gastrointestinal mucosa. Further metabolism also occurs in the liver, plasma, erythrocytes and synovial fluid. Only 1% of an oral dose of aspirin is excreted unchanged in the urine. The remainder is excreted in urine as salicylate and its metabolites.

USES

The types of pain eased by aspirin are varied, usually of low intensity and range from bone and joint pain, headache and toothache to acute rheumatic fever. Aspirin is usually the drug of first choice in rheumatoid arthritis, but it is of relatively little help in the treatment of acute gout and severe ankylosing spondylitis. Aspirin may be used in individual doses of 600 mg to 1 g as required, purely as an analgesic. However, to exert an anti-inflammatory effect, regular dosage every 3–4 hours is necessary, the total dosage being 4–6 g daily. The aim is to use the lowest effective dose which is often the highest tolerated. Only about half the patients who tolerate a lower dosage will continue at a higher dosage of 4–6 g for any length of time and many of these experience troublesome adverse reactions.

ADVERSE DRUG REACTIONS

Headaches, dizziness and tinnitus are common particularly at continued high dosage. Other side effects include difficulty in hearing, dimness of vision, mental confusion, hyperventilation, sweating, thirst and worsening of gout.

Overdosage with salicylates initially causes overbreathing with increased respiration rate followed by respiratory alkalosis. In infants and children this may easily be missed.

Hypersensitivity reactions are not common but may be severe and even fatal, e.g. acute asthma and anaphylactic reactions. Aspirin hypersensitivity may occur after taking only small amounts of the drug.

DRUG INTERACTIONS

Aspirin may enhance the activity of coumarin anticoagulants (warfarin) and sulfonylurea hypoglycaemic agents. The activity of methotrexate may be markedly enhanced and its toxicity increased by co-administration of aspirin.

Aspirin diminishes the effects of uricosuric agents such as probenecid and sulfinpyrazone. As aspirin can be taken by the patient without prescription, it is important to know the potential interactions. Some potential drug interactions are listed in Table 22.1.

TABLE 22.1   Potential drug interactions with aspirin

Drug	Possible Interaction
Alcohol	Increased gastrointestinal irritation with risk of gastric haemorrhage
Ammonium chloride Ascorbic acid	Increased salicylate levels due to decreased urinary clearance
Antacids	Decreased plasma salicylate levels due to increased urinary clearance. Therapeutic plasma levels may not be maintained
Anticoagulants	Increased risk of gastric haemorrhage with both oral anticoagulants and heparin
Antidiabetic drugs (oral)	Increased hypoglycaemic effect with sulfonylureas and large doses of aspirin
Corticosteroids	Accumulation of salicylate with toxicity when long-term steroid therapy is withdrawn and dose of aspirin is not reduced
Methotrexate	Activity of methotrexate enhanced and toxicity increased
Uricosuric agents	Low doses of aspirin inhibit uricosuric action of probenecid and sulfinpyrazone
Valproic acid	Aspirin significantly increases plasma levels of unbound valproic acid and should be avoided in patients taking valproic acid

22

MUSCULOSKELETAL DISORDERS

PRECAUTIONS AND CONTRAINDICATIONS

Aspirin should not be administered to patients with haemophilia, asthma or those with an intolerance to aspirin. It should be given with extreme caution to patients prone to dyspepsia or known to have a lesion of the gastric mucosa. Aspirin should be used with caution in patients with impaired renal function and particularly in dehydrated children. It should only be given to pregnant patients if the potential benefit justifies the potential risk to the fetus. Aspirin and other salicylates are excreted into breast milk in low concentrations and therefore should be used cautiously by women who are breast feeding.

Diflunisal

Diflunisal is a derivative of salicylate with higher potency, longer duration of action and better tolerance than aspirin.

TRADE NAMES

Diflunisal: *Dolobid*.

MECHANISM OF ACTION

The exact mode of action of diflunisal is not known; however it is a prostaglandin synthetase inhibitor which may explain its analgesic and anti-inflammatory actions. It appears to act peripherally with no central nervous system effects.

USES

Diflunisal is a useful analgesic for short-term relief of postoperative, dental and post-traumatic pain, and it is also useful in long-term treatment of osteoarthritis and rheumatoid arthritis. The initial dose is 500 mg twice daily, and then adjusted to individual patient's requirements. The maximum daily dose is 1 g. Tablets should be swallowed whole. Diflunisal is available as 250 mg and 500 mg tablets.

PHARMACOKINETICS

Diflunisal is completely absorbed after oral administration with peak plasma levels attained in about 2 hours. It is metabolised in the liver (88%). It is highly protein bound (98%–99%) and its excretion is mainly renal.

ADVERSE DRUG REACTIONS

Side effects are relatively uncommon with diflunisal, with gastrointestinal upsets the most frequent. Skin rashes and pruritus are uncommon. Gastrointestinal bleeding has been reported.

DRUG INTERACTIONS

Diflunisal may cause some prolongation of prothrombin times when given with oral anticoagulants. Patients receiving such a combination should be closely monitored.

PRECAUTIONS AND CONTRAINDICATIONS

Diflunisal should not be administered to patients with salicylate hypersensitivity or to patients with active gastrointestinal bleeding. It should be used with caution in patients with impaired renal function and hypertension. Diflunisal should not be given to pregnant or breast feeding women.

Indomethacin

TRADE NAMES

Indomethacin: *Indocid*; *Arthrexin*.

MECHANISM OF ACTION

Indomethacin inhibits the synthesis of prostaglandins. It is one of the most potent non-steroidal anti-inflammatory agents available and will, if tolerated, reduce inflammatory swelling and lessen pain in the inflammatory arthropathies.

PHARMACOKINETICS

Indomethacin is rapidly absorbed following oral administration. Peak plasma levels are attained in approximately 2 hours. The rate of absorption following rectal administration is generally more rapid than that following oral administration while the bioavailability is comparable to, or slightly less than, that following oral administration. Indomethacin is extensively bound to plasma proteins (99%) and is metabolised in the liver to metabolites that do not possess anti-inflammatory activity. Excretion of indomethacin and its metabolites is via the kidneys (~60%) and faeces (~33%).

USES

Indomethacin is indicated in the active stages of rheumatoid arthritis, osteoarthritis, degenerative joint disease of the hip, ankylosing spondylitis and gout. It is also indicated for treatment of acute musculoskeletal disorders such as bursitis, low back pain, and inflammation, pain and oedema following orthopaedic surgical procedures. The recommended dosage of indomethacin is 50–200 mg daily (in divided doses, 2–3 times daily). In patients with persistent night pain and/or morning stiffness, a dose of up to 100 mg at bedtime may be used. It is rarely necessary to exceed a daily dose of 200 mg. Indomethacin is available as 25 mg capsules and 100 mg suppositories.

ADVERSE DRUG REACTIONS

Headaches, vertigo, lightheadedness, confusion and a number of other cerebral sensations are dose related and diminish or disappear with reduction of dosage. Gastrointestinal symptoms, abdominal pain, vague discomfort, anorexia or peptic ulceration may occur at any time on any dose. Blood dyscrasias have been reported but are rare. Severe depression, hallucinations and even psychoses have been reported. The use of suppositories may diminish, but not entirely prevent, gastrointestinal irritation.

DRUG INTERACTIONS

As indomethacin is highly protein bound, interactions may occur with oral anticoagulants, phenytoin, salicylates, sulfonamides and sulfonylureas.

Indomethacin significantly reduces the renal clearance of, and therefore increases plasma levels of lithium.

Renal elimination of methotrexate is inhibited by indomethacin, therefore it should be avoided in patients receiving methotrexate. Renal function should be closely monitored in patients receiving NSAIDs and cyclosporin.

PRECAUTIONS AND CONTRAINDICATIONS

Indomethacin should not be used in patients in whom asthmatic attacks, urticaria or rhinitis are precipitated by salicylates and other NSAIDs.

It should not be given to patients with active peptic ulcer or with a history of recurrent gastrointestinal ulceration. The suppositories are contraindicated in patients with a recent history of proctitis. Since indomethacin is eliminated primarily by the kidneys, patients with impaired renal function should be closely monitored. Indomethacin may cause fluid retention and should be used with caution in patients with compromised cardiac function or hypertension.

Indomethacin should not be used during pregnancy or given to women who are breast feeding.

Sulindac

Sulindac is a derivative of indomethacin. It appears to have similar effects without some of the characteristic adverse reactions.

TRADE NAMES

Sulindac: *Clinoril*; *Aclin*.

PHARMACOKINETICS

Sulindac is approximately 90% absorbed after oral administration. It undergoes metabolism to active and inactive metabolites. The active metabolite is a potent inhibitor of prostaglandin synthesis. Peak concentrations of the active metabolite are achieved in about 2 hours when sulindac is administered in the fasting state and in about 3–4 hours when administered with food. Sulindac and its metabolites are extensively (90%–98%) bound to plasma proteins. The primary route of excretion for both sulindac and its inactive metabolite is via the urine with some excreted via the faeces and bile.

USES

Sulindac is as effective as aspirin in rheumatoid arthritis. It is more effective than ibuprofen, comparable to naproxen and is a useful alternative to indomethacin. A dose of 200 mg twice daily is usually required in severe rheumatoid arthritis. The dose can often be reduced to 200 mg daily in milder conditions and should be given in the lowest effective maintenance dose. It is also indicated in the treatment of osteoarthritis, ankylosing spondylitis, acute gouty arthritis and periarticular diseases such as bursitis, tendonitis and tenosynovitis. It is available as 100 mg and 200 mg tablets.

ADVERSE DRUG REACTIONS

Sulindac is generally well tolerated. Those adverse effects which occur tend to be mild and seldom lead to withdrawal of treatment. Constipation, epigastric pain, nausea and diarrhoea are the most common side effects, occurring in 25% of patients.

DRUG INTERACTIONS

The concomitant administration of aspirin with sulindac is not recommended as aspirin depresses the plasma levels of the active metabolite. Patients taking oral anticoagulants and oral hypoglycaemics should be monitored as a possible interaction exists between these drugs and sulindac.

PRECAUTIONS AND CONTRAINDICATIONS

Sulindac should not be used in patients in whom acute asthmatic attacks have been precipitated by aspirin or other NSAIDs. The drug should not be given to patients with active gastrointestinal bleeding and should be avoided in patients with a history of gastrointestinal haemorrhage or ulcers.

Sulindac should be used with caution in patients with impaired renal function. Abnormalities in liver function tests have been reported and should be monitored until they return to normal. Sulindac is a moderate to weak inhibitor of platelet function and patients who may be adversely affected by this should be monitored closely.

Sulindac should not be given to women who are pregnant or to those who are breast feeding.

Propionic Acid Derivatives

The propionic acid derivatives (ibuprofen, naproxen, ketoprofen, tiaprofenic acid, mefenamic acid, diclofenac sodium, piroxicam and tenoxicam) are useful in a wide range of rheumatic disorders. They are used to suppress pain when there is evidence of inflammation, i.e. heat, redness and swelling. The spectrum of effects and side effects of propionic acid derivatives are similar, although patients respond individually to them in terms of both pain relief and adverse reactions.

Ibuprofen

TRADE NAMES

Ibuprofen: *Brufen*.

MECHANISM OF ACTION

It is postulated that ibuprofen produces an anti-inflammatory effect in part by inhibiting prostaglandin synthetase.

PHARMACOKINETICS

Ibuprofen is well absorbed after oral administration. Peak serum levels occur 45 minutes after administration on an empty stomach and at 1–1.5 hours if taken after food. Ibuprofen is highly protein bound (99%) and is metabolised to two metabolites both devoid of anti-inflammatory and analgesic activity. The kidney is the major route of excretion for both the metabolites and ibuprofen.

USES

Ibuprofen is indicated for treatment of rheumatoid arthritis, osteoarthritis and relief of acute and/or chronic pain states in which there is an inflammatory component.

The recommended initial dose is 1200–1600 mg daily in three or four divided doses. For acute exacerbations in patients already taking ibuprofen, a maximum daily dose of 2400 mg may be prescribed reverting to a maximum of 1600 mg daily once the patient is stabilised. Ibuprofen is available as 200 mg and 400 mg tablets.

ADVERSE DRUG REACTIONS

Toxic amblyopia has been reported with ibuprofen but responds rapidly to drug withdrawal. Gastrointestinal side effects are the most common, including nausea, epigastric pain, heartburn, abdominal distress, vomiting, diarrhoea and constipation. Other side effects include those common to other NSAIDs.

DRUG INTERACTIONS

Due to its extensive protein binding, ibuprofen could theoretically potentiate the effect of coumarin anticoagulants, sulfonylurea antidiabetic agents and some antiepileptic drugs. If corticosteroids are reduced or discontinued during ibuprofen therapy the dose of ibuprofen should be reduced gradually.

PRECAUTIONS AND CONTRAINDICATIONS

Ibuprofen is contraindicated in patients sensitive to aspirin and other NSAIDs. It should not be used when active gastrointestinal bleeding is present. It should be used with caution in patients with impaired liver function, cardiac failure, and coagulation defects.

Ibuprofen should not be given to pregnant women or to those who are breast feeding.

Naproxen

TRADE NAMES

Naproxen: *Inza*; *Naprosyn*, *Naprosyn SR*.

MECHANISM OF ACTION

The exact mechanism of naproxen's anti-inflammatory and analgesic action is not entirely clear. It has, however, been shown to inhibit the synthesis and release of prostaglandins.

PHARMACOKINETICS

Naproxen is completely absorbed from the gastrointestinal tract following oral administration peak plasma levels being attained within 2–4 hours. It is extensively bound (99.9%) to albumin. Metabolism occurs in the liver to form inactive compounds. Excretion is mainly via the kidneys, with a small proportion via the faeces.

USES

Naproxen is indicated for the treatment of rheumatoid arthritis and osteoarthritis. The dosage range of naproxen is 375 mg to 1 g daily in two divided doses. It is available as 250 mg and 500 mg tablets, 750 mg and 1000 mg sustained release tablets, 125 mg/5 mL suspension and 500 mg suppositories.

ADVERSE DRUG REACTIONS

The most frequently reported side effects are stomatitis and effects related to the gastrointestinal tract (constipation, abdominal pain, nausea, dyspepsia, diarrhoea). Central nervous system side effects include headache, dizziness, drowsiness, lightheadedness and vertigo.

DRUG INTERACTIONS

Patients taking coumarin anticoagulants should be monitored for an increase in prothrombin time. Caution should be exercised in patients taking lithium or methotrexate as naproxen has the potential to reduce the clearance of both these drugs. Naproxen may also increase the effect of sulfonamides and sulfonylureas.

PRECAUTIONS AND CONTRAINDICATIONS

Naproxen should not be administered to patients who are hypersensitive to NSAIDs or to patients with active gastrointestinal bleeding. The suppositories should not be used in patients with any inflammatory lesions of the rectum or anus or in patients with a recent history of rectal or anal bleeding.

Naproxen should be used with caution in patients with hypertension or heart failure because of its propensity to cause fluid retention. Patients with impaired renal function and liver failure should be closely monitored if taking naproxen.

Naproxen should be avoided in women who are pregnant or breast feeding.

22 MUSCULOSKELETAL DISORDERS

Ketoprofen

TRADE NAMES

Ketoprofen: *Orudis, Orudis SR.*

MECHANISM OF ACTION

Ketoprofen acts by inhibiting prostaglandin synthesis.

PHARMACOKINETICS

Ketoprofen is readily absorbed from the gastrointestinal tract, peak plasma concentrations occurring at 0.5–2.0 hours after administration. Absorption is retarded in the presence of food. Metabolism occurs in the liver and excretion is mainly via the urine with a small proportion via the faeces.

USES

Ketoprofen is indicated for treatment of rheumatoid arthritis and osteoarthritis. Initial dosage is 50 mg three times daily increased to 200 mg daily in divided doses depending on the patient's weight and the severity of the symptoms.

It is available as 50 mg and 100 mg capsules and a sustained release preparation is available as 100 mg and 200 mg capsules (*Orudis SR*). The dosage range for the sustained release formulation is 100–200 mg once daily. All oral formulations of ketoprofen should be taken with food. Ketoprofen is also available as a 100 mg suppository which is appropriate for controlling overnight symptoms. The dosage is 100 mg at night.

ADVERSE DRUG REACTIONS

The most frequently observed adverse reactions are gastrointestinal.

Drug interactions, precautions and contraindications are similar to those with other NSAIDs.

Tiaprofenic Acid

TRADE NAMES

Tiaprofenic acid: *Surgam.*

MECHANISM OF ACTION

Tiaprofenic acid inhibits the biosynthesis of prostaglandins and is a non-selective antagonist of bradykinin, prostaglandin E_2, serotonin, histamine and acetylcholine. These actions produce analgesic, anti-inflammatory and antipyretic effects.

PHARMACOKINETICS

Tiaprofenic acid is rapidly and completely absorbed after oral administration, probably from the duodenum. Peak plasma levels occur 0.5–1 hour after administration. Food decreases the bioavailability by 10% to 20% and increases the time required to reach maximum plasma levels. It is highly bound to plasma proteins (98%). Tiaprofenic acid is metabolised to a limited extent, metabolites accounting for less than 5% of the excreted drug. Excretion of the drug and it metabolites is predominately renal, the remainder being via the bile.

USES

Tiaprofenic acid is an effective anti-inflammatory and analgesic agent in the treatment of osteoarthritis, rheumatoid arthritis and acute pain states resulting from minor surgery or trauma. Studies have demonstrated tiaprofenic acid to be a suitable alternative to aspirin, diclofenac, ibuprofen, indomethacin, naproxen, piroxicam and sulindac in rheumatoid arthritis and osteoarthritis and to aspirin in acute pain states. The usual starting and maintenance dose is 200 mg three times daily. Some patients can be maintained on 300 mg daily. Tiaprofenic acid is available as 200 mg and 300 mg tablets.

ADVERSE DRUG REACTIONS

The most common adverse effects are gastrointestinal with peptic ulcer the most severe. Other side effects include indigestion, nausea, heartburn and epigastric pain.

Dizziness, drowsiness and headache occur to a lesser extent. Rash, erythema, pruritus and photosensitivity occur rarely. As with other NSAIDs fluid retention and oedema have been observed.

DRUG INTERACTIONS

Tiaprofenic acid is extensively bound to serum albumin (98%). Therefore caution should be observed when the drug is used concurrently with anticoagulants, sulfonylurea hypoglycaemic agents, sulfonamides, and phenytoin. The renal clearance of drugs such as lithium and methotrexate may be reduced during concomitant therapy with NSAIDs. Caution should therefore be exercised if these combinations are used.

PRECAUTIONS AND CONTRAINDICATIONS

Tiaprofenic acid may cause fluid retention and should be used with caution in patients with compromised cardiac function, hypertension or other conditions predisposing to fluid retention. The anti-inflammatory actions of tiaprofenic acid may mask the signs and symptoms of infection.

Tiafrofenic acid should not be given to pregnant women or those who are breast feeding.

Mefenamic Acid

Mefenamic acid belongs to the fenemate group of drugs which possess analgesic, anti-inflammatory and antipyretic properties.

TRADE NAMES

Mefenamic acid: *Ponstan.*

MECHANISM OF ACTION

Mefenamic acid inhibits the enzymes of prostaglandin synthesis and also antagonises the actions of prostaglandin at receptor sites.

PHARMACOKINETICS

Mefenamic acid is slowly absorbed from the small intestine and peak blood levels are attained 2–4 hours after oral administration. It is extensively bound to plasma proteins.

Metabolism occurs in the liver and excretion of the drug and its metabolites occurs principally in the urine (~50%) with about 20% recovered from the faeces.

USES

Mefenamic acid is used mainly as an analgesic agent to relieve pain arising in rheumatic conditions. It is also indicated for short-term relief of mild to moderate pain, e.g. dysmenorrhoea, dental and soft tissue pain. Mefenamic acid is available as 250 mg capsules. Dosage is 500 mg three times daily with food.

ADVERSE DRUG REACTIONS

Gastrointestinal irritation is common. Dyspepsia, abdominal discomfort and diarrhoea are the most frequently reported side effects. Rashes occur rarely. Mefenamic acid has been reported to cause haemolytic anaemia. In aspirin sensitive patients it may cause bronchoconstriction.

DRUG INTERACTIONS

Mefenamic acid binds strongly to plasma protein and may potentiate the activity of coumarin anticoagulants. It should therefore be used with caution in patients receiving warfarin.

PRECAUTIONS AND CONTRAINDICATIONS

Mefenamic acid is contraindicated in patients showing evidence of gastrointestinal inflammation and/or ulceration, patients in whom aspirin and other NSAIDs have induced symptoms of bronchospasm and those with impaired renal function. Mefenamic acid should not be given to pregnant or breast feeding women.

The drug should be promptly discontinued if diarrhoea occurs or a rash develops.

Diclofenac Sodium

Diclofenac sodium is a non-steroidal compound, which exhibits marked anti-inflammatory, analgesic, and antipyretic activity.

TRADE NAMES

Diclofenac sodium: *Fenac*; *Voltaren*.

MECHANISM OF ACTION

It is a potent inhibitor of prostaglandin synthesis.

PHARMACOKINETICS

Diclofenac is well absorbed following oral administration peak plasma levels occurring in 1–2 hours. It is extensively metabolised in the liver to inactive metabolites and is highly bound to serum albumin (99%). Approximately two-thirds of a dose is excreted in the urine, the remainder via the bile.

USES

Diclofenac is indicated for the treatment of rheumatoid arthritis and osteoarthritis and for relief of acute and chronic pain states in which there is an inflammatory component.

Initial dosage is 75–150 mg daily, depending on the severity of the condition, given in two or three divided doses. For long-term therapy, 75–100 mg daily in divided doses, is usually sufficient. It is available as 25 mg and 50 mg enteric coated tablets and these should be swallowed whole.

ADVERSE DRUG REACTIONS

Diclofenac is generally well tolerated. Gastrointestinal symptoms (eructation, nausea, epigastric pain, diarrhoea) are the most common but are mild and transient. Peptic ulcer or gastrointestinal haemorrhage has been reported but usually in patients with a history of such disorders. Less common reactions include drug rash, eczema, peripheral oedema, blood dyscrasias, headache, dizziness and tiredness.

DRUG INTERACTIONS

Diclofenac may reduce the clearance of lithium and methotrexate and therefore increase the risk of toxicity. Due to its extensive protein binding, diclofenac may potentiate the effect of anticoagulants.

PRECAUTIONS AND CONTRAINDICATIONS

Patients hypersensitive to salicylates or who have a peptic ulcer or gastrointestinal bleeding should not be given diclofenac. Care should be exercised when treating patients with severe hepatic or renal disease and patients on long-term therapy should have regular blood counts.

Diclofenac should be avoided in pregnant or breast feeding women.

Piroxicam

Piroxicam is a non-steroidal anti-inflammatory agent which possesses analgesic and antipyretic properties.

TRADE NAMES

Piroxicam: *Feldene*.

MECHANISM OF ACTION

Piroxicam inhibits biosynthesis of prostaglandins and collagen induced platelet aggregation.

PHARMACOKINETICS

Piroxicam is well absorbed following oral administration. Peak plasma levels occur 2 hours after administration. It is extensively metabolised in the liver and excreted in the urine. It is highly protein bound (99%).

USES

Piroxicam is indicated for the symptomatic treatment of rheumatoid arthritis, osteoarthritis and ankylosing spondylitis and for relief of acute and/or chronic pain states in which there is an inflammatory component.

The recommended starting dose is 10 mg daily, increased to 20 mg as a single dose. Administration of doses higher than 20 mg daily are not recommended. It is available as 10 mg and 20 mg capsules.

ADVERSE DRUG REACTIONS

More common reactions include abdominal discomfort and pain, flatulence, nausea, constipation, diarrhoea, dizziness and headache. Other side effects reported include tinnitus, vertigo, deafness, hypertension, tachycardia, palpitations, skin rashes, sedation, drowsiness, and oedema. Peptic ulceration and gastrointestinal haemorrhage may occur.

DRUG INTERACTIONS

As with other NSAIDs, piroxicam decreases platelet aggregation and prolongs bleeding time. Patients receiving anticoagulants should be closely monitored. Dosage requirements of anticoagulants and other drugs that are highly protein bound should be closely monitored. Care should be taken when patients receive methotrexate or lithium in conjunction with piroxicam.

PRECAUTIONS AND CONTRAINDICATIONS

Piroxicam should not be administered to patients with a known hypersensitivity to aspirin and other NSAIDs or to patients with peptic ulcer disease or a history of it. It should be used with caution in patients with impaired hepatic function as abnormalities in liver function tests have been reported. As with other NSAIDs, piroxicam may mask the symptoms of infection. Patients with compromised cardiac function should be monitored as sodium retention is a side effect common to most NSAIDs.

Piroxicam should not be given to pregnant or breast feeding women.

Tenoxicam

TRADE NAMES

Tenoxicam: *Tilcotil*.

MECHANISM OF ACTION

The exact mechanism of action of tenoxicam is not known but appears to be associated with inhibition of prostaglandin synthesis.

PHARMACOKINETICS

After oral administration, tenoxicam is completely absorbed in its unchanged form. Peak plasma concentrations occur 1–2 hours after administration in fasted subjects. When taken with a meal absorp-

tion is the same but occurs at a slower rate. In the blood, over 99% of the drug is bound to serum albumin. Tenoxicam is entirely metabolised in the body before its excretion. Up to two-thirds of the metabolites are excreted in the urine, the rest via the bile.

USES

Tenoxicam is indicated for the symptomatic treatment of rheumatoid arthritis, osteoarthritis, ankylosing spondylitis and for relief of acute and/or chronic pain states in which there is an inflammatory component.

The recommended starting dose is 10 mg daily and if necessary this can be increased after two weeks to 20 mg daily. Daily doses higher than 20 mg should be avoided since this increases the possibility of adverse effects without significantly increasing efficacy. Tenoxicam is available as 10 mg tablets.

ADVERSE DRUG REACTIONS

Gastrointestinal effects include epigastralgia, nausea and heartburn. Central nervous system effects include headache, dizziness, tiredness, and sleeping disturbances. Dermatological effects which may occur are erythema, urticaria and itching. As with other NSAIDs, severe skin reactions such as Stevens-Johnson syndrome, Lyell's syndrome and photosensitivity reactions may occur in rare instances.

DRUG INTERACTIONS

Tenoxicam decreases platelet aggregation and prolongs bleeding times. Patients should be closely monitored when anticoagulants are being used. Tenoxicam is highly protein bound and therefore might be expected to displace other protein bound drugs such as oral antidiabetic agents. Dosage requirements of these drugs should be closely monitored when given with tenoxicam. Renal clearance of lithium may be decreased in presence of tenoxicam and therefore lithium plasma concentrations should be monitored.

MUSCULOSKELETAL DISORDERS

22

Extreme care should be exercised in giving methotrexate to patients taking tenoxicam because of the possibility that NSAIDs inhibit the renal clearance of methotrexate.

Tenoxicam should be given under close supervision in patients with a history of impaired hepatic function as abnormalities in liver function tests have been reported. The anti-inflammatory, antipyretic and analgesic effects of tenoxicam may mask the signs of infection.

Sodium retention may occur with all NSAIDs and therefore tenoxicam should be used with caution in patients with compromised cardiac function or hypertension.

PRECAUTIONS AND CONTRAINDICATIONS

Tenoxicam should not be administered to patients known to be hypersensitive to the drug or to patients in whom salicylates or other NSAIDs induce symptoms of asthma, rhinitis and urticaria.

Patients who are suffering or have suffered from severe inflammatory diseases of the upper gastrointestinal tract, including gastritis, gastric and duodenal ulcer and active gastrointestinal bleeding, should not be given tenoxicam.

The drug should be avoided in patients who are undergoing anaesthesia or surgery because of an increased risk of acute renal failure and the possibility of impaired haemostasis. Tenoxicam should be used with caution in patients with impaired renal function.

The drug should not be given to pregnant or breast feeding women.

NURSING IMPLICATIONS

ASSESSMENT

Prior to the administration of NSAIDs to patients with rheumatoid arthritis, the nurse should assess the patient's history for any indication of allergy, peptic ulceration, other intestinal lesions or previous gastrointestinal bleeding. Concurrent use of drugs which may interact with the NSAID (especially anticoagulants and sulfonylurea hypoglycaemic drugs) should also be determined. In all of these cases the drug should be withheld and the physician informed. If the potent anti-inflammatory drugs (e.g. indomethacin) are to be used, the patient's history should also exclude evidence of renal or hepatic impairment and blood dyscrasias. Baseline observations of the degree of joint pain, swelling and movement should be documented.

ADMINISTRATION

To reduce irritation to the intestinal mucosa all these drugs are best given with food. Antacids can reduce plasma salicylate levels. Slow release or enteric coated formulations should not be dissolved or crushed.

EVALUATION

When aspirin is being used in rheumatic disorders it must be remembered that high doses are needed to obtain the anti-inflammatory effect required. There is often a fine line between the therapeutic and toxic levels of the drug. These patients therefore need to be observed closely for signs of salicylate toxicity, e.g. hyperventilation, tinnitus, dimness of vision, confusion, headache, sweating, thirst, nausea, vomiting and diarrhoea.

All patients should be observed for signs of drug effectiveness, i.e. relief of pain, reduction of swelling and improved joint mobility.

All patients on NSAIDs are at risk of gastrointestinal upset and bleeding, therefore the nurse needs to be alert for signs of these. Patients taking indomethacin should be observed for central nervous system effects.

Evaluation of patients who have been taking aspirin for a long time should also include observations for tarry stools, haematemesis, petechiae and bruising, which could occur as aspirin reduces prothrombin levels and platelet adhesiveness.

PATIENT EDUCATION

The patient should be taught the importance of taking the correct dose regularly to maintain blood levels necessary for therapeutic effect and to evaluate for adverse effects or toxicity and report these if they occur. To reduce the risk of gastrointestinal upset patients should be advised to take their medication with food or milk.

It should be stressed to patients taking the potent anti-inflammatory drugs the need to report immediately a sore throat or any other symptoms of blood dyscrasias to their doctor. If on long-term therapy these patients should be made aware of the importance of keeping regular appointments to have their blood count monitored. It may be necessary to explain to patients taking aspirin why such large doses are needed. The importance of keeping these drugs out of the reach of children should be stressed.

DISEASE MODIFYING AGENTS

D-Penicillamine

D-Penicillamine is a degradation product of penicillin. It does not possess any antibacterial activity.

TRADE NAMES

D-Penicillamine: *D-Penamine.*

MECHANISM OF ACTION

The mechanism of action of D-penicillamine in the treatment of rheumatoid arthritis is not known but may be related to inhibition of collagen formation. D-Penicillamine also combines with copper and it is this mechanism of action which is utilised in the treatment of Wilson's disease.

PHARMACOKINETICS

D-Penicillamine is readily absorbed from the gastrointestinal tract, peak blood concentrations being attained at 1 hour. It is thought that the drug is metabolised in the liver and excreted in the urine and faeces.

USES

D-Penicillamine is used in the treatment of severe, active rheumatoid arthritis. Its use should be reserved for those patients with active rheumatoid arthritis who have failed to respond to an adequate trial of conventional therapy. Response is slow, usually taking about three months for the first signs of remission to occur and maintenance therapy may be indefinite. Administration of D-penicillamine alone is not a complete treatment for rheumatoid arthritis and the drug should only be used as one part of a complete program of therapy.

Dosage is 125–250 mg daily for one month, increasing by the same amount at intervals of one to three months according to the patient's response and tolerance. Maximum recommended daily dose is 1–1.5 g in divided doses. No more than 500 mg should be administered at any one time. D-Penicillamine should be given on an empty stomach, at least 1 hour before or 2 hours after food. D-Penicillamine is available as 125 mg and 250 mg tablets.

ADVERSE DRUG REACTIONS

Reported adverse drug reactions are numerous and often serious. They include haematological changes, gastrointestinal, hepatic and renal effects and allergic reactions. Myasthenia gravis syndrome has been reported rarely and in most cases was reversible when D-penicillamine was discontinued. Loss of taste is a very common side effect.

DRUG INTERACTIONS

Food, aluminium hydroxide (antacids) and ferrous sulfate reduce the absorption of D-penicillamine and therefore therapy with these agents should be separated by at least one hour. Severe adverse reactions have been reported when D-penicillamine has been given in conjunction with gold. D-Penicillamine potentiates the effects of isoniazid.

MUSCULOSKELETAL DISORDERS

22

PRECAUTIONS AND CONTRAINDICATIONS

D-Penicillamine should be used with caution in patients with a history of penicillin allergy. It should not be used in patients receiving gold therapy or antimalarial drugs.

The drug should only be given to pregnant women if the benefits outweigh the potential risks to the fetus and it should not be given to women who are breast feeding.

Sodium Aurothiomalate

Gold in the form of sodium aurothiomalate is parenterally administered.

TRADE NAMES

Sodium aurothiomalate: *Myocrisin.*

MECHANISM OF ACTION

Sodium aurothiomalate suppresses the disease process of rheumatoid arthritis by penetrating into joint cavities and affecting the lysosomal membranes. It also binds with plasma proteins and thereby inactivates lysosomal enzymes within the cell.

PHARMACOKINETICS

Sodium aurothiomalate solutions are rapidly absorbed following intramuscular injection, with peak serum concentrations occurring in 3–6 hours. The metabolic fate of parenteral gold compounds is obscure but it is thought that the drug is not broken down to an elemental form of gold. Excretion is via the urine (70%) and faeces (30%).

USES

The use of gold is limited to patients with active, progressive rheumatoid arthritis which cannot be satisfactorily controlled with NSAIDs alone. Sodium aurothiomalate is injected intramuscularly into the upper outer quadrant of the gluteal region. It is usually administered at weekly intervals. The usual initial dose is 10 mg followed by 25 mg for the second dose, then 25–50 mg weekly until gold toxicity or substantial clinical improvement occurs or a cumulative dose of 1 g has been administered.

It is available as 10 mg, 20 mg and 50 mg ampoules.

ADVERSE DRUG REACTIONS

Minor reactions such as rashes are frequent but must not be taken lightly as they may be early signs of toxicity. The most serious and frequent complication is renal failure. Blood disorders may also occur.

DRUG INTERACTIONS

Gold formulations should not be given in conjunction with D-penicillamine.

PRECAUTIONS AND CONTRAINDICATIONS

Gold treatment is contraindicated in patients with gross renal or hepatic disease, diabetes, marked toxaemia, a history of blood dyscrasias or exfoliative dermatitis.

It is also contraindicated in women who are pregnant or breast feeding.

Auranofin

Auranofin is a synthetic gold compound which is administered orally.

TRADE NAMES

Auranofin: *Ridaura.*

MECHANISM OF ACTION

Auranofin acts by enhancing cell mediated immunity, inhibiting antibody dependent cellular cytotoxicity, inhibiting release of lysosomal enzymes and inhibiting platelet aggregation.

PHARMACOKINETICS

Approximately 25% of the dose of auranofin is absorbed from the gastrointestinal tract following oral administration. Absorption occurs mainly from the small intestine and to a lesser extent from the large intestine. Peak plasma concentrations occur at 2 hours. The exact nature of metabolism of auranofin is unclear although it has been suggested that the drug may undergo metabolism by deacetylation in the gastrointestinal mucosa. Excretion of gold from auranofin is via the urine (5% within 10 days and 15% over six months) and via the faeces (75% in 10 days and 85% over six months).

USES

Auranofin is used in the management of the active stage of classical or definite rheumatoid arthritis in adults who have not responded to an adequate trial of NSAIDs. It should not be used alone but as one part of a comprehensive treatment program.

ADVERSE DRUG REACTIONS

The highest incidence of adverse effects is during the first six months of therapy. However, reactions may occur after many months of treatment. Most common side effects include diarrhoea, abdominal pain, nausea, vomiting, rash, pruritus and stomatitis.

More severe reactions have been reported and include blood dyscrasias, hepatic jaundice, interstitial pneumonitis, peripheral neuropathy, nephrotic syndrome and membranous glomerulonephritis.

DRUG INTERACTIONS

The concomitant use of auranofin and D-penicillamine, antimalarials, immunosuppressants, cytotoxic agents, levamisole and high dose corticosteroids should be undertaken with extreme caution due to the potential of these drugs to cause blood dyscrasias or some other additive toxicity.

PRECAUTIONS AND CONTAINDICATIONS

Auranofin is contraindicated in any patient who has exhibited previous toxicity to parenteral gold or to other heavy metals. It is also contraindicated in patients with progressive renal disease, severe active hepatic disease, a history of bone marrow toxicity, severe haematological disorders and severe chronic forms of dermatitis. Care should be exercised in prescribing auranofin to any patient with inflammatory bowel disease because of the possibility of inducing diarrhoea.

The drug should be avoided in pregnant or breast feeding women.

Sulfasalazine

TRADE NAMES

Sulfasalazine: *Salazopyrin.*

MECHANISM OF ACTION

After absorption, sulfasalazine is split into sulfapyridine and 5-aminosalicylic acid (5-ASA). Sulfapyridine is believed to be the active moiety in the treatment of rheumatoid arthritis, possibly reducing antigen absorption from the gut while the 5-ASA moiety has only modest anti-inflammatory activity.

PHARMACOKINETICS

Sulfasalazine is absorbed from the gastrointestinal tract. Only 10%–15% is absorbed as unchanged drug, the remainder of an oral dose passes into the colon where intestinal flora cause breakdown into sulfapyridine and 5-ASA. Sulfasalazine is rapidly absorbed from the colon. Peak plasma concentrations of sulfapyridine occur within 6–24 hours. After an oral dose of enteric coated sulfasalazine, peak plasma concentrations of sulfapyridine occur within 12–24 hours. Patients who are slow acetylators tend to have higher serum concentrations of sulfapyridine. Most of a dose of sulfasalazine is excreted in the urine with a small amount in the faeces.

USES

Sulfasalazine is mainly used in the treatment of ulcerative colitis and Crohn's disease but it is also used to treat rheumatoid arthritis which has failed to respond to NSAID therapy. Dosages of 1–3 g daily in divided doses should be given (four times daily for plain tablets and two to three times daily for enteric coated tablets). Both oral formulations come in 500 mg tablets and should be taken after food. A 500 mg suppository is available and these are usually administered morning and night.

ADVERSE DRUG REACTIONS

Most common side effects are nausea, vomiting, diarrhoea, dizziness and abdominal

22 MUSCULOSKELETAL DISORDERS

pain. Less common reactions include skin rashes. Serious haematological reactions have been reported but are rare.

DRUG INTERACTIONS

The drug inhibits folic acid absorption, interferes with folic acid metabolism and may result in folic acid deficiency. It also shares the potential drug interactions of the sulfonamides, See Chapter 30 Infectious Diseases.

PRECAUTIONS AND CONTRAINDICATIONS

Sulfasalazine should not be given to patients hypersensitive to salicylates or those with intestinal or urinary obstruction. See also Chapter 30 Infectious Diseases.

The benefits of sulfasalazine therapy must be weighed against the potential risk to the fetus in pregnant patients and it should be avoided in breast feeding women.

Chloroquine, Hydroxychloroquine

TRADE NAMES

Chloroquine: *Chlorquin*.
Hydroxychloroquine: *Plaquenil*.

MECHANISM OF ACTION

The exact mode of action of the 4-aminoquinolones, chloroquine and hydroxychloroquine, in the treatment of rheumatoid arthritis is unknown.

PHARMACOKINETICS

The 4-aminoquinolones are absorbed very rapidly and almost completely from the gastrointestinal tract. They are metabolised in the liver and excreted in the urine.

USES

Chloroquine and hydroxychloroquine are indicated in the treatment of acute and chronic rheumatoid arthritis in patients who do not respond adequately to other less toxic antirheumatics. They may be used in addition to NSAIDs. Dosages of 250 mg of chloroquine phosphate once a day are used and may be increased to up to 750 mg daily. Tablets of 250 mg are available. Dosages of hydroxychloroquine are 200 mg twice to three times daily until the desired response is obtained. It is available as a 200 mg tablet. Both preparations should be taken with meals or milk to minimise the gastrointestinal irritation.

ADVERSE DRUG REACTIONS

Side effects of the 4-aminoquinolones are usually dose related. They include diarrhoea, loss of appetite, nausea, vomiting, dizziness, headache, nervousness and skin rash or itching. A blue black discolouration of the skin, fingernails or inside of the mouth has been reported. Irreversible retinal damage may be more likely to occur when the daily dosage equals or exceeds the equivalent of 150 mg of chloroquine and the total dosage exceeds the equivalent of 100 g of chloroquine. It is recommended that all patients have an initial ophthalmological examination, repeated at 3-month intervals during therapy. Other serious side effects although rare, include convulsions, mood changes and blood dyscrasias.

DRUG INTERACTIONS

Kaolin and magnesium trisilicate reduce the bioavailability of chloroquine and therefore should not be taken concomitantly. Alcohol should be avoided.

PRECAUTIONS AND CONTRAINDICATIONS

Chloroquine and hydroxychloroquine are contraindicated in patients with known hypersensitivity to the 4-aminoquinolone compounds and those who have demonstrated retinal or visual field changes attributed to any of the 4-aminoquinolone compounds. These drugs should be used with caution in patients with liver disease.

The 4-aminoquinolones should not be given to pregnant or breast feeding women.

NURSING IMPLICATIONS

ASSESSMENT

Prior to administration of disease modifying agents to patients with rheumatoid arthritis the nurse should assess the patient's history for evidence of renal impairment or blood dyscrasias. The urine should be tested for protein.

EVALUATION

Patients receiving these drugs will usually have regular appointments at their rheumatology clinic for checks on their dosage regimen, administration of gold injections and evaluation of improvement in their condition or adverse effects. The nurse should test the urine for protein and report the result to the medical officer. Nursing evaluation should also include observation of the patient for any other signs of adverse drug effects, including signs of skin reactions, evidence of blood dyscrasias (e.g. bruising, haematuria or evidence of infection) and reports of tiredness and lethargy.

PATIENT EDUCATION

Patients need to be reassured that these drugs are slower acting than other anti-inflammatory drugs they may have taken in the past and that it may take some time for benefit to be apparent. The patient should be asked to report skin rashes, mouth ulcers or evidence of bleeding or infection to the physician. The importance of keeping regular appointments for urine tests, blood tests and assessment of dosages and progress should be stressed.

DRUGS USED IN GOUT ▉▉▉▉▉▉▉

Gout is a clinical syndrome characterised by recurrent attacks of acute monoarticular arthritis which is associated with an elevation of serum urate (hyperuricaemia) and abnormal accumulation of urate within the body. The upper limit of normal for the serum urate concentration is usually defined as 0.42 mmol/L in males and 0.36 mmol/L in females.

The hyperuricaemia which invariably precedes gouty arthritis is due to either metabolic overproduction of urate or a reduced ability of the kidney to excrete urate. Precipitation of urate crystals into joints, renal tubules and tissues may result in acute arthritis, renal calculi and tophi.

NSAIDs and colchicine are used for the treatment of acute attacks of gout, while long-term treatment is based on the use of uricosuric agents and agents preventing uric acid formation. It is important that urate lowering drugs are not started during an acute attack as they may prolong the acute attack and convert it into chronic inflammatory arthritis.

TREATMENT OF THE ACUTE ATTACK

Non-Steroidal Anti-Inflammatory Drugs

Among the NSAIDs, the greatest experience has been with indomethacin, and this is regarded by many as the drug of choice. Other NSAIDs have been found to be effective in acute gout, e.g. naproxen, piroxicam and sulindac. The most important factor in their use is employing a suitably large dose which is usually greater than that given as maintenance in other forms of arthritis. Indomethacin can be given in doses of up to 100 mg every 4 hours until the pain is relieved, whereupon dose and frequency of administration can be

MUSCULOSKELETAL DISORDERS

22

reduced each day. These higher doses are generally tolerated by patients with gouty arthritis. Sulindac, which is structurally related to indomethacin, may cause less gastrointestinal irritation.

Colchicine

The alkaloid colchicine has been used for centuries to counteract the pain of acute gout.

TRADE NAMES

Colchicine: *Colgout.*

MECHANISM OF ACTION

Colchicine's exact mode of action is unclear, but the drug appears to reduce the inflammatory response to deposition of monosodium urate crystals in joint tissue. It also interferes with sodium urate deposition by decreasing lactic acid production.

PHARMACOKINETICS

Colchicine is absorbed from the gastrointestinal tract and metabolised by the liver. Colchicine and its metabolites are excreted primarily in faeces and lesser amounts in the urine.

USES

Colchicine is the drug of choice for the relief of acute gouty arthritis. It may also be used with prophylactic treatment in recurrent gouty arthritis. The initial dose is 1 mg followed by 500 micrograms every 2–3 hours until control is attained or toxicity develops. The total course of therapy for an acute attack is 4–8 mg. A maintenance dose of 500 micrograms 2–3 times daily may be necessary in some patients. Colchicine is available as a 500 microgram tablet.

ADVERSE DRUG REACTIONS

The most common side effects of colchicine therapy are nausea, abdominal discomfort, vomiting and diarrhoea. Therapy should be discontinued if these symptoms occur as they are the early signs of toxicity.

DRUG INTERACTIONS

Colchicine may enhance the response to sympathomimetic agents and central nervous system depressants.

PRECAUTIONS AND CONTRAINDICATIONS

Colchicine should be used with caution in geriatric or debilitated patients because of possible cumulative effects. It is contraindicated in patients with serious gastrointestinal, renal or cardiac disorders.

The drug should be avoided in pregnant or breast feeding women.

LONG-TERM TREATMENT

Long-term treatment of gout is aimed at reducing the uric acid in the body either by increasing renal excretion with uricosuric drugs or by decreasing its synthesis in the tissues by the use of allopurinol. This may take many months. Success is shown by a reduction in acute attacks, a lowering of serum uric acid and absorption of tophi. Long-term treatment may be given concurrently with treatment for an acute attack. Treatment can be continued indefinitely.

Allopurinol

TRADE NAMES

Allopurinol: *Capurate*; *Progout*; *Zyloprim.*

MECHANISM OF ACTION

Allopurinol reduces the formation of uric acid from purines by inhibiting the enzyme xanthine oxidase.

PHARMACOKINETICS

Following oral administration, up to 90% of a dose of allopurinol is absorbed from the gastrointestinal tract. Peak plasma levels are attained 2–6 hours after each dose. It is metabolised in the liver and excreted in the urine.

USES

Allopurinol is used to lower serum and urinary uric acid concentrations in the management of primary and secondary gout. The drug is indicated in patients with frequent disabling attacks of gout. Dosage range is 200–600 mg daily. It is available as 100 mg and 300 mg tablets.

ADVERSE DRUG REACTIONS

Adverse reactions to allopurinol are uncommon. The incidence is higher in the presence of renal and/or hepatic failure. Skin reactions are the most common effect and allopurinol should be withdrawn immediately if they occur.

DRUG INTERACTIONS

When mercaptopurine or azathioprine are given concurrently with allopurinol, the dose of mercaptopurine and azathioprine should be reduced to one-quarter of the usual dose.

Large doses of salicylates or uricosuric agents may decrease the therapeutic activity of allopurinol.

PRECAUTIONS AND CONTRAINDICATIONS

Extra caution should be exercised if renal function is poor. Allopurinol should not be given to pregnant or breast feeding women.

Probenecid

TRADE NAMES

Probenecid: *Benemid.*

MECHANISM OF ACTION

Probenecid is a uricosuric agent which promotes the urinary excretion of uric acid thereby reducing serum urate concentrations.

PHARMACOKINETICS

Probenecid is completely absorbed after oral administration and peak plasma concentrations are reached in 2–4 hours. It is metabolised in the liver to metabolites that also have uricosuric activity. It is excreted via the urine.

USES

Probenecid is used to lower serum urate concentrations in the treatment of chronic gouty arthritis and tophaceous gout. It is indicated in patients with frequent disabling attacks of gout. Therapy should be initiated at 250 mg twice daily for one week and increased by weekly increments of 250 mg until a daily dose of 2 g is achieved. It is available as a 500 mg tablet.

ADVERSE DRUG REACTIONS

The common side effects of probenecid are gastrointestinal distress and skin rashes. These occur more often when higher doses are used. Serious adverse reactions such as nephrotic syndrome, bone marrow depression and hepatic necrosis are rare.

DRUG INTERACTIONS

Concomitant administration of aspirin is not advised as it antagonises the uricosuric action of probenecid. Care should be exercised if methotrexate is prescribed with probenecid as probenecid has been reported to decrease the tubular secretion of methotrexate and potentiate its toxicity. Probenecid decreases the renal excretion of other drugs and it is important to know of the potential interactions.

PRECAUTIONS AND CONTRAINDICATIONS

Probenecid should be used with caution in patients with renal impairment and in those patients with a history of peptic ulcer. Probenecid has been used during pregnancy without producing adverse effects; however, the anticipated benefits should be weighed against possible hazards. There is no data available on its use in breast feeding women.

Sulfinpyrazone

TRADE NAMES

Sulfinpyrazone: *Anturan.*

MECHANISM OF ACTION

Sulfinpyrazone has a uricosuric action and promotes the excretion of urates by inhibition of renal tubular reabsorption.

MUSCULOSKELETAL DISORDERS

22

PHARMACOKINETICS

It is well absorbed after oral administration; its uricosuric effect persisting for as long as 10 hours. It is extensively bound to plasma proteins (95%–99%). Most of the drug (90%) is excreted unchanged in the urine, the remainder is eliminated as a metabolite which also possesses uricosuric activity.

USES

Sulfinpyrazone is indicated for the treatment of chronic gout. The initial dose is 100–200 mg daily. After the first week, the dose may be gradually increased until a satisfactory lowering of plasma uric acid is achieved and maintained. Maximum daily dose is 400 mg (divided into 2–4 doses) but some resistant patients may require up to 800 mg daily. It is available as 100 mg tablets. Administration with food is advised.

ADVERSE DRUG REACTIONS

Gastrointestinal irritation is the most common side effect and is often dosage related. Skin rashes are also common.

DRUG INTERACTIONS

Concomitant administration with salicylates must be avoided as salicylates antagonise the effect of sulfinpyrazone. Care should be exercised if the patient is also receiving anticoagulant drugs, antidiabetic agents (including insulin), penicillins and sulfonamides.

PRECAUTIONS AND CONTRAINDICATIONS

Sulfinyprazone should be used with extreme caution in patients with a history of peptic ulcer. Patients with a history of impaired renal function, renal calculi or renal colic should be closely observed. Periodic blood counts are recommended during therapy with sulfinpyrazone.

It is recommended that sulfinpyrazone not be prescribed during the first three months of pregnancy unless its use is considered mandatory. There is no information on its use in breast feeding women.

Salicylates

Salicylates (aspirin and sodium salicylate) in large doses of 5–6 g daily increase

TABLE 22.2 Drug interactions which may occur with drugs used in the treatment of gout

Drug	May interact with	Potential result
Allopurinol	Ampicillin	Increased incidence of skin rash
	Thiazide diuretics	Therapeutic efficacy of allopurinol inhibited
	Azothiaprine Mercaptopurine	Activity of antineoplastic agent increased (reduce dose to 25% of usual dose)
	Anticoagulants (coumarin) e.g. warfarin	Activity of coumarin anticoagulants increased
Probenecid	Salicylates Thiazide diuretics	Therapeutic efficacy of probenecid inhibited
Sulfinpyrazone	Salicylates Thiazide diuretics Anticoagulants (coumarin) e.g. warfarin	Therapeutic efficacy of sulfinpyrazone inhibited Activity of coumarin anticoagulants increased

serum urate levels by inhibiting renal tubular reabsorption of uric acid. (*Note*: salicylates in low doses of 1–2 g daily have the reverse effect and decrease urate secretion by inhibiting tubular secretion.) However, the adverse effects of salicylates in high doses are frequent and limit their use in the treatment of gout.

The uricosuric action of probenecid and sulfinpyrazone is antagonised by the salicylates, and they should not be used in combination. See aspirin and salicylates in the NSAIDs section.

Drug interactions which may occur with the drugs used in the treatment of gout are listed in Table 22.2.

NURSING IMPLICATIONS

ASSESSMENT

Initially the nurse should establish baseline observations of joint pain, swelling and frequency of attacks. Depending on which type of drug is used the patient's history should be checked for liver impairment, renal impairment, ulcerative gastrointestinal disorders, pregnancy, renal calculi and known hypersensitivity to the drug.

ADMINISTRATION

As gastric irritation and upset is often a problem with these drugs they should always be given with food.

EVALUATION

Evaluation is primarily concerned with observing for therapeutic effects of the drug such as relief of pain, reduction of swelling and return of serum urate levels to normal. The nurse should also observe for adverse effects such as allergic reactions and gastrointestinal upsets including nausea, vomiting, diarrhoea and abdominal pain. Severe gastrointestinal disturbance is a sign of toxicity with colchicine and will necessitate discontinuing the drug. Reports of retroperitoneal pain may indicate the presence of kidney stones which are especially likely to occur with uricosuric drugs as the increased clearance of uric acid by these drugs tends to promote stone formation. As the effects of the oral hypoglycaemic drugs are enhanced by the uricosuric agents diabetic patients taking these drugs should be watched for signs of hypoglycaemia.

PATIENT EDUCATION

If the patient is to take colchicine for acute attacks, they should be advised to initiate therapy at the earliest indication of the attack and to continue therapy until relief is obtained. However, if signs of toxicity such as nausea, vomiting or diarrhoea occur, they must discontinue taking the drug and seek advice from the physician.

It should be stressed to patients taking any of these drugs that a high fluid intake (at least 3 L daily), is vitally important to prevent formation of kidney stones and the formation of new deposits of uric acid.

Patients taking uricosuric drugs or allopurinol should be advised that they may initially experience transient attacks as the uric acid is being mobilised from the joints, but that this will pass once serum urate levels approach normal.

Patients taking a uricosuric drug should also be advised to avoid aspirin or over the counter preparations which contain it, as this will reduce the effect of the drug.

MUSCULOSKELETAL DISORDERS

22

MUSCLE RELAXANTS

Muscle relaxant drugs can be divided into four main groups: neuromuscular blocking agents; centrally acting muscle relaxants; directly acting skeletal muscle relaxants; and indirectly acting muscle relaxants. The first of these groups, the neuromuscular blocking agents, is discussed in Chapter 24 Drugs Used in Anaesthesia.

CENTRALLY ACTING MUSCLE RELAXANTS

Centrally acting muscle relaxants act on the central nervous system. They are used mainly for relieving painful muscle spasms or spasticity occurring in musculoskeletal and neuromuscular disorders.

Methocarbamol

TRADE NAMES

Methocarbamol: *Robaxin*.

MECHANISM OF ACTION

Methocarbamol is a potent skeletal muscle relaxant which has a selective action on the central nervous system resulting in a diminution of skeletal muscle hyperactivity without concomitant alteration in normal muscle tone.

PHARMACOKINETICS

The drug is rapidly and almost completely absorbed from the gastrointestinal tract after oral administration and peak serum concentrations are attained in approximately 1–2 hours. Methocarbamol is metabolised in the liver. The drug and its metabolites are excreted rapidly and almost completely in the urine.

USES

Methocarbamol is indicated for treatment of acute skeletal muscle hyperactivity secondary to acute musculoskeletal injuries or surgical procedures. The initial oral dosage is 1.5 g four times daily for 2–3 days. For maintenance therapy, the dosage can be decreased to 4.0–4.5 g daily in 3–6 divided doses. Tablets of 500 mg are available.

ADVERSE DRUG REACTIONS

The most frequent adverse effects are drowsiness, dizziness and lightheadedness. Blurred vision, headache, fever, and anorexia may occur.

DRUG INTERACTIONS

Additive central nervous system depression may occur when methocarbamol is administered concurrently with other central nervous system depressants including alcohol. The drug should also be used with caution in patients with myasthenia gravis receiving anticholinesterase agents.

PRECAUTIONS AND CONTRAINDICATIONS

Patients should be warned that methocarbamol may impair their ability to perform hazardous activities requiring mental alertness or physical coordination such as operating machinery or driving a motor vehicle.

The drug is not recommended during pregnancy unless the benefits outweigh the possible risks. There is no information on its use during lactation.

Orphenadrine Citrate

TRADE NAMES

Orphenadrine Citrate: *Norflex*.

MECHANISM OF ACTION

Orphenadrine citrate reduces skeletal muscle spasm through an atropine-like central action on cerebral motor centres.

PHARMACOKINETICS

Orphenadrine is absorbed from the gastrointestinal tract but the metabolic fate of the drug has not been fully determined. At least eight metabolites are known and the drug and its metabolites are excreted in the urine.

USES

Orphenadrine citrate is used alone or in combination with aspirin as an adjunct to rest, physical therapy and other measures for the relief of discomfort associated with acute painful musculoskeletal disorders. Dosage is 100 mg twice daily, increased to 300 mg daily when necessary. Tablets of 100 mg orphenadrine citrate are available.

ADVERSE DRUG REACTIONS

Side effects include dry mouth, blurred vision, urinary hesitancy or retention, mydriasis, drowsiness, headache, weakness, palpitations and tachycardia. Gastrointestinal disturbances may also occur.

DRUG INTERACTIONS

Concomitant administration of orphenadrine and propoxyphene may produce additive central nervous system effects.

PRECAUTIONS AND CONTRAINDICATIONS

Orphenadrine should be used with caution in patients with conditions in which anticholinergic effects are undesirable. Its use in pregnancy should be avoided unless the benefits outweigh the risks. No adverse effects have been reported on its use during lactation.

Benzodiazepines

TRADE NAMES

Diazepam: *Antenex*; *Ducene*; *Valium*.
Lorazepam: *Ativan*.

MECHANISM OF ACTION

The exact mode of action of the benzodiazepines as muscle relaxants has not been fully elucidated. The drug appears to act at the limbic, thalamic and hypothalamic levels of the central nervous system producing anxiolytic, sedative, hypnotic, skeletal muscle relaxant and anticonvulsant effects.

USES

Benzodiazepines such as diazepam and lorazepam have central muscle relaxant properties. They are used as an adjunct for the relief of acute, painful musculoskeletal conditions, and to manage skeletal muscle spasticity such as reflex spasm secondary to local pathology. They are also used in the treatment of spastic cerebral palsy.

Dosage of benzodiazepines must be carefully individualised and the smallest effective dosage should be used to avoid oversedation. Initially, they are usually administered three or four times daily.

For details on dosage, adverse drug reactions, interactions, precautions and contraindications, see Chapter 26 Psychiatric Disorders.

DIRECTLY ACTING SKELETAL MUSCLE RELAXANTS

Dantrolene

TRADE NAMES

Dantrolene: *Dantrium*.

MECHANISM OF ACTION

Dantrolene produces relaxation and reduces contraction of skeletal muscle by decreasing the amount of calcium released from the sarcoplasmic reticulum. It does not alter neuromuscular transmission.

PHARMACOKINETICS

About 35% of an oral dose of dantrolene is absorbed from the gastrointestinal tract, peak plasma concentrations occurring about 5 hours after administration. Dantrolene is metabolised in the liver to metabolites which are less active than the parent drug. It is excreted in the urine mainly as metabolites.

USES

Dantrolene is used for the symptomatic treatment of skeletal muscle spasm due to multiple sclerosis, spinal cord injury, cerebral palsy and stroke. Dantrolene is not indicated for muscle spasm associated with rheumatoid disorders. Initial oral dosage is 25 mg once daily, increased to 25 mg twice, three or four times daily, and then increased by increments of 25 mg up to 100 mg twice, three or four times daily if necessary. Dosage increases should be made at 4–7 day intervals until desired response is achieved or adverse effects prevent further increases. It is available as 25 mg and 50 mg capsules.

ADVERSE DRUG REACTIONS

Side effects are seen in the gastrointestinal system (nausea and diarrhoea); nervous system (drowsiness, dizziness, lightheadedness, speech and visual disturbances, mental depression and confusion); urogenital system (urinary frequency, incontinence, nocturia and urinary retention); and in the cardiovascular system (tachycardia and erratic blood pressure).

DRUG INTERACTIONS

Caution should be observed if patients are given oestrogen and dantrolene therapy together as hepatotoxicity has been reported. Dantrolene should be used with caution in patients with impaired pulmonary function or severe myocardial disease. The central effects of dantrolene may be enhanced by sedative drugs or antianxiety drugs.

PRECAUTIONS AND CONTRAINDICATIONS

The drug is contraindicated in patients with active hepatic disease and upper motor neuron disorders. It should be used with caution in patients with severely impaired cardiac function. It should not be used in patients who must utilise spasticity to maintain upright posture and balance in moving.

Dantrolene should only be used during pregnancy if the potential benefits outweigh the risks. There is no information on its use during lactation.

INDIRECTLY ACTING MUSCLE RELAXANTS

Baclofen

TRADE NAMES

Baclofen: *Clofen; Lioresal.*

MECHANISM OF ACTION

Baclofen is an indirect muscle relaxant and antispasticity agent which acts at the spinal level. Although the mode of action is not fully known, its major effect is presynaptic inhibition.

PHARMACOKINETICS

Baclofen is rapidly and almost completely absorbed from the gastrointestinal tract, peak plasma concentrations occurring at 2–3 hours. Onset of therapeutic effect may vary from hours to weeks. Only about 15% of the drug is metabolised in the liver; 70%–80% is excreted in the urine as metabolites and parent drug, the remainder in the faeces.

USES

Baclofen is indicated for suppression of voluntary muscle spasms in conditions such as multiple sclerosis and lesions of the spinal cord. Patients must be hospitalised during the initiation of treatment in order to monitor usage and adverse reactions. Initial dose is 5 mg three times daily. Daily dose may be increased by 15 mg at three-day intervals until optimum effect is achieved (usually 40–80 mg daily). Some patients may benefit from a four times daily drug regimen. Whenever baclofen is discontinued, daily dosage should be reduced slowly; abrupt withdrawal may precipitate hallucinations and/or seizures and acute exacerbation of spasticity. The drug is available as 10 mg and 25 mg tablets.

ADVERSE DRUG REACTIONS

Side effects are likely to be encountered early in therapy if the initial dose is too high. The incidence appears to be higher in elderly patients and in patients with cerebral forms of spasticity. The more common adverse reactions are: gastrointestinal system (nausea, vomiting, diarrhoea and dyspepsia); musculoskeletal system (asthenia, muscle weakness, hypotonia, muscle incoordination and tremors); nervous system (day-time sedation, lethargy, vertigo, headache and dizziness).

DRUG INTERACTIONS

Care should be exercised in administering baclofen in conjunction with psychotropic or other neurotropic drugs. However, diazepam and nitrazepam appear to be compatible with baclofen.

PRECAUTIONS AND CONTRAINDICATIONS

Baclofen is contraindicated in patients with a history of epilepsy or convulsive disorders. As baclofen is excreted largely in the urine, a reduction in dosage may be necessary for patients with impaired renal function. It should be used with caution in patients with a history of gastric and duodenal ulcer, severe psychiatric disorders and in patients receiving antihypertensive therapy.

The drug should be avoided during pregnancy and by women who are breast feeding as there is no information on its use in these groups of patients.

NURSING IMPLICATIONS

ASSESSMENT

A comprehensive physical assessment should be performed prior to commencing the medication. A baseline of physical inactivity should be established and recorded along with the presence of other indications of physical disability.

EVALUATION

The patient should be monitored carefully for signs of drug effectiveness and adverse effects.

PATIENT EDUCATION

Patients should be advised that motor incoordination, drowsiness and other central nervous system effects may occur and that they should take extra care when negotiating stairs and performing daily activities to avoid falls and subsequent injury.

MUSCULOSKELETAL DISORDERS

22

COUNTERIRRITANTS AND RUBEFACIENTS

There is probably little difference between the counterirritant effects produced by physical and chemical methods. Pain, whether superficial or deep seated, is relieved by any method which produces irritation of the skin. Counterirritation is comforting in painful lesions of the muscles, tendons and joints and in non-articular rheumatism. A large number of substances have been and still are used as counterirritants. Essentially they act through the same mechanism.

The essential oils, when applied to the intact skin, have irritant and rubefacient actions causing a sensation of warmth and smarting, followed by a mild local anaesthesia. For this reason they are used as counterirritants and cutaneous stimulants in the treatment of chronic inflammatory conditions and to relieve neuralgia and rheumatic pains. Clove oil, eucalyptus oil, thyme oil and turpentine oil are commonly used in counterirritation formulations.

Other pharmaceuticals used in these formulations include camphor, methyl salicylate and capsicum. Camphor is applied externally and acts as a rubefacient and mild analgesic and is employed in liniments as a counterirritant in fibrositis and neuralgia. Methyl salicylate is employed only for cutaneous counterirritation in ointments and liniments. Capsicum is used as a counterirritant in lumbago, neuralgia and rheumatism.

A wide range of proprietary preparations of this nature is available. Although the formulations vary, their action is similar. They include *Dencorub, Finalgon, Metsal, Deep Heat* and *Capsig.*

TOPICAL ANAESTHETICS ▄▄▄▄▄▄▄

Topical anaesthetics are compounds which produce insensitivity by preventing transmission of impulses along nerve fibres and at nerve endings. The effects are reversible. In general, loss of pain (analgesia) occurs before loss of sensory and autonomic function (anaesthesia) and loss of motor function (paralysis).

Surface or topical anaesthesia blocks the sensory nerve ending in the skin or mucous membranes, but to reach these structures the drug must have good powers of penetration. There are a number of special uses for topical anaesthesia, including anaesthetising the cornea during ophthalmological procedures and the throat and larynx before intubation and bronchoscopy. However, application to the skin may give rise to allergic reactions; such reactions may be avoided by changing to a local anaesthetic of the alternative chemical type.

There are two chemical types of topical anaesthetics: the ester type which includes amethocaine, benzocaine, cocaine and procaine, and the amide type which includes bupivacaine, cinchocaine, lignocaine, mepivacaine and prilocaine.

ESTERS

Amethocaine

A potent local anaesthetic whose action is greater than that of lignocaine. It is mainly used as a surface anaesthetic in ophthalmology and otorhinolaryngology. A 1%–3% ointment is used in painful conditions of the anus or rectum.

Benzocaine

Benzocaine is used in concentrations of 5%–10% in ointments and dusting powders as a local anaesthetic applied to ulcerated surfaces, burns or wounds or for the relief of intractable pruritus. Proprietary preparations include *Caligesic, Hemorex, Rectinol* and *Dermoplast.*

Cocaine

A surface anaesthetic which is used almost entirely in ophthamology and otolaryngology.

Procaine

Procaine is not effective as a surface anaesthetic because of its poor penetration of intact mucous membranes and so is used chiefly by injection.

AMIDES

Bupivacaine

Bupivacaine is a long-acting local anaesthetic used mainly by injection for different types of nerve block, see Chapter 24 Drugs Used in Anaesthesia.

Cinchocaine

This is a local anaesthetic with a longer duration of action than lignocaine and can therefore be used in lower concentrations. A 1% cream or ointment has been used for the relief of painful skin conditions.

Proprietary preparations include *Scheriproct, Ultraproct* and *Proctosedyl*.

Lignocaine

Lignocaine is a widely used local anaesthetic. Anal or genital pruritus and painful haemorrhoids may be relieved with suppositories or a 5% ointment or cream. A 2% gel may also be applied prior to cystoscopy or catheterisation, and a 4% solution may be used before bronchoscopy. Proprietary preparations include *Xylocaine, Xyloproct, Xylotox* and *Paxyl*.

Mepivacaine

This is a local anaesthetic used for different types of nerve blocks; it is not used in cream or ointment preparations. See Chapter 24.

Prilocaine

This local anaesthetic is used for surface anaesthesia as well as for nerve blocks. A 4% topical solution is used for surface anaesthesia of mucous membranes in bronchoscopy and minor surgery of the mouth, nose and throat. The proprietary preparation is known as *Citanest*. See Chapter 24.

ENZYME PREPARATIONS

Enzyme preparations are often used in treating trauma of the soft tissues, such as sprains and bruises. Some are available in oral form while others are applied topically. While the mode of action of proteolytic enzymes has not been fully established, it seems most probable that breakdown of fibrin and permeability modifications of venules and lymphatics underlie the action.

Enzyme preparations are used in the treatment of traumatic injuries (contusions, sprains, ecchymoses and haematosis); infections and other inflammatory disorders (abscesses and other local infections; phlebitis and thrombophelebitis, thrombotic and postpartum haemorrhoids, varicose ulcers and bursitis); allergic reactions (allergic rhinitis, urticaria and angioneurotic oedema); and for induced trauma (resulting from dental, obstetrical and general surgical procedures, including instrumentation).

TOPICAL PREPARATIONS

Fibrinolysin with Desoxyribonuclease

The combination of these two enzymes is marketed as *Elase* and is based on the observations that purulent exudates consist largely of fibrinous material and nucleoprotein. Desoxyribonuclease attacks the DNA, and fibrinolysin attacks principally fibrin of blood blots and fibrinous exudates. It is indicated for topical use as a debriding agent in a variety of inflammatory and infected lesions.

Local application should be repeated at intervals for as long as enzyme action is desired. After application *Elase* ointment becomes rapidly and progressively less active and for practical purposes is ineffective after 24 hours. Adverse drug reactions attributable to the enzymes have not been a problem at the dose used.

Heparinoid Compounds

Heparinoid compounds may be applied topically for their anticoagulant and anti-inflammatory effects. They should be gently massaged into the affected areas several times daily, avoiding any areas of broken skin. Slight reddening of the skin is a favourable response and indicates an improvement in local blood flow. Examples of this type of product include *Hirudoid, Lasonil, Movelat* and *Pergalen*.

MUSCULOSKELETAL DISORDERS

22

NURSING IMPLICATIONS

Topical Enzyme Preparations

The type of lesion to which the substance is to be applied should be assessed and appropriate equipment organised. Before fresh ointment is applied the area should be cleaned thoroughly and debrided as necessary. Fresh ointment should be applied avoiding healthy skin areas. Enzyme preparations should be applied at least once daily. The patient should be evaluated for effectiveness of treatment, allergic reactions noted and progress and results documented.

Heparinoid Compounds

The area to be treated should be assessed and any areas where skin is broken noted. The compound is applied by gently massaging into the skin, avoiding any broken areas. The patient should be evaluated for effectiveness of treatment.

FURTHER READING

American Hospital Formulary Service (1994) American Society of Hospital Pharmacists, Bethesda.

Gilman, A.G., Rall, T.W., Nies, A.S., Taylor, P., eds, (1990), *Goodman and Gilman the pharmacological basis of therapeutics*, 8th ed. Pergamon Press, New York.

TEST YOUR KNOWLEDGE

1. Which of the following drugs are used in musculoskeletal diseases: pheniramine, aspirin, ibuprofen, chlorthalidone, indomethacin, D-penicillamine, phenmetrazine?

2. List one disease state for which the following drugs are used: (a) sodium aurothiomalate, (b) lignocaine, (c) methyl salicylate, (d) baclofen, (e) probenecid, (f) naproxen.

3. List two adverse effects often seen with the following drugs: (a) indomethacin, (b) baclofen, (c) colchicine, (d) sulindac.

4. Write brief notes on the nursing implications for the use of: (a) non-steroidal anti-inflammatory drugs (NSAIDs), (b) drugs used for the treatment of gout, (c) topical enzyme preparations.

5. List four drugs or drug groups with actions that may be altered by concomitant administration of aspirin.

TABLE 22.3   Summary table — drug treatment of musculoskeletal disorders

DRUG GROUP Drug Name	Use	Action	Adverse Reactions	Nursing Implications
NON-STEROIDAL ANTI-INFLAMMATORY DRUGS (NSAIDs) Aspirin Sodium salicylate	Anti-inflammatory analgesic, used in inflammatory diseases and conditions; antipyretic, used to reduce fever; and reduces platelet aggregation	Central and peripheral analgesic action, inhibition of prostaglandin synthesis in inflamed tissue	Headache, dizziness, tinnitus, GI bleeding, worsening of gout	**Assess:** History of previous allergy, intestinal lesions, dyspepsia, peptic ulceration, anticoagulant therapy, use of hypoglycaemic drugs and uricosurics, for kidney or liver disease, pregnancy, lactation, coagulation disorders or bleeding tendencies; establish baseline description of joint pain, inflammation and degree of mobility **Administer:** With meals at times ordered. **Evaluate:** For relief of pain, inflammation and improved mobility, signs of allergy, GI distress, increased bleeding, tenderness, signs of salicylate toxicity **Educate:** Self-evaluation for side effects and toxicity, need for compliance in maintaining adequate blood levels to achieve therapeutic benefit, to take with food or milk and not to break or dissolve enteric coated or slow release formulations
Diflunisal	Analgesic, anti-inflammatory	Prostaglandin inhibition	Relatively uncommon, include GI upset, GI bleeding and rash	As for salicylates

22   MUSCULOSKELETAL DISORDERS

TABLE 22.3 continued

DRUG GROUP Drug Name	Use	Action	Adverse Reactions	Nursing Implications
Indomethacin	Anti-inflammatory, uricosuric	Prostaglandin inhibition, promotes excretion of uric acid	Headache, vertigo, confusion, GI discomfort, GI peptic ulceration, blood dyscrasias, depression	**Assess:** History for previous allergy or sensitivity, dyspepsia, peptic ulceration, renal or hepatic dysfunction, asthma, bleeding tendencies, concurrent use of anticoagulants and uricosurics; establish baseline documentation of inflammation and immobility **Administer:** oral, with food; suppositories per rectum, usually at night **Evaluate:** For relief of pain, inflammation and improved mobility, for adverse effects such as rash, GI disturbances, GI bleeding, dizziness, increased bleeding tendencies, blood dyscrasias and CNS side effects **Educate:** Self-evaluation for adverse effects, potential danger of driving or working with power tools and industrial machinery (due to CNS effects); to take with food
Sulindac	Anti-inflammatory, uricosuric	Prostaglandin inhibition, promotes excretion of uric acid	Constipation, epigastric pain, nausea	As for indomethacin
Ibuprofen Naproxen Ketoprofen Tiaprofenic acid	Anti-inflammatory, uricosuric	Prostaglandin inhibition, promote excretion of uric acid	GI disturbances, GI bleeding, rash, headache, lightheadedness	**Assess:** As for aspirin **Administer:** As for aspirin **Evaluate:** For relief of pain, inflammation and improved mobility, for signs of allergy, GI distress, increased bleeding tendencies

TABLE 22.3 continued

DRUG GROUP Drug Name	Use	Action	Adverse Reactions	Nursing Implications
Mefenamic acid	Analgesic, anti-inflammatory	Prostaglandin inhibition	GI irritation, rash, haemolytic anaemia, bronchoconstriction	**Educate**: Self-evaluation for side effects, the need for compliance in maintaining adequate blood levels to achieve therapeutic benefit, to take with food or milk **Assess**: History of previous allergy to fenemates or aspirin; pregnancy, lactation, dyspepsia, peptic ulceration, concurrent use of coumarin type anticoagulants, e.g. warfarin; establish baseline description of pain and degree of mobility **Administer**: With food **Evaluate**: For drug effectiveness, e.g. relief of pain and improved mobility; for adverse effects including allergy (rash, asthma, bronchoconstriction), GI upset and bleeding **Educate**: Self-evaluation for side effects, the need for compliance to achieve therapeutic benefit; to take with food or milk
Diclofenac Piroxicam Tenoxicam	Analgesic, anti-inflammatory	Prostaglandin inhibition	Relatively uncommon, may include GI upset, rash, GI bleeding	As for salicylates
DISEASE MODIFYING AGENTS Sodium aurothiomalate	Rheumatoid arthritis	Mechanism of action is unclear, but can control active, progressive disease	Renal failure, blood disorders, rash	**Assess**: For pregnancy, lactation, history of renal insufficiency, previous hypersensitivity; test urine for protein; establish baseline observations of degree of joint function, mobility and pain; baseline blood count may be required

22 MUSCULOSKELETAL DISORDERS

TABLE 22.3 continued

DRUG GROUP Drug Name	Use	Action	Adverse Reactions	Nursing Implications
				Administer: By intramuscular injection, dose as ordered at proper intervals **Evaluate**: For improvement in clinical condition; monitor laboratory reports including ESR and blood counts; observe for adverse effects such as pruritus, exfoliative dermatitis, mouth ulcers, bone marrow suppression, renal impairment; test urine for protein; watch for post injection vasomotor reactions such as flushing, anxiety or palpitations **Educate**: Self-evaluation for improvement and adverse effects; stress importance of keeping appointments for regular checks on urine and blood count and to report adverse effects to physician
D-penicillamine	Rheumatoid arthritis	Appears to suppress disease activity	Haematological changes, GI upsets, allergic reactions, renal failure	**Assess**: As for sodium aurothiomalate. **Administer**: Orally, low dose increasing to daily maintenance dose as ordered **Evaluate**: As for sodium aurothiomalate. **Educate**: As for sodium aurothiomalate
Auranofin	Rheumatoid arthritis	Mechanism of action is unclear	Blood disorders, renal failure, liver failure, GI disturbances	**Assess**: For previous history of allergies to sodium aurothiomalate or to heavy metals other than gold **Administer**: With food **Evaluate**: For improvement in clinical condition, blood count, monthly urinalysis, liver function test

TABLE 22.3 continued

DRUG GROUP Drug Name	Use	Action	Adverse Reactions	Nursing Implications
Sulfasalazine	Rheumatoid arthritis	Possible reduction in antigen absorption and mild anti-inflammatory activity.	GI, CNS disturbances	**Assess:** For history of allergy to sulfonamides, sensitivity to salicylates, pregnancy, lactation, renal or hepatic failure, uraemia, glucose-6-phosphate dehydrogenase (G-6-PD) deficiency. **Administer:** After meals. Enteric coated tablet should be swallowed whole. **Evaluate:** For improvement in clinical condition, monitor blood count
AMINOQUINOLONES Chloroquine Hydroxychloroquine	Rheumatoid arthritis	Mechanism of action unknown	Diarrhoea, nausea, vomiting dizziness, nervousness, skin rash. A blue-black discolouration of skin, fingernails and mouth. Convulsions, mood changes and blood dyscrasias. Irreversible retinal damage	**Assess:** For previous history of hypersensitivity to aminoquinolone compounds, liver disease and retinal or visual field changes **Administer:** With milk or food
ANTIGOUT PREPARATIONS Colchicine	High dose for acute gout attack; low dose for long-term prophylaxis	Uricosuric, promotes renal excretion of uric acid	Nausea, diarrhoea	**Assess:** For history of renal, liver or heart disease, ulcerative gastrointestinal disorders; document baseline observations of joint swelling and pain and frequency of attacks **Administer:** With food at prescribed intervals until relief is obtained

22 MUSCULOSKELETAL DISORDERS

TABLE 22.3 continued

DRUG GROUP Drug Name	Use	Action	Adverse Reactions	Nursing Implications
				Evaluate: For relief of joint pain and swelling; for signs of toxicity (nausea, diarrhoea, abdominal pain); fluid intake and output **Educate**: To initiate therapy at earliest indication of acute attack: to maintain high fluid intake; to self-evaluate for adverse effects and to discontinue therapy when pain is relieved or there are signs of toxicity
Allopurinol	Long-term gout prophylaxis	Suppresses synthesis of uric acid by inhibition of xanthine oxidase	Rash, fever, nausea, diarrhoea, abdominal pain, bone marrow depression in patients with renal disease	**Assess**: For pregnancy, renal dysfunction **Administer**: With food **Evaluate**: For skin rash, drowsiness, GI upsets **Educate**: That transient initial increase in attacks may occur and that drug effectiveness may require several weeks; to self-evaluate for adverse effects; to maintain high fluid intake; warn that drowsiness may occur initially and to avoid driving or using power equipment during this time
Probenecid Sulfinpyrazone	Long-term gout prophylaxis	Increased renal excretion of uric acid	*Probenecid*: Headache, GI upset, urinary frequency, anaphylaxis, flushing, dizziness, haemolytic anaemia *Sulfinpyrazone*: GI bleeds, rash, anaemia, blood dyscrasias (rare)	**Assess**: For history of renal calculi, renal disease, hypersensitivity, use of hypoglycaemic drugs or aspirin; establish baseline observations of joint pain, swelling frequency and severity of attacks **Administer**: With meals **Evaluate**: For adverse effects, especially signs of renal calculi (observe urine for calculi; report complaints of retroperitoneal pain); monitor effects of drug (improvement in condition and/or further attacks)

TABLE 22.3 continued

DRUG GROUP Drug Name	Use	Action	Adverse Reactions	Nursing Implications
				Educate: To drink at least 3 L fluid per day; may experience fleeting attacks of gout initially as drug starts to take effect; to continue taking drug as prescribed at regular intervals unless otherwise instructed by physician; not to take aspirin or other over-the-counter medication without consulting physician
CENTRALLY ACTING MUSCLE RELAXANTS Methocarbamol Orphenadrine Benzodiazepines (e.g. diazepam)	Painful muscle spasm, spasticity	Act on CNS	Drowsiness, confusion (benzodiazepines)	*Methocarbamol* **Assess**: Degree of physical incapacity and current disease state, pregnancy, history of liver, renal, neurological dysfunction **Evaluate**: For drug effectiveness, for adverse effects such as drowsiness, dizziness, blurred vision, weakness, lethargy, ataxia and nystagmus **Educate**: Self-evaluation for adverse effects, that motor coordination may be impaired and to take appropriate precautions *Orphenadrine* **Assess**: Degree of physical incapacity and current disease state; establish baseline observations relating to degree of muscle spasm; general assessment as for anticholinergic drugs **Evaluate**: For drug effectiveness (improvement in spasm); for anticholinergic side effects

MUSCULOSKELETAL DISORDERS

22

TABLE 22.3 continued

DRUG GROUP Drug Name	Use	Action	Adverse Reactions	Nursing Implications
DIRECTLY ACTING MUSCLE RELAXANTS Dantrolene	Painful muscle spasm, spasticity	Reduces amount of calcium released in muscle	Nausea, diarrhoea, drowsiness, dizziness, speech and visual disturbances, depression, confusion, urinary problems, tachycardia, erratic blood pressure	**Assess:** History for cardiopulmonary insufficiency, concurrent use of anxiolytic or sedative drugs; pregnancy, renal or hepatic disease, degree of muscle spasm **Evaluate:** For relief and adverse effects, e.g. GI upset; check blood pressure and pulse regularly, urine output for signs of retention or frequency; observe for CNS side effects **Educate:** As for methocarbamol
INDIRECTLY ACTING MUSCLE RELAXANTS Baclofen	Muscle relaxant, spasticity	Presynaptic inhibition of impulses	Nausea, vomiting, diarrhoea, dyspepsia, asthenia, muscle weakness, hypotonia, tremor, sedation, lethargy, vertigo, headache	**Assess:** History for convulsive disorders, psychiatric disorders, renal dysfunction, gastric or duodenal ulceration; establish age, pregnancy, lactation, concurrent use of antihypertensive drugs; establish baseline observations for blood pressure, degree of muscle spasm and disability **Evaluate:** For drug effectiveness and monitor for adverse effects related to GI, muscle weakness, ataxia, and CNS effects **Educate:** As for methocarbamol

Pain Relief

RHONDA FIGGIS CLOSE

O B J E C T I V E S

At the conclusion of this chapter the reader should be able to:

1. Define the term analgesic;

2. Describe how peripherally acting analgesics and opioid analgesics exert their effect;

3. List the different types of analgesics and give examples of each group;

4. Discuss the common adverse drug reactions and contraindications of analgesic drugs and the signs of overdose for each class of analgesic drug;

5. Decribe the principles to be followed in giving analgesia to the palliative care patient; and

6. Write brief notes describing the nursing implications of analgesic drugs.

PAIN

Pain has been defined as 'a disturbed sensation causing suffering or distress'. The degree of pain experienced by any one person is dependent not only on the stimulus and its perception but also on its interpretation by the sufferer, and this may be entirely different for any two people.

In the first century AD, Marcus Aurelius wrote: 'If thou art pained by any external thing, it is not this thing that disturbs thee, but thy own judgement about it'. Each patient should be assessed individually. A stereotyped approach to the degree of painfulness of a condition and bias to the usefulness or otherwise of analgesics should be avoided. It is extremely difficult to measure pain and any assessment of it must necessarily be subjective.

The use of analgesic substances in the control of pain has been known since the time of Hippocrates who recommended the use of the leaves of the willow to alleviate the pain of childbirth.

The use of salicylate containing barks, leaves and fruits for therapeutic purposes has been referred to throughout the early Christian era, the Middle Ages and the Renaissance. In 1763 the President of the Royal Society, the Reverend Edward Stone, reported using salicylate as an antipyretic agent, though its use in home remedies had no doubt predated this.

ANALGESICS

Analgesics are usually divided into two main groups: the mild, simple or weak analgesics; and the strong or opioid analgesics.

The mild analgesics include: aspirin and the salicylates, paracetamol, the non-steroidal anti-inflammatory drugs (NSAIDs), and the weak opioids (narcotics), including codeine and dextropropoxyphene.

Aspirin, paracetamol and the NSAIDs exert their action peripherally by influencing the production of pain producing substances at the site of injury or inflammation. The weak opioids act centrally.

Opioid analgesics are the strong (narcotic) substances which exert their analgesic effect through the central nervous system. They reduce the patient's ability to perceive the sensation of pain and alter their emotional reaction to pain, probably by acting on the cerebral cortex. Drugs in this group include morphine and pethidine.

MILD ANALGESICS

Aspirin and the Salicylates

Aspirin (acetylsalicylic acid) was first prepared by Van Gerhardt in 1853. Salicylic acid became available in 1874 but it was not until alternatives for long-term use were researched that the advantages of aspirin were noticed. In 1899 Wohlgemut Dreser used aspirin in the treatment of rheumatic disease and its powerful analgesic effect was soon noted. So it took more than half a century after aspirin was first prepared for it to be utilised clinically.

Salicylates are more widely used for pain relief than any other class of drug and aspirin is the most important drug in this group. It is analgesic, antipyretic and anti-inflammatory in action. Estimates have been made that between 10 000 and 20 000 tons of aspirin are consumed annually in the USA. It is non-addictive and chronic use will not lead to dependence. Its toxicity is less than most other analgesics. Notwithstanding this, over 10 000 cases of serious intoxication occur in the USA every year. It is not the harmless household remedy it is often thought to be. Because of its ready availability it tends to be underestimated as an analgesic. In double blind cross over studies, 650 mg of aspirin was found to be more effective than eight other oral analgesics in the management of cancer pain.

MECHANISM OF ACTION

ANALGESIC ACTION

Aspirin acts peripherally. It is thought to exert its effect by influencing the production of prostaglandins, pain producing substances released at the site of injury or disease. The inhibition of prostaglandin synthesis by aspirin and related drugs has been postulated as an explanation of the many actions and side effects of this class of analgesic. These actions and side effects include the analgesic, antipyretic and anti-inflammatory effects, gastric irritation and ulceration, sodium retention, effect on reproductive function, and perhaps even the observed prevention of cholera induced diarrhoea.

ANTIPYRETIC ACTION

Moderate doses of aspirin reduce elevated body temperature by means of a predominantly central effect. The drug influences the hypothalamus, the body's 'thermostat'. Aspirin has no effect on normal body temperature. The antipyretic effect appears to be due, not to a direct effect on the hypothalamic neurons, but rather to involve inhibition of prostaglandin synthesis. Toxic doses of aspirin produce a rise in body temperature, or a 'pyretic' effect, due to increased oxygen consumption and metabolic rate. This results in sweating and enhances the dehydration of salicylate intoxication characterised by rapid breathing, vomiting, headache, irritability, ketosis, hypoglycaemia and, in severe cases, convulsions and respiratory failure.

ANTI-INFLAMMATORY ACTION

Aspirin and salicylates have long been used by rheumatologists to reduce inflammation. It is thought that they exert their effect by the inhibition of cyclo-oxygenase (prostaglandin synthetase) an enzyme involved in the synthesis of prostaglandins. For further information see Chapter 22 Musculoskeletal Disorders.

OTHER ACTIONS

Other actions of salicylates include the increase of urinary excretion of urates when salicylates are given in large doses, while small doses may cause a decrease in urate excretion resulting in precipitation of gout attacks in susceptible individuals.

Aspirin inhibits the aggregation of platelets and prolongs bleeding times (see Chapter 13 Blood Disorders).

High doses of salicylates can cause a reduction in the plasma level of factor VII and an increase in prothrombin time especially when the body's metabolic rate is increased by fever.

PHARMACOKINETICS

Absorption of aspirin occurs in the stomach and also in the small intestine. It is rapidly hydrolysed to salicylate. Both compounds are therapeutically active.

Aspirin and the salicylates are distributed rapidly to all body tissues. The analgesic effect begins within 30 minutes and lasts for 3–6 hours. Excretion is mainly by the kidney.

USES

Aspirin is used for its analgesic effect in the treatment of pain. The drug is particularly suitable for the relief of less severe types of pain such as headaches, toothache, myalgias, neuritis, joint and muscle pains, pain in febrile illness and other pain from peripheral or superficial sites. It is not particularly useful for pain of visceral origin. It is also used for its antipyretic effect in reducing body temperature in fever and for its anti-inflammatory as well as its analgesic effect in rheumatoid arthritis and other rheumatic complaints.

Aspirin also inhibits platelet aggregation and is used to prevent transient ischaemic

PAIN RELIEF

23

attacks, myocardial infarction, deep venous thrombosis and vascular occlusion (see Chapter 13 Blood Disorders).

Aspirin is available as plain tablets, soluble tablets (three times more quickly absorbed than plain aspirin) and tablets with glycine (which dissolve more rapidly than plain aspirin). Mixtures are no longer recommended because aspirin rapidly decomposes in aqueous solutions. Soluble aspirin tablets can be dissolved and taken immediately or used as a gargle for sore throats.

The usual dose of aspirin as an analgesic and antipyretic ranges from 300 mg to 1 g repeated every 4 hours if necessary up to a maximum of 4 g per day. For acute rheumatic disorders 4–8 g daily in divided doses may be used although doses up to 5.4 g daily in divided doses may be sufficient for the chronic disorder. Aspirin should be taken after food to reduce gastric irritation. Preparations containing aspirin are listed in Table 23.1.

ADVERSE DRUG REACTIONS

The most common adverse effects are gastrointestinal and include nausea, vomiting, ulceration and bleeding. Ingestion of aspirin produces a measurable blood loss from the alimentary tract, probably due to an alteration in platelet adhesiveness. This blood loss is mostly insignificant but patients with a history of abnormal bleeding (e.g. after minor surgery, tooth extraction), gastric ulceration or alcoholic gastritis, should not take aspirin.

Salicylates can displace bilirubin from plasma binding sites producing a raised level of free bilirubin which may lead to kernicterus in neonates and subsequent mental retardation.

Aspirin may cause hypersensitivity reactions. Bronchospasm is the most common reaction, however, urticaria and angioedema may also occur. Studies in the USA have shown that aspirin intolerance occurs in about 0.9% of normal subjects and in about 4.3% of asthmatic patients. Allergy appears more likely in those over the age of 50 years and occurs more often in women than in men.

DRUG INTERACTIONS

Aspirin enhances the anticoagulant effect of warfarin and increases the risk of bleeding from warfarin.

Sulfonylureas (e.g. tolbutamide) may be displaced from serum albumin binding sites by salicylates thus releasing more free tolbutamide and resulting in a hypoglycaemic reaction. Salicylates may cause a reduction in blood sugar, so possibly an additive effect is involved. Salicylates compete with probenecid in the renal tubule and so antagonise the uricosuric effect of this drug.

The more common drug interactions with aspirin are listed in Table 22.1, Chapter 22 Musculoskeletal Disorders.

PRECAUTIONS AND CONTRAINDICATIONS

Aspirin should be used with caution in patients with a history of gastrointestinal bleeding or ulceration.

It is contraindicated in patients with bleeding disorders and a known hypersensitivity to salicylates and other non-steroidal anti-inflammatory agents.

Aspirin appears to increase the risk of children developing Reye's syndrome if it is administered during a viral illness such as influenza or chickenpox. It should therefore not be used to treat acute febrile illnesses in children or teenagers. Reye's syndrome is characterised by vomiting, fever, delirium and coma. Pathologically it consists of encephalopathy and fatty degeneration of the liver and other viscera. It can be fatal and survivors may have permanent brain damage. It is recommended that paracetamol be used as the first-line antipyretic for these illnesses in children and young adults.

TABLE 23.1   Preparations containing aspirin

Trade name	Form	Contents (mg)			
		Aspirin	Paracetamol	Codeine phosphate	Other
Alka-Seltzer	S	325			
Aspalgin	S	300		8	
Aspirin	T, S	300			
Aspro	T, C, S	300			
Bayer Aspirin	T	300			
Bex	P	650			
	T	325			
Bufferin	B, T	250			
Codiphen	T	250		9	
Codis	S	500		8	
Codox	S	300			Dihydrocodeine tartrate 7.5
Codral Forte*	T	325		30	
Decrin	P	650		10	
Disprin	S, C	300			
Disprin Direct	T	300			Glycine
Disprin Forte	S	300		9.5	
Doloxene Co*	C	325			Dextropropoxyphene napsylate 100
Ecotrin	E	650			
Morphalgin*	S	250			Morphine hydrochloride 5
Percodan*	T	224	160		Oxycodone 4.83
Solcode	S	500		8	
Solprin	S	300			
Solvin	T	300			Glycine
Spren	T	300			
Veganin	T	325		8	
Vincent's	P	500			
Winsprin	C	325			

B = buffered; C = capsule; E = enteric coated; P = powder; S = soluble or dispersible tablet;
T = tablet
*Prescription only

PAIN RELIEF

23

NURSING IMPLICATIONS

ASSESSMENT

The patient should be assessed for a history of previous allergy, gastrointestinal bleeding or ulceration, or use of anticoagulant drugs.

During physical assessment the skin should be inspected for bruising or other signs which may be related to coagulopathy. If there are any signs of haemorrhaging or coagulopathy the patient should be assessed by a doctor before the dose is administered.

ADMINISTRATION

Aspirin should be taken with food or milk to minimise the risk of gastrointestinal discomfort and ulceration. Soluble tablets should be dissolved in water.

EVALUATION

The patient should be evaluated for pain relief, reduction in fever, signs of allergy, toxicity or gastrointestinal distress and signs of bleeding tendency after prolonged use.

PATIENT EDUCATION

As most aspirin is purchased on a non-prescription basis to treat self-diagnosed illness, the primary nursing implications are those involved with patient education. Because of its ready availability many do not regard aspirin as a drug. Nurses should be certain that patients are familiar with the adverse effects and contraindications of aspirin. Persons who experience mild dyspepsia should be instructed to take aspirin with milk or food. If this fails to give relief then paracetamol could be suggested instead. Those with a history of gastrointestinal bleeding or ulceration, bleeding disorders or who are taking anticoagulant drugs should be advised that aspirin is contraindicated in these instances. If they require analgesia they should seek advice from their doctor or pharmacist. Paracetamol is usually considered a safe alternative.

Patients should be informed of the signs of salicylate toxicity, i.e. tinnitus, dimness of vision, dizziness and confusion, and that they should reduce or cease their dose if these effects are observed.

Nurses need to be familiar with other medications their patients may be taking so that they can correctly advise them about any potential drug interactions with aspirin (see Chapter 22).

Aspirin should be stored in a cool dry place and not in warm moist conditions, e.g. bathroom cabinets. In warm moist conditions aspirin (acetylsalicylic acid) will decompose into its components, acetic acid and salicylic acid. Tablets which smell of vinegar (from decomposition to acetic acid) or show crystals on the surface (salicylic acid) should not be used. Aspirin should be kept out of the reach of children due to the high incidence of accidental overdose which has occurred with this product.

Paracetamol

Paracetamol has analgesic and antipyretic properties. It has a similar mechanism of action to aspirin and is an alternative analgesic when aspirin is contraindicated. It does not have the marked anti-inflammatory effect of aspirin.

Paracetamol is known as acetaminophen in the USA.

PHARMACOKINETICS

Paracetamol is rapidly absorbed from the gastrointestinal tract, metabolised in the liver and rapidly excreted in the urine, 3% as unchanged drug and the rest in a conjugated form. Paracetamol has a half life of 1–3.5 hours.

USES

Paracetamol is used as an antipyretic and as an analgesic. It is available as plain and soluble tablets, capsules, suppositories and paediatric

TABLE 23.2 Preparations containing paracetamol

Trade name	Form	Contents (mg)				
		Paracetamol	Codeine	Doxylamine	Dextro-propoxyphene hydrochloride	Promethazine
Capadex*	C	325			32.5	
Codalgin	T	500	8			
Codral Pain Relief	T	500	8			
Digesic*	T	325			32.5	
Dymadon**	T	500				
Dymadon Co	T	500	8			
Dymadon Forte*	T	500	30			
Dymadon P	T	500				
Fiorinal	T	500	8	5		
Fiorinal-Dental	C	500	10	2		
Mersyndol	T	450	9.75	5		
Mersyndol Forte*	T	450	30	5		
Panadeine	T, C, S	500	8			
Panadeine Forte*	T	500	30			
Panadol**	T, C, S, Su	500				
Panalgesic	T	500	8	5		
Panamax	T	500				
Panamax Co	T	500	8			
Panquil**	T	250				25
Paradex*	T	325			32.5	
Paralgin	T	500				
Setamol	T	500				
Tylenol**	T, C	500				

B = buffered; C = capsule; E = enteric coated; P = powder; S = soluble or dispersible tablet; Su = suppository; T = tablet.
*Prescription only **Paediatric preparations available

drops and syrup. The usual adult dose is 1 g every 4 hours to a maximum of 8 tablets a day. The usual paediatric dose is 12.5 mg/kg body weight every 4 hours up to four times a day. It is also available in compound products such as *Panadeine* (paracetamol and codeine), see Table 23.2.

ADVERSE DRUG REACTIONS
Paracetamol is normally well tolerated, although gastric irritation and haemorrhage have occasionally been reported. Side effects are not common.

PAIN RELIEF

23

PRECAUTIONS AND CONTRAINDICATIONS

Paracetamol should be given with caution to patients with impaired kidney and liver function.

OVERDOSAGE

Overdosage with paracetamol is dangerous and can cause irreversible liver damage which can be fatal unless treatment is commenced within 12 hours of ingestion. The observed liver toxicity is due to the formation of a toxic metabolite of paracetamol which causes liver necrosis. Overdose is treated with acetylcysteine which protects the liver cells by acting as a substrate for the toxic metabolite (see Chapter 9 Poisonings and Their Treatment).

NURSING IMPLICATIONS

Paracetamol is a widely used over the counter medication. Nursing implications relate mainly to patient and community teaching. Paracetamol has been a vehicle for attempted suicide which may in fact be unintentionally successful if treatment is not commenced promptly. It should be noted that an overdose victim may present without any symptoms and in the past people have been sent home without treatment. Such action can lead to disastrous consequences. Because the effects of overdose can be irreversible and fatal, emphasis must be placed on preventing children from having easy access to this drug. For this reason the attractively coloured paediatric elixirs should have childproof tops.

ASSESSMENT

The patient should be assessed for a history of previous allergy and a base-line description of the pain and fever should be established.

ADMINISTRATION

Paracetamol should be administered orally or rectally. The paediatric suppositories can be moistened to make insertion easier. In the treatment of chronic pain the drug should be given regularly every four hours.

EVALUATION

The patient should be evaluated for relief of pain and fever.

PATIENT EDUCATION

Patients should be educated on the dangers of overdose and the importance of keeping the medication out of reach of children.

ANALGESIC ABUSE

Chronic analgesic abuse has led to a high incidence of nephropathy associated with a history of large doses over a period of years.

In mild cases withdrawal of the analgesics has led to reversal of the condition. However, in more severe cases, the initial papillary necrosis leads on to secondary atrophic changes in the renal cortex and renal function continues to deteriorate despite the withdrawal of the analgesics.

Renal complications include haematuria, urinary tract infection, renal colic and reduced urine concentrating ability. The high rate of analgesic nephropathy caused by the abuse of compound analgesics in Australia, dating back 20–30 years, has led to the development of expertise in this country which is recognised internationally in the field of renal medicine.

ANALGESIC SEDATIVE COMBINATIONS

Sedatives have no analgesic activity and compound sedative analgesic preparations have a high abuse potential, especially combined preparations containing barbiturates.

In most instances, analgesic preparations alone are adequate to dispel aches and pains, thereby allowing relaxation and the development of a normal sleep pattern without the need for a hypnotic.

Specialists in pain relief all agree that there is no place for barbiturates in the management of pain. In small doses barbiturates are hyperalgesic and increase the reaction to painful stimuli. In view of the poor clinical record of barbiturates and barbiturate–analgesic combinations and the abuse of such products in the community, combinations such as paracetamol–codeine–pentobarbitone (*Nembudeine*, *Pentalgin*) have been removed from the market in Australia. Sedation does not override pain. If sufficient analgesia is given to relieve pain, most people do not require further sedation. For those who do require additional sedation one of the benzodiazepine compounds (e.g. nitrazepam, temazepam) can be prescribed.

NON-STEROIDAL ANTI-INFLAMMATORY DRUGS

Mefenamic Acid, Naproxen Sodium, Ibuprofen

There are a large number of non-steroidal anti-inflammatory drugs (NSAIDs) available on the Australian market. These compounds are widely used for the symptomatic relief of pain and inflammation in musculoskeletal disorders including arthritis, rheumatoid arthritis and gout, see Chapter 22 Musculoskeletal Disorders.

All the NSAIDs have analgesic, anti-inflammatory and antipyretic properties. Drugs which merit mention in this chapter are: mefenamic acid 250 mg (*Ponstan*, *Mefic*); naproxen sodium 275 mg (*Naprogesic*);

ibuprofen 200 mg (*Nurofen*) and ketorolac (*Toradol*).

USES

Because of their peripheral analgesic properties these drugs have found a niche in the treatment of dysmenorrhoea, headache, dental pain and other pain of a musculoskeletal origin.

The half-life of naproxen is between 12 and 15 hours and twice daily dosage is, therefore, adequate. Ibuprofen and mefenamic acid have much shorter half-lives (2.5 and 3.5 hours respectively) and need more frequent dosing.

Care must be taken in using NSAIDs in patients with a history of gastrointestinal bleeding or ulceration. Caution is also needed in congestive heart failure and/or hypertension due to possible deterioration of renal function and salt and water retention. The elderly are particularly at risk because of their age related changes in renal function.

For information on the mechanism of action, pharmacokinetics, adverse drug reactions, drug interactions and precautions and contraindications of NSAIDs see Chapter 22.

NURSING IMPLICATIONS

NSAIDs should be given with food wherever possible to reduce the risk of gastrointestinal upset.

The possibility of drug interactions, particularly with diuretics (e.g. thiazides, loop, and potassium sparing diuretics) and antihypertensive drugs (e.g. β blocking drugs) where a loss of blood pressure control may result especially in the elderly, must be considered.

PAIN RELIEF

23

Ketorolac

Ketorolac is a new analgesic NSAID that is available as an injection and tablets. It is more effective as an analgesic than as an anti-inflammatory agent.

TRADE NAMES

Ketoraloc: *Toradol.*

MECHANISM OF ACTION

Like other NSAIDs it exerts its activity by inhibiting prostaglandin synthesis.

PHARMACOKINETICS

Absorption of ketorolac is rapid with plasma concentrations reaching a maximum at 45–50 minutes after intramuscular injection or 30–40 minutes after oral dosage.

Ketorolac is extremely highly protein bound (more than 99%). It is mainly metabolised by glucuronic acid conjugation and is excreted mainly in the urine (90%), the remainder in the faeces (10%). The elimination half-life is said to be around 4–6 hours and is longer in the elderly and in the presence of renal dysfunction.

USES

Ketorolac is used for the relief of moderate or severe postoperative pain following general, orthopaedic and oral surgery and for short-term pain relief (for up to 2 days) in other forms of acute pain. It is currently the only analgesic NSAID available in injectable form (10 mg and 30 mg). It is also available for oral use (10 mg tablets).

Ketorolac 30 mg is said to be comparable in efficacy to morphine 12 mg and pethidine 100 mg given intramuscularly. The usual dose for adults under 65 years of age is 30 mg intramuscularly initially, then 10–30 mg intramuscularly every 4–6 hours to a maximum of 120 mg per day. For the elderly an initial dose of 10 mg is suggested followed by 10–30 mg every 4–6 hours as required to a maximum of 60 mg per day. In all patients administration of ketorolac injection should not exceed 2 days. With the tablets the maximum duration of therapy is 7 days. For adults under 65 years of age the usual oral dose is 10 mg every 4–6 hours to a maximum of 40 mg per day. The elderly may take 10 mg every 6–8 hours to a maximum of 30–40 mg per day.

As a non-narcotic analgesic ketorolac has the advantages of not depressing the central nervous system or causing respiratory depression and lacks the potential for physical and psychological dependence. It has been used in combination with opioid analgesics for postoperative pain.

It is not recommended for long term use.

ADVERSE DRUG REACTIONS

As with other NSAIDs the adverse drug reactions are less frequent with short-term use and after low doses. The most frequently reported adverse reactions are gastrointestinal effects (e.g. dyspepsia, nausea, gastrointestinal pain) and central nervous system reactions (e.g. headache).

The most serious reactions are acute renal failure, hypersensitivity reactions and gastrointestinal ulceration and bleeding.

Other reactions include dermatological effects (rash, pruritus) and cardiovascular reactions (oedema, flushing, palpitations, hypotension, syncope).

DRUG INTERACTIONS

Ketorolac may prolong bleeding time and should be used with caution in patients receiving anticoagulants (e.g. warfarin and heparin).

The dose of ketorolac should be reduced when the drug is given with high dose aspirin or probenecid.

The diuretic response to frusemide is reduced by approximately 20%. The effect of non-depolarising muscle relaxants may be enhanced.

PRECAUTIONS AND CONTRAINDICATIONS

The precautions to be taken with the use of ketorolac are the same as those for other NSAIDs.

The drug should be used with caution in elderly and debilitated patients; patients with impaired renal or hepatic function; those with active or a history of gastrointestinal bleeding or ulceration; and those with coagulation disorders.

Ketorolac should not be used in patients with bronchospastic reactivity (e.g. asthma) or other allergic reactions to aspirin or other NSAIDs. It should not be used in patients with a previously demonstrated hypersensitivity to ketorolac or those with nasal polyps or angioedema.

WEAK OPIOID ANALGESICS

The opioids (narcotics, opiate agonists) are a group of naturally occurring, semisynthetic and synthetic compounds that are opium or morphine-like in their properties. They exert their analgesic effect through action on receptors in the central nervous system. Although generally regarded as powerful analgesics, several compounds in this class have only mild analgesic properties, whilst others such as dextromoramide and morphine are extremely strong analgesics. All opioids have analgesic, antitussive and constipating effects to some degree, and all are potentially dependence producing.

Those opioids which can be classified as mild analgesics are dextropropoxyphene, codeine phosphate and dihydrocodeine.

Dextropropoxyphene

Dextropropoxyphene is a synthetic analgesic structurally related to methadone. However, it is less analgesic, antitussive and dependence producing than methadone. When used alone it is only marginally more effective as an analgesic than placebo.

TRADE NAMES

Dextropropoxyphene: *Doloxene*.

PHARMACOKINETICS

Dextropropoxyphene is readily absorbed from the gastrointestinal tract but the first-pass metabolism effect through the liver is considerable. It is distributed rapidly and is concentrated in the lungs, liver and kidneys. Excretion is by the kidney with the drug appearing in the urine, mainly as metabolites.

The analgesic effect occurs within in 15–60 minutes and lasts for 4–6 hours.

USES

Dextropropoxyphene is mainly used combined with other analgesics such as aspirin or paracetamol for the treatment of mild to moderate pain.

It is available as dextropropoxyphene 100 mg capsules (*Doloxene*), dextropropoxyphene with aspirin (*Doloxene Co*) and dextropropoxyphene with paracetamol (*Di-Gesic, Capadex, Paradex*). It is more effective when administered as a combination preparation.

The usual adult dose of dextropropoxyphene 100 mg capsules and dextropropoxyphene–aspirin preparations is one capsule every four hours as necessary. For dextropropoxyphene–paracetamol combinations the dosage is two tablets every four hours.

ADVERSE DRUG REACTIONS

Adverse reactions to the drug are similar to those of morphine although less marked. The most common side effects are gastrointestinal (abdominal pain and constipation). Other effects include headache, drowsiness, dizziness, insomnia and habituation. Liver impairment has also been reported.

Prolonged use may lead to dependence of the morphine type. It has become a much abused drug and despite early claims that it was not dependence producing, the actual incidence of dependence is about the same as that for codeine phosphate. Overdosage has led to a large number of deaths both intentional and unintentional. In the USA, the Food and Drug Administration estimates that 1000 to 2000 deaths each year are associated with dextropropoxyphene. Overdosage symptoms are similar to those of morphine and characterised by respiratory depression. Additionally, pulmonary oedema, cardiac arrhythmias, convulsions or psychotic reactions may be experienced.

PAIN RELIEF

23

DRUG INTERACTIONS

Dextropropoxyphene may cause an increase in serum concentrations of carbamazepine leading to toxicity. It may also potentiate the effects of warfarin.

PRECAUTIONS AND CONTRAINDICATIONS

These are similar to those for morphine. Alcohol and other central nervous system depressants may enhance the hazards of dextropropoxyphene. Severely depressed patients should use another analgesic. Central nervous system stimulants may enhance the convulsant action of high doses of dextropropoxyphene.

NURSING IMPLICATIONS

As mixed analgesics containing dextropropoxyphene are widely used, the nurse needs to be fully aware of the individual properties of each drug contained in these compound formulations so that appropriate assessment, evaluation and patient education can be carried out.

Due to the narcotic activity of dextropropoxyphene there is potential for abuse of products containing the drug. In Australia, all compounds containing dextropropoxyphene are restricted and available only on prescription.

Patients should be warned not to take alcohol with dextropropoxyphene as the central nervous system depressant effects of both substances will be greatly potentiated. They should also be warned of the consequences of overdosage and instructed to take the drug as directed by the doctor.

Nurses should be aware that *Doloxene Co* contains aspirin *not* codeine, and that all nursing implications for aspirin will also apply to *Doloxene Co*.

Constipation can be a problem for patients taking compounds containing dextropropoxyphene.

Codeine Phosphate

Codeine phosphate is a weak opioid. It is active orally and is approximately two-thirds as effective when given orally as when given by injection. It has all the pharmacological properties of the opioid class although weight for weight it is far less potent than morphine. Hence it has become regarded as one of the mild analgesics.

Codeine phosphate 30 mg is equivalent in analgesic potency to aspirin 600 mg.

PHARMACOKINETICS

Codeine is well absorbed from the gastrointestinal tract with peak plasma levels occuring in about one hour. Codeine is about two-thirds as effective orally as parenterally. It is metabolised in the liver to morphine and norcodeine. Excretion is almost entirely by the kidney. The plasma half-life is between 3 and 4 hours.

USES

Codeine phosphate is particularly effective in treating pain of visceral origin. For somatic pain it is commonly given in combination with aspirin or paracetamol (see Table 23.3), and the combined analgesic effect is said to be synergistic. It is also used as an antitussive as Linctus Codeine and in the treatment of diarrhoea.

It is available as 30 mg tablets, injections of 50 mg/mL and in a number of combination tablet forms (see Table 23.3). The adult analgesic dose is 15–60 mg every four hours as necessary.

ADVERSE DRUG REACTIONS

These are the same as for other opioids — nausea, anorexia, confusion, sweating and constipation. The constipating effect of codeine phosphate is frequently exploited therapeutically to treat severe diarrhoea.

DRUG INTERACTIONS

Enhanced central nervous system depressant effects are experienced when codeine is taken with alcohol and other depressants such as the butyrophenones, sedatives and the phenothiazines.

TABLE 23.3 Commonly used analgesics containing codeine

Trade Name	Contents (mg)			
	Codeine	Paracetamol	Aspirin	Doxylamine
Aspalgin	8		300	
Codiphen	9		250	
Codis	8		500	
Codral Forte*	30		325	
Decrin Powders	10		650	
Disprin Forte	9.5		500	
Solcode	8		500	
Veganin	8		325	
Codalgin	8	500		
Codral Pain Relief	8	500		
Dymadon Co	8	500		
Dymadon Forte*	30	500		
Fiorinal	8	500		5
Fiorinal-Dental	10	500		2
Mersyndol	9.75	450		5
Mersyndol Forte*	30	450		5
Panadeine	8	500		
Panadeine Forte*	30	500		
Panalgesic	8	500		5
Panamax Co	8	500		

*Prescription only

PRECAUTIONS AND CONTRAINDICATIONS
As codeine has a depressant effect on the central nervous system patients should be warned of impairment of skills such as driving.

Dihydrocodeine

Dihydrocodeine tartrate (or bitartrate) is related to codeine phosphate and is an analgesic and antitussive which may produce morphine like dependence in susceptible in-dividuals. The usual analgesic dose is 30–60 mg (60 mg being equi-analgesic to 10 mg of morphine).

Forms available include: *Codox* tablets — 7.5 mg dihydrocodeine with 300 mg aspirin, for use as an analgesic; and *Tuscodin* lozenges — 7.5 mg dihydrocodeine with chlorhexidine (an antiseptic) and lignocaine (a local anaesthetic), for use as an analgesic and an antitussive. Dihydrocodeine is also used as an ingredient of some cough mixtures, e.g. *Rikodeine*.

ADVERSE DRUG REACTIONS

Adverse reactions are the same as those of other opioids.

OPIOID ANALGESICS

The term *opioid* is used to designate those drugs with a morphine-like action. Opioid analgesics are also known as *opiate agonists* and *narcotic* analgesics.

Analgesia with the opioid analgesics is produced through an interaction between the drug and opiate receptors in the central nervous system. Analgesia probably occurs through a change in the patient's perception of pain and an alteration in the emotional reaction to the painful stimulus.

Opioids have some of the properties of naturally occurring peptides such as the enkephalins and the endorphins which are widely distributed in the central nervous system and appear to act, amongst other functions, as modulators of neurotransmission or as neurotransmitters.

Stimulation of the opiate receptors, of which there are several types, can lead to various responses including analgesia, euphoria, respiratory depression, nausea and vomiting, physical dependence, sedation, dysphoria, hallucinations and vasomotor stimulation, depending on the receptors stimulated.

Opioids can be classified according to their effects on the receptors. Agonists are purely stimulating in their effects; antagonists may block the receptor and therefore the activity of other agents; whilst agonist/antagonists can stimulate one receptor type while blocking another. (See Table 23.4.)

Opioids are the most important agents used in the management of postoperative pain and may be administered continuously by infusion or intermittently in small doses injected at regular intervals by intravenous, intramuscular or subcutaneous injection. They appear to be more effective against dull continuous pain than sharp intermittent pain. Treatment of visceral pain with narcotic analgesics is especially effective.

TABLE 23.4   Opioid analgesics

Opioid type	Example
Agonist	Methadone, fentanyl, morphine, oxycodone, pethidine, phenoperidine
Agonist/antagonist	Buprenorphine, pentazocine
Pure antagonist	Naloxone

Opioids can also produce a state of mild sedation with analgesia called neuroleptanalgesia when combined with a neuroleptic agent such as droperidol. This type of anaesthesia enables patient cooperation during minor procedures.

The main disadvantages of the opioids are depression of respiration (which is mostly dose related), constipation, tolerance and dependence with repeated usage. In some individuals the use of opioids for a period longer than a few days may produce psychic and physical dependence. The hallucinogenic and euphoric effects of these drugs are factors which can lead to abuse.

Opium, which contains a number of alkaloids including morphine, has been known in medical practice for many centuries. Thomas Sydenham in 1680 wrote: 'Among the remedies which it has pleased almighty God to give man to relieve his suffering, none is so universal and so efficacious as opium'.

Opium is obtained by cutting the seed head of the opium poppy and collecting the dried exudate. The alkaloids derived from opium include morphine, codeine, papaverine and noscapine. Papaveretum is a purified mixture of these alkaloids.

Morphine

Morphine is the most potent derivative of opium. It acts on the central nervous system as a depressant, leading to analgesia, drowsiness, respiratory depression and depression of the cough reflex, and as a stimulant leading to vomiting, miosis, convulsions and some hyperactive spinal cord reflexes. It can stimulate smooth muscle leading to spasm of the biliary and urinary tracts. It decreases gut motility, thereby causing constipation.

PHARMACOKINETICS

Morphine is absorbed from the gastrointestinal tract but undergoes considerable first-pass metabolism in the liver. The effects are not as predictable as when the drug is administered by the subcutaneous or intramuscular route. It is only about one-third as effective when given orally as when given by subcutaneous, intramuscular or intravenous injection. Peak analgesia occurs around 60 minutes after an oral dose; 20–60 minutes after a rectal dose; 50–90 minutes after subcutaneous injection; 30–60 minutes after intramuscular injection; and 20 minutes after intravenous injection. The analgesic effect lasts around four hours.

It is distributed throughout the body but especially in the lungs, liver, spleen and kidneys. About 90% of the dose is excreted in the urine while 10% is excreted into the faeces through the bile.

USES

Morphine is administered as a surgical pre-medication, for the relief of postoperative pain when a reasonably long acting preparation is required; for alleviation of the pain of terminal diseases such as cancer; and for the treatment of severe acute pain resulting from trauma, burns and myocardial infarction. It was formerly used as a cough suppressant (Linctus Morphine).

It is the analgesic of choice in the treatment of severe pain following myocardial infarction and it relieves the dyspnoea associated with severe left ventricular failure and pulmonary oedema.

With its oral activity and 4-hour duration of action morphine is the drug of choice for management of the pain of advanced malignant disease. In cases of continuous pain a 4-hourly regimen is the optimum balance between pain relief, practical convenience and side effects. It is important that mor-phine is administered regularly to these patients. Regular dosing gives far better pain control than administration of the drug on an 'as needed' basis. The risk of addiction should not be viewed as a problem in the terminally ill. (See section on drugs used in palliative care in this chapter.)

Morphine may be given by intramuscular, intravenous or subcutaneous injection, by intravenous infusion, intrathecally, epidurally or orally as mixture or tablets.

Morphine mixtures are commonly used in the management of terminal pain. Patients who have a reaction to the preservative in the readily obtainable morphine mixture can have a fresh mixture tailor made. Most patients do better on plain morphine dissolved in water if they get nauseous with the syrup or flavouring agents commonly added to the mixtures.

These simple mixtures have largely replaced the old 'Brompton's cocktail', a mixture of morphine, cocaine, alcohol and chloroform water which has largely fallen into disrepute due to side effects such as the psychosis caused by cocaine, impaired judgment and coordination, burning in the throat (caused by the high alcohol content) and nausea (caused by the syrup content).

Morphine is also available as controlled release tablets in 10 mg, 30 mg, 60 mg and 100 mg strengths (*MS Contin*); as controlled release pellets in capsules in 20 mg, 50 mg and 100 mg strengths (*Kapanol*); and in a combination of 5 mg morphine with 250 mg aspirin (*Morphalgin* tablets). Morphine sulfate is available in strengths up to 30 mg/mL for intravenous, intramuscular and subcutaneous injection and morphine tartrate in strengths of 120 mg and 400 mg for subcutaneous injection.

Morphine may be administered in doses of 2–5 mg diluted in glucose injection or normal saline injection by the epidural route for chronic intractable pain. Pain relief generally occurs within 15 minutes of epidural administration and has been reported to last from 6–24 hours after a single epidural dose. No more than a total of 10 mg should be administered epidurally over 24 hours.

PAIN RELIEF

23

It may also be administered intrathecally in very small doses of 0.2–1.0 mg. Such doses can provide adequate analgesia for up to 24 hours.

Note: When administering morphine by the intrathecal or epidural routes, preservative free injectable preparations of morphine must be used.

ADVERSE DRUG REACTIONS

The most important reactions are respiratory depression, nausea, vomiting, constipation and dependence.

Hypotension and bradycardia may occur through stimulation of the vagal centre and impairment of the sympathetic vascular reflexes, particularly in those patients who are taking antihypertensive drugs.

DRUG INTERACTIONS

Additive central nervous system depressant effects are experienced when morphine is administered with other central nervous system depressants such as alcohol, butyrophenones, sedatives and phenothiazines and, it is thought by some researchers, with MAOIs and tricyclic antidepressants.

Morphine may also enhance the repiratory depressant effects of neuromuscular blocking agents.

PRECAUTIONS AND CONTRAINDICATIONS

Overdosage with morphine may lead to death due to severe respiratory depression.

Extreme care needs to be exercised in giving morphine to newborn or premature infants. It is not usually given preoperatively to children under one year of age. It should also be given with care and the dose reduced in elderly or debilitated patients.

It is contraindicated in head injuries, acute alcoholism and conditions in which intracranial pressure is raised except in the acute care situation where patients can be closely monitored. It is also contraindicated after operations on the biliary tract, in the presence of excessive bronchial secretions and in respiratory depression. It should not be given in any respiratory related disease such as bronchial asthma or heart failure secondary to chronic lung disease.

It should be given in reduced doses or with great caution in patients with prostatic hypertrophy, shock, impaired liver function, adrenocortical insufficiency, hypothyroidism, or with obstructive or inflammatory bowel disorders.

Pethidine

Pethidine (meperidine (*Demerol*) in the USA) is a synthetic strong analgesic which was introduced in 1939. It has morphine-like properties but causes less constipation and urinary retention than morphine and does not have the cough suppressant activity of morphine.

PHARMACOKINETICS

Pethidine is readily absorbed from the gastrointestinal tract and is metabolised in the liver. It is less than half as effective when given orally as when given by intravenous or intramuscular injection. It has a more rapid onset of action and a shorter duration of action than morphine. Its analgesic effect only lasts 2–4 hours.

It crosses the placenta and also appears in breast milk.

USES

Pethidine is useful for the treatment of pain requiring stronger analgesia than that provided by drugs such as codeine phosphate but where the potency of morphine may not be required. On a weight for weight basis 100 mg of pethidine has equal analgesic potency to 10 mg morphine.

Pethidine may be given orally, although it is less effective when given by this route than when given by injection. Its short duration of action makes it unsuitable for the treatment of prolonged painful episodes or chronic pain.

Its major usefulness is as a premedication prior to surgery and in the treatment of postoperative pain. It is particularly useful following abdominal surgery as it is less likely to cause urinary retention and constipation than morphine. For these reasons and because it does not diminish the force of contraction of the uterus it has also been quite widely used in obstetric analgesia. However, it should be used with caution as it may prolong labour and cause respiratory depression in the newborn.

ADVERSE DRUG REACTIONS

These are essentially the same as those of morphine. Pethidine may cause vomiting, dry mouth and blurred vision, but the psychic effects are not as marked as with morphine.

Constipation and urinary retention occur less often than with morphine. Following high doses by mouth or in intolerant persons, stimulation of the central nervous system and convulsions may occur.

Local reactions often occur after injection. However, hypersensitivity reactions are rare.

Overdose can result in death from respiratory depression.

DRUG INTERACTIONS

Administration with MAOIs has caused serious and sometimes fatal reactions. With central nervous system depressants there is a combined depressant effect. Combination with phenothiazines has led to hypotension and prolonged respiratory depression.

PRECAUTIONS AND CONTRAINDICATIONS

Administration with, or within 14 days of administration of, MAOIs should be avoided.

Papaveretum

Papaveretum acts on the central nervous system. It is a purified mixture of the opium alkaloids (anhydrous morphine, codeine, noscapine and papaverine). It has the analgesic and narcotic properties of morphine.

PHARMACOKINETICS

See morphine.

USES

Papaveretum is a convenient means of administering the total alkaloids of opium by injection and may be used in all cases in which morphine is indicated. It is commonly used with hyoscine for preoperative medication.

For adverse drug reactions, drug interactions, precautions and contraindications see morphine, although it is claimed to produce fewer side effects than morphine.

Diamorphine (Heroin)

Diamorphine is not available for therapeutic use in Australia or many other countries, although it is still available to doctors in the United Kingdom. It is used illicitly in many countries including Australia. It is a semisynthetic drug first made from morphine (to which it is metabolised in the body) in 1874 in London. It was first introduced 24 years later (1898) as a remedy for cough and for morphine addiction. It was some time before it was realised that its efficiency in treatment of the latter was by substitution of one dependence producing drug for another. It is commonly said that heroin is the most potent of all dependence producing drugs. Orally it is 1.5 times more potent than morphine but no more efficaceous.

ADVERSE DRUG REACTIONS

These are similar to those of morphine although it causes less vomiting, restlessness and fidgeting.

Methadone

Methadone (*Physeptone*) is a synthetic morphine-like compound with properties similar to those of morphine including its abuse potential. It is, however, much more active orally than morphine.

PHARMACOKINETICS

Methadone is absorbed from the gastrointestinal tract and distributed widely in the tissues. It is metabolised by the liver and excreted in the bile and the urine. It crosses the placenta.

Its high potency and long duration of action (its plasma half-life is 22–72 hours) means that the danger of accumulation in

PAIN RELIEF

23

the elderly or debilitated patient is great. It should not, therefore, be given more often than once every six hours.

USES

It has been used in the treatment of postoperative pain, as a cough suppressant and as a strong oral analgesic in terminal pain. Methadone has had a place in the past few years in the treatment of heroin and morphine addiction.

ADVERSE DRUG REACTIONS

Adverse reactions include vomiting, sedation and dependence, which is less severe than with morphine and heroin. Because of its dependence producing properties, its use in the treatment of long-term chronic pain that is not terminal should be avoided.

DRUG INTERACTIONS

Rifampicin, phenytoin and other liver enzyme inducing drugs cause a drop in plasma concentrations of methadone and symptoms of narcotic withdrawal in persons on a methadone maintenance program.

PRECAUTIONS AND CONTRAINDICATIONS

Methadone should be used with caution in elderly or debilitated patients because of the risk of accumulation. It is not recommended for use in labour because its prolonged action increases the risk of neonatal depression. Babies born to methadone dependent mothers must be closely monitored and if necessary, treated for withdrawal symptoms.

Fentanyl, Phenoperidine

Fentanyl (*Sublimaze*) and phenoperidine (*Operidine*) are potent synthetic opioid agonists with a rapid onset and short duration of action.

Fentanyl is 100 to 150 times more potent than morphine on a weight basis and phenoperidine is 75 times more potent.

PHARMACOKINETICS

The onset of action of fentanyl is almost immediate following intravenous injection and the analgesic effect lasts 30–60 minutes. The repiratory depressant effects last longer.

USES

Fentanyl and phenoperidine are used for analgesia of short duration during anaesthesia and in the immediate postoperative period. They are combined with a neuroleptic agent such as droperidol to produce neuroleptanalgesia.

Fentanyl has been combined with the local anaesthetic bupivicaine and administered by epidural infusion to control postoperative pain.

Phenoperidine is also used as a respiratory depressant in patients on prolonged assisted ventilation.

Adverse drug reactions, drug interactions, precautions and contraindications are the same as for morphine. As a precaution resuscitation equipment and naloxone should be readily available to manage severe respiratory depression.

Dextromoramide

Dextromoramide (**Palfium**) is a narcotic analgesic which is claimed to be as equally effective by the oral route as by injection. It has been used as a potent analgesic in terminal pain.

It is claimed to be twice as potent as morphine but produces short lasting analgesia of about two hours which limits its use in chronic terminal pain. It is sometimes used to relieve exacerbations of acute and chronic pain (breakthrough pain) in terminal illnesses.

Oxycodone

This is a useful analgesic which has about equal potency to morphine. It is marketed as tablets either alone (*Endone*), in combination with aspirin and paracetamol (*Percodan*) and as suppositories (*Proladone*). It has a relatively long half-life of about six hours, fewer side effects than morphine and is effective orally. It is therefore a useful

TABLE 23.5 Equivalent doses of analgesics

Analgesic	Dose	Equivalent doses*
Mild analgesics		
Aspirin	600 mg	Approximately equivalent to:
Paracetamol	1 g	morphine 1.5 mg IM, 3–9 mg orally
Codeine	30 mg	dextromoramide 1.5 mg orally
Pentazocine	30 mg	methadone 3 mg orally
Dextropropoxyphene	60 mg	oxycodone 4.5 mg orally
Strong analgesics		
Morphine	10 mg IM	20–60 mg orally
Methadone	10 mg IM	20 mg orally
Oxycodone	15 mg IM	30 mg orally
Pethidine	75 mg IM	Unsatisfactory orally
Dextromoramide	5 mg IM	10 mg orally

*These data are useful only as a starting point when changing analgesics as there is much variation between individual patients, results of studies and half-lives of the various agents

alternative to morphine in the treatment of moderate pain in terminal illness.

Buprenorphine

Buprenorphine (*Temgesic*) has agonist/antagonist activity. That is, it both stimulates and blocks the opiate receptors in the central nervous system.

It is well absorbed sublingually, about 0.4 mg being equianalgesic with 10 mg of morphine. It is thought to have less abuse potential than morphine. It also appears to have a lower incidence of side effects and psychotomimetic effects than pentazocine, and about double the duration of action of morphine.

Pentazocine

Pentazocine (*Fortral*) is a synthetic analgesic of about one-third the potency of morphine. It is also an opiate antagonist and can therefore induce withdrawal symptoms in addicts.

It can cause dependence as it also has partial opiate agonist activity, but the potential for producing dependence is less than with other morphine-like drugs. It may need to be given more frequently than morphine (e.g. every three hours) and is available for injection and for oral use.

ADVERSE DRUG REACTIONS

Adversed reactions include nausea, vomiting, hypertension, sweating, dizziness, palpitations, tachycardia and central nervous system disturbances (euphoria, restlessness, hallucinations, delusions, distorted body image, depersonalisation, nightmares and depression).

Equivalent doses of the mild and strong analgesics are listed in Table 23.5.

NURSING IMPLICATIONS

ASSESSMENT

The nursing care of the patient in pain involves more than just giving the ordered analgesic. An holistic approach to the patient as an individual should always be used. Full assessment of the patient should include documenting the type and frequency of pain, the underlying cause, the patient's psychological reaction to the pain and the type of drug to be used for its relief.

PAIN RELIEF

23

The patient may not verbalise his or her pain and the nurse needs to be able to recognise the various signs that the individual patient may manifest when experiencing pain, e.g. increased pulse rate and respiratory rate, facial expression, posture, guarding muscular action, restlessness, sweating or pallor.

The nurse should also realise that some patients may not desire to have their awareness reduced by drugs and this right should be respected. Alternative measures such as the application of heat or cold or massage should not be overlooked. Sometimes such simple nursing measures as changing the position of the patient, loosening a tight dressing, a back rub or talking with the patient may do a great deal to promote comfort and alleviate anxieties and fears. Psychological support can often assist in pain relief.

Pain is what the person experiencing it says it is, and carers should avoid having fixed ideas about what they think the patient is experiencing. People, especially those with a terminal illness, should be given adequate analgesia as required. It is not appropriate to withhold pain relief either in this class of patient or those in the acute postoperative period because of fear of addiction.

The nursing implications are essentially the same for all opioid analgesics. Prior to administration the patient's drug profile should be assessed for concurrent use of drugs such as alcohol, barbiturates, phenothiazines, sedatives or antidepressants, as the combined use of any of these with a narcotic will cause cumulative central nervous system depressant effects.

Patients whose histories reveal chronic respiratory disease, liver disease, convulsive disorders, Addison's disease or myxodoedema, are at increased risk of adverse effects and should therefore be subject to close monitoring following administration.

Where it is vitally important to monitor the patient's neurological state (e.g. in raised intracranial pressure, head injuries, diabetic ketoacidosis), the administration of potent opioids will usually be contraindicated as they will mask the true neurological state of the patient.

ADMINISTRATION

Opioids are most effective if they are administered to the patient before the pain reaches its greatest level of intensity. Administration should be scheduled so that the peak effect is reached when painful procedures are being performed. The syringe should be aspirated carefully before injecting intramuscular or subcutaneous doses to avoid accidental intravenous administration. Opioids should not be mixed with other drugs in the same syringe or infusion, as physical and chemical drug incompatibilities can occur.

Morphine mixture may be diluted with milk, fruit juice or flavouring to make it more palatable.

Note: The majority of opioid drugs are classified in Schedule 8 of the Poisons Act. Nurses must strictly observe the rules relating to the administration of Schedule 8 drugs. All narcotic drugs must be ordered by a medical officer (who must specify and limit the amount of the drug which can be given on any particular order). Any breakage or loss must be reported to the appropriate person as defined by the law in the particular State — usually the chief pharmacist in a hospital.

EVALUATION

Following administration the nurse must assess the efficacy of the drug used for degree and duration of pain relief. Tools such as visual analogue scales or pain charts may be used to assess pain and to evaluate the efficacy of analgesic agents being used. The patient should be monitored carefully for signs of adverse effects and toxicity. Respiration should be checked regularly and narcotics should not be given if the respiration rate falls below 10 per minute. Blood pressure and pulse rate should also be monitored closely. The patient should be watched for abdominal and bladder distention and constipation and impaction prevented, especially in terminal care patients. The nurse should be alert for signs of dependence and tolerance, such as coryza and an itching nose, which usually will appear 24 to 28 hours after the last administered dose. Patients should be assisted to the sitting position slowly due to the postural hypotension which can occur with opioids.

PATIENT EDUCATION

Patients should be reassured that the side rails are for their protection against falling due to narcotic induced altered sensory perceptions. They must be encouraged to deep breathe, cough and change position regularly as the antitussive and respiratory depressant properties of most narcotics can produce other respiratory complications.

OPIOID ANTAGONISTS

Nalorphine

Nalorphine (*Lethidrone*) is used to reverse overdosage of the opioids with which it competes at the site of action. It was often used in an attempt to avoid respiratory depression caused by the narcotic analgesics in both mother and child at childbirth. The introduction of the antagonist to the narcotic is complex and great care is needed in combining the two so that the respiratory depression is not made worse. It is closely related to morphine with some of the same actions (e.g. analgesia), but it has tended to become obsolete as it produces unpleasant abnormalities of mood and hallucinations. It is of no use in reducing the respiratory depression of other drugs such as the barbiturates.

Naloxone

Naloxone (*Narcan*) has, to a great extent, replaced nalorphine. It is a pure opiate antagonist and reverses the action of relatively large doses of all opioids including the respiratory depressant effect. It is the only specific antagonist to pentazocine.

USES

Naloxone is available in two strengths, a 400 micrograms/mL injection for use in adults to reverse postoperative opiate depression and in opioid overdosage and a neonatal preparation of 20 micrograms/mL given into the umbilical vein of the newborn baby to reverse respiratory depression following administration of opioid analgesia to the mother.

For information on pharmacokinetics, adverse drug reactions, precautions and contraindications see Chapter 9 Poisonings and Their Treatment.

NURSING IMPLICATIONS

Nursing assessment includes documenting the extent of opioid induced respiratory depression and the determination of any existing addiction.

Evaluation following administration focuses on monitoring the patient's respiration and level of consciousness.

Since the duration of action of some narcotics may exceed that of naloxone repeat doses of naloxone may be necessary.

When naloxone is administered to narcotic addicts to reverse the effects of overdose signs of withdrawal may be expected.

PAIN RELIEF

23

PREVENTION OF POSTOPERATIVE PAIN ▆▆▆▆▆▆▆▆▆▆

There is a close relationship between injury response and acute pain and its treatment.

It is important to prepare the patient for pain before the surgery takes place. Patients who are prepared prophylactically for pain before surgery do better than those who are not. Studies show that by producing a profound blockade of pain before the injury is produced a significant decrease in morbidity is achieved. For example, a study of the beneficial effect of preventive analgesia on patients who had a limb removed demonstrated that a group of patients given epidural analgesia for 72 hours preoperatively had a much lower incidence of phantom limb pain at six months and one year after surgery.

It is also known that acute pain causes adverse effects on the cardiovascular system and that this can be prevented with good pain relief.

As a matter of normal practice, therefore, good patient care should include preventive treatment of expected pain including regular administration of intermittent intramuscular injections postoperatively.

ANALGESICS AND ADJUVANT DRUGS USED IN PALLIATIVE CARE ▆▆▆▆▆▆▆▆

The chronic pain experienced in cancer is not like the acute pain experienced after trauma. It generally appears unending or worsening and can be totally consuming, substantially isolating patients from those around them and their surroundings. Additionally, the pain experienced can be exacerbated by anxiety and depression.

Treatment of the pain is the first priority but it is also very important to look for other causes of immediate discomfort so that they can be relieved. If this is done then the need for analgesia may be substantially lessened.

One of the causes of discomfort can be constipation. A patient who is receiving an opioid will become constipated and it is essential to treat this at the onset of therapy and not after it becomes a problem. A faecal softener with a peristaltic stimulant such as *Coloxyl with Senna* can be used as a starting point. Suppositories and enemas may also be necessary. Important points to remember are that the patient should be kept well hydrated, eat a high fibre diet and be as active as possible. Other symptoms which may occur, either because of the progression of the disease or the treatment, include nausea, dry or painful mouth, dysphasia, anorexia and insomnia.

Prochlorperazine (*Stemetil*), chlorpromazine (*Largactil*), haloperidol (*Serenace*), metoclopramide (*Maxolon, Pramin*) and domperidone (*Motilium*) may be used for short-term treatment when nausea and vomiting become a problem. The last two drugs should not be given to patients with obstructions as they may worsen colic. Ondansetron (*Zofran*) is a potent agent which blocks the initiation of a vomiting reflex caused by cytotoxic chemotherapy and radiotherapy. It is used when nausea and vomiting become intractable.

Other symptoms, such as dry and painful mouth, dysphasia due to painful lesions and anorexia should be treated according to the underlying cause of the symptoms.

The cause of insomnia needs to be ascertained. It is no use giving a hypnotic if the patient is still in pain as no amount of sedative will override the pain. The patient who is no longer in pain may no longer have insomnia. Other symptoms which may be related to insomnia include: joint stiffness and night sweats, which can be treated with an NSAID such as indomethacin; cramps which may respond to quinine; fear of incontinence for which a condom may be appropriate; and early wakening or depression which may respond to amitriptyline. If a hypnotic is still required then a short acting benzodiazepine such as temazepam is usually satisfactory. Unless a prolonged anxiolytic effect is required long acting benzodiazepines such as diazepam or nitrazepam are best avoided. Chlormethiazole (*Hemineurin M*) can be given as a hypnotic if the patient is elderly or confused.

Anxiety and depression can be treated by first taking into account the natural sadness of the dying for which emotional and spiritual support may be helpful. Anxiolytic drugs such as the benzodiazepines and phenothiazines may be used depending on the individual patient response, while clinical depression can be treated by amitriptyline.

If the symptom of the pain is caused directly by the cancer then it is likely to be continuous and should be treated regularly and not on an as necessary (prn) basis. The symptoms need to be checked regularly and the dose constantly reviewed as the situation may change rapidly. The correct dose of analgesic is the lowest which achieves pain control.

About 70% of cancer patients will experience significant pain and it is the symptom most feared by patients. If the cause of the pain is carefully diagnosed it may be found that other therapy is available so that analgesia may be avoided or at least given in lower doses.

Adjuvant therapy may be used. Radiotherapy or a nerve block may be indicated. NSAIDs may be added for bone pain; corticosteroids may help with nerve compression pain, raised intracranial pressure or a large tumour mass; and muscle relaxants and other drugs may be useful in pain control. When the pain is severe and due to nerve involvement anticonvulsants such as valproic acid or carbamazepine may be appropriate.

MORPHINE

Oral Morphine

The use of oral morphine has revolutionised the management of terminal pain. In cancer patients it is only rarely necessary to give morphine by injection, e.g. for intractable vomiting or if the patient is in a coma or unable to swallow. If the need arises to convert from oral morphine administration to parenteral administration the dosage should be halved.

Conversely when converting from parenteral morphine to oral therapy the injection dose should be doubled and if this is ineffective it may need to be trebled.

In the management of severe pain in advanced terminal disease, dose escalation may be necessary. Each dosage increment should be sufficient to have increased analgesic effect otherwise patient confidence in the drug will be lost. In the hospital setting the following dosage increments have been recommended: 5 mg to 10 mg, 15 mg, 20 mg, 30 mg, 40 mg, 60 mg, 80 mg, 100 mg, 120 mg, 160 mg, 200 mg, 240 mg, 300 mg, 360 mg. At home, the increments are usually around 50% or as low as 33% of the previous dose. The dosage should only be increased once in a 24-hour period.

Important points which should be remembered in dose escalation are:

- Escalation of doses is unlimited;

- Doses must be given regularly (at least every 4 hours);

- Constipation and nausea should be treated as soon as they become apparent;

- Addiction is not a problem;

- Sedation will not normally be a problem after the first few days therapy; and

- If oral therapy is not feasible subcutaneous morphine is quite easily managed even in the home and is less traumatic to the patient than an intravenous infusion.

It is important to keep a record of the initial dose of oral morphine given and the

PAIN RELIEF

23

resulting pain and consciousness level. A pain relief chart should be used.

An initial dose for a patient who has not received opioid analgesics before and whose pain is not particularly severe, is 5–10 mg. This may be titrated upwards in 5 mg increments until the dose is sufficient to give adequate pain relief for 4–5 hours. Pain which occurs before this time is an indication of an inadequate dose. *If this occurs the dose should be increased until the pain is controlled but the interval between doses should not be reduced.* Too frequent doses accelerate the production of tolerance and disturb the patient unnecessarily. *Prn doses should never be used.*

The standard morphine mixture contains 2 mg/mL but morphine is very soluble and can be made up in much greater strengths if required. Stronger mixtures can be very bitter and may need the addition of some syrup, either added to the morphine or taken separately. Some patients tolerate the morphine better without syrup or preservative and this factor needs to be taken into account when necessary.

Once a patient has been stabilised on morphine mixture it may be more convenient to replace the mixture with long acting tablets (*MS Contin*) or long acting capsules (*Kapanol*) which only need to be taken twice a day. The dose of *MS Contin* or *Kapanol* required is determined by calculating the total dose of morphine mixture required over a 24-hour period and dividing by two.

Subcutaneous Morphine

When the oral route for pain relief becomes unsatisfactory for any reason, e.g. lack of pain control, persistent nausea and vomiting, inability to swallow or the patient is semiconscious, parenteral morphine may become necessary.

Regular 4-hourly bolus subcutaneous morphine injection is preferred to the more painful intramuscular injection or the intravenous route.

Advantages of regular subcutaneous morphine include:

- A constant level of analgesia;
- Relatively painless administration compared with the pain and tissue irritation of repeated intramuscular injections;
- Usefulness in cachetic patients with reduced muscle mass; and
- No loss of mobility, i.e. the patient is not attached to an intravenous pole.

DOSAGE

When converting from an oral dose of morphine to subcutaneous administration, one-half the oral dose is a useful place to begin.

If converting from an intravenous morphine infusion to an intermittent subcutaneous dose, the total dose of morphine delivered by the intravenous route over 4 hours is equivalent to the subcutaneous dose given 4-hourly, e.g. an intravenous dose of 20 mg/hour would be given as 80 mg every 4 hours by the subcutaneous route with the first dose given as soon as intravenous administration is ceased.

Continuous subcutaneous infusion is possible but not usually necessary. The hourly dose would be equivalent to that delivered hourly by an intravenous infusion.

Intravenous Morphine

Intravenous administration is useful for the short-term control of severe pain. Long-term use is not recommended.

A continuous infusion pump should be used. If this is not available a paediatric drip chamber must be used and a maximum of a 2-hour dose added to the chamber at any one time.

Epidural Morphine

The usual starting dose by this route is 5 mg in 10 mL normal saline, given twice daily. Elderly and debilitated patients may be adequately controlled with smaller doses. The drug can be administered either by intermittent injection or by infusion.

Note: *The aim at all times with the dosage of analgesics is to provide adequate pain control whilst maintaining patient alertness.*

DRUG DEPENDENCE

Dependence on opioids will occur to some extent after as little as one week of continuous therapy with these drugs. Dependence is pharmacologically related to tolerance. If a patient is becoming tolerant to the opioid and requiring larger doses then it is likely that dependence is also developing. However, this is not usually a problem clinically as doses can be gradually lowered as the cause of the pain is removed and if the opioid is prescribed judiciously and not for chronic conditions such as back pain, headaches, pancreatitis and chronic renal colic. Dependence is seen more as a behavioural pattern in some people where there is complete involvement with the use and procurement of the drug. See also Chapter 1 Pharmacodynamics.

TREATMENT AND WITHDRAWAL

Withdrawal of the drug may be the first step on the long road of rehabilitation to recovery. It can be extremely unpleasant and results are often disappointing in persons who are addicted as the circumstances which led to the dependency in the first place may not be changed leading to a high rate of relapse.

Withdrawal can be abrupt, provided that steps are taken to deal with the side effects of withdrawal as they occur, or slow and gradual over a period of 10 days or longer.

The initial symptoms of withdrawal from opioids are restlessness, rhinorrhoea, yawning, perspiration, gooseflesh and mydriasis. These are followed by kicking movements, adbominal and muscle cramps, nausea, vomiting and diarrhoea.

In Australia, opioid dependent persons attempting to overcome their addiction may have the opportunity to participate in the Methadone Program. In this program methadone is substituted for the heroin or opioid on which the user has become dependent, then the dose is adjusted and slowly lowered.

Methadone is the favoured substitute for withdrawal from the opioid causing the addiction because it can be given by the oral route and its long half-life allows the drug to be given once a day.

MAINTENANCE THERAPY

When it is ascertained that an addict is unable to completely withdraw from narcotics, maintenance therapy with methadone may be undertaken particularly with those addicts who otherwise lead a fairly normal life. However, the advantage of the less invasive oral route over the inherent risks of using the intravenous route is not necessarily seen by the addict who hankers for the immediate 'high' of the intravenous route. Addicts taking part in a methadone program are closely monitored and are required to give urine samples which are checked for the presence of other drugs. If treated addicts on the program are found using other drugs they lose their place on the program.

PAIN RELIEF

23

FURTHER READING

Analgesic Guidelines 2nd Ed. (Jan. 1992.) Prepared by the Analgesic Sub-Committee, Victorian Drug Usage Advisory Committee.

Presley R.W., Cousins M.J. (1992) 'Current Concepts in Chronic Pain Management' In *Current Therapeutics* June, 51–60.

Twycross, R.G. (1978) 'Relief of Pain' In *The Management of Terminal Disease*, C. Saunders (ed.) London: Edward Arnold 65–92.

TEST YOUR KNOWLEDGE

1. Define the terms analgesic and antipyretic.

2. What are the major contraindications to paracetamol?

3. List the uses of codeine.

4. What advice would you give to a patient who has been prescribed dextropropoxyphene?

5. List the naturally occurring opium derivatives commonly used and the synthetic opioids.

6. State the nursing implications of giving narcotic drugs.

7. To which class of drug does ketorolac belong? Where and how does this class of drug exert its effect?

8. State the most important principles in the use of analgesia in the patient requiring palliative care.

TABLE 23.6 Summary table — analgesics

DRUG GROUP Drug Name	Use	Action	Adverse Reactions	Nursing Implications
MILD ANALGESICS Aspirin Salicylates	Relief of minor pain, fever, inflammatory conditions; prevention of platelet aggregation	Analgesic, anti-inflammatory, antipyretic, antiplatelet	GIT bleeding, allergy especially in asthmatics, vomiting, diarrhoea, angioneurotic oedema	**Assess:** For history of previous allergy, intestinal lesions, dyspepsia, peptic ulceration, anticoagulant therapy, use of oral hypoglycaemic drugs and uricosurics, kidney or liver disease, pregnancy, lactation, coagulation disorders or bleeding tendencies. Establish and document baseline observations of location and degree of pain and fever **Administer:** As required or as ordered, preferably with food or milk to reduce risk of GIT irritation **Evaluate:** For relief of pain, reduction in pyrexia, signs of allergy, toxicity, GIT distress, bleeding tendencies with long-term use **Educate:** To self-evaluate for side effects, toxicity, potential drug interactions; to take with food or milk; not to break or dissolve enteric coated or slow release formulations; to keep out of reach of children
Paracetamol	Relief of mild to moderate pain (e.g. myalgia, toothache, headache)	Analgesic (peripheral action), antipyretic (acts on hypothalamus)	Rare: Haematological reactions, rash. In acute overdosage may cause potentially fatal liver failure (symptoms are jaundice, hypoglycaemia, metabolic acidosis) which may take 3 days to develop, treat with acetylcysteine	**Assess:** For history of analgesic nephropathy or previous hypersensitivity **Administer:** 1–2 tablets every 3–4 h; maximum, 8 tablets daily **Evaluate:** For relief of pain, reduction in pyrexia **Educate:** To keep out of reach of children; paracetamol is *not* a harmless drug in overdosage

23 PAIN RELIEF

TABLE 23.6 continued

DRUG GROUP Drug Name	Use	Action	Adverse Reactions	Nursing Implications
NSAIDs Mefenamic acid Naproxen sodium Ibuprofen	Relief of mild to moderate pain, e.g. dental pain, dysmenorrhoea, menstrual pain	NSAIDs which inhibit prostaglandin synthesis	Drowsiness, dizziness, headache, nausea, rash. Ulceration of gut, severe diarrhoea, bleeding, haematemesis	**Assess:** For history of asthma, pregnancy (effects on fetus unknown), concurrent use of oral anticoagulants (additive effect), previous diarrhoea with drug, impaired renal function, age **Administer:** With food; mefenamic acid, 500 mg 3 times a day; naproxen, 275 mg every 6–8 h; ibuprofen, 200–400 mg every 4 h; ketorolac, 10–30 mg IM every 4–6 h for acute pain **Evaluate:** For relief of pain **Educate:** To take with food
Ketorolac	Relief of moderate or severe postoperative pain; short-term relief of acute pain			
OPIOID ANALGESICS Morphine Pethidine Papaveretum Methadone Fentanyl Phenoperidine Pentazocine Dextromoramide Oxycodone Buprenorphine	Severe pain, e.g. in terminal disease, postoperative	CNS depressant	Respiratory depression, nausea, vomiting, hypotension, bradycardia, constipation, suppression of cough reflex	**Assess:** For concurrent use of alcohol and other CNS depressant drugs, history of chronic respiratory disease, liver disease, convulsive disorders, Addisons disease, myxoedema, head injury, raised intracranial pressure, severe debilitation, pregnancy, lactation; Establish base line observations of vital signs especially respiratory rate; document extent and severity of pain **Administer:** Before development of severe pain; observe legal/hospital policy requirements; IV—by slow injection or dilute infusion; IM or SC—aspirate syringe to avoid accidental IV administration **Evaluate:** For relief of pain and analgesic effect, hypersensitivity, toxicity and side effects, developing dependence; monitor vital signs especially respiratory rate; institute measures to prevent and/or treat constipation **Educate:** To ambulate with assistance; that side rails are used for safety; not to smoke while under the influence of the drug; to cough, deep breathe and change position regularly
Codeine phosphate Dextropropoxyphene Dihydrocodeine	Weaker opioids for less severe pain			

Drugs Used in Anaesthesia

ROSS D. MacPHERSON

O B J E C T I V E S

At the conclusion of this chapter the reader should be able to:

1. Name the groups of drugs commonly used by the anaesthetist;

2. Understand the reasons for their administration;

3. Describe the pharmacology of the drugs used in anaesthesia and their undesirable side effects;

4. Assist the anaesthetist with the anaesthetic and with preoperative and postoperative care; and

5. Give factual and helpful information to patients who require anaesthesia and/or pain relief.

ANAESTHESIA

General anaesthesia requires not only that the patient be unconscious, but also free of pain and usually with a degree of skeletal muscle relaxation. In earlier times, a single drug such as ether was used to produce all these effects. A variety of agents, combined in varying proportions, are now used to provide the right balance of loss of pain, loss of consciousness and muscle relaxation. This anaesthesia can be delivered by a number of routes with injection and inhalation being the most common.

OXYGEN

Oxygen is the most important agent used in anaesthesia. No procedure can be performed without it. Atmospheric air contains just over 20% oxygen which provides a partial pressure of oxygen adequate to almost fully saturate our haemoglobin and provide an oxygen content in blood of approximately 20 mL/100 mL, taking into account the small quantity dissolved in plasma. Usually concentrations of 30% or greater are used in anaesthesia with the balance being either air or nitrous oxide.

In anaesthesia oxygen is needed not only to supply normal metabolic needs but also to correct any mild hypoxia which might occur as a result of the depressant effect of anaesthetic drugs or stresses associated with prolonged surgical procedures. On the anaesthetic machine, oxygen delivery is controlled by flowmeters and a variety of visual and auditory fail-safe devices are incorporated to alert the anaesthetist to any failure of the system. In the recovery room and elsewhere oxygen can be delivered in varying concentrations using either masks or nasal prongs and adequate oxygenation monitored by measurement of either blood gasses or, more commonly, by oxygen saturation usually using pulse oximetry.

PREMEDICATION

Premedication serves a number of purposes: to allay fear and anxiety; to reduce secretions of the respiratory tract; and as an adjunct to other pharmacological agents. The most usual combination is either a narcotic, a benzodiazepine or a phenothiazine given with an anticholinergic drug, see Tables 24.1 and 24.2.

The anticholinergic drugs atropine and hyoscine are often employed as premedication for two reasons. In response to procedures such as tracheal intubation or the administration of drugs the parasympathetic nervous system is stimulated resulting in an increase in secretions and a decrease in heart rate. Both these responses are mediated by the vagus nerve. Anticholinergic agents antagonise these undesirable responses by peripheral postsynaptic blockade of muscarinic receptors. Some groups of patients, especially children and young adults, often exhibit a reflex tachycardia in response to anticholinergic drug administration as they have a relatively high degree of vagal tone.

Although anticholinergic agents employed as premedication are used because their effects are primarily peripheral, central effects are sometimes seen evidenced by either drowsiness or excitability. Cutaneous vasodilatation, leading to facial flushing is another side effect.

Most premedications are administered intramuscularly approximately 30–60 minutes prior to operation. Benzodiazepines can be given orally (with a sip of water) or intravenously, immediately prior to procedures such as endoscopy.

TABLE 24.1   Some drugs used for premedication

Drug group	Drug	Trade names	Action*
Barbiturates**	Pentobarbitone	*Nembutal*	Sedative, hypnotic
	Amylobarbitone	*Amytal*	
Benzodiazepines	Diazepam	*Valium*	
	Lorazepam	*Ativan*	
	Oxazepam	*Serepax*	
	Temazepam	*Normison, Euhypnos,*	
		Temaze	
Phenothiazines	Promethazine	*Phenergan*	Neuroleptic,
	Trimeprazine	*Vallergan*	antipsychotic,
Butyrophenones	Haloperidol	*Serenace*	antiemetic, sedative
	Droperidol	*Droleptan*	
Opioids (natural)	Papaveretum		Narcotic, analgesic
	Morphine		
	Codeine		
Opioids (synthetic)	Pethidine		
	Pentazocine	*Fortral*	
Anticholinergics	Atropine	*Scopolamine*	Prevent bradycardia,
	Hyoscine		antisialogogue,
			antiemetic

*See Chapter 23 Pain Relief and Chapter 26 Psychiatric Disorders.
**Barbiturates are not as popular since the introduction of benzodiazepines

TABLE 24.2   Dosages of some drugs used for premedication

Drug	Average healthy adult		Small or sick adult		Child	
	Dose (mg)	Route	Dose (mg)	Route	Dose (mg/kg body weight)	Route
Pentobarbitone	200	Oral	100	Oral	3	Oral
Diazepam	15	Oral	7	Oral	0.2	Oral
Promethazine	50	IM	25	IM	1	Oral
Papaveretum	20	IM	10	IM	0.1	IM
Morphine	15	IM	7.5	IM	0.2	IM
Pethidine	100	IM	50	IM	1.4	IM
Atropine	0.5	IM	0.3	IM	0.01	IM
Papaveretum	20	IM	10	IM	–	–
+ hyoscine*	+ 0.4		+ 0.2			

*Papaveretum and hyoscine are available in the one ampoule.
Note: Dosage of premedication drugs varies with the age, weight and health of the patient.

DRUGS USED IN ANAESTHESIA

24

Benzodiazepines especially are well known for their amnesic effects. Patients may have impaired memory of events following drug administration (antegrade amnesia) and of events or instructions preceeding the injections (retrograde amnesia). This often has medicolegal implications and instructions to patients, e.g. those returning home following day surgery, should be in writing.

In general, the use of premedication as routine procedure has declined in recent years and its use often depends on the personal preference of the anaesthetist. Its use tends to be avoided especially in day surgery where the object is to minimise drug usage and to have the patient awake and alert as soon after the procedure as possible.

Patients are generally fasted for six hours prior to surgery, however, patients taking regular oral medication, e.g. antihypertensive agents, can still take their medication with a sip of water during this period.

GENERAL ANAESTHESIA

The conduct of general anaesthesia is divided into three phases. The first phase is induction, when the patient is taken from a state of wakefulness or semiwakefulness to unconsciousness; the second phase is maintenance during which the surgical procedure is performed; and the third phase is recovery when the anaesthetic is ceased or reversed and the patient allowed to regain consciousness.

During induction the aim is to render the patient unconscious as rapidly as possible as, initially, there is some degree of physical excitation, manifest by skeletal muscle activity (trismus, stridor and limb rigidity) and autonomic nervous system stimulation (sweating, salivation). To induce anaesthesia quickly drugs are administered intravenously and reach high concentrations in the brain within a few seconds following injection. General anaesthesia is usually maintained with inhalational agents which are mixed with oxygen prior to delivery to the patient. The fact that the patient has lost consciousness does not mean that they are free of pain and anaesthesia may need to be supplemented by narcotic analgesics. Skeletal muscle relaxants may also be required to provide loss of muscle tone.

At the conclusion of the procedure the anaesthetic gases are stopped and, if needed, the effects of muscle relaxants are reversed (see below). The patient slowly regains consciousness and is transferred to the recovery room for a period of close observation.

THEORIES OF GENERAL ANAESTHESIA

General anaesthesia is not mediated by drugs interacting at specific receptor sites within the central nervous system. Examination of the molecular structures of anaesthetic agents shows them to be a structurally diverse group, including substances such as carbon tetrafluoride, ethylene and inert gases such as xenon. It is likely that their effects are mediated by a non-specific physicochemical interaction with neurones of the central nervous system.

The most satisfactory explanation to date is that the anaesthetic molecules, by virtue of their high lipid solubility, cross the blood brain barrier relatively easily and become incorporated in the neuronal membrane. Once in place they prevent or reduce transmission of impulses entering the brain from peripheral and central sources along the neurone by disrupting eit er the passage of ions aross the membrane or the internal environment of the nerve. Without input of neuronal traffic to centres in the brainstem, consciousness is lost.

The ideal intravenous anaesthetic should be water soluble and stable in solution, non-irritant to tissues and not painful on injection, have no adverse psychological or muscular effects, act predictably and be rapidly metabolised and excreted as inactive products. It should also have a low incidence of allergic reactions, nausea and vomiting.

The attributes of the ideal inhalational agent are quite different. Such a drug should be non-flammable and chemically stable, pleasant and non-irritant to inhale, effective at low concentrations, have low toxicity and a low incidence of nausea and vomiting, act rapidly and have minimal effects on cardiovascular and respiratory status.

INTRAVENOUS ANAESTHETIC AGENTS

Barbiturates: Thiopentone, Methohexitone

The barbiturates were once widely prescribed for use as sedatives, hypnotics and antiepileptic agents. Apart from their use in some forms of epilepsy they are now most commonly used as agents for the induction and maintenace of anaesthesia, the two most popular agents being sodium thiopentone and methohexitone.

Thiopentone

Thiopentone sodium remains the most widely used agent in the world for the induction of anaesthesia.

TRADE NAMES

Thiopentone sodium (thiopental): *Pentothal*.

MECHANISM OF ACTION

Thiopentone produces loss of consciousness by inhibiting the release of central nervous system neurotransmitters, depressing the transmission of impulses along neurones and reducing the movement of both sodium and potassium ions across the nerve membrane.

PHARMACOKINETICS

Thiopentone is a very lipid soluble molecule which is non-ionised at physiological pH and so crosses the blood brain barrier easily. Following intravenous injection thiopentone reaches the brain and causes unconsciousness within seconds. It can also be administered rectally (this route is usually reserved for children), in which case it acts within 20 minutes. Due to its high lipid solubility it is rapidly redistributed to other tissues, especially fat and muscle. Therefore, after a single bolus its duration of action is relatively brief (usually less than 5 minutes) and, if anaesthesia is to be maintained using this drug alone, repeated injections are necessary. Thiopentone is metabolised relatively slowly in the liver and excreted via renal mechanisms.

USES

Thiopentone is used for induction of anaesthesia. A 2.5% or 5% solution is generally used and the dose for induction of anaesthesia is calculated on the basis of approximately 5 mg/kg.

ADVERSE DRUG REACTIONS

The solution is highly alkaline with a pH of around 10.6 and extravasation of the injection must be avoided as damage to tissues will result. Inadvertent intra-arterial injection may result in removal of endothelial cells lining the artery and an intense arteritis, sometimes causing ischaemia and gangrene of the limb which may need to be amputated.

PRECAUTIONS AND CONTRAINDICATIONS

Thiopentone depresses both the respiratory centre, which can result in apnoea, and cardiovascular function resulting in a decrease in both cardiac output and blood pressure. For these reasons it is only administered under conditions where both personnel and equipment are available to deal with these potential problems.

DRUGS USED IN ANAESTHESIA

24

Methohexitone

Methohexitone is another barbiturate used for the induction of anaesthesia.

TRADE NAMES

Methohexitone: *Brietal Sodium.*

MECHANISM OF ACTION

As for thiopentone.

PHARMACOKINETICS

Methohexitone passes rapidly across the blood brain barrier after intravenous administration and, if the drug is used alone, the patient will reawaken in 3–4 minutes due to redistribution of the drug into muscle-fat storage sites. Methohexitone is extensively metabolised with less than 1% of the drug being excreted unchanged in the urine.

USES

For induction methohexitone can be given intravenously and rectally, it can also be administered by the intramuscular route.

ADVERSE DRUG REACTIONS

One important difference between thiopentone and methohexitone is that methohexitone administration can cause epileptic seizures in susceptible patients, especially children. It can also cause excitement during administration. There is a greater incidence of pain on injection with methohexitone than with thiopentone.

Methohexitone is now infrequently used. Its duration of action after a single dose is much shorter than that of thiopentone and its main use was for very brief procedures such as anaesthesia for electroconvulsive therapy.

PRECAUTIONS AND CONTRAINDICATIONS

As for thiopentone.

Propofol

Propofol is a relatively recent anaesthetic agent. It is chemically unrelated to any other group and has gained popularity for both induction and maintenance of anaesthesia.

TRADE NAMES

Propofol: *Diprivan.*

MECHANISM OF ACTION

The mechanism by which propofol causes unconsciousness is unclear but it most likely impairs ionic movements across the nerve membrane.

PHARMACOKINETICS

Propofol causes loss of consciousness within 30 seconds following intravenous administration. It is not given by any other route. It is extensively protein bound, metabolised in the liver by conjugation and excreted. As with other highly lipid soluble drugs it is rapidly redistributed to other tissues following administration.

USES

Propofol is used for induction and maintenance of anaesthesia. Because of its low aqueous solubility it is supplied dissolved in a soya bean/water emulsion. For induction it is administered intravenously at a dose of 2 mg/kg and for maintenance at a slightly higher rate per hour. It is supplied in 20 mL ampoules and 50 mL and 100 mL vials for maintenance infusion. The vials are not for multi-use as they contain no preservative.

ADVERSE DRUG REACTIONS

There are reports of considerable pain on injection especially when injected into small veins and some anaesthetists add a small amount of lignocaine 1% to the injection to reduce this pain. Propofol also causes significantly more hypotension than other induction agents, primarily by peripheral dilatation resulting in a reduction in peripheral resistance and attenuation of the myogenic response of vascular smooth muscle. Bronchospasm may also occur in susceptible patients, e.g. asthmatics.

PRECAUTIONS AND CONTRAINDICATIONS

Propofol is physically incompatible with the neuromuscular blocking drug atracurium.

Benzodiazepines: Diazepam, Midazolam

MECHANISM OF ACTION

The benzodiazepines, diazepam and midazolam, are known to act at specific receptor sites in the central nervous system. As a result of benzodiazepines interacting at these receptors there is a conformational change in another set of receptors, those normally stimulated by the endogenous inhibitory neurotransmittor γ aminobutyric acid (GABA). This change results in an increased sensitivity to GABA which, by promoting the influx of chloride ions into the cell, make the receptors more negative (hyperpolarised) and more difficult to activate. Therefore neurones become more inhibited.

Diazepam

TRADE NAMES

Diazepam: *Valium*; *Diazemuls*.

PHARMACOKINETICS

Diazepam is best administered parenterally by the intravenous route as absorption from the intramuscular route is very variable and can result in local abscess formation. The metabolism of diazepam is of great importance. It is metabolised into at least three active metabolites, the most important being *N*-desmethyldiazepam (or nordiazepam). Almost all the diazepam metabolites have pharmacological activity and long half-lives (the half-life of *N*-desmethyldiazepam can be greater that 100 hours). When given orally absorption is excellent with bioavailability approaching 90%.

USES

Diazepam is rarely used as a sole induction agent for general anaesthesia but is often employed to provide hypnosis and amnesia prior to endoscopic procedures. It is often given orally as a premedication. The intravenous dose is usually between 10 mg and 20 mg, but higher doses are sometimes necessary. However, with higher doses respiratory depression and, occasionally, brief periods of apnoea may occur.

ADVERSE DRUG REACTIONS

The intravenous injection is often painful, although this is less of a problem with the emulsion formulation. Prolonged sedation, which may be still evident 24 hours after the injection, is primarily due to the presence of the active metabolites. When the drug is used for day surgery cases, patients should be specifically cautioned to avoid driving or operating machinery following the procedure and that they may still be impaired for up to 48 hours following injection.

DRUG INTERACTIONS

The excretion of benzodiazepines has been reportedly slowed in patients taking either cimetidine or oral contraceptives.

PRECAUTIONS AND CONTRAINDICATIONS

Diazepam has low water solubility and for parenteral use is formulated as a solution in propylene glycol and an oil in water emulsion. Care must be used when diluting the drug to prevent its precipitation. Dilution of diazepam (*Valium*) injection is *not recommended*. If dilution of diazepam emulsion injection (*Diazemuls*) is undertaken the diluent used should be either *Intralipid* or 5% dextrose. It can be injected directly into intravenous lines of normal saline. The rate of injection should not exceed 5 mg/minute to avoid apnoea.

Midazolam

TRADE NAMES

Midazolam: *Hypnovel*.

PHARMACOKINETICS

Midazolam is a short acting benzodiazepine. In contrast to diazepam, it has a

DRUGS USED IN ANAESTHESIA

24

very short half-life (approximately 2 hours) because of its rapid metabolism to only one active metabolite which is conjugated and excreted renally. It can be given intramuscularly when used as premedication.

USES

Because of its short duration of action midazolam is particularly useful as the sole agent for endoscopy and other brief procedures. It is much more effective when given in combination with a narcotic such as morphine or fentanyl. In the intensive care setting it is often given by continuous intravenous infusion at a rate of 1–8 mg per hour and the patient's level of consciousness can be rapidly altered. The time taken for drowsiness to occur is longer than with barbiturate agents, up to 3–5 minutes following intravenous injection.

Hypnovel injection is a solution of midazolam in water for injections, buffered to an acidic pH of 3.3 at which the drug is water soluble. At physiological pH (7.4) the molecule becomes lipid soluble instead of water soluble. Hence, after injection the drug gains rapid access to the central nervous system.

ADVERSE DRUG REACTIONS

Pain on injection is the most commonly reported adverse reaction and occurs following both intravenous and intramuscular administration. Common adverse effects reported subsequent to injection are headache, nausea and vomiting, coughing and prolonged drowsiness. Generally the cardiovascular system is minimally affected by benzodiazepines, with systolic and diastolic pressures falling by between 5% and 10% as a result of peripheral vasodilatation.

DRUG INTERACTIONS

The activity of most sedative drugs, including the benzodiazepines, is accentuated by co-administration of other central nervous system depressant drugs. Consumption of ethanol preceeding midazolam can also prolong and intensify the response.

PRECAUTIONS AND CONTRAINDICATIONS

There is a high incidence of respiratory depression and apnoea following midazolam administration, especially in the elderly and in those with significant pre-existing disease states. In these patients the usual dosage for induction, 10–15 mg by slow intravenous injection, may need to be reduced by up to 25%. To produce conscious sedation for endoscopy the dose is considerably less, usually in the range 2.5 mg to 5 mg (total).

The product information for midazolam has recently been revised, stressing the dangers of respiratory depression, apnoea and respiratory arrest which could be unnoticed by staff and result in hypoxia and perhaps death. After high doses it can take several hours for the drug to be eliminated and vigilance is essential following its administration. The benzodiazepine antagonist flumazenil (*Anexate*) has been used to reverse benzodiazepine induced sedation.

Midazolam administration usually results in significant anterograde amnesia, again an important consideration in day surgery or short stay cases. The patient may be having a perfectly lucid conversation with you, perhaps two hours after the procedure, but the next day has no recollection at all of the conversation ever taking place.

INHALATIONAL ANAESTHETIC AGENTS

In 1846 the American dentist William Morton first successfully demonstrated ether anaesthesia. The following year, chloroform, which had been synthesised over a decade earlier was also shown to have anaesthetic properties by Doctors David Waldie and James Young Simpson. Ether and chloroform were introduced to Australia within 12 months of their initial discovery. One of our early surgeons, Mr Charles Nathan, along with dentist John Belisario share the honour of introducing ether anaesthesia to NSW, while at the same time William Pugh, surgeon to St John's Hospital in Launceston, Van Diemen's Land, first used ether in

Tasmania. Since then a number of inhalational agents have come and gone. Chloroform is no longer used owing to a high incidence of liver dysfunction, while ether, still used in some countries, is highly inflammable and considered too dangerous.

Inhalational anaesthetic agents are traditionally divided into gases and volatile agents. The word volatile actually means 'changeable' as these agents are liquids under standard conditions but are delivered to the patient in the gaseous state by means of special vapourisers mounted on the anaesthetic machine. Halothane, isoflurane, enflurane and methoxyflurane are examples of volatile anaesthetic agents. Of the gaseous agents only nitrous oxide is in current use.

Enflurane, Halothane, Isoflurane, Methoxyflurane

TRADE NAMES

Enflurane: *Ethrane.*
Halothane: *Fluothane.*
Isoflurane: *Forthane.*
Methoxyflurane: *Penthrane.*

PHARMACOKINETICS

The inhaled agent must move through a number of phases before reaching its site of action, the brain. Initially it must move from the anaesthetic machine into the patient's lungs and from there equilibrate with plasma. The rate at which this equilibration occurs is determined by the solubility of the gas in plasma, and the lower the solubility of the gas (the blood/gas partition coefficient) the more rapidly will this equilibration occur. Conversely, the more soluble the agent, the longer the time needed for the equilibration process. The onset of anaesthesia is directly related to the solubility, or blood/gas partition coefficient. Poorly soluble agents, such as nitrous oxide, equilibrate rapidly with plasma and therefore have a rapid onset of anaesthetic action (induction). Such agents also leave the plasma

rapidly once the gas supply is stopped so recovery is also rapid.

The potency of inhaled anaesthetic agents is described using another convention. Since these agents are gases they cannot be compared on a weight basis in the same way we can compare, for example, morphine and pethidine. The potency of an inhaled agent is expressed in terms of its minimum alveolar concentration (MAC). The MAC is generally defined as the minimum amount of gas in volume/% required to be administered to a patient such that there is no reflex response to a skin incision in 50% of subjects. Thus, very potent anaesthetic agents such as halothane have low MACs, in this case 0.76 which means that, at equilibrium, if alveolar air contains only 0.76% halothane, that will be sufficient to cause anaesthesia in 50% of patients. As the potency of anaesthetic agents decreases so the MAC becomes larger.

In summary, the blood/gas coefficient of a gas, reflected in its solubility, determines the speed of induction and recovery, while the MAC is a measure of the relative potency of gases and is mainly determined by their lipid solubility or oil/gas partition coefficient, see Table 24.3.

The main features of commonly used volatile anaesthetic agents are listed in Table 24.4 as well as some details of obsolete agents provided for comparison. One point that should be noted is that, although they have potent anaesthetic qualities, some of these agents are only minimally analgesic and supplementation with either narcotic analgesics or nitrous oxide is required.

Sevoflurane and desflurane are two new volatile anaesthetics not yet available in Australia. However, when they do become available they should prove popular as they have very low blood/gas solubilities and are taken up and eliminated quickly.

An unusual feature of most inhalational anaesthetic drugs is their relative inertness. That is to say that they undergo minimal metabolism in the body and, with one exception — methoxyflurane, are excreted essentially unchanged.

DRUGS USED IN ANAESTHESIA

24

TABLE 24.3 Partition coefficients and MACs of some inhalational anaesthetic agents

Agent	Type	Year introduced	Partition coefficients		MAC	Rate of induction
			Blood:gas	Oil:gas		
Diethyl ether*	Volatile	1842	12	65	1.9	Slow
Chloroform*	Volatile	1847	8.4	400	0.5	Slow
Methoxyflurane	Volatile	1960	13	950	0.16	Slow
Halothane	Volatile	1956	2.4	220	0.8	Medium
Enflurane	Volatile	1968	1.9	98	1.8	Medium
Isoflurane	Volatile	1980	1.4	0.6	1.15	Medium
Nitrous oxide	Gas	1844	0.47	1.4	>100	Rapid
Cyclopropane*	Gas	1933	0.55	11.5	9.6	Rapid

*Not currently used in Australia.

ADVERSE DRUG REACTIONS

One continuing problem with the chloroform-like drugs (the halogenated hydrocarbons) is their propensity to cause hepatic dysfunction. Halothane also has a propensity to cause an allergic hepatitis and, although it has been the most popular volatile anaesthetic agent for many years, its use is now declining, being replaced by agents with less potential for hepatic adverse reactions.

Nitrous Oxide

USES

This agent is commonly used not only in anaesthetic practice but also in emergency medicine and obstetrics.

Nitrous oxide is an odourless non-flammable gas, supplied in cylinders painted a distinctive blue. From a pharmacological perspective, this gas has some unique properties. It has excellent analgesic properties with a 25% concentration comparable with morphine for postoperative analgesia. The concentration of nitrous oxide delivered to the patient is controlled by the anaesthetist by mixing pure nitrous oxide with oxygen. Under these circumstances concentrations of 60%–70% can be used in combination with 30%–40% oxygen. The MAC for nitrous oxide is greater than 100, which means that even if pure nitrous oxide were deliverd to a patient anaesthesia could not be assured. Therefore, nitrous oxide is often referred to as an excellent analgesic but a poor anaesthetic. In routine anaesthetic practice nitrous oxide–oxygen mixture is used to provide analgesia and is combined with one of the volatile agents to achieve loss of consciousness. When nitrous oxide is used as part of the anaesthetic procedure the MACs of most volatile agents are significantly reduced.

For dental, obstetric and emergency procedures nitrous oxide is supplied pre-mixed with oxygen in equal concentrations as *Entonox* (the cylinders are blue with a white top). This 50:50 mixture combines sufficient oxygen to prevent hypoxia with a nitrous oxide concentration sufficient to provide reliable analgesia. Because of its low solubility (evidenced by a blood/gas partition co-efficient of 0.47) the onset of response to, and recovery from, the effects of nitrous oxide are quite rapid.

TABLE 24.4 Pharmacological profiles of some inhaled anaesthetic agents

Agent	Advantages	Disadvantages
Diethyl ether	Potent volatile anaesthetic which provides some analgesia; full surgical anaesthesia and muscle relaxation possible; circulation and respiration adequately maintained; relatively easy to administer and still used in developing countries; cheap.	Forms explosive mixture with air and oxygen making it too dangerous to use in modern operating theatres; irritant to respiratory tract which can cause problems during induction phase; stimulates bronchial secretions; vomiting during procedure and after recovery is a hazard.
Chloroform	Potent volatile agent which provides anaesthesia and analgesia; non-explosive.	Now obsolete because of unacceptably high incidence of hepatic dysfunction; very low safety margin; has caused cardiac arrest.
Halothane	Potent volatile anaesthetic, rapid induction, some muscle relaxation; has suppressant effect on bronchial secretions; relatively cheap; non-explosive. Least irritating to the airways and can be used to induce anaesthesia in children.	Sensitises myocardium to circulating catecholamines (may lead to arrhythmias); hepatic complications (may be irreversible) are a problem and have resulted in decreased use; weak analgesic properties.
Enflurane	Volatile anaesthetic with some stimulant activity; causes less myocardial sensitisation to catecholamines than halothane; not associated with hepatic damage; non-flammable.	Epileptic seizures in some patients during induction and recovery phases; metabolised to a small degree (~5%) to flouride which can cause renal damage.
Isoflurane	Volatile anaesthetic similar to enflurane; does not sensitise myocardium to catecholamines; non-flammable, non-explosive. Probably the most commonly used inhalational agent.	Convulsive episodes have occurred; some respiratory tract irritation.
Methoxyflurane	Exceptionally potent volatile anaesthetic (MAC 0.16%) with significant analgesic properties; less uterine relaxation; does not sensitise myocardium to catecholamines.	Undergoes extensive metabolism to fluoride which can reach potentially toxic concentrations in plasma after 1–2 hours of use resulting in renal failure; induction and recovery are slow.
Nitrous oxide	Gaseous anaesthetic with excellent analgesic properties and rapid onset of action; wide margin of safety; does not cause significant depression of respiratory or cardiovascular function provided it is mixed with adequate oxygen; non-explosive and relatively safe to use.	Not potent enough to be used as sole agent; prolonged administration can result in bone marrow depression and interference with folate metabolism; increased incidence of nausea and vomiting.

DRUGS USED IN ANAESTHESIA

24

ADVERSE DRUG REACTIONS

Nitrous oxide–oxygen mixtures are relatively safe and the drug has minimal effects on respiratory and cardiovascular function (unlike the potent volatile agents) although in 10%–15% of patients nausea and vomiting have been reported. However, adverse effects including inactivation of vitamin B_{12}, bone marrow depression and megaloblastic anaemia, have been reported, especially after prolonged exposure.

It is of paramount importance that adequate oxygen is always supplied when using nitrous oxide.

MUSCLE RELAXANTS

The introduction of drugs capable of producing relaxation of skeletal muscle has contributed to reducing the risk associated with early general anaesthesia. For many operations, especially those on the thorax and abdomen, skeletal muscles must be adequately relaxed. To achieve this using anaesthetic drugs alone an almost toxic dose would be needed. When muscle relaxation is required it is now achieved by the use of muscle relaxants combined with sufficient intravenous or inhalational agents to provide loss of pain and loss of consciousness.

There are three types of muscle in the body, smooth, cardiac and skeletal, and the mechanism of stimulation of each type is quite different. In skeletal muscle, contraction is produced by the release of the neurotransmitter acetylcholine from presynaptic vesicles, which pass across the synaptic cleft and stimulate nicotinic receptors on the muscle membrane. As a result of this interaction depolarisation occurs and calcium is released. The calcium combines with troponin on the actin filament and initiates a muscle contraction. The acetylcholine molecules are rapidly broken down by enzymes such as acetylcholine esterase.

The administration of neuromuscular blocking drugs results in a paralysis of skeletal muscles, including the diaphragm and the muscles of respiration. Smooth muscle, under the control of the autonomic nervous system, and cardiac muscle are unaffected. It is usual to consider these drugs in two groups: depolarising agents; and non-depolarising agents. Details of the neuromuscular blocking drugs are summarised in Table 24.5.

DEPOLARISING MUSCLE RELAXANTS

Suxamethonium

TRADE NAMES

Suxamethonium (succinylcholine): *Scoline*; *Anectine*.

MECHANISM OF ACTION

Suxamethonium is the only depolarising neuromuscular blocking drug in current use. Suxamethonium initially depolarises the membrane resulting in a brief period of muscle contraction, evidenced by transient muscle fasciculations, and followed by blockade and paralysis. The depolarisation occurs because the shape of the molecule resembles acetylcholine so closely that it initially stimulates the receptor site in the same manner. However, following this phase the suxamethonium molecule remains at the receptor site but does not cause further stimulation.

PHARMACOKINETICS

Suxamethonium is broken down rapidly in the peripheral circulation by a group of enzymes called pseudocholinesterases which rapidly deactivate much of the drug before it even reaches the neuromuscular junction. It has been estimated that only 20%–30% of an intravenously administered dose actually

TABLE 24.5   Muscle relaxants

Group	Drug	Year introduced	Approximate duration (minutes)	Presentation (storage*)	Occasional side effects
Depolarising agents (No antidote)	Suxamethonium	1951	5	2 mL, 50 mg/mL (2–8°C)	Bradycardia, afterpains, prolonged block
Non-depolarising agents (competitive blockers) (Antidote: neostigmine)	Tubocurarine	1945	20–30	2 mL, 10 mg/mL (20°C)	Histamine release, hypotension, allergy
	Alcuronium	1961	20–30	2 mL, 5 mg/mL (20°C)	Allergy
	Pancuronium	1967	30	2 mL, 2 mg/mL (2–8°C)	Tachycardia
	Vecuronium	1980	15	4 mg powder, 1 mL diluent; 10 mg powder (unstable after reconstitution)	
	Atracurium	1980	20	2.5 mL, 5 mL, 10 mg/mL (2–8°C)	Histamine release, allergy

*20°C—room temperature; 2–8°C—refrigerator

reaches the target tissue. The onset of muscle relaxation following suxamethonium administration is fast, usually within 30 seconds, and its duration of action short, approximately five minutes.

USES

Because of its pharmacokinetic characteristics, suxamethonium is of no use for procedures requiring prolonged muscle relaxation but is particularly useful for very short procedures (e.g. electroconvulsive therapy) or to produce muscle relaxation to facilitate endotracheal intubation.

ADVERSE DRUG REACTIONS

Use of suxamethonium can result in a rise in serum potassium levels which may cause problems in patients with renal failure or burns.

Muscle pains are common following suxamethonium administration and this reaction can be delayed until the third or fourth postoperative day. The mechanism is not known but it is not thought to be due to the initial muscle fasciculations. In some groups of patients — females, the unfit and middle aged — this reaction occurs with greater frequency.

DRUGS USED IN ANAESTHESIA

24

DRUG INTERACTIONS

Suxamethonium is physically incompatible with thiopentone.

PRECAUTIONS AND CONTRAINDICATIONS

The main problem faced with use of sux-amethonium lies in its metabolism. In some patients the pseudocholinesterases respon-sible for the removal of the drug may be reduced. Some people have a genetically determined reduction in cholinesterase con-centration. In others the concentration is lowered because of pre-existing diease states, e.g. liver or renal disease and thyro-toxic conditions, or by concomitant drug treatment with lithium salts, ketamine, or cytotoxic agents. When suxamethonium is administered to these patients apnoea may persist for hours. The effects of sux-amethonium cannot be pharmacologically reversed and for this reason it is sometimes referred to as a 'non-competitive' neuromus-cular blocking drug, as it does not actually compete with acetylcholine for the receptor site. If the activity of suxamethonium is pro-longed for any reason the only realistic treatment is that the patient be maintained on assisted ventilation until the drug is eventually excreted.

NON-DEPOLARISING MUSCLE RELAXANTS

Alcuronium, Atracurium, Pancuronium, Tubocucarine, Vecuronium

TRADE NAMES

Alcuronium: *Alloferin.*
Atracurium: *Tracrium.*
Pancuronium: *Pavulon.*
Tubocucarine: *Tubarine.*
Vecuronium: *Norcuron.*

MECHANISM OF ACTION

Non-depolarising muscle relaxants are chemically and pharmacologically different from the depolarising group and are re-ferred to as competitive neuromuscular blockers. They are large molecules, too large to actually occupy the acetylcholine binding site on the skeletal muscle end-plate. Rather, they compete directly with the released acetylcholine and prevent its at-tachment to the nicotinic binding site. The activity of the non-depolarising neuromuscu-lar blocking drugs can be antagonised by in-creasing the concentration of the molecule with which they are competing (i.e. acetyl-choline) at the neuromuscular junction.

The enzyme responsible for the degrada-tion of acetylcholine is cholinesterase and the activity of this enzyme can be reduced substantially by anticholinesterase drugs, such as neostigmine. Therefore, near the end of a procedure during which non-depo-larising agents have been used to provide muscle relaxation it is usual to 'reverse' the blockade by injection of neostigmine. The result is a dramatic increase in acetylcholine concentration and the neuromuscular block-ade is overcome. The administration of neo-stigmine alone, however, results in the accumulation of a large amount of acetyl-choline at muscarinic receptor sites which would cause undesirable effects such as an increase in secretions and bradycardia. To circumvent this the antimuscarinic agent atropine is routinely co-administered.

PHARMACOKINETICS

Following administration the onset of neuromuscular paralysis is relatively slow (within 1–5 minutes) and the duration of paralysis is dependent on the individual agent. Likewise, the metabolism and excre-tion of these agents show great individual variation but, importantly, they utilise hepatic and renal means and their removal is not dependent on pseudocholinesterase.

USES

These drugs have relatively long durations of action, and are used to provide muscle paralysis during surgical procedures. Of the agents listed in Table 24.5, atracurium and vecuronium have been released relatively recently and are probably the most popular agents at present. Their duration of action is somewhat shorter than earlier agents, their reversal with anticholinesterase agents is more reliable, they are less dependent on renal mechanisms for their excretion and generally have a better adverse effect profile, causing less cardiovascular side effects.

NEW MUSCLE RELAXANTS

A number of new muscle relaxants will shortly become available. Pipecuronium is an agent similar to pancuronium, possessing a long duration of action but without the cardiovascular effects, e.g. tachycardia.

Rocuronium and mivacurium are both short acting agents. The latter is used as a continuous infusion, a change from the usual mode of repeated intravenous injections. Like suxamethonium both agents have a rapid onset of action but do not have the annoying side effects so often seen with this agent.

NARCOTIC ANALGESICS IN ANAESTHESIA ▐███████████

Phenoperidine (*Operidine*), fentanyl (*Sublimaze*), alfentanil, carfentanyl and sufentanil are strong narcotic analgesic drugs modelled on the pethidine molecule. In terms of relative potency they are considerably more potent than morphine. Their use, however, is limited because of their very short half-lives and the fact that they all produce intense respiratory depression and apnoea and therefore cannot be employed unless assisted ventilation is available.

Fentanyl and phenoperidine are currently the only agents available. They are used in combination with intravenous or inhalational agents in general anaesthesia to produce apnoea and analgesia. Potent analgesics such as fentanyl can also be administered by the epidural route to provide postoperative analgesia.

NEUROLEPTANALGESIA

The other main application of potent narcotic analgesics is the production of neuroleptanalgesia (also referred to as neuroleptanaesthesia). The term, first used in 1959, describes the state of patients following injection of one of the potent analgesics mentioned above concomitantly with a sedative drug of the butyrophenone category such as droperidol (*Droleptan*) or haloperidol (*Serenace*). The state of neurolepsis has been variously described as being a state of artificial hiberna-tion, an indifference to surroundings or a condition of profoundly reduced anxiety. The patient, who is insensitive to pain, is not necessarily 'asleep' and can respond to commands. The process is not as popular nowadays, principally because of medico-legal difficulties. Patients have reported awareness during the procedure, which is both disturbing at the time and after discharge from hospital.

DRUGS USED IN ANAESTHESIA

24

KETAMINE AND DISSOCIATIVE ANAESTHESIA ▰

In the 1960s a substance called phencyclidine (PCP) was synthesised and investigated as an anaesthetic agent. While it proved very effective as an intravenous anaesthetic it was soon withdrawn because of a high incidence of hallucinations associated with its use. It is still used overseas in veterinary medicine and is popular as a drug of abuse, known to users as 'angel dust'. Manipulation of the molecule eventually resulted in the synthesis of an analogue, ketamine.

Ketamine is used to produce a state known as dissociative anaesthesia. The term 'dissociative anaesthesia' was coined to describe the nature of ketamine induced anaesthesia which was as if two areas of the brain (the limbic and neocortical systems) had been dissociated from one another. Others have taken the definition to mean that the patient is dissociated from their surroundings, which is a good description of the response to the drug. Patients are able to maintain respiration, the eyes are often open, yet they are unaware of their surroundings.

KETAMINE

TRADE NAMES
Ketamine: *Ketalar*.

MECHANISM OF ACTION

Ketamine has specific effects on particular regions of the brain and prevents the transmission of afferent signals, especially from pain pathways.

PHARMACOKINETICS

Ketamine can be administered intravenously or intramuscularly. It is extensively metabolised in the liver to an active metabolite. Some induction of hepatic microsomes occurs after repeated administration, which might explain the tolerance associated with continued use.

USES

Ketamine has excellent analgesic properties and is particularly useful as an anaesthetic/analgesic for procedures such as burns dressings and orthopaedic manipulations. It is particularly useful in children who respond well to the drug and are less likely to suffer from hallucinogenic and emergence phenonoma. It is occasionally used as the sole agent for minor operations.

An important feature of ketamine is that it has a stimulant rather than a depressant action on the cardiovascular system, making it particularly useful for patients in whom hypotension must be avoided. The mechanism of this response is unclear but is almost certainly due to central nervous system stimulation rather than any direct end organ action.

ADVERSE DRUG REACTIONS

The main limitation to the use of ketamine is the problem of unpleasant dreams and occasionally true hallucinations. A number of strategies have been suggested to reduce the incidence of these adverse reactions. These include allowing the patient to awaken from the anaesthetic without excessive stimulation, using small amounts of benzodiazepines in combination with the drug and even psychotherapy prior to the operation.

LOCAL ANAESTHESIA ▮▮▮▮▮▮

LOCAL ANAESTHETIC AGENTS

Amethocaine, Bupivacaine, Cinchocaine, Cocaine, Lignocaine, Mepivacaine, Prilocaine, Procaine

TRADE NAMES

Bupivacaine: *Marcain.*
Cinchocaine: *Nupercaine.*
Lignocaine: *Xylocaine.*
Mepivacaine: *Carbocaine.*
Prilocaine: *Citanest.*

MECHANISM OF ACTION

Information about pain, pressure and temperature is transmitted from peripheral receptors via nerves to the spinal cord where the information is processed and relayed to higher centres in the brain. The transmission of this information is by action potentials which themselves depend on the movement of ions across nerve membranes.

Inside the nerve fibres the cation potassium is present in high concentrations (approximately 112 mmol/L), while outside sodium is the predominant cation (135 mmol/L). As an electrical impulse passes along a neurone its propagation is maintained by the passage of sodium ions from the outside of the neurone to the inside, down a concentration gradient. This movement of sodium occurs through specialised sodium channels, specifically designed to facilitate the process. Local anaesthetics act in two ways. They suppress the general activity of the nerve fibre in a non-specific manner similar to general anaesthetic agents, making it less likely to respond to an impulse. More importantly, they exert a specific effect on the sodium channels specifically blocking the rate and degree of opening of sodium channels, thus reducing the capacity of nerves to transmit afferent signals.

Details of local anaesthetic agents are given in Table 24.6. The agents can be divided into two categories based on their chemical structure, whether they possess an amide (e.g. lignocaine) or ester structure (e.g. procaine). There is no difference in the mechanism of action of either group, but the distinction is useful in patients who demonstrate an allergic reaction to a local anaesthetic, a member of the other group can be chosen for future use.

PHARMACOKINETICS

When local anaesthetics are used to provide topical, infiltration or regional anaesthesia their effects are terminated by diffusion away from the site by capillary vessels, an event which can be reduced by the judicious use of vasoconstrictor agents. Their eventual removal from the body is dependent on their chemical structure. Members of the amide group are mainly metabolised in the liver, often to active metabolites, while members of the ester group are hydrolysed relatively rapidly in the plasma by cholinesterase enzymes.

USES

Local anaesthetic agents can be injected at a number of sites so that efferent, and in some cases afferent, signals to and from the spinal cord can be interrupted.

It is possible to anaesthetise surfaces by the direct application of anaesthetic drugs, i.e. topical anaesthesia. *EMLA Cream* (a preparation containing prilocaine and lignocaine) if applied in sufficient quantity under an occlusive dressing for a long enough period will produce topical anaesthesia of skin surfaces. This method is used particularly in children prior to venepuncture. Mucous membranes, such as those lining the mouth, nasal passages and the ocular conjunctivae, are quite sensitive to local anaesthetic agents which can be applied directly to those surfaces. Cocaine has been traditionally used by ear, nose and throat surgeons for topical anaesthesia.

DRUGS USED IN ANAESTHESIA

24

TABLE 24.6 Common local anaesthetics

Group	Drug	% Concentration required (g/100 mL)				Maximum dose with adrenalin* (mg/kg)	Onset and duration of action
		Topical	Infiltration	Plexus, epidural	Spinal		
Esters	Procaine	—	1	2	2	10	Slow onset, short acting (30–45 min)
	Amethocaine	1	0.1–0.2	0.25	1	2	Slow onset, long acting (4–6 hours)
	Cocaine	Too toxic for injection; 5%–10% still used for topical anaesthesia; has vasoconstrictor action on its own					
Amides	Lignocaine	2–10	0.5–1.0	1.5–2.0	5	7	Rapid onset, medium acting (1–2 hours)
	Mepivocaine	—	1	1.5–2.0	—	7	Slow onset, medium acting (1–2 hours)
	Prilocaine	—	0.5–1.0	2–3	—	10	Slow onset, medium acting (1–2 hour)
	Bupivacaine	—	0.25	0.25–0.5	0.5**	3	Slow onset, long acting (4–8 hours or longer)
	Cinchocaine	Very toxic; used only for subarachnoid blocks as 0.5% solution; 6% glucose already added to make solution heavier than cerebrospinal fluid (hypobaric)					

*Reduce maximum dose by half if vasoconstrictor not added.   **Bupivacaine 0.5% is isobaric, with 8% glucose is hypbaric

The most common use of local anaesthetic drugs is in providing local, i.e. infiltration, anaesthesia. The anaesthetic agent is injected, usually using multiple injections, in and around the desired site. This technique is used to provide anaesthesia prior to wound debridement and suturing or for removal of skin lesions. It must be remembered that peripheral sensory nerves carry a variety of information to the central nervous system. Not only are pain signals transmitted, but also impulses subserving cold, warmth, touch and deep pressure. After the anaesthetic is injected all these sensations can be affected to a greater or lesser degree depending on the location of the injection and the amount of local anaesthetic used. The reason for their different sensitivities lies in the varying sizes of the neurones and whether they utilise myelinated fibres or not. The progressive loss of sensations follows the order given above; that is, pain is the first sensation to be lost, deep pressure the last. The clinical importance of this fact is that patients must be told that they may still feel sensations of pushing and movement but that there should be no pain.

Local anaesthetics usually take 2–4 minutes to take effect. The duration of action can be prolonged by the addition of vasoconstrictor agents such as adrenaline. This has the dual advantage of not only prolonging the duration of anaesthesia but allowing smaller amounts to be used. Local anaesthetics containing vasoconstrictors are never used in procedures involving the extremities (fingers and toes) as they can cause digital ischaemia and necrosis.

Larger areas of the body can be anaesthetised by injecting anaesthetic agents into progressively larger nerves. This is called regional anaesthesia and can be used as part of a general anaesthetic technique or alone. For example, in the emergency treatment of fractures of the lower limb, local anaesthetic can be injected around the femoral nerve in the inguinal area, thus effectively reducing pain. By knowing the sensory distribution of nerves, and their anatomical locations, almost any part of the body can be successfully anaesthetised using a regional technique. The result of the block and whether autonomic function and motor function are affected is dependent on the nature of the nerve, its physical diameter and the amount of anaesthetic used.

Even larger areas of the body can be anaesthetised by the injection of local anaesthetics into spaces about the spinal cord. The most common techniques being extradural (epidural) and spinal anaesthesia. In extradural anaesthesia a needle is inserted between vertebrae and anaesthetic agents injected into the narrow space between the dura and the bony spinal canal. This area contains mainly fat and connective tissue as well nerve roots and associated blood vessels. Only small amounts of drug are needed, however, the actual height of analgesia produced is very variable. Lignocaine, bupivacaine and amethocaine are all employed in extradural anaesthesia. The technique is extensively used for the relief of pain following surgical procedures, as part of a general anaesthetic technique, or for pain relief during labour. It has the advantage that a small plastic catheter can be left in place and 'top up' injections given from time to time.

For spinal analgesia, solutions of local anaesthetic drugs are injected directly into the cerebrospinal fluid within the subarachnoid space. Special solutions of local anaesthetic mixed with glucose are sometimes used, so increasing the specific gravity of the solution. By placing patients in suitable positions on the operating table, and taking into account that the anaesthetic solution will fall within the cerebrospinal fluid due to the effects of gravity and because it has a higher specific gravity, anaesthesia of a range of regions can be undertaken. Spinal anaesthesia can be used for amputations, obstetric cases and in urological and prostatic procedures. The patient is effectively anaesthetised with relaxation of skeletal muscle, yet, if correctly positioned, has spontaneous respirations and is awake throughout the procedure.

The usual concentration of lignocaine used in anaesthetics is between 0.5% and 2%,

DRUGS USED IN ANAESTHESIA

24

with concentrations of 5% being used in spinal anaesthesia.

ADVERSE DRUG REACTIONS

Local anaesthetics are particularly dangerous if large amounts are allowed to reach the systemic circulation as cardiovascular collapse and central nervous system stimulation can follow. Epileptic seizures can occur following the injection of high doses, presumably because inhibitory fibres are suppressed allowing excitatory impulses to predominate. Following these excitatory events, central nervous system depression occurs, manifested by drowsiness, cardiovascular and respiratory depression and, eventually, coma.

Cardiac arrhythmias induced by local anaesthetic agents can be particularly difficult to treat and are often fatal. The risks of major adverse reactions with local anaesthetics is directly related to the dosage employed. Regional and epidural techniques employ large volumes and are most likely to cause difficulties if a large proportion of the dose inadvertently finds its way into the systemic circulation.

NURSING IMPLICATIONS

Patients scheduled for surgery and anaesthesia may be considered in terms of preoperative, intraoperative and postoperative care. Several groups of nursing staff are involved so accurate and consistent records are essential.

PREOPERATIVE CARE IN THE WARD

A nursing history should provide information about the following:

- Past and present illness; degree of limitation of activity; particular reference should be made to cardiovascular and respiratory systems.

- Present drug therapy, especially antihypertensives, corticosteroids, insulin, diuretics, digoxin, antianginal drugs, anticoagulants.

- Past surgical and anaesthetic experiences; previous deep venous thrombosis, nausea and vomiting, allergic reactions, pulmonary complications, 'collapse', familial problems with anaesthetics.

- Assessment of behaviour and habits; smoking, alcohol, drug addiction, biohazards, emotional state, availability of next of kin, recent ingestion of fluid or food.

Certain measurements and tests are carried out in the ward by the nursing staff and provide valuable information about the patient:

- Recording of pulse (rate and regularity) and blood pressure.

- Spirometry to record vital capacity (VC) and forced expiratory volume in one second (FEV_1).

- All patients should be weighed. Many anaesthetic drugs are administered on a body weight basis.

- Body temperature. Pyrexia may be the first indication of underlying or coexisting infection.

- Urinalysis. The presence of protein, blood or glucose may indicate an unexpected systemic disease.

The nursing staff plays a vital role in preoperative preparation:

- Psychological — friendly reassurance. Allaying anxiety and assisting with informed consent and its documentation.

- Supervision of preoperative instructions about fasting, drug therapy, physiotherapy, anticoagulants, identity labels for allergy and biohazard.

- Accurate administration of premedicant drugs and observing their effects, particularly the degree of central nervous system depression, repiratory and/or cardiovascular depression. These drugs may be ordered at a specific time or 'on call' to theatres. When there is nursing concern about preoperative instructions and/or their legibility, the medical staff should be consulted as soon as possible. Patients should remain in bed after premedication as these agents cause hypotension and patients may faint causing themselves injury.

- Intravenous infusions should be continued or set up as ordered, e.g. in diabetics a glucose/insulin infusion may be required.

INTRAOPERATIVE CARE IN THE THEATRE

- All the patient's papers for the current and past admissions should be available in the theatre for the anaesthetist.

- The identity of the patient should be checked carefully in theatre reception and again in the anaesthetic room.

- Intravenous lines should be checked with preoperative instructions and rate adjusted accordingly. The anaesthetist should be informed immediately about any problems.

- Transportation in theatres should be smooth. The patient should be reassured and made comfortable.

- The anaesthetic machine should be checked for accurate performance — correct coupling of oxygen and nitrous oxide, functioning rotameters, gas tight breathing system, vapourisers primed and turned off, disconnect alarm and scavenging available.

- Required anaesthetic drugs should be drawn up and labelled.

- Monitors should be connected — pulse monitor, pulse oximeter, sphygmomanometer, ECG 'dots' and leads.

- If not already in situ an intravenous infusion is set up. For major operations arterial and central venous cannulations may be required. Reserved blood should be in theatres.

- With urgent operations a rapid sequence induction requires preoxygenation and cricoid pressure (Sellick's manoeuvre) prior to endotracheal intubation.

- The anaesthetised patient must be protected from injury particularly during movement and positioning for operation. Careless movement and/or head up tilt may lead to marked hypotension.

- During local anaesthesia continued reassurance is essential.

POSTOPERATIVE CARE IN RECOVERY

- Oxygen therapy is frequently required.

- Vital signs are charted — level of consciousness, pulse, blood pressure, ECG, urinary output.

- Patient's colour, respiratory rate, depth and pattern are monitored to ensure the anaesthesia has been adequately reversed.

- Anomalies which may be related to the anaesthetic, e.g. laryngospasm, and inadequate reversal should be reported to the anaesthetist for prompt treatment.

- Site of operation and drainage tubes should be observed for bleeding.

DRUGS USED IN ANAESTHESIA

24

- The patient is reassured. Narcotics and/or antiemetics may be required.

- Depending on the climate and the patient, facilities should be available to warm or cool.

- Restless patients should be protected from injury. Unexplained restlessness may be due to hypoxia and the medical staff should be consulted before giving a narcotic.

- Patients who have had dissociative anaesthesia, especially children who have received ketamine, should be handled gently and not disturbed unnecessarily to avoid triggering hallucinations.

FURTHER READING

Atkinson, R.S., Rushman, G.B., Lee, J.A. (1992) *A synopsis of anaesthesia*, 11th edn. Wright, Bristol.

Bowman, W.C., Rand, M.J. (1980) *Textbook of pharmacology*, 2nd edn. Blackwell Scientific, Oxford.

Gilman, A.G., Rall, T.W., Nies, A.S., Taylor, P. (1991) *Goodman and Gilman's the pharmacological basis of therapeutics*, 8th edn. Maxwell MacMillan, New York.

Lunn, J.N. (1986) *Lecture notes on anaesthetics*, 3rd edn. Blackwell Scientific, Oxford.

TEST YOUR KNOWLEDGE

I. Isoflurane and enflurane are examples of commonly used volatile anaesthetic agents. True or false?

2. Most volatile agents are extremely inflammable. True or false?

3. Giving a patient 100% nitrous oxide is a common way to give the drug. True or false?

4. Halothane is known to occasionally have an adverse effect on the liver and cause a form of hepatitis. True or false?

5. The duration of action of suxamethonium is about 30 minutes. True or false?

6. Muscle twitching (fasciculations) is usually observed after the administration of atracurium. True or false?

7. Most skeletal muscle relaxant drugs used today are of the depolarising type. True or false?

8. The duration of action of thiopentone injection is short. This is because it is rapidly metabolised by the liver. True or false?

9. Accidental injection of thiopentone into an artery can result in major complications such as gangrene and limb loss. True or false?

10. Peripheral nerve stimulators are a useful way of monitoring the effectiveness of skeletal muscle relaxants. True or false?

11. Local anaesthetics can be divided into two chemical groups, the esters and amides. True or false?

12. Pain, light touch, pressure and movement are all equally affected by injection of local anaesthetic agents. True or false?

13. Adrenaline is added to some local anaesthetic preparations to increase their duration of action. True or false?

14. Preparations containing lignocaine and adrenaline should not be used to anaesthetise fingers and toes. True or false?

15. Large doses of local anaesthetic agents if accidentally given intravenously can cause cardiac arrhythmias and convulsions. True or false?

16. Muscle aches and pains are common after using vecuronium. True or false?

17. Papaveretum and hyoscine are sometimes used together as a premedication. True or false?

18. Isoflurane can be safely administered from a halothane vapouriser. True or false?

19. Ether is (a) no longer used in Australia; (b) highly flammable; (c) a volatile anaesthetic; (d) still used in some overseas countries; or (e) all of the above.

20. Propofol (a) is dissolved in water in the ampoule; (b) causes unconsciousness for about 1 hour after a single injection; (c) sometimes causes pain on injection; (d) has the trade name *Hypnovel*; or (e) all of the above.

21. Flumazenil reverses action of drugs such as (a) diazepam (benzodiazepines); (b) morphine (opiates); (c) thiopentone (barbiturates); or (d) general anaesthetic agents.

22. Local anaesthetics act by (a) increasing the movement of sodium into the neurone; (b) decreasing the movement of sodium into the neurone; (c) increasing the movement of potassium into the neurone; (d) decreasing the movement of potassium into the neurone; or (e) primarily affecting calcium movement.

23. The transmitter chemical at the neuromuscular junction is (a) noradrenaline; (b) adrenaline; (c) nicotine; (d) muscarine; or (e) acetylcholine.

24. Which of the following side effects is not associated with morphine use (a) histamine release; (b) sedation; (c) nausea; (d) hypertension; or (e) vomiting.

25. Neostigmine acts by (a) increasing the amount of acetylcholine at the neuromuscular junction; (b) increasing the amount of noradrenaline at the neuromuscular junction; (c) decreasing the amount of acetylcholine at the neuromuscular junction; (d) decreasing the amount of noradrenaline at the neuromuscular junction; or (e) increasing the concentrations of both noradrenaline and acetylcholine at the neuromuscular junction.

DRUGS USED IN ANAESTHESIA

24

Neurological Disorders

RHONDA FIGGIS CLOSE

O B J E C T I V E S

At the conclusion of this chapter the reader should be able to:

1. Define the terms epilepsy, migraine, and parkinsonism;

2. Differentiate between the various types of each of these diseases;

3. List the drugs used in each of these diseases and their common side effects; and

4. List the nursing implications associated with medication given in each of these diseases.

EPILEPSY

Epilepsy has been around for a very long time. It was probably first described in ancient Egyptian writings about 2000 years BC and was frequently discussed by Roman and Greek scholars. It was known as the 'falling sickness' or the 'sacred disease' and was thought to be the manifestation of action by the gods and spirits.

SYMPTOMATIC EPILEPSY

Symptomatic (secondary) epilepsy may be due to *intracranial factors* such as infection (e.g. meningitis, encephalitis, neurosyphilis, abscess, tuberculosis), trauma (e.g. at birth or from head injury, vascular lesions, cerebral degeneration and tumours; or *extracranial factors* such as anoxia, poisons (e.g. alcohol, ethyl chloride, lead, cocaine), metabolic disturbances (e.g. with uraemia, alkalosis, liver failure, hypoglycaemia) and withdrawal of medications (e.g. hypnotics, opiates).

IDIOPATHIC EPILEPSY

Epilepsy is classified as idiopathic (primary) epilepsy when no cause (such as those listed above) is present. It should be noted that all living brains have the capacity to produce a seizure if the stimulus is sufficient. Some individuals have spontaneous seizures without any provocative stimuli, others may be affected by such stimuli as flickering light, excessive alcohol intake or severe fatigue, while others may require an electroconvulsive shock before a seizure develops. The degree of stimulus needed to produce a seizure in a particular individual is the 'seizure threshold' of that person.

Both symptomatic and idiopathic epilepsy can produce several types of seizures. Several of the more common seizures are discussed below.

Tonic-clonic Seizures

In this type of seizure the patient loses consciousness and falls to the ground in a state of tonic rigidity. During this state the familiar 'epileptic cry' is heard, air being forced out through the tightly adducted vocal chords. The rigidity of the muscles is followed by generalised jerking, which is then replaced by the limbs becoming flaccid. The patient may regain consciousness in about five to 15 minutes, may be confused for a further 15 minutes or so and may then go into a deep sleep. Preceding the seizure there may be a prodromal phase, usually only a mood change lasting for hours or several days, and a brief aura, with varying signs including vague apprehension and turning of the head or eyes.

These seizures are also known as major or grand mal seizures.

Absence Seizures

These occur only in children, who may have 'little absences' of about 10–15 seconds when they stare straight ahead, sometimes blinking.

Focal or Partial Epilepsy (Jacksonian Epilepsy)

Hughlings Jackson first described seizures originating in the cortex in 1888. These seizures may remain localised and affect the appropriate part of the body. For example, a seizure in the motor cortex results in violent movements of a limb or part of a limb; in the sensory cortex, abnormal sensations appear in the other side of the body; and in the occipital region, impairment of vision such as brief flashes of light or confused visual hallucinations may occur. The seizures may also spread to adjacent areas producing a grand mal convulsion.

Complex Partial Seizures (Temporal Lobe Epilepsy)

This is a particular kind of focal seizure generally arising in the temporal lobe. It is the most common form of minor epilepsy seen in adults, accounting for one-third of all varieties of epilepsy. The following symptoms are usual: hallucinations involving the senses of taste, smell, hearing and vision; visceral sensations; disorders of memory (deja vu); dreamy states; and automatic behaviour which may be violent.

Status Epilepticus

This is a medical emergency in which seizures follow one another with no intervening periods of consciousness. Grand mal status epilepticus may persist for hours or days and can be fatal. Status epilepticus may occur spontaneously or may be precipitated by a too rapid withdrawal of anticonvulsants.

INTERNATIONAL CLASSIFICATION OF EPILEPTIC SEIZURES

The International Classification of Epileptic Seizures classifies seizures into partial seizures which begin locally and generalised seizures which begin symmetrically without a focal point. Partial seizures may spread throughout the brain and become secondary generalised seizures. (See Table 25.1).

TABLE 25.1 International Classification of Epileptic Seizures*

I. Partial seizures (seizures beginning locally)
A. *Simple partial seizures (generally without impairment of consciousness)*
  1. With motor symptoms (includes Jacksonian seizures)
  2. With special sensory or somatosensory symptoms (e.g. tingling, buzzing)
  3. With autonomic symptoms or signs (e.g. sweating, pallor)
  4. Compound forms, e.g. with psychic symptoms (disturbance of higher cerebral function)

B. *Complex partial seizures (generally with impairment of consciousness)*
(temporal lobe or psychomotor seizures)
  1. Simple partial onset followed by impairment of consciousness
  2. With impairment of consciousness at onset of cognitive symptoms
  3. Affective symptoms
  4. Psychosensory symptoms
  5. Psychomotor symptoms (automatisms)

C. *Partial seizures evolving to generalised seizures*

II. Generalised (bilaterally symmetrical, convulsive and non-convulsive and without local onset) seizures
A. *Absences (petit mal, stare)*
B. *Myoclonic seizures (sudden, brief jerks)*
C. *Infantile spasms*
D. *Clonic seizures (muscle contraction and relaxation)*
E. *Tonic seizures (muscle contraction)*
F. *Tonic-clonic seizures (grand mal)*
G. *Atonic seizures (drop attack)*
H. *Akinetic seizures*

III. Unilateral seizures (or predominantly)

IV. Unclassified epileptic seizures (due to incomplete data, e.g. neonatal seizures)

*From Commission on Classification and Terminology of the International League Against Epilepsy

25 NEUROLOGICAL DISORDERS

DRUGS FOR MAJOR SEIZURES AND COMPLEX PARTIAL SEIZURES

Phenytoin

TRADE NAMES

Phenytoin (Diphenylhydantoin, DPH): *Dilantin.*

MECHANISM OF ACTION

The drug is thought to inhibit the spread of the seizure discharge through the brain and to decrease the intracellular sodium concentration.

PHARMACOKINETICS

Phenytoin is almost completely but slowly absorbed from the gastrointestinal tract, mostly from the upper gastrointestinal tract. The rate of absorption is thought to be increased by food. Different brands and formulations can have different bioavailability. Absorption from the gastrointestinal tract is faster and more complete than that from an intramuscular injection.

Metabolism occurs in the liver where phenytoin is converted to its inactive metabolite. The rate of metabolism appears to be influenced by the patient's genetic and racial characteristics. The metabolism of phenytoin becomes saturated with increasing dosages. Dosage increments should be small and plasma levels measured 1–2 weeks after any dosage changes. Phenytoin is recycled by the liver and is excreted in the urine as its metabolite. Phenytoin is highly protein bound (about 90%), widely distributed, and has a long half-life of about 22 hours after steady state is reached, although this may take several weeks. Plasma levels of the drug are frequently ordered as an aid to assessing the level of control.

Phenytoin crosses the placenta and small amounts are excreted into breast milk.

USES

Phenytoin is used to control tonic-clonic (grand mal) and partial (focal) seizures. It is also used prophylactically to prevent seizures following severe head trauma and during or after neurosurgery.

Doses are adjusted according to the needs of the individual patient so that constant monitoring is necessary until steady state is reached. Levels between 10 and 20 micrograms/mL (40–80 micromol/L) are usually sufficient although sometimes levels outside this range may be necessary. A loading dose is sometimes given to 'short cut' the route to steady state which might otherwise take several weeks to attain. The initial oral dose is usually 300 mg daily which may be increased to 600 mg if necessary. Increments are made in periods ranging from one week to one month. The maintenance dose is usually 300–400 mg daily. Because of its long half-life (about 22 hours) the daily dose may be given twice daily or as a single dose. This greatly helps with compliance. Taking the drug with or after food and with at least a half glass of water lessens gastric irritation.

Although different formulations may be the same strength they may have different degrees of bioavailability. It is therefore important that patients, once stabilised on one formulation, should not be changed to another without being closely monitored.

Any change from another anticonvulsant drug to phenytoin should be done gradually by decreasing the dosage of the other drug and increasing the dosage of phenytoin. Similarly, while changing from phenytoin to another drug the reverse process takes place. It is considered better to use one drug wherever possible rather than combination therapy, although taking more than one drug to cope with different sorts of epilepsy is sometimes necessary.

Intravenous phenytoin sodium is usually given after intravenous diazepam in the treatment of tonic-clonic status epilepticus as a loading dose of 10–15 mg per kg body weight. It is extremely important that it be given slowly at a constant rate of not more than 50 mg per minute. Deaths have occurred from the too rapid intravenous injection of phenytoin. Maintenance doses of 100 mg either by mouth or intravenously are then given every 6–8 hours.

Phenytoin sodium given by intramuscular injection is erratically absorbed and is usually only used to maintain blood levels when the patient is unconscious or otherwise unable to take doses by mouth. It is rarely used. When transferring from oral to intramuscular administration the dose should be increased by 50%; when transferring back to oral administration the oral dose should be reduced by 50% for the same amount of time the patient was receiving the intramuscular injection to allow for absorption of any residual drug in the muscle tissues.

Phenytoin has also been used as an antiarrhythmic drug, particularly for arrhythmias associated with digitalis toxicity.

ADVERSE DRUG REACTIONS

Adverse reactions with phenytoin are fairly common and include moroseness, vomiting, constipation, mental confusion, headache, dizziness, insomnia, transient nervousness, slurred speech, ataxia, diplopia and nystagmus (oscillatory movements of the eyeballs).

Some adverse reactions, e.g. nystagmus, muscular incoordination and vertigo, are due to phenytoin toxicity and are therefore dose related. These effects may remit following a lowering of the dose for two or three days after which the patient is reassessed.

Gum hypertrophy often occurs. It is sometimes necessary to change to another anticonvulsant if this reaction takes place. It may possibly be corrected by dental hygiene, if this does not work dental surgery may be necessary.

Fetal hydantoin syndrome, which may include cleft palate, has been noted when the mother has taken phenytoin during pregnancy. However, other drugs have also been implicated.

Dermatitis sometimes occurs, and this may be accompanied by fever and a blood disorder (eosinophilia). Unusual and excessive hair growth (hirsutism) has been reported and acne is common. Other less well known drug reactions with long-term phenytoin use include various blood disorders such as leucopenia, agranulocytosis and thrombocytopenia.

DRUG INTERACTIONS

The metabolism of phenytoin may be affected significantly by the concomitant use of other drugs.

Barbiturates and carbamazepine may enhance the metabolism of phenytoin by microsomal liver enzyme induction, resulting in lowered blood levels of phenytoin. Phenytoin is a strong inducer of liver enzymes and induces the metabolism of a number of drugs including some antibiotics (e.g. doxycycline), corticosteroids, quinidine, oral contraceptives and other sex hormones, leading to the possibility of greatly reduced blood levels and effects.

Coumarin anticoagulants, amiodarone, trimethoprim, sulfonamides, disulfiram, isoniazid and chloramphenicol may inhibit the metabolism of phenytoin resulting in signs of phenytoin toxicity.

Because phenytoin is a highly protein bound drug it can be displaced by other drugs (e.g. aspirin and salicylates, sulfonamides, tolbutamide, valproic acid) which compete at the binding sites. However, as phenytoin is so widely distributed, metabolised and excreted, the concentration of free active drug remains about the same, provided there is no hepatic impairment, this interference by other drugs is not clinically significant.

PRECAUTIONS AND CONTRAINDICATIONS

Toxic concentrations of phenytoin may develop in patients receiving drugs which inhibit hepatic metabolism (see Drug Interactions) and in patients with impaired liver function.

NEUROLOGICAL DISORDERS

25

Carbamazepine

Carbamazepine can be included in the miscellaneous group of drugs used in the treatment of epilepsy.

TRADE NAMES

Carbamazepine: *Tegretol*; *Teril*.

MECHANISM OF ACTION

The drug's mode of action in epilepsy is not fully understood but it resembles phenytoin in some of its actions.

PHARMACOKINETICS

Carbamazepine is completely but slowly absorbed from the gastrointestinal tract. It is largely metabolised in the liver with one of its metabolites having about a third of the antiepileptic activity of carbamazepine itself. It is widely distributed throughout the body and is excreted in the urine in the form of its metabolites.

Carbamazepine is about 75% bound to plasma proteins. It is able to induce its own metabolism so that previously untreated patients may have lower plasma levels on repeated administration. Because of this property it is advisable to regularly monitor plasma levels as an aid to control.

Carbamazepine crosses the placenta and is excreted in breast milk.

USES

Carbamazepine may be given to control tonic-clonic (grand mal) and partial (focal) seizures or may be combined with other drugs for patients who are resistant to treatment. It is of particular use in the treatment of partial complex seizures, especially when associated with disturbed behaviour. Retarded children have been shown to benefit in some studies, both in the control of their epilepsy and in behaviour disturbances. Carbamazepine has been successfully used in the treatment of tic doloureux and is the drug of first choice in the treatment of trigeminal neuralgia. It has also been used in glossopharynygeal neuralgia and for manic depressive psychoses not responding to lithium.

The initial oral dose should be low to minimise side effects, usually 100–200 mg once or twice daily. The dose is then increased in increments of 200 mg to a maintenance dose of 0.8–1.2 g daily or occasionally up to 1.6 g daily given in two to four doses. Because of the drug's long half-life the daily dose may be divided and be given in two doses. Twice daily dosage aids considerably in compliance. The time and manner of taking the drug should be standardised to avoid fluctuations in plasma levels and possible precipitation of seizures.

Changing to another antiepileptic or withdrawing the drug should be undertaken slowly to minimise precipitating a seizure.

ADVERSE DRUG REACTIONS

Dizziness, drowsiness and ataxia can occur in the early stages of treatment so it is important to start with a low dose. Drowsiness, ataxia, nystagmus and diplopia (double vision) have been associated with high plasma levels and may disappear with a reduction in dosage.

Gastrointestinal symptoms are less commonly reported. Generalised rashes, Stevens-Johnson syndrome, blood disorders including agranulocytosis and aplastic anaemia, headache and heart block have also been reported.

DRUG INTERACTIONS

Erythromycin, isoniazid and danazol have been shown to inhibit the metabolism of carbamazepine thus causing raised blood levels leading to toxicity. Cimetidine has also been shown to inhibit carbamazepine metabolism.

Carbamazepine is a liver enzyme inducer and induces the metabolism of some other drugs including antibiotics, e.g. doxycycline, anticoagulants and oral contraceptives.

Carbamazepine may also induce its own metabolism. When prescribed with phenytoin each drug may induce the other's metabolism.

Because of its similarity in structure to the tricyclic antidepressants it has been suggested that the drug should not be prescribed with the MAOIs or within 14 days of their use.

Carbamazepine intoxication has occurred when the drug was given concomitantly with benzodiazepines and calcium antagonists.

PRECAUTIONS AND CONTRAINDICATIONS

Carbamazepine should be administered with caution to patients with a history of hepatic, renal or cardiac disease or blood disorders. Caution should also be observed in patients with elevated intraocular pressure because of the drug's mild anticholinergic properties.

Carbamazepine should be avoided in patients with some cardiac problems (e.g. atrioventricular conduction abnormalities) unless they have a pacemaker.

Sodium Valproate, Semisodium Valproate

TRADE NAMES

Sodium valproate: *Epilim*; *Valpro*.
Semisodium valproate: *Valcote*.

MECHANISM OF ACTION

Sodium valproate is thought to maintain levels of γ amino butyric acid (GABA) in the brain by inhibiting the enzyme GABA transaminase which causes the breakdown of GABA.

PHARMACOKINETICS

The salts of valproic acid (i.e. sodium valproate and semisodium valproate) are quickly and completely absorbed from the gastrointestinal tract. Administration with or after food causes a delay in the rate but not the extent of absorption.

The drugs are largely metabolised in the liver, metabolism being enhanced by drugs which induce hepatic microsomal enzymes (e.g. phenytoin, barbiturates). However, the valproates do not seem to enhance their own metabolism as do the liver enzyme inducing drugs previously mentioned. Excretion is via the urine, mostly as metabolites.

The valproates are about 90% bound to the plasma protein. Reported half-lives range from 5 to 20 hours depending on whether they are prescribed alone or with other antiepileptic drugs which induce liver enzymes and so speed up metabolism of the valproate.

The valproates cross the placenta and small amounts are secreted in the breast milk.

USES

The valproates have been shown to be effective in the treatment of temporal lobe epilepsy, petit mal, grand mal, mixed epilepsy and myoclonic seizures. They are used in primary generalised epilepsy, simple and complex absence seizures and as an adjunct in multiple seizure epilepsy. Children generally perform better at school when taking these drugs because they have less sedative effect than other anticonvulsant drugs.

A suggested initial adult dose of sodium valproate is 600 mg daily in divided doses increased every three days by 200 mg daily, to a range of 1–2 g daily. This dosage may be increased to 2.5 g daily if adequate control has not been achieved.

A suggested initial dose for children weighing more than 20 kg is 400 mg daily in divided doses, gradually increasing until control is achieved, with a usual range of 20–30 mg/kg daily. Children weighing less than 20 kg may be given 20 mg/kg daily although this may be increased in some cases.

Sodium valproate should be taken with or after food. A low initial dose is recommended to avoid gastric intolerance. It should be taken at the same time each day to avoid inappropriate fluctuations in plasma concentrations.

In adults the recommended initial dose of semisodium valproate is 15 mg/kg/day increasing at one week intervals by 5–10 mg/kg/day until seizures are controlled or side effects prevent further increases. The maximum recommended dosage is 60 mg/kg/day.

For children, adult doses are usually given. In severe cases, the dose may be

NEUROLOGICAL DISORDERS

25

increased to 40 mg/kg/day but careful monitoring needs to take place.

The tablets should not be chewed but swallowed whole with milk or water. If gastric irritation occurs, they should be taken with food.

ADVERSE DRUG REACTIONS

Adverse reactions include nausea, vomiting, gastrointestinal irritation, increased appetite and excessive weight gain, drowsiness, oedema, ataxia (incoordination of muscle action) and transient hair loss with regrowth of curly hair. High doses have led to tremor, prolongation of bleeding time (reversible) and thrombocytopenia.

Liver dysfunction leading to hepatic failure and death have been reported. Monitoring of liver function at least monthly is advised in patients taking the drug, until six months after the controlling dose is reached. The position may be then reviewed and less frequent monitoring may be appropriate. Patients should be instructed to report any unusual bleeding or abdominal pain. Pancreatitis has also been reported.

Congenital malformations, e.g. neural tube defects, have been reported in infants born to women who received valproate during pregnancy. However, the causal effect has been debated as these women were frequently taking other antiepileptic medication.

DRUG INTERACTIONS

Sodium valproate inhibits the hepatic metabolism of phenobarbitone, primidone and diazepam causing a rise in plasma concentrations which may lead to toxicity. The combined use of sodium valproate and clonazepam has been associated with the development of absence seizures.

As the valproates are extensively bound to plasma proteins they can be displaced by drugs such as phenytoin competing for protein binding sites thus liberating more free (pharmacologically active) valproate into the plasma. This could lead to much higher and potentially toxic blood levels. Administration of hepatic enzyme inducers such as phenytoin, carbamazepine, phenobarbitone and primidone concomitantly with a valproate may enhance the metabolism of the valproate. The interaction between valproate and phenytoin is complex and involves inhibition of phenytoin metabolism as well as competition for the protein binding sites.

Valproates may cause false positive results of urine tests for diabetes because of its partial excretion as ketone bodies.

PRECAUTIONS AND CONTRAINDICATIONS

Diabetic patients should be warned that sodium valproate may cause false positive results of urine tests for ketones.

Valproates may affect bleeding time and caution should be observed when valproate is administered with other drugs such as aspirin or warfarin which affect blood coagulation.

To avoid fatal liver failure in patients taking valproate the following has been advised: polytherapy in children under 3 years of age should be avoided if possible; when there is a family history of childhood hepatic disease, use should be avoided; as low a dose as possible should be used; salicylates should be avoided; valproate should not be given to fasting children with intercurrent illness; careful surveillance should be maintained for untoward symptoms, especially after febrile illness.

Collective data from 13 study groups indicate that exposure to valproic acid in the first trimester of pregnancy is causally associated with a considerably increased risk of neural tube defects and that its use during pregnancy should be avoided.

Barbiturates: Phenobarbitone, Methylphenobarbitone

Members of this group are derived from barbituric acid and are closely related in structure. They include phenobarbitone (tablets and injection) and methylphenobarbitone (tablets) which is metabolised to phenobarbitone. Another drug in this group is primidone which is metabolised to two other drugs, a compound known as PEMA (phenylethylmalonamide) and phenobarbitone.

TRADE NAMES

Methylphenobarbitone: *Prominal.*

MECHANISM OF ACTION

Barbiturates depress the central nervous system, i.e. the cerebral cortex and the reticular formation.

PHARMACOKINETICS

Barbiturates are absorbed readily from the gastrointestinal tract and begin their action within half an hour. Phenobarbitone is more lipid soluble and may take an hour or longer to act although the sodium salts act more quickly.

Barbiturates are metabolised in the liver by liver enzymes and secreted by the kidney. The duration of action of individual barbiturates is dependent on the time taken for this process. Phenobarbitone is only partially metabolised in the liver and about 25% is secreted unchanged in the urine. It is about 40% bound to plasma proteins while its half-life may be as long as 75 hours in children and 100 hours in adults. This can be increased in the presence of renal or hepatic disease, overdosage or the elderly. Control can be assessed by plasma concentration monitoring.

Phenobarbitone crosses into the placenta and small amounts enter the breast milk.

USES

The barbiturates have come into some disrepute as sedatives but as anticonvulsants they have a long and proven history of efficacy. These drugs have been used for the treatment of major seizures of all kinds and are still used in paediatrics for febrile convulsions.

Phenobarbitone and other barbiturates can be used to control tonic-clonic (grand mal) and partial (focal) seizures. The dose is generally 60–180 mg daily, usually taken at night and adjusted to the needs of the patient to achieve control of seizures. This usually requires plasma concentrations of 10–40 micrograms per mL. Phenobarbitone has been used in the treatment of status epilepticus as an alternative to diazepam and phenytoin. It may be given intravenously no faster than 100 mg per minute.

However, its intravenous use is not without hazards even with diluted solutions and very careful monitoring should take place. Delayed blood levels may result from intramuscular use. Subcutaneous administration can cause tissue necrosis.

Phenobarbitone has also been used to reduce hyperbilirubinaemia in neonates as it stimulates the microsomal liver enzymes which metabolise bilirubin.

ADVERSE DRUG REACTIONS

The barbiturates have a sedative effect and in some children produce irritability and aggravate any tendency to excessive movement associated with muscle spasm (hyperkinesia). Other well recognised side effects are incoordination of muscle action (ataxia) and rashes.

These drugs tend to produce tolerance and severe withdrawal effects. Other reactions include sedation, respiratory depression, allergic reactions particularly skin reactions (1%–3% with phenobarbitone) and photosensitivity. Occasionally Stevens-Johnson syndrome, exfoliative dermatitis, purpura and toxic epidermal necrolysis have been reported.

Hyperexcitability and irritability have occurred, particularly in children and the elderly. Ataxia and nystagmus may occur with excessive doses. Hepatitis and cholestasis have been reported.

DRUG INTERACTIONS

Because these drugs are inducers of liver enzymes they cause increased metabolism and therefore decrease the effect of any other drugs which are metabolised by liver enzymes, given concomitantly. Such drugs include carbamazepine, cyclosporin, metronidazole, phenytoin, quinidine, doxycycline, warfarin, tricyclic antidepressants, theophylline and steroid hormones, including oral contraceptives.

The central nervous system and respiratory depressant effects of the barbiturates are enhanced by the concurrent administration of other central nervous system depressants such as alcohol. The lethal dose

NEUROLOGICAL DISORDERS

25

of the barbiturates is lowered by alcohol because of this synergistic effect. Rises in blood levels of phenobarbitone and primidone have been reported with the concurrent administration of valproic acid.

PRECAUTIONS AND CONTRAINDICATIONS

Phenobarbitone and other barbiturates are contraindicated in patients with acute intermittent porphyria. They should be given with care to children, the elderly and patients with impaired respiratory, renal or hepatic function. When the impairment is severe, these drugs should be avoided.

Primidone

Primidone is an a antiepileptic drug which is partially metabolised to phenobarbitone. It therefore exhibits all the properties of phenobarbitone including uses, adverse drug reactions, drug interactions, precautions and contraindications. Some additional points are noted below.

TRADE NAMES

Primidone: *Mysoline.*

PHARMACOKINETICS

Primidone has a short half-life compared with its main metabolites phenobarbitone and phenylethylmalonamide (PEMA). It also exhibits only partial plasma protein binding (20%–25%). It crosses the placenta and is present in breast milk.

USES

Primidone is an antiepileptic agent used for tonic-clonic (grand mal) and partial (focal) seizures and for some other forms of epilepsy.

It is available as tablets for oral use and is given initially at a dose of 125 mg daily. The dose is then increased in increments of 125 mg in children and up to 250 mg in adults every three days up to a total of 1.5–2 g daily until seizures are controlled. The usual maintenance dose in adults and children over nine years is 0.75–1.5 g daily.

ADVERSE DRUG REACTIONS

These include vertigo, nausea, vomiting, visual disturbances, headache, weakness or fatigue as well as those listed under phenobarbitone.

Benzodiazepines: Diazepam, Nitrazepam, Lorazepam, Clonazepam, Clobazam

Drugs in this group are used in the treatment of various kinds of epilepsy.

TRADE NAMES

Diazepam: *Antenex; Diazemuls; Ducene; Valium.*
Nitrazepam: *Alodorm; Mogadon.*
Lorazepam: *Ativan; Emoten.*
Clonazepam: *Rivotril.*
Clobazam: *Frisium.*

MECHANISM OF ACTION

Benzodiazepines seem to act by facilitating the synaptic actions of γ-aminobutyric acid (GABA), a major inhibitory neurotransmitter in the brain.

USES

Diazepam given intravenously is an extremely useful drug in the treatment of status epilepticus although it does not act as a potent anticonvulsant when given orally. In status epilepticus 5–10 mg is given by slow intravenous injection, repeated in 10–15 minutes until a total of 30 mg is given. For children the dose is 200–300 micrograms/kg body weight or 1 mg per year of age. When the seizures are controlled repeat occurrences may be prevented with intravenous phenytoin sodium or a slow infusion of diazepam (maximum dose: 3 mg/kg over 24 hours). Diazepam can also be given rectally, the dose being the same.

Nitrazepam has been of use in achieving initial control of refractory myoclonic seizures in some children. However, its long-term efficacy is not clear and must be balanced against the evidence of impairment of motor and cognitive development associated with nitrazepam treatment.

Clonazepam is a benzodiazepine which has been shown to have marked antiepileptic properties. It has been used in a wide range of epilepsies, including status epilepticus, in adults and children. However, its use is sometimes limited by the development of tolerance and sedation. Treatment is usually begun with small doses which are gradually increased to the optimum for the patient. The daily dosage, which is usually divided into three or four doses, is normally 0.5–1.0 mg for infants, 1–3 mg for children and 4–8 mg for adults. The usual dose in status epilepticus is 500 micrograms for infants and children and 1 mg for adults, given by slow intravenous injection over about 30 seconds. It may also be given by slow intravenous infusion in sodium chloride 0.9% or glucose solutions. Transition to another type of antiepileptic treatment or withdrawal from clonazepam should be slow to avoid precipitating more seizures.

Lorazepam is unlike other benzodiazepines in that it is well absorbed intramuscularly as well as orally. It should be given in reduced dosage to elderly or debilitated patients.

Clobazam has been used in doses of 20–30 mg daily, given in divided doses or as a single dose at night, as adjunctive therapy in the management of epilepsy. In children over 3 years not more than half the recommended adult dose may be given.

For information on pharmacokinetics, adverse drug reactions and drug interactions see section on benzodiazepines, Chapter 26 Psychiatric Disorders.

PRECAUTIONS AND CONTRAINDICATIONS

Intravenous injections of diazepam should be administered slowly using a large lumen vessel, e.g. the antecubital vein, as diazepam can cause thrombophlebitis. Rapid injection can cause hypotension and respiratory depression. See also Chapter 26.

Vigabatrin

TRADE NAMES

Vigabatrin: *Sabril.*

MECHANISM OF ACTION

Vigabatrin is a selective irreversible inhibitor of GABA transaminase, the enzyme responsible for the metabolism of GABA. Treatment with vigabatrin leads to an increase in brain levels of GABA.

PHARMACOKINETICS

Vigabatrin is rapidly absorbed from the gastrointestinal tract following oral administration. Absorption is largely unaffected by food.

Vigabatrin is widely distributed and has a half-life of 5–8 hours. No major metabolites have been identified. The drug is excreted unchanged by the kidney. Estimations of plasma levels as a guide to efficacy have not been found necessary in clinical use as there appears to be no correlation between serum and cerebrospinal fluid concentrations of vigabatrin.

USES

Vigabatrin is indicated for the treatment of epilepsy which is not satisfactorily controlled by other antiepileptic drugs. It is given orally once or twice daily and may be taken before or after meals.

The recommended adult starting dose is 2 g which is added to the patient's current therapeutic regimen. The dose may be increased or decreased in 0.5 g or 1.0 g increments depending on clinical response and tolerability. Increasing the daily dose above 4 g does not usually result in improved efficacy. The duration of the effects of the drug is dependent on the rate of resynthesis of GABA transaminase rather than the concentration of the drug in the plasma.

The recommended daily starting dose is 1 g in children aged 3–9 years and 2 g in older children. In the elderly a reduction in dosage may be necessary in patients with impaired renal function.

ADVERSE DRUG REACTIONS

Adverse drug reactions are central nervous system related and are probably a result of the increased GABA levels caused by vigabatrin.

NEUROLOGICAL DISORDERS

25

The following effects, although not yet established as caused by vigabatrin, have been reported: drowsiness and fatigue, dizziness, nervousness, irritability, depression, headache and, less commonly, psychosis, confusion, memory disturbances and vision complaints, e.g. diplopia (double vision). The sedative effect of vigabatrin decreases with continuing treatment.

Other adverse reactions reported include minor gastrointestinal side effects and weight gain. Excitation and agitation have been seen in children.

As with other antiepileptic drugs, some patients (especially those with myoclonic seizures) may experience an increase in seizure frequency with vigabatrin. There is no evidence of neurotoxicity in humans.

DRUG INTERACTIONS

As vigabatrin is not metabolised or protein bound and does not induce hepatic metabolising enzymes it is thought that interactions with other drugs are unlikely. However, a gradual reduction of about 20% in plasma phenytoin concentration has been observed when used with vigabatrin. The mechanism of this is not understood but it is thought unlikely to be of therapeutic significance.

No clinically significant interactions have been seen with phenobarbitone, carbamazepine or sodium valproate in clinical trials.

PRECAUTIONS AND CONTRAINDICATIONS

As vigabatrin is eliminated by the kidneys caution should be observed when administering to elderly patients with reduced renal function.

Vigabatrin has caused intramyelinic oedema in the brain white matter tracts in animal studies. While there is no evidence to suggest that this happens in humans it is recommended that patients treated with vigabatrin should be closely observed for adverse effects including those of neurological function.

Drowsiness has been observed in clinical trials and patients should be warned of this possibility and advised against driving a motor vehicle, operating machinery or performing any hazardous tasks.

Lamotrigine

Lamotrigine is a new antiepileptic drug. Chemically it is a phenyltriazine compound unrelated to other drugs presently used for epilepsy.

TRADE NAMES

Lamotrigine: *Lamictal.*

MECHANISM OF ACTION

Lamotrigine acts by stabilising neuronal membranes and inhibiting neurotransmitter release, especially glutamate, the excitatory amino acid which plays a key role in the generation of epileptic seizures.

PHARMACOKINETICS

Lamotrigine is rapidly and completely absorbed from the gastrointestinal tract. Its elimination half-life is 29 hours. Lamotrigine induces its own metabolism leading to a 25% decrease in its elimination half-life.

It is metabolised in the liver and 94% is excreted in the urine. Of this, 65% is the major metabolite and 8% is unchanged lamotrigine. Lamotrigine is 55% bound to plasma proteins.

USES

Lamotrigine is used in the treatment of partial seizures and generalised tonic-clonic seizures not satisfactorily controlled with other antiepileptic drugs.

It is available as tablets in strengths of 25 mg, 50 mg, 100 mg and 200 mg. The dosage in adults and children over 12 years of age is 50 mg twice a day for the first two weeks. The usual maintenance dose is:

Patients taking enzyme inducing antiepileptic drugs (e.g. carbamazepine, phenytoin, phenobarbitone and primidone): 200–400 mg per day given in two individual doses;

Patients taking sodium valproate as well as enzyme inducing antiepileptic drugs:

100–200 mg per day given in two individual doses; and patients taking sodium valproate alone: 100–200 mg per day given in two individual doses. However, because of limited experience the dosage for this group of patients should be chosen with great caution.

Use in children under 12 years of age is not recommended as there is, as yet, insufficient information for this patient group.

ADVERSE DRUG REACTIONS

Skin rashes, usually maculopapular in appearance, occurred in 10% of patients taking this drug in clinical trials. These resolved on withdrawal of the drug. Very rarely the skin rashes included angiodema and Stevens-Johnson syndrome.

Other adverse reactions have included dizziness, headache, diplopia, ataxia, somnolence, nausea, asthenia, amblyopia, vomiting, rhinitis and pharyngitis.

DRUG INTERACTIONS

Antiepileptic drugs (e.g. phenytoin, carbamazepine, phenobarbitone and primidone) which induce drug metabolising liver enzymes, enhance the metabolism of lamotrigine. Sodium valproate, which inhibits drug metabolising liver enzymes, reduces the metabolism of lamotrigine.

PRECAUTIONS AND CONTRAINDICATIONS

Elderly patients should be treated with caution and monitored closely. Due to insufficient data it is recommended that lamotrigine should not be used in pregnancy unless the potential benefits of treatment of the mother outweigh any possible risk to the developing fetus.

Gabapentin

TRADE NAMES

Gabapentin: *Neurontin.*

MECHANISM OF ACTION

Gabapentin has an unknown mechanism of action which is apparently not like that of the other antiepileptic drugs. Although it is a structurally related analogue of the neuro-transmitter GABA and was specifically designed with increased lipophilicity to enable its penetration of the blood brain barrier. It does not exert its antiepileptic effect via GABA related mechanisms. It is thought it may bind to a site linked to L-amino acid transport.

PHARMACOKINETICS

Gabapentin is widely distributed in body tissues and has a large volume of distribution. It is not bound to human plasma proteins.

The drug is not metabolised and is eliminated by renal clearance. Drug clearance is reduced in renal impairment, raising plasma gabapentin levels.

The elimination half-life of gabapentin is about 5–7 hours after a single oral dose of 200–400 mg.

The drug is not protein bound and does not induce liver enzymes. Absorption is not affected by food.

USES

Gabapentin has proved useful as add-on therapy in patients with partial epilepsy resistant to conventional treatment. Gabapentin appears particularly useful to patients with complex partial seizures and partial seizures secondarily generalised. Experience with the drug in other seizure types is limited at this time.

The usual does is 900–1800 mg of gabapentin daily divided into three doses given every eight hours. Dosages up to 2400 mg/day may be necessary and are usually well tolerated. In patients with impaired renal function, reduced dosage is necessary.

Withdrawal of the drug or the addition of other antiepileptic drugs should be achieved slowly to avoid rebound seizures.

ADVERSE DRUG REACTION

Somnolence, dizziness, ataxia and fatigue are the most common adverse effects observed during therapy.

DRUG INTERACTIONS

Because of the absence of metabolic clearance, inability to induce liver enzymes and

NEUROLOGICAL DISORDERS

25

lack of protein binding, drug interactions with other antiepileptic drugs have not been a problem. The pharmacokinetics of gabapentin are not modified by antiepileptic drugs and the pharmacokinetics of antiepileptic drugs such as valproate, phenobarbitone, carbamazepine, phenytoin and oral contraceptives are not influenced by gabapentin.

DRUGS FOR ABSENCE SEIZURES

Succinimides: Ethosuximide, Methsuximide, Phensuximide

The succinimide drugs were developed for use in petit mal in the search for drugs with minimal side effects. This group includes ethosuximide (the best known drug in the group), methsuximide and phensuximide.

TRADE NAMES

Ethosuximide: *Zarontin.*
Methsuximide: *Celontin.*
Phensuximide: *Milontin.*

MECHANISM OF ACTION

The mode of action of the succinimides is not fully understood.

PHARMACOKINETICS

Ethosuximide is readily absorbed from the gastrointestinal tract and hydroxylated in the liver to a metabolite which is thought to be inactive. About one-fifth of the drug is secreted unchanged in the urine with the rest excreted in the form of metabolites.

The drug is widely distributed throughout the body and not significantly bound to plasma proteins. The half-life is reported to be about 60 hours in adults and 30 hours in children. It has been suggested that monitoring plasma levels is of help in maintaining control.

Ethosuximide crosses the placenta and is secreted in breast milk.

USES

The succinimides are used in the treatment of petit mal (absence) seizures. They may be used in conjunction with other antiepileptics when other kinds of seizures are present but, as they may may cause an increase in tonic-clonic seizures, the dose of the other drug may need to be adjusted.

Methsuximide and phensuximide are generally similar to ethosuximide, however, phensuximide is reported to be less effective while methsuximide has some action in complex partial seizures.

The dosage for ethosuximide is: under 6 years: initially 250 mg orally daily in two divided doses; then increase dose by 250 mg every 4–7 days to 1 g daily until control of seizures is obtained; 6 years and over: initially 500 mg daily; then increase dose by 250 mg every 4–7 days to 1.5–2.0 g until control of seizures is obtained. At higher doses strict monitoring is necessary.

The dosage for methsuximide is: initially 300 mg daily as a single oral dose increasing by 300 mg at weekly intervals until control of seizures is obtained. Maximum recommended daily dose is 1.2 g.

The dosage for phensuximide is: 0.5–1 g, two to three times daily orally.

ADVERSE DRUG REACTIONS

These drugs may induce major seizures if there is a tendency to this condition so it may be necessary to combine them with another drug effective against major epilepsy.

Adverse drug reactions include gastrointestinal effects such as nausea, vomiting, anorexia, gastric upset and abdominal pain.

Other effects reported are lethargy, drowsiness, headache, dizziness, euphoria and hiccup. Abnormal values for liver and renal function, personality changes, depression, psychosis, skin rashes, lupus erythematosis, various blood disorders including pancytopenia, leucopenia and (rarely) bone marrow depression have also been reported.

DRUG INTERACTIONS

An interaction has been reported with isoniazid.

PRECAUTIONS AND CONTRAINDICATIONS
The succinimides should be used with extreme caution in the presence of hepatic or renal failure.

Sodium Valproate

Sodium valproate and semisodium valproate are effective in the treatment of absence seizures (petit mal), see earlier section on sodium valproate.

DRUGS FOR STATUS EPILEPTICUS

Diazepam, Clonazepam, Phenytoin, Paraldehyde, Thiopentone Sodium, Chlormethiazole

Status epilepticus is a medical emergency. Immediate management involves ensuring ventilation, establishing an intravenous line and terminating seizure activity. Intravenous diazepam 5–10 mg should be given over 1–2 minutes. The seizures may stop by the time the injection is completed. The dose may be repeated at 10–15 minute intervals until a total of 30 mg has been given. In children, doses of 1 mg every 2–5 minutes may be given up to a maximum of 10 mg in children more than five years of age, with about half this dose being given to children under five years. As the effect of diazepam may be of short duration phenytoin should also be given intravenously as a loading dose of 10–15 mg/kg at a rate of 50 mg/minute for adults. Doses for children vary according to weight.

Clonazepam (1–4 mg intravenously) is sometimes given instead of diazepam. It has a longer effect than diazepam but side effects such as respiratory depression and sedation may be more pronounced than with diazepam. Intramuscular paraldehyde has been used but it is not favoured because of its toxicity and odour.

If these methods fail to control status epilepticus, short acting barbiturate anaesthesia with thiopentone sodium may be tried. In refractory cases, chlormethiazole infusion has been used with success.

POST-TRAUMATIC EPILEPSY

Seizures may begin any time up to 24 months after trauma. This applies in about 10% of severe closed head injuries and 40% of penetrating head wounds. Patients with such injuries should receive prophylactic anticonvulsants (e.g. phenytoin 100 mg three times daily) for up to three years to reduce the risk of seizures. Anticonvulsants (e.g. phenytoin 300–400 mg per day) may be given after skull fractures to protect against seizures.

Osmotic diuretics (urea, mannitol, glycerol) given intravenously to reduce cerebral oedema should be reserved for preoperative use in patients with haematomas or those whose condition is deteriorating. The benefit of corticosteroid therapy is questionable.

NURSING IMPLICATIONS

ADMINISTRATION

The use of anticonvulsants is aimed at controlling seizures. Several types of anticonvulsants may be administered concurrently in an effort to obtain stability. The nurse should ensure that the drugs are given at the prescribed times to avoid inappropriate fluctuations in plasma concentrations. It is essential that therapeutic blood levels be reached and maintained. This may take several days or weeks and the length of time required will vary depending on the drug. The nurse should ensure that blood samples are taken at the correct time, usually immediately before a dose. Anticonvulsants should not be suddenly withdrawn.

25 NEUROLOGICAL DISORDERS

EVALUATION

Patients should be monitored closely for control of seizures and adverse reactions to anticonvulsant therapy. If a particular anticonvulsant is causing an adverse effect a different drug should be considered.

PATIENT EDUCATION

Many epileptics have experienced rejection, socially, from potential employers or, if the patient happens to be a child, from parents who cannot understand why their child has been afflicted in this way. There are still enormous misconceptions about epilepsy in the community which on the whole regards the disease as a mental disorder. Nurses can do much to educate patients, their relatives and the community about epilepsy.

When a patient is taking anticonvulsants it is essential that the following points be stressed:

- Most seizures are caused by non-compliance with medication regimens. It is therefore important that patients being treated for epilepsy know to take their medication as ordered and that they be given encouragement to do so. The reduction in the frequency of attacks will add immeasurably to their quality of life. It should also be stressed that the dose should not be altered without consulting a medical officer, that sudden discontinuation may induce seizures and in some cases status epilepticus, and that they should maintain an adequate supply of medication at all times.

- Although it is usually preferable to continue anticonvulsant medication during pregnancy (the risk to both mother and fetus of uncontrolled seizures may be more serious than the effects of the drug) women taking anticonvulsants should discuss the risks associated with pregnancy with their physician prior to attempting conception.

- Regular blood tests for therapeutic blood levels of anticonvulsants and haematological disorders should be carried out.

- The patient and relatives should be informed of known adverse and toxic effects and advised to see a physician should these occur.

- If drowsiness occurs, patients should avoid activities which are potentially hazardous such as driving a motor vehicle or using machinery. Patients should be advised about driving and licensing requirements in different States. If taking barbiturates the patient should be advised to rise slowly from the recumbent position.

- The urine may change colour with the use of phenytoin.

- Patients should be informed of the many potential drug interactions between anticonvulsants and other medications that may be administered concurrently. The concurrent use of alcohol is usually contraindicated as alcohol is known to lower the seizure threshold.

- Patients receiving anticonvulsant medication should wear or carry a medical identification tag.

PARKINSONISM

Parkinsonism is a neurological disorder which manifests as disturbances of posture, rigidity, tremor and hypokinesia (abnormally decreased muscular movement). It has been recognised as a disease entity for over 150 years and is a fairly common disorder. It has been said that it may affect as many as one in every 100 of the population over 70 years of age, although this figure has been disputed.

The disease symptoms are due to changes in the brain, i.e. a reduction of dopamine receptors and cell loss in the substantia nigra. The two systems controlling movement become out of balance so that the dopaminergic system is defective and the cholinergic system is dominant. Drug treatment can therefore be utilised to restore the dopaminergic system (with levodopa, bromocriptine, selegiline, amantadine) or depress the cholinergic system (with anticholinergic drugs, e.g. benzhexol, benztropine).

DRUGS FOR PARKINSONISM

Levodopa

Levodopa (L-dopa) is the drug of first choice in the treatment of parkinsonism. Dopamine is not effective as it is poorly absorbed from the gut and does not cross the blood-brain barrier, whereas levodopa, the immediate precursor to dopamine in the biochemical chain leading to noradrenaline, does.

TRADE NAMES

Levodopa with benserazide: *Madopar Q*; *Madopar M*; *Madopar, Madopar HBS*. Levodopa with carbidopa: *Sinemet*; *Sinemet-M*; *Sinemet 100/25*; *Sinemet-CR*.

MECHANISM OF ACTION

Levodopa (L-dopa) is acted on by the enzyme decarboxylase to produce dopamine. (See Figure 25.1)

Levodopa acts by replenishing dopamine in the corpus striatum. The beneficial response is related to the amount of dopamine present. Levodopa does not cure the disease. It acts as replacement therapy much the same as insulin in diabetes. Levodopa tablets have been taken off the market in Australia. It is now only available in combination with decarboxylase inhibitors.

Decarboxylase inhibitors combined with levodopa provided an advance in the treatment of parkinsonism. Carbidopa is a decarboxylase inhibitor which does not pass the blood-brain barrier. By combining it with levodopa, the peripheral breakdown of levodopa to dopamine by the enzyme decarboxylase does not take place. This conversion then cannot occur until the drug reaches the brain where the carbidopa is excluded by the blood-brain barrier.

As levodopa is not acted on until it reaches its target organ (the brain) a much smaller dose is needed (approximately only 20% of that required if levodopa was taken alone). This leads to a corresponding reduction in some side effects, e.g. nausea and vomiting. This particular combination of drugs is marketed as *Sinemet*. Benserazide, another decarboxylase inhibitor, is used in the combination product *Madopar*.

NEUROLOGICAL DISORDERS

25

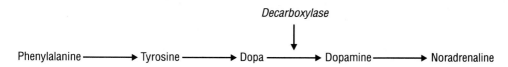

FIGURE 25.1 Levodopa acted upon by the enzyme decarboxylase

PHARMACOKINETICS

Levodopa is absorbed from the gastrointestinal tract, mainly from the small intestine, only a small amount (about 2%) being excreted in the faeces. It is decarboxylated rapidly to dopamine and is about 80% excreted in the urine mainly as metabolites. Some levodopa is metabolised to 3-O-methyldopa and noradrenaline. Levodopa is actively transported across the blood brain barrier but, because of its rapid peripheral decarboxylation, very little finds its way into the central nervous system unless it is given with a decarboxylase inhibitor.

USES

Levodopa is generally more effective in the treatment of hypokinesia (abnormally decreased muscular movement) than in the treatment of rigidity and tremor. Although the majority of patients benefit from the use of levodopa, improvement in mobility is often lost after two years or so as the disease progresses.

Levodopa should be taken after meals. A suggested initial dose is 125 mg orally twice daily, increased gradually every four days according to response to a dose between 1 g and 8 g daily in divided doses. Some patients need shorter dose intervals than others to avoid fluctuations in mobility.

Levodopa is now routinely given with a peripheral decarboxylase inhibitor so that lower doses may be used. Patients on the combination drugs need careful monitoring as both the beneficial and adverse effects tend to occur more rapidly than with levodopa alone.

A dose of 75 mg of carbidopa daily has been recommended for full inhibition of peripheral dopa decarboxylase. The initial dose of levodopa given with carbidopa should be about 20% of the dose of levodopa previously taken alone. The levodopa–carbidopa combination is available in three strengths: levodopa 250 mg + carbidopa 25 mg (*Sinemet*), levodopa 100 mg + carbidopa 25 mg (*Sinemet 100/25*), levodopa 100 mg + carbidopa 10 mg (*Sinemet-M*), and as a controlled release formulation containing levodopa 200 mg + carbidopa 50 mg (*Sinemet-CR*) for use in patients with greatly fluctuating symptoms.

With the levodopa–benserazide combination the ratio given is usually one part of benserazide base to four parts of levodopa. The initial dose of levodopa should be about 15% of that taken alone. The suggested initial dose is benserazide 25 mg with levodopa 100 mg, increasing to a maintenance dose according to response. It is rarely necessary to exceed benserazide 250 mg and levodopa 1 g daily. The levodopa–benserazide combination is available in three strengths: levodopa 50 mg + benserazide 12.5 mg (*Madopar Q*), levodopa 100 mg + benserazide 25 mg (*Madopar M*), levodopa 200 mg + benserazide 50 mg (*Madopar*) and as a controlled release capsule containing levodopa 100 mg + benserazide 25 mg (*Madopar HBS*).

ADVERSE DRUG REACTIONS

Adverse effects include gastrointestinal effects, especially anorexia, nausea and vomiting, postural hypotension, involuntary movements of face and lips, cardiac arrhythmias and psychiatric symptoms which occur commonly in the elderly. Other effects include anxiety, agitation, euphoria, insomnia, drowsiness and depression.

More serious effects which may lead to withdrawal of levodopa or reduction in dosage include aggression, hallucinations, delerium, paranoid delusions, severe depression with possible suicidal behaviour and unmasking of dementia.

DRUG INTERACTIONS

Monoamine oxidase inhibitors (MAOIs) decrease dopamine and noradrenaline degradation resulting in an increase of these amines, possibly leading to dangerous hypertension. It is advised that levodopa not be given for at least 14 days after ceasing the MAOI.

Anticholinergics, when administered in sufficiently large doses, may decrease gastric motility and inhibit levodopa absorption, thereby reducing its efficacy. Metoclopramide accelerates gastric emptying and has been reported to increase the rate of absorption of levodopa.

Tranquillisers such as phenothiazines (e.g. chlorpromazine), phenothiazine antihistamines (e.g. promethazine), butyrophenones (e.g. haloperidol) and tetrabenazine diminish the effect of levodopa by acting as dopamine inhibitors in the central nervous system.

Antihypertensive agents may cause additive hypotension. Clonidine has been reported to inhibit the therapeutic effect of levodopa. Benzodiazepines and phenytoin may reduce the effect of levodopa. The mechanism whereby this occurs is not fully understood.

Pyridoxine lowers the therapeutic effect of levodopa, acting as a coenzyme in the decarboxylation of levodopa to dopamine in the peripheral circulation hence leaving less levodopa to penetrate the brain. However, pyridoxine does not appear to antagonise levodopa in the presence of decarboxylase inhibitors.

PRECAUTIONS AND CONTRAINDICATIONS

Levodopa therapy should be administered with caution to patients receiving cardiovascular drugs. Such patients should be monitored closely at the beginning of therapy. It should also be administered with caution to patients with diabetes mellitis, psychiatric disturbances, open angle glaucoma or duodenal ulcers.

Tests for cardiovascular, haematological, renal or hepatic function should be performed periodically.

It has been recommended that levodopa not be given to patients with a history of malignant melanoma. The activation of malignant melanoma by levodopa is only suspected.

Patients who benefit from levodopa should be warned to resume normal activities gradually to avoid accidents. If therapy is to be withdrawn, it should be done gradually.

Levodopa is contraindicated in patients with closed angle glaucoma.

Bromocriptine

Bromocriptine has been widely used in the treatment of Parkinson's disease. It is an ergot derivative with a direct stimulating effect on dopaminergic receptors.

TRADE NAMES

Bromocriptine: *Parlodel.*

MECHANISM OF ACTION

Bromocriptine is a dopamine agonist acting at receptors in the central nervous system, cardiovascular system, pituitary and hypothalamic axis and gastrointestinal tract.

PHARMACOKINETICS

Bromocriptine is absorbed incompletely from the gastrointestinal tract, metabolised in the liver and excreted mainly in the bile.

USES

Because of its dopaminergic activity bromocriptine is used in the treatment of idiopathic or postencephalitic Parkinson's disease. It also inhibits the secretion of prolactin from the anterior pituitary and has been used for the suppression of physiological lactation and infertility (see Chapter 20 Drug Therapy in Pregnancy and Labour and Chapter 21 Contraception and Infertility).

USES

A bromocriptine dosage of 3.5–10 mg daily is approximately as effective as 100 mg of levodopa plus a decarboxylase inhibitor. However, some patients may need doses of up to 40 mg daily. The combined use of bromocriptine with a levodopa–decarboxylase inhibitor is very effective. When being introduced into a levodopa–decarboxylase regimen the dose of bromocriptine should be increased gradually while decreasing the dose of levodopa until an optimum response is obtained.

ADVERSE DRUG REACTIONS

High doses of bromocriptine may lead to nausea, vomiting and dyskinesia. Patients showing evidence of loss of higher integrative

NEUROLOGICAL DISORDERS

25

function or dementia are prone to the side effects of mental clouding and confusion. These are usually dose related. If the drug is stopped and a more gradual increase in dosage is instigated these side effects may resolve.

Nausea may be lessened by taking the drug with food. Cardiovascular side effects include vasospasm in the fingers and toes induced by cold and cramps (bromocriptine is a vasoconstrictor), severe hypotension, arrhythmias and exacerbation of angina.

Other adverse effects include dyskinesias, nasal congestion, headache, drowsiness, dryness of mouth, constipation, diarrhoea and altered liver function tests.

PRECAUTIONS AND CONTRAINDICATIONS

Patients who drive or operate machinery should be warned of the possibility of dizziness and fainting during the first few days of treatment with bromocriptine.

Bromocriptine should be given with caution to patients with cardiovascular disease, liver disease or a history of psychotic disorders. For patients receiving long-term therapy, liver function tests and annual check-ups for postmenopausal women have been recommended.

Selegiline Hydrochloride

TRADE NAMES

Selegiline hydrochloride: *Eldepryl*.

MECHANISM OF ACTION

Selegiline at therapeutic doses is a selective inhibitor of cerebral monoamine oxidase type B (MAO-B). It does not normally cause MAO-A hypertensive reactions such as the 'cheese reaction' (see MAOIs Chapter 26 Psychiatric Disorders). MAO-B constitutes about 80% of the total human brain MAO activity resulting in the breakdown of dopamine. By inhibiting this breakdown selegiline increases the amount of dopamine available.

There is some evidence that selegiline may also act through other mechanisms such as inhibition of dopamine re-uptake.

PHARMACOKINETICS

Absorption of selegiline from the gastrointestinal tract is relatively rapid with peak metabolite serum concentrations reached in 0.5–2.0 hours. The metabolites are measured as the concentration of the parent drug in the serum or urine is too low to be detected by currently available analytical methods.

The drug is distributed rapidly and extensively, crosses the blood brain barrier with ease and is 94% bound to plasma proteins at therapeutic concentrations. Selegiline is extensively metabolised, mainly in the liver, and 86% is excreted as metabolites in the urine of patients with Parkinson's disease.

USES

With the progression of Parkinson's disease the response to a given dose of sustained levodopa treatment 'wears off' over a period of years and side effects develop. This is thought to be due to the inability of the decreasing neurones to synthesise and release adequate amounts of dopamine. Selegiline, by inhibiting MAO-B, increases the pool of dopamine available. The breakdown of dopamine by MAO-B has been shown to be reduced by a mean of 92% in patients with Parkinson's disease receiving selegiline as well as levodopa when compared with those receiving levodopa alone. Thus, selegiline has been found to be of great benefit as an adjunct to levodopa therapy as the response to levodopa begins to lessen.

Selegiline appears to be of benefit in 70% of cases. It is particularly useful in treating the end-of-dose disturbances such as akinesia, early morning and nocturnal akinesia, and the 'on-off' phenomenon experienced after long-term treatment with levodopa.

The recommended oral dose of selegiline is 5 mg twice daily, with breakfast and at midday to avoid possible insomnia, nausea and dizziness. A reduction in levodopa dosage of about 10%–30% may be possible without losing control of symptoms. The daily dosage of 10 mg should not be exceeded without restricting intake of tyramine containing substances such as cheese or common cold remedies because of non-specific MAO inhibition leading to a hypertensive crisis.

ADVERSE DRUG REACTIONS

Selegiline is generally well tolerated. Most adverse reactions are probably caused by increased dopaminergic activity and can often be managed by a reduction in levodopa dosage. Side effects have included increased dyskinesias, nausea, dizziness, confusion, hypotension, insomnia, vivid dreams, anxiety, akathisia, hallucinations, dry mouth and psychosis.

DRUG INTERACTIONS

Selegiline combined with other non-selective MAOIs may cause severe hypotension.

Ataxia, agitation, shivering and mania have been reported with the concomitant use of selegiline and fluoxetine. Because of the long half-life of fluoxetine and its active metabolite at least five weeks should be allowed between discontinuation of fluoxetine and initiation of selegiline therapy. When discontinuing selegiline therapy and initiating therapy with fluoxetine, a two week period would be sufficient because of the short half-life of selegiline and its active metabolites.

Delirium, stupor, agitation and muscular rigidity have been reported with the concomitant use of selegiline and pethidine. Although the mechanism of this possible interaction is poorly understood, it is advisable to avoid the use of selegiline concurrently with pethidine.

PRECAUTIONS AND CONTRAINDICATIONS

Some patients may experience exacerbation of levodopa side effects when also taking selegiline. These effects may often be alleviated by reducing the dose of levodopa by 10%–30%.

Selegiline should be given cautiously to patients with peptic or duodenal ulcer, cardiac arrhythmias, severe angina pectoris, labile hypertension or psychosis.

Selegiline should not be used at daily doses exceeding those recommended (10 mg per day) because of the risks associated with non-selective inhibition of MAO. The selectivity for MAO-B may not be absolute, even at the recommended daily dose of 10 mg per day, and selectivity is further diminished as daily doses are increased.

Selegiline is contraindicated in patients with a known hypersensitivity to the drug and whenever levodopa therapy is contraindicated.

Amantadine

Amantadine is an antiviral drug which was discovered to be of benefit in parkinsonism when given to a parkinsonian patient for influenza.

TRADE NAMES

Amantadine: *Symmetrel*; *Antadine*.

MECHANISM OF ACTION

Amantadine is thought to act by increasing dopamine synthesis.

PHARMACOKINETICS

Amantadine is readily absorbed from the gastrointestinal tract and peak blood concentrations are observed in about four hours. It is distributed widely into body tissues and fluids, including the cerebrospinal fluid. It is mainly excreted unchanged in the urine. It is also excreted in breast milk. The drug has an average half-life of 15 hours.

USES

Amantadine is used in the early stages of Parkinson's disease when symptoms of dysarthria (impairment of articulation, stammering), loss of manual dexterity and disorders of gait predominate. It has a relatively limited usefulness.

Treatment is usually started with 100 mg daily, increasing to 100 mg twice daily after a week. Doses up to 400 mg have occasionally been used.

ADVERSE DRUG REACTIONS

Most adverse reactions are fairly mild and are dose related. They may be reversed by withdrawing the drug but often resolve if the drug is continued. Parkinsonian patients receiving amantadine commonly experience blue or purple mottling of the skin, sometimes associated with ankle oedema. Central nervous system symptoms such as nervousness, inability to concentrate, dizziness, insomnia and mood changes may occur while psychotic reactions such as confusion and hallucinations have been reported, especially in patients with impaired renal function.

DRUG INTERACTIONS

Amantadine given to patients on anticholinergic drugs such as benzhexol or orphenadrine has caused increased adverse anticholinergic effects including hallucinations. The combination of amantadine and central nervous system stimulants (e.g. dexamphetamine, caffeine) can result in increased central nervous system stimulant effects and is best avoided.

PRECAUTIONS AND CONTRAINDICATIONS

Caution should be exercised when amantadine is given to patients with cardiovascular or liver disease, impaired renal function, psychosis, recurrent eczema and in elderly patients. Amantadine therapy should not be stopped abruptly.

The dose of anticholinergic drugs such as benzhexol and orphenadrine needs to be reduced when prescribed with amantadine to reduce the adverse effects.

The use of amantadine is contraindicated in patients with severe renal disease or a history of epilepsy or gastric ulceration and in pregnant women and nursing mothers.

Anticholinergic Agents: Benzhexol, Biperiden, Benztropine, Orphenadrine, Procyclidine

Anticholinergic therapy for Parkinson's disease is the oldest form of drug therapy, introduced by Charcot in 1867.

TRADE NAMES

Benzhexol: *Artane.*
Biperiden: *Akineton.*

Benztropine: *Cogentin.*
Orphenadrine: *Norflex, Disipal.*
Procyclidine: *Kemadrin.*

MECHANISM OF ACTION

These drugs reduce cholinergic activity, thereby reducing the dominance of the cholinergic system present in parkinsonism. They act by blocking acetylcholine in the central nervous system. When symptoms are mild (rigidity and tremor with little or no gait disorder or akinesia) anticholinergics may be useful.

PHARMACOKINETICS

These drugs tend to be readily absorbed from the gastrointestinal tract, distributed in the tissues and are excreted in the urine. The bioavailability varies, e.g. biperiden is 29% bioavailable while procyclidine is 72.5% bioavailable.

USES

These drugs are used mainly for the symptomatic treatment of parkinsonism. The extrapyramidal syndrome induced by phenothiazines and other drugs may also be treated with this group of drugs. However, they are of no use in the slow and impaired power of voluntary movement often seen in parkinsonism.

Biperiden has more antinicotinic properties than benzhexol, while benztropine and orphenadrine have additional antihistaminic and local anaesthetic properties. Procyclidine controls rigidity more effectively than it controls tremor.

The dosage of these drugs must be built up or withdrawn gradually in the treatment of parkinsonism. Therapy should never be terminated suddenly. It is usual when changing from one drug to another to build up one drug while withdrawing the other gradually.

ADVERSE DRUG REACTIONS

Adverse reactions may occur from accumulation of the drug leading to a toxic state with confusion, which may be wrongly attributed to the disease. Incipient glaucoma may be precipitated. Other side effects include dryness of mouth, urinary hesitancy or retention, nausea and drowsiness.

Reactions common to this whole group of drugs include dilation of pupils and loss of accommodation and photophobia, dryness of mouth with difficulty in swallowing and talking, thirst, transient tachycardia, palpitations and arrhythmias, urinary urgency, retention, and reduction of tone of the gastrointestinal tract leading to constipation.

Mental confusion, excitement, nausea and vomiting have also been reported. Elderly and brain damaged patients may exhibit confusion. For minor reactions the dosage may be reduced until tolerance has developed. With more severe reactions the drug should be discontinued for several days and then treatment resumed with the same or another drug.

These drugs have been abused by young schizophrenic patients. Acute brain syndrome has been reported in several patients.

DRUG INTERACTIONS

The effects of this group of drugs are enhanced by other drugs with a similar effect, e.g. amantidine, some antihistamines, phenothiazines, butyrophenones and tricyclic antidepressants. Absorption of other drugs may be reduced because of the reduction in gastric motility caused by anticholinergic agents.

PRECAUTIONS AND CONTRAINDICATIONS

Caution should be exercised when giving these drugs to children and the elderly, patients with diarrhoea, fever, conditions characterised by tachycardia (such as thyrotoxicosis, cardiac insufficiency) or in cardiac surgery where an increase in heart rate would be deleterious. Patients with atherosclerosis are more likely to have severe mental disturbances.

Anticholinergics are contraindicated in patients with known hypersensitivity to these drugs.

Extreme caution should be exercised when these drugs are given to patients with myasthenia gravis.

These drugs are contraindicated in patients with closed angle glaucoma or a narrow angle between the iris and the cornea, in ambient high temperatures, and in patients with acute myocardial infarction.

NURSING IMPLICATIONS

ASSESSMENT

Assessment should begin with a review of the patient's history for the diagnosed cause of the parkinsonian symptoms. Dopaminergic drugs should not be administered to patients whose parkinsonian symptoms are secondary to the use of neuroleptic drugs. Also, confirmation of the order from the prescriber should be sought if the history shows evidence of psychoses of any kind, confusional states, postural hypotension, endocrine, cardiac, renal or hepatic impairment, diabetes or glaucoma. The patient's drug use should be reviewed for concurrent use of MAOIs, tricyclic antidepressants or other sympathomimetic type drugs. Antipsychotic agents are contraindicated because of possible interactions.

Physical assessment should include establishing baseline observations of blood pressure (standing and lying), pulse rate, features of parkinsonism (degree of joint movement, tremor, rigidity, ambulation, daily living activities and emotional state) and colour and temperature of extremities.

ADMINISTRATION

To avoid unpleasant gastrointestinal side effects, dopaminergic drugs are best given with food.

EVALUATION

Evaluation should include documentation of drug effectiveness, i.e. both subjective and objective signs of improvement of parkinsonian symptoms. The patient

NEUROLOGICAL DISORDERS

25

should be observed for adverse effects such as postural hypotension, cardiac arrhythmias, poor peripheral circulation and urinary retention. Observations include monitoring blood pressure (lying and standing), pulse rate, colour and temperature of extremities and urinary output. Observation of the patient's mood and behaviour is essential for prompt identification of any undesirable emotional effects from the drug.

PATIENT EDUCATION

Education should involve the patient and the family. They should be taught the indications of drug effectiveness and adverse effects, and advised to report the latter to their physician. Over the counter cough and cold preparations containing sympathomimetic decongestants should be avoided in patients taking levodopa preparations. The patient and family also need to be advised that the urine and perspiration may become darkened and that the full effects of the drug may not be experienced for several months. Such advice provides reassurance and enhanced compliance.

Patients receiving doses of selegiline greater than 10 mg per day should be advised to avoid foods containing tyramine (see MAOIs Chapter 26 Psychiatric Disorders).

MIGRAINE

Migraine can be a disabling affliction and affects approximately 20% of the population, occurring on average in twice as many women as men and causing the loss of a large number of working days in the year. Migraine is usually a sudden form of headache which is associated with nausea, vomiting and photophobia. According to the National Health Survey 1989–90, in terms of lost activity, headache is five times more debilitating than all other neurological disorders together.

Migraine differs from the other forms of headache such as tension headaches which are not as severe or paroxysmal. It is a chronic, dull pressing sensation which may go on day after day. Sufferers may have a combination of the two kinds of headache, a dull continuous headache punctuated by episodes of the more severe migraine attacks. The insidious progression of headaches of increasing severity together with other neurological symptoms should be investigated for the possibility of intracranial tumour.

Following the recommendation of the International Headache Society in the 1980s, the old terms 'common migraine' and 'classical migraine with aura' were abandoned in favour of 'migraine without aura' and 'migraine with aura' respectively. These are now internationally recognised definitions.

Migraine with aura is often anteceded by visual disturbances such as blank flashing spots in the vision (fortification spectra), dysphasia and paraesthesia on one side of the body. Migraine without aura does not produce these symptoms. Migraine occurs most commonly in adults, between puberty and 65 years. It does, however, occur in children and in this group is often anteceded by abdominal pain and vomiting.

Trigger factors are wide ranging and may be emotional (e.g. stress or relaxation after stress), physical (exertion, head injury), hormonal (premenstrual) or even brought on by foods (e.g. cheese or red wine). Other factors are intrinsic body substances such as serotonin, bradykinin and histamine.

Non-drug treatment may include avoidance of precipitating factors (certain foods, situations and so on) and use of psychotherapy, physiotherapy and, in some cases, acupuncture. Drug treatment of migraine may be divided into long-term management and prevention and treatment of the acute attack.

DRUGS FOR LONG-TERM MANAGEMENT AND PREVENTION

Prophylactic drug treatment may be indicated if attacks occur more than twice each month. Drugs used are those which alter catecholamine action, antiserotonin drugs and others.

β Blocking Drugs

The β blocking drugs alter the effects of catecholamines and are used in the treatment of hypertension. During treatment of hypertension in patients who were migraine sufferers it was observed that some no longer seemed to have migraine attacks. Since then propranolol (*Inderal*) and pindolol (*Visken*) have been shown in clinical trials to be useful for prevention of migraine.

MECHANISM OF ACTION

These drugs were thought to act on the β adrenergic receptors. However, it has been shown that propranolol has an affinity for some 5-HT-like receptors, it is thought that this could be significant in their action in the prevention of migraine.

USES

The β adrenergic blocking drugs which have no intrinsic sympathomimetic activity, such as propranolol, atenolol, timolol, metoprolol, have proved beneficial for some patients in the prophylaxis of migraine.

For information on pharmacokinetics, adverse drug reactions, drug interactions, precautions and contraindications see β blocking drugs Chapter 12 Cardiovascular Diseases.

Clonidine

Clonidine alters the effects of catecholamines and is normally used to treat hypertension but has been used in small doses (25 micrograms) as *Dixarit* for long-term therapy of migraine.

MECHANISM OF ACTION

Clonidine appears to act centrally, by stimulating the α_2 adrenergic receptors, as well as peripherally.

USES

Clonidine (*Dixarit*) is sometimes used in small doses (25 micrograms) as long-term therapy for the prevention of migraine. It has been given a different trade name in the 25 micrograms dosage form from its counterpart used in hypertension (*Catapres* 150 micrograms) to avoid confusion. If a person taking *Catapres* for hypertension also has migraine it is of no value to give *Dixarit* as well.

For information on pharmacokinetics, adverse drug reactions, drug interactions, precautions and contraindications see clonidine Chapter 12 Cardiovascular Diseases.

Tricyclic Antidepressants

Tricyclic antidepressant drugs (e.g. amitriptyline) increase available 5-HT (serotonin) by blocking its uptake. There have been some encouraging results in reducing migraine using doses of 10–60 mg given at night. They are also useful for patients with both migraine and tension headache. Amitriptyline and dothiepin are thought to be the most effective.

For information on pharmacokinetcs, adverse drug reactions, drug interactions, precautions and contraindications see tricyclic antidepressants Chapter 26 Psychiatric Disorders.

Monoamine Oxidase Inhibitors

MAOIs (e.g. phenelzine, tranylcypromine) act by preventing the breakdown of both noradrenaline and serotonin (5-HT), thus making more of both of these neurotransmitters available. They have been shown in some studies to be useful in the prevention of migraine but unfortunately there are a large number of potentially dangerous side effects associated with the use of these drugs. They should probably only be tried after all other therapy has failed.

NEUROLOGICAL DISORDERS

25

For information on pharmacokinetics, adverse drug reactions, drug interactions, precautions and contraindications see MAOIs, Chapter 26 Psychiatric Disorders.

Antiserotonin Antihistamines: Cyproheptadine, Methdilazine, Pizotifen Malate

This group of drugs has proved helpful to some patients in the control of migraine attacks.

TRADE NAMES

Cyproheptadine: *Periactin*.
Methdilazine: *Dilosyn*.
Pizotifen malate: *Sandomigran*.

MECHANISM OF ACTION

These drugs are predominantly antagonists of the 5-HT$_2$ receptors.

PHARMACOKINETICS

These drugs are readily absorbed from the gastrointestinal tract, metabolised in the liver and excreted, usually as metabolites, in the urine. Small amounts may be excreted in the faeces.

USES

These drugs are used as prophylactic therapy. They have been given during the day but because of drowsiness they are now often given as a single dose at night. Usual doses are cyproheptadine: 4–8 mg three times daily; methdilazine: 8 mg twice daily; pizotifen malate: 0.5 mg three times daily.

ADVERSE DRUG REACTIONS

Cyproheptadine and pizotifen malate have appetite stimulating properties. This is possibly advantageous to some but disadvantageous to others and are best avoided in patients who tend to put on weight.

Other side effects common to all antihistamines include drowsiness, inability to concentrate, lassitude, dizziness, hypertension, muscle weakness and incoordination. Other effects may be gastrointestinal and include nausea, vomiting, diarrhoea or constipation and colic.

DRUG INTERACTIONS

Central nervous system depressants such as alcohol, barbiturates, hypnotics, narcotics or sedatives will enhance the sedative effect of these antihistamines. MAOIs will enhance the adverse antimuscarinic effects.

PRECAUTIONS AND CONTRAINDICATIONS

These drugs must be used with great care in conditions such as narrow angle glaucoma, urinary retention and prostatic hypertrophy. Patients should not drive or operate machinery and should abstain from alcohol whilst taking antihistamines.

Methysergide

Methysergide (*Deseril*) is an antiserotonin drug. It is a derivative of ergot and has been used effectively in the prophylactic treatment of migraine.

TRADE NAMES

Methysergide: *Deseril*.

MECHANISM OF ACTION

Methysergide is a 5-HT$_2$ antagonist with mixed actions on 5-HT receptors, being a partial agonist in some situations and an antagonist in others.

USES

Methysergide is a useful agent in the prophylactic treatment of migraine. It is ineffective in the treatment of the acute migraine attack.

Dosage is 2–6 mg methysergide base daily in divided doses, taken with meals. Dosage may be started at 1 mg at bedtime and built up gradually over two weeks to the minimum effective dose. It is suggested that courses of methysergide should be intermittent (e.g. one month off in every four to six). The drug should be used with extreme care and close monitoring.

ADVERSE DRUG REACTIONS

Gastrointestinal tract effects such as nausea, vomiting and abdominal pain are common. Central nervous system effects include dizziness, drowsiness, ataxia, insomnia, confusion, weakness, restlessness, euphoria, hallucinations and light headedness. Weight gain and joint and muscle pain have been reported.

A rare and serious adverse reaction is retroperitoneal fibrosis (obstructive renal disease) and peritoneal fibrosis, which may develop after prolonged use.

DRUG INTERACTIONS

An interaction between methysergide and a high parenteral dose of ergotamine has been reported. Methysergide and propranolol taken together have been implicated in causing gangrene.

PRECAUTIONS AND CONTRAINDICATIONS

In the presence of peptic ulcer the drug should be used with great caution. If fibrosis or arterial spasm develop methysergide should be withdrawn.

Methysergide is contraindicated in valvular heart disease, collagen and pulmonary diseases and in debilitated states.

Phenytoin

Phenytoin (*Dilantin*) is generally of little use except in migraine in children, when it can be extremely efficacious, and in adults with a rare type of migraine which has an aura of unilateral sensory symptoms or aphasia.

For information on pharmacokinetcs, adverse drug reactions, drug interactions, precautions and contraindications see the section on phenytoin and anticonvulsants.

Anxiolytics

Anxiolytics (e.g. benzodiazepines) can be useful for some people but generally do not appear to have much place in the treatment of migraine. There is little evidence to show they are any better than placebos.

For information on pharmacokinetics, adverse drug reactions, drug interactions, precautions and contraindications see benzodiazepines Chapter 26 Psychiatric Disorders.

Sex Hormones

Although it has been observed that migraine prone patients do not have migraine attacks while pregnant, the results of the use of oestrogens have proved disappointing. The increased risk of stroke with oestrogen therapy is another deterrent to therapy.

For information on pharmacokinetics, adverse drug reactions, drug interactions, precautions and contraindications see oestrogens Chapter 19 Endocrine Diseases.

When using these drugs for the prevention of migraine it is necessary to try the drug for a few weeks. If no response is obtained a larger dose should be used before another drug is tried. Dosage must be tailored to the individual patient's needs.

DRUGS FOR THE ACUTE ATTACK

Treatment of the acute attack of migraine may be divided into drug and non-drug treatment. A therapeutic atmosphere should be provided for the patient who is encouraged to sleep. Most patients respond well if they do so. Drug therapy of the acute attack of migraine can be divided into two broad categories: non-specific therapy to relieve the pain and specific therapy designed to abort the attack.

Analgesics: Aspirin, Paracetamol

Aspirin's action as an analgesic and antiprostaglandin agent is utilised in the treatment of migraine. It should be given in a dose of 900 mg (three tablets) using the soluble form for better and more rapid absorption. Paracetamol should be given in a dose of 1 g (2 tablets) using the soluble form. It is important that both aspirin and paracetamol be given in the soluble form as absorption is impaired during the acute attack of migraine because of gastric stasis.

Other mild analgesics, e.g. codeine, may be used in combination with aspirin or paracetamol.

For further information on these drugs see Chapter 23 Pain Relief.

Antiemetics: Metoclopramide, Prochlorperazine, Meclozine Hydrochloride

Metoclopramide (*Maxolon*) is the antiemetic of choice as it stimulates gastric motility and so counteracts gastric stasis encountered during an attack. It has central nervous effects but little effect on a normal stomach. It has been found to be of benefit in a migraine attack if a 10 mg dose is given by injection 10 minutes before a dose of aspirin or paracetamol. The absorption of the analgesic then becomes almost normal.

Other antiemetics used include prochlorperazine (*Stemetil*) and meclozine hydrochloride (*Ancolan*).

For further information on these drugs see Chapter 17 Gastrointestinal Disorders.

Ergotamine Tartrate

Ergot related substances have been used in the treatment of migraine for more than 60 years.

MECHANISM OF ACTION

Ergotamine has marked vasoconstrictor effects and so is helpful in migraine in constricting the blood vessels in the brain. It also causes peripheral vasoconstriction and nausea, as well as having a powerful effect on the uterus.

PHARMACOKINETICS

Ergotamine is incompletely absorbed from the gastrointestinal tract and there is considerable variation in the bioavailability of the drug. It is reported to be extensively metabolised in the liver and along with most of its metabolites is excreted in the bile. Ergotamine and its metabolites are reported to be secreted in breast milk.

USES

Ergotamine has been used in the treatment of the acute attack of migraine although it is not used as frequently now that prophylactic treatment of migraine has become more popular. However, it still has a place for patients with infrequent severe attacks.

If ergotamine is to be used it should be given as early in the attack as possible for best effect using as small a dose as possible. In subsequent attacks the total effective dose may be given immediately. The usual dose is 1–2 mg, repeated if necessary in one hour. The maximum total daily dose is 6 mg with a maximum of not more than 10 mg in a week.

Absorption by the various routes is variable in different individuals. Concurrent administration of caffeine is said to enhance the effect of ergotamine, so some dose forms are combined with this drug.

Preparations include: *Ergodryl Mono* capsules contain 1 mg ergotamine; *Cafergot* tablets contain 1 mg ergotamine combined with 100 mg caffeine, *Ergodryl* capsules contain the same combination plus an antihistamine; *Migral* tablets contain 2 mg ergotamine, 100 mg caffeine and an antihistamine; *Medihaler Ergotamine* as an aerosol delivery of 0.36 mg ergotamine per valve depression; *Dihydergot* is an injection containing dihydroergotamine 1 mg/mL.

ADVERSE DRUG REACTIONS

Adverse drug reactions include nausea, vomiting, paraesthesia and pain and weakness in the extremities. Peripheral vasoconstriction may occur at therapeutic doses in sensitive individuals.

Combinations of ergotamine and caffeine should be avoided at night as central nervous system stimulation may result from the caffeine content.

DRUG INTERACTIONS

A few reports of interactions have occurred with the concurrent administration of ergotamine and β blocking drugs. Ergotism has been reported with concurrent administration of ergotamine and erythromycin.

PRECAUTIONS AND CONTRAINDICATIONS

The vasoconstriction effects of ergotamine are enhanced by sympathomimetic agents such as adrenaline and ephedrine.

Ergotamine should not be given prophylactically as prolonged use may give rise to gangrene of the extremities.

OVERDOSAGE

No more than 6 mg per 24 hours or 10 mg per week of ergotamine should be taken. Patients should be warned to keep within the recommended dosage and that numbness or tingling of the extremities indicates toxicity and that generally ergotamine should be discontinued if these effects occur.

Symptoms of acute overdose include nausea, vomiting, diarrhoea, thirst, coldness, pruritus, rapid pulse, tachycardia, dizziness, numbness and tingling of the extremities and ultimately confusion and coma.

Treatment is symptomatic and includes gastric lavage, prevention of further absorption by administration of activated charcoal and treatment of arterial spasm with vasodilators such as sodium nitroprusside.

Long-term administration of doses exceeding 10–20 mg per week results in protracted headache and continued vasoconstriction (particularly of the extremities) which can ultimately lead to gangrene.

Sedatives

Most patients respond to treatment of the acute attack if they can go to sleep. This may be aided by use of a sedative such as diazepam 5–10 mg.

Sumatriptan

A recent breakthrough in the treatment of migraine attacks is the development of sumatriptan. It is claimed that 6 mg administered subcutaneously will relieve over 80% of migraine attacks and that a 100 mg dose taken orally will reliably and quickly relieve the acute attack in 50%–66% of patients.

TRADE NAMES

Sumatriptan: *Imigran.*

MECHANISM OF ACTION

During research on migraine patients in Sydney in the 1970s it was observed that platelet 5-HT (serotonin) dropped rapidly at the start of a migraine attack, that the urinary excretion of the major metabolite of serotonin increased and that intravenous administration of 5-HT would abort a spontaneous or response induced headache. Based on this research sumatriptan was designed to exert its effect as a highly selective and potent 5-HT-like receptor agonist.

The 5-HT receptor is found predominantly in cranial blood vessels and it has been shown in animals that sumatriptan selectively constricts the carotid arterial circulation which supplies blood to the extracranial and intracranial tissues such as the meninges. It is thought that the dilation of these vessels is the underlying cause of migraine in man.

Clinical response begins within 10 to 15 minutes following subcutaneous injection and around 30 minutes following oral administration of sumatriptan.

PHARMACOKINETICS

Peak serum concentrations occur within 25 minutes following a subcutaneous dose. The elimination half-life is 2 hours. Sumatriptan is rapidly absorbed from the gut, 70% of the maximum concentration occurring within 45 minutes. However the oral bioavailability is only about 14% due to first pass metabolism and incomplete absorption. The pharmacokinetics of the drug do not appear to be significantly affected by food. Sumatriptan is eliminated mainly by metabolism, while its major metabolite is excreted primarily in the urine.

USES

Sumatriptan is indicated for the acute intermittent relief of migraine with or without aura and cluster headache. It should not be used prophylactically. It acts quickly, within a few minutes of injection.

Sumatriptan is available as film coated tablets of 100 mg sumatriptan base or pre-filled syringes of 6 mg. An autoinjection device is also available. The oral form of the drug should be taken at the onset of an attack but is still effective when taken later. A second tablet may be necessary within 24 hours because of its short half-life. No more than three tablets may be taken in any 24 hour period. The subcutaneous injection of 6 mg may be repeated once only in a 24 hour period.

ADVERSE DRUG REACTIONS

Most common adverse drug reactions are a full flushed sensation (particularly in the head), chest pain and tightness (not associated with ECG changes). Other side effects include sensations of tingling, heaviness, pressure, heavy headedness or headache and light headedness. A most frequently reported symptom following subcutaneous injection is transient pain at the injection site. Also reported are mild transient nausea, vomiting and an odd taste sensation. Symptoms are usually transient and mild.

DRUG INTERACTIONS

A possible interaction with MAOIs has been suggested. There is little information available on interactions and no evidence of interactions with dihydroergotamine, pizotifen, alcohol or propanolol.

PRECAUTIONS AND CONTRAINDICATIONS

Additive vasospastic effects may occur if sumatriptan is given with ergotamine and concomitant use should be avoided.

In rare cases the transient chest pain which occurs after sumatriptan administration can be the result of coronary vasospasm. Patients with chest pain of possible cardiac origin should seek medical help immediately. Sumatriptan is not recommended for patients with recent cardiac arrhythmias or cerebrovascular accidents.

Sumatriptan is contraindicated in patients with symptomatic ischaemic heart disease, previous myocardial infarction, Prinzmetal's angina or uncontrolled hypertension.

NURSING IMPLICATIONS

The drugs used in the treatment of migraine may be considered in terms of management of the acute attack and long-term management and prevention. It is important to assess the headache profile, including family history, description of signs of the approaching attack, precipitating factors, duration, temporal profile and relieving factors.

Baseline vital signs such as blood pressure, pulse rate and weight should be considered. A history of vascular, hepatic, renal or cardiac disease should form part of the assessment. Current pregnancy, infection or hypertension must be recorded.

ADMINISTRATION

In an acute attack ergotamine or sumatriptan should be administered as early in the attack as possible.

A maximum dose of 6 mg ergotamine per day and 10 mg per week should not be exceeded.

No more than three tablets of sumatriptan should be taken in any 24 hour period and the injection should only be repeated once in a 24 hour period.

Ergotamine and sumatriptan should not be used prophylactically.

EVALUATION

It is important to evaluate the therapeutic effects of these drugs. The blood pressure (lying and standing) should be recorded. The patient should be observed for non-transient claudication, coldness of extremities, nausea, vomiting, anorexia, dysuria, backache, chest pain and depression. If any of these effects occur they should be reported.

PATIENT EDUCATION

Patients should be advised to avoid precipitating factors associated with the headache.

In the treatment of an acute migraine attack patients should be advised to start their sumatriptan or egotamine preparation early in the attack.

Patients taking ergotamine must be warned not to take more than 6 mg per day or 10 mg per week and to stop the drug if they experience numbness or tingling of the extremities and seek medical advice.

Those patients prescribed sumatriptan need to be warned not to take more than three tablets of sumatriptan in a 24 hour period or to repeat the injection only once in 24 hours.

The patient should learn to recognise side effects of their medication and seek medical advice if necessary. Patients prescribed sumatriptan must be instructed to seek medical help immediately should they develop chest pain.

Patient education should also include advising those patients prescribed drugs causing hypotension to rise slowly from the lying position to avoid postural hypotension.

Drugs administered for long-term management and prevention include drugs which alter catecholamine action, e.g. clonidine, β blockers, tricyclic antidepressants and MAOIs. β blockers may prolong insulin induced hypoglycaemia and are probably best avoided in diabetic patients. The diet of patients taking MAOIs should be assessed and adequate instruction about necessary dietary restrictions given (see Chapter 26).

Antiserotonin drugs may also be used for long-term management and patients should be informed of the adverse gastrointestinal and central nervous system effects of these drugs, including a possible increase in appetite.

The nursing implications for analgesics are listed in Chapter 23.

TEST YOUR KNOWLEDGE

1. Define the term 'epilepsy'.

2. List extracranial factors which may lead to secondary epilepsy.

3. List three drugs used in the treatment of major seizures and complex partial seizures.

4. State the nursing implications of giving phenytoin by IV injection.

5. What is the new terminology for classical and common migraine?

6. Describe three classes of drugs used in the long-term management of migraine and list the drugs in each class.

7. List the drugs used in an acute attack of migraine.

8. What is the new drug used in the treatment of migraine?

9. State any nursing implications of drugs used in migraine.

10. Why may it be of benefit to give IM metoclopramide 10 minutes before other medication in the acute migraine attack?

11. What adverse effect does prolonged use of ergotamine have?

12. Describe Parkinson's disease.

13. Describe how a decarboxylase inhibitor added to levodopa benefits the patient.

14. List other drugs used in parkinsonism.

NEUROLOGICAL DISORDERS

25 ■

TABLE 25.2 Summary table — drugs used in neurology

DRUG GROUP Drug Name	Use	Action	Adverse Reactions	Nursing Implications
DRUGS FOR EPILEPSY Major seizures and complex partial seizures				
Phenytoin sodium	All types of epilepsy except petit mal	Alters CNS electrolyte concentrations and inhibits spread of seizure discharge	Gum hypertrophy, fetal hydantoin syndrome, hirsutism, acne, nystagmus, vertigo, incoordination	**Assess:** Baseline vital signs, BP, pulse rate, presence of pregnancy or lactation, epilepsy profile and number of seizures, concurrent medications and alcohol use, previous drug reaction, history of head injury, alcohol abuse, allergic reaction, cardiac disease, hypertension or diabetes mellitus **Administer:** Orally with meals to prevent GIT irritation; may be given in suspension form, shake bottle well before administration. Parenteral: do not give IM, do not mix with other drugs; IV give slowly at dose not exceeding 50 mg/min, not advisable to administer phenytoin (*Dilantin*) with IV solutions other than normal saline; administered with an IV infusion it may be given into a fastrunning infusion of normal saline via a Y injection site, or in a burette at a concentration no greater than 10 mg/mL; should be administered carefully as sudden hypotension or cardiac arrhythmias may occur **Evaluate:** BP, pulse rate, therapeutic effectiveness by reduction in number of seizures; adverse effects involving CNS (drowsiness, ataxia, nystagmus); regular blood screening for folic acid depletion, megaloblastic anaemia and hyperglycaemia; diabetic patients may need to increase insulin dose

TABLE 25.2 continued

DRUG GROUP Drug Name	Use	Action	Adverse Reactions	Nursing Implications
				Educate: Correct dosage regimen; self-evaluation for side effects, signs of toxicity and therapeutic effect; to maintain adequate supply of medication and not to alter dose without consulting medical officer; to avoid use of alcohol
Carbamazepine	Tonic-clonic (grand mal) and partial (focal) seizures	Believed to stabilise the seizure threshold and to limit the spread of seizure activity	Dizziness, drowsiness, ataxia, diplopia (may disappear with reduced dosage); blood disorders, GI symptoms, rash	**Assess:** Epileptic profile and number of seizures; concurrent medication (should not be administered concurrently with barbiturates); previous drug reactions; presence of pregnancy or lactation; history of kidney, liver, cardiovascular disease, bone marrow depression **Administer:** Orally with food **Evaluate:** Therapeutic effectiveness (by reduction in seizure number or severity); adverse reactions (e.g. haematological disorders, ensure regular blood screening); CNS depression resulting in drowsiness
Sodium valproate Semisodium valproate	Temporal lobe epilepsy, grand mal, mixed seizures, myoclonic seizures	Inhibits GABA transaminase	Indigestion, vomiting, drowsiness, bleeding, alopecia, liver dysfunction	**Assess:** Epilepsy profile and number of seizures; concurrent medications; previous drug reactions; presence of pregnancy or lactation; history of diabetes mellitus or liver disease **Administer:** Orally with food; capsule should be swallowed whole and not chewed as this has been known to induce mouth ulcers and throat irritation **Evaluate:** Therapeutic effectiveness (by reduction in number and severity of seizures); diabetics for false positive ketones on urinalysis; may be an increased bleeding time when administered concurrently with aspirin; liver function tests

25 NEUROLOGICAL DISORDERS

TABLE 25.2 continued

DRUG GROUP Drug Name	Use	Action	Adverse Reactions	Nursing Implications
Barbiturates: Phenobarbitone Methylphenobarbitone Primidone	All major seizures, paediatric febrile convulsions, status epilepticus	Inhibits spread of seizure discharge	Sedation, irritability, ataxia, rashes, tolerance, liver enzyme induction	Assess: Baseline vital signs, BP, temperature, respiration, weight and sleep pattern; epilepsy profile and number of seizures; previous drug reactions and alcohol intake; presence of pregnancy or lactation **Administer:** According to legal requirements; ensure compliance; orally or parenterally according to manufacturer's instructions; observe for hypotension and respiratory depression **Evaluate:** Therapeutic effectiveness (by reduction in number of seizures); adverse effects especially CNS manifestations (e.g. drowsiness to which tolerance usually develops); slurred speech, ataxia or vertigo
Benzodiazepines: Diazepam Nitrazepam Clonazepam Lorazepam Clobazam	Status epilepticus, myoclonic epilepsy	Prevent seizure discharge	Drowsiness, sedation, ataxia, behavioural instability, tolerance	**Assess:** Epileptic profile and vital signs, number of seizures, respiration rate, alcohol intake, previous drug reaction, history of respiratory disease in small children **Administer:** Orally or parenterally **Evaluate:** Therapeutic effectiveness (by reduction in number or severity of seizures); adverse reactions especially CNS problems (e.g. behavioural disorders in children, psychosis and neurological signs (ataxia, drowsiness) in adults)

TABLE 25.2 continued

DRUG GROUP Drug Name	Use	Action	Adverse Reactions	Nursing Implications
Vigabatrin	Epilepsy not controlled by other drugs	Irreversible inhibition of the enzyme which metabolises the neurotransmitter GABA	CNS related (drowsiness, dizziness, nervousness, irritability)	**Assess:** Epileptic profile and number of seizures; concurrent medication; previous drug reactions; history of renal disease **Administer:** Once daily before or after meals **Evaluation:** Therapeutic effectiveness (by reduction in seizure numbers or severity); adverse reactions especially CNS effects (e.g. drowsiness, dizziness, visual disturbances) **Educate:** Correct dosage regimen; to avoid driving or operating machinery if drowsy
Lamotrigine	Partial and generalised tonic-clonic seizures not controlled by other drugs	Stabilises neuronal membranes and inhibits neurotransmitter release	Skin rashes, Stevens-Johnson syndrome (rare), ataxia, somnolence, diplopia, nausea	**Assess:** Epileptic profile and number of seizures; concurrent medication; previous drug reactions; presence of pregnancy or lactation **Administer:** Twice daily **Evaluate:** Therapeutic effectiveness (by reduction in seizure numbers or severity); adverse reactions e.g. skin rashes, CNS effects (ataxia, drowsiness); monitor elderly patients closely
Absence seizures Succinimides: Ethosuximide Methsuximide Phensuximide	Absence seizures (petit mal)	Prevents seizure discharge	Anorexia, nausea, vomiting, induction of major seizures, bone marrow depression	**Assess:** Epilepsy profile and number of seizures; previous drug reactions; history of kidney or liver disease or psychiatric disturbances **Administer:** Orally with meals to reduce GIT irritation. Evaluate: Therapeutic effectiveness (by reduction in number or severity of seizures); adverse effects e.g. gum hypertrophy or haematological problems; CNS depression, psychiatric disturbances and drowsiness
Sodium valproate (see above)				

25 NEUROLOGICAL DISORDERS

TABLE 25.2 continued

DRUG GROUP Drug Name	Use	Action	Adverse Reactions	Nursing Implications
DRUGS FOR PARKINSONISM Dopaminergics Levodopa + decarboxylase inhibitor	Parkinsonism	Replenishes dopamine in corpus striatum	Anorexia, nausea, vomiting, postural hypotension, involuntary movement of face and lips, cardiac arrhythmias	**Assess:** For history of parkinsonism secondary to use of neuroleptic drugs, dementia, memory loss, confusion, psychoses, postural hypotension, endocrine, renal, cardiac, hepatic impairment, diabetes, glaucoma; concurrent use of other drugs which can interact with levodopa (e.g. MAOIs may cause dangerous hypertension with levodopa); establish baseline BP (lying and standing), colour and temperature of extremities, urinary output; document baseline observations of parkinsonian symptoms and emotional state **Administer:** With food **Evaluate:** For therapeutic effect; sympathomimetic effect, i.e. BP, pulse rate, colour and temperature of extremities, urinary output; psychological behaviour **Educate:** To change position slowly to avoid postural hypotension; that urine and perspiration may darken; drug efficacy may not occur for several months
Bromocriptine	Parkinsonism	Enhances dopaminergic activity		**Assess:** For history of parkinsonism and document baseline observation of symptoms **Administer:** With food **Evaluate:** For therapeutic effect (improvement in symptoms); dyskinesia; confusion

TABLE 25.2 continued

DRUG GROUP Drug Name	Use	Action	Adverse Reactions	Nursing Implications
Selegiline	When Parkinson's disease progresses and effects of levodopa wear off	Selective inhibitor of MAO-B, thereby increasing dopamine available	Mostly due to increased dopaminergic activity and include: nausea, dizziness, confusion, insomnia	**Assess:** For history of parkinsonism and document baseline observation of symptoms; concurrent medication (should not be administered with other MAOIs, pethidine, fluoxetine); history of GIT disease, cardiac disease, psychosis, contraindication to levodopa **Administer:** Orally twice daily with breakfast and lunch (to avoid insomnia) **Evaluation:** As for levodopa, for exacerbation of levodopa side effects **Education:** To take medication at breakfast and lunchtime, to avoid tyramine containing food (e.g. ripe cheese, *Vegemite*) and cough and cold remedies if taking more than 10 mg per day
Amantadine	Parkinsonism, antiviral	Enhances dopaminergic activity	Hallucinations; skin pigmentation; confusion; difficulty in concentration; slurred speech; orthostatic hypotension; depression; lethargy; insomnia	**Assess:** For history of parkinsonism, hypotension, urinary output **Administer:** By mouth **Evaluate:** For improvement in hypokinesia and rigidity. Has little effect on tremor

25 NEUROLOGICAL DISORDERS

TABLE 25.2 continued

DRUG GROUP Drug Name	Use	Action	Adverse Reactions	Nursing Implications
Anticholinergics agents: Benzhexol Biperiden Benztropine Orphenadrine Procyclidine	Parkinsonism	Reduces dominance of cholinergic system	Dryness of mouth, difficulty in swallowing and talking, thirst, reduced bronchial secretions, other anticholingeric effects	**Assess:** History of parkinsonism, these drugs can be used in all forms of parkinsonism **Administer:** Usually in divided doses according to needs and tolerance of patient **Evaluate:** For improvement in tremor and rigidity
DRUGS FOR MIGRAINE Long-term management and prevention β blockers e.g. propranolol, pindolol	Long-term prevention of migraine	Block β effects of adrenaline	Generally well tolerated, bradycardia, hypotension, nausea, vomiting, diarrhoea, lassitude, visual disturbances, nightmares, hallucinations, rashes, parasthesia, hypoglycaemia, bronchoconstriction	**Assess:** Heart rate, blood pressure, asthma. **Administer:** Taper off when therapy ceased, check hospital policy for withdrawal before general anaesthesia **Evaluate:** Heart rate, arterial pressure, for signs of heart failure, bronchospasm **Educate:** Early signs of heart failure, hypotension, bradycardia; not to miss doses or stop treatment suddenly

TABLE 25.2 continued

DRUG GROUP Drug Name	Use	Action	Adverse Reactions	Nursing Implications
Clonidine	Long-term prevention of migraine	Reduces outflow of catecholamines from sympathetic nervous system	Dry mouth, sedation, constipation, fluid retention, rebound hypertension on withdrawal, headache, weakness, orthostatic hypotension, bradycardia, nasal stuffiness, dry mouth, GIT disturbances, impotence.	**Assess:** Baseline arterial pressure; likelihood of compliance; elderly patients more likely to suffer adverse effects **Administer:** Establish and reinforce regular pattern of administration; do not cease therapy suddenly **Evaluate:** Lying, sitting, standing BP for hypotension; signs of hypotension, ischaemia; for other adverse effects **Educate:** Consequences of non-compliance; not to stop therapy suddenly; not to miss doses or catchup
Tricyclic antidepressants e.g. amitriptyline, nortriptyline	Long-term management and prevention of migraine	Block neuronal uptake of noradrenaline thus making more available	Sedation, anticholinergic effects, postural hypotension, cardiac effects, skin rashes, blood dyscrasias, jaundice, weight gain, sweating, paradoxical manic excitement	**Assess:** Baseline vital signs, lying and standing BP, pulse rate, respiration rate, weight, sleep pattern and bowel habits; previous drug reactions, concurrent medications especially alcohol intake; presenting disease symptoms pattern; history of behavioural disturbances, convulsions, glaucoma, thyroid, liver, renal disease **Administer:** Ensure compliance **Evaluate:** Therapeutic effectiveness; adverse effects such as dermatological reactions, postural hypotension and altered sleep pattern; changes in bowel habits; weight gain; changes in pulse rate, blood dyscrasias, jaundice, and urinary retention **Educate:** Expected therapeutic and adverse effects, and appropriate measures to be taken to avoid adverse effects; risk of sedation

25 NEUROLOGICAL DISORDERS

TABLE 25.2 continued

DRUG GROUP Drug Name	Use	Action	Adverse Reactions	Nursing Implications
MAOIs e.g. phenelzine, tranylcypromine	Long-term management and prevention of migraine	Inhibit enzymatic breakdown of noradrenaline	Severe hypertension, liver damage, hypotension, insomnia, gastric upset, dizziness, dry mouth, muscle weakness, cardiac arrhythmias, disturbances of colour vision. *Note*: care with tyramine containing foods and over the counter medications for cough and cold	**Assess:** Baseline vital signs, such as lying and standing BP, pulse rate, weight, and hydration status; current medications and alcohol intake; history of hypertension, glaucoma, cardiac or cerebrovascular disease, liver or renal disease; diet or any recent changes in diet **Administer:** Usually orally **Evaluate:** Therapeutic effectiveness, adverse effects, BP (lying and standing), constipation and behavioural changes **Educate:** Importance of recognising deviations from therapeutic effect and presentation of adverse effects; to avoid tyramine containing foods and over the counter remedies
Antiserotonin antihistamines: Cyproheptadine Methdilazine Pizotifen malate	Long-term management and prevention of migraine	Antiserotonin	Cyproheptadine and pizotifen stimulate appetite. Drowsiness, lack of concentration, lassitude, dizziness, hypertension, weakness, incoordination, nausea, vomiting, diarrhoea, colic, constipation	**Assess:** Migraine profile; baseline vital signs, BP (lying and standing), pulse rate and weight, present medications, previous drug reactions. Methysergide — history of peripheral vascular disease, cardiac disease or hypertension **Administer:** Methysergide — with drug holiday, e.g. one month off in every 4–6 months; monitor regimen carefully **Evaluate:** Therapeutic effectiveness, BP (lying and standing) and adverse effects **Educate:** To recognise adverse effects and to seek medical advice if any occur; to rise slowly from lying position
Methysergide	Long-term management and prevention of migraine	Antiserotonin	Retroperitoneal fibrosis, fibrosis of heart and pleura of lung	

TABLE 25.2 continued

DRUG GROUP Drug Name	Use	Action	Adverse Reactions	Nursing Implications
Acute attack Analgesics: Aspirin Paracetamol Codeine	Treatment of pain in acute attack	Analgesic and antiprostaglandin effects	See Chapter 23 Pain Relief	Use soluble forms of analgesics in treatment of acute migraine attack. See Chapter 23
Antiemetics: Metoclopramide Prochlorperazine Meclozine hydrochloride	Treatment of nausea and vomiting in acute migraine attack	Antinauseant, antiemetic	See Chapter 17 Gastrointestinal Disorders	Use suppository forms or administer by injection if necessary. See Chapter 17
Ergot Alkaloids: Ergotamine tartrate	Treatment of acute attack of migraine	Vasoconstrictor	Nausea; vomiting; paraesthesia; pain and weakness of extremities; peripheral vasoconstriction; insomnia if combinations of ergotamine and caffeine taken at night; ergot toxicity; tachycardia; bradycardia; hypertension or hypotension	**Assess:** For onset of acute migraine attack; history of hypertension; pregnancy; impaired hepatic or renal function; concurrent medications **Administer:** Orally, sublingually or rectally (in suppository form); 1–2 mg may be given at onset of attack and repeated every 0.5–1.0 hour up to total of 6 mg per day. No more than 10 mg should be taken per week **Evaluate:** For alleviation of symptoms; BP changes; nausea; weakness; signs of ergot toxicity **Educate:** Recognition of onset of attack and to commence therapy quickly; maximum daily and weekly doses allowed; signs of toxicity; to lie down in darkened room; concurrent use of analgesics, emetics, sedatives as required

25 NEUROLOGICAL DISORDERS

TABLE 25.2 continued

DRUG GROUP Drug Name	Use	Action	Adverse Reactions	Nursing Implications
Sedatives Diazepam	To reduce anxiety and promote sleep during acute phase	Antianxiety, sedation	See Chapter 26 Psychiatric Disorders	See Chapter 26
Serotonin₁ (5-HT₁) Agonists: Sumatriptan	Acute attack of migraine	5-HT like receptor agonist.	Usually transient: chest pain, flushed sensation, nausea, vomiting, odd taste; increased BP	**Assess:** For onset of acute migraine attack; history of ischaemic heart disease, myocardial infarction, uncontrolled blood pressure **Administer:** Orally or by SCI at onset of attack, no more than 3 tablets within 24 hours, repeat SCI only once in 24 hours; first dose to be given by or under direct supervision of physician **Evaluate:** For alleviation of symptoms, chest pain, BP changes **Educate:** To start medication at onset of attack, not to exceed 3 tablets a day; not to use prophylactically; to report if attacks do not respond

Psychiatric Disorders

STUART J. BAKER

O B J E C T I V E S

At the conclusion of this chapter the reader should be able to:

1. List the different classes of drugs used in the treatment of psychiatric disturbances;

2. List the basic pharmacological actions of each class of drugs;

3. Identify which classes of drugs are used to treat the major psychiatric disorders; and

4. Itemise the more important adverse effects and the toxic effects of each class of drugs.

PSYCHOPHARMACOLOGY

Psychotropic drugs treat a variety of conditions including schizophrenia, mania, depressive illness, anxiety and insomnia. Generally, they are palliative not curative. Antidepressants are an exception as they reduce the duration of a depressive illness. Consequently, psychotropic drugs should be used in conjunction with other forms of therapy such as psychotherapy, group therapy and relaxation therapy.

When commencing psychotropic drugs small doses should be used initially to minimise side effects and to enable a gradual build up to the optimum dose for the individual. Psychotropics can be used on a long-term or intermittent basis depending on the type or severity of the psychiatric disorder.

Patients suffering from some psychiatric disorders may have difficulty complying with complicated drug treatment regimens; many of the psychotropics have long half-lives and can be given orally in a once daily dose which aids in improving compliance. Many drugs used to treat physical illness can induce psychiatric symptoms such as depression, mania, hallucinations and delusions. This may happen (rarely) when they are used in therapeutic doses but is more common when they are abused. Elderly patients are particularly sensitive to these effects. Some examples of such drugs are the centrally acting antihypertensive agents (e.g. methyldopa, clonidine), anticholingeric agents (e.g. atropine eye drops, benztropine), antianxiety drugs and histamine H_2 antagonists (e.g. cimetidine).

A common classification of psychotropic drugs is shown in Table 26.1; their uses, actions, and adverse effects are summarised in Table 26.9 at the end of the chapter.

TABLE 26.1   Classification of psychotropic drugs

Antipsychotics (formerly major tranquillisers or neuroleptics)
Definition: drugs with therapeutic effects on psychoses such as schizophrenia
    Phenothiazines, e.g. chlorpromazine
    Butyrophenones, e.g. haloperidol
    Thioxanthenes, e.g. thiothixene
    Diphenylbutylpiperidines, e.g. pimozide
    Dibenzodiazepines, e.g. clozapine

Antidepressants
Definition: drugs effective in the treatment of pathological depressive states
    Tricyclics, e.g. amitriptyline
    Tetracyclics, e.g. mianserin
    Monoamine oxidase inhibitors (MAOIs), e.g. moclobemide
    Selective serotonin reuptake inhibitors, e.g. fluoxetine

Antimanic Drugs
Definition: drugs effective in the treatment of manic states
    Lithium
    Carbamazepine
    Clonazepam

Psychostimulants
Definition: drugs which temporarily increase alertness
    Amphetamines
    Caffeine
    Methylphenidate
    Cocaine

Anxiolytics (formerly minor tranquillisers or sedatives)
Definition: drugs which reduce pathological anxiety, tension and agitation
    Benzodiazepines, e.g. diazepam
    Azaspirones, e.g. buspirone

Hypnotics
Definition: drugs which are used to induce sleep
    Benzodiazepines
    Barbiturates
    Miscellaneous

ANTIPSYCHOTIC DRUGS ▮▮▮▮▮

The antipsychotic drugs are used to alleviate the symptoms of major psychiatric illnesses, that is, they are used to treat psychoses rather than neuroses. Antipsychotic drugs are palliative not curative.

PHENOTHIAZINES

Chlorpromazine, Thioridazine, Trifluoperazine, Fluphenazine, Perphenazine, Pericyazine

TRADE NAMES

Chlorpromazine: *Largactil*.
Fluphenazine: *Anatensol*.
Pericyazine: *Neulactil*.
Perphenazine: *Trilafon*.
Thioridazine: *Melleril*.
Trifluoperazine: *Stelazine*.

BUTYROPHENONES

Haloperidol

TRADE NAMES

Haloperidol: *Serenace*.

THIOXANTHENES

Thiothixene

TRADE NAMES

Thiothixene: *Navane*.

DIPHENYLBUTYLPIPERIDINES

Pimozide

TRADE NAMES

Pimozide: *Orap*.

MECHANISM OF ACTION

All classes of antipsychotics are believed to act by blocking the action of the neuro-transmitter dopamine in the mesolimbic and mesocortical areas of the brain.

The antipsychotics have three different therapeutic actions:

- **A tranquillising action** — calming and reducing agitation within a few minutes (after intramuscular injection) or a few hours (after oral medication).

- **An antipsychotic action** — reducing mainly the hallucinations, delusions and thought disorder of psychosis, in two weeks to two months after starting antipsychotic drugs.

- **A sedative action** — producing drowsiness. This action is best seen as a side effect and may or may not occur depending on the antipsychotic (e.g. chlorpromazine is more sedating than haloperidol) and the dose.

All antipsychotics, except thioridazine, are also antiemetics.

PHARMACOKINETICS

Oral antipsychotics are variably absorbed. The same oral dose of a specific drug in different patients can give nearly 90-fold variations in peak plasma concentrations. Intramuscular administration gives 2–10 times higher and more reliable plasma concentrations than oral administration. An intramuscular injection of 2 mg haloperidol is equivalent to an oral dose of 4–20 mg. Antipsychotic drugs have plasma half-lives of 10–20 hours and are present even longer in the brain. Maintenance treatment with oral antipsychotics can often be given in a single daily dose (usually at bedtime) once the correct dose is established.

Antipsychotics persist in the body for some weeks after oral doses and up to six

PSYCHIATRIC DISORDERS

26

months after depot injections. Even though the drug is detectable in the body for a long time it does not necessarily mean that either the therapeutic effect or side effects last that long. In general, the correlation between plasma concentrations and clinical efficacy is poor. Regular monitoring of plasma levels is not clinically useful.

Antipsychotics are metabolised by the microsomal enzymes in the liver to (mainly) inactive metabolites and these metabolites are excreted primarily in the urine (and also in the bile). Metabolism and excretion are greatest in healthy young people. Doses are usually decreased in children, the elderly and people with markedly reduced liver function. However, these lower doses are usually a result of good clinical practice (i.e. individualised doses) rather than pharmacokinetic principles as the individual variation in plasma and brain levels is so pronounced.

USES

Schizophrenia is the major condition in which antipsychotics are used. About 1% of the population is estimated to be suffering from one of the schizophrenias. The antipsychotics reduce the relapse rate and enable the patient to function within the community. Other conditions which respond to antipsychotic therapy include schizoaffective and schizophreniform disorders, mania, psychotic depression, organic delusional disorder and sometimes substance induced mental disorders.

Chlorpromazine was the first antipsychotic drug and when it was introduced in 1952 it revolutionised the treatment of psychotic patients. Before chlorpromazine psychotic patients were institutionalised and had very little hope of rehabilitation or recovery. Drug treatment of these patients was limited to massive doses of sedatives such as bromides and barbiturates.

Chlorpromazine belongs to a class of chemically related substances called phenothiazines. Following the introduction of chlorpromazine a number of other phenothiazines were marketed as well as a number of non-phenothiazines which were also discovered to have antipsychotic activity (see Table 26.2).

TABLE 26.2 Equivalent doses and daily dose ranges for the antipsychotic drugs

Drug	Equivalent dose (mg)	Daily dose range (mg)
Phenothiazines		
Chlorpromazine	100	50–1200
Thioridazine	100	50–800
Trifluoperazine	5	4–40
Fluphenazine	2	1–20
Perphenazine	10	8–64
Pericyazine	10	5–60
Butyrophenones		
Haloperidol	2	2–100
Thioxanthenes		
Thiothixene	3	6–60
Diphenylbutylpiperidines		
Pimozide	2	2–30
Dibenzodiazepine		
Clozapine	50	150–450

Occasionally, experienced psychiatrists will use doses greater than the maximum doses listed in Table 26.2. High doses should be the exception rather than the rule because benefits to the patient taper off with increasing dose but side effects are more likely to occur.

The antipsychotics are usually given orally as tablets or liquids. Liquids (syrups or suspensions) are messy and their only advantage is to ensure that the patient has swallowed the dose instead of hiding a tablet in the cheek for disposal later.

Some of the antipsychotics are also available in injectable form. Particularly important are the slow release injectable forms of fluphenazine decanoate (*Modecate*), haloperidol decanoate (*Haldol*) and flupenthixol decanoate (*Fluanxol*). These oil-soluble depot preparations are administered intramuscularly, usually at 2–4 week intervals. The active drug is gradually released over 2–4 weeks. They are useful in patients who are poor compliers (because it is at least known when they miss a dose) or those who have poor absorption of orally administered drugs.

Intramuscular chlorpromazine is not a depot injection and should be given by deep intramuscular injection because the solution is extremely irritating (oily injections like the depot antipsychotics are not irritating). There is also a non-depot haloperidol injection which is widely used as either an intramuscular or intravenous injection. In general injection solutions should not be mixed in the same syringe (to avoid chemical and physical incompatibility).

A technique known as 'rapid neuroleptisation' has been used to rapidly control violent or dangerous behaviour. This involves single or repeated intramuscular or intravenous administration of haloperidol, alone or in combination with intravenous diazepam. This technique is now rarely used and it should be used only in physically healthy patients with close clinical observation maintained for emergence of cardiovascular and neurological side effects. Dosage schedules will vary depending upon the clinical circumstances.

ADVERSE DRUG REACTIONS

The antipsychotic drugs act on many organ systems and numerous side effects may be expected. These adverse effects occur to varying degrees with the different compounds available.

Sedation is more likely with chlorpromazine and thioridazine but tolerance can develop and sedation may be less of a problem in long-term treatment.

Anticholinergic effects, including dry mouth, blurred vision, constipation and urinary hesitation or retention, occur particularly with thioridazine and chlorpromazine. Sometimes dry mouth and blurred vision improve two weeks or so after starting antipsychotics.

Endocrine effects are more common in women and include breast enlargement and lactation and alterations in the menstrual cycle, e.g. amenorrhea.

Dermatological effects, e.g. photosensitivity especially in fair skinned patients, may be a problem with chlorpromazine.

Ocular effects such as deposits of pigment in the retina, cornea and lens are possible with thioridazine and chlorpromazine. Pigmentary retinopathy with loss of visual acuity may occur with thioridazine in doses exceeding 800 mg/day over an extended period, this dose should never be exceeded.

Hepatic effects such as altered liver function and jaundice may occur. The problem is most common with chlorpromazine.

Haemopoietic effects such as depression of white cell count are possible, although extremely rare with antipsychotics.

Cardiovascular effects such as hypotension, especially in elderly patients on high doses, may be a problem. Changes in ECG readings are usually benign. Thioridazine and chlorpromazine have been implicated most often. Haloperidol may also cause hypotension when administered intravenously.

Seizures may occur as all antipsychotics, especially in high doses, have the potential to lower the seizure threshold in epileptic and non-epileptic patients. The risk of seizures is increased in epileptic patients.

PSYCHIATRIC DISORDERS

26

Extrapyramidal effects are caused by all antipsychotics to varying degrees. This is due to their mechanism of action, the blockade of dopaminergic transmission. Extrapyramidal effects may show within a few hours or up to several months after commencing therapy. The effects seen are akinesia, akathisia, acute dystonic reactions and drug induced parkinsonism; all these are different forms of abnormal muscle movements. They may be reduced or eliminated by dose reduction of the antipsychotic or by administration of antiparkinsonian medications such as benzhexol, benztropine, procyclidine, orphenadrine, biperiden and amantadine, see Chapter 25 Neurological Disorders.

Tardive dyskinesia (i.e. late onset dyskinesia) may occur in some patients following treatment with antipsychotics for more than one year. Tardive dyskinesia consists of choreiform movements of the tongue, jaw and face and sometimes the extremities. It may occur with any of the currently available drugs and is more prevalent in elderly patients. In some cases tardive dyskinesia may be irreversible even on discontinuation of antipsychotics and no effective treatment is available. Hence, antipsychotics should only be used to treat psychoses and not chronic anxiety or nau-

sea. All patients on long-term antipsychotic drugs should be regularly reviewed for the emergence of orofacial or limb dyskinesias and when these occur medication should be discontinued if possible.

Neuroleptic malignant syndrome (NMS) is a rare syndrome occuring in approximately 0.2% of patients taking antipsychotics. The syndrome is characterised by fever, rigidity, stupor and autonomic signs (e.g. excessive sweating, tachycardia) and can be fatal (about 10% of cases). Recognition is vital as the main treatment is withdrawal of the antipsychotic. Dantrolene and bromocriptine may be of benefit. Patients who have had neuroleptic malignant syndrome should not be re-challenged with antipsychotics for at least two weeks after the syndrome has subsided.

Sedation, hypotension, anticholinergic and extrapyramidal adverse effects are the most commonly occurring and troublesome adverse effects seen with the antipsychotics. Table 26.3 is a guide to the relative incidence of these effects with the more commonly used antipsychotics.

DRUG INTERACTIONS

The sedative effects of central nervous system depressant drugs and alcohol may be enhanced by antipsychotics.

TABLE 26.3 Adverse effects of antipsychotics

Drug	Extrapyramidal Effects	Sedative Effects	Hypotensive Effects	Anticholinergic Effects
Chlorpromazine	+	+++	+++	++
Thioridazine	+	+++	++	+++
Fluphenazine	+++	++	+	+
Perphenazine	+++	+	+	+
Trifluoperazine	+++	+	+	+
Thiothixene	+++	+	+	+
Haloperidol	+++	+	+	+
Pimozide	++	+	+	+
Clozapine	q	+++	++	+++

q minimal
+ low
++ moderate
+++ high

Phenothiazines may reverse the antihypertensive property of guanethidine and serious rises in diastolic blood pressure may occur. Chlorpromazine may interfere (rarely) with the metabolism of phenytoin leading to phenytoin toxicity. Phenothiazines also block the effects of adrenaline and may impair the metabolism of tricyclic antidepressants.

Antacids may interfere with the absorption of phenothiazines so doses should be spaced about two hours apart.

Levodopa will not reverse the parkinsonian symptoms induced by phenothiazines because dopamine receptor sites are already occupied by phenothiazines and the addition of more dopamine will therefore have no effect. Also, levodopa may induce psychosis. Anticholinergic drugs may add to the autonomic adverse effects of antipsychotics.

Sedative and anticholinergic interactions are the most common clinically significant drug interactions.

PRECAUTIONS AND CONTRAINDICATIONS

Intramuscular phenothiazines should be administered by deep intramuscular injection. Staff handling phenothiazines should take care not to spill solutions onto the skin.

Abrupt withdrawal of phenothiazines is associated with nausea, vomiting, insomnia and headache. Phenothiazine drugs and any accompanying antiparkinsonian drugs should be withdrawn slowly. However, the high frequency of non-compliance means that withdrawal is most often initiated abruptly by the patient despite advice to continue treatment.

Contraindications include known phenothiazine hypersensitivity, hypotensive states, coma and serious head injury. The antipsychotics should be used with caution in patients with a history of liver dysfunction or bone marrow depression, in the elderly, and in patients with Parkinson's disease or epilepsy.

Clozapine

Clozapine (*Clozaril*) is an antipsychotic which was introduced in the early 1970s. It was withdrawn in most countries in 1975 after 16 cases of agranulocytosis (eight were fatal) were reported in Finland.

It has been recently reintroduced because it has advantages over other antipsychotics, e.g. fewer extrapyramidal side effects (including tardive dyskinesia) and some benefit in patients resistant to other antipsychotics.

Agranulocytosis occurs with other antipsychotics but it is about 10 times more common with clozapine (1%–2% of patients versus about 0.1% of patients taking chlorpromazine). Patients can only receive clozapine if their blood is strictly monitored. Other side effects are listed in Table 26.9 at the end of the chapter.

Risperidone

Risperidone (*Risperdal*) is an antipsychotic drug which is a potent antagonist of serotonin S2 receptors and a relatively weak antagonist of dopamine D2 receptors. It is at least as effective as other antipsychotics and it may improve the negative symptoms of schizophrenia. In general it has fewer adverse effects than other antipsychotics. Orthostatic hypotension is the most troublesome effect. Drug interactions are assumed to be the same as those with other antipsychotics.

The initial dose is 0.5 mg twice daily in the elderly and 1 mg twice daily in most other patients. The dose should be gradually increased and not exceed 3–4 mg twice daily. Doses higher than 5 mg twice daily are no more efficacious and any advantage of risperidone (e.g. fewer extrapyramidal effects) is then lost.

NURSING IMPLICATIONS

ASSESSMENT

A medication history of therapeutic drugs, alcohol intake and previous drug hypersensitivity should be taken. Previous seizure activity should be noted. A history of

PSYCHIATRIC DISORDERS

26

diseases will be age dependent, but previous cardiovascular disease, glaucoma, myasthenia gravis and benign prostatic hypertrophy are important. Baseline vital signs, cardiac function, weight and blood pressure (lying and standing) should be recorded prior to administration of antipsychotics. Postural hypotension can occur with chlorpromazine and thioridazine.

ADMINISTRATION

The person administering intramuscular chlorpromazine should be careful when handling the drug as contact dermatitis can occur. Nursing staff should avoid spilling the non-oily injections on their skin. If a spill occurs the area should be washed with water to reduce skin irritation.

Observation of the patient for non-compliance is important. Abrupt withdrawal of antipsychotic drugs may result in nausea, vomiting, headache and insomnia, so medications should be tapered off slowly when ceasing therapy.

EVALUATION

Management and evaluation of a patient who is taking antipsychotic medication mainly involves observing for therapeutic effects and appropriate intervention should adverse effects occur. Interactions may occur when antipsychotic drugs are taken concurrently with alcohol or other central nervous system depressants. If seizures occur the dose of antipsychotic may need to be reduced, the drug replaced by another or an anticonvulsant introduced.

Postural hypotension can be a problem. Patients experience dizziness on standing from a lying or sitting position. Measurement of lying and standing blood pressure as well as asking patients how they feel after getting up will provide a good indication of any changes in blood pressure.

Drowsiness may occur so the patient's activities may need to be supervised initially while in hospital. New behaviours should be evaluated carefully. The emergence of dystonias can be a major problem in the younger age group and tardive dyskinesia in the older age group may indicate the need to maintain as low a therapeutic dose as possible. Akathisia is characterised by constant pacing movements and may indicate the need to reduce the dose or withdraw the drug. Pseudoparkinsonism with rigidity and dyskinesia may indicate a need to lower the dose of antipsychotic drugs, although tolerance may develop in some situations.

It is especially important that the nurse knows the signs and symptoms of extrapyramidal side effects and that these effects sometimes occur after even one dose of an antipsychotic. It is important to remember that these effects can occur when least expected, e.g. when the drug is being used as an antiemetic in a non-psychiatric situation.

Extrapyramidal and other side effects can be distressing and can make patients reluctant to take the medication. It should be remembered that the patient has the right to be informed and to refuse his or her medication. It is often the nurse's role to listen to the patient and counsel appropriately.

Antipsychotics should be used with caution in glaucoma and blurred vision should be reported. Nurses should anticipate the sudden presentation of cardiac toxicity and ensure that resuscitation equipment is adequate. Regular blood screening may be required but observation for bruising, bleeding, lethargy or mouth ulcers is more important as they may indicate leucopenia or agranulocytosis. Darkening of the skin may occur. Regular liver function tests are necessary as any abnormality may necessitate cessation or change of medication. Regular weighing should take place and weight gain may be helped by encouraging a balanced diet and adequate exercise. Regular gynaecological check-ups for lactation and menstrual abnormalities may be necessary for women. In men the development of gynaecomastia may indicate the need to change or cease the antipsychotic medication.

PATIENT EDUCATION

Patient education is vitally important and a fundamental process for discharge protocols. The patient should be advised not to suddenly discontinue the medication and to be wary of taking over-the-counter medications concurrently, especially antihistamines. Driving or using machinery may be a risk if drowsiness occurs (and even if it does not). Rising slowly from the lying position will help to avoid postural hypotension. The hypotensive patient should be advised to avoid taking hot baths. The onset of fatigue, sore throat or bruising indicates the need to consult a medical officer. A transient decrease in libido and ejaculatory failure may occur in some male patients.

The family should be involved in the patient education program. Patient information materials should be used to help educate the patient and family. Information concerning adverse effects is important, and gaining the cooperation of family members may help avoid non-compliance. Patients should be advised not to become too cold in the winter or too hot in the summer as their body temperature may parallel the ambient temperature. To prevent photosensitivity the patient should be advised to avoid overexposure to sunlight and to use 15+ UV-blocking sunscreens.

ANTIMANIC DRUGS

Lithium Carbonate

Lithium carbonate is the only specific antimanic drug known. Its antimanic properties were discovered in 1949 by the Australian psychiatrist, John Cade. Carbamazepine and clonazepam have recently been used in manic patients resistant to lithium and these two drugs have been helpful either alone or combined with lithium but lithium remains the first-line treatment. (The side effects of these two drugs are briefly listed in Table 26.9 at the end of this chapter.) Lithium carbonate is the only form used in Australia, lithium citrate is also used in other countries. Dose forms of lithium carbonate are shown in Table 26.4.

TRADE NAMES

Lithium carbonate: *Lithicarb*; *Priadel*.

PHARMACOKINETICS

Although lithium carbonate is administered it is the lithium ion which is the active drug. It is fully absorbed after oral administration. After single doses peak plasma levels are reached in 2–4 hours (6–8 hours after the sustained release tablet) and complete absorption takes about 8 hours. Lithium is not used parenterally. After about three to eight days of lithium treatment the plasma lithium level will accurately reflect total body lithium and can be used to monitor treatment.

PSYCHIATRIC DISORDERS

26

TABLE 26.4   Daily dose range of lithium carbonate

Dose form	Trade names	Usual daily dose range (mg)
250 mg tablet	*Lithicarb*	500–2000
400 mg sustained release tablet	*Priadel**	400–2000

* These tablets must be swallowed whole and not crushed or dissolved

Lithium is an element and cannot be metabolised. It is excreted by the kidneys (95%) with small amounts excreted in the sweat and faeces.

There is a lag between starting lithium therapy and showing improvement. About 80% of patients respond 5–10 days after therapeutic blood levels are reached. Therapeutic blood levels take 5–14 days to build up so most patients will respond about two weeks after starting lithium.

Therapeutic blood levels required in the treatment of acute mania range from 0.8–1.2 mmol/L. In the long-term maintenance treatment of manic depressive disorder effective levels are lower and lie between 0.6 mmol/L and 0.8 mmol/L. Maintaining patients at levels higher than 0.6–0.8 mmol/L only makes toxicity more likely. The patient should be maintained at the lowest level consistent with optimum therapeutic effects. Serious toxic effects are more likely above levels of 1.5–2.0 mmol/L.

All patients should have their serum lithium levels monitored frequently, perhaps weekly during the start of therapy and about every six months during maintenance therapy. Blood samples must be taken 12 hours (± 30 minutes) after the previous dose, e.g. if the previous dose is taken at 9.00 p.m. then the blood sample must be taken between 8.30 and 9.30 a.m. the next morning. Samples taken outside this time can give misleading results. Lithium is usually administered in the morning and the evening.

The sustained release formulation offers no substantial advantage over plain tablets. However, there is a trend towards once daily dosing (usually at night) with lithium and the sustained release tablet is usually preferred. This is because the slower time to peak plasma level may reduce initial toxicity from the larger doses given once daily. Twelve-hour plasma levels are about 25% higher. For example, if 500 mg twice daily gives a plasma level of 0.6 mmol/L then 1000 mg at night would give about 0.75 mmol/L. The dose does not have to be reduced, it is the patient who is treated not the plasma level.

USES

Administration of lithium has no noticeable psychotropic action in normal subjects. Lithium is used in the treatment of the manic phase of manic depressive illness, and for long-term maintenance therapy where it reduces the frequency and/or severity and duration of manic and depressive episodes. The duration of lithium therapy may vary from 2–3 years to indefinitely.

Lithium has been used in other psychiatric conditions with variable results. It is of modest value in the primary treatment of the depressive phase of manic depressive illness; antidepressant drugs or electroconvulsive therapy should be used first in this phase.

ADVERSE DRUG REACTIONS

Polydipsia (excessive thirst) resulting from polyuria (excessive urinary loss) can be troublesome initially. It is reversible on discontinuation of therapy but this is not usually necessary as symptoms may subside within a few weeks. Patients should be reassured.

Skin reactions such as acne may appear during the first few weeks of therapy but may disappear spontaneously.

In a small percentage of patients lithium may cause enlargement of the thyroid gland and some degree of hypothyroidism. These symptoms are reversed on discontinuation of lithium therapy or when thyroxine is given. Thyroid function should be assessed before starting lithium therapy and yearly during long-term treatment.

Lithium is eliminated primarily via the kidney and any impairment of renal function will alter lithium clearance. Acute lithium toxicity may result in kidney damage which may in turn predispose the patient to further episodes of toxicity. A nephrogenic diabetes insipidus-like syndrome may occur in a small percentage of patients and will require a thorough renal evaluation if lithium is to be continued. Between 10% and 20% of patients report a persistent increase in urine volume and thirst during lithium treatment. However, prospective studies of renal function in patients maintained on lithium at therapeutic plasma levels do not show evidence of progressive renal impairment.

Lithium crosses the placenta and the incidence of congenital malformations (especially cardiac) in the children of mothers receiving lithium is greater than in the general population. Lithium is generally contraindicated during the first trimester of pregnancy but if discontinuation of lithium would seriously compromise the mother's health, it may be used with great caution and frequent blood level estimations. Lithium is excreted in breast milk so mothers should be encouraged not to breast feed.

TOXICITY

At blood levels above 1.5 mmol/L the patient is likely to exhibit signs of toxicity. Acute toxicity is seen at concentrations of 2.0 mmol/L or greater. There is no specific antidote to lithium poisoning. Treatment consists of withdrawing the drug, giving adequate fluid and electrolyte replacement and aiding renal excretion of lithium by the administration of sodium bicarbonate. Haemodialysis is the treatment of choice for severe lithium poisoning. When the plasma level exceeds 3.0–4.0 mmol/L, anuria is suspected or there is evidence of shock or coma, the patient should be dialysed. Prolonged severe toxicity may lead to irreversible neurological damage or death.

Early signs of toxicity include sluggishness, lethargy, fine tremor (particularly of the hands), nausea, vomiting, anorexia, abdominal discomfort and diarrhoea. At very high blood levels ataxia, slurred speech and a marked tremor occur. Finally, seizures, loss of consciousness from cerebral anoxia, shock and cardiac impairment (due to electrolyte imbalance), and ultimately death may occur.

Causes of high blood levels are multiple and include: excessive dosage; reduction in lithium excretion (which occurs when renal damage is present); low sodium intake (from special or sometimes 'fad' diets) or increased sodium loss (e.g. after excessive sweating or diuretic therapy); dehydration; and drug interactions.

DRUG INTERACTIONS

Drugs which increase lithium blood levels and may produce toxicity are thiazide diuretics, chlorthalidone and anti-inflammatory drugs such as indomethacin and ibuprofen.

Drugs which reduce lithium blood levels are sodium bicarbonate, sodium chloride, and possibly aminophylline, theophylline and acetazolamide.

High doses of lithium and haloperidol given together have occasionally been reported to cause neurotoxicity. Lithium may prolong the neuromuscular blockade produced by suxamethonium or pancuronium. Lithium may also prolong recovery time after barbiturate anaesthetic induction with thiopentone.

PRECAUTIONS AND CONTRAINDICATIONS

Cardiac and renal disease are contraindications to lithium therapy and, generally, lithium should not be used during pregnancy and breast feeding.

NURSING IMPLICATIONS

ASSESSMENT

Assessment of lithium levels within 12 hours of the last dose (except in situations of acute toxicity) is extremely important. Use of concurrent medications, especially diuretics, should be noted. A reduced sodium diet also should be noted. Evaluation of baseline vital signs such as weight, sleep patterns and fluid balance is important. A history of cardiac or cerebrovascular disease, cerebral organic dementia, and renal or thyroid disease is relevant. Thyroid function should be assessed.

ADMINISTRATION

The management of the patient taking lithium is mainly concerned with the maintenance of adequate lithium blood levels.

PSYCHIATRIC DISORDERS

26

Drug interactions have been described above. The concurrent use of drugs high in sodium (e.g. *Citravescent* and *Dexsal*) should be avoided as it will result in decreased lithium blood levels. Other drugs such as frusemide (*Lasix*) or methyldopa (*Aldomet*) may possibly increase lithium blood levels. An extremely low dietary sodium intake will result in increased lithium blood levels. Adequate hydration should also be maintained.

EVALUATION

It is important to observe the patient for therapeutic effectiveness. Observation of behavioural parameters should be noted. Dietary sodium intake should be monitored and signs of fluid and electrolyte imbalance (characterised by polyuria and polydipsia) should be reported. Skin reactions may occur during the first few weeks of treatment. Thyroid function should be observed, especially in relation to hypothyroidism.

PATIENT EDUCATION

Patient education involves informing the patient of expected therapeutic effects and assisting them in recognising any deterioration. They should be taught the signs of lithium toxicity and encouraged to visit a medical practitioner should these occur. If drowsiness occurs the patient should be discouraged from driving a vehicle or using machinery. Dietary advice about salt intake should be given and regular blood screening for lithium levels carried out. The patient should be instructed to avoid over-the-counter drugs which contain sodium, e.g. *Dexsal*.

ANXIOLYTICS ▮▮▮▮▮▮▮▮▮▮

Anxiolytic is the name given to those compounds which are effective in alleviating the symptoms of anxiety. The benzodiazepines are the most widely used anxiolytic agents but before their introduction barbiturates, bromides and meprobamate were used. (Anxiolytics were formerly known as minor tranquillisers or sedatives.)

BARBITURATES

The barbiturates were first used early this century. They, along with the bromides, enjoyed wide use in the treatment of anxiety states before the introduction of meprobamate and then the benzodiazepines. Today, they are considered unsuitable for continuing therapy in the treatment of the anxious patient because of their dependence potential, profound sedative effect and the fact that they interact with a considerable number of drugs. Their use is mainly restricted to the treatment of convulsive disorders and as induction agents in anaesthesia.

NURSING IMPLICATIONS

The long-term use of barbiturates should be restricted to those patients who are dependent and cannot cease their use. The principal aim of nursing management should be to discourage any new patients from regularly taking barbiturates.

ASSESSMENT

In the assessment of a patient taking barbiturates, it is important to consider age as the elderly may have an increased sensitivity to the drug. Abuse potential (including suicidal tendency) should be recorded. A history of allergic states or dermatological reactions is important.

Current medication and the presence of pregnancy or lactation should be noted. Renal and liver function should be assessed. Baseline vital signs such as blood pressure, pulse rate, weight and sleep patterns and blood screening tests are necessary.

ADMINISTRATION

It is important to comply with legal requirements in relation to the administration and recording of these drugs.

EVALUATION

If administering these drugs continuously careful monitoring is essential. The dose should always be tapered off and never ceased abruptly as withdrawal seizures may occur. Concurrent use of barbiturates with other central nervous system depressants should be avoided. The presentation of drowsiness or ataxia may necessitate the patient being supervised during certain activities. Dermatological reactions should be reported as they may indicate systemic lupus erythematosis. Patients should be weighed regularly, their sleep patterns evaluated and blood pressure (lying and standing) should be recorded. Dependence may be a problem with the long-term administration of these drugs.

PATIENT EDUCATION

Patients should be taught to identify adverse reactions. They should avoid situations which require alertness or concentration when drowsy or dizzy, such as driving a motor vehicle or operating machinery. Education concerning compliance and the effects of sudden withdrawal of the drug should be stressed. Alcohol and other central nervous system depressants should not be used concurrently. The presentation of sore throat or mouth ulcers necessitates a visit to their medical officer. Patients should be educated to rise slowly from the lying position and to avoid hot baths in case of hypotension. Although it is preferable that warfarin not be prescribed concomitantly with barbiturates this may be unavoidable in some instances. Patients should be instructed to comply carefully with dosage regimens in these cases.

BENZODIAZEPINES

Alprazolam, Bromazepam, Chlordiazepoxide, Clobazam, Clonazepam, Clorazepate, Diazepam, Flunitrazepam, Flurazepam, Lorazepam, Midazolam, Nitrazepam, Oxazepam, Temazepam

TRADE NAMES

Alprazolam: *Xanax.*
Bromazepam: *Lexotan.*
Chlordiazepoxide: *Librium.*
Clobazam: *Frisium.*
Clonazepam: *Rivotril.*
Clorazepate: *Tranxene.*
Diazepam: *Antenex*; *Valium*; *Ducene.*
Flunitrazepam: *Rohypnol.*
Flurazepam: *Dalmane.*
Lorazepam: *Ativan.*
Midazolam: *Hypnovel.*
Nitrazepam: *Alodorm*; *Mogadon.*
Oxazepam: *Serepax*; *Murelax.*
Temazepam: *Normison*; *Euhypnos*; *Temaze.*

A number of benzodiazepines are marketed. They are commonly divided into two broad categories as shown in Table 26.5 but this is an overly simplistic classification.

MECHANISM OF ACTION

The site of action of the benzodiazepines is unclear. Proposed sites include the reticular activating system, median forebrain bundle and hypothalamus. Benzodiazepine receptors closely located to γ aminobutyric acid (GABA) receptors have been identified in the brain. Benzodiazepine actions are produced by potentiating the action of GABA.

PSYCHIATRIC DISORDERS

26

PHARMACOKINETICS

There has been more nonsense written about benzodiazepine pharmacokinetics than those of any other drug group. This nonsense has followed from the following generalisations which are *incorrect*:

1. The onset of action is related to the time taken to reach peak plasma levels.

This is incorrect as invariably the clinical effect (anxiolytic or hypnotic) occurs before peak levels are reached. About all that can be said is that oral oxazepam takes about two hours to act and the rest act in about one hour.

2. Benzodiazepines can be classified as short, intermediate, or long acting based on their half-lives of elimination after single oral doses.

This is incorrect as it is the distribution phase (after absorption and before elimination) which is the critical phase. For example, diazepam is short acting after a single dose because it is rapidly distributed around the body and its elimination half-life of up to 100 hours is irrelevant. It is a little different with continuous dosing. If benzodiazepines are taken regularly two or three times daily steady state levels are reached in the blood and the antianxiety effect will be continuous.

TABLE 26.5 Categories of benzodiazepines

Long acting (half-life exceeds 10 hours)
Alprazolam
Bromazepam
Chlordiazepoxide
Clobazam
Clonazepam
Clorazepate
Diazepam
Flunitrazepam
Flurazepam
Lorazepam
Nitrazepam

Short acting (half-life less than 10 hours)
Midazolam
Oxazepam
Temazepam

3. Long acting benzodiazepines will accumulate when given on a long-term basis and cause increasing sedation.

This is incorrect as it has been shown that long-term users (average 58 months use) continue to have beneficial antianxiety effects through the day and these are slightly enhanced after each dose. These people do not have sedation or performance impairment (even immediately after a dose) but they can have short periods of memory impairment after, but not before, each dose.

Hence the onset and duration of action of benzodiazepines should not be oversimplified. As long-term use is usual, the facts in the previous paragraph are far more clinically useful than all of the simplistic generalisations about pharmacokinetics. Their metabolism can be stated simply. Lorazepam, oxazepam and temazepam do not have active metabolites, the others do and all benzodiazepines are excreted renally after metabolism. Reduced liver or kidney function may slightly increase the plasma drug level but this is not usually clinically significant.

USES

The benzodiazepines are regarded as the drugs of choice in the treatment of anxiety states. They have numerous other uses including treatment of convulsive disorders, insomnia, night terrors and somnambulism in children, and are employed in obstetrics and in the treatment of acute alcohol withdrawal. Although it is a common belief that benzodiazepines are muscle relaxants, they do not relax skeletal muscle in humans.

In 1980 the Committee on the Review of Medicines (UK) found all benzodiazepines to be efficacious as short-term treatment of anxiety and insomnia, with no agent being more effective than another. The usual division of benzodiazepines into rigid treatment categories of anxiolytic agents (e.g. diazepam) and hypnotics (e.g. nitrazepam) is not based on the known pharmacological and clinical properties of the group.

The major issue concerning benzodiazepines is dependence (see Adverse Drug Reactions, below). Physical dependence can occur and benzodiazepine use should be restricted to either intermittent therapy over two to three weeks or used as part of an overall management plan in chronic severe anxiety disorders. The two uses to avoid are firstly, minor anxiety symptoms (i.e. not severe enough to rate a diagnosis of anxiety disorder) and secondly, sole treatment for any condition. Benzodiazepines only alleviate anxiety, they do not remove or cure anxiety or treat any cause of anxiety.

Short acting compounds are generally used to treat anxiety, insomnia and other appropriate conditions in elderly patients and those with renal or hepatic impairment. The short acting compounds are also suitable for the treatment of insomnia in patients who do not have accompanying anxiety and in whom daytime alertness is required.

The benzodiazepines are administered as tablets, capsules or liquids. Diazepam, clonazepam and midazolam are available in Australia in injectable form. All may be administered intravenously. Diazepam injection is prepared in a non-aqueous solvent and is incompatible with many intravenous fluids and other drugs; advice should be sought before mixing diazepam injections with other drugs or intravenous fluids. Diazepam is poorly absorbed when injected intramuscularly (except for the *Diazemuls* preparation); intramuscular injection is ineffective for status epilepticus. Some hospital pharmacy departments prepare a rectal diazepam preparation which is well absorbed and can be used for status epilepticus when intravenous administration is not feasible.

ADVERSE DRUG REACTIONS

Adverse reactions are extensions of the general pharmacology of the group and are more likely in elderly patients. They include sedation, ataxia, dizziness, vertigo, dysarthria, incoordination, muscle weakness and blurred vision. After excessive dosage or when accumulation has occurred,

there may be impairment of intellectual function, motor performance, coordination and reaction. There is some evidence that hip fractures are increased in elderly patients who take benzodiazepines. Skin reactions and paradoxical excitement are uncommon. Fortunately, adverse drug reactions to benzodiazepines occur remarkably rarely but care should be exercised by patients who operate machinery or drive motor vehicles.

The benzodiazepines are comparatively safe in overdose and fatalities are rare, even after gross overdosage. Intensive care may be required to prevent complications such as inhaled vomitus and obstructed airways. Rapid reversal of benzodiazepine intoxication can be achieved with the antagonist flumazenil.

DEPENDENCE POTENTIAL

Recent studies have confirmed that many patients taking benzodiazepines on a long-term basis (i.e. for periods longer than four months) may experience withdrawal symptoms. This physical dependence may occur even at therapeutic dose levels. Withdrawal symptoms occur earlier and are more severe with the short acting compounds. To diminish the risk of dependence, benzodiazepines should generally be used for short term treatment only.

Withdrawal symptoms may appear within 24 hours after abrupt withdrawal of short acting drugs and in 3–10 days after abrupt withdrawal of longer acting compounds. Symptoms include anxiety, apprehension, tremor, insomnia, nausea and vomiting. Seizures may occur after long-term use. Therefore, all continuous benzodiazepine therapy (i.e. unless given on an occasional basis only) should be withdrawn gradually over weeks or months.

DRUG INTERACTIONS

Benzodiazepines have relatively few clinically significant drug interactions except for the expected potentiation of the sedative properties of other central nervous system depressants, e.g. alcohol, antipsychotics, antidepressants, antihistamines and other

PSYCHIATRIC DISORDERS

26

hypnotics and sedatives. It should be noted that unexpected interactions (e.g. blackout) with alcohol may occur during the day or evening following the nocturnal use of long acting benzodiazepines. Cimetidine inhibits the metabolism of diazepam and will increase the plasma levels and may potentiate the sedative effects of diazepam.

Care should be exercised in the administration of benzodiazepines to the elderly and to patients with liver and kidney disease as outlined above. These drugs are not suitable for use in disorders such as depression, tension headache and dysmenorrhea (occurring in the absence of anxiety) or in the treatment of psychotic disturbances. Benzodiazepines are without analgesic or antidepressant activity.

Except for myasthenia gravis, there are no absolute contraindications for the benzodiazepines. It is advisable to avoid use in children wherever possible.

Buspirone

Buspirone is a non-sedating anxiolytic.

TRADE NAMES

Buspirone: *Buspar*.

MECHANISM OF ACTION

Buspirone is different to the benzodiazepines in a number of ways. It has no anticonvulsant or muscle relaxant properties; it does not affect GABA transmission but does affect serotonergic, noradrenergic and dopaminergic activity; and it has, so far, low potential for abuse or dependence (i.e. withdrawal effects have not been reported).

PHARMACOKINETICS

Buspirone is orally absorbed. It usually takes 1–2 weeks after starting therapy for the anxiolytic effect to occur. The maximum anxiolytic effect may take 4–6 weeks.

USES

Buspirone is useful in chronic anxiety, anxious patients with a history of substance abuse and in situations where sedation may be dangerous to an anxious patient. The anxiolytic dose range is 15–45 mg daily in divided doses.

Buspirone is safe in overdose but its most important feature is that it is not effective on a 'prn' (when necessary) basis.

ADVERSE DRUG REACTIONS

Headache, dizziness, lightheadedness, nervousness, fatigue, paraesthesia and gastrointestinal upset occur in about 10% of patients.

DRUG INTERACTIONS

Drug interactions are not a major concern but increased blood pressure has been reported with buspirone–MAOI combinations and buspirone can inhibit the metabolism of haloperidol.

NURSING IMPLICATIONS

ASSESSMENT

Regardless of the benzodiazepine prescribed the implications for nursing care remain the same. Assessment should begin with checking the patient's history for any evidence of previous hypersensitivity to benzodiazepines. The patient's employment and lifestyle should also be considered as people who operate power machinery or who drive a car need to be informed of the sedative effect of the drugs. Baseline measures of vital signs and blood pressure will need to be taken to form an objective measure of the anxiety state. Nursing staff should be especially aware that the elderly and those with renal and/or hepatic insufficiency will be less capable of metabolising and excreting the drugs and therefore accumulation and toxicity can occur.

ADMINISTRATION

In hospitals this requires the usual procedure for administration of restricted drugs. If the patient shows signs of toxicity (such

as excessive sedation, ataxia and so on) the nurse should withhold the drug and seek further orders.

As a general rule, parenteral preparations of diazepam should not be diluted with other solutions or mixed in the same syringe or bottle with other drugs. Intravenous injections should be given slowly and directly into the vein (not diluted) and the patient's blood pressure checked regularly. The vein should be flushed with normal saline after intravenous administration of diazepam.

The majority of benzodiazepines, however, are self-administered in the home and the misuse and abuse of these drugs has reached alarming proportions. Nurses who work in general practice surgeries should be alert for patients who frequently request renewal of prescriptions for these medications. Community health nurses should be alert for patients who are less able to cope or who subscribe to the belief that 'there's a pill to cure everything'. These people may be actual or potential benzodiazepine abusers.

EVALUATION

The nurse should note the patient's subjective reports of reduced anxiety. The monitoring of vital signs can give objective signs of reduced anxiety, i.e. lower blood pressure, pulse and respiratory rates. Patients should be observed for adverse effects, including rashes, and signs of toxicity, e.g. excessive sedation and ataxia. The nurse should supervise elderly patients who may be at risk of falling, especially in bathrooms or on stairs.

PATIENT EDUCATION

Patient education should include instructions regarding the criteria for determining the effectiveness of therapy and identifying adverse effects. Warnings should be given concerning the sedative effects of the drug and of the dangers of driving cars or operating machinery. Patients should be advised of the potentiating effects of alcohol and other tranquillising drugs. Patients and the community in general should be informed concerning the potential for physical dependence with these drugs. Such information can help prevent irresponsible use and abuse. It is important that patients taking benzodiazepines are counselled that abrupt withdrawal following prolonged use can result in severe withdrawal effects.

It should be emphasised that these drugs, while they relieve the symptoms of anxiety, do not resolve the source of the anxiety. Proper counselling of these patients should be employed and may reduce or eliminate the need for this type of drug.

ANTIDEPRESSANTS ██████████

26

Antidepressant drugs are effective in the treatment of depressive disorders and include three major classes of compound: heterocyclic antidepressants, serotonin selective reuptake inhibitors and monoamine oxidase inhibitors (MAOIs). Antidepressant drugs relieve depression by elevating the mood of the patient but they are not central nervous system stimulants (i.e. they are not like the amphetamines).

Depression must be viewed as a distinct clinical entity. Depression is different to everyday sadness or unhappiness. The major difficulty in diagnosis is distinguishing between various states of low mood, e.g. unhappiness (everyone is occasionally unhappy), depressive symptoms related to an event such as bereavement, a depressive disorder related to the person's personality (dysthymia), or a major depressive illness. There is no easy test to correctly diagnose among these or other possibilities. The important point is that antidepressant drugs are most beneficial in major depressive illness, can be helpful in dysthymia but are usually not appropriate for other states of lowered mood.

Treatment of depression may be multiple and involve psychotherapy or electroconvulsive therapy. It must be remembered that depressive patients can be suicidal and the risk of suicide must be taken into account when selecting therapy.

Heterocyclic antidepressants is a name devised to embrace the well known tricyclic antidepressants and newer antidepressants which are not tricyclic in chemical structure but have similar actions in depression, e.g. mianserin. Heterocyclic antidepressants may be administered orally in daily divided doses or as a single large daily dose at bedtime. Elderly patients often cannot tolerate a single large dose and are best treated by divided dose regimens.

The advantages of a single daily dose are threefold. Firstly, it optimises the sedating effects thus obviating the need for a hypnotic (sleep disturbances are a part of depressive illness). Secondly, it encourages compliance. Thirdly, it reduces the incidence of most of the troublesome side effects as these are most intense during the first few hours after administration and the patient will therefore sleep through them.

There are some small differences between tricyclic antidepressants and mianserin so the tricyclics will be discussed first, followed by a brief summary of the advantages and disadvantages of mianserin.

TRICYCLIC ANTIDEPRESSANTS

Amitriptyline, Clomipramine, Desipramine, Dothiepin, Doxepin, Imipramine, Nortriptyline, Trimipramine

TRADE NAMES

Amitriptyline: *Tryptanol*; *Endep*; *Laroxyl*.
Clomipramine: *Anafranil*.
Desipramine: *Pertofran*.
Dothiepin: *Prothiaden*.
Doxepin: *Deptran*; *Sinequan*.
Imipramine: *Tofranil*.
Nortriptyline: *Allegron*; *Nortab*.
Trimipramine: *Surmontil*.

MECHANISM OF ACTION

The antidepressant activity of the tricyclics is thought to be due to their ability to block neuronal uptake of amines such as noradrenaline and serotonin, and thus increase the effective concentrations of these substances in the synapse. The tricyclics have a number of pharmacological actions in addition to their antidepressant activity, including anticholinergic, antiserotonin and antihistamine actions.

PHARMACOKINETICS

Tricyclic antidepressants are rapidly and completely absorbed after oral use with peak plasma concentrations occurring within 2–8 hours. They are also rapidly metabolised by the liver (first-pass effect) sometimes to active metabolites. For example, imipramine is metabolised to desipramine and a blood level measurement should measure both drugs.

Generally, plasma drug measurement is not useful (poor correlation with clinical effect) except for nortriptyline which has its maximum antidepressant effect at levels between 50 ng/mL and 150 ng/mL.

Elimination half-lives vary greatly from one individual to another (e.g. nortriptyline 15–90 hours) but they are all sufficiently long acting to make single daily doses possible if that is convenient to the patient. Tricyclics are eliminated more slowly in the elderly who should receive about one-third to one-half of a younger adult's dose.

Tricyclics are 90%–95% protein bound and are widely distributed outside the blood stream. They are very toxic in overdose and extracorporeal dialysis is ineffective in removing them because of this extravascular reservoir.

USES

The tricyclic antidepressants are the drugs of first choice for those forms of depression which respond to drug therapy. Treatment should be initiated with low doses and gradually built up until a response is obtained. It may take 7–21 days after therapeutic doses are reached to obtain a response. A usual therapeutic dose for a physically healthy adult is at least 150 mg daily (see Table 26.6). If a patient fails to respond to tricyclic therapy and electroconvulsive therapy is considered unsuitable, the MAOIs are usually the next choice.

TABLE 26.6 Average daily doses for tricyclic antidepressants

Drug	Average daily doses (mg)
Amitriptyline	100–250
Clomipramine	100–250
Desipramine	100–250
Dothiepin	100–200
Doxepin	100–300
Imipramine	100–250
Nortriptyline	50–150
Trimipramine	100–300

ADVERSE DRUG REACTIONS

Sedation is common, especially during initial therapy. Anticholinergic effects also occur frequently and include dry mouth, blurred vision, constipation and urinary hesitancy or retention. Other anticholinergic drugs potentiate these effects.

Cardiovascular effects include postural hypotension, which is common particularly in elderly patients or those on high doses. AV conduction time may be prolonged. Tachycardia and extrasystoles may occur, especially at high doses. Care must be taken if cardiac disease is present.

Skin rashes, blood dyscrasias, jaundice, weight gain and sweating are less common adverse effects.

After overdose toxic reactions are mainly anticholinergic, cerebral or cardiac. Tricyclics can easily be fatal in overdose and are the most common prescription drug involved in fatal overdoses.

DRUG INTERACTIONS

Antipsychotics, cimetidine, methylphenidate and steroid preparations (including oral contraceptives) can interfere with the metabolism of tricyclics, thereby enhancing their adverse effects.

Barbiturates increase the liver metabolism of tricyclics and decrease their action. Prescribing barbiturates (also potentially fatal in overdose) to someone who is depressed can rarely, if ever, be justified.

Tricyclics enhance the effects of alcohol and other sedatives.

The anticholinergic effects of tricyclics are potentiated by combining them with other anticholinergic compounds such as some of the antiparkinsonian drugs.

Tricyclics potentiate the action of sympathomimetic amines such as noradrenaline. Tricyclics inhibit the action of the antihypertensive agents, guanethidine and debrisoquine. The central antihypertensive effect of clonidine may be blocked by tricyclics.

Severe central nervous system toxicity leading to coma is possible when tricyclics and MAOIs are combined. However, although this is an extremely severe reaction it is very rare and cautious combined use by experienced clinicians can be life saving.

PRECAUTIONS AND CONTRAINDICATIONS

Because of their adverse cardiac effects, tricyclics should not be used during the acute recovery period after myocardial infarction.

Mianserin

TRADE NAMES

Mianserin: *Tolvon*.

Mianserin is a tetracyclic antidepressant. Its dose range is 30–120 mg daily and its mechanism of action is thought to be similar to the tricyclics. It appears to be less cardiotoxic, much safer in overdose and to have fewer undesirable autonomic properties than tricyclics. Mianserin is associated with an increased risk of neutropenia, agranulocytosis and arthralgia.

SELECTIVE SEROTONIN REUPTAKE INHIBITORS

Fluoxetine

TRADE NAMES

Fluoxetine: *Prozac*.

MECHANISM OF ACTION

Fluoxetine blocks the reuptake of serotonin, it does not affect noradrenaline or other neurotransmitters. It is a selective serotonin reuptake inhibitor (SSRI) antidepressant.

PHARMACOKINETICS

Fluoxetine is orally absorbed and very long acting. If the dose is increased it may take 3–4 weeks for side effects to appear. Generally, doses should not be increased more frequently than monthly.

USES

Fluoxetine is as effective in depression as the tricyclics, mianserin or MAOIs, but has some advantages in its side effect profile. For example, it does not have the typical tricyclic side effects of sedation, autonomic effects (dry mouth, blurred vision, constipation) or cardiovascular effects.

The standard dose is a single 20 mg capsule in the morning. Doses are not increased gradually as happens with other antidepressants.

ADVERSE DRUG REACTIONS

The most common side effects with fluoxetine are nervousness, insomnia, nausea, diarrhoea, headache and tremor. Most patients (90%–95%) can take 20 mg daily without these side effects being severe enough for treatment to be stopped.

Suicidal ideas have appeared in a few patients treated with fluoxetine. This also happens with other antidepressants but suicidal thoughts should be especially monitored in patients taking fluoxetine. An allergic syndrome of rash, fever, joint pain and respiratory symptoms occurs in about 1% of patients.

DRUG INTERACTIONS

Fluoxetine should not be combined with MAOIs (some fatal interactions have occurred). MAOIs must be stopped for two weeks before starting fluoxetine, or fluoxetine must be stopped for five weeks before starting MAOIs. Fluoxetine also interacts to some degree with all other psychotropic drugs.

Paroxetine

TRADE NAMES

Paroxetine: *Aropax*.

Paroxetine is as effective as fluoxetine and is used in depression. Its adverse effects and drug interactions should be the same as those of fluoxetine. It differs in its pharmacokinetics having a shorter half-life (mean of ≃ 24 hours) and it does not have an active metabolite. Overall, paroxetine is removed from the body more quickly and only two weeks cessation is needed before starting an MAOI. Reducing the dose in response to an adverse effect (e.g. nausea or agitation) may alleviate the adverse effect more quickly than would happen with fluoxetine. Withdrawal effects may occur in 1–4 days if the drug is stopped abruptly.

Most patients respond to 20 mg daily, taken in the morning with food. Some patients may respond to dose increases of 10 mg weekly up to a maximum dose of 50 mg daily (40 mg in the elderly).

Sertraline

TRADE NAMES

Sertraline: *Zoloft*.

Sertraline is similar to paroxetine, is also shorter acting than fluoxetine and has an average half-life of 26 hours. It has a slightly active metabolite that is probably unimportant. It interferes less with the metabolism of some other drugs (e.g. tricyclic antidepressants) than paroxetine and fluoxetine. Most of the time this is not clinically relevant because SSRIs and tricyclics are not used together.

MONOAMINE OXIDASE INHIBITORS

The monoamine oxidase inhibitors (MAOIs) were introduced in the mid 1950s after it was noticed that depressed, tubercular patients receiving the antitubercular drug iproniazid (also an MAOI) showed an improvement in mood.

Phenelzine, Tranylcypromine

TRADE NAMES

Phenelzine: *Nardil.*
Tranylcypromine: *Parnate.*

MECHANISM OF ACTION

These drugs inhibit the enzyme monoamine oxidase (MAO) which is responsible for the breakdown of neurotransmitters such as serotonin and noradrenaline. If MAO is inhibited then serotonin and noradrenaline accumulate in the brain.

PHARMACOKINETICS

These drugs are only given by the oral route and are well absorbed. They begin to exert their action within 5–10 days after starting therapy.

USES

The MAOIs are not drugs of first choice in the treatment of depression but should be reserved for cases where other drug treatments and therapy regimens have been inadequate, i.e. if heterocyclic antidepressants fail and electroconvulsive therapy is unsuitable. It may take several days before a response is evident.

The average daily dose ranges for the MAIOs are listed in Table 26.7.

TABLE 26.7 Average daily dose ranges for the MAOIs

Drug	Dose range (mg)
Moclobemide	300–600
Phenelzine	45–90
Tranylcypromine	10–40

ADVERSE DRUG REACTIONS

Transient hypertension occurs occasionally and hypertensive crisis, characterised by headache, palpitations, nausea and vomiting, may occur. Hypertensive crisis may occasionally lead to subarachnoid or intracranial haemorrhage. It may be precipitated by the ingestion of certain foods or drugs (see Drug Interactions).

Liver damage has been reported with phenelzine.

Hypotension is the most common troublesome side effect and is probably due to the ganglion blocking effects of these drugs.

Tranylcypromine in particular has a rapid and direct central nervous system stimulant action in addition to its ability to inhibit MAO. In order to avoid insomnia it should not be given later than midafternoon. Phenelzine is usually sedating but daytime somnolence has been reported with both phenelzine and tranylcypromine.

Other less common effects are gastric upsets, dizziness, dry mouth, muscle weakness, cardiac arrhythmias and disturbances in red and green colour vision.

DRUG INTERACTIONS

Drugs which can interact with MAOIs to cause a hypertensive crisis or a serotonergic syndrome are: sympathomimetic amines (e.g. adrenaline, ephedrine, phenylephrine, methoxamine, phenylpropanolamine, metaraminol, isoprenaline, tyramine and dopamine); appetite suppressants (e.g. diethylpropion, fenfluramine, dexfenfluramine, amphetamine and dexamphetamine); and methylphenidate, methyldopa, levodopa and pethidine.

PSYCHIATRIC DISORDERS

26

Foods which can interact to cause a hypertensive crisis are cheese, yeast extracts (*Vegemite, Marmite, Bonox, Bovril*), pickled herrings, broad bean pods, banana peel, sauerkraut and any aged meat, poultry or egg products. For some other foods the evidence is weaker but in general all food should be fresh, stored properly and eaten soon after purchase. Alcohol use should be minimised in depression anyway but chianti and home brew beer are the drinks which should be avoided. Two standard glasses of other alcoholic drinks are permitted occasionally.

Tricyclic antidepressants, pethidine and reserpine can interact with MAOIs to cause severe serotonergic reactions (sometimes fatal) including delirium, rigidity, seizures and hypo- or hypertension.

MAOIs inhibit the metabolism of many drugs (by inhibiting liver microsomal enzymes) and so potentiate their action. Some examples are central nervous system depressants including alcohol, barbiturates, opiates, benzodiazepines and anaesthetic agents; atropine; cocaine; antihistamines; tricyclic antidepressants; oral hypoglycaemic agents; antihypertensive drugs; and muscle relaxants (e.g. tubocurarine).

Moclobemide

Moclobemide is a new MAOI antidepressant which is very unlikely to cause the food interactions which are a problem with the older MAOIs. For example, more than 1 kg of some cheeses and up to 70 g of *Marmite* can be taken safely with moclobemide at a dose of 200 mg three times daily after meals. It is also safe in overdose.

TRADE NAMES

Moclobemide: *Aurorix.*

PHARMACOKINETICS

Moclobemide is absorbed rapidly and completely after oral administration. It is sufficiently lipophilic (i.e. fat soluble) to efficiently cross the blood-brain barrier.

About 20% of an administered dose is rapidly metabolised in the liver (first-pass effect) and protein binding is relatively low (about 50%).

Like other antidepressants moclobemide does not act immediately, it may take about 10 days for onset. Moclobemide is a reversible inhibitor of monoamine oxidase-A (RIMA) which means that its side effects subside a couple of hours after treatment is stopped. The effects of older MAOIs, which are irreversible, last 10–14 days after treatment is stopped.

Moclobemide is completely metabolised to inactive metabolites and has an elimination half-life of 1–2 hours. No dosage decrease is needed in the elderly or in patients with reduced renal function.

USES

Moclobemide should be started at a dose of 150 mg twice daily taken at the end of a meal and increased at 2-weekly intervals up to a maximum of 600 mg daily.

ADVERSE DRUG REACTIONS

Side effects are insomnia, dizziness, nausea, dry mouth, constipation, diarrhoea, anxiety and restlessness.

DRUG INTERACTIONS

Moclobemide interacts with cimetidine and the moclobemide dose should be halved if cimetidine is being used. Some sources state that moclobemide does not interact with the same drugs as other MAOIs. This is probably incorrect. Like other MAOIs, moclobemide probably inhibits liver microsomal enzymes and it should be assumed that it will interact with pethidine, tricyclic antidepressants, sympathomimetic amines and the other drugs listed under MAOI drug interactions above.

Moclobemide has the advantage over other MAOIs of not interacting with foods containing tyramine and the advantage over both the tricyclics and other MAOIs of being safe in overdose.

NURSING IMPLICATIONS

ASSESSMENT

Depression should be accurately assessed. Medications and socially acceptable drugs such as alcohol should be noted. The presence of pregnancy or lactation should be recorded. A history of cardiovascular disease, hypertension, epilepsy, diabetes mellitus, glaucoma, constipation, organic brain disease or liver disease is relevant. Baseline blood pressure, pulse rate, weight, bowel habits and sleep patterns should be noted and an ECG taken to compare with later changes should they present.

ADMINISTRATION AND EVALUATION

The therapeutic effect of antidepressant drugs may take up to three weeks to manifest. As the patient's depression begins to improve, the risk of suicide may paradoxically increase, due to an increased drive and will on the patient's part to carry out an attempt. Patients should be observed for abnormal behaviour during this time.

When stopping therapy with the tricyclic antidepressants, the dose should be tapered gradually to avoid withdrawal symptoms. The diet of the patient should be adequate to prevent constipation. Nurses should also observe and report other anticholinergic effects such as dry mouth, blurred vision and urinary retention or hesitancy. Blood pressure (lying and standing) should be monitored and any observation of tachycardia or cardiac arrhythmias reported.

The administration of MAOIs necessitates monitoring of blood pressure (lying and standing) and observing for postural hypotension. Hypertensive crises may occur and are usually indicated by the onset of headache. Atropine-like effects such as constipation may occur. Euphoria may present and should be reported. Toxic overdose may present as psychosis or coma, so changes in behaviour or consciousness should be noted and reported. Dietary considerations include the withdrawal of all tyramine containing foods. Sympathomimetic amines should not be administered concurrently. The monitoring of liver function is essential with phenelzine.

PATIENT EDUCATION

Patient education for antidepressant drugs includes teaching about the expected therapeutic effect and the recognition of deviations from this effect. Also, the signs of adverse effects should be taught. Exercise and an appropriate diet should be encouraged to prevent weight gain. A list of foods containing tyramine should be given to patients receiving MAOIs and the possible effects of tyramine rich foods explained. As with most other drugs which act on the central nervous system, situations which require alertness or concentration should be avoided if the patient is dizzy or drowsy. Patients should be educated to rise slowly from the lying position to avoid postural hypotension. With MAOIs the patient should understand that a headache may indicate the onset of a hypertensive crisis and should not be treated with analgesics. Generally patients should avoid taking over-the-counter medications concurrently, especially cough and cold preparations. Dry mouth caused by tricyclic antidepressants may be alleviated to some degree by sucking hard sugarless sweets or chewing gum to stimulate salivation.

PSYCHOSTIMULANTS

Psychostimulants are drugs which increase the level of alertness. Since many of these drugs produce dependence only a few remain on the market and these are strictly controlled by legislation, which may vary slightly from State to State.

Dexamphetamine

Dexamphetamine is a powerful central nervous system stimulant. In addition to its effects on the central nervous system it also elevates blood pressure, increases pulse rate and diminishes the appetite. Due to its central effects it stimulates respiration and reverses the effect of central nervous system depressant drugs (e.g. anaesthetics and hypnotics).

USES

Dexamphetamine has been used for a number of indications including to increase wakefulness and diminish fatigue, mild cases of depression, apathetic or withdr wn senile behaviour, to reverse the effects of anaesthetics and overdoses of hypnotic agents, and to increase response to psychotherapy. It has also been employed to diminish appetite and in the treatment of narcolepsy and hyperkinetic states in children arising from minimal brain dysfunction. Strict legislative controls now restrict its use to the treatment of narcolepsy and childhood hyperkinetic states.

Dexamphetamine is available as 5 mg tablets. The normal dose range is 2.5–5.0 mg administered orally three times daily.

ADVERSE DRUG REACTIONS

Central effects include restlessness, dizziness, tremor, talkativeness, tenseness, irritability, weakness, insomnia, euphoria, fever, confusion, delirium, panic and hallucinations.

Cardiovascular effects include headache, pallor or flushing, palpitations, cardiac arrhythmias, hypertension or hypotension and sweating.

Gastrointestinal effects include dry mouth, anorexia, nausea, vomiting, diarrhoea and abdominal cramping.

PRECAUTIONS

Tolerance to doses of dexamphetamine develops easily, leading to increasing doses of the drug being required to produce the desired physiological effect.

ABUSE POTENTIAL

True physical addiction to amphetamines can occur and on discontinuation of therapy the patient will experience a withdrawal syndrome characterised by prolonged sleep, lassitude and fatigue, increased appetite and occasional profound depression. There is an amphetamine induced toxic syndrome characterised by vivid visual, auditory and tactile hallucinations, skin excoriation and paranoia.

Caffeine

Caffeine is not used therapeutically in psychiatric practice. Some combined analgesic preparations contain small doses of caffeine designed to give mild central nervous system stimulation and mood elevation. If administered in therapeutic doses caffeine stimulates the central nervous system and minimises drowsiness and fatigue. It produces a diuresis, stimulates cardiac muscle, relaxes the smooth muscle of the bronchioles and blood vessels causing dilation and stimulates gastric secretion.

Methylphenidate

Methylphenidate is a mild central nervous system stimulant with effects predominantly on mental rather than motor activity. Its properties are essentially the same as dexamphetamine and it is intermediate in action between dexamphetamine and caffeine.

TRADE NAMES

Methylphenidate: *Ritalin*.

USES

Methylphenidate has been used for the same indications as dexamphetamine but, like dexamphetamine, its use is now restricted to the treatment of narcolepsy and hyperkinetic states in children.

Methylphenidate is available as 10 mg tablets. The oral dose is 10–20 mg administered three times daily before food. The most common use is in children with attention deficit disorder with hyperactivity (sometimes called minimal brain dysfunction or hyperactivity). For children, the average daily dose range is 10–40 mg with 20 mg daily or less usually being sufficient.

ADVERSE DRUG REACTIONS

These include nervousness, insomnia, anorexia, nausea, dizziness, palpitations, headache, skin rash and occasionally changes in blood pressure and pulse rate.

DRUG INTERACTIONS

Methylphenidate may inhibit the metabolism of warfarin, anticonvulsants and tricyclic antidepressants. The toxicity of these drugs may be increased when used concurrently with methylphenidate. Neither methylphenidate nor dexamphetamine should be combined with MAOIs as a hypertensive crisis may ensue.

PRECAUTIONS AND CONTRAINDICATIONS

Methylphenidate should be used with care in hypertensive patients and those with convulsive disorders (the drug may aggravate convulsive tendencies).

The abuse potential of methylphenidate is probably less than that of dexamphetamine but it should be used with caution especially if therapy may be long term or if the patient is emotionally unstable.

Patients suffering from the following conditions should generally not be given methylphenidate therapy: severe depression, anxiety and tension states, thyrotoxicosis, tachyarrhythmias, severe angina, glaucoma or epilepsy.

The safety of methylphenidate in pregnancy is not established.

Cocaine

The most clinically important action of cocaine is its ability to block nerve conduction when locally applied (i.e. its local anaesthetic properties). However, cocaine is also a powerful central nervous system stimulant which has often been used to lessen the sense of fatigue and increase capacity for work. Cocaine stimulates emesis, respiration, the cardiac muscle (in moderate doses) and causes a rise in body temperature. It may be used topically as a local anaesthetic, particularly in ophthalmic and ear, nose and throat work, and has been used as a component of narcotic analgesic mixtures for pain alleviation in the terminally ill (e.g. Brompton's Mixture). These analgesic mixtures normally contain morphine, alcohol and cocaine, the cocaine being used to counteract to some degree the central depressant actions of morphine and alcohol. The use of cocaine for this purpose should be discouraged and has reduced significantly in recent years.

Cocaine has no legitimate psychiatric use.

NURSING IMPLICATIONS

ASSESSMENT

Psychostimulants are used therapeutically for two reasons: the management of narcolepsy and hyperkinesis in children. It is therefore important to note for which condition the patient is being treated. In children it is important to assess weight, height, sleep patterns and motor activity. A history of epilepsy, psychological disorders or diabetes mellitus should be recorded. Nurses should establish baseline vital signs such as blood pressure, pulse rate and weight, and note the presence of pregnancy or lactation.

PSYCHIATRIC DISORDERS

26

ADMINISTRATION

Nurses should be aware of legislative controls which apply to stimulant drugs and should record drugs appropriately.

EVALUATION

Regular weighing is an important feature of management. This is mainly because appetite suppression will occur, even though these drugs are no longer used to treat obesity. Psychostimulants should not usually be administered to people with a history of depression or alcohol abuse. During treatment nursing staff should observe and report abnormal motor activity such as dyskinesia. The medication should not be ceased suddenly as withdrawal may occur. It is important to note the presence of adverse effects such as skin rash, bruising, diarrhoea, constipation, visual disturbances or behavioural changes. Patients receiving methylphenidate in conjunction with warfarin and anticonvulsant drugs should be monitored carefully as the toxicity of these drugs may be increased in the presence of methylphenidate.

PATIENT EDUCATION

Patient education involves teaching the patient about the expected therapeutic effect and how to recognise deviations from this in terms of adverse effects. The patient should be informed that if they miss a dose not to take an extra dose to 'catch up'. In some cases situations which require alertness or concentration should be avoided if visual disturbances are present.

HYPNOTICS ▮▮▮▮▮▮▮▮▮▮

The word hypnotic is derived from the Greek hypnos, meaning sleep. Hypnotics are drugs which will induce sleep. Over the years many agents have been used such as alcohol, opium, belladonna and bromides. Today a variety of compounds are used.

BENZODIAZEPINES

Nitrazepam, Temazepam

TRADE NAMES

Nitrazepam: *Alodorm*; *Mogadon*.
Temazepam: *Euhypnos*; *Normison*; *Temaze*.

BARBITURATES

Amylobarbitone, Butobarbitone, Pentobarbitone

TRADE NAMES

Amylobarbitone: *Amytal Sodium*.
Butobarbitone: *Soneryl*.
Pentobarbitone: *Nembutal*.

MISCELLANEOUS AGENTS

Chloral Hydrate, Chlormethiazole

TRADE NAMES

Chloral hydrate: *Dormel*; *Noctec*.
Chlormethiazole: *Hemineurin*.

MECHANISM OF ACTION

All hypnotics depress the central nervous system but the different agents vary in their degree of selectivity of action on different parts of the central nervous system.

Workers in sleep laboratories have identified five stages of sleep during the sleep cycle: 'dreaming time' or rapid eye movement (REM) sleep followed by successive stages of deepening sleep culminating in stage 4, the deepest sleep. These stages are repeated in cycles throughout the night.

There is more stage 4 sleep in the early hours of sleep and more dreaming time during the latter stages of sleep. The young have more stage 4 sleep than the old. Suppression of dreaming time can produce emotional disturbances.

While all hypnotics depress the amount of REM sleep, the barbiturates depress the REM stage of sleep rather more than the benzodiazepines. Cessation of drugs which suppress REM sleep can cause a rebound increase in dreaming time, often producing disturbing nightmares.

PHARMACOKINETICS

The benzodiazepine hypnotics most commonly used are temazepam and nitrazepam. Temazepam is quickly absorbed (20 minutes to reach 80% of peak plasma concentration) from the soft capsule formulation used in Australia. It has no active metabolites and is renally excreted as the inactive glucuronide metabolite. It has an elimination half-life of 6–8 hours. Although it is short acting and does not cause morning 'hangover', its hypnotic effect wears off after a couple of weeks of continuous use. This occurs with all short acting benzodiazepine hypnotics.

Nitrazepam is well absorbed orally with peak plasma levels occurring 40–80 minutes after administration. It is mainly eliminated by metabolism rather than excretion and has an elimination half-life of about 30 hours. Therefore, it may produce morning 'hangover' and is more slowly eliminated if liver function is reduced. However, long acting benzodiazepine hypnotics have been shown to be continually effective for six months or more and long-term users are often not troubled by day time sedation. So, the question must be 'Is long-term hypnotic use beneficial for this patient?'. If the answer is yes, then there is more clinical evidence to support the use of nitrazepam rather than temazepam. However, considerable care and regular monitoring of long-term use of nitrazepam in the elderly is required as not only sedation but cognitive impairment and falls may occur.

Chloral hydrate is an inactive drug that must be metabolised to an active metabolite (trichloroethanol). Peak levels of trichloroethanol occur 20–60 minutes after oral administration of chloral hydrate and its elimination half-life is 7–9.5 hours.

Barbiturates have no place as hypnotics because of their long duration of action and their adverse effects. The place of chlormethiazole as a hypnotic is also doubtful (see adverse drug reactions).

The hypnotics are usually given orally as tablets, capsules or liquids. When a rapid hypnotic effect is desired, e.g. in extreme psychiatric disturbances, some hypnotics may be administered parenterally combined with an antipsychotic.

USES

Hypnotics are used to relieve insomnia. There are three major types of insomnia: difficulty falling asleep; difficulty staying asleep; and early morning waking. Just as the anxiolytic agents do not relieve the cause of anxiety, the hypnotics do not relieve the cause of insomnia. No drug produces a true physiological sleep but some hypnotics disturb the physiology of sleep to a lesser extent than others. Hypnotics should be prescribed in as low a dose as possible and for short periods only.

Hypnotics should be taken on retiring. They must not be taken too early as the patient may become drowsy and disoriented and have some form of accident or forget they have taken it and 'double up' on their dose. Hypnotics should not be administered routinely as it can quickly lead to physical dependence. They should be taken only when really necessary and after other methods have been tried, e.g. hot bath, listening to soothing music, relaxation techniques, hot drinks or a small nightcap. Hypnotics should be used with great caution in the elderly as the ageing brain is more sensitive to their action. It is easy to produce a toxic confusional state resembling dementia or organic brain disease by long-term administration of hypnotics.

The usual dose ranges for the hypnotic agents are listed in Table 26.8.

PSYCHIATRIC DISORDERS

26

TABLE 26.8 Dose ranges for hypnotic agents

Drug	Usual dose range (mg)
Benzodiazepines	
Nitrazepam	5–10
Temazepam	10–20
Barbiturates	
Amylobarbitone	200–400
Butobarbitone	100–200
Pentobarbitone	50–100
Miscellaneous agents	
Chloral hydrate	500–1000
Chlormethiazole	200–400

ADVERSE DRUG REACTIONS

Benzodiazepines may cause nightmares, confusion or rashes but these only occur rarely. Long acting benzodiazepines produce a hangover effect. The benzodiazepines are, however, the hypnotic agents of choice due to their low incidence of adverse reactions and low toxicity.

Barbiturates may cause disorientation, dizziness, ataxia, depression, sleep disturbances and altered dreaming patterns. Paradoxical excitement can occur in children and the elderly. Hangover is common due to the long duration of action of many barbiturates. A rare adverse effect is the development of systemic lupus erythematosis (SLE).

Chloral hydrate may cause gastric irritation, skin rashes and itching. It is relatively free of adverse reactions and is often considered suitable for the very young and very old.

Chlormethiazole occasionally may cause sneezing and rhinitis in younger patients, and gastrointestinal disturbances. There have been many cases of rapidly acquired dependence especially in alcoholics and those with a history of drug abuse. Hypotension and bronchorrhea can occur during intravenous infusion. In the treatment of alcohol withdrawal chlormethiazole should be reserved for inpatient use.

DRUG INTERACTIONS

The hypnotics will have additive sedating effects with other drugs possessing central nervous system depressant activity.

Barbiturates stimulate liver microsomal enzymes and therefore increase the metabolism and decrease the efficacy of a number of drugs, e.g. phenytoin, warfarin and low dose oral contraceptives.

Chloral hydrate enhances the anticoagulant effect of warfarin and concurrent use may lead to haemorrhage. When combined with alcohol, chloral hydrate may produce an unpleasant vasodilating reaction, characterised by reflex tachycardia, palpitations and facial flushing.

PRECAUTIONS AND CONTRAINDICATIONS

Hypnotics should be used with great caution or not at all in patients with compromised liver function as a prolongation of central nervous depression may occur.

Barbiturates should never be given to patients suffering from porphyria as an acute attack may be precipitated.

Chloral hydrate is contraindicated in patients with peptic ulcer due to its gastric irritant properties.

NURSING IMPLICATIONS

ASSESSMENT

The hypnotics include the benzodiazepines (discussed previously), the barbiturates and a variety of other compounds including chloral hydrate and chlormethiazole.

The important assessment parameters are similar to those for the groups of drugs previously discussed under psychopharmacology. It is important to assess the current medication regimen for possible interactions, especially with other central nervous system depressants. Assessment of liver function is essential as decreased function will lead to an increased length of central nervous system depression.

An important function of the nurse is proper assessment of the reason for a patient's insomnia before resorting to the use of drugs. Often, simple nursing measures can be instituted which may avoid the need to use drugs altogether. For example, listening to the patient's anxieties and counselling appropriately may do far more to promote proper rest than a drug induced sleep from which the patient wakes only to face the original anxiety once more. Simple physical measures to promote comfort (such as position change, a back rub or an extra blanket) should not be overlooked.

ADMINISTRATION

Administration is usually oral although some hypnotics may be given parenterally. To avoid the unpleasant taste, chloral hydrate mixture may be chilled or it may be given in capsule form. Both chloral hydrate and chlormethiazole should be given with food or milk to avoid gastric irritation. Hypnotics should be administered later (rather than earlier) in the evening as drowsiness during activities while preparing for sleep may lead to accidents. Care and supervision of the elderly person taking hypnotics is essential and bedrails may be needed to protect the patient during the night.

Dependence may be a problem with routine administration. The medication must be tapered off and never stopped abruptly as severe withdrawal convulsions may occur.

Care must be taken with parenteral infusion of chlormethiazole as profound hypotension and respiratory obstruction may occur.

Dermatological reactions such as an irritating rash may be observed in patients taking chloral hydrate.

EVALUATION

Evaluating the therapeutic effect of these drugs is essential. Adverse reactions should be noted, especially states resembling dementia. Note should also be taken of the length of time over which the medication has been administered.

PATIENT EDUCATION

Patient education, especially of the elderly, may prevent serious adverse effects and accidents. Teaching relatives about the therapeutic and adverse effects will also be beneficial to the patient. Such education should include the adverse effects of combining hypnotics with central nervous system depressants, especially alcohol, and of suddenly ceasing the medication.

The patient should be advised to take the medication immediately on retiring and to avoid situations that require alertness and concentration after taking the medication. The patient should also be advised not to take extra medication if a dose is missed. Supervision may be needed for the confused elderly patient.

PSYCHIATRIC DISORDERS

26

FURTHER READING

Gelenberg A.J., Bassuk E.L., Schoonover S.C. (1991) *The Practitioner's Guide to Psychoactive Drugs*, 3rd edn, Plenum Medical, New York.

Perry P.J., Alexander B., Liskow B.I. (1991) *Psychotropic Drug Handbook*, 6th edn, Harvey Whitney Books, Cincinnati.

Psychotropic Guidelines Subcommittee. (1992) *Psychotropic Drug Guidelines*, 2nd edn, Victorian Drug Usage Advisory Committee, Melbourne.

Patient information cards and leaflets, written in simple language, are available at low cost from Drug-Wise, Psychiatric Services, Health and Community Services, 555 Collins St, Melbourne, (03) 616 7003.

TEST YOUR KNOWLEDGE

1. It is advisable to recommend the use of a sunscreen agent to patients taking which one of the following drugs: methaqualone, chlorpromazine, benztropine, droperidol, temazepam, lithium carbonate?

2. Tardive dyskinesia is an adverse reaction brought about by which two of the following drugs: lithium carbonate, oxazepam, chlorpromazine, perphenazine, chlordiazepoxide, trimipramine, doxepin, amitriptyline?

3. With which of the following drugs should tyramine rich foods be avoided: amitriptyline, tranylcypromine, phenelzine, haloperidol, thioridazine?

4. A 52-year-old process worker presents with a 6-month history of insomnia. There is no history of anxiety or depressive illness. The physician decides to prescribe a hypnotic drug. Which of the following would be the most suitable drug: nitrazepam, oxazepam, temazepam, chlorpromazine, chloral hydrate? Give the reasons for your choice.

5. Why is the antiparkinsonian agent L-dopa unsuitable for counteracting extrapyramidal side effects caused by chlorpromazine?

6. A 45-year-old manic depressive patient who has had uneventful lithium carbonate therapy for seven years develops the following symptoms: lethargy, confusion and a slight tremor of the hands. On taking a history the psychiatrist discovers that in recent months the patient has been placed on the following therapy: glibenclamide 5 mg in the morning for mild diabetes and methyldopa 250 mg three times daily and chlorothiazide 500 mg in the morning for hypertension. Which of the newly prescribed drugs may have caused the patient's symptoms and by what mechanism?

7. Antipsychotic agents are useful in the treatment of insomnia and anxiety states. Is this statement true or false?

8. Methylphenidate is used for the treatment of which two of the following conditions: manic depressive illness, narcolepsy, childhood hyperkinetic states, tardive dyskinesia?

9. Tricyclic antidepressants are most useful in the treatment of which one of the following types of depression: depression associated with manic depressive illness, major depressive illness, depression secondary to organic brain disease, depression secondary to personal loss?

10. Describe the nursing procedure you would follow after the administration of an intravenous dose of diazepam.

TABLE 26.9 Summary table — psychotropic drugs

DRUG GROUP Drug Name	Use	Action	Adverse Reactions	Nursing Implications
ANTIPSYCHOTICS Low potency— Chlorpromazine Pericyazine Perphenazine Thioridazine	Palliative treatment of psychoses, e.g. schizophrenia, mania	Blocks central action of dopamine	Sedation; anticholinergic effects; breast enlargement, lactation, menstrual difficulties in women; photosensitivity; pigmentation of cornea, retina, lens; jaundice; depression of white cell count; ECG changes; hypotension; lowered seizure threshold; weight gain; extrapyramidal side effects, tardive dyskinesia	**Administer:** Chlorpromazine injections irritate the skin, avoid spillage; avoid abrupt withdrawal **Evaluate:** For non-compliance; monitor regularly for extrapyramidal side effects and postural hypotension **Educate:** Patient and family about side effects
High potency— Phenothiazines: Fluphenazine Trifluoperazine Butyrophenones: Haloperidol Droperidol Thioxanthenes: Thiothixene Diphenylbutylpiperidines: Pimozide	As above	As above	As above but extrapyramidal side effects (acute dystonias, akinesia, parkinsonism, akathisia) more likely; other adverse effects less likely; tardive dyskinesia	As above

26 PSYCHIATRIC DISORDERS

TABLE 26.9 continued

DRUG GROUP Drug Name	Use	Action	Adverse Reactions	Nursing Implications
Dibenzodiazepines: Clozapine	Treatment of resistant schizophrenia	Blocks dopamine and serotonin	Agranulocytosis (1%–2% of patients); constipation; dizziness; headache; hyperthermia; hypertension; nausea, vomiting; salivation; sedation; seizures; syncope; tachycardia; weight gain	As above
ANTIMANIC DRUGS Lithium	Treatment of manic phase and long-term maintenance therapy of manic depressive illness (bipolar disorder)	Reduces frequency and/or severity of manic and depressive episodes	Polydipsia, polyuria; skin rashes; hypothyroidism; nephrogenic diabetes insipidus. Signs of acute toxicity: nausea, vomiting, lethargy, tremor, anorexia, abdominal discomfort, diarrhoea, ataxia, slurred speech, loss of consciousness, electrolyte imbalance, cardiac impairment	**Evaluate:** Measure serum lithium levels every 6 months or if toxicity possible (levels must be measured within 12 hours of last dose); check polyuria is not increasing **Educate:** Patients about early signs of lithium toxicity; patients and families about side effects
Carbamazepine	Acute mania and prophylaxis of bipolar disorder; adjunct to lithium	As above	Dizziness, drowsiness, ataxia, blurred vision, headache, tremors, blood dyscrasias, rash, hyponatraemia, hypothyroidism; many drug interactions	

TABLE 26.9 continued

DRUG GROUP Drug Name	Use	Action	Adverse Reactions	Nursing Implications
Clonazepam	Acute mania. Adjunct to lithium or antipsychotics	As above	Ataxia, drowsiness, salivation, benzodiazepine withdrawal symptoms possible but uncommon	**Assess:** Each patient must be carefully assessed; avoid value judgements about dependence and whether individual patients need benzodiazepines; discourage barbiturate use if possible **Administer:** Avoid abrupt withdrawal **Educate:** Patient and family about side effects; warn about use of alcohol and possible effects of these drugs on driving and operating machinery
ANXIOLYTICS Barbiturates	No longer considered appropriate treatment	CNS depression	Hypotension, decreased heart rate, respiratory depression, dizziness, ataxia, rash, decreased gastric secretions, habituation and tolerance, liver enzyme induction, withdrawal symptoms, contraindicated in patients with porphyria. Many drug interactions	
Benzodiazepines Alprazolam Bromazepam Chlordiazepoxide Clonazepam Clorazepate Diazepam Flunitrazepam Flurazepam Lorazepam Nitrazepam Oxazepam Temazepam	Anxiety states, convulsive disorders, insomnia, alcohol withdrawal	Potentiates GABA	Habituation, tolerance, sedation, ataxia, dizziness, vertigo, dysarthria, incoordination, muscle weakness, skin rash, blurred vision	

26 PSYCHIATRIC DISORDERS

TABLE 26.9 continued

DRUG GROUP Drug Name	Use	Action	Adverse Reactions	Nursing Implications
ANTIDEPRESSANTS Heterocyclics: Amitriptyline Clomipramine Desipramine Dothiepin Doxepin Imipramine Nortriptyline Trimipramine	Pathological depression	Mood elevation. Increase action of noradrenaline, serotonin	Sedation, anticholinergic effects (dry mouth, blurred vision, urinary retention, constipation), postural hypotension, cardiac effects, skin rashes, blood dyscrasias, jaundice, weight gain, sweating	**Administer:** Avoid abrupt withdrawal **Assess:** Monitor suicide risk especially during first month of treatment (overdose is potentially fatal with tricyclic antidepressants and MAOIs); monitor postural hypotension with tricyclics and MAOIs (especially in elderly) **Educate:** Patient and family about side effects
Mianserin	As above	Mood elevation	Similar to tricyclics but fewer cardiac and anticholinergic effects; increased risk of agranulocytosis and neutropenia	
SSRIs: Fluoxetine Paroxetine Sertraline	As above	Increase action of serotonin	Nervousness, insomnia, nausea, diarrhoea, headache, tremor, rash, fever, joint pain	As above

TABLE 26.9 continued

DRUG GROUP Drug Name	Use	Action	Adverse Reactions	Nursing Implications
MAOIs: Moclobemide Phenelzine Tranylcypromine	As above	Inhibit MAO and allow accumulation of noradrenaline and serotonin in the brain	Severe hypertension, liver damage, hypotension, insomnia, gastric upset, dizziness, dry mouth, muscle weakness, cardiac arrhythmias	Educate: As above; avoid drug–food interactions which could cause hypertensive crisis; care required with tyramine containing foods and OTC cough and cold preparations, low risk of this interaction with moclobemide
PSYCHOSTIMULANTS Dexamphetamine	Narcolepsy; attention deficit disorder (hyperkinesia) in children	CNS stimulation	Restlessness, dizziness, tremor, tenseness, irritability, euphoria, fever, confusion, panic, hallucinations, headache, pallor, flushing, cardiac arrhythmias, sweating, hypertension or hypotension, dry mouth, anorexia, nausea, vomiting, diarrhoea, abdominal cramps	Administer: Avoid abrupt withdrawal Evaluate: Monitor weight in children

26 PSYCHIATRIC DISORDERS

TABLE 26.9 continued

DRUG GROUP Drug Name	Use	Action	Adverse Reactions	Nursing Implications
Methylphenidate	As above	As above	Nervousness, insomnia, anorexia, nausea, dizziness, palpitations, headache, rash, unstable blood pressure	
Cocaine	Occasionally in morphine based mixtures for pain in severe or terminally ill patients; usually as local anaesthetic in eye and ENT procedures	Blocks nerve conduction, counteracts CNS depression caused by morphine	As for other stimulant drugs. Cocaine has no legitimate psychiatric or analgesic use	
HYPNOTICS Barbiturates Benzodiazepines	See anxiolytics See anxiolytics			
Chloral hydrate Chlormethiazole	Insomnia	CNS depressant	Gastric irritation, rash, hypotension, paradoxical excitement, hangover, visual blurring, confusion, toxic convulsions, delirium, habituation and tolerance, withdrawal symptoms	**Administer:** Avoid abrupt withdrawal **Evaluate:** Periodically assess sleep and need for medication and discuss with doctor **Educate:** Patient about good sleep habits; the effects of alcohol; to take drug immediately on retiring

Eye Disorders

MARGARET P. SHAW

O B J E C T I V E S

At the conclusion of this chapter the reader should be able to:

1. List the pharmacological actions, uses and side effects of drugs used in ophthalmology; and

2. List the correct storage, dosage and method of instillation of eye medications.

PREPARATIONS USED IN EYE DISORDERS

The following types of preparations may be used in treating the eye:

- **Eye drops** (for quick local penetration, suitable for day time use).
- **Minims or maxims** (single dose eye drops without preservative).
- **Eye ointments** (suitable for night time use, the medication is more slowly released and therefore longer acting).
- **Subconjunctival injections** (give optimum local effect, e.g. with antibiotics and steroids).
- **Retrobulbar injection** (for local anaesthetics and alcohol).
- **Oral drugs** (e.g. antibiotics, steroids).
- **Parenteral drugs** (e.g. antibiotics, antifungals and antivirals for sight threatening infections).

STANDARDS FOR TOPICAL EYE PREPARATIONS

Topical eye preparations should be formulated to ensure sterility and stability.

Sterility

Sterility is necessary to stop the growth of bacteria. The methods used are: steam sterilising (if the drug is heat stable); filtration through a membrane filter (if the drug is heat labile); aseptic technique (if the drug is insoluble, e.g. hydrocortisone).

The addition of a preservative such as benzalkonium or chlorhexidine, delays the growth of bacteria once the bottle has been opened. After opening, drops with preservative may be used by an outpatient for one month and by an inpatient for one week. Drops without preservative should be refrigerated and discarded three days after opening.

Stability

Stability ensures that the drug keeps its full strength, and is comfortable on instillation into the eye. It is achieved by adjusting the pH with a buffer, usually borate or phosphate. Drugs unstable to heat should be refrigerated, e.g. penicillin.

HOW TO INSTILL EYE DROPS

When an eye drop is instilled, four things may occur:

1. It may run out of the eye and be lost;
2. It may be diluted by tears and lose its effect;
3. It may run down the tear duct and throat into the stomach to give systemic side effects; or
4. It may be absorbed into the eye to give the desired effect.

Therefore, correct method of instillation is important. When using eye drops the patient's head should be tilted slightly backwards and the lower lid pulled down to form a pocket. The bottle should be held so that it does not touch the patient's eye or eye lids and one drop instilled into the pocket. The patient should then gently close the eye. Pressure over the puncta will prevent systemic side effects of the more potent drops, e.g. mydriatics and timolol. When using eye ointment 1 cm is inserted inside the lower lid. The tube should then be carefully pulled down over the lid to break off the dose of ointment. The cap should be replaced immediately.

Figures 27.1 and 27.2 illustrate the correct methods for installation of eye drops and eye ointment.

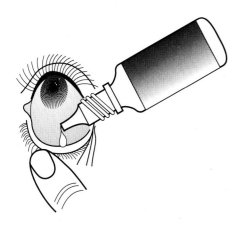

FIGURE 27.1   Instillation of eye drops.

Reproduced with permission from Fildes Pty Ltd,
28–32 George Street, Sandringham, Victoria.

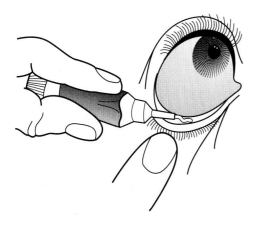

FIGURE 27.2   Instillation of eye ointment.

Reproduced with permission from Fildes Pty Ltd.

NURSING IMPLICATIONS

ASSESSMENT

Initially ophthalmic patients should be assessed for any existing visual disability to establish a baseline for observations plus appropriate nursing actions to assist them where necessary. Before the administration of any ophthalmic preparations a check should be made for any previous allergic reactions to the drug to be used. Of vital importance is the correct and careful identification of the patient.

The nurse should be fully conversant with the patient's ophthalmic diagnosis and history, the presence or history of other diseases and the action of the drug to be administered. For example, if a pupil is dilated in error this could precipitate a glaucoma attack in patients with narrow iridocorneal angles. Not only is correct identification of the patient important but the nurse must make doubly sure which eye is to be treated.

ADMINISTRATION

When using eye drops the patient's head should be tilted slightly backwards and the lower lid pulled down to form a pocket. The bottle should be held so that it does not touch the patient's eye or eye lids and one drop instilled into the pocket. The patient should then gently close the eye. Pressure over the puncta will prevent systemic side effects of the more potent drops. When using eye ointment 1 cm is inserted inside the lower lid. The tube is then carefully pulled down over the lid to break off the dose of ointment. The cap should be replaced immediately.

Because of the delicate nature of the eye great care must be taken to avoid infection. Precautions to be observed during administration relate to keeping the medication from becoming contaminated and avoiding cross infection between patients. For this reason the medication container should not be allowed to come into contact with the patient's eye or eyelid; lids on containers should be promptly replaced; individual medication for each patient should be used; preparations should be stored according to the manufacturer's directions; and expiry dates should be checked and drops discarded one month

EYE DISORDERS

27

after opening or according to the hospital's policy.

Correct administration procedure is important as it not only prevents infection but also ensures maximum effect of the medication.

The nurse should ensure that the patient receives the correct drug and correct dose. Ophthalmic drugs are often available in a variety of strengths so names and strengths of preparations should be checked carefully. Medications in suspension should be shaken before use.

To ensure that the drug is given at the correct time the dosage schedules should be checked carefully. If the patient is to receive more than one medication in the same eye, administration may need to be spaced two or more minutes apart to ensure the correct effect with each preparation. The medications should generally be given in the following order:

(i) soluble drops (e.g. atropine eye drops, chloramphenicol eye drops);

(ii) suspensions (e.g. *Prednefrin Forte* eye drops); and

(iii) ointments (e.g. chloramphenicol eye ointment).

EVALUATION

Evaluation should include observation of the patient for the required effect of the drug, local signs of allergy and optic or systemic side effects. If it is expected that the drug will have some effect on the patient's vision (e.g. photophobia, accommodation difficulties or decreased visual field) the nurse should ensure the patient understands this and take appropriate nursing measures to assist when applicable.

PATIENT EDUCATION

The nurse should ensure that the patient (or carer) understands the correct way to instil eye drops or ointment, the dosage regimen and, if using multiple drops, which one to instil first and the correct time to wait between each instillation. The patient should be instructed to report to their doctor any untoward local or systemic effects which could be due to the drug.

AUTONOMIC CONTROL OF OCULAR FUNCTION ▬▬▬▬▬

SYMPATHETIC NERVOUS SYSTEM

Noradrenaline and adrenaline released at nerve endings contract the dilator pupillae to produce **mydriasis** (dilation of the pupil). Drugs which have the same action are termed sympathomimetic, e.g. adrenaline, phenylephrine.

Drugs can also be used to block the action of adrenaline at its α and β receptors. The drug most commonly used is the β blocker timolol.

PARASYMPATHETIC NERVOUS SYSTEM

Acetylcholine released at nerve endings contracts the sphincter pupillae to produce **miosis** (constriction of the pupil). Drugs which have the same action are termed parasympathomimetic or cholinergic, e.g. pilocarpine and carbachol.

The action of acetylcholine is terminated by the enzyme cholinesterase. If a drug is used to combine with or destroy cholinesterase an accumulation of naturally produced acetylcholine occurs thus producing prolonged miosis. Such drugs are called anticholinesterases, e.g. ecothiopate. Drugs that block acetylcholine at its receptors are called anticholinergics, e.g. atropine, homatropine, cyclopentolate and tropicamide.

These drugs dilate the pupil and are also cycloplegic (i.e. they paralyse the muscles of accommodation).

MYDRIATIC DRUGS

ANTICHOLINERGICS

Atropine, Homatropine, Cyclopentolate, Tropicamide

This group of drugs block the action of acetylcholine and produce mydriasis and cycloplegia. They are used to dilate the pupil both before and after surgery, after trauma, in the treatment of inflammatory eye conditions such as iritis and uveitis, and to relax the ciliary muscle and aid healing.

The naturally occurring anticholinergic is atropine. It is extracted from *Atropa belladonna* (deadly nightshade). Its action may last for up to 14 days and is too strong to be reversed by a miotic. It is available as 0.5% and 1% drops. Dosage varies from once or twice a day to four times daily for severe inflammation.

Diagnostically the drops are sometimes used for three days before ocular refraction is measured in children up to 12 years old. The dose used is one drop 2–3 times a day. However, cyclopentolate drops instilled at the time of refraction are now preferred.

A related but shorter acting drug is homatropine (2% and 5% drops). Its effect lasts for 24–48 hours and it may be used when a patient is sensitive to the toxic effects of atropine.

Other mydriatics include cyclopentolate 1% drops (*Cyclopen*) and tropicamide 0.5% and 1% drops (*Mydriacyl*). (Note: 0.5% tropicamide is not a cycloplegic). Because of their quick onset and shorter duration of action (up to 24 hours and 9 hours respectively) they are used when adult refraction is measured. The dosage is one drop, repeated in 10 minutes if required. Side effects are much less common than with atropine.

Cyclopentolate is also used therapeutically when a patient is allergic to atropine or a shorter acting mydriatic is required.

ADVERSE DRUG REACTIONS

Local reactions include redness, swelling, photophobia and increased intraocular pressure. Systemic effects include dry mouth, nausea, tachycardia, restlessness and confusion.

NURSING IMPLICATIONS

The anticholinergics are a potent group of drugs, therefore correct and careful identification of the patient is vitally important. The administration of anticholinergic drops to a patient who has glaucoma could have disastrous consequences.

The nurse should be aware of the duration of action of the drug used. If the effect is not to be reversed the nurse should ensure that the patient understands that the drug will affect vision and accommodation. Appropriate nursing measures to help the patient cope with these effects should be taken when necessary. When the pupil is dilated photophobia can be distressing and the use of sunglasses can help alleviate this discomfort.

Systemic side effects of the longer acting mydriatics can be minimised by putting pressure on the puncta during administration. Only one drop should be instilled.

EYE DISORDERS

27

SYMPATHOMIMETICS

Adrenaline, Dipivefrin, Phenylephrine

This group of drugs are weak mydriatics and do not produce cycloplegia. They lower intraocular pressure by decreasing the production of aqueous humour and in lower strengths act as vasocontrictors.

Adrenaline (*Eppy-N* 1%, *Epifrin* 1% and 2%) is used in the treatment of open angle glaucoma. The usual dosage is one drop twice daily. Solutions must be protected from air and light and discarded if coloured brown.

Dipivefrin (*Propine* 0.1%) is a newer prodrug. It is not active until converted to adrenaline in the aqueous humour. Local and systemic side effects are less common with this drug.

Phenylephrine 10% decreases intraocular pressure in the normal and glaucomatous eye. It is especially effective for breaking down synechiae (adhesions) in the eye and is used in combination with other mydriatics for intensive dilation. Drops containing 0.125% (*Isoptofrin*, *Prefrin*) produce a blanching effect only on a red eye. This drug will sting the eye on instillation. The dosage for both strengths of phenylephrine is up to four times a day.

ADVERSE DRUG REACTIONS

Systemic side effects of the sympathomimetics include nausea, dizziness, headache, tachycardia and increased blood pressure. Prolonged use may cause a brown discolouration of conjunctiva and lens.

PRECAUTIONS AND CONTRAINDICATIONS

Adrenaline is contraindicated in narrow angle glaucoma as the mydriatic effect could precipitate angle closure. It should be used with caution in hypertension.

NURSING IMPLICATIONS

The nurse should ensure that one drop only is correctly instilled to prevent systemic side effects. Adrenaline drops should not be used if they have turned brown.

DRUGS FOR GLAUCOMA

Glaucoma is a condition in which there is increased intraocular pressure due to excessive retention of aqueous humour. This is accompanied by a decrease of visual field, and changes in the optic disc.

The causes of glaucoma are: obstruction of the flow of aqueous humour in the trabecular meshwork; narrowing or closure of the filtration (iridocorneal) angle; congenital; and secondary to injury or drugs (mydriatics or steroids). If glaucoma is not treated blindness will result. The aim of treatment is to increase the outflow of aqueous humour or to decrease aqueous humour production.

SYMPATHOMIMETICS

See Mydriatic Drugs, adrenaline and dipivefrin.

MIOTIC DRUGS

Cholinergics: Pilocarpine, Carbachol

The cholinergic (parasympathomimetic) group of drugs simulate the action of acetylcholine. They constrict the pupil to produce miosis and contract the ciliary muscles to increase the outflow of aqueous humour. Accommodation is also increased. Their main use is in open angle glaucoma and to reverse the action of mydriatics more rapidly (with the exception of atropine).

Pilocarpine 0.5%–6% is used for chronic open angle glaucoma. A two week trial will indicate which strength is suitable. The dose is 1 drop every 6 hours. In acute glaucoma crises it is used every 15 minutes for 1–2 hours; every hour for the next 4–6 hours; then every 4 hours for 12 hours to help lower pressure prior to surgery.

Carbachol 1.5% and 3% is slightly stronger than pilocarpine and may be used when a patient does not respond or has become sensitive to pilocarpine.

ADVERSE DRUG REACTIONS

Ocular side effects include brow ache, headache, accommodative spasm if close work is undertaken within two hours of instillation and decreased visual field. Systemic side effects include nausea, diarrhoea, weakness, salivation, sweating and asthma.

CONTRAINDICATIONS

These drugs are contraindicated in acute iritis and narrow angle glaucoma.

NURSING IMPLICATIONS

If a cholinergic eye drop is used with adrenaline the adrenaline should be instilled at least 5 minutes after the cholinergic. The slight mydriatic effect of adrenaline decreases the miotic effect of the cholinergic to give better vision and at the same time prevents the pain due to the stimulation of opposing ocular muscles.

The patient should be identified carefully, e.g. it would be dangerous to administer a miotic to a patient with acute iritis.

The nurse should ensure that the patient understands the effects the drug may have

on vision and that appropriate nursing action is taken to help the patient cope should these effects occur.

Anticholinesterases: Ecothiopate

Ecothiopate is an anticholinesterase which allows the accumulation of naturally occurring acetylcholine by preventing its destruction by cholinesterase. Like the cholinergics it produces miosis and increases the outflow of aqueous humour but is longer acting. It is used for more resistant cases of open angle glaucoma and in the treatment of accommodative strabismus.

Ecothiopate (*Phospholine Iodide*) is available as 0.03%, 0.06%, 0.125% and 0.25% drops. The dosage is one drop twice a day and the effect lasts for up to four weeks. The drops should be freshly prepared. They last for one month under refrigeration.

ADVERSE DRUG REACTIONS

Side effects are the same as those of the cholinergics. In addition ecothiopate can cause pupillary cysts (due to prolonged constriction) and cataracts. The cysts can be prevented by instilling phenylephrine 2.5% eye drops.

PRECAUTIONS AND CONTRAINDICATIONS

Exposure to organophosphate compounds (e.g. compounds used in crop dusting) should be avoided. Use should be discontinued for six weeks before a general anaesthetic as the effect can be fatal if succinylcholine is used in conjunction with an anticholinesterase. It is contraindicated in narrow angle glaucoma.

β BLOCKING DRUGS

Timolol, Betaxolol, Levobunolol

The β blocking drugs used in open angle glaucoma are timolol 0.25% and 0.5% (*Timoptol*), betaxolol 0.25% (*Betoptic S*) and 0.5% (*Betoptic*), levobunolol 0.25% and 0.5%

EYE DISORDERS

27

(*Betagan*). These drugs act mainly by decreasing aqueous production. The dosage is 1 drop once or twice a day. They differ from previous glaucoma therapy in that there is no change in pupil size. The half-life of levobunolol is twice that of timolol. β blocking drugs may be used alone or in conjunction with a miotic or acetazolamide. If instilled before adrenaline the mydriatic effect of adrenaline is prevented.

ADVERSE DRUG REACTIONS

Ocular side effects are rare. Systemic side effects include asthma and bradycardia.

PRECAUTIONS AND CONTRAINDICATIONS

Timolol is contraindicated in severe heart disease and asthma. Betaxolol is cardioselective and may be used with caution in asthmatics.

CARBONIC ANHYDRASE INHIBITORS

Acetazolamide, Dichlorphenamide, Methazolamide

Carbonic anhydrase is an enzyme which regulates bicarbonate reabsorption. In the eye bicarbonate is necessary for the production of aqueous humour. If its reabsorption is suppressed the amount of aqueous humour produced decreases and the intraocular pressure is lowered.

Acetazolamide (*Diamox*), dichlorphenamide (*Daranide*) and methazolamide (*Neptazane*) inhibit the action of carbonic anhydrase thereby decreasing the production of aqueous humour and lowering the intraocular pressure. A transient diuresis also occurs.

PHARMACOKINETICS

After oral administration all three drugs are absorbed from the gastrointestinal tract. After administration acetazolamide tablets begin to reduce intraocular pressure in one hour and their duration of action is 8–12 hours. After intravenous administration the onset of action of acetazolamide is rapid,

with a reduction in intraocular pressure occurring in about 2 minutes. Dichlorphenamide tablets exert their effect in 30–60 minutes and it lasts for 6–12 hours.

USES

Carbonic anhydrase inhibitors are used in all types of glaucoma, usually in combination with a miotic or adrenaline. In glaucoma crises, when a rapid effect is needed, acetazolamide 500 mg is given by intravenous or intramuscular injection. Other uses include decreasing raised intraocular pressure after injury or secondary to drugs, e.g. mydriatics and corticosteroids.

Usual oral dosages are: acetazolamide, up to a maximum 1 g per day in divided doses; dichlorphenamide, in glaucoma crises 200 mg at once then 100 mg every 12 hours until a response is obtained, maintenance dose 25–50 mg up to three times a day; methazolamide, 50–100 mg two or three times a day. Gastric irritation is prevented by giving the tablets after food.

ADVERSE DRUG REACTIONS

Adverse reactions include nausea, vomiting, diarrhoea and hypokalaemia which may present as tingling in the extremities. A potassium supplement may be needed. Hypersensitivity reactions common to sulfonamides can occur in patients receiving carbonic anhydrase inhibitors.

PRECAUTIONS AND CONTRAINDICATIONS

Carbonic anhydrase inhibitors are contraindicated in acidosis and renal failure.

NURSING IMPLICATIONS

Because these drugs are derivatives of the sulfonamides it is important to check for a history of allergy to any drugs in this group.

The nurse should also be aware of the effect of carbonic anhydrase inhibition on the electrolyte and acid–base balance of the individual. If the drug is to be used for

more than one or two doses there may be increased potassium excretion leading to hypokalaemia and increased bicarbonate excretion (due to retention of hydrogen ions). This can cause systemic acidosis and alkaline urine, which may predispose the patient to stone formation. To avoid gastric irritation these drugs should be given after food.

OSMOTIC DIURETICS

Osmosis occurs when water is drawn through a semipermeable membrane from a region of lower concentration to a region of higher concentration. When an osmotic agent enters the blood stream it draws water from the aqueous and vitreous humours and reduces intraocular pressure. Osmotic diuretics are used to treat glaucoma crises and to restore a flat anterior chamber after operation.

Glycerol

PHARMACOKINETICS

Glycerol is rapidly absorbed following oral administration and intraocular pressure begins to decline within 10–30 minutes. The effect may last for 4–8 hours.

USES

Glycerol is given orally as a 50% flavoured mixture. The dosage is up to 1–1.5 g/kg body weight. It should be stored in the refrigerator and administered cold as it is very unpleasant to take.

ADVERSE DRUG REACTIONS

Adverse reactions include dizziness, headache, nausea and diarrhoea. Glycerol may raise blood sugar in diabetics.

Mannitol

PHARMACOKINETICS

Mannitol is not absorbed orally and must be administered by intravenous infusion. Intraocular pressure is lowered within 40 minutes and the effect persists for 5–6 hours.

USES

For a rapid diuresis a 20% solution of mannitol is given intravenously. The dosage is 1.5–2 g/kg body weight. If the solution crystallises it can be redissolved by warming before use. Catheterisation may be necessary in some patients.

ADVERSE DRUG REACTIONS

Adverse reactions include acidosis, headache, nausea and electrolyte imbalance.

FIBROBLAST SUPPRESSANTS

A new use for the cytotoxic drug fluorouracil is the suppression of fibroblasts after a filtering operation for glaucoma. The drug stops the healing of the bleb and formation of scar tissue. It is given as a subconjunctival injection at a dose of 5 mg/0.2 mL once a day for seven days or for a shorter period if there are any signs of corneal toxicity.

EYE DISORDERS

27

DRUGS FOR EYE INFECTIONS ▮▮▮▮▮

Eye infections may be bacterial, viral or fungal in origin. A mild infection should be treated topically only, while severe infections and trauma require the addition of systemic medication.

ANTIBACTERIALS

Chloramphenicol, Gentamicin, Neomycin, Polymyxin, Bacitracin, Penicillin, Cephalothin, Ciprofloxacin, Tobramycin

Chloramphenicol (*Chloromycetin*) has good intraocular penetration and a broad spectrum of activity. It is used for conjunctivitis, before and after surgery, and after foreign body removal. Drops should be stored in the refrigerator.

Gentamicin (*Genoptic*) and tobramycin (*Tobrex*) are used for pseudomonal endophthalmitis. The drops are used every 1–2 hours. Tobramycin is also available as an ointment.

Neomycin is a broad spectrum antibiotic. Combined with polymyxin and bacitracin, it is available as *Neosporin* eye drops and ointment and is effective against most Gram positive and Gram negative infections. It is also used before and after surgery.

Polymyxin B acts by restricting cell membrane function and is used for pseudomonal corneal ulcers. It is combined with chloramphenicol in *Chloromyxin* eye drops and ointment to give a broader spectrum of activity. Drops should be stored in the refrigerator.

Penicillin and bacitracin act on the bacterial cell wall structure. Penicillin drops are rarely used as they often cause allergies.

Ciprofloxacin (*Ciloxan*) drops are used for pseudomonal corneal ulcers. Initially the drug is given every 0.5–1 hour decreasing to every 4 hours.

SEVERE INFECTIONS

Bacterial endophthalmitis presents a sight threatening situation and should be treated promptly with topical and systemic antibiotics.

A common treatment is cephalothin eye drops 5% and gentamicin eye drops 0.9% used alternately every half hour, with systemic administration of cephalothin injection 1 g every 6 hours and gentamicin injection 3–5 mg/kg body weight daily in divided doses. (*Note*: cephalothin eye drops must be kept refrigerated at all times).

Flucloxacillin, 1 g every 6 hours, may be used for penicillinase sensitive staphylococci infections. Benzylpenicillin is used in large doses for streptococcal and pneumococcal infections.

ADVERSE DRUG REACTIONS

Side effects of topical antibacterial eye treatment are mainly allergic but precautions should be taken with those drugs that could have systemic side effects. Although rare, chloramphenicol can cause aplastic anaemia.

Sulfacetamide

The sulfonamides are bacteriostatic and act by interfering with the synthesis of folic acid. The only drug in this group used in the eye is sulfacetamide (*Acetopt*). In conjunctivitis the drops are instilled every 4–6 hours. Sulfacetamide is also used before and after surgery and after foreign body removal.

ADVERSE DRUG REACTIONS

The main side effects are redness, swelling, watering and stinging of the eyes.

ANTIVIRAL AGENTS

The virus, herpes simplex, affects the cornea producing superficial punctate keratitis and later dentritic ulcers. The lesions may become chronic and result in scarring which may impair vision.

Idoxuridine, Vidarabine

To prevent the initial or epithelial stage spreading, idoxuridine (*Stoxil*, *Herplex*) drops are used every 1–2 hours by day and the ointment applied at night for a maximum of 21 days.

Intraocular penetration is poor and for stromal or deeper lesions vidarabine (*Vira A*) can be used. The ointment is instilled five times a day. It penetrates the vitreous humour as the metabolite Ara-hypoxanthine and terminates the viral chain.

PRECAUTIONS AND CONTRAINDICATIONS

Idoxuridine should be used with caution in pregnancy.

Acyclovir

Acyclovir (*Zovirax*) is used in the treatment of herpes simplex and herpes zoster ophthalmicus. It differs from the other antiviral agents in that it only penetrates viral cells, thus avoiding toxicity to other tissue.

Topical application of the 3% ointment five times a day promotes healing of keratitis caused by the herpes simplex virus. The drug can also be given orally in a dose of 200 mg five times a day for 7 days.

Acyclovir eye ointment is also beneficial in herpes zoster infections but if the infection is severe systemic therapy should be used as well. The usual dose is 800 mg orally five times a day for 7 days. Treatment needs to be commenced within 48 hours of the initial symptoms to be effective in preventing postherpetic pain. Intravenous administration is not usually necessary as the oral form of the drug is well absorbed and adequate levels are reached in the aqueous humour.

ADVERSE DRUG REACTIONS

Transient stinging may occur following application of the ointment. For further information on adverse drug reactions and contraindications to systemic administration see Chapter 30 Infectious Diseases.

Trifluorothymidine

Trifluorothymidine (*Viroptic*) eye drops 1% are used for keratoconjunctivitis and epithelial keratitis due to herpes simplex virus types 1 and 2. The dosage is one drop every 2 hours to a maximum of nine doses per day. If there is no sign of improvement after 14 days alternative treatment should be tried. Trifluorothymidine should not be used for longer than 21 days.

ADVERSE DRUG REACTIONS

Possible side effects are stinging, hypersensitivity, hyperemia and increased intraocular pressure.

PRECAUTIONS AND CONTRAINDICATIONS

Trifluorothymidine should not be given to pregnant women or nursing mothers unless the benefits outweigh the risks.

NURSING IMPLICATIONS

Cephalothin and other preservative free antibiotic drops should be refrigerated. Sulfacetamide may sting on instillation.

ANTIFUNGAL AGENTS

Fungi can penetrate the eye via the cornea or posterior chamber. The most common causes of fungal infections are garden matter and cosmetics and the use of contaminated needles by drug addicts. Fungal eye infections are difficult to treat as both topical and systemic penetration into the eye is poor and the fungus continues to spread even after the corneal wound has healed. Antifungal agents act by binding to a sterol in the membrane of the fungal cell.

Natamycin

Natamycin (*Natacyn*) eye drops are available as a 5% sterile suspension and are used

27 EYE DISORDERS

in *Candida* and *Aspergillis* sp. infections. The drug also has some antiviral properties. The drops should be shaken before use and instilled every 1–2 hours.

The suspended particles in the drops tend to cause some eye discomfort.

Miconazole

Miconazole may be given by intravenous infusion at a dosage of up to 3600 mg/day in three divided doses.

The main side effects are rash, chills, fever and nausea.

Flucytosine

Flucytosine (*Ancotil*) is available as 500 mg tablets and as an infusion. It is used for candidal and cryptococcal infections.

The dose is 50 mg/kg body weight given at 6-hour intervals. Regular monitoring of blood and liver function should be performed.

Ketoconazole

Ketoconazole (*Nizoral*) is a fungistatic agent used where other treatment has failed. It penetrates the aqueous humour relatively well. The dosage is 200 mg daily as a single dose or 200 mg twice daily for severe infection. This drug should not be given with antacids.

Amphotericin

In the case of fungi penetrating the eye quite deeply an intravitreal injection of amphotericin 5–10 micrograms may be needed.

For further information on antifungal agents see Chapter 30 Infectious Diseases.

MISCELLANEOUS EYE PREPARATIONS

CORTICOSTEROIDS

Hydrocortisone, Fluorometholone, Prednisolone, Dexamethasone

Anti-inflammatory corticosteroids used topically inhibit redness, swelling and capillary dilation in the eye. They also inhibit deposits of collagen, a protein substance that can cause scarring of the cornea after chemical burns or trauma. Minor inflammation such as contact dermatitis or allergy is treated with hydrocortisone 0.5% and 1% (*Hycor*) drops and ointment. Iritis, uveitis and chemical burns may require a stronger agent such as fluorometholone (*FML*), prednisolone 0.5% (*Predsol*) or dexamethasone (*Maxidex*). Prednisolone 1% is combined with the vasoconstricting agent phenylephrine 0.125% in the preparation *Prednefrin Forte*. With the exception of *Predsol* these preparations are all suspensions and should be shaken before use.

With higher doses side effects are more likely so dosage of topical eye preparations should be kept to the minimum dose which produces a satisfactory response. Corticosteroids are also given systemically in large doses for optic neuritis, temporal arteritis and as immunosuppressants in sympathetic ophthalmia and thyroid exophthalmos.

ADVERSE DRUG REACTIONS

Adverse reactions include thinning of the cornea, raised intraocular pressure and with long-term usage, cataracts.

PRECAUTIONS AND CONTRAINDICATIONS

Corticosteroids can mask infection and delay wound healing. Antibiotic cover should be added if there is any risk of infection. They should never be used in herpes simplex infections but may be used with caution in herpes zoster infections once ulceration is controlled. Corticosteroids must be used with great care in glaucoma patients.

LOCAL ANAESTHETICS

Cocaine, Amethocaine, Proparacaine, Benoxinate, Lignocaine

Local anaesthetics act by blocking the conduction of superficial nerves. They also increase the permeability of the cornea. This aids the absorption of other drugs, e.g. homatropine and fluorescein. They are used to anaesthetise the cornea before Schiotz tonometry (a test for intraocular pressure), before the removal of foreign bodies, and for some minor operations.

Cocaine 1%–4% acts in 10 minutes and superficial anaesthesia lasts about 2 hours. It is also a mydriatic and blanches the sclera.

Amethocaine is not quite as long acting. It is used before surgery and for foreign body removal. The shorter acting proparacaine (*Ophthetic*) acts within 13 seconds and lasts up to 20 minutes. It is used before Schiotz tonometry and foreign body removal. The dosage may be repeated up to six times in 30 minutes for minor operations.

Benoxinate (*Novesine*) 0.4% is similar in action but less damaging to the cornea. Combined with fluorescein (*Fluress*) it is used to aid foreign body detection.

Lignocaine (*Xylocaine*) 4% can be used for welding burns up to six times in 24 hours. The patient should be hospitalised for observation as anaesthetic drops can damage the cornea. They also cause loss of blink reflex so a foreign body may easily enter the eye. If the eye is rubbed this will cause further damage. Always tell the patient never to rub their anaesthetised eye. Lignocaine is also used as a retrobulbar injection for local anaesthesia before surgery. The addition of adrenaline prolongs the anaesthetic effect.

STAINING AGENTS

Fluorescein, Rose Bengal

Fluorescein is a phthalein dye that has intense fluorescence in dilute solution. It stains tissues not protected by living epithelium. It is available as 0.25%, 1% or 2% minims or sterile impregnated strips. The strips are inserted into the conjunctival cul de sac to release the drug.

It is used to diagnose abrasions and foreign bodies in the cornea, to check the fit of hard contact lenses and to check the lachrymal system. After examination the eye is irrigated with normal saline eye lotion. Fluorescein injection is used intravenously to examine retinal blood flow and to diagnose retinal detachments.

Adverse drug reactions include transient nausea and occasionally urticaria and anaphylactic reactions following intravenous injection.

Bengal Rose has more affinity for staining destabilised conjunctival cells. It is available as minims or strips and is used to detect keratoconjunctivitis sicca.

CONJUNCTIVAL DECONGESTANTS

Phenylephrine, Naphazoline, Zinc Sulfate

Decongestants are used to constrict superficial blood vessels of the eye due to minor irritation or allergy. A red eye rapidly regains its white look.

Phenylephrine 0.125% (*Isoptofrin*) may be instilled three or four times a day but should be used with caution, as even this strength may cause mydriasis. Naphazoline (*Privine*) is used for the same purpose. Prolonged use of decongestants may cause rebound redness.

Zinc sulfate 0.25% is an astringent and antiseptic drop used to soothe non-specific irritation. Sometimes it is combined with phenylephrine as a vasoconstrictor

EYE DISORDERS

27

(*Zincfrin*). The dosage is one drop instilled 3 or 4 times a day.

ANTIALLERGY PREPARATIONS

Antazoline, Sodium Cromoglycate

Antazoline (*Antistine, Albalon*) is an antihistamine which is often combined with the vasoconstrictor naphazoline in preparations such as *Antistine Privine Eye Drops* and *Albalon-A*. It should not be used for longer than 14 days without medical advice because of possible sensitivity to the antihistamine.

Sodium cromoglycate (*Opticrom*) is prescribed prophylactically to prevent allergies. It acts by stopping the mast cells from rupturing and releasing histamine and is effective for treating vernal (spring) keratoconjunctivitis.

Both preparations may be used four times a day.

LUBRICANTS

Hypromellose, Polyvinyl Alcohol

Lubricants are used to soothe dry eyes. This can result from lack of tears, prolonged periods of unconsciousness or the inability of the eye lids to close properly due to facial palsy or thyrotoxicosis. Lack of treatment could lead to the formation of corneal ulcers. Drops used include hypromellose (*Lacril, Methopt, Isopto Tears, Tears Naturale, Polytears*) and polyvinyl alcohol (*Liquifilm, Tears Plus*). Non-preserved single use drops include *Refresh* and the more viscous *Celluvisc*. The drops may be used as often as required. For longer contact or night time use the ointment *Lacrilube* can be used.

ENZYME PREPARATIONS

Urokinase

Urokinase is used to dissolve clots in retinal arteries or veins. It should be refrigerated and protected from light. For further information on urokinase see Chapter 13 Blood Disorders.

CHELATING AGENTS

EDTA, Desferrioxamine

These drugs remove heavy metal ions by forming a complex with them. This is necessary if the metal is imbedded in the cornea and cannot easily be extracted or washed away. Calcium deposits after lime burns may also be treated with EDTA (ethylene diamine tetra-acetate sodium). Desferrioxamine (*Desferal*) chelates iron deposits.

MUCOLYTICS AND COLLAGENASE INHIBITORS

Acetylcysteine

Acetylcysteine is a mucolytic used to decrease viscid secretions. In the eye a 10% solution is used four times a day to treat chronic ulcerative keratitis.

Another use for acetylcysteine eye drops is as a collagenase inhibitor. Collagenase is an enzyme which can break down collagen in the epithelium of the eye causing ulceration. It is released after trauma such as chemical burns, especially lime burns. The newly forming epithelium becomes changed in nature and the fibrous tissue formed causes scarring. To prevent this, treatment with acetylcysteine drops should start within 24–48 hours of the trauma. The dosage is one drop every two hours reducing to four times a day.

PROSTAGLANDIN INHIBITORS

Indomethacin

Indomethacin 1% as eye drops (*Indoptol*) is

instilled preoperatively before extracapsular surgery to decrease surgically induced miosis. It inhibits the release of prostaglandin resulting from irritation of the iris during surgery.

SYSTEMIC DRUGS WHICH CAUSE OCULAR SIDE EFFECTS

Some drugs taken in large doses over a prolonged period have the potential to cause ocular side effects. In most cases this will be reversible if the dosage is reduced or the drug withdrawn.

The phenothiazines can cause corneal and lens pigmentation and impair vision especially thioridazine and chlorpromazine. Phenothiazines can also cause an oculogyric crisis (the eyes roll back in the head and fixate upwards).

The benzodiazepines, e.g. diazepam, and the tricyclic antidepressants, e.g. amtriptyline and nortriptyline, because of their anticholinergic effects, can increase intraocular pressure. These two groups of drugs should be used with caution in glaucoma patients. Monoamine oxidase inhibitors cause blurred vision.

The sedative chloral hydrate can cause diplopia (double vision) and miosis. Barbiturates used long term can paralyse extraocular muscles. In early barbiturate poisoning the pupils are constricted but react to light, in later stages the pupils are dilated.

The antiarrhythmic drug amiodarone causes corneal microdeposits in 90% of patients. These deposits usually do not cause any visual disturbances and clear on withdrawal of the drug.

FURTHER READING

Bartlett, J.D., Jaanus, S.D. (1984) *Clinical ocular pharmacology*, 2nd edn. Butterworth, Stoneham, M.A.

Fraunfelder, T.F, Roy, F. (1985) *Current ocular therapy*, 2nd edn, vol. 2. Saunders, Philadelphia, P.A.

Grant, W. Morton. (1974) *Toxicology of the eye*, 2nd edn. Charles C. Thomas, Springfield, Illinois.

EYE DISORDERS

27

TEST YOUR KNOWLEDGE

1. What is the action of homatropine on the eye?

2. Name two ocular and two systemic side effects of atropine?

3. What are the main contraindications for timolol?

4. What are the side effects of *Diamox*?

5. Which drop should be instilled first: (a) adrenaline or pilocarpine; (b) adrenaline or timolol?

6. How long should you keep eye drops (a) with preservative and (b) without preservative once opened?

7. When is fluorouracil used as a subconjunctival injection?

8. Give the name of an antifungal eye drop and its dosage.

9. What are the storage requirements for cephalothin eye drops?

10. What is the dosage of acyclovir tablets in herpes zoster ophthalmicus?

TABLE 27.1 Summary table — drugs used in ophthalmology

DRUG GROUP Drug name	Use	Action	Adverse reactions	Nursing implications
MYDRIATIC DRUGS Anticholinergics Atropine Homatropine Cyclopentolate Tropicamide	Pupil dilation	Block acetylcholine to produce mydriasis and cycloplegia (NB tropicamide 0.5% is not cycloplegic)	*Ocular:* redness, swelling, photophobia, increased intraocular pressure. *Systemic:* Dry mouth, nausea, tachycardia, restlessness, confusion (see Chapter 10)	**Assess:** Correct patient, eye, drug, dose and strength; for history of glaucoma, urinary retention; concurrent use of other anticholinergic drugs **Administer:** Dose as ordered; use correct technique; compress puncta to avoid systemic side effects **Evaluate:** For drug effectiveness in relation to purpose for which it was given; for systemic side effects such as dry mouth, tachycardia, restlessness or confusion **Educate:** Make sure the patient understands the effects of the drug and to report any systemic side effects if they occur; instruct on correct administration technique if patient to administer medication themself
Sympathomimetics Phenylephrine	Combined with a cyclopegic for intensive dilation to break synechiae	Weakly mydriatic, not cyclopegic	*Systemic:* Nausea, dizziness, headache, tachycardia, hypertension	**Assess:** Correct patient, eye, drug, dose and strength; pulse rate and blood pressure **Administer:** Dose as ordered, use correct technique **Evaluate:** For efficacy; for systemic side effects **Educate:** See anticholinergics

27 EYE DISORDERS

TABLE 27.1 Continued

DRUG GROUP Drug name	Use	Action	Adverse reactions	Nursing implications
DRUGS FOR GLAUCOMA				
Sympathomimetics Adrenaline Dipivefrin	Decrease production of aqueous humour to lower intraocular pressure in glaucoma	Weakly mydriatic, not cyclopegic	*Systemic:* Nausea, dizziness, headache, tachycardia, hypertension	**Assess:** Correct patient, eye, drug, dose and strength; pulse rate and blood pressure **Administer:** Dose as ordered, use correct technique **Evaluate:** For efficacy; for systemic side effects **Educate:** See anticholinergics
Miotics Pilocarpine Carbachol	Pupil constriction, miosis, open angle glaucoma, reversal of mydriatics	Stimulates acetylcholine, contracts ciliary muscle, increases aqueous humour outflow	*Ocular:* Brow ache and headache, accommodative spasm *Systemic:* nausea, diarrhoea, weakness, salivation, sweating, asthma. Ecothiopate can cause pupillary cysts and cataracts	**Assess:** Correct patient, eye, drug, dose and strength **Administer:** As ordered, check dosage regimen and timing of doses carefully, use correct technique **Evaluate:** For efficacy; ocular and systemic side effects; duration of action **Educate:** Correct dosage and administration technique if patient to self-administer; to understand effect of drug on accommodation and visual field; to report any untoward local or systemic effects
Ecothiopate	Resistant open angle glaucoma, accommodative strabismus	Prevents enzymatic destruction of acetylcholine causing miosis and increased aqueous outflow		

TABLE 27.1 Continued

DRUG GROUP Drug name	Use	Action	Adverse reactions	Nursing implications
β Blocking drugs Timolol Betaxolol Levobunolol	Open angle glaucoma, ocular hypertension (betaxolol suitable for most asthmatics)	Decreases aqueous humour production	*Ocular:* rare *Systemic:* see Chapter 12	**Assess:** Correct patient, eye, drug and dose; history of asthma or heart failure; establish baseline pulse rate **Administration:** Dose as ordered, use correct technique **Evaluate:** For efficacy; note no change in pupil size with timolol; for asthma and bradycardia **Educate:** Correct administration technique; to report systemic side effects
Carbonic anhydrase inhibitors Acetazolamide Dichlorphenamide Methazolamide	Lower intraocular pressure in open angle glaucoma, secondary glaucoma, preoperatively in narrow angle glaucoma	Inhibit carbonic anhydrase so modifying bicarbonate absorption	Nausea, vomiting, diarrhoea, gastric irritation, hypokalaemia, tingling of extremities	**Assess:** Hypersensitivity to sulfonamides, pregnancy, weight, intraocular pressure, hepatic or renal disease, fluid and electrolyte balance, cardiac disease **Administer:** Dose as ordered, give oral doses after food to prevent gastric irritation **Evaluate:** Efficacy; urinary pH; adequate fluid intake to prevent stone formation (long-term use); signs of hypokalaemia (paraesthesia, muscle weakness, cardiac irregularities); acidosis (fatigue, confusion, hyperventilation); drowsiness and gastric irritation may occur **Educate:** To avoid activities requiring full alertness as drowsiness may occur; to replace potassium in diet

27 EYE DISORDERS

TABLE 27.1 Continued

DRUG GROUP Drug name	Use	Action	Adverse reactions	Nursing implications
Osmotic diuretics Glycerol	Glaucoma crisis	Draws water by osmosis from aqueous and vitreous humours	May raise blood sugar levels; dehydration and electrolyte imbalances if therapy too vigorous	**Assess:** Fluid and electrolyte balance; intraocular pressure; weight; urine for sugar, history of diabetes **Administer:** Orally as 50% flavoured mixture, 1–1.5 g/kg; store in refrigerator and give cold **Evaluate:** Reduction in intraocular pressure; tolerance to unpleasant taste; urine output; dehydration, hypokalaemia, dizziness, headache, nausea **Educate:** Reason for therapy; urine output will increase
Mannitol	See glycerol	See glycerol	Dehydration and electrolyte imbalances if therapy too vigorous	**Assess:** Fluid and electrolyte balance; intraocular pressure; weight **Administer:** IV as ordered **Evaluate:** See glycerol **Educate:** See glycerol
DRUGS FOR EYE INFECTIONS Antibacterials Chloramphenicol Gentamicin Tobramycin Neomycin Polymyxin Bacitracin Penicillin Cephalothin Ciprofloxacin	Bacterial eye infections	Antibacterial (see Chapter 30)	Mainly allergic reactions; systemic effects (e.g. aplastic anaemia with chloramphenicol, renal and 8th cranial nerve damage with gentamicin and tobramycin)	**Assess:** History of hypersensitivity to drug; correct eye, drug, dose and dosage regimen **Administer:** Use correct technique, dosage regimen and storage **Evaluate:** Efficacy (reduction in signs of infection); for signs of allergy or systemic side effects **Educate:** Correct administration technique, dosage regimen and storage precautions

TABLE 27.1 Continued

DRUG GROUP Drug name	Use	Action	Adverse reactions	Nursing implications
Sulfonamides Sulfacetamide	Bacterial eye infections	Antibacterial (see Chapter 30)	Redness, watering, swelling, stinging	**Assess:** See antibacterials **Administer:** See antibacterials **Evaluate:** Efficacy; signs of allergy or irritation **Educate:** See antibacterials; drops may sting on application
Antivirals Idoxuridine Vidarabine Acyclovir Trifluorothymidine	Viral eye infections	Antiviral (see Chapter 30)	Local stinging	**Assess:** See antibacterials; caution in pregnancy **Administer:** See antibacterials **Evaluate:** Efficacy **Educate:** See antibacterials
Antifungals Natamycin Miconazole Flucytosine Ketoconazole Amphotericin	Fungal eye infections	Antifungal (see Chapter 30). Penetration of the eye is poor after topical, IV and oral administration	See Chapter 30	**Assess:** See antibacterials **Administer:** See antibacterials; shake suspensions before use **Evaluate:** See antibacterials **Educate:** See antibacterials; to shake suspensions

27 EYE DISORDERS

TABLE 27.1   Continued

DRUG GROUP Drug name	Use	Action	Adverse reactions	Nursing implications
MISCELLANEOUS EYE PREPARATIONS Corticosteroids Hydrocortisone Fluorometholone Prednisolone Dexamethasone	Redness, swelling, capillary dilation, after burns and trauma to prevent corneal scarring, minor inflammation, allergy	Anti-inflammatory (see Chapter 19)	Corneal thinning after long-term use, raised intraocular pressure, masking of infection, delayed wound healing, may be systemically absorbed	**Assess:** Intraocular pressure, for glaucoma, infection, herpes simplex; correct patient, eye, drug and dose **Administer:** As ordered, use correct technique, shake suspensions before use and instil last if other drops being used **Evaluate:** Reduction in inflammation (lessening of redness, swelling and capillary dilation); for signs of infection, raised intraocular pressure, visual impairment **Educate:** To use only as ordered and to report any unusual visual effects, e.g. pain, visual impairment
Local anaesthetics Cocaine Amethocaine Proparacaine Benoxinate Lignocaine	Anaesthesia of eye	Block conduction along superficial nerves, increase corneal permeability	*Ocular:* Corneal damage, loss of blink reflex *Systemic:* excitement, confusion, headache, nausea, convulsions, respiratory arrest	Assess: Correct patient, eye and reason for use **Administer:** Use correct technique, at ordered intervals when applicable; be aware of type and duration of action of drug; protect eye with pad **Evaluate:** For required effect; ensure cornea protected as blink reflex will be lost and cornea can be damaged; observe for systemic side effects **Educate:** Not to rub anaesthetised eye as cornea could be damaged

TABLE 27.1 Continued

DRUG GROUP Drug name	Use	Action	Adverse reactions	Nursing implications
Staining agents Fluorescein	Diagnosis of abrasions and foreign bodies in cornea, to check lachrimal system; IV to examine retinal blood flow	Stains tissues not protected by living epithelium	*Ocular:* rare *Systemic:* after IV use transient nausea, urticaria, collapse	**Assess:** Local application: correct patient, eye and dose. IV use: baseline vital signs and skin colour **Administer:** Local: as ordered, after examination irrigate eye with normal saline. IV: as ordered, use freshly prepared solutions **Evaluate:** IV use: vital signs, observe for nausea, allergy, yellowing of skin **Educate:** Yellowing of skin may occur but will fade after 24 h
Rose Bengal	Detection of keratoconjunctivitis sicca	Stains destabilised conjunctival cells	Rare	**Assess:** Correct patient, eye and dose **Administer:** As ordered, after examination irrigate eye with normal saline
Mucolytic Acetylcysteine	Keratoconjunctivitis sicca	Decreases viscid secretions Inhibits collagenase	Stinging, redness, sensitisation	**Assess:** Correct patient, eye, drug and dose **Administer:** Before instilling, wipe excess mucus from eye using normal saline, check expiry date **Evaluate:** Tear film should gradually become more stable **Educate:** Long-term use prevents adhesion of dried mucus strands to cornea; to use only as ordered

27 EYE DISORDERS

TABLE 27.1 Continued

DRUG GROUP Drug name	Use	Action	Adverse reactions	Nursing implications
Conjunctival decongestants Phenylephrine Naphazoline	Reduction of redness due to minor irritation or allergy	Sympathomimetic, constrict superficial blood vessels	*Ocular*: slight stinging on instillation. *Systemic*: as for sympathomimetics	**Assess:** Correct patient, eye, dose and strength; baseline pulse rate and blood pressure **Administer:** Correct dose and interval as ordered, use correct technique **Evaluate:** For desired effect, mydriasis, increased intraocular pressure, systemic effects, e.g. tachycardia, raised blood pressure **Educate:** Correct technique, to only use as ordered and for limited period
Antiallergy preparations Antazoline Sodium cromoglycate	Allergic eye conditions	Antazoline is an antihistamine; sodium cromoglycate prevents mast cell rupture and histamine release	Rare except hypersensitivity	**Assess:** See decongestants **Administer:** See decongestants **Evaluate:** For desired effect **Educate:** See decongestants
Lubricants Hypromellose Polyvinyl alcohol	Soothing	Tear replacement	Rare	**Assess:** Correct patient, eye and degree of dryness **Administer:** As often as required, use ointment at night **Evaluate:** For desired effect **Educate:** Correct technique
Enzyme preparation Urokinase	Dissolves clots	Lyses clots		

TABLE 27.1   Continued

DRUG GROUP Drug name	Use	Action	Adverse reactions	Nursing implications
Chelating agents EDTA Desferrioxamine	Dissolves heavy metals and calcium deposits			
Prostaglandin inhibitor Indomethacin	Decreases surgically induced miosis			

27 EYE DISORDERS

Skin Diseases

MARIE THÉRÈSE ROSENBERG

O B J E C T I V E S

At the conclusion of this chapter the reader should be able to:

1. State the difference between creams, ointments and lotions;

2. Describe the conditions under which these different types of external preparations are used;

3. Identify the various classes of drugs used for topical application;

4. List some drugs used systemically in the treatment of skin diseases;

5. List the untoward effects of some topical applications, particularly the corticosteroids; and

6. State precautions needed when retinoids are taken systemically.

DERMATOLOGY

Throughout the history of dermatology a large number of therapeutic agents has been tried in the treatment of skin diseases. The text from a fragment of papyrus dating from about the time of Rameses II, 1250 BC, directs the physician to take the talons of a falcon and the shell of a tortoise, and after pronouncing a magic incantation over them, to boil them in oil and apply the oil to the site of a wound. This was claimed to be a reliable remedy, proven a million times over.

The Ebers Papyrus described the benefits of the castor oil plant; the husk crushed in water and applied to the head cures headache, the plant crushed and worked into a mass with lard and applied to the scalp promotes the growth of hair; the oil from the seeds, incorporated into an ointment and applied early in the morning for 10 days will heal wounds that have an evil smelling discharge.

Galen, a Roman physician who lived in the second century, invented cold cream, a mixture of oils, wax and water. When applied to the skin the water evaporated, producing a cooling sensation, hence the name 'cold' cream. This is still used today.

The discovery that hydrocortisone acetate had an anti-inflammatory action when applied to areas of eczema and dermatitis completely altered the management of non-infective skin disorders. In 1960 triamcinolone acetonide was developed and found to be 10 times more potent than hydrocortisone. Since then, hundreds of corticosteroids have been synthesised, and they are the most commonly used and misused topical skin preparations available.

Skin ailments may be caused by trauma (cuts, blisters, burns); inflammatory reactions to contact with irritant substances; allergic reactions; alteration of normal function (e.g. acceleration of growth leading to thickened skin and scaling); or by reactions to drugs.

TYPES OF PREPARATIONS

Just as a drug to be taken systemically is incorporated into a suitable dosage form such as a mixture, tablet or injection, so a drug to be applied to the skin is usually incorporated into a vehicle, the type being dependent on the effect desired. The vehicles applied to the skin consist of the basic elements water, oil or grease and powder in varying proportions, and derivatives of ethylene oxide of differing molecular weights, called macrogols.

WATER

Water is used in the form of wet compresses as a means of heating or cooling the skin. The effect depends on the degree of exposure of the dressing to the air. Closed moist dressings, such as those covered with a sheet of plastic and sealed round the edges with adhesive tape, heat up rapidly, even if applied cold. They remain moist and may be left undisturbed for many hours. Thick, crusted lesions, e.g. those of psoriasis, are sometimes treated in this way. Open wet dressings are used when a cooling effect is desired, e.g. in the treatment of superficial inflammation.

WATER SOLUBLE BASES

Water is used in the preparation of bases which are water soluble and therefore can be easily removed with water. Such preparations are particularly suitable for use on hairy areas of the body. They may be gels prepared from substances which absorb water and swell, e.g. methylcellulose in *Xylocaine Jelly*, or mixtures of macrogols. Macrogols, also called polyethylene glycols, are mixtures of condensation polymers of ethylene oxide and water.

OILS AND GREASES

Oils and greases are used to soften rough, dry skin. Oils are frequently applied by putting a quantity of oil into the bath. A solubilising agent is used to disperse the oil in the water. This leaves a fine film of oil all over the body, an effect which is extremely difficult to achieve making an application by hand. Grease has a softening, protective action on the skin, retaining heat and moisture. The most frequently used grease is soft paraffin, sometimes called petroleum jelly or *Vaseline*. A grease is used on dry and scaling areas. It should not be used on weeping areas as it does not absorb moisture and keeps the area warm, leading to maceration of the skin. It is usually difficult to apply on a wet area as it slides off. Grease and grease based preparations are called ointments.

POWDERS

Dusting powders form a loose thin layer on the skin so that active medicaments contained in them have a limited action. Fine powders provide lubrication between opposing skin surfaces thus preventing irritation caused by friction. Powders should not be used on any badly weeping surface as they absorb moisture and the exudate may cement the powder into coarse granules which irritate the skin.

WATER PLUS POWDER

These preparations are called shake **lotions** because the powder, being in suspension, settles on the bottom of the container which must be shaken before use. After application, the water evaporates rapidly with a cooling effect and the powder is left as a film on the skin. This is really only a modified version of the application of a dusting powder. Lotions are used for superficial inflammatory reactions and for slightly oozing conditions. They tend to dry the skin unless the environment has a high humidity. They are unsuitable for use in hairy areas.

GREASE PLUS POWDER

Ointments usually contain one or more powders mixed with grease. They are not readily absorbed into the skin, and their function is mainly protective. They usually have the consistency of butter.

Pastes are mixtures of grease and a high concentration of powder, usually 50% or more. They are very stiff and difficult to apply, particularly in cold weather. Pastes do absorb some moisture because of their high powder content while the grease base helps to keep the skin from drying out.

WATER PLUS OIL OR GREASE

By the use of an emulsifying agent, grease (or oil) and aqueous liquid can be made to form a stable emulsion called a **cream**. An *aqueous cream* is an oil in water emulsion, i.e. a suspension of oil globules in an aqueous medium. An *oily cream* is a water in oil emulsion, i.e. a suspension of water globules in an oily medium. Oily creams are protective and emollient, while aqueous creams mix readily with skin secretions and a high degree of absorption of active medicament may be expected. Powders may be mixed in with them but not in high concentration as creams are relatively unstable. High concentrations of medicaments cause the emulsion to crack, i.e. revert to its original two layers of grease and aqueous liquid.

Creams are the most widely used dermatological preparations. They are useful in inflammatory conditions and may be used on

SKIN DISEASES

28

weeping areas and hairy areas. They are simple to apply and are easily removed by washing with water, in contrast to ointments which are difficult to remove by washing. Creams are not suitable for chronic scaling skin diseases where a protective effect is required.

Creams are subject to contamination by moulds and to dehydration if stored for any length of time. A dehydrated cream should not be used as the concentration of medicament may have risen and may cause damage to the skin.

SOOTHING AND PROTECTIVE PREPARATIONS

Soothing and protective preparations include lotions, solutions, creams, powders, ointments and oils.

Calamine lotion is a suspension of calamine and zinc oxide in water containing 0.5% phenol. Calamine is a basic zinc carbonate coloured pink with ferric oxide. The colour can vary depending on the amount of ferric oxide present. The calamine and zinc oxide protect the skin and the evaporation of the water cools it. Phenol is readily absorbed through the skin and in adequate concentration paralyses the sensory nerve endings. In the low concentration present in calamine lotion phenol has this effect, but to a much lesser degree, and therefore acts as a local anaesthetic to relieve itching. It also has a mild antiseptic action.

Coal tar solution is sometimes used to relieve generalised itch, 30 mL is added to 90 L (about half a bathtub full) of tepid water (37°C) and the patient soaks in it for 10–15 minutes and is then patted dry with a soft towel. Coal tar contains a number of substances including phenol, and the solution contains a solubilising agent, polysorbate 80, to enable dispersion of the coal tar.

Aqueous cream and **cetomacrogol cream aqueous** consist of a mixture of waxes and fats emulsified in water. They are soothing to dry skin and, having a high water content, can replace much of the moisture which has been lost. Cetomacrogol cream aqueous is also called *sorbolene cream*. They are frequently used alone as moisturisers or as bases for the application of other medicaments.

Oily glycerin cream is used for excessively dry skin, e.g. in the treatment of ichthyosis.

Barrier creams are formulated to protect the skin from contaminants such as acids, alkalis, oils, paints and tars, and their ingredients vary according to the type of contaminant. A Worksafe Australia sponsored study found that occupational skin diseases cost New South Wales about $12 million each year. Most barrier creams contain a dimethicone. The dimethicones are a range of water repellent liquids which have a low surface tension, and form part of the group of substances known as silicones. Dimethicones are resistant to most chemical substances except concentrated acids. *Dermafilm* and *Silcon Cream* both contain 10% dimethicone; *Silic 15* contains 15%. These creams are often used around ileostomies and colostomies to prevent maceration of the skin. *Dimethicream* containing 10% dimethicone is a low viscosity cream which provides good skin lubrication for massage.

Talcum powder is used to lubricate surfaces which rub together and so prevents chafing. Talc is purified native magnesium silicate and contains spores so it is usually sterilised before use. Some commercial talcum powders contain boric acid. These should not be used lavishly on raw surfaces such as a baby's diaper area, as enough boric acid may be absorbed to cause systemic poisoning. Any talcum powder should be used with care in the vicinity of infants as inhalation of the powder can cause severe respiratory problems, even death. There were 80 reported cases of powder accidents in Victoria during 1990. *Prantal* powder contains the anticholinergic agent diphemanil methylsulfate and is used to control excessive sweating.

Soft paraffin (*Vaseline*, petroleum jelly), **hard paraffin** (paraffin wax) and **liquid paraffin** are often used together with **beeswax** in varying proportions to produce an ointment of a desired consistency. Soft paraffin may also be used on its own. It comes in two forms, white and yellow. White soft paraffin has been bleached with sulfur dioxide and is therefore not suitable for use in eye ointments. The paraffins are all bland, non-sensitising and protective, but are also occlusive.

Wool fat is the natural grease from the wool of sheep. It absorbs water to produce lanolin, a form in which it is often used as a moisturising agent and to protect skin from drying. In 1986 the Victorian Department of Health confirmed the presence of organophosphorus pesticide residues in samples of lanolin. This was widely publicised and led to great concern that lanolin containing products could cause cancer. In March 1987 the National Health and Medical Research Council issued a statement on lanolin products recommending an interim limit of 40 ppm (parts per million) total organophosphorus pesticide residues as this level posed no hazard to human health. It further recommended that efforts be made to reduce this level even further, a goal which most manufacturers of wool fat containing products achieved, e.g. down to 9 ppm in wool fat and therefore less in lanolin and even less in products which contain only a proportion of lanolin. Wool fat may cause sensitivity reactions.

Bath oils, as their name implies, are added to the bath or applied to the wet skin after a shower. They contain oils, liquid paraffin, wool fat extracts and dispersants. After the bath the skin is patted dry. In this way a fine film of oil can be applied easily to the whole body. *Alpha-Keri Oil, Derma-oil* and *Rikoderm Bath Oil* are commercial examples. Some bath oils contain tars to allay itching, e.g. *Pinetarsol* and *Q.V. Tar.*

CLEANSERS AND KERATOLYTICS ▬▬

CLEANSERS

Soap

The modern practice of hygiene encourages the frequent use of soap. This may be quite damaging to the skin, as soap is caustic, causing swelling and disintegration of the keratin layer. Unless there is considerable exudate it is unnecessary to wash off a previous application of cream or ointment before applying another. Cleansing creams are cosmetically acceptable alternatives to soap for cleansing the face. *Cetaphil Lotion* and *Q.V. Bar* are soap substitutes.

Medicated soaps and scrubs may be useful in some conditions to reduce the number of skin bacteria, e.g. in acne.

Hydrogen Peroxide

Hydrogen peroxide is used to cleanse open wounds and ulcers. The solution releases oxygen on contact with organic matter and the effervescent action loosens debris.

Benzoyl Peroxide

Benzoyl peroxide 10% in a lotion or cream base is used in the treatment of acne. When applied to the skin, benzoyl peroxide releases oxygen which penetrates into the sebaceous follicle and suppresses the organism *Corynebacterium acnes*. Benzoyl peroxide is potentially a contact sensitiser. It may also bleach coloured garments if it comes in contact with them. Care should be taken to avoid contact with eyes, lips and mouth.

SKIN DISEASES

28

KERATOLYTICS

Keratolytic agents are sometimes desirable therapy when accumulation of keratinised cells causes flaking and scaling.

Salicylic Acid

Salicylic acid is used in varying concentrations and in different vehicles. For mild scaling, 1%–2% in soft paraffin keeps the skin warm and moist, which assists in the scaling process; 2%–5% in a cream base can be used for more advanced lesions. Salicylic acid is used also for the removal of common warts. Up to 20% may be used, usually dissolved in flexible collodion, which forms a flexible skin on drying. Care must be taken that the skin surrounding the wart is protected. This can be done by smearing soft paraffin on the skin up to the edge of the wart. The salicylic acid paint is applied directly to the wart which is then covered with an occlusive dressing such as *Elastoplast*. This causes maceration of the keratin layer and so increases the effect of the salicylic acid. The dressing should be removed, the paint reapplied and the wart covered, twice a day.

Resorcinol

Resorcinol is frequently added to salicylic acid in hair lotions. It aids in removing the scale of dandruff and is also antipruritic. It causes darkening of the hair, a process which is intensified in the presence of alkali.

Podophyllum Resin

Podophyllum resin dissolved in compound benzoin tincture in concentrations up to 25% is used in the topical treatment of condylomata acuminata (soft genital warts). Podophyllum is very irritating to normal skin which should always be protected during application of the paint. Podophyllum can be absorbed through the skin and can cause systemic toxicity, characterised by haematological and neurological complications. Any unusual symptoms occurring in a patient who has been treated with podophyllum should be reported to the medical officer immediately. *Posalfilin* ointment contains podophyllum resin 20% and salicylic acid 25% and is indicated in the treatment of plantar warts. *Posalfilin* paint contains podophyllum resin 20% and salicylic acid 10% and is recommended for common warts. Treatment should be ceased at the first sign of inflammation. The use of podophyllum is contraindicated in pregnancy.

BUF-PUF

A *BUF-PUF* is an abrasive pad made of inert polyester fibres. It contains no medication and achieves its effect by removing dead skin cells by abrasion.

Urea

Urea 10% in a cream base is used to promote hydration of the skin. It increases the uptake of water by the stratum corneum, giving it a high water binding capacity. Urea cream is used in treatment of ichthyosis and other chronic dry skin conditions. Urea cream darkens on storage. A number of commercial preparations are available, e.g. *Aquacare-HP* and *Aquadrate*.

RETINOIDS

Vitamin A (retinol) has long been known to be essential for healthy skin. Deficiency gives rise to hyperkeratotic skin changes with lowered resistance to minor skin infections. Treatment with vitamin A has been tried for conditions such as psoriasis but has failed because high dose long-term treatment is needed and hypervitaminosis A develops before the skin condition clears. In an attempt to overcome this disadvantage many synthetic derivatives of vitamin A have been produced (over 1500 in the last few years) and several have come into clinical use. Each derivative appears to have a slightly different specificity.

Tretinoin

The first retinoid was tretinoin. However, it was found to have the same disadvantages as vitamin A when given systemically but proved effective on local application.

TRADE NAMES

Tretinoin: *Airol; Retin-A.*

USES

It is used as a cream, lotion, gel or alcoholic paint for the treatment of acne and other conditions characterised by thickening of the skin, e.g. ichthyosis. Its action in acne is two-fold. It loosens the comedones which block the outlet of the pilosebaceous follicles and induces proliferation of the follicular epithelium. Shortly after treatment is commenced the acne appears to be worse. Within a week the skin becomes red and scaly and pustules sometimes form. This is due to small plugs of dried sebum being expelled from deep within the follicle. Perseverance with treatment is rewarded with a marked improvement in 8–12 weeks.

ADVERSE DRUG REACTIONS

Topical application of tretinoin increases the susceptibility of the skin to sunlight by thinning the stratum corneum. Its main adverse effect is an irritant dermatitis which may be severe. This is more common with the alcoholic paint.

Etretinate

Etretinate is used orally in the treatment of dermatoses characterised by severe disorders of keratinisation.

TRADE NAMES

Etretinate: *Tigason.*

MECHANISM OF ACTION

The exact mechanism of action of etretinate is not fully understood. It reverses the epidermal proliferation and increased keratinisation seen in hyperkeratotic disorders.

PHARMACOKINETICS

About 40% of an oral dose is absorbed but there is a large variation between patients. Maximum plasma levels are reached in 2–5 hours. Etretinate undergoes significant first pass metabolism. It is highly bound to tissues. With the usual treatment regimen involving multiple doses of the drug there is progressive accumulation of etretinate in the body, probably in body fat, and after cessation of treatment this accumulated drug is slowly released.

Etretinate is metabolised by enzymes in the gut wall and by the liver to an active metabolite, acitretin, which is then further metabolised to inactive compounds. About 60% of a dose is excreted unchanged in the faeces and the remainder in the faeces and urine as metabolites. The half-life of a single dose is 6–12 hours. However, because of the accumulation in the body following multiple dosing, plasma levels have been detected 140 days after ceasing therapy. The elimination half-life has been estimated at 100 days.

USES

Etretinate is used in the treatment of severe intractable psoriasis and in other severe forms of keratinisation disorders, e.g. ichthyosis, keratosis follicularis (Darier's disease), lichen planus and pityriasis rubra pilaris.

Because of interpatient variation in bioavailability all doses must be individually titrated under close clinical supervision. The maximum daily dose is 1 mg/kg body weight, administered in two or three divided doses. Some authorities recommend a starting dose of 0.75 mg/kg body weight, increased to 1 mg/kg if therapeutic response is inadequate. If side effects occur the dose is reduced to 0.3–0.6 mg/kg body weight depending on the dose the patient can tolerate. Once a response has been achieved the dose is reduced to 0.5 mg/kg body weight daily. When the patient appears to be experiencing no further improvement in the condition, the treatment is ceased

SKIN DISEASES

28

and if exacerbations of the disease occur future treatment is given intermittently. Some patients experience such a short remission that maintenance therapy is continued at the lowest dose that prevents recurrence. *Tigason* is available in capsules containing 10 mg and 25 mg.

ADVERSE DRUG REACTIONS

Etretinate is teratogenic. Most patients experience some erythema, burning, itching and dryness of the lips and mucosae, thinning and increased fragility of the skin, and desquamation of the skin particularly of the palms and soles. Hair thinning and alopecia may occur, usually 4–8 weeks after commencing therapy. Dryness of the eyes and conjunctivitis may occur. Biochemical abnormalities include elevated serum triglycerides and/or cholesterol. Less commonly, liver function tests return abnormal values. Platelet count is sometimes decreased. Up to 20% of patients experience increased sweating, chills and thirst. The side effects are usually reversible.

DRUG INTERACTIONS

A high fat meal increases the absorption of etretinate to a significant degree. Vitamin A containing products should not be taken concurrently because the similarity in mode of action may lead to hypervitaminosis A. The risk of hepatotoxicity may be increased in chronic alcohol abuse. Etretinate displaces phenytoin from its binding sites in plasma to a minor degree.

PRECAUTIONS AND CONTRAINDICATIONS

Liver function tests should be performed at commencement of therapy and at 3-monthly intervals during therapy. Serum lipid levels should also be estimated before and at regular intervals during therapy and, if necessary, after cessation of therapy. The skin may be more susceptible to sunburn and appropriate measures should be taken.

Special care should be exercised if treatment is required in children as skeletal changes and premature closure of the epiphyses have been seen in young animals treated with etretinate.

Etretinate is contraindicated in pregnancy and in women of childbearing potential unless the condition is life threatening and alternative therapy is ineffective. Because of the long storage of the drug in the body pregnancy must be avoided for two years after cessation of treatment. It is not known if etretinate is excreted in breast milk and therefore it is not recommended for nursing mothers.

Isotretinoin

TRADE NAMES

Isotretinoin: *Roaccutane.*

MECHANISM OF ACTION

The exact mechanism of action is unknown. Sebaceous gland size is reduced and differentiation of sebaceous gland cells and keratinocytes is inhibited. There is a decrease in sebum production with consequent alteration of the skin surface lipid composition. Cohesion between cells in the stratum corneum is reduced resulting in increased desquamation and skin fragility. The inhibition of keratinisation and increased desquamation in the pilosebaceous duct prevents the duct obstruction which is characteristic of cystic acne.

PHARMACOKINETICS

There is considerable interpatient variation in blood levels following administration of isotretinoin. Peak plasma levels occur in 1–4 hours. The presence of food in the stomach while delaying slightly the absorption of isotretinoin nevertheless increases the bioavailability of the drug. Isotretinoin appears in most tissues of the body. It is highly bound to plasma albumen. The drug is metabolised in the liver and both drug and metabolites undergo enterohepatic recycling. Isotretinoin and its metabolites are excreted in both the urine and the faeces. The apparent half-life of the drug varies between patients, but in some is up to 50 hours.

USES

Isotretinoin is used in the treatment of severe cystic acne and usually a single course is sufficient to obtain prolonged remission of the disease. The dose must be individually titrated according to the patient's response and tolerance to the drug.

Initially, 0.5–1 mg/kg body weight per day is given, either as a single daily dose or divided into two doses per day, and continued for 2–4 weeks. If little or no response is obtained, the dose is increased up to a maximum of 2 mg/kg body weight per day. The acne appears to get worse during initiation of treatment, but usually settles down in a week or 10 days. Treatment is continued for 16 weeks. Improvement usually continues after cessation of treatment, therefore if a second course is considered necessary, an interval of eight weeks should elapse before beginning the second course. Isotretinoin is available in 10 mg and 20 mg capsules.

ADVERSE DRUG REACTIONS

Almost all patients experience cheilitis, dry mouth and nose, facial dermatitis and pruritus. In higher doses the drug causes elevation of serum triglycerides, cholesterol and liver enzymes, reversible on lowering the dose. Occasionally more serious reactions occur, such as benign intracranial hypertension and/or corneal opacities, which require immediate cessation of the drug and suitable treatment.

DRUG INTERACTIONS

Products containing vitamin A should not be taken during treatment as they may potentiate toxicity. Alcohol and oestrogens may potentiate the rise in serum triglyceride levels. Tetracyclines, like isotretinoin, may rarely cause intracranial hypertension and are therefore contraindicated.

PRECAUTIONS AND CONTRAINDICATIONS

As with etretinate, pregnancy is an absolute contraindication for treatment with isotretinoin. Because of the drug's long half-life, pregnancy should be avoided for at least four weeks following cessation of therapy. Care must be exercised in treating young adolescents as the drug may cause premature closure of the epiphyses.

NURSING IMPLICATIONS

ASSESSMENT

Nurses caring for patients with skin disorders should ensure that they understand the different functions of the products to be used. For example, an ointment should not be substituted for a cream or vice versa. The area to be treated should be assessed for the extent and type of lesion and whether the skin is dry, cracked, moist, weeping or hairy. Baseline observations of the condition of the skin should be documented.

APPLICATION

Bath oils

The nurse should ensure that the correct strength of preparation is used. The temperature of the water should be checked to avoid burning or hypothermia, particularly if the patient is to be kept in the bath for a long time. Elderly and debilitated patients should be assisted.

Lotions

Lotions should be used sparingly as overuse leads to drying and cracking of the skin.

Wet dressings

The nurse should ensure that open wet dressings are kept moist and renewed or remoistened regularly.

Powders

Powders should be used sparingly. They should not be used on weeping or hairy areas.

Ointments

As ointments do not penetrate, only a thin smear should be used. It is not necessary

SKIN DISEASES

28

to wash off ointment before making a new application. Ointments should not be applied to oozing lesions where drainage is required but are valuable in acute and chronic lesions where there are crusts to soften. Application to hairy areas causes matting. Prolonged application to hairy areas may cause folliculitis. Application following the direction of hair growth will lessen folliculitis.

Creams

Exudates are absorbed freely with creams and drainage is not inhibited. Creams are not suitable for chronic scaling skin diseases where a protective effect is required. They may be used on hairy or weeping areas. A cream which is hard or has a cracked surface should not be used as this indicates dehydration of the cream and the concentration of the medication will have increased.

Keratolytics and cleansers

The nurse should ensure that these preparations are used only when indicated. They soften horny layers and reduce thickening of the skin. Salicylic acid and, in particular, podophyllum resin preparations should be applied carefully and healthy skin protected. When applying hair lotion containing resorcinol the nurse should ensure that the hair is free of soap and warn fair haired patients of probable darkening of the hair.

Retinoids

The nurse should be aware of the side effects which may occur and notify the doctor immediately if the patient complains of severe headache or disturbance of vision.

EVALUATION

Patients should be observed for signs of improvement or deterioration in their skin conditions. When powders, lotions and/or baths are being used the skin should be checked for drying or cracking. Elderly or debilitated patients should be watched for hypothermia during baths or if large areas are being treated with wet dressings.

PATIENT EDUCATION

If patients are to apply the medication they should be taught the correct procedure, any precautions to observe during application and any adverse effects to watch for. Most patients with skin problems should be advised against the use of soap and it should be stressed that excessive washing of the skin may be harmful. Patients using hair lotions containing resorcinol need to be advised to wash their hair free of soap before application, especially if they have fair hair.

All patients with peripheral vascular disease or diabetes mellitus should be warned against the unsupervised use of keratolytic agents lest skin irritation results in an ulcer.

Patients being treated with topical retinoids should be warned to avoid direct exposure to sunlight. The *Standard for the Uniform Scheduling of Drugs and Poisons*, published by the National Health and Medical Research Council, restricts the prescribing of oral retinoids to specialist physicians and dermatologists. Patients prescribed oral retinoids should be given an information leaflet about their treatment. The nurse should tactfully impress upon patients the dangers inherent in the use of these drugs so they are not tempted to pass on any capsules to a friend or neighbour who appears to have the same condition.

The nurse should ensure that the patient understands that applications to skin should be applied gently as vigorous application could aggravate the existing condition. Even a *BUF-PUF*, used for the purpose of abrading dead cells from the outer layer of skin, should be soaped well and used gently. Patients should be advised concerning any product which may stain the skin or clothing (e.g. clioquinol) so that appropriate precautions can be taken.

Finally, it should be borne in mind that conditions of the skin are often accompanied by disfigurement, feelings of rejection and a poor self-image. Emotional support of patients is therefore important. Nurses must be careful to avoid showing any sign of repulsion and should encourage patients to the best of their ability.

ANTI-INFECTIVE PREPARATIONS ▉▉▉

Most bacterial skin infections are caused by staphylococci or streptococci. Antibiotics which are used systemically in the treatment of bacterial infection should not, as a general rule, be applied topically. It has been found that this practice encourages the development of resistant bacterial strains because of the low antibiotic plasma concentration which results. Moreover, topical use of antibiotics, especially penicillins, frequently causes contact dermatitis.

TOPICAL TREATMENT OF BACTERIAL SKIN INFECTIONS

Triclosan

Triclosan is an antibacterial agent which is very effective against most species of staphylococci commonly found on the skin. It is effective against some Gram negative organisms but not against *Pseudomonas* sp., yeasts or fungi. When used regularly it has a cumulative antimicrobial effect on the skin and is used in medicated soaps (*Sapoderm*), face washes and scrubs (*pHisohex, Clearasil Daily Face Wash, Novaderm R*) in the adjunctive treatment of infected lesions.

Chlorhexidine

Chlorhexidine is effective against a wide range of bacteria, yeasts, some fungi and some viruses. It is ineffective against spores except at high temperatures. It is used mainly in aqueous solution (which must be sterilised) for treatment of infected wounds, and in alcoholic solution in preparation of the skin before surgery. Chlorhexidine is incompatible with soap. Chlorhexidine is commercially available as *Hibitane*.

Povidone Iodine

Povidone iodine is widely used for disinfection of cuts and abrasions, minor burns, blisters and skin infections such as impetigo and tinea. It kills bacteria, viruses, protozoa and fungi and is effective against spores. It is available in a number of forms as *Betadine* preparations, including a surgical scrub, an alcoholic solution for skin preparation prior to surgery, an antiseptic liquid, impregnated gauze pads, a paint and an ointment. For further information on chlorhexidine and povidone iodine see Chapter 35 Antiseptics, Disinfectants and Infection Control.

Metronidazole

Metronidazole is an antiprotozoal and anaerobic antibacterial agent. It is available as a 0.75% gel (*Rozex*) for treating the inflammatory papules, pustules and erythema of rosacea. Its mode of action in this disease is not known. There is minimal absorption from topical application and so plasma levels are insignificant. Local reactions occur in a small number of patients and include eye irritation and redness and dryness of the skin. The area to be treated should be washed and dried and a thin film of ointment applied and rubbed in twice daily.

SKIN DISEASES

28

Antibiotics

The antibiotics **neomycin, bacitracin** and **polymyxin** are frequently used in combination in an ointment base for superficial infections such as impetigo. There are a number of commercial preparations of this type, *Neosporin Topical, Mycitracin Ointment* and *Spersin Ointment*. This combination has the advantage that these antibiotics are rarely used systemically.

Neomycin acts by interfering with bacterial protein synthesis, bacitracin by interfering with bacterial cell wall synthesis, and polymyxin by binding to and changing the permeability of the bacterial cytoplasmic membrane. Thus there is a three-fold attack on the bacteria. The combination also retards the development of bacterial resistance. Neomycin and bacitracin can cause sensitivity reactions following prolonged application. Persistence or recurrence of inflammation in spite of or following treatment with ointments containing neomycin or bacitracin should arouse suspicion that a sensitivity reaction has occurred and should be drawn to the attention of the doctor. Extensive impetigo not responding readily to topical therapy may need treatment with systemic antibiotics.

Framycetin has a similar action to that of neomycin and is available as *Sofra-Tulle*, a sterile paraffin gauze dressing impregnated with 1% framycetin. The dressing is used for burns, ulcers and in plastic surgery. *Soframycin Ointment* contains 1.5% framycetin plus 0.005% gramicidin, another antibiotic. **Gramicidin** alters the function of the bacterial plasma membrane. Like neomycin, framycetin often causes a sensitivity reaction.

Gentamicin interferes with bacterial protein synthesis and is very effective against Gram negative bacteria as well as many Gram positive bacteria. However, because of its frequent systemic use it is not often used as a drug of first choice in topical therapy.

Mupirocin is an antibiotic developed for topical use only. It acts by inhibiting bacterial protein synthesis. It is the active ingredient in *Bactroban* and in *Bactroban Nasal*.

Each contains 2% mupirocin. *Bactroban Nasal* is recommended for the elimination of nasal carriage of staphylococci, and the ointment for treatment of mild impetigo. A few patients experience itching, burning and dryness at the site of application.

SYSTEMIC TREATMENT OF BACTERIAL SKIN INFECTIONS

Infected skin conditions frequently require systemic treatment with antibiotics to combat the infection, followed or accompanied by specific treatment for the underlying condition. Another reason systemic antibiotics may be required in hospitalised patients is that hospital organisms, because of constant exposure to antibiotics, may be resistant to them in the concentrations used for topical application.

Since the organisms most often involved are staphylococci and streptococci, one of the oral penicillins is usually adequate but other systemic antibiotics may be used depending on the sensitivity of the organism. Tetracycline is frequently used in the long-term treatment of acne. It is given once or twice daily, often for several years.

For further information on these agents see Chapter 30 Infectious Diseases.

ANTIVIRAL AGENTS

Idoxuridine

Idoxuridine is incorporated into viral DNA instead of thymidine thus inhibiting replication of the virus. It is available as *Stoxil Topical* containing 0.5% idoxuridine in a water miscible ointment base. This is applied to the lesion every hour for the first 24 hours then every four hours until the lesion is healed. For the use of idoxuridine in dendritic ulcers of the eye see Chapter 27 Eye Disorders.

Acyclovir

TRADE NAMES

Acyclovir: *Zovirax*.

MECHANISM OF ACTION

In herpes infected cells acyclovir is converted by viral thymidine kinase and other cell enzymes to acyclovir triphosphate, which is the pharmacologically active form of the drug. The acyclovir triphosphate is incorporated into the viral DNA molecule instead of the physiological deoxyguanosine triphosphate. DNA synthesis, and viral replication is brought to an end.

PHARMACOKINETICS

Only about 20% of an oral dose is absorbed probably because the transport mechanism in the gut is saturable, since the fraction absorbed decreases with increasing dosage. Peak plasma concentrations occur within 1.5–2.5 hours. Food does not appear to affect absorption. Acyclovir is widely distributed in body tissues including cerebrospinal fluid and saliva. It crosses the placenta and is excreted in breast milk. Up to 33% is bound to plasma proteins. Metabolism takes place in the herpes virus infected cells. About 60% of the drug is excreted unchanged by the kidneys by glomerular filtration and tubular secretion, and about 10%–15% as an inactive metabolite. The half-life is 2.5–2.9 hours.

USES

The intravenous infusion is used for acute clinical manifestations of mucocutaneous herpes simplex virus infections, especially in immunocompromised patients. *Zovirax* intravenous infusion contains 250 mg of acyclovir sodium. It is reconstituted with 10 mL of either water for injection or sodium chloride 0.9% injection. It is given in a dose of 5 mg/kg body weight every eight hours by slow intravenous infusion over a one-hour period to avoid renal tubular damage. The prepared solution may be further diluted if desired. The nurse diluting the solution should refer to the package insert which accompanies the product to elicit the details of dilution.

Zovirax Tablets contain either 200 mg or 400 mg of acyclovir. Oral treatment is used for initial attacks of genital herpes and to manage recurrent episodes. It is also given orally for the treatment of acute attacks of non-ophthalmic herpes zoster infection (shingles). For initial genital herpes, 200 mg is given five times a day at approximately 4-hourly intervals for 10 days. For recurrent attacks, 200 mg is given two or three times a day for up to six months. High dose is used for herpes zoster infections, 800 mg being given five times a day, commencing as early as possible in the attack and continuing for seven days. Dosage adjustment is required in renal impairment.

ADVERSE DRUG REACTIONS

Local inflammation or phlebitis may occur at the injection site and skin rashes and hives sometimes occur. The main side effect is renal damage and rapid increases in blood urea and creatinine may be found. The patient should be monitored for this side effect.

Nausea and vomiting and headache are the most frequent side effects experienced during oral administration.

DRUG INTERACTIONS

Concomitant administration of probenecid prolongs the half-life of acyclovir by about 20%.

PRECAUTIONS AND CONTRAINDICATIONS

The patient must always be well hydrated as dehydration increases the risk of renal damage.

It is known that acyclovir crosses the placenta. There have not been any well controlled studies to evaluate the effect of acyclovir on the human fetus, and therefore it should not be used during pregnancy unless the potential benefit outweighs the risk.

For use of acyclovir in the eye see Chapter 27 Eye Disorders. For further information on acyclovir see Chapter 30 Infectious Diseases.

SKIN DISEASES

28

ANTIFUNGAL AGENTS

Just as there are a great many bacteria, each group reacting differently to various antibiotics, so too there are many fungi and several different kinds of antifungal preparations are necessary. Some of these are used systemically, e.g. griseofulvin, some topically, e.g. tolnaftate, and some both systemically and topically, e.g. miconazole.

Magenta

Magenta is a dye which is effective in the treatment of paronychia and superficial dermatophytoses, especially in moist areas when dermatitis is present. It is contained in *Castellani's Paint* which is painted on twice a day.

Griseofulvin

MECHANISM OF ACTION

The main action of griseofulvin is disruption of the mitotic spindle structure of the fungal cell thus arresting cell division in metaphase.

PHARMACOKINETICS

Griseofulvin is administered orally and absorption depends on the particle size of the griseofulvin in the product. Microsize, consisting predominantly of particles 4 μm in diameter, is irregularly absorbed, while ultramicrosize, consisting mainly of particles 1 μm in diameter is almost completely absorbed. Absorption is increased if a high fat meal is taken concomitantly. However, there is no clinical evidence that one form is more effective than the other.

Griseofulvin is concentrated in skin, hair, nails, liver, fat and skeletal muscles. It is deposited in keratin precursor cells and is tightly bound to new keratin. Its distribution into skin is very rapid but the concentration falls equally rapidly when the drug is ceased. Griseofulvin is metabolised in the liver to an inactive metabolite. It is excreted in both urine and faeces. Its half-life is in the order of 9–24 hours.

USES

Griseofulvin is available as *Grisovin* (microsize) 500 mg tablets and as *Griseostatin* (ultramicrosize) 330 mg tablets. In each case, one tablet is taken daily for as long as necessary to shed the infected keratin. For infection of soft tissue, such as the palms of the hands, this may be up to four weeks, for nails, six months therapy is usually required.

ADVERSE DRUG REACTIONS

The incidence of serious side effects with griseofulvin is very low. Hypersensitivity reactions may occur, e.g. skin rash and urticaria. Gastrointestinal disturbances, dry mouth, headache, dizziness, fatigue and vertigo are sometimes experienced.

DRUG INTERACTIONS

Griseofulvin decreases the activity of warfarin and the dose of warfarin may need to be increased. Barbiturates decrease levels of griseofulvin. Alcohol may interact with griseofulvin resulting in headache, breathlessness, nausea, giddiness and facial flushing. Griseofulvin may reduce the effectiveness of oral contraceptives.

PRECAUTIONS AND CONTRAINDICATIONS

Griseofulvin is classified as B3 in the Australian Categorisation of Medicines in Pregnancy, that is, studies in animals have shown evidence of an increased occurrence of fetal damage but the significance of this is considered uncertain in humans. Therefore the use of griseofulvin should be avoided during pregnancy. It is not known if griseofulvin is excreted in breast milk.

Griseofulvin is contraindicated in patients with porphyria or with liver failure.

Terbinafine

MECHANISM OF ACTION

Terbinafine (*Lamisil*) is fungicidal. It inhibits an enzyme, squalene oxidase, in the fungal cell membrane. This causes a block in sterol synthesis, and squalene accumulates in the fungal cell resulting in cell death.

PHARMACOKINETICS

Less than 5% is absorbed after topical application of the cream. When given orally terbinafine is rapidly absorbed and distributed mainly to lipophilic tissues. It concentrates in the skin and nails. It is secreted in sebum, thus achieving a high concentration in hair follicles. Although it accumulates in the lipophilic retinal and choroidal tissues no ophthalmological abnormalities have so far been reported in humans. Terbinafine is metabolised in the liver to inactive products which are excreted mainly in the urine. The half-life is about 17 hours but may be longer in patients with hepatic or renal impairment.

USES

Terbinafine is available as a 1% cream and as 250 mg tablets. It is used for the treatment of dermatophyte infections such as tinea corporis, tinea cruris, tinea pedis and onychomycosis. Oral treatment is given when the site, severity or extent of the infection warrants it. Dosage is one 250 mg tablet daily. Skin infections usually respond in 2–6 weeks, nail infections in 6–12 weeks. Clinical improvement continues after therapy is completed.

ADVERSE DRUG REACTIONS

About 10% of patients experience some reactions, mainly gastrointestinal disturbance and skin erythema and pruritus. Occasionally transient increases in liver enzymes and serum creatinine occur and there have been isolated cases of Stevens-Johnson syndrome and hepatobiliary dysfunction.

PRECAUTIONS

Oral dosage should be halved in patients with renal disease. Patients with hepatic or renal disease should be monitored carefully during treatment. Contact of the cream with the eyes should be avoided. Terbinafine should not be given during pregnancy unless the expected benefits outweigh the potential risks.

Nystatin

Nystatin (*Mycostatin, Nilstat*) is effective against yeast and yeast-like fungi, including *Candida albicans*. It is available as a cream, ointment and gel for candida infections of the skin, and also as a vaginal cream and pessaries for local treatment of vulvovaginal candidiasis. The cream or ointment is used two or three times daily and the vaginal cream and pessaries once or twice daily. Treatment is continued until the symptoms abate.

Tolnaftate

Tolnaftate (*Tinacidin, Tinaderm*) is used as a 1% solution or cream in the treatment of various species of tinea. It is not active against *Candida* sp.

Miconazole, Econazole, Clotrimazole, Isoconazole, Ketoconazole

Miconazole, econazole, clotrimazole, isoconazole and ketoconazole are closely related antifungal agents used for topical treatment of dermal infections such as tinea pedis, tinea cruris and tinea corporis. They are effective also against candida infections, including paronychia, cutaneous candidiasis and external genital candidiasis. Side effects include burning, stinging, pruritus, urticaria and general irritation, particularly in children. The topical creams are used also in the treatment of pityriasis versicolor, being applied twice daily for three weeks.

For further information see Chapter 30 Infectious Diseases.

ANTIPARASITICS

Lindane

Lindane has been the favoured treatment for lice and scabies for a number of years. It was formerly used as an agricultural

SKIN DISEASES

28

pesticide but has recently received much adverse publicity because of residues in meat from grazing animals. Its use in pediculosis and scabies is short term and is generally considered safe. However, some authorities consider that alternative treatment should be used in infants, children and perhaps pregnant women.

Quellada Head Lice Treatment contains 1% lindane in a shampoo base. It is effective against lice and their eggs (nits). It is applied to dry hair, using sufficient to thoroughly wet the hair (about 25 mL for short hair, more for longer hair) and rubbed vigorously through the hair for at least four minutes, making sure that all parts of the hair and scalp are treated. The hair is then washed with water and dried with a towel. A fine-tooth comb is used to remove the dead lice and nits. If difficulty is experienced in removing the nits, which are cemented to the hairs by a hard secretion, the comb should be dipped in vinegar, which dissolves the cement. One application is usually sufficient, but it may be repeated in 24 hours if necessary. It should not be repeated more than twice in one week.

Lindane 1% lotion may be used for body lice. Clothing must be disinfected. Cottons may be boiled. One way of ridding clothing of lice is to enclose it in a plastic bag and leave it for four weeks, since the lice can live only on the host.

For scabies, lindane 1% cream (*Quellada Cream*) is applied thinly to the whole body except the head and washed off after 8–12 hours. One application is usually sufficient but a second application may be made a week later if necessary.

Pyrethrins

Pyrethrins are a group of insecticidal substances obtained from the pyrethrum flower which act as nerve poisons against head lice. They are usually used in combination with piperonyl butoxide which increases their efficiency. This combination is available as *Banlice* mousse. The foam is applied at several sites and massaged into the hair and scalp in sufficient quantity to wet the head thoroughly and left on for 10 minutes. The hair is then well washed with shampoo. Dead lice and nits are removed with a fine-tooth comb. The treatment may be repeated after 8–10 days if necessary. Pyrethrins can cause irritation of the skin and eyes.

Permethrin

Permethrin is a synthetic analogue of pyrethrins and is used in the treatment of scabies. It is available as *Lyclear Scabies Cream* containing 5% permethrin. Prior to treatment the skin should be clean, dry and cool. The cream is applied over the whole body except the head and gently rubbed in, particular care being taken to work it into folds in the skin. The whole body is well washed 8–24 hours later. Recommended applications are up to 30 g for adults and children over 12 and lesser quantities for children according to their size. Children under 2 years and adults over 70 should be treated under medical supervision. Because children under 2 years are unlikely to be able to indicate the site of infestation it is recommended that the face, neck and head be treated in this age group. One application is usually sufficient but a second application may be made after 8–10 days if necessary.

Maldison

Maldison (malathion) is an organophosphate used as a 0.5% lotion for head lice in a similar manner to lindane. It is available as *Cleensheen* or *Lice Rid*. Maldison can be absorbed through the skin and is therefore unsuitable for treatment of body lice.

Benzyl Benzoate

Benzyl benzoate is used for scabies as a 25% emulsion. The patient has a hot bath, is dried, and the benzyl benzoate emulsion applied over the whole body surface from the neck down. The application may be repeated the following day.

Crotamiton

Crotamiton is used for scabies as a 10% cream (*Eurax*). As with other treatments the patient takes a warm bath and the cream is then rubbed in all over the body from the neck down, particular care being taken to work it into folds in the skin. A second application is made the following day. Crotamiton is considered preferable for infants and very young children.

With all treatments for scabies a complete change of clothing and bed linen must be made and a bath taken the day after the final treatment.

NURSING IMPLICATIONS

ASSESSMENT

The patient's history should be reviewed for any previous episodes of allergic reaction to the substance to be used. The area to be treated should be assessed and observations concerning the appearance and extent of skin lesions documented.

ADMINISTRATION

To avoid sensitisation, antibiotic preparations should be applied topically for as short a time as reasonable. To minimise further trouble if sensitisation does occur the drug used should, wherever possible, be one that is unlikely to be needed for systemic administration in the future.

EVALUATION

The skin should be observed for signs of lessening of the infection. Where antibiotic preparations have been used the nurse should watch closely for signs of persistent or recurrent inflammation which could indicate a sensitivity reaction. If neomycin is applied to large lesions or for a prolonged period of time the nurse should be alert for complaints of tinnitus, dizziness or deafness, which could indicate absorption and subsequent ototoxic effects.

PATIENT EDUCATION

Patients should be advised to discontinue treatment and seek medical advice if inflammation persists or recurs when using topical antibiotic preparations. The nurse should make sure patients are aware of the need to disinfect all clothing, bed linen and any other articles such as brushes and combs following treatment for pediculosis or scabies.

BURNS

Current treatment of burns is with silver sulfadiazine cream available as *Silvazine* cream containing 1% silver sulfadiazine and 0.2% chlorhexidine. The chlorhexidine acts as a prophylactic against staphylococcal infection. Silver sulfadiazine is effective against *Pseudomonas* organisms, which are very common contaminants in large burns. The cream itself causes no pain on application. The nurse scrubs up, dons cap, sterile gown and gloves and applies the cream thickly with a gloved hand. There have been reports of sensitivity reactions to the cream.

SUNBURN

Sunburn is frequent in all parts of Australia, especially in tropical and subtropical areas. It is treated in a similar way to any other burn. Frequent and prolonged exposure to the sun causes premature ageing of the skin and skin cancer, notably melanoma. Ultraviolet radiation from the sun is divided into two categories, UV-A and UV-B. Both

SKIN DISEASES

28

bands cause skin damage but the immediate erythema and burning as a result of exposure are caused by UV-B radiation. The efficacy of a particular sunscreen is expressed as its sun protection factor (SPF) and this is calculated in relation to its protection against UV-B radiation, maximal protection being given by an SPF of 15+. Methods of evaluating the efficacy of sunscreens against UV-A radiation are more difficult and have not yet been fully developed. Because sunscreens, which are now widely used, prevent the immediate erythema, people tend to stay in the sun for prolonged periods and may unknowingly suffer the effects of UV-A radiation. Disorders largely exclusive to UV-A radiation are photosensitisation to drugs, fragility and blistering of the skin and many photodermatoses.

TOPICAL CORTICOSTEROIDS

Corticosteroids applied topically suppress inflammation and allergic reactions, produce a prolonged vasoconstriction and have a preventive effect in cell division. It is suggested that they decrease membrane permeability and inhibit release of toxic substances by attaching themselves to tissue receptors. In addition, their vasoconstrictive action decreases serum extravasation, swelling and discomfort, including itching. They are also immunosuppressive and may inhibit allergic reactions by preventing the production of antigen–antibody complexes.

The effectiveness of topical corticosteroids appears to be related to the potency of the drug and to the concentration achieved in the cutaneous tissues. Percutaneous absorption or penetration depends on the extent of skin damage, the relative concentration of the corticosteroid preparation, the vehicle, the type of dressing and the characteristics of the specific steroid. In general, fluorinated steroids and acetonides have increased potency. The preparations listed as potent in Table 28.1 have about 360 times the activity of hydrocortisone 1% on the skin.

TABLE 28.1   Potency of topical corticosteroids

Potency	Generic Name	Strength	Trade Name
Very potent	Fluocinolone acetonide	0.2%	—
Potent	Betamethasone dipropionate	0.05%	*Diprosone*
	Betamethasone valerate	0.1%	*Betnovate, Celestone-V*
	Fluclorolone acetonide	0.025%	*Topilar*
	Fluocinolone acetonide	0.025%	—
	Fluocortolone	0.5%	*Ultralan*
	Halcinonide	0.1%	*Halciderm*
	Triamcinolone acetonide	0.1%	*Aristocort, Aristocomb*
Moderately potent	Alclometasone dipropionate	0.05%	*Logoderm*
	Betamethasone valerate	0.05%	*Betnovate 1/2, Celestone-V 1/2*
	Fluocortolone	0.2%	*Ultralan D*
	Triamcinolone acetonide	0.05%	*Aristocort 0.05%, Kenalone 0.05%*
	Betamethasone valerate	0.02%	*Betnovate 1/5, Celestone-M*
	Triamcinolone acetonide	0.02%	*Aristocort 0.02%, Kenalone 0.02%*
Weak	Hydrocortisone acetate	1%	*Cortef, Dermacort, Egocort, Sigmacort*
		0.5%	*Cortaid, Cortic 0.5%, Derm-Aid*

Topical corticosteroids are recommended as a supplement to but not a substitute for preparations used conventionally in the management of dermatoses. It is most important to realise that dermatoses are controlled but not healed by these agents. Most dermatoses, particularly the eczematous group, respond to topical or systemic administration of corticosteroids. Other skin conditions such as those associated with systemic collagen disease, pemphigus, sarcoidosis, drug induced eruptions and urticaria may respond to systemic but not to topical therapy.

Topical corticosteroids are recommended in the treatment of acute and chronic dermatoses (including atopic, seborrheic, contact and some types of chronic eczematous dermatitis) and in infantile eczema, neurodermatitis, intertriginous dermatitis and anogenital pruritus.

Topical corticosteroids are ineffective in the treatment of sunburn or other burns.

ADVERSE DRUG REACTIONS

Sodium retention and transient inhibition of pituitary adrenal function have been reported when large areas have been treated for prolonged periods of time with topical corticosteroids. Prolonged facial application, especially of fluorinated steroids, may result in rosacea-like dermatitis, diffuse erythema, perioral dermatitis or acne.

PRECAUTIONS AND CONTRAINDICATIONS

Potent corticosteroids appear to clear lesions of solar malignancies (sunspots) on the face while being applied. However, in reality they produce epidermal atrophy with a diffuse and ill-defined spread of the malignant lesion into the surrounding tissues and leave the skin very fragile should future surgery be necessary.

There are several contraindications to the use of topical corticosteroids. The stronger, more potent fluorinated preparations are associated with a higher incidence of side effects. Local complications include atrophy of the epidermis and dermis with striae and secondary haemorrhage into the tissues. For this reason, fluorinated corticosteroids should not be used on the face. Tachyphylaxis is a recognised problem, that is, corticosteroids are less effective the greater their strength and the longer and more frequent their usage. The use of corticosteroids topically masks the inflammation of bacterial and fungal infections. Particular care should be taken with children having large areas treated, as absorption of the corticosteroid may occur giving rise to unwanted systemic effects.

NURSING IMPLICATIONS

ASSESSMENT

Before applying a topical corticosteroid the nurse should assess the skin condition and site of application. If the skin shows signs of infection, malignancy or atrophy, medical advice should be sought before making the application.

APPLICATION

It is important that the nurse checks the type of corticosteroid and the strength before applying the preparation. Topical corticosteroids should be applied with an applicator or gloves as continued contact with the fingers may cause cutaneous atrophy.

EVALUATION

The patient should be observed for improvement in the skin condition. Children having large areas treated should be closely watched for signs of systemic absorption. The skin should be watched for evidence of infection or atrophy of the dermis.

PATIENT EDUCATION

Education should emphasise the proper application of topical corticosteroids. Only a thin application is necessary. Patients who have been using corticosteroid preparations for prolonged periods should be advised to taper off their use as sudden cessation may result in rebound exacerbation of the skin

SKIN DISEASES

28

condition. They should also be taught self-evaluation for local or systemic effects, such as atrophy of the skin, infection or oedema. It is important that patients be warned that these are potent preparations which should not be used indiscriminately or without first seeking medical advice.

NON-STEROIDAL ANTIPRURITICS ▮▮▮▮

Pruritus is a symptom, not a disease, but the intense discomfort it can produce should not be underestimated. All wet dressings and shake lotions have some antipruritic effect but certain substances have a specific action.

Phenol present in calamine lotion decreases itch by anaesthetising the cutaneous nerve endings.

Camphor and **menthol** are often added to calamine lotion in concentrations of 1% to 3% as mild antipruritics.

Coal tar baths are used for generalised itching, see Soothing and Protective Preparations.

Crotamiton (*Eurax*) has been shown to relieve itching for periods of up to 10 hours. It is available as a 10% cream and lotion. It should not be allowed to come into contact with the eyes and should not be applied to acutely inflamed and weeping skin conditions. It should be rubbed gently into the area two or three times daily and is generally well tolerated.

Local anaesthetics such as benzocaine and lignocaine and topical antihistamines are best avoided as they are frequent causes of sensitivity.

NURSING IMPLICATIONS

ASSESSMENT

Assessment of the patient with pruritus involves firstly establishing the underlying cause so that appropriate therapy may be initiated. Where local applications are to be used for symptomatic relief the patient's history should be checked for previous allergy to the substance and the skin examined for signs of excessive dryness, cracking, or weeping.

APPLICATION

Any precautions specific to the substance being used should be observed, e.g. taking care not to allow crotamiton to come in contact with the eyes or mucous surfaces. Treatment of eruptions caused by the use of a drug should preferably be systemic as topical applications often make the condition worse.

EVALUATION

The patient should be observed for relief of the pruritus and any adverse effects of the treatment, especially hypersensitivity and drying or cracking of the skin.

PATIENT EDUCATION

The patient should be instructed on the correct method of application and advised to refrain from scratching or rubbing. This tends to damage the epidermis and sets up a cycle of lesion, more scratching and further damage.

PIGMENTATION DISORDERS ▬▬▬

VITILIGO

Methoxsalen, Trioxsalen

Methoxsalen (*Oxsoralen*) and trioxsalen (*Trisoralen*) are used in the treatment of vitiligo and other pigmentation deficiencies of the skin. Methoxsalen is available as capsules of 10 mg for oral use and as a 1% lotion for topical use. Trioxsalen is available only as 5 mg tablets for oral use.

These drugs are inactive in themselves but sensitise the skin to sunlight or artificial UV light so that formation of melanin pigments is increased following exposure. The photosensitivity is apparent about one hour after a dose, peaks at about two hours and then gradually decreases until it is completely lost after about eight hours.

Overexposure to sunlight or UV light after taking these drugs may result in serious burning with blistering of the skin and the photosensitivity may persist for several days, therefore all exposed areas must be protected from the sun. The eyes must be protected and glasses which filter out UV light should be worn for 24 hours after ingestion of these drugs. Ordinary sunglasses may not provide the protection required and advice should be obtained from the manufacturer as to the properties of the lens. Lips should also be protected with a sunscreen.

Methoxsalen is given in a dose of 20 mg and trioxsalen in a dose of 10 mg about two hours before exposure to the source of UV light. Exposure times should be short at first, and increased according to response. Forty-eight hours should be allowed between exposures.

Topical application of methoxsalen is usually more severe in its effects than oral administration. The 1% topical lotion may need to be diluted before application to prevent excessive reactions. The lotion is applied and followed with a one-minute exposure to UV light. Exposure time may be increased cautiously according to response. Treatments should not be more often than once a week.

Photosensitivity reactions are of two types, phototoxic and photoallergic. Phototoxic reactions are usually dose dependent and affect only the area of the skin exposed to the light. Photoallergic reactions bear no relationship to the dose of the drug and may be generalised.

Foods such as carrots, celery, parsley, parsnips and mustard contain psoralens which are photosensitisers. These foods can cause phototoxic reactions. Drugs such as tetracyclines, phenothiazines, sulfonamides, nalidixic acid and topically applied antihistamines may cause phototoxic reactions. Photoallergic reactions can result from ingestion of sulfonamides, thiazides, griseofulvin and phenothiazines. All of these foods and drugs should be avoided during therapy with methoxsalen or trioxsalen.

Cover Creams

Regular cosmetics very often do not cover the lesions of pigmentation disorders but special cover creams are available from manufacturers of cosmetics. *Dermacolor*, *Covermark* and *Keromask* all contain titanium dioxide to produce the opaque covering. Each brand is available in a number of different shades and patients who need such cosmetics usually find which cream suits them best by trial and error.

NURSING IMPLICATIONS

28

SKIN DISEASES

ADMINISTRATION

Methoxsalen and trioxsalen, whether oral or topical, should always be administered under close supervision. The topical lotion should not be given to the patient to take home.

EVALUATION

During treatment with these drugs evaluation is mainly concerned with observing the patient's skin for signs of burning. If this occurs the patient must be removed from the source of UV light immediately. Pruritus may be the first sign of burning.

PATIENT EDUCATION

Patients must be warned of the possibility of sunburn and of the need to protect lips and eyes and all exposed skin for 24 hours after taking these drugs.

PSORIASIS

Psoriasis is a skin disease of unknown aetiology characterised by silvery, scaly patches. When the scale is removed erythematous papules are revealed, usually showing several bleeding points. The basic pathology is a disturbance in the proliferation of epidermal cells. The disease follows an unpredictable course with spontaneous remissions and exacerbations, but there is no known cure and the condition is therefore life long.

Topical therapy is the mainstay in the treatment of psoriasis and keratolytics and softening agents such as glycerin oily cream are extensively used. In severe cases corticosteroids are used systemically and topically. However, there is a high rate of relapse following treatment with systemic steroids and they should be used only for short periods. Contemporary therapy includes the careful use of topical and systemic antimitotic drugs.

Dithranol

Dithranol combines with DNA thus inhibiting the synthesis of nucleoprotein and so diminishing cellular proliferation. It is available as *Dithrocream* in concentrations ranging from 0.1% to 2%. The lowest effective strength should be used. *Dithrasal H.P. Ointment* contains dithranol and salicylic acid in a washable base.

Dithranol preparations are applied to the affected areas only, left on for 10 minutes initially and then washed off with water. Contact time is increased gradually up to 30 minutes. Dithranol is a powerful irritant and must not be used on inflamed areas or near the eyes. Dithranol stains the skin and hair (reversible on cessation of therapy), clothes and other materials, e.g. plastic and tiles. Staining of baths and shower recesses can be avoided by removing dithranol preparations with paraffin oil prior to washing. Some patients are hypersensitive to the drug.

Methotrexate

Methotrexate, a folic acid antagonist, also inhibits cellular proliferation.

Methotrexate is available as 2.5 mg tablets (*Ledertrexate, Methoblastin*). It is given orally for severe disabling psoriasis which does not respond to other therapy. Many oral dosage regimens are followed. Two regimens used are: 25–37.5 mg once weekly; or 5–15 mg/cm^2 of body surface once weekly. Methotrexate is also applied topically as weak soaks using a 0.015% solution.

For further information on methotrexate see Chapter 31 Cancer Chemotherapy.

Retinoids

Vitamin A derivatives are also used in the treatment of psoriasis (see etretinate).

PUVA

PUVA is a regimen combining oral methoxsalen and long range UV light. The mechanism of action is inhibition of DNA synthesis. The treatment must be closely supervised to prevent serious burns (see methoxsalen).

Calcipotriol

Calcipotriol is a vitamin D derivative which induces differentiation and suppresses proliferation of epidermal cells. It is available for topical application as *Daivonex*. It is applied morning and evening until satisfactory improvement has occurred, when application may be reduced to once daily or ceased until the condition recurs. Excessive systemic absorption of calcipotriol may result in hypercalcaemia, therefore it is recommended that *Daivonex* not be used in severe extensive psoriasis and that the quantity applied not exceed 100 g per week. The ointment should not be used concurrently with calcium or vitamin D supplements. The ointment base sometimes causes itching and erythema and contact with the face chould be avoided.

NURSING IMPLICATIONS

APPLICATION

Application of dithranol containing preparations should be preceded by a preliminary test for sensitivity on a small area of disease affected skin.

EVALUATION

The skin should be observed for improvement in the condition or any untoward effects. When dithranol is used the patient should be watched for allergic reactions. When etretinate is used the patient should be observed for mucosal dryness, palmoplantar desquamation, pruritus, thinning of the skin or alopecia.

PATIENT EDUCATION

Patients receiving dithranol treatment should be advised that the skin and hair may darken in colour and that clothes, plastics and tiles will be stained.

Patients receiving etretinate should be instructed to avoid direct exposure to sunlight and to use a suitable sunscreen when necessary.

Patients receiving methotrexate should be warned to contact their doctor promptly should they have any signs of infection, fever, severe diarrhoea or unusual bleeding. They should also be advised not to take any other medication without the approval of their doctor.

Patients receiving calcipotriol should be warned not to take calcium or vitamin D supplements during treatment, and to wash their hands after application to avoid inadvertant transfer of the ointment to the face.

HEPARINOID PREPARATIONS

28

Heparinoid, as its name suggests, is a substance with heparin-like activity. Heparinoids possess anticoagulant and anti-inflammatory properties and promote fibrinolysis. They therefore increase local blood and lymph flow and accelerate reabsorption of local oedema and infiltrations. Heparinoids appear to be effectively absorbed through the skin.

Hirudoid cream contains heparinoid equivalent to 25 000 units of heparin in each 100 g. Each 100 g of *Lasonil* ointment contains heparinoid equivalent to 5000 units of heparin plus 15 000 IU of hyaluronidase which assists absorption and dispersion by breaking down hyaluronic acid.

These products are used in the treatment of sprains, contusions and haematomata and for superficial thromboses and varicose ulcers. They are also effective in softening scar tissue. Bruising after venepuncture is dissipated more rapidly by their use.

The earlier treatment is begun, the better the results that may be expected. Depending on the extent of the lesion, 3–5 cm of the cream or ointment should be applied two or three times daily. In certain cases more may be necessary. In thrombosis and thrombophlebitis it should be applied on gauze to the affected area, but in varicose ulcers it should be massaged into the skin around the ulcer in the direction of the venous return, from below the ulcer upwards. For the treatment of haematomata and scars, the cream may be massaged into the skin.

Heparinoid preparations should not be applied to bleeding areas. In suppurative processes they should not come in contact with the infected area.

NURSING IMPLICATIONS

Treatment should be commenced as soon as possible. Contact of these preparations with broken skin should be avoided.

ULCERS

The commonest ulcers encountered are those of the leg secondary to vascular disorders. When stasis occurs in the blood vessels the first noticeable effect is oedema, generally on the inner aspect of the ankle. This is frequently followed by an itchy dermatitis. The skin becomes red and fragile and any slight trauma such as scratching or a knock breaks the skin and an ulcer forms. These ulcers are sometimes difficult to heal and the primary aim of treatment must be to restore blood flow. This is done by correct bandaging or the wearing of a suitable elastic stocking and exercise. Local therapy is aimed at keeping the ulcer site clean and preventing further damage. Because of the oedema the ulcer is usually wet and oozing at the beginning of treatment.

Topical antibiotics are best avoided. If gross infection is present a systemic antibiotic should be given according to the sensitivity of the infecting organism.

Kaltostat is an absorbent, haemostatic wound dressing consisting of calcium alginate fibres. If the ulcer is deep it is packed with the dressing and then covered with another dressing. Unless exudate is excessive the dressing should be changed only on alternate days and, as healing progresses, once or twice weekly. *Kaltostat* is not used in the treatment of dry wounds.

Dextranomer, a chemical modification of dextran, can absorb up to four times its own weight of fluid. It is available as spherical beads (*Debrisan*) which, after the ulcer is washed with water or saline, are spread over the wet ulcer bed to a depth of at least 3 mm. Capillary action draws the exudate up into the layer of beads. When the layer becomes saturated it forms a hard mass and therefore needs to be changed before saturation occurs, usually once or twice daily. The old beads are removed by a stream of normal saline and a new application made. No other topical treatment should be used at the same time.

Proteolytic enzymes are sometimes used to soften hard slough. Preparations available are *Elase*, a mixture of fibrinolysin and desoxyribonuclease, and *Varidase*, a combination of streptokinase and streptodornase. The former is supplied as a soft ointment, the latter as a dry powder which must be reconstituted with normal saline and applied as a wet dressing. *Varidase* solution must be stored in a refrigerator and used within seven days as it loses potency rapidly at room temperature.

Other methods of removing exudate and slough are daily soaks with normal saline or a surface active agent such as cetrimide.

NURSING IMPLICATIONS·

Patients who are ambulant should be watched and reminded not to stand in one place except for very short periods. If the patient is wearing a pressure stocking or bandage walking should be encouraged as it improves circulation. When dressing an ulcer all crusts should be removed as crusts under a pressure bandage may cause further damage to the tissue. Dressings should not be changed too often as it frequently damages healing tissue. *Kaltostat* dressings frequently develop an unpleasant odour; this is to be expected and is not a reason to change the dressing.

FURTHER READING

Burton, J.L. (1990), *Essentials of Dermatology*, Churchill Livingstone, London.

Marks, J., Rawlins, M.D. (1987) 'Skin diseases', *Avery's Drug Treatment*, 3rd Edition.

Sams, W.M. and Lynch, P.J., (1990), *Principles and Practice of Dermatology*, Churchill Livingstone, New York.

Wargon, O. (1989), 'Managing psoriasis', *Current Therapeutics*, Vol 30, No. 6, pp 79-93.

Willsteed, E. (1989), 'Choice of vehicle for topical therapy', *Current Therapeutics*, Vol. 30, No. 1, pp 57-60.

TEST YOUR KNOWLEDGE

1. A cream consists of: (a) an oily substance dispersed in water; (b) an aqueous substance dispersed in oil; (c) a white powder evenly suspended in an aqueous vehicle; (d) (a) and (b); (e) (a), (b), and (c).

2. Photosensitivity is: (a) an abnormal fear of being photographed; (b) a burn caused by contact with photographic chemicals; (c) damage to the skin as a result of exposure to sunlight or artificial light.

3. The doctor has ordered betamethasone cream to be applied to a small weeping lesion on the patient's arm. You are unable to obtain cream but can obtain betamethasone ointment. What is likely to be the effect on the lesion if you use it?

4. A friend asks for advice about the 'tinea' lesion between her toes. The lesion is red and weeping and the skin is cracked. Would it be better to apply an antifungal powder or cream? Why?

5. The doctor has ordered salicylic acid 20% paint for a young woman with several warts on her hand. What instructions would you give the patient for its use?

6. You have been applying neomycin soaks to a large infected area on the back. The lesion is healing rapidly, then for no apparent reason it again becomes inflamed and this inflammation persists in spite of continuing treatment. What would you suspect has happened?

7. An extensive infected leg ulcer has been irrigated with a solution of neomycin 0.5% for 10 days and, while the infection seems to be clearing, there is as yet little evidence of healing. The appropriate action is to: (a) continue the treatment; (b) change to another treatment to speed up the healing process; (c) draw to the attention of the attending medical officer that prolonged treatment with neomycin may have serious side effects.

SKIN DISEASES

28

TABLE 28.2   Summary table — drugs used in dermatology

DRUG GROUP Drug Name	Use	Action	Adverse Reactions	Nursing Implications
Retinoids Tretinoin (topical)	Severe acne, keratitis, psoriasis	Affects differentiation of epithelial tissue	Increased susceptibility of skin to sunlight	**Assess:** History for previous adverse effects to drug; document baseline observations of lesions and general condition of skin **Administer:** Local application **Evaluate:** For improvement; observe for signs of photosensitivity **Educate:** To avoid direct exposure to sunlight during treatment and to protect treated area with clothing or suitable sunscreen
Etretinate (oral)	Disorders of keratinisation, e.g. psoriasis, ichthyosis, lichen planus	Affects differentiation of epithelial tissue	Cheilitis, mucosal dryness, palmoplantar desquamation, pruritus, thinning of skin, alopecia, headache, elevated liver enzymes; embryotoxic and teratogenic	**Assess:** Age, as should be used with caution in women of childbearing potential; pregnancy; history for previous adverse effects to drug; document baseline observations of lesions and general condition of skin **Administer:** Orally as ordered **Evaluate:** For signs of improvement in skin condition; for adverse effects, e.g. mucosal dryness, palmoplantar desquamation, pruritus, thinning of skin, alopecia
Isotretinoin (oral)	Severe nodulocystic acne			

Anti-infective preparations
See Chapter 30 Infectious Diseases

TABLE 28.2 continued

DRUG GROUP Drug Name	Use	Action	Adverse Reactions	Nursing Implications
Topical Corticosteroids Alclometasone dipropionate Betamethasone dipropionate Betamethasone valerate Fluocinolone acetonide Fluclorolone acetonide Flumethasone pivalate Fluocortolone hexanoate Fluocortolone pivalate Halcinonide Hydrocortisone acetate Triamcinolone acetonide	Control of acute and chronic dermatoses	Suppression of inflammation and allergy, production of vasoconstriction, prevention of cell division	Epidermal atrophy, spread of malignant lesions, rosacea-like facial dermatitis, erythema and acne; systemic absorption a distinct possibility leading to systemic side effects, see Chapter 19 Endocrine Diseases	**Assess:** Skin condition and designated site of application; skin for signs of infection, malignancy or atrophy **Administer:** Use sterile technique and applicator or gloves to minimise risk of atrophy **Evaluate:** Efficacy; for development of overlying infection, temperature, dermal atrophy, striae, thinning of epidermis, rebound effect, systemic absorption **Educate:** Proper application; self-evaluation for efficacy, local and systemic side effects; to taper off use gradually; to avoid indiscriminate use; to seek medical advice when appropriate
Preparations for pigmentation disorders Methoxsalen Trioxsalen	Vitiligo and other pigmentation disorders	Sensitises skin to UV light so formation of melanin pigments is increased	Burning, blistering of skin and eyes	**Assess:** Area to be treated (local applications); document baseline observations of skin lesions **Administer:** Vitiligo—Topically or orally followed by exposure of skin to sunlight or artificial UV light. Psoriasis—usually orally followed by exposure to UV light. Topical treatment must always be performed under strict medical supervision, the lotion should never be given to the patient to take home

28 SKIN DISEASES

TABLE 28.2 continued

DRUG GROUP Drug Name	Use	Action	Adverse Reactions	Nursing Implications
				Evaluate: For improvement and signs of burning; if burning occurs patient must be immediately removed from source of light **Educate:** Warn of possibility of sunburn, to protect lips with sunscreen
Preparations for psoriasis Dithranol	Psoriasis	Combines with DNA and diminishes cell proliferation	Burning sensation, eye irritation, skin staining	**Assess:** For previous hypersensitivity to drug; document baseline description of skin lesions **Administer:** Perform preliminary test on small area of skin to check for sensitivity before applying for treatment; keep away from eyes **Evaluate:** For improvement in lesions, allergic response **Educate:** That burning sensation may occur when first applied, that skin and hair may darken

Antihistamines

ROSS W. HOLLAND

O B J E C T I V E S

At the conclusion of this chapter the reader should be able to:

1. Describe how antihistamine drugs are thought to act;

2. List common adverse reactions to antihistamines;

3. List the conditions for which antihistamines are effective; and

4. Identify antihistamines from a list of drugs.

HISTAMINE AND ALLERGIES ■

Histamine is a naturally occurring substance whose normal function in the body is in tissue growth and repair, control of gastric secretion and probably as a chemical transmitter in the brain.

It is stored in mast cells, found particularly in the skin and mucosal lining of the nose, lungs and gastrointestinal tract. Under some circumstances (e.g. when mast cells are damaged by chemicals, drugs, heat or trauma) abnormally large amounts of histamine are released causing a localised or widespread allergic-type reaction.

An example of a local reaction is the characteristic 'triple response' resulting from an insect bite. First, a red spot develops due to local dilation of the capillaries in response to histamine release. Second, a brighter red flare, extending about 1 cm beyond the original spot, develops as a result of more widespread dilation of neighbouring arterioles. Third, localised oedema forms a wheal. An example of a more extreme hypersensitivity reaction would be anaphylactic shock in response to contact with an allergen.

It is thought that histamine, once released, acts at specific receptor sites in various tissues. These receptors are classified into H_1, H_2 and H_3 subgroups. Activation of H_1 receptors causes smooth muscle contraction, increases vascular permeability, increases the production of mucus and activates sensory nerves to induce pruritus and reflexes such as sneezing. Drugs that block this response are discussed in this chapter. The H_2 receptors appear to be confined to the control of gastric secretions. Drugs that act on the H_2 receptors are called H_2 receptor antagonists and are discussed in Chapter 17 Gastrointestinal Disorders. Because their action is on gastric secretion, these drugs are primarily used in the treatment of gastric ulceration. H_3 receptors are located in the brain. Drugs acting on these receptors are discussed in Chapter 26 Psychiatric Disorders.

ANTIHISTAMINE THERAPY ■

Antihistamines come from several different chemical classes. Theoretically, if a drug from one class does not work, one from another class can be tried. However, in practice the only real indication to change is if the adverse effects of a particular antihistamine, perhaps drowsiness or irritability, are unacceptable.

COMMON ANTIHISTAMINES

Astemizole, Azatadine, Chlorpheniramine, Cyproheptadine, Dimenhydrinate, Diphenhydramine, Dexchlorpheniramine, Loratadine, Mebhydrolin, Pheniramine, Promethazine, Terfenadine

TRADE NAMES

Astemizole: *Hismanal.*
Azatadine: *Zadine.*

Chlorpheniramine: *Piriton.*
Cyproheptadine: *Periactin.*
Dimenhydrinate: *Andrumin; Dramamine.*
Diphenhydramine: *Benadryl.*
Dexchlorpheniramine: *Polaramine.*
Loratadine: *Claratyne.*
Mebhydrolin: *Fabahistin.*
Pheniramine: *Avil.*
Promethazine: *Phenergan.*
Terfenadine: *Teldane.*

MECHANISM OF ACTION

Drugs that block the action of histamine at H_1 receptors are called antihistamines.

They appear to occupy receptor sites to the exclusion of histamine. Thus they antagonise most of the effects of histamine, reducing the intensity of allergic and anaphylactic reactions. It had been thought that they did not prevent the release of histamine from mast cells but recent evidence suggests that azatadine, at least, may have this added action. They have no action on H_2 receptors.

Antihistamines antagonise the important vasodilator effects of histamine, reduce capillary permeability and the consequent formation of oedema. They greatly diminish the itching that accompanies allergic reactions. Other effects include depression of the central nervous system, sedation and suppression of nausea and vomiting. Most antihistamines have anticholinergic activity which accounts for the dryness of the mouth experienced by some patients. In addition, a local anaesthetic effect has been noted with all these drugs. The exceptions are terfenadine, loratadine and astemizole.

PHARMACOKINETICS

In general, antihistamines are absorbed rapidly after oral administration and begin to provide symptomatic relief within 15–30 minutes. They are detectable in serum for 3–6 hours but it has been noted that the duration of effects is longer than might be anticipated from their pharmacokinetics.

The older antihistamines have short half-lives and must be given at 4–6 hour intervals. The newer drugs are longer acting, two having a 12-hour dose interval (azatadine and terfenadine) and one being taken only once a day (astemizole).

USES

Antihistamines have a place in the treatment of allergic reactions where histamine is the mediator. They are most useful in treating urticaria and pruritus, insect bites and stings, allergic rhinitis (hay fever) and in sinusitis because of their drying effect. They may also be used for allergic-type drug reactions and in the treatment of anaphylactic shock.

Antihistamines are not used in the treatment of asthma. Histamine is no longer believed to be the major cause of asthmatic symptoms. It is now thought the roles of macrophages and eosinophils are more important in sustaining the underlying chronic inflammation. Antihistamines are occasionally used in cough mixtures for their antitussive effect. However, this use is undesirable as their anticholinergic drying effect can produce thickening of mucus within the lungs, leading to an unproductive cough.

The sedative effects are often used to advantage, although tolerance usually develops after a few days. For this purpose short-term use only is advocated, particularly for children. Occasionally, the sedative effect is utilised when an antihistamine is used alone or in conjunction with narcotics as a preoperative medication.

Those antihistamines which effectively suppress nausea and vomiting (pheniramine, dimenhydrinate) may be used to prevent motion sickness and are present in several commercial preparations. Some have been used to prevent morning sickness. However, their use in morning sickness has declined over the past few years with increasing awareness of the adverse effects of drugs on the developing fetus.

It is particularly important to take into account the wide and differing durations of action of these substances. Astemizole is taken only once daily. Terfenadine and azatadine are taken twice a day, as are the sustained and time-release forms of some other antihistamines. Others need to be administered three or four times a day. It should also be noted that antihistamines which come in more than one dose form cannot be substituted for each other. For example three *Polaramine* 2 mg tablets taken together will not have the same effect as one *Polaramine* 6 mg tablet. This is because the 6 mg tablet is a repeat action formulation designed to be taken at intervals of 12 hours, whereas the 2 mg tablet does not have this repetitive action and must be administered more frequently. As with all drugs, strengths should be checked before administration.

ANTIHISTAMINES

29

It is worth remembering that should skin allergy tests be required to determine susceptibility to a particular allergen — it is necessary to cease taking any antihistamines prior to testing. The decision as to when to cease the medication is dependent on the half-life of the medication.

The chemical class, sedative effect and dosage schedules of the antihistamines are shown in Table 29.1.

ADVERSE DRUG REACTIONS

Adverse reactions to this group of substances are closely related to their pharmacological effects but there is considerable individual variation in response. Most prominent effects are drowsiness and dry mouth, however, with the newer compounds azatadine, terfenadine and astemizole, drowsiness is not considered a problem because these drugs do not pass readily into the brain at normal doses. Apart from their sedating and drying effects H_1 antihistamines have a relatively low incidence of adverse effects. These include dizziness, blurred or double vision, loss of appetite, muscle weakness, lassitude and, when given by the intravenous route, hypotension. When high doses are given paradoxical stimulation of the central nervous system sometimes occurs resulting in wakefulness and hyperactivity, particularly in children. When antihistamines are applied to the skin an allergic type dermatitis can occur, so topical application is not generally recommended.

DRUG INTERACTIONS

Because of the potential to cause drowsiness, which principally occurs with some older type antihistamines, care should be taken not to consume alcohol, drive motor vehicles or operate machinery while taking these medications. Concurrent administration with some other medications, e.g. tranquillisers, antianxiety drugs and hypnotics, may lead to an additive anticholinergic or sedative action. Also, it should be remembered that many over the counter cold and hay fever remedies contain antihistamines. Concurrent use may lead to an additive effect, particularly with drowsiness.

TABLE 29.1 Chemical class, sedative effect and dosage schedules of antihistamines

Chemical class	Drug name	Sedation	Usual adult dose
Alkylamine	Chlorpheniramine	+	4 mg four times a day
	Dexchlorpheniramine	+	2 mg four times a day 6 mg Repetab twice a day
	Pheniramine	+	25–50 mg three times a day
Ethanolamine	Dimenhydrinate	++	50 mg three times a day
	Diphenhydramine	+++	50 mg three times a day
Phenothiazine	Promethazine	+++	25 mg three times a day
Piperidine	Azatadine	++	1 mg twice a day
	Cyproheptadine	+	4 mg three times a day
	Loratadine	+/−	10 mg once daily
Miscellaneous	Astemizole	+/−	10 mg once daily
	Terfenadine	+/−	60 mg twice a day

NURSING IMPLICATIONS

ASSESSMENT

Because of the frequent occurrence of sedation with antihistamine therapy the patient's need to be fully alert should be assessed. Interactions with other drugs and alcohol in particular (which may be taken inadvertently in cough medicine) are common, potentially dangerous and should be avoided. It should be remembered that the anticholinergic effect of antihistamines can cause respiratory secretions to become thick and sticky and this could lead to respiratory complications in situations where a productive loose cough is desirable. Some antihistamines belong to the phenothiazine group of drugs and therefore there is the possibility of extrapyramidal side effects occurring.

ADMINISTRATION

A large number of doses and forms are available so orders for antihistamines should be checked carefully against container labels. Lower doses may be given to avoid sedation. Sustained release tablets should be swallowed whole and not crushed. Crushing will alter the anticipated long acting slow release effect. The exact form and strength of tablet ordered should always be given. Tablets of a different strength should not be substituted to 'make up' the dose.

EVALUATION

The effectiveness of the drug in reducing the allergic response, causing sedation and producing unwanted side effects should be evaluated. Allergic reactions to antihistamines can develop. Allergic dermatitis can occur with topical use. Any change in blood pressure after intravenous injection should be reported immediately.

ACUTE POISONING

Acute poisoning may occur especially in children because of the common usage of antihistamine drugs. Signs of acute toxicity include central nervous system effects such as excitement, lack of coordination and convulsions. The pupils may become dilated and fixed, the face flushed and fever may occur. Cardiorespiratory collapse and subsequent death can occur within 24 hours of the ingestion of 20 to 30 tablets by a young child. The treatment is symptomatic since there is no specific antidote.

PATIENT EDUCATION

Patients must be made aware of the possibility of drowsiness and the dangers when driving a motor vehicle or operating machinery, and of the possible potentiation of sedative effects when taken with other drugs, particularly tranquillisers and alcohol. Patients taking antihistamines should be instructed to inform their doctor, dentist or pharmacist that they are having these medications before taking other medications which may be prescribed or purchased at a pharmacy. Parents should be aware of the toxic effects and the need to keep antihistamines out of the reach of children.

ANTIHISTAMINES

29

TEST YOUR KNOWLEDGE

1. Describe how antihistamines are thought to act.

2. Which of the following drugs are antihistamines: (a) phenylbutazone (*Butazolidin*); (b) diphenhydramine (*Benadryl*); (c) promethazine (*Phenergan*); (d) phenytoin (*Dilantin*); (e) dexchlorpheniramine (*Polaramine*); (f) dextropropoxyphene (*Doloxene*)?

3. List four conditions for which antihistamines may be used.

4. (a) What are the two most prominent adverse reactions to antihistamines? (b) List two others.

5. Name two non-sedating antihistamines.

6. Which of the following antihistamines are long-acting: (a) terfenadine; (b) dexchlorpheniramine; (c) astemizole; (d) azatadine; (e) mebhydrolin.

TABLE 29.2 Summary table — antihistamines

Drug Group	Use	Action	Adverse Reactions	Nursing Implications
Antihistamines (H₁ receptor antagonists)	Allergic reactions mediated by histamine, e.g. urticaria, pruritus, insect bites, drug reactions, anaphylaxis, rhinitis	Block action of histamine at H₁ receptors	Drowsiness; dry mouth; dizziness; visual blurring; loss of appetite; muscle weakness; lassitude; hypotension	**Assess:** For known hypersensitivity; establish baseline blood pressure (IV use); concurrent use of other anticholinergic-like drugs and CNS depressants, including alcohol **Administer:** Check labels carefully; lower doses to avoid sedation where necessary; give oral doses with food **Evaluate:** Reduction of signs of allergy; sedative effect; allergic dermatitis with topical application; blood pressure changes with intravenous use; signs of toxicity, especially in children **Educate:** Warn that drowsiness and dry mouth may occur and advise of potential dangers when driving a motor vehicle and operating machinery and of potentiation of sedative effects with other sedative-type drugs, including alcohol

29 ANTIHISTAMINES

CHAPTER

30

Infectious Diseases

JEFFERY D. HUGHES

O B J E C T I V E S

At the conclusion of this chapter the reader should be able to:

1. Describe the parameters on which the selection of an anti-infective agent is based;

2. Describe, in general terms, the mode of action of the various groups of anti-infective agents;

3. List those anti-infective agents used to treat infections due to Gram positive organisms, Gram negative organisms, fungi, malarial parasites, trichomonads, tubercle bacilli and viruses;

4. Differentiate between the various anti-infective agents in each group with respect to dosage, route and administration, major side effects and uses; and

5. List the anti-infective agents that must be given by deep intramuscular injection to avoid or reduce pain, those that should be administered slowly intravenously or by infusion to minimise venous irritation and thrombophlebitis, and those that should be administered orally on an empty stomach.

DRUG THERAPY ▋

The goal of drug therapy in the treatment of infectious diseases is to assist the body in ridding itself of the infecting organism. This is accomplished by use of an anti-infective agent which, while not seriously impairing the normal defence mechanisms of the patient, is 'selectively toxic' to the causative organism.

The terms 'anti-infective' and 'antimicrobial' are used in this chapter to mean all chemotherapeutic agents used against microorganisms.

HISTORY

Since ancient times people have used agents empirically for the treatment of infections. The ancient Greeks used male fern as an intestinal anthelmintic and the ancient Hindus treated leprosy with chaulmoogra (the oil from the ripe seeds of the *Hydnocarpus* species). The history of modern anti-infective therapy did not, however, begin until the late 19th century when salvarsan (an arsenical used to treat syphilis) was discovered.

The present anti-infective era dates from the demonstration by Florey, Chain and others in 1940 that penicillin, discovered by Fleming in 1929, exerts a powerful systemic antibacterial effect. The success of this drug led to a search for other similar substances, and now a wide range of naturally occurring and synthetic anti-infective agents is available.

ANTI-INFECTIVE THERAPY ▋

GENERAL PRINCIPLES

For the treatment of each infection there is generally one drug or occasionally a combination of drugs, that is likely to be a better choice than other drugs or drug combinations. When an infection does not respond to a first-choice drug or the patient cannot tolerate it, there is usually a preferred order of choice among alternative drugs.

The Medical Letter on Drugs and Therapeutics.
Handbook of Antimicrobial Therapy. New York: The
Medical Letter Inc., 1984.

The choice of when to commence antimicrobial therapy is dependent on the clinical status of the patient, the site of infection, the probable infecting organism and possible outcome if treatment is not commenced. In patients who are otherwise healthy and have only a mild illness, therapy may be delayed until a firm diagnosis is made. In other patients, therapy should be commenced immediately once a history has been taken, physical examination completed and laboratory assessment made. Situations which require immediate treatment are febrile episodes in neutropenic patients, possible acute endocarditis, septicaemia and focal infections (e.g. urinary tract infections, pneumonias) where the patient is moderately to severely ill.

Once the decision to commence therapy has been made the choice of an anti-infective agent is either empirical or definitive. In the first case the physician must select a drug which will be active against the most likely pathogen(s) on the basis of the site of infection and the clinical status of the patient. In the second case the physician knows the identity of the infecting microorganism and the choice of antimicrobial is made on the basis of known or tested sensitivities.

Appropriate specimens must be collected to identify the infecting organisms. The specimen taken is dependent on the site of infection and suspected pathogens (e.g. early morning urine samples for tuberculosis, midstream urine samples for urinary tract infections, sputum samples for pneumonias). Appropriate samples must be taken before antimicrobial therapy is commenced. The first tests carried out to identify infecting organisms are: (a) **microscopy,** looking at cell size, shape and grouping; and (b) **staining,** to differentiate between Gram positive and Gram negative bacteria. These tests will often give sufficient information on which to base the choice of antimicrobial. The organism can then be cultured and further identified on the basis of biochemical tests. Antimicrobial sensitivities should also be carried out. In some instances the above methods of identification are ineffective or inappropriate. In these cases serological testing may be carried out to identify the infecting organism (e.g. hepatitis B and C, Q fever).

Once the organism has been identified the patient should receive the narrowest spectrum antimicrobial possible. In choosing the appropriate antimicrobial consideration must be given to both host and drug related factors. The immune status of patients, their ability to eliminate drugs, the drug's ability to penetrate the site of infection and its toxicity all influence the dosage schedule and route of administration chosen.

In patients who are immunocompromised the types of infections encountered often reflect the particular immune defect (e.g. impaired cell mediated immunity predisposes to fungal infections), hence the range of most likely pathogens is increased. Impaired immune function decreases the effectiveness of certain antimicrobials (e.g. aminoglycosides are ineffective when used alone in profoundly neutropenic patients). Treatment of infections in immunocompromised patients requires special consideration.

Ability of the antimicrobial to penetrate the site of infection is a critical factor. Not only must the drug reach the site of infection, it must do so in sufficient concentration to inhibit the growth of the microorganism. Penetration of the drug into a particular site can be influenced both by the route of administration of the drug and the dose administered. For example, penicillins penetrate the blood brain barrier poorly and oral phenoxymethylpenicillin is ineffective for the treatment of pneumococcal meningitis, yet intravenous benzylpenicillin given in high doses is the treatment of choice for this condition.

Absorption of antimicrobials and hence drug levels achieved at the site of infection may be influenced by the clinical status of the patient. Seriously ill patients may not absorb orally administered agents. In patients with hypotension or decreased circulation, even intramuscularly administered drugs may not provide adequate serum and tissue levels. Intravenous therapy is preferred for the seriously ill. Oral therapy is generally used for minor infections (e.g. urinary tract infections, bronchitis), to complete a course of therapy following parenteral antimicrobials or for chronic infections (e.g. tuberculosis, chronic osteomyelitis).

Drug toxicity is also an important issue. The more toxic antimicrobial agents should be reserved for the treatment of serious infections which are unresponsive to less toxic alternatives (e.g. flucloxacillin should be used in preference to vancomycin except in those instances where the patient is hypersensitive to penicillins or the staphylococcus is resistant to flucloxacillin).

The dose of the chosen antimicrobial is made on the basis of the type of infection to be treated. It should, however, be modified in those patients who have a reduced ability to eliminate the drug (e.g. patients with renal impairment given aminoglycosides or fluoroquinolones). In these instances, the dose and/or dosage interval may need to be adjusted. In some cases dosage modifications can be made on the basis of antimicrobial serum concentrations (e.g. aminoglycosides, vancomycin, flucytosine).

It is fundamental to the successful treatment of an infectious disease process that the correct drug, dose route and frequency

INFECTIOUS DISEASES

30

of administration are selected for the particular patient. Inadequate dosage may lead to the development of bacterial resistance, and inadequate length of treatment may lead to relapse. Systemic anti-infective agents should not be used to treat trivial, self-limiting infections.

In summary, the choice of an appropriate anti-infective agent is based on:

1. the **clinical diagnosis**;

2. the **identification of the infecting organism**;

3. the **result of in vitro sensitivity tests** indicating those drugs that are active against the organism isolated from the specimen;

4. **drug characteristics** — ability of the drug to penetrate to the site of infection, toxicity, interaction or incompatibility with other drug therapy, and cost; and

5. **patient factors** — age, hepatic and renal function, history of drug sensitivity and the status of the patient's immune response.

When the desired response to therapy does not occur as expected, the following questions should be asked when reconsidering therapy:

1. Is the isolated organism the true pathogen?

2. Is a previously unsuspected infection present?

3. Is the antimicrobial therapy adequate (i.e. correct drug, dosage and route of administration)?

4. Is the antimicrobial penetrating the site of infection?

5. Is drainage/debridement required?

6. Have resistant organisms or superinfection developed?

7. Is the persistent fever due to another cause such as underlying illness, iatrogenic complications (e.g. phlebitis) or drug reaction?

Mechanism of Action

Anti-infective agents inhibit or kill invading organisms by interfering with their metabolic processes or disrupting vital cell structures. The five principal sites of antimicrobial action are:

1. the **cell wall** — agents, such as the penicillins, cephalosporins and vancomycin, interfere with the osmotic defences of the cell wall so that the cell absorbs water and bursts.

2. the **lipoprotein cell membrane** (inside the cell wall) — disorientation of the molecules of the cell membrane, similar to the action of a detergent at the oil–water interface, results in the membrane becoming permeable and vital cellular components escaping. Amphotericin B, colistin and polymyxin B interfere with the integrity of the cell membrane.

3. **ribosomes and nucleic acid metabolism** — aminoglycosides, chloramphenicol, erythromycin, lincomycin, clindamycin and the tetracyclines interfere with protein synthesis controlled by ribosomes.

4. **DNA** (deoxyribonucleic acid) — interference with the synthesis of the major nucleic acid, DNA, in the nucleus inhibits cell replication. For example, griseofulvin disrupts the cell's mitotic spindle structure, thus arresting the metaphase of cell division; nalidixic acid and the new quinolones inhibit the enzyme, DNA-gyrase, which is necessary for bacterial DNA replication and some aspects of transcription, repair, recombination and transposition.

5. **intermediary metabolism** — the agent interferes with the synthesis of essential cellular components (antimetabolite action). For example, folic acid is required for growth in bacterial cells, and its metabolism is inhibited by sulfonamides, trimethoprim and pyrimethamine.

(See Figure 30.1.)

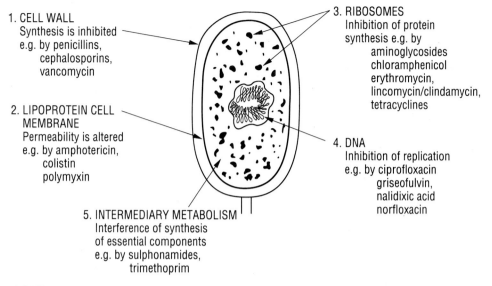

1. CELL WALL
   Synthesis is inhibited
   e.g. by penicillins,
      cephalosporins,
      vancomycin

2. LIPOPROTEIN CELL
   MEMBRANE
   Permeability is altered
   e.g. by amphotericin,
      colistin
      polymyxin

5. INTERMEDIARY METABOLISM
   Interference of synthesis
   of essential components
   e.g. by sulphonamides,
      trimethoprim

3. RIBOSOMES
   Inhibition of protein
   synthesis e.g. by
      aminoglycosides
      chloramphenicol
      erythromycin,
      lincomycin/clindamycin,
      tetracyclines

4. DNA
   Inhibition of replication
   e.g. by ciprofloxacin
      griseofulvin,
      nalidixic acid
      norfloxacin

FIGURE 30.1   Principal sites of action of anti-infective agents

Anti-infective agents may be described as 'cidal' or 'static' in action. Cidal (bactericidal, fungicidal, viricidal) agents kill the infecting organism. In many cases the cidal activity of an agent (e.g. penicillins, cephalosporins) is dependent on the microorganism being in a state of active division. Static (bacteriostatic, fungistatic, viristatic) agents inhibit the growth of but do not kill the microorganism. The effectiveness of these agents is dependent on the existence of adequate host defence mechanisms. The activity of all antimicrobial agents is influenced to some degree by the concentration of drug achievable at the site of infection and the duration of exposure of the organism to the drug.

Combination Therapy

Most infections are or should be treated with a single agent, selected on the basis of the microorganism isolated and its pattern of antimicrobial sensitivities. However, there are situations in which the use of combination therapy is justified. The use of multiple antimicrobial agents is indicated when synergy is clearly advantageous in definitive therapy. Synergy seems to be important in the treatment of infections caused by the following microorganisms:

- *Cryptococcus neoformans* infection is treated with amphotericin B plus flucytosine

- *Pseudomonas aeruginosa* infection is treated with an aminoglycoside plus piperacillin

- Enterococcal infection is treated with benzylpenicillin plus an aminoglycoside

- Enterobacteriaceae infection is treated with a β-lactamase resistant β-lactam antibiotic plus an aminoglycoside.

Combination agents are also used to prevent the emergence of resistant organisms, e.g. in the treatment of tuberculosis. Polymicrobial infections, such as those which may follow bowel perforation or associated with diabetic foot ulcers, often require treatment with two or more antimicrobial agents. However, the introduction of broad spectrum agents such as imipenem may allow single drug therapy in these situations.

Whilst the addition of one antimicrobial agent to another may result in synergistic activity in some instances, more often additive or indifferent effects are seen. Occasionally the combination of two anti-infective agents may result in antagonism.

INFECTIOUS DISEASES

30

One drug should always be used unless there is a clear indication that multiple therapy will be more effective. It should be realised that the use of combination therapy carries with it a greater risk of adverse effects, superinfections, increased expense and changes to the natural microflora ecology. The latter has implications not only for the individual patient, but also the entire ward and hospital population and the community at large.

Resistance

Microorganisms may be inherently resistant or acquire resistance to the action of individual and/or groups of antimicrobial agents. Resistance may arise through the following mechanisms:

- **Alteration in the target site**, e.g. penicillins — altered or new penicillin binding proteins; acyclovir — absence of thymidine kinase; quinolones — altered DNA-gyrase

- **Production of detoxifying enzymes**, e.g. penicillins — β-lactamases; aminoglycosides — acetyltransferases, phosphotransferases and nucleotidyl-transferases

- **Decreased antimicrobial uptake** due to either (a) diminished permeability, e.g. β-lactams — alteration in outer membrane proteins, or (b) active efflux, e.g. tetracycline — active transport of the agent out of the cell.

Such resistance may result from mutation of the microorganism or acquisition of genetic material from other resistant microorganisms.

Transfer of genetic material from one organism to another may be achieved by one of the following mechanisms:

- *Conjugation* involves the transfer of extranuclear particles of genetic material (DNA), known as plasmids, while the bacteria are in direct contact with one another. Clinically conjugation is the most important process for the transfer of

resistance. It occurs in Gram negative organisms.

- *Transduction* occurs when Gram positive organisms, particularly *Staphylococcus aureus*, acquire resistance by being infected with some genetic material carried by a virus (bacteriophage).

- *Transformation* occurs when fragments of genetic material released from a bacterial cell as a result of lysis are engulfed by another cell, and thus confer on the latter cell characteristics (resistance) encoded in the transferred material.

(See Figure 30.2.)

Continued exposure of microorganisms to antimicrobials can produce selective pressure, resulting in the proliferation of resistant subgroups of the organisms. In this instance effectiveness of the anti-infective agents is reduced as the percentage of resistant strains increases.

Antimicrobial resistance can be avoided or reduced through the appropriate use of antimicrobials. It may also be overcome by the structural modification of existing antibiotics, the use of detoxifying enzyme inhibitors, the introduction of new classes of antimicrobials and the use of combination therapy.

Hazards

The administration of an antimicrobial agent poses three major hazards to the patient: drug toxicity, hypersensitivity or allergic reactions, and superinfection.

DRUG TOXICITY

No antimicrobial is completely free of toxic effects, even those administered topically to the skin. Details of the major toxicities of commonly administered antimicrobials are discussed under the individual agents.

HYPERSENSITIVITY

Hypersensitivity or allergic reactions pose a major problem in the use of antimicrobial agents. It has been estimated that allergic reactions to penicillins occur in 2%–5% of

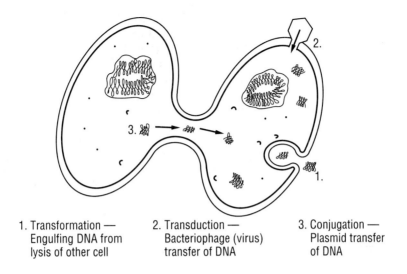

1. Transformation —
   Engulfing DNA from
   lysis of other cell

2. Transduction —
   Bacteriophage (virus)
   transfer of DNA

3. Conjugation —
   Plasmid transfer
   of DNA

FIGURE 30.2   Mechanisms of bacterial transfer of resistance

the general population. These range from mild skin reactions to potentially fatal anaphylactoid reactions.

Sensitisation to a particular antimicrobial may occur during therapy or through exposure to other sources (e.g. food products). Once sensitised to a particular agent the patient may experience an allergic reaction on subsequent exposure to that drug or a related drug. Allergic reactions are divided into four groups.

The first group, Type I, is mediated by IgE antibodies and includes both immediate and accelerated reactions. Immediate reactions occur within 60 minutes of drug administration. The patient generally experiences itching of the palms or axilla, apprehension, weakness, coughing, sneezing, shortness of breath or a sudden rise in body temperature. However, these allergic reactions may be manifested only as flushing, generalised pruritus or urticaria. They may also be anaphylactoid in nature and involve vascular collapse, shock, cardiac arrest, bronchospasm, laryngeal oedema and respiratory depression or arrest. Accelerated reactions occur 60 minutes to 72 hours after drug administration and include fever, pruritus and urticaria. They are generally

not life threatening except when laryngeal spasm occurs.

Type II and III reactions are less common and are mediated by IgG and IgM antibodies. Type II reactions include haematological reactions such as haemolytic anaemia while Type III reactions manifest as drug fever, interstitial nephritis and allergic vasculitis. A serum sickness-like reaction may occur with penicillins.

Delayed, Type IV reactions are mediated by IgG antibodies and may develop days, and occasionally weeks, after use of the causative agent. Skin rashes, including erythema, urticaria, bullous eruptions, exfoliative dermatitis, contact dermatitis and Stevens-Johnson syndrome may develop.

Management of allergic reactions is dependent on the type of reaction. For example, anaphylactic reactions require immediate treatment, whilst delayed reactions may only require drug withdrawal and observation.

When a patient has a history of allergic reactions or experiences an allergic reaction to a particular antimicrobial, an agent which does not exhibit cross-reactivity should be used. In rare instances the patient may need to be desensitised so that the offending agent can be used again.

30 INFECTIOUS DISEASES

SUPERINFECTION

Superinfection may result from substitution of resistant organisms for the original sensitive microorgansm at the initial site of infection. It may also occur where there is overgrowth of resistant organisms, often gut flora, at other sites within the body. The use of broad spectrum antibiotics carries with it the greatest risk of superinfection. These agents are capable of suppressing gut flora and allowing overgrowth of resistant bacteria and fungi.

DURATION OF THERAPY

The duration of antimicrobial therapy should be such that it ensures cure, without the risk of relapse, and does not expose the patient unnecessarily to the hazards of antimicrobial therapy. Different infections may require different durations of treatment. For example, urinary tract infections require three days of therapy compared with endocarditis which requires six weeks. When used for surgical prophylaxis, antimicrobials should be given as a single dose whenever possible, and in most cases prophylaxis should not extend beyond 24 hours.

ADMINISTRATION

Preparation

In the hospital setting antimicrobials are often given parenterally. Many of these agents are only available as a sterile powder requiring reconstitution prior to administration. When instructions for dilution are not provided by the prescriber the nurse should refer to the product literature and/or parenteral drug administration guidelines to determine the correct diluent and correct volume of diluent to use. The nurse should ensure that strict aseptic technique is followed when reconstituting the drug.

If the dose required is less than that contained in the reconstituted solution, the nurse should check carefully the prescribed dose, calculate the volume (millilitres) of solution required to give the dose, then request a second nurse to check the calculation. An incorrect dose may result in inadequate treatment (dose too low) or drug toxicity (dose too high).

Although many reconstituted antimicrobials are stable when stored in the refrigerator for up to 24–48 hours, it is advisable to discard any unused solution after each dose. This eliminates the risk of contamination of the solution and possible deterioration during storage.

Methods of Administration

The drug should be administered in accordance with the prescriber's directions. If these conflict with the recommendations made in the product literature or parenteral administration guidelines, the nurse should check with the prescriber before giving the drug.

When given intramuscularly, antimicrobials should be administered deep into the muscle mass to reduce the incidence of pain and sterile abscess formation. Drugs given as an intravenous bolus should be administered over 2–5 minutes, to minimise the risk of adverse effects. When a small volume of drug (e.g. an aminoglycoside) is to be injected, it should be further diluted with 10 mL of sodium chloride 0.9% solution to facilitate slow injection. A number of antimicrobials are administered as infusions (e.g. acyclovir, imipenem, amphotericin B, vancomycin) because of solubility problems and/or to reduce the incidence of adverse effects. The nurse should ensure that the anti-infective is compatible with the diluent and that the final solution is compatible with any other fluid or drugs being administered concurrently. If there is uncertainty about the correct method of administration the nurse should check with the pharmacy department in the hospital.

Many orally administered antimicrobials are given on an empty stomach to facilitate absorption. If the prescriber fails to endorse when the drug should be given in relation to food, the nurse should refer to the product literature or pharmacy department to ascertain the appropriate time of administration.

Storage

Antimicrobials should be stored in accordance with the manufacturer's instructions. Many of these agents degrade rapidly when stored under unfavourable conditions. The nurse should check carefully that the drug has been stored under the correct conditions and that its expiry date has not been exceeded before giving the drug.

NURSING IMPLICATIONS

ASSESSMENT

The patient should be assessed for any history of anaphylactic reaction or allergy to the anti-infective to be used; possible interactions with other drugs, food and intravenous fluids; and renal and hepatic function. Specimens for culture and sensitivity testing should be taken prior to commencement of treatment and baseline temperature and signs of infection recorded.

ADMINISTRATION

Prior to administration the nurse should check that the agent has been stored and reconstituted according to the manufacturer's directions; whether oral doses are to be given with or without food; the compatibility of intravenous doses with fluid; recommended dilution and rate of administration; and with intramuscular orders if the drug can be given via this route and likely side effects (e.g. pain, induration, abscess formation). Time schedules must be adhered to to maintain serum concentrations and the prescribed course completed but not exceeded.

EVALUATION

The nurse should observe the patient for signs that the infection is abating and whether superinfection is occurring. Toxic effects, such as gastrointestinal disturbances and allergic reactions (immediate, accelerated or delayed), and signs of local irritation or phlebitis with intravenous therapy should be watched for. Blood samples should be taken to determine serum trough and peak levels where appropriate.

PATIENT EDUCATION

Patients should be advised of possible adverse effects and signs of allergy; food and drug interactions; the dose schedule and the importance of completing the prescribed course.

The nursing implications for individual agents are listed under the specific drug or group and in the table at the end of the chapter.

INFECTIOUS DISEASES

30

ANTIBACTERIAL AGENTS

This section covers those groups of anti-infective agents commonly used for the treatment of bacterial infections. These agents include the β-lactams — penicillins, cephalosporins (including cephamycins and oxa-β-lactams), monobactams, and carbapenems; the aminoglycosides; the tetracyclines; the macrolides — erythromycin; clindamycin and lincomycin; and chloramphenicol.

PENICILLINS

Penicillin was isolated from *Penicillium notatum* by Fleming in 1929 and was first used as an anti-infective agent by Chain and Florey in 1940. Penicillin used by early workers was an amorphous compound containing impurities and was a mixture of several penicillin compounds. Of these natural penicillins benzylpenicillin (penicillin G) was found to be the most suitable for general use.

Today a wide range of penicillins is available. These are broadly classified as natural penicillins and semisynthetic penicillins. The semisynthetic penicillins are prepared by adding different side chains to the penicillin nucleus (6-aminopenicillanic acid, 6-APA), and have differing properties and antibacterial activity. The 6-APA nucleus of the penicillins contains a β-lactam ring, thus these antibiotics are referred to as β-lactams. They are structurally and pharmacologically related to other β-lactam antibiotics including the cephalosporins, cephamycins, oxa-β-lactams, monobactams and carbapenems.

Natural Penicillins: Benzylpenicillin, Phenoxymethylpenicillin

These two so-called natural penicillins, benzylpenicillin (penicillin G) and phenoxymethylpenicillin (penicillin V), are produced biosynthetically by fermentation from *Penicillium chrysogenum*.

TRADE NAMES

Benzylpenicillin: *Bicillin All-Purpose*; *Benzylpenicillin*.
Phenoxymethylpenicillin: *Abbocillin V, VK*; *Cilicaine V, VK*; *LPV*; *PVK*.

Benzathine penicillin: *Bicillin All-Purpose*.
Procaine penicillin: *Bicillin All-Purpose*; *Cilicaine*.

MECHANISM OF ACTION

All β-lactams (penicillins, cephalosporins, monobactams, carbapenems) are believed to act in the same way. They attach to a number of different proteins on the cell membrane known as penicillin binding proteins. These proteins are all believed to have enzymatic functions. The binding of penicillins and other β-lactam antibiotics to specific penicillin binding proteins results in inhibition of cell wall synthesis and cell division. The bactericidal action of β-lactams occurs as a result of cell lysis.

PHARMACOKINETICS

Benzylpenicillin is acid-labile and hence is destroyed in the low pH of the stomach. It is therefore generally given parenterally. When given as either the sodium or potassium salt, absorption after intramuscular injection is rapid. If, however, it is administered in the form of procaine penicillin G or benzathine penicillin G absorption is delayed and serum levels remain higher longer.

Phenoxymethylpenicillin is acid-stable and therefore may be given orally. Oral absorption is rapid but incomplete; it is impaired when the drug is given with or after food.

All penicillins are widely distributed in the body attaining therapeutic concentrations in the serum and urine, and synovial, pleural and pericardial fluids. Penetration into the cerebrospinal fluid is limited when the meninges are not inflamed. Both drugs cross the placenta.

Benzylpenicillin and phenoxymethylpenicillin are rapidly cleared from the body (their half-lives are 0.7 hours and 0.5 hours respectively). Like all penicillins they are excreted primarily by the kidney. Dosage reduction is therefore required in patients with renal failure.

SPECTRUM OF ACTIVITY

Benzylpenicillin and phenoxymethylpenicillin are highly active against many Gram positive cocci, in particular *Streptococcus pneumoniae, Streptococcus pyogenes,* viridans streptococci, *Streptococcus bovis* and non-penicillinase producing *Staphylococcus aureus.* The natural penicillins are less active against Gram negative bacteria, however, benzylpenicillin still remains the treatment of choice for infections due to *Neisseria meningitidis* and *Pasteurella multocida,* and is an important agent in the treatment of gonorrhoea and syphilis.

Anaerobes including *Clostridium, Fusebacterium* and *Bacteriodes* sp. (except *Bacteroides fragilis*) are sensitive to these agents.

USES

The principal uses of benzylpenicillin are the treatment of bacterial meningitis, endocarditis, cellulitis, erysipelas, pneumonia (including aspiration pneumonia), gonorrhoea, syphilis, gangrene and tetanus, caused by the organisms listed above. It is also the treatment of choice for anthrax, leptospirosis, diphtheria, actinomycosis and Lyme disease. The dosage range for benzylpenicillin is 2.4 million to 24 million units daily dependent on the severity of the disease. Long acting procaine penicillin G is usually given in a dose of 1–1.5 million units intramuscularly daily. The dose of benzathine penicillin G depends on the indication for use.

Phenoxymethylpenicillin is used to treat less serious infections such as pharyngitis, minor oral infections and skin infections due to susceptible organisms, or to complete a parenteral course of therapy. The usual adult dose ranges from 250–500 mg 6-hourly. Low dose phenoxymethylpenicillin (250 mg 12-hourly) may be given for prophylaxis against rheumatic fever.

ADVERSE DRUG REACTIONS

The penicillins are amongst the safest antibiotics in use today. Adverse drug reactions are reported in 1% to 10% of patients with hypersensitivity reactions being the most troublesome. Hypersensitivity reactions to penicillins may be divided into four groups.

Immediate reactions vary in intensity from wheezing and urticaria to hypotension, shock and death. Accelerated reactions include fever, pruritus and urticaria. They are generally not life threatening except when laryngeal spasm occurs. Delayed reactions are the most common form of penicillin allergy, accounting for over 80% of cases. A morbilliform eruption is typical of this type of reaction. Less common reactions are Type II and III reactions such as haemolytic anaemia, interstitial nephritis, drug fever, vasculitis and blood dyscrasias. For details on these four reaction types see Hypersensitivity section earlier in this chapter.

Phenoxymethylpenicillin is usually well tolerated but may cause gastrointestinal upset with high doses.

Neurotoxicity may occur when very high doses of penicillin (more than 20 million units/day) are given, particularly in patients with renal impairment.

Procaine penicillin G must never be given intravenously as it may cause toxicity or even death. Toxic reactions seen with this agent are in part due to the procaine component and include convulsions, respiratory paralysis and hypotension.

DRUG INTERACTIONS

The bactericidal activity of penicillins and aminoglycosides may be additive or synergistic when the drugs are administered concurrently. Benzylpenicillin and aminoglycosides are, however, physically and/or chemically incompatible and therefore should not be mixed prior to or during administration. Probenecid inhibits the tubular secretion of penicillins thus excretion is delayed and serum levels enhanced. Clavulanic acid is a β-lactamase inhibitor, which when co-administered with penicillins prevents their destruction by these enzymes.

Benzylpenicillin in combination with clavulanic acid has shown synergism against some strains of *Neisseria gonorrhoeae, Staphylococcus aureus* and *Bacteroides fragilis.*

PRECAUTIONS AND CONTRAINDICATIONS

These agents are contraindicated in patients with a history of penicillin allergy. Procaine benzylpenicillin is contraindicated in patients with a history of procaine hypersensitivity.

Penicillinase Resistant Antistaphylococcal Penicillins: Methicillin, Cloxacillin, Flucloxacillin

Following the introduction of benzylpenicillin resistance amongst staphylococci soon became apparent. Today over 80% of clinical isolates of *Staphylococcus aureus* and most strains of *Staphylococcus epidermidis* are capable of destroying penicillin through the production of penicillinase (a β-lactamase). In 1960, the first of the penicillinase-resistant penicillins, methicillin, was introduced. Antistaphylococcal penicillins now available are methicillin, nafcillin and the isoxazolyl penicillins (oxacillin, cloxacillin, dicloxacillin and flucloxacillin).

TRADE NAMES

Cloxacillin: *Alclox; Austrastaph.*
Flucloxacillin: *Flopen; Floxapen; Flucil; Staphylex.*

MECHANISM OF ACTION

Inhibition of cell wall synthesis, see natural penicillins.

PHARMACOKINETICS

Methicillin is acid-labile and hence must be given parenterally to achieve therapeutic concentrations. Flucloxacillin and cloxacillin, however, are acid-stable and therefore may be given either parenterally or orally.

Following oral administration both drugs are rapidly absorbed from the small intestine with peak concentrations achieved within 30–60 minutes. Absorption is delayed in the presence of food and both drugs should be administered on an empty stomach.

All three drugs are widely distributed in the body, however they exhibit poor penetration into the central nervous system. They all cross the placenta and may be detected in breast milk. All are renally excreted and, as for the natural penicillins, dosage reduction is necessary in renal dysfunction.

SPECTRUM OF ACTIVITY

These agents are active against penicillinase-producing staphylococci. Whilst they are active against other Gram positive bacteria including streptococci, they are generally less active than benzylpenicillin which remains the agent of choice.

USES

Antistaphylococcal penicillins are indicated for infections due to penicillinase producing staphylococci such as osteomyelitis, endocarditis, septicaemia, abscesses, mastitis, skin infections and toxic shock syndrome.

The dose of flucloxacillin or cloxacillin used is dependent on the type and severity of the infection and for adults ranges between 4 g and 12 g daily in divided doses parenterally, and 1 g and 4 g daily orally. Both agents are irritant to the vein when administered intravenously and therefore should be given well diluted (1 g/20 mL) and injected slowly. Doses greater than 1 g are best given in 50–100 mL of sodium chloride 0.9% solution as a 30-minute infusion.

ADVERSE DRUG REACTIONS

Antistaphylococcal penicillins have a similar spectrum of adverse effects to natural penicillins. Methicillin use has been associated with development of interstitial nephritis. Flucloxacillin has recently been implicated as a cause of hepatotoxicity, in particular cholestatic jaundice. While similar reactions have also been reported with other antibiotics used in the treatment of staphylococcal infections, monitoring of liver function tests is advised for patients receiving flucloxacillin.

DRUG INTERACTIONS

Probenecid decreases renal tubular secretion and increases plasma penicillin levels. Aminoglycosides and antistaphylococcal penicillins have synergistic activity when administered concurrently.

PRECAUTIONS AND CONTRAINDICATIONS

Use of these drugs in patients with a history of allergy to penicillins should be avoided.

Flucloxacillin should be used with caution in patients with hepatic dysfunction and liver function tests should be monitored during therapy. In patients with renal impairment dosage reduction may be necessary.

Aminopenicillins: Amoxycillin, Ampicillin

Amoxycillin and ampicillin are the most important, members of this group. They have an extended spectrum of activity against Gram negative organisms by virtue of an improved ability to penetrate the outer membranes of these organisms and to gain access to the penicillin binding proteins.

TRADE NAMES

Amoxycillin: *Amoxil*; *Cilamox*; *Moxacin*; *Fisamox*; *Alphamox*.
Ampicillin: *Ampicyn*; *Austrapen*; *Penbritin*; *Alphacin*.

MECHANISM OF ACTION

Inhibition of cell wall synthesis, see natural penicillins.

PHARMACOKINETICS

Ampicillin and amoxycillin can be given orally or parenterally. Amoxycillin is approximately 95% absorbed from the gastrointestinal tract compared with 40% for ampicillin. Given in similar doses amoxycillin produces plasma levels twice those of ampicillin. Peak concentrations following oral administration are seen within two hours.

Ampicillin and amoxycillin are widely distributed in the body. They are eliminated by renal excretion and have similar half-lives (approximately 60 minutes).

SPECTRUM OF ACTIVITY

Amoxycillin and ampicillin are active against most organisms inhibited by benzylpenicillin. They are slightly less active against streptococci, but more active against enterococci and *Listeria monocytogenes*. The aminopenicillins are highly active against non-penicillinase producing *Haemophilus influenzae*, *Escherichia coli*, *Proteus mirabilis* and *Salmonella* and *Shigella* sp. Ampicillin exhibits better activity against *Shigella* sp. than amoxycillin, however, amoxycillin is more active against *Salmonella* sp. Both agents are inactive against penicillinase producing staphylococci and *Proteus* and *Klebsiella* sp. Most strains of *Pseudomonas* sp. are resistant.

USES

Ampicillin and amoxycillin are used to treat urinary tract infections, pneumonia, acute and acute on chronic bronchitis, otitis media, acute sinusitis, venereal disease, shigellosis and salmonellosis.

They may also be used alone or in combination with other antibiotics for the treatment of bacterial meningitis including infections caused by *Listeria monocytogenes*, endocarditis due to group D streptococci, peritonitis and pelvic inflammatory disease. Aminopenicillins have also been used in the treatment of typhoid fever.

The dose of amoxycillin or ampicillin used varies dependent on the site and severity of infection. The usual oral dose for amoxycillin ranges from 250 mg 8-hourly for urinary tract infections to 500 mg 8-hourly for respiratory tract infections. For more severe infections amoxycillin is given parenterally in a dose ranging from 3 g to 12 g daily in divided doses. For gonococcal

INFECTIOUS DISEASES

30 ■

urethritis due to non-penicillinase producing *Neisserria gonorrhoeae* a single 3 g oral dose of amoxycillin may be used.

Doses for ampicillin are similar to those for amoxycillin, however, the drug must be administered 6-hourly compared to 8-hourly for amoxycillin.

ADVERSE DRUG REACTIONS

The adverse effects are similar to those of natural penicillins, although the incidence of maculopapular, erythematous rashes appears somewhat higher. These agents should not be administered to patients with known or suspected glandular fever as over 90% of patients with this condition will develop a rash with these drugs.

Gastrointestinal adverse effects are common with these agents, particularly ampicillin. Both have been associated with the development of pseudomembraneous colitis.

DRUG INTERACTIONS

An increased risk of severe skin reactions has been reported in patients given an aminopenicillin concurrently with allopurinol. Whilst evidence to support this claim appears to be lacking, caution is advised when using the combination. Clavulanic acid and sulbactam extend the spectrum of amoxycillin and ampicillin against many β lactamase producing bacteria. Probenecid inhibits renal secretion and increases plasma levels of aminopenicillins.

PRECAUTIONS AND CONTRAINDICATIONS

Aminopenicillins are contraindicated in patients with a history of hypersensitivity reaction to penicillin and known or suspected glandular fever. These agents should be used with caution in patients receiving concurrent allopurinol treatment. Dosage reduction is necessary in patients with renal dysfunction.

Extended Spectrum Penicillins: Carbenicillin, Ticarcillin, Azlocillin, Mezlocillin, Piperacillin

These agents fall into two groups — the carboxypenicillins (carbenicillin, ticarcillin) and the acylaminopenicillins (azlocillin, mezlocillin, piperacillin). They are all semi-synthetic penicillins which have increased activity against Gram negative bacteria. Notably all have clinical activity against *Pseudomonas aeruginosa*.

TRADE NAMES

Azlocillin: *Securopen*.
Piperacillin: *Pipril*.
Ticarcillin: *Tarcil; Ticillin*.

MECHANISM OF ACTION

Inhibition of cell wall synthesis, see natural penicillins.

PHARMACOKINETICS

Azlocillin, mezlocillin, piperacillin, carbenicillin and ticarcillin are not appreciably absorbed from the gastrointestinal tract and must be given parenterally. Following intramuscular injection, they are readily absorbed with peak concentrations attained 30 minutes to two hours after injection. Carbenicillin in the form of carbenicillin indanyl sodium (carindacillin) is acid stable and may be given orally, absorption being rapid but incomplete.

Extended spectrum penicillins are widely distributed into body fluids and tissues. The drugs attain concentrations in the bile several to one hundred times that of plasma. Like other penicillins, penetration into the cerebrospinal fluid is low in the absence of inflamed meninges. All cross the placenta and all are distributed into breast milk at low concentration.

Extended spectrum penicillins are metabolised to varying degrees. The parent drugs and their metabolites are rapidly excreted, principally in the urine. Biliary excretion also plays a role in their elimination and this is diminished in biliary obstruction. Their half-lives are short, ranging from 0.6 hours to 1.3 hours.

SPECTRUM OF ACTIVITY

Carbenicillin exhibits significant activity against *Pseudomonas aeruginosa*. It is also active against some strains of *Proteus, Enterobacter* and *Serratia* sp. and *Bacteroides fragilis* that are not sensitive to the penicillins previously discussed. Its activity against other Gram negative bacilli is comparable to amoxycillin, however it is somewhat less active against streptococci. Ticarcillin has a similar spectrum of activity to carbenicillin but is more active against *Pseudomonas aeruginosa*.

Piperacillin is more active than either ticarcillin or carbenicillin against some Enterobacteriaceae (particularly *Klebsiella* sp.), *Bacteroides fragilis* and *Pseudomonas aeruginosa*. Mezlocillin is the least active against *Pseudomonas aeruginosa*, but exhibits a similar spectrum of activity to piperacillin against Enterobacteriaceae. Azlocillin has similar activity against *Pseudomonas aeruginosa* to piperacillin, but reduced activity against Enterobacteriaceae.

Extended spectrum penicillins are degraded by many of the β lactamases produced by Gram negative bacilli.

USES

Extended spectrum penicillins are primarily used in the treatment of serious infections due to *Pseudomonas aeruginosa* and amoxycillin-resistant strains of *Proteus* sp., usually in combination with an aminoglycoside. They are also used as a component of combination regimens in febrile neutropenic patients. The usual adult dosages for the extended spectrum penicillins are shown in Table 30.1.

ADVERSE DRUG REACTIONS

The extended spectrum penicillins may provoke any of the reactions that occur with natural penicillins.

Gastrointestinal reactions may occur following parenteral administration and include nausea, vomiting, flatulence, loose stools, diarrhoea and altered taste. Hypokalaemia, sometimes associated with metabolic alkalosis, has been reported and is thought to be due to an increase in renal potassium loss. All the extended spectrum penicillins are formulated as sodium salts and all have been associated with the development of hypernatraemia. The acylaminopenicillins contain less than half the sodium in commercially available carboxypenicillin products.

Carbenicillin and ticarcillin may cause abnormal platelet aggregation and have been reported to cause prolongation of bleeding times. Other disturbances of coagulation have also been reported with extended spectrum penicillins.

TABLE 30.1 Dosages for extended spectrum penicillins

Drug	Route	Dose Range (Adults, normal renal function)	Frequency of Dosing
Azlocillin	IV	2–4 g	8-hourly
Carbenicillin	IV	2.5–5 g	4–6-hourly
Mezlocillin	IV	2–4 g	8-hourly
Piperacillin	IM	1–2 g	4–6-hourly
	IV	2–4 g	4–6-hourly
Ticarcillin	IV, IM	1.5–3 g	4–6-hourly

INFECTIOUS DISEASES

30

DRUG INTERACTIONS

The activity of extended spectrum penicillins and aminoglycosides is additive or synergistic in vitro against some strains of *Pseudomonas aeruginosa*. When mixed, extended spectrum penicillins can inactivate aminoglycosides in solution; the rate of inactivation being dependent on concentration of penicillin present, duration of exposure and temperature. For this reason penicillins and aminoglycosides should not be mixed in the same syringe or intravenous container.

The combination of clavulanic acid with carbenicillin, ticarcillin or piperacillin, results in a synergistic bactericidal effect against many β-lactamase producing bacteria.

Probenecid inhibits the renal excretion of penicillins resulting in higher and prolonged plasma levels. Probenecid has also been shown to reduce the volume of distribution of azlocillin, mezlocillin and piperacillin which may contribute to their higher plasma levels.

Neuromuscular blockade induced by vecuronium bromide may be prolonged by as much as 55% by the intra-operative administration of acylaminopenicillins. Patients receiving lithium who are prescribed carbenicillin disodium or ticarcillin disodium should have their lithium levels monitored closely as the resultant increased sodium intake may affect lithium elimination.

PRECAUTIONS AND CONTRAINDICATIONS

Extended spectrum penicillins are contraindicated in patients with a known allergy to penicillins. Dosage reduction is necessary in renal and hepatic dysfunction. Carbenicillin and ticarcillin should be used with caution in patients with bleeding tendencies, particularly those with impaired renal function.

Periodic monitoring of serum potassium and sodium levels is advised during therapy with extended spectrum penicillins.

Penicillin–β-Lactamase Inhibitor Combinations: Amoxycillin–Clavulanic Acid, Ticarcillin–Clavulanic Acid

A number of techniques have been developed to prevent enzymatic degradation of penicillins. One approach has been to alter their structure making them less susceptible to β-lactamase hydrolysis. Another approach is to combine the penicillin with a second agent which has less or no intrinsic antibacterial activity but which is a potent inhibitor of β-lactamases, thereby protecting the penicillin from degradation and facilitating its lethal effects.

A number of β-lactamase inhibitors have been developed; the most widely studied being clavulanic acid, tazobactam and sulbactam. These agents primarily inhibit plasmid mediated β-lactamases of many Gram positive and Gram negative bacteria. Gram negative bacilli such as *Enterobacter, Citrobacter* and *Serratia* sp*., Pseudomonas aeruginosa* and indole-positive *Proteus* sp. produce β-lactamases which are less susceptible to these agents. It should be stressed that these inhibitors do not enhance the penicillin's activity against bacteria inherently resistant to the penicillin.

Clavulanic acid and sulbactam have been shown to improve the efficacy of a number of β-lactams when used in combination, including ampicillin, amoxycillin, ticarcillin, azlocillin, carbenicillin and cefoperazone.

TRADE NAMES

Amoxycillin–clavulanic acid: *Augmentin*. Ticarcillin–clavulanic acid: *Timentin*.

SPECTRUM OF ACTIVITY

The combining of amoxycillin with clavulanic acid extends the spectrum of amoxycillin to include β-lactamase producing *Escherichia coli, Klebsiella* sp*., Staphylococcus aureus, Haemophilus influenzae* and *Bacteroides fragilis*.

Similar improvements in the spectrum of ticarcillin are achieved when it is combined with clavulanic acid. This combination is also active against *Pseudomonas aeruginosa* which possesses plasmid mediated β-lactamases.

USES

Amoxycillin–clavulanic acid is used in the treatment of urinary tract infections (dose 250 mg–125 mg 8-hourly), respiratory tract infections, otitis media, skin infections and bites (dose 500 mg–125 mg 8-hourly). The combination of ticarcillin–clavulanic acid may be used in the treatment of a similar range of infections as ticarcillin. Additionally, it has proven an effective single agent in the treatment of febrile neutropenic patients.

ADVERSE DRUG REACTIONS

Adverse drug reactions to the combinations are similar to those seen with the parent penicillins. In the case of amoxycillin–clavulanic acid, gastrointestinal intolerance is greater than with amoxycillin alone. In addition, the use of the combination has been associated with the development of cholestatic jaundice.

DRUG INTERACTIONS

Whilst probenecid inhibits the renal excretion of penicillins it does not interfere with the elimination of clavulanic acid.

PRECAUTIONS AND CONTRAINDICATIONS

Precautions and contraindications are the same as those for the penicillin components. In addition patients receiving amoxycillin–clavulanic acid should be monitored for the development of hepatotoxicity, which may arise even after cessation of the drug.

CEPHALOSPORINS

The cephalosporins were first discovered in 1945. They were obtained from a mould cultured from a seawater sample taken near a Sardinian sewage outfall. All cephalosporins are synthetic derivatives of cephalosporin C, a compound produced by the *Cephalo-*

sporium fungus. As such, they all contain a common β-lactam nucleus, 7-aminocephalosporanic acid, which confers a similar mode of action to the penicillins.

Cephalosporins are generally grouped into generations dependent on their spectrum of activity.

First generation cephalosporins include cephalothin, cephazolin, cephradine and cephalexin.

The **second generation cephalosporins** include cephamandole, cefuroxime, cefaclor and the two cephamycins cefoxitin and cefotetan.

Third generation cephalosporins include latamoxef (a β-oxalactam), cefotaxime, ceftriaxone, ceftazidime and cefixime.

The important differences between these agents are discussed below but, as a general rule, first generation cephalosporins have the greatest activity against Gram positive bacteria and third generation agents the greatest activity against Gram negative organisms.

TRADE NAMES

First generation cephalosporins
Cephalexin: *Ceporex*; *Keflex.*
Cephalothin: *Keflin.*
Cephazolin: *Cefamezin*; *Kefzol.*

Second generation cephalosporins
Cefaclor: *Ceclor.*
Cefotetan: *Apatef.*
Cefoxitin: *Mefoxin.*
Cephamandole: *Mandol.*

Third generation cephalosporins
Cefotaxime: *Claforan.*
Ceftriaxone: *Rocephin.*
Ceftazidime: *Fortum.*

MECHANISM OF ACTION

Inhibition of cell wall synthesis, see natural penicillins.

PHARMACOKINETICS

Only cephalexin, cefaclor, cephradine, cefuroxime axetil and cefixime are absorbed from the gastrointestinal tract, all the other cephalosporins listed above must be given parenterally. Absorption of most oral cephalosporins, except cefuroxime axetil, is delayed by the administration of food.

Cephalosporins are widely distributed in the body following absorption, with therapeutic concentrations attained in tissues and fluids including synovial fluid, pleural fluid and bone. Ceftriaxone, cefoperazone, cephazolin, cephamandole and cefotaxime achieve therapeutic levels in the bile whilst third generation cephalosporins penetrate the central nervous system. Cephalosporins readily cross the placenta and are found in breast milk in low concentrations.

The cephalosporins show considerable variability in their rate of elimination from the body (half-lives: cephalothin 0.5 hours, cefotetan 3.1 hours, ceftriaxone 8 hours). The principal route of elimination for cephalosporins is renal excretion. Therefore clearance is delayed in the presence of renal failure with resultant higher serum levels.

SPECTRUM OF ACTIVITY

FIRST GENERATION CEPHALOSPORINS: CEPHALEXIN, CEPHALOTHIN, CEPHAZOLIN

The first generation cephalosporins have a spectrum of activity which includes *Escherichia coli*, *Klebsiella pneumoniae*, *Proteus mirabilis* and most Gram positive cocci. They are not active against enterococci, methicillin-resistant staphylococci, *Bacteroides fragilis* or *Pseudomonas aeruginosa* and possess only moderate activity against *Haemophilus influenzae*.

SECOND GENERATION CEPHALOSPORINS: CEFACLOR, CEFOXITIN, CEFOTETAN, CEPHAMANDOLE

The second generation agents have improved activity against Gram negative bacilli, but are generally less active than first generation cephalosporins against Gram positive bacteria.

Cephamandole is more active against *Enterobacter* sp., indole-positive *Proteus* sp. and other Enterobacteriaceae than first generation agents. It also possesses good activity against *Haemophilus influenzae* and comparable activity to cefazolin against Gram posi-

tive organisms. Cefaclor has a similar spectrum of activity to cephalexin but is more active against *Haemophilus influenzae*.

The cephamycins, cefoxitin and cefotetan, both have appreciable activity against anaerobes including *Bacteroides fragilis*. Compared to cephamandole, cefoxitin has a broader Gram negative spectrum including activity against gonococci and *Serratia* sp., however it has inferior activity against *Haemophilus influenzae* and no activity against *Enterobacter* sp. Cefotetan is more active than cefoxitin against Enterobacteriaceae. However, none of the second generation cephalosporins have activity against enterococci or *Pseudomonas aeruginosa*.

THIRD GENERATION CEPHALOSPORINS: CEFOTAXIME, CEFTAZIDIME, CEFTRIAXONE

The third generation cephalosporins exhibit the greatest activity against Gram negative bacteria.

Ceftriaxone and cefotaxime exhibit similar spectra of activity. They have excellent activity against *Escherichia coli*, *Serratia*, *Proteus*, *Providencia*, *Morganella*, *Citrobacter*, *Klebsiella*, *Enterobacter*, *Salmonella* and *Shigella* sp., *Neisseria gonorrhoeae* and *Haemophilus influenzae* including many β-lactamase producing strains. *Pseudomonas aeruginosa* and *Acinetobacter* sp. exhibit a high level of resistance. Both agents are active against Gram positive organisms, with cefotaxime being more active against staphylococci than ceftriaxone, but less active than cephamandole. Cefotaxime is active against some strains of *Bacteroides fragilis*, but less so than cefoxitin or cefotetan. Neither agent is effective for enterococcal infections or listeriosis.

Ceftazidime's major advantage over other currently available third generation agents is clinically significant activity against *Pseudomonas aeruginosa*.

USES

Despite a limited number of first-line indications, cephalosporins represent the most commonly prescribed group of antibiotics in hospitals.

First generation cephalosporins can be used in place of penicillins to treat *Staphylococcus aureus* infections, except meningitis. Methicillin resistant staphylococci are, however, generally resistant to cephalosporins. First generation agents are useful in treatment of staphylococcal osteomyelitis and septic arthritis, whilst second and third generation drugs can be used for such infections caused by Gram negative organisms.

Both upper and lower respiratory tract infections may be treated with cephalosporins since all cephalosporins possess good activity against pneumococci. Second and third generation agents may be used for *Haemophilus influenzae* infections.

Third generation cephalosporins are used to treat infections such as pneumonia, septicaemia, endocarditis and meningitis caused by Gram negative bacilli. In meningitis the third generation cephalosporins are now recommended for initial treatment in both children and adults. While they are effective in infections due to *Haemophilus influenzae, Neisseria meningitidis* and *Streptococcus pneumoniae* (the three commonest pathogens) they are ineffective in *Listeria monocytogenes* infections.

Ceftriaxone has become the treatment of choice in many centres for gonorrhoea. Cefoxitin and cefotetan may be used as single agents in the treatment of pelvic inflammatory disease.

Cephalosporins are the most commonly prescribed antibiotics for surgical prophylaxis. Cefoxitin or cefotetan may be used where anaerobes are likely to be encountered.

Table 30.2 provides details of dosage recommendations for commonly prescribed cephalosporins.

ADVERSE DRUG REACTIONS

Allergic reactions are the most frequently encountered adverse effect of cephalosporins; between 5% and 15% of patients allergic to penicillins will show cross-reactivity with cephalosporins. Other adverse effects include thrombophlebitis, pain on intramuscular injection, diarrhoea, pseudomembranous colitis and disturbances of renal, hepatic and haematological function.

Cephalosporins possessing an N-methylthiotetrazole side chain (cephamandole, cefotetan and latamoxef) may cause hypoprothrombinaemia, with or without bleeding. They may also produce a disulfiram-like reaction (flushing, intense nausea and headache) following ingestion of alcohol.

TABLE 30.2 Dosages for cephalosporins

Drug	Route	Dosage Schedule (Adults, normal renal function)	Frequency of Dosing
1st Generation			
Cephalexin	Oral	250–500 mg	6-hourly
Cephalothin	IV, IM	1–2 g	4–6-hourly
Cephazolin	IV, IM	500 mg–1 g	6–8-hourly
2nd Generation			
Cefaclor	Oral	250–500 mg	8-hourly
Cefotetan	IV	1–2 g	12-hourly
Cefoxitin	IV, IM	1–2 g	8-hourly
Cephamandole	IV, IM	1–2 g	6–8-hourly
3rd Generation			
Cefotaxime	IV, IM	1–2 g	6–12-hourly
Ceftriaxone	IV, IM	1–2 g	12–24-hourly
Ceftazidime	IV	1–2 g	8-hourly

INFECTIOUS DISEASES

30

Diarrhoea is more common following administration of cefoperazone and ceftriaxone, however all cephalosporins have been associated with the development of pseudomembraneous colitis. Ceftriaxone in high doses has been reported to cause biliary sludge (biliary pseudolithiasis) and symptoms resembling cholelithiasis. Cefaclor used in children may cause a serum sickness-like illness.

DRUG INTERACTIONS

The combination of aminoglycosides and cephalosporins may produce additive or synergistic activity, particularly against Gram negative bacilli. Combination therapy is often used for pseudomonal infections. The use of first generation cephalosporins and aminoglycosides may result in additive nephrotoxicity, hence close monitoring of renal function is recommended.

Probenecid will increase the serum concentrations of those cephalosporins which are eliminated by tubular secretion (e.g. cephamandole, cephalexin, cefaclor).

Disulfiram-like reactions may occur when alcohol is ingested during or within 48–72 hours of administration of β-lactams containing an N-methylthiotetrazole side chain. However administration of the first dose of these antibiotics to patients intoxicated with alcohol does not produce this reaction.

PRECAUTIONS AND CONTRAINDICATIONS

Cephalosporins are contraindicated in patients with a history of allergy to these drugs. They should also be used with extreme caution in patients with a history of penicillin allergy, particularly anaphylaxis.

Prolonged use of these agents may result in the overgrowth of non-sensitive organisms with resultant superinfection. In any patient developing diarrhoea whilst receiving a cephalosporin *Clostridium difficile* infection should be excluded.

Patients who have received cephalosporins containing an N-methylthiotetrazole side chain should be advised not to ingest alcohol for at least 72 hours after ceasing therapy.

Patients receiving ceftriaxone should be monitored closely for the development of symptoms of cholelithiasis. Patients, particularly the elderly, malnourished or debilitated and those with renal or hepatic dysfunction, receiving cephalosporins containing the N-methylthiotetrazole side chain should have their coagulation profile monitored regularly. Prophylactic vitamin K is indicated in these high risk patients who are to receive more than two days therapy with these agents.

NEWER β-LACTAMS

Monobactams: Aztreonam

Monobactams represent a unique family of β-lactams which lack the two-ring configuration of the penicillins and cephalosporins and have in its place a monocyclic nucleus (3-aminobactamic acid). Monobactams, discovered in 1979, are natural products of bacteria. However, naturally occurring monobactams have only modest antimicrobial activity and this has lead to the development of synthetically prepared agents. Aztreonam is the first of the monobactams to become commercially available.

TRADE NAMES

Aztreonam: *Azactam*.

MECHANISM OF ACTION

Aztreonam interferes with bacterial cell wall biosynthesis in a similar manner to natural penicillins. It has an affinity for penicillin binding protein 3, which affords it activity against Gram negative bacteria.

PHARMACOKINETICS

Aztreonam is poorly absorbed orally and therefore must be given parenterally. Following intramuscular injection it is well absorbed, giving levels comparable to intravenous administration after one hour.

Aztreonam is widely distributed into body fluids and tissues including the cerebrospinal fluid. The drug crosses the placenta and is distributed into the amniotic fluid. It is eliminated primarily by the kidney. Its half-life is about 1.9 hours in patients with normal renal function.

SPECTRUM OF ACTIVITY

Aztreonam exhibits excellent activity against a wide range of aerobic Gram negative bacteria including the Enterobacteriaceae, *Pseudomonas aeruginosa, Haemophilus influenzae* and *Neisseria gonorrhoeae*, including β-lactamase producing strains. The drug is highly resistant to enzymatic inactivation by β-lactamases. Aztreonam exhibits comparable activity against Enterobacteriaceae to cefotaxime. It has, however, virtually no activity against Gram positive or anaerobic organisms.

USES

Aztreonam, with its excellent activity against Gram negative aerobic bacteria, is a potential alternative to the use of aminoglycosides. It may be used alone or in combination in the treatment of bone and joint infections; lower respiratory tract infections; intra-abdominal and gynaecological infections; skin and soft tissue infections; urinary tract infections; and septicaemia and meningitis due to susceptible organisms. Because of its lack of cross-reactivity with other β-lactam antibiotics (see Adverse Drug Reactions) it may be used to treat such infections in patients with a history of penicillin and/or cephalosporin allergy. The dose of aztreonam varies from 500 mg to 1 g 12-hourly for urinary tract infections to 2 g 6–8-hourly for serious infections.

ADVERSE DRUG REACTIONS

Aztreonam exhibits low toxicity. Adverse reactions are similar to those of other β-lactams, with hypersensitivity reactions posing the greatest problem. Rash, with or without eosinophilia, occurs in 1%–2% of patients given the drug. Cross-reactivity between aztreonam and other β-lactams, however, appears to be negligible.

Gastrointestinal upset, nausea, diarrhoea and alteration in taste sensation have been reported.

DRUG INTERACTIONS

Aztreonam given in combination with aminoglycosides and certain β-lactam antibiotics exhibits additive or synergistic activity against some strains of *Pseudomonas aeruginosa* and the Enterobacteriaceae.

PRECAUTIONS AND CONTRAINDICATIONS

Aztreonam is contraindicated in patients with a known allergy to the drug. It should be used with caution in patients with known allergies to other β-lactams, particularly immediate hypersensitivity reactions, although the risk of cross-reactivity appears extremely low. Dosage reduction is required in patients with renal impairment.

Carbapenems: Imipenem

Thienamycin, the first of the carbapenems, was isolated from cultures of *Streptomyces cattleya* in the early 1970s. Imipenem is an N-formimidyl derivative of thienamycin. The carbapenems unlike penicillins and cephalosporins contain a fused β-lactam and five-membered ring system. This structural difference affords imipenem increased antibacterial activity and stability against most β-lactamases.

Imipenem is readily hydrolysed by renal dehydropeptidases. For this reason it has been formulated with cilastatin, a dehydropeptidase inhibitor (1:1 ratio). This prevents renal breakdown of imipenem and protects against possible nephrotoxicity.

TRADE NAMES

Imipenem–cilastatin: *Primaxin*.

MECHANISM OF ACTION

Imipenem interferes with cell wall synthesis in a similar manner to the naturally occurring penicillins. It is bactericidal.

30 INFECTIOUS DISEASES

PHARMACOKINETICS

Neither imipenem nor cilastatin are appreciably absorbed following oral administration and hence the combination is given parenterally. Following administration as an intravenous infusion imipenem is distributed widely in body tissues and fluids. Both drugs enter the cerebrospinal fluid, cross the placenta and are distributed into cord blood and amniotic fluid. Imipenem is excreted in breast milk.

The mean half-lives for imipenem and cilastatin are about one hour. Approximately 70% of imipenem is excreted unchanged in the urine when given with cilastatin, the remainder appears in the hydrolysed form. Less than 1% of the drug is excreted in the bile or recovered in the faeces.

In the presence of renal dysfunction, imipenem can be cleared by extrarenal mechanisms, however, cilastatin cannot.

SPECTRUM OF ACTIVITY

Imipenem is the first antibiotic to exhibit marked activity against virtually all clinically important bacteria frequently resistant to other β-lactams, e.g., staphylococci, enterococci, *Pseudomonas aeruginosa*, multidrug resistant Enterobacteriaceae, *Bacteroides fragilis* and β-lactamase producing strains of *Haemophilus influenzae* and *Neisseria gonorrhoeae*. Microorganisms intrinsically resistant to imipenem include methicillin-resistant staphylococci, *Enterococcus faecium*, *Xanthomonas maltophilia*, *Chlamydia trachomatis* and *Mycobacterium tuberculosis*.

USES

Imipenem–cilastatin is indicated for the treatment of serious infections such as septicaemia, endocarditis, peritonitis, pneumonia, pelvic inflammatory disease, osteomyelitis, septic arthritis and skin and soft tissue infections. Imipenem, because of its broad spectrum of activity, is an ideal agent for empiric use in patients with polymicrobial infections or patients with infection of unknown origin. The dosage range is 250–500 mg 6–8-hourly to 1 g 6-hourly dependent on the severity of the infection.

Imipenem–cilastatin must be given by intravenous infusion, usually diluted in sodium chloride 0.9% solution and given over 30–60 minutes.

ADVERSE DRUG REACTIONS

Untoward effects seen with imipenem–cilastatin are similar to those reported with other β-lactam antibiotics. The most common adverse effects are phlebitis or pain at the site of infusion, nausea and vomiting. Seizures have been reported in patients receiving the combination, more commonly in those with renal impairment receiving high doses. Superinfection with resistant organisms, particularly *Xanthomonas maltophilia* and fungi, may occur.

DRUG INTERACTIONS

The combination of imipenem and aminoglycosides may produce additive or synergistic activity against some Gram positive bacteria including staphylococci, *Enterococcus faecalis* and *Listeria* sp.

The combination of ganciclovir and imipenem–cilastatin has been associated with a higher incidence of seizures and should be used with caution.

PRECAUTIONS AND CONTRAINDICATIONS

Imipenem–cilastatin is contraindicated in patients with a known hypersensitivity to the combination. Since cross-reactivity has been demonstrated between imipenem and other β-lactams the combination should be used with caution in patients with a history of penicillin and/or cephalosporin allergy.

Adverse central nervous system reactions such as confusional states, myoclonus and seizures have been reported with imipenem–cilastatin particularly in the presence of high serum concentrations. The combination should therefore be used with caution in patients with a history of central nervous system disorders and/or renal impairment. Dosage reduction is indicated in patients with renal impairment.

AMINOGLYCOSIDES

Amikacin, Gentamicin, Netilmicin, Neomycin, Kanamycin, Framycetin, Streptomycin, Tobramycin, Sissomicin

The aminoglycosides are a group of antibiotics obtained from cultures of *Streptomyces* or *Micromonospora* sp. The first of the aminoglycosides, streptomycin, was discovered in 1944. Since that time a number of others have been introduced into clinical practice including neomycin (1944), kanamycin (1957), gentamicin (1964), tobramycin (1971), and more recently netilmicin, amikacin and sissomicin. In general these later agents show more resistance to bacterial enzyme degradation.

The suffix 'mycin' is used to distinguish those aminoglycosides produced by a *Streptomyces* sp. (e.g. neomycin) from those produced by *Micromonospora* sp. (e.g. gentamicin) which are given a 'micin' suffix.

TRADE NAMES

Amikacin: *Amikin.*
Framycetin: *Soframycin.*
Gentamicin: *Cidomycin*; *Garamycin.*
Neomycin: *Neosulf.*
Netilmicin: *Netromycin.*
Tobramycin: *Nebcin.*

MECHANISM OF ACTION

Aminoglycosides in most instances are bactericidal. They act by binding to the 30S subunit of bacterial ribosomes, causing misreading of the messenger RNA. The subsequent synthesis of abnormal or non-functional proteins results in cell death.

PHARMACOKINETICS

Aminoglycosides are poorly absorbed from the gastrointestinal tract. Following intramuscular injection, absorption is very good, however, the time to achieve peak serum concentrations and the levels achieved show considerable variation. Topical administration such as irrigation of wounds, debrided skin or joints, may result in substantial drug absorption. Administration in the form of nebulisation also results in rapid drug absorption.

Aminoglycosides distribute rapidly into body fluids including ascitic, pericardial, peritoneal, pleural, synovial and abscess fluids. Penetration into the cerebrospinal fluid is limited (5% when meninges are not inflamed). The drugs also show low penetration into sputum, requiring the use of high serum levels to ensure adequate lung concentrations. Aminoglycosides cross the placenta with fetal serum concentrations about half those of the mother.

Aminoglycosides are eliminated via the kidney by glomerular filtration. In patients with normal renal function the half-lives of all aminoglycosides are in the range 2–4 hours.

SPECTRUM OF ACTIVITY

Aminoglycosides have limited activity against Gram positive bacteria, primarily staphylococci. They do, however, exhibit synergistic activity when administered with penicillin against enterococci, viridan streptococci and other streptococci. They are not active against *Streptococcus pneumoniae*.

Aminoglycosides exhibit good activity against a wide range of aerobic Gram negative bacteria including Enterobacteriaeceae (e.g. *Escherichia coli, Klebsiella* and *Proteus* sp.), and *Pseudomonas, Acinetobacter* and *Providencia* sp.

USES

Oral aminoglycosides are used to decontaminate the gastrointestinal tract to either diminish the risk of infection (e.g. preoperatively) or reduce ammonia production in the gut (e.g. hepatic encephalopathy). Topically, they are used in the treatment of minor skin infections and eye and ear infections.

However, aminoglycosides are primarily used parenterally either as single agents or in combination with a β-lactam antibiotic for the treatment of Gram negative bacterial infections. Gentamicin remains the agent of choice for such infections unless resistance is proven. Tobramycin is intrinsically more active against *Pseudomonas aeruginosa* than gentamicin and may be preferred when treating pseudomonal infections. Aminoglycosides are also combined with penicillins or vancomycin to treat

INFECTIOUS DISEASES

30 ■

enterococcal and staphylococcal endocarditis. Amikacin, which demonstrates the greatest resistance to bacterial enzymatic degradation, should be reserved for infections due to bacteria with proven resistance to both gentamicin and tobramcyin.

Streptomycin and kanamycin administered intramuscularly can be used as part of the initial treatment of tuberculosis and other mycobacterium infections.

Dosage schedules for commonly used aminoglycosides are shown in Table 30.3. Aminoglycosides may be given 2–3 times daily (multidose schedule) or once a day. The serum concentrations differ between the two regimens.

ADVERSE DRUG REACTIONS

Ototoxicity and nephrotoxicity are the major problems associated with aminoglycoside usage. Ototoxicity may be either vestibular (vertigo, dizziness, ataxia) or auditory (tinnitus, roaring in the ears, hearing loss). Although all aminoglycosides are capable of producing both forms of ototoxicity, vestibular toxicity is more common with streptomycin, gentamicin and tobramycin, and auditory damage with amikacin, kanamycin and neomycin.

Aminoglycosides are concentrated in the renal cortex and high concentrations may be associated with tubular necrosis. Nephrotoxicity has been shown to be associated with sustained high trough serum levels, thus when aminoglycosides are used serum levels should be monitored for evidence of drug accumulation. Co-administration of other potentially nephrotoxic drugs (e.g. cephalosporins, cisplatin) may enhance the nephrotoxicity of aminoglycosides.

Aminoglycosides may also induce a number of electrolyte disturbances including hypokalaemia, hypomagnesaemia, hypocalcaemia and hyponatraemia.

High doses of aminoglycosides may cause neuromuscular blockade. Neomycin and netilmicin having the greatest potential to cause this adverse effect. Aminoglycosides have also been reported to cause hypersensitivity reactions (e.g. rash, urticaria, eosinophilia), gastrointestinal disturbances and blood dyscrasias.

DRUG INTERACTIONS

Aminoglycosides when used in combination with a number of β-lactam antibiotics produce either additive or synergistic antimicrobial activity (see β-lactams).

The combination of an aminoglycoside with other potentially neurotoxic, ototoxic or nephrotoxic drugs enhances the risk of aminoglycoside toxicity, therefore patients on such combinations should be monitored closely for adverse effects.

When combined with general anaesthetics or neuromuscular blocking drugs, aminoglycosides may potentiate neuromuscular

TABLE 30.3 Dosages for aminoglycosides

Aminoglycoside	Dose	Serum concentrations			
		Multidose regimen		Single dose regimen	
		Peak	Trough	Peak*	Trough
Amikacin	30 mg/kg/day	15–30 mg/L	< 5 mg/L	> 55 mg/L	< 5 mg/L
Gentamicin	5 mg/kg/day	4.5–10 mg/L	< 2 mg/L	> 16 mg/L	< 1 mg/L
Netilmicin	5 mg/kg/day	4.5–10 mg/L	< 2 mg/L	> 16 mg/L	< 1 mg/L
Tobramycin	5 mg/kg/day	4.5–10 mg/L	< 2 mg/L	> 16 mg/L	< 1 mg/L

*Peak levels usually not measured

blockade and respiratory paralysis. Use of these combinations requires careful monitoring of the patient.

PRECAUTIONS AND CONTRAINDICATIONS

Aminoglycosides are contraindicated in patients with a previous history of aminoglycoside hypersensitivity. Cross-reactivity occurs amongst this group of drugs and an allergy to one aminoglycoside may contraindicate the use of another.

In patients with a history of tinnitus, vertigo, hearing loss or renal impairment, aminoglycosides should be used with extreme caution. Dosage reduction is necessary in patients with renal impairment. Monitoring of serum drug levels is essential to ensure drug accumulation with its inherent risk of increased toxicity does not occur.

Neuromuscular blockade induced by aminoglycosides may worsen muscle weakness in patients with Parkinson's disease, myasthenia gravis and other neuromuscular disorders.

MONITORING OF SERUM
AMINOGLYCOSIDE LEVELS

Monitoring of aminoglycoside serum levels is essential to ensure therapeutic efficacy and minimise the risk of toxicity (notably ototoxicity and nephrotoxicity). It has been clearly demonstrated that response rate is dependent on the ratio between the peak concentration and the minimal inhibitory concentration (MIC); the higher the ratio the greater the cure rate. Whilst it has long been believed that the ototoxicity is associated with excessively high peak concentrations (e.g. >10 mg/L for gentamicin) and nephrotoxicity with high trough levels (e.g. >2 mg/L for gentamicin) recent evidence suggests that it is the trough level which is critical to the development of both.

When monitoring serum aminoglycoside levels samples for 'peak' concentrations should be taken 30 minutes after an intravenous bolus injection, 30 minutes after the completion of a 30 minute infusion, and 60 minutes after an intramuscular

injection. Blood for trough levels should be taken just prior to the administration of the next dose.

All patients receiving aminoglycosides should have serum levels monitored. The critically ill, the very young, the very old, patients with changing renal function and poor responders require more frequent monitoring.

TETRACYCLINES

Tetracycline, Doxycycline, Methacycline, Minocycline, Rolitetracycline, Oxytetracycline, Chlortetracycline

The tetracyclines are a closely related family of broad spectrum antibiotics. The first tetracycline, chlortetracycline, was isolated from *Streptomyces aurefaciens* in 1948. Oxytetracycline followed in 1950 and in 1953 tetracycline, a derivative of chlortetracycline and oxytetracycline, was produced. Since that time a number of other tetracyclines have been developed. However, emergence of resistance to these drugs since their introduction has led to a decrease in their clinical usefulness.

TRADE NAMES

Chlortetracycline: *Aureomycin.*
Doxycycline: *Doryx; Doxylin; Vibramycin.*
Methacycline: *Rondomycin.*
Minocycline: *Minomycin.*
Rolitetracycline: *Reverin.*
Tetracycline: *Achromycin; Hostacycline P; Hydracycline; Latycin; Tetrex; Mysteclin.*

MECHANISM OF ACTION

Tetracyclines bind to certain subunits of bacterial ribosomes and inhibit binding of transfer RNA complexes. This in turn results in inhibition of protein synthesis. Tetracyclines may also have some effect on the bacterial cell membrane resulting in leakage of cell contents. In general tetracyclines are bacteriostatic, but at high dosage they may exert a bactericidal action.

INFECTIOUS DISEASES

30

PHARMACOKINETICS

Following oral administration tetracyclines are absorbed incompletely from the stomach and small intestine. Absorption is greatest when the drugs are administered on an empty stomach and is impaired in the presence of food, milk, iron salts and antacids containing aluminium, magnesium or calcium. The absorption of minocycline and doxycycline, however, is not significantly affected by food or milk.

Tetracyclines diffuse well into most body tissues and fluids, with the exception of the blood brain barrier where cerebrospinal fluid concentrations are less than 30% of those in the serum. The drugs are concentrated in bone (especially growing bone) and teeth (during the early stages of calcification) causing yellow fluorescence. Tetracyclines cross the placenta giving fetal serum concentrations of about 50%–75% of those in the mother. They are also excreted in high concentrations in the breast milk.

All tetracyclines are distributed into bile and undergo some degree of enterohepatic recirculation (i.e. reabsorption following excretion in the bile). Concentrations attained in the bile may be 20 times those in the serum in the absence of biliary obstruction.

Tetracycline, methacycline and oxytetracycline are excreted unchanged in the urine by glomerular filtration. Doxycycline and minocycline, however, are eliminated by non-renal mechanisms. Doxycycline may undergo metabolism in the gut wall, whilst minocycline appears to undergo metabolism in the liver. A proportion of all tetracyclines is excreted in the faeces.

SPECTRUM OF ACTIVITY

At the time of their introduction tetracyclines were active against many strains of Gram positive and Gram negative, aerobic and anaerobic bacteria. Plasmid mediated resistance has, however, significantly reduced their efficacy. Apart from activity against these bacteria, tetracyclines are also active against the mycoplasmas, *Rickettsiae* sp., *Ureaplasma urealyticum, Chlamydia* sp., spirochetes (e.g. *Treponema pallidum, Leptospira* sp.), protozoa and chloroquine-resistant malaria parasites.

USES

Tetracyclines are considered the drug of choice for the treatment of chlamydial infections (psittacosis, trachoma, pelvic inflammatory disease, urethritis and lymphogranuloma venereum), mycoplasma pneumonia, rickettsial infections (Q fever, Rocky Mountain spotted fever, typhus), brucellosis, non-specific urethritis, cholera, relapsing fever and granuloma inguinale. They may also be used as an alternative in the treatment of gonorrhoea, syphilis and Lyme disease. Other common uses include treatment of bronchitis, prostatitis and acne (oral and/or topical treatment). Common dosage schedules for tetracyclines are shown in Table 30.4.

Doxycycline given in a dose of 100 mg daily may be used as a prophylactic agent for malaria. It has also been used to prevent traveller's diarrhoea, but its clinical efficacy has yet to be proven. Tetracycline 250 mg 6-hourly is often given in combination with quinine to treat patients with falciparum malaria due to organisms which show multi-drug resistance.

ADVERSE DRUG REACTIONS

The most common adverse effect of tetracyclines is gastrointestinal upset including nausea, vomiting and diarrhoea. This may in part be reduced by administering the drugs with a light meal.

Tetracyclines may adversely affect bone and teeth development in children up to the age of 8 years and in the fetus. Brown discolouration of the teeth and hypoplasia of the enamel may occur and there may be retardation of bone growth.

Hepatotoxicity can occur, and is a particular problem during pregnancy. The administration of out of date tetracyclines may cause a Fanconi-like syndrome (a renal proximal tubule deformation). Tetracyclines, particularly in patients with renal impairment, may induce protein catabolism with a resultant increase in serum urea.

TABLE 30.4 Dosages for tetracyclines

Drug	Route	Dose Schedules (Adults, normal renal function)	Frequency of Dosing
Doxycycline	Oral	100 mg	Daily
Methacycline	Oral	150–300 mg	6–12-hourly
Minocycline	Oral	100 mg	12-hourly
Rolitetracycline	IV	275 mg	Daily
Tetracycline	Oral	250–500 mg	6-hourly

Other untoward effects reported include skin rashes, phototoxic reactions, urticaria, angioedema, eosinophilia, fever, serum sickness, black coated tongue and raised intracranial pressure. Minocycline has been associated with a high incidence of vestibular symptoms (dizziness, vertigo, ataxia). Staphylococcal enteritis is a serious complication of these agents.

DRUG INTERACTIONS

Antacids containing aluminium, calcium or magnesium, and iron salts significantly reduce the absorption of tetracyclines by producing non-absorbable complexes in the gut. Co-administration of these agents should be avoided.

Tetracyclines have been reported to potentiate the effects of warfarin; patients receiving the combination require more frequent monitoring of their prothrombin times. Conversely, the efficacy of oestrogen containing oral contraceptives may be reduced by the administration of tetracyclines.

Through their bacteriostatic action tetracyclines may antagonise the activity of bactericidal drugs, and some clinicians suggest that the combination should not be used. However, there is little clinical evidence to support this view.

PRECAUTIONS AND CONTRAINDICATIONS

Tetracyclines may cause fetal toxicity and their use in pregnant women should be restricted to those situations where no other alternative exists. They should not be used in children under the age of 8 years because of their adverse effects on bone and tooth development. Since they are excreted in breast milk their use is best avoided in nursing mothers. Alternatively, the mother should be advised to cease breast feeding whilst taking the drug.

With the exception of doxycycline, tetracyclines should not be used in patients with renal dysfunction as they may accumulate and worsen azotaemia.

Patients receiving these antibiotics should be warned of the possibility of phototoxic reactions and be advised to avoid excessive sun exposure and to stop taking the drug if erythema occurs.

Tetracyclines are irritant substances and oesophageal ulceration and perforation has occurred secondary to capsules sticking in the throat. For this reason, tetracyclines should always be taken with adequate amounts of fluids with the patient in an upright position.

MACROLIDES

Erythromycin

Erythromycin, an antibiotic produced by *Streptomyces erythreus*, was introduced into clinical practice in 1952. Since that time it has been used as a substitute for penicillin

INFECTIOUS DISEASES

30

in patients with penicillin allergies. Today, it is considered one of the least toxic antibiotics in clinical use.

TRADE NAMES

Erythromycin base: *EMU-V; Eryc; Erythrocin IM.*
Erythromycin stearate: *Erythrocin.*
Erythromycin lactobionate: *Erythrocin IV.*
Erythromycin estolate: *Ilosone.*
Erythromycin ethylsuccinate: *EES.*

MECHANISM OF ACTION

Erythromycin acts to inhibit protein synthesis by binding to the 50S subunit of bacterial ribosomes. In general it is bacteriostatic in action, but in high concentrations against a low inoculum of bacteria it may be bactericidal.

PHARMACOKINETICS

Erythromycin is available in a number of forms — erythromycin base, erythromycin stearate, erythromycin estolate, erythromycin lactobionate and erythromcyin ethylsuccinate.

When given orally, erythromycin is absorbed primarily from the duodenum. The rate and extent of absorption varies dependent on the formulation administered, acid-stability of the derivative, presence of food and gastric emptying time. Although erythromycin is absorbed following intramuscular injection, this method of administration is extremely painful and therefore not recommended.

Following absorption, erythromycin distributes widely into body tissues and fluids, producing concentrations equal to or greater than those obtained in the serum. The cerebrospinal fluid is an exception, with concentrations rarely exceeding 10% of serum levels. Erythromycin crosses the placenta with fetal concentrations reaching 10% of maternal levels. The drug is also excreted in the breast milk in concentrations of 50% of those in the serum.

Elimination of erythromycin is mainly via the bile. It is partly metabolised in the liver to inactive metabolites. Only 15% of the drug is excreted unchanged in the urine. In patients with normal renal function it has a half-life of 1.5–2 hours. Dosage adjustment is not necessary in patients with renal impairment.

SPECTRUM OF ACTIVITY

Erythromycin demonstrates a similar spectrum of activity against Gram positive organisms to that of benzylpenicillin. It is also active against some strains of Gram negative bacilli (including *Haemophilus influenzae* and *Legionella, Pasteurella* and *Brucella* sp.) and Gram negative cocci (*Neisseria* sp.). Enterobacteriaceae and *Pseudomonas aeruginosa* are resistant. Erythromycin also inhibits some *Chlamydia* and *Actinomyces* sp., *Mycoplasma pneumoniae, Rickettsiae* sp., *Ureaplasma urealyticum* and *Treponema* sp.

USES

Erythromycin is commonly used as an alternative to penicillin in patients with penicillin allergy. It is an effective agent for the treatment of streptococcal infections (e.g. lower respiratory tract, skin or soft tissue infections) and staphylococcal infections (e.g. boils, carbuncles, wound infections). It may also be used to treat bronchitis and otitis media where *Haemophilus influenzae* may be a pathogen, although it is less effective than penicillins or cephalosporins.

Erythromycin is considered the drug of choice in the treatment of atypical pneumonias caused by *Legionella* and *Chlamydia* sp., *Mycoplasma pneumoniae* and Q fever. It is also first-line therapy for whooping cough, diphtheria and *Campylobacter* sp. infections, although for the last, fluoroquinolones may be more effective.

For serious infections such as pneumonias, erythromycin should be given parenterally. It should be well diluted before administration and administered slowly to avoid local irritation and thrombophlebitis. Doses greater than 300 mg should be diluted in at least 100 mL of glucose 5% or sodium chloride 0.9% solution and infused over 30–60 minutes. Oral doses of erythromycin for adults generally range from 250–500 mg 6-hourly, whilst intravenous doses may be as high as 1 g 6-hourly, dependent on the severity of the infection.

ADVERSE DRUG REACTIONS

Gastrointestinal distress and diarrhoea are common untoward effects of erythromyin. It increases motilin levels in the gut resulting in increased gastrointestinal motility. These effects may be reduced by administering the drug with meals.

Hypersensitivity reactions (e.g. rash, eosinophilia, fever) occur rarely. Cholestatic jaundice may occur with all forms of erythromycin, but appears more common with the estolate. High doses of parenteral erythromycin may produce transient deafness.

Intravenous administration is commonly associated with local irritation and thrombophlebitis.

DRUG INTERACTIONS

Erythromycin inhibits the cytochrome P450 system in the liver resulting in decreased clearance of carbamazepine, theophylline, warfarin and cyclosporin, and potentiation of the effects of these drugs. Frequent monitoring of serum levels of these drugs and prothrombin times in the case of warfarin are recommended during concurrent use. Erythromycin may increase serum digoxin concentrations by inhibiting destruction of the drug by intestinal bacteria. Patients commenced on erythromycin whilst taking digoxin should have their digoxin levels monitored closely.

PRECAUTIONS AND CONTRAINDICATIONS

Erythromycin is contraindicated in patients with a history of hypersensitivity to the drug.

Patients receiving erythromycin, particularly the estolate preparation, should have their hepatic function monitored regularly.

Newer Macrolides: Roxithromycin, Clarithromycin, Azithromycin

Problems of erratic absorption, gastrointestinal intolerance, limited spectrum of antimicrobial activity and short half-life have hindered the widespread use of erythromycin. However, there are now a number of new macrolides which have been released for general use or are undergoing clinical trials. These agents include roxithromycin, clarithromycin, flurithromycin, xithromycin, azithromycin and dirithromycin. All these agents are said to be associated with less gastrointestinal intolerance and all have longer half-lives facilitating once daily (e.g. azithromycin) or twice daily (e.g. roxithromycin, clarithromycin) dosing.

Roxithromycin is an ether oxime derivative of erythromycin. It is orally absorbed and has a longer half-life than the parent drug. It has a similar spectrum of antimicrobial activity to erythromycin. Clarithromycin is a 6-O-methyl derivative of erythromycin. It is absorbed orally and has a similar spectrum of activity to erythromycin. However, clarithromycin is converted to a 14-hydroxy metabolite in the body and this compound is twice as active against *Haemophilus influenzae* as the parent drug. Clarithromycin also possesses significant activity against *Mycobacterium avium-intracellulare*. Both roxithromycin and clarithromycin are concentrated in human phagocytes.

Azithromycin is one of a new class of macrolides known as azalides. It is reported to be less active against Gram positive organisms than erythromycin but more active against *Haemophilus influenzae and Legionella* sp. It is also active against *Toxoplasma gondii* and *Mycobacterium avium-intracellulare*. The drug has a long half-life (68 hours) and is given once daily.

TRADE NAMES

Roxithromycin: *Rulide*; *Biaxin*.
Clarithromycin: *Klarid*.

MISCELLANEOUS AGENTS

Lincomycin, Clindamycin

Lincomycin was isolated from the actinomycete, *Streptomyces lincolnensis*, in 1962. It was later shown to have a unique structure,

30 INFECTIOUS DISEASES

allowing its use in patients with penicillin allergy. Minor modifications to the chemical structure of lincomycin produced clindamycin, an antibiotic with improved antibacterial activity and gastrointestinal absorption when compared with lincomycin. In recent years clindamycin has virtually replaced lincomycin in clinical use.

TRADE NAMES

Lincomycin: *Lincocin.*
Clindamycin: *Dalacin C.*

MECHANISM OF ACTION

Like erythromycin and chloramphenicol, clindamycin and lincomycin inhibit protein synthesis by binding to the 50S subunit of the bacterial ribosome. Lincomycin is generally bacteriostatic, whereas clindamycin may be bactericidal or bacteriostatic, depending on the sensitivity of the organism, inoculum size and the concentration of the antibiotic.

PHARMACOKINETICS

Lincomycin and clindamycin are both absorbed from the gastrointestinal tract, however, clindamycin is almost 100% bioavailable whilst lincomycin is only 40% bioavailable. Following absorption both drugs are widely distributed into body tissues and fluids, including bone, sputum, bile and pleural fluid. Lincomycin penetrates into the cerebrospinal fluid when the meninges are inflamed but clindamycin does not. Both drugs cross the placenta producing significant concentrations in the fetal circulation (clindamycin 100% of maternal concentrations, lincomycin 50%), and both are found in breast milk.

Both drugs undergo hepatic metabolism. Only 10% of clindamycin and 10%–30% of lincomycin are excreted unchanged in the urine. Dosage reduction of these drugs is only necessary in patients with severe renal dysfunction or hepatic disease. The normal half-life of clindamycin is about 2–3 hours and for lincomycin about 5 hours.

SPECTRUM OF ACTIVITY

Clindamycin and lincomycin share similar spectra of activity, however clindamycin is intrinsically more active. Clindamycin is active against most Gram positive bacteria including staphylococci, pneumococci and other streptococci (except *Enterococcus faecalis*). It possesses excellent activity against anaerobes and microaerophilic organisms including *Bacteroides*, *Clostridium*, and *Fusobacterium* sp. It is virtually inactive against Gram negative aerobic bacteria. Cross-resistance exists between clindamycin and lincomycin, and partial cross-resistance occurs between erythromycin and clindamycin.

USES

Clindamycin is effective in the management of anaerobic infections, particularly those associated with *Bacteroides fragilis* such as appendicitis, peritonitis, post-partum infections, septic abortions and pelvic inflammatory disease. In these infections it should be combined with an agent effective against Gram negative bacilli (e.g. amoxycillin, cephalosporins, aminoglycosides). Clindamycin shows excellent penetration into lung tissue and is considered by some clinicians to be the agent of choice in the management of aspiration pneumonia.

Both lincomycin and clindamcyin may be used as alternatives to penicillins in the treatment of Gram positive infections due to staphylococci, pneumococci or streptococci, e.g., infections of the lower respiratory tract, skin and soft tissue and the oral cavity. Because of their propensity to concentrate in bone they may be used to treat osteomyelitis. The usual oral dose of clindamycin for adults is 150–300 mg 6-hourly, and the intravenous dose is 600–1200 mg 6–8-hourly as a 30-minute infusion. The adult dose of lincomycin varies according to the severity of the infection. The intravenous dose range is 600 mg–1 g 8–12-hourly as a 30-minute infusion.

ADVERSE DRUG REACTIONS

Untoward effects with both clindamycin and lincomycin are more commonly seen when the drugs are given orally. Diarrhoea and pseudomembranous colitis (which may be fatal) are particularly troublesome. Patients developing diarrhoea whilst receiving these agents should have their stools tested for the presence of *Clostridium difficile* and its endotoxin. If found, the drug should be ceased and, if diarrhoea persists, therapy instituted with either metronidazole (400 mg orally 8-hourly) or vancomycin (125 mg orally 6-hourly) for 5–10 days. Glossitis, stomatitis, skin rashes, vaginitis and thrombocytopenia have also been reported.

DRUG INTERACTIONS

Clindamycin possesses mild neuromuscular blocking activity and it should be used with caution with other neuromuscular blocking agents.

PRECAUTIONS AND CONTRAINDICATIONS

The use of clindamycin or lincomycin is contraindicated in patients with a history of hypersensitivity to either agent. Patients with a history of gastrointestinal disease, particularly colitis, should avoid the unnecessary use of these antibiotics. In patients who develop diarrhoea whilst receiving these antibiotics the drug should be ceased if possible and the patient treated as outlined above.

In patients with severe renal impairment and/or hepatic failure, serum clindamycin concentrations should be monitored if high-dose therapy is used. Periodic liver function tests and full blood counts are recommended for patients receiving these antibiotics for prolonged periods.

Chloramphenicol

Chloramphenicol was isolated in 1947 from *Streptomyces venezueles*. It was the first of the broad spectrum antibiotics with activity against aerobic and anaerobic Gram positive and Gram negative bacteria. Unfortunately, its use has been associated with serious, sometimes fatal, blood dyscrasias which have lead to its limited systemic use.

TRADE NAMES

Chloramphenicol: *Chloromycetin*; *Chlorsig*.

MECHANISM OF ACTION

Chloramphenicol inhibits bacterial protein synthesis by binding to the 50S subunit of the bacterial ribosome. Chloramphenicol may also inhibit mammalian protein synthesis, although this is thought to be due to an effect on mitochondrial function.

PHARMACOKINETICS

Chloramphenicol is well absorbed following oral administration (bioavailability 75%–90%) with peak serum levels attained after 1–3 hours. The drug is widely distributed into most body tissues and fluids including saliva, ascitic fluid, pleural fluid, synovial fluid and the aqueous and vitreous humours of the eye. Chloramphenicol penetrates into the cerebrospinal fluid even in the absence of inflammation. The drug crosses the placenta in high concentration and is also distributed into breast milk.

Chloramphenicol undergoes hepatic metabolism. The inactive metabolites are excreted in the urine by tubular secretion and the active drug (5%–15% of the dose) by glomerular filtration.

SPECTRUM OF ACTIVITY

Chloramphenicol is active against a wide range of aerobic and anaerobic Gram positive bacteria, including staphylococci, *Streptococcus pneumoniae* and other streptococci. In addition, the drug is active against a wide range of Gram negative bacteria including many strains of Enterobacteriaceae, *Haemophilus influenzae*, *Neisseria meningitidis* and *Salmonella* and *Shigella* sp. *Rickettsiae*, *Chlamydia* and *Mycoplasma* sp. are also sensitive to chloramphenicol.

Resistance to chloramphenicol, both natural and acquired, has been demonstrated in some strains of staphylococci, *Salmonella* and *Shigella* sp., *Escherichia coli*, *Haemophilus influenzae* and *Pseudomonas aeruginosa*.

USES

Topically, chloramphenicol is commonly used to treat eye infections. For use in the eye it is available as either drops or ointment.

INFECTIOUS DISEASES

30

Systemic use is generally restricted to the treatment of serious infections due to susceptible organisms where potentially less toxic drugs are ineffective or contraindicated. Chloramphenicol is often used empirically in the treatment of bacterial meningitis either alone or in combination with amoxycillin, ampicillin or a third generation cephalosporin, particularly when *Haemophilus influenzae* infection is suspected. However, the clinical efficacy of third generation cephalosporins in these infections may relegate chloramphenicol to a second-line drug. Chloramphenicol is also a useful agent for the treatment of other forms of meningitis in patients allergic to penicillins. Brain abscesses which are often polymicrobial are another indication for chloramphenicol. In anaerobic infections, particularly those due to *Bacteroides fragilis*, chloramphenicol may be used in place of clindamycin or metronidazole.

Chloramphenicol has long been considered the agent of choice for the treatment of severe *Salmonella typhi* infections, however the increasing incidence of resistance and the introduction of the fluoroquinolones has diminished its role. Oral chloramphenicol should be used in preference to parenteral therapy wherever possible as it results in higher serum levels. The usual dose of chloramphenicol is 50–80 mg/kg daily in divided doses, but serum levels should be monitored and the dose adjusted accordingly to avoid toxicity.

ADVERSE DRUG REACTIONS

Bone marrow toxicity is the most important adverse effect of chloramphenicol. It may take two forms.

Dose related bone marrow suppression is the most common form and is usually reversible. Patients at risk are those receiving high doses of chloramphenicol (>4 g daily), those on prolonged therapy and those in whom chloramphenicol serum levels exceed 25 mg/L. This form of toxicity may result in anaemia, reticulocytopenia and neutropenia. Withdrawal of the drug usually results in complete recovery within two weeks.

Non-dose related, irreversible bone marrow depression occurs rarely (1 in 25 000–40 000 courses) generally manifesting as aplastic anaemia. It is associated with a 50% mortality rate. Aplastic anaemia may occur following a single dose of chloramphenicol, but more commonly develops weeks to months after the drug has been ceased. This adverse effect has been reported following the use of chloramphenicol eye drops.

The use of chloramphenicol in premature infants and babies less than 2 weeks old can result in the development of the so-called grey baby syndrome. The inability of young infants to conjugate and excrete chloramphenicol can lead to accumulation of the drug. The grey baby syndrome usually develops 2–9 days after commencing therapy. Early symptoms include failure to feed, abdominal distension and vomiting. These may progress to pallor, cyanosis and vasomotor collapse with accompanying respiratory distress. Death may ensue within hours. Withdrawal of chloramphenicol at the first sign of symptoms may avert the syndrome. Similar syndromes have been reported in children up to 2 years old.

Other adverse effects include optic neuritis, gastrointestinal upset (nausea, vomiting, diarrhoea, stomatitis, glossitis) and hypersensitivity reactions (rashes and fever).

DRUG INTERACTIONS

Chloramphenicol is capable of inhibiting microsomal enzymes and thus inhibiting metabolism and potentiating the effects of drugs such as phenytoin, tolbutamide, chlorpropamide and warfarin.

The concurrent use of chloramphenicol with other myelosuppressive agents should be avoided because of possible additive toxicity. Chloramphenicol use should be avoided in patients receiving antianaemia therapy as the drug may interfere with the efficacy of such therapy.

PRECAUTIONS AND CONTRAINDICATIONS

Chloramphenicol is contraindicated in patients with a history of allergy to the drug.

Its use should be avoided in patients with pre-existing anaemia, leucopenia or thrombocytopenia as it may worsen such conditions. Patients receiving chloramphenicol should have their blood count monitored before the commencement of therapy and every two to three days whilst on the drug. Serum levels should be monitored to ensure they do not exceed 25 mg/L.

The drug should not be used in premature infants and in the first two weeks of newborn life, except in extreme life-threatening situations, because of the risk of the grey baby syndrome.

GLYCOPEPTIDE ANTIBIOTICS

Vancomycin

Vancomycin is a tricyclic glycopeptide antibiotic unrelated to other commercially available agents. It is obtained from cultures of *Nocardia orientalis*.

TRADE NAMES

Vancomycin: *Vancocin*; *Vancoled*.

MECHANISM OF ACTION

Vancomycin binds to the bacterial cell wall causing blockade of glycopeptide polymerisation. This results in immediate inhibition of cell wall synthesis. Vancomycin is generally bactericidal in action. It acts at a different site to the penicillins and other β-lactams and therefore exhibits no cross-resistance with these antibiotics.

PHARMACOKINETICS

Vancomycin is not absorbed from the intact gastrointestinal tract and must be given parenterally for systemic infections.

Following intravenous infusion the drug distributes widely into body tissues and fluids including ascitic, pericardial, pleural and synovial fluids. Vancomycin attains low concentrations in cerebrospinal fluid in patients with meningitis. The drug readily crosses the placenta, but diffusion into breast milk is low.

Vancomycin is excreted primarily in the urine by glomerular filtration. The half-life of the drug in patients with normal renal function is 4–6 hours. Drug accumulation occurs in patients with renal impairment.

SPECTRUM OF ACTIVITY

Vancomycin is clinically active only against Gram positive bacteria, particularly aerobes. It is active against both penicillin sensitive and penicillin resistant organisms including *Staphylococcus aureus, Staphylococcus epidermidis*, group A streptococci, *Streptococcus pneumoniae*, viridans streptococci, enterococci, *Corynebacterium diptheriae* and *Clostridia* sp. The drug is active against methicillin resistant staphylococci.

USES

Oral vancomycin may be used to treat *Clostridium difficile* associated colitis, in a dose of 125 mg 6-hourly. The drug may also be given orally to treat staphylococcal enteritis.

Parenterally, vancomycin is used to treat serious infections caused by susceptible organisms, which cannot be treated with other effective, less toxic antimicrobials.

Vancomycin is the drug of choice for the treatment of methicillin resistant staphylococcal infections. In patients with penicillin allergy it is the treatment of choice, in combination with an aminoglycoside, for *Enterococcus faecalis* endocarditis.

The usual parenteral dose of vancomycin is 2 g daily given in divided doses. The dose should be adjusted in accordance with the patient's renal function to attain peak serum concentrations in the range 20–40 mg/L and trough levels of 5–10 mg/L. The drug must be given as an infusion over 60 minutes to avoid the development of the 'red-man syndrome' (see Adverse Drug Reactions).

ADVERSE DRUG REACTIONS

Rapid infusion of vancomycin may result in the so-called 'red-man' or 'red-neck' syndrome. It is characterised by a sudden and

30 INFECTIOUS DISEASES

possibly severe fall in blood pressure which may be accompanied by flushing and/or a maculopapular rash on the face, neck, chest and upper extremities. The latter features may occur in the absence of hypotension. The reaction is, in part, thought to be due to histamine release.

Ototoxicity and nephrotoxicity are the most serious adverse effects associated with vancomycin. Ototoxicity appears to occur more commonly in patients in whom serum levels exceed 80 mg/L, but it can occur at lower drug levels. Vancomycin generally affects the auditory branch of the eighth nerve, however, cases of permanent deafness are rare. Nephrotoxicity, like ototoxicity, is more likely to occur in patients with elevated serum levels. Co-administration of aminoglycosides may potentiate the nephrotoxicity of vancomycin.

Apart from the red-man syndrome, vancomycin may cause other skin reactions, with rashes occurring in about 5% of patients. Intravenous administration may cause phlebitis and the drug should be adequately diluted before administration. Haematological toxicity (neutropenia, eosinophilia, thrombocytopenia) has also been reported during vancomycin therapy.

DRUG INTERACTIONS

Concurrent administration of potentially ototoxic or nephrotoxic drugs (e.g. aminoglycosides) may have an additive effect. Wherever possible these combinations should not be used.

PRECAUTIONS AND CONTRAINDICATIONS

Vancomycin is contraindicated in patients with a previous allergy to the drug. It should be used with caution in patients with renal impairment or hearing loss. Regular monitoring of serum levels must be carried out, as well as periodic urinalysis and renal function tests.

Patients receiving prolonged courses of vancomycin or who have received other drugs which may cause blood dyscrasias should have periodic full blood pictures performed.

Teicoplanin

Teicoplanin is a glycopeptide antibiotic complex structurally related to vancomycin. It is a fermentation product obtained from *Actinoplanes teichomyceticus*. It exhibits a similar mode of action and spectrum of activity to vancomycin, being active against Gram positive aerobic and anaerobic bacteria. Like vancomycin it is active against methicillin-resistant *Staphylococcus aureus* and *Staphylococcus epidermidis*, and is not destroyed by β-lactamases.

Teicoplanin is poorly absorbed orally. It has a long half-life (60 hours) and thus need only be administered once daily. The drug is eliminated both renally (approximately 50%) and non-renally.

Unlike vancomycin, it may be given intramuscularly or by intravenous bolus injection. The red-man syndrome has not been reported following administration of teicoplanin. The usual dose is 200 mg daily, however this dose should be reduced in renal failure.

With the exception of the red-man syndrome, teicoplanin exhibits a similar spectrum of adverse effects to vancomycin.

CEPHALOSPORIN P ANTIBIOTICS

Fusidic Acid

Fusidic acid (sodium fusidate) is a steroid antibiotic derived from the fungus *Fusidium coccineum*. Fusidic acid is structurally related to cephalosporin P.

TRADE NAMES

Fusidic acid: *Fucidin*.

MECHANISM OF ACTION

Fusidic acid is bactericidal. Unlike penicillins and cephalosporins, it acts to inhibit protein synthesis rather than cell wall synthesis. Therefore cross-resistance between β-lactams and fusidic acid is not seen.

PHARMACOKINETICS

Fusidic acid is well absorbed orally, with peak concentrations occurring after 2–4 hours. Following absorption it is widely distributed into body tissues and fluids achieving therapeutic concentrations in bone, soft tissue, synovial fluid, pus, vitreous and aqueous humours, the cerebrospinal fluid, sputum, burn crusts and serum. Fusidic acid crosses the placenta and may be detected in breast milk.

Fusidic acid is concentrated and excreted in the bile. Little drug is found in the urine. The drug also undergoes substantial metabolism.

SPECTRUM OF ACTIVITY

Staphylococci, including penicillinase producing strains and methicillin resistant strains, are sensitive to fusidic acid. Other Gram positive cocci appear less sensitive, whereas Gram negative bacteria are generally resistant.

Development of resistance is a problem when fusidic acid is used alone. Therefore combination therapy with another anti-staphylococcal agent (e.g. flucloxacillin, rifampicin) is recommended.

USES

Fusidic acid may be used to treat localised as well as generalised staphylococcal infections such as abscesses, osteomyelitis, pneumonia, peritonitis, septicaemia, wound infections and enteritis.

Fusidic acid in combination with rifampicin may be used as an alternative to vancomycin in patients unable to tolerate that drug or who require oral therapy.

The drug is available as an oral suspension (250 mg/5 mL), tablets (as sodium fusidate 250 mg) and as an intravenous infusion (as diethanolamine fusidate 580 mg equivalent to 500 mg sodium fusidate). The usual dose of fusidic acid is 500 mg 8-hourly. When given intravenously it should be diluted in 250–500 mL of sodium chloride 0.9% solution and infused over 2–4 hours.

ADVERSE DRUG REACTIONS

Fusidic acid demonstrates little toxicity. The most common adverse effect are mild gastrointestinal disturbances (e.g. dyspepsia, nausea and vomiting). Jaundice has been reported following the use of fusidic acid, however it is reversible.

Cross-reactivity does not occur in patients with penicillin hypersensitivity.

DRUG INTERACTIONS

Fusidic acid should be administered with caution in combination with other antibiotics excreted similarly in the bile (e.g. lincomycin and rifampicin).

PRECAUTIONS AND CONTRAINDICATIONS

Fusidic acid is contraindicated in patients with a history of allergy to the drug. Liver function tests should be performed periodically.

RIFAMYCIN B ANTIBIOTICS

Rifampicin

Rifampicin is a semisynthetic derivative of rifamycin B, an antibiotic produced by *Streptomyces mediterranei*. Although, principally used for the treatment of tuberculosis, the drug may also be used for a number of other bacterial infections.

TRADE NAMES

Rifampicin: *Rifadin*; *Rimycin*.

MECHANISM OF ACTION

Rifampicin interferes with RNA synthesis by inhibiting DNA dependent RNA polymerase. It may be bactericidal or bacteriostatic, depending on the concentration of the drug attained at the infection site and the susceptibility of the organism.

PHARMACOKINETICS

Rifampicin is well absorbed following oral administration. Food may delay and reduce oral absorption of the drug and it is generally given on an empty stomach.

INFECTIOUS DISEASES

30

The drug is lipid soluble and following absorption is widely distributed into most body tissues and fluids including the lungs, liver, pleural fluid, prostate, seminal fluid, bile, bone, saliva and tears. Rifampicin reaches levels in the cerebrospinal fluid around 10%–20% of concurrent serum levels. The drug crosses the placenta and may be detected in the breast milk.

Rifampicin is deacetylated in the liver to an active metabolite. The parent drug and its metabolite are excreted in the bile. The half-life of the drug is about 3 hours, but this becomes shorter during long-term therapy.

SPECTRUM OF ACTIVITY

Rifampicin is active against most Gram positive bacteria (e.g. staphylococci and streptococci). It is active against *Neisseria meningitidis, Neisseria gonorrhoeae* and *Haemophilus influenzae*, as well as some enteric Gram negative organisms. *Legionella pneumophilia* is also sensitive to rifampicin.

Most strains of *Mycobacterium tuberculosis* are sensitive to rifampicin, but the sensitivity of *Mycobacterium* sp. is variable. *Chlamydia trachomatis* and many other *Chlamydia* sp. are sensitive to rifampicin.

USES

The principal use of rifampicin is in the treatment of tuberculosis where it is used in combination with at least one other anti-tubercular drug. The adult dose in this instance is 450–600 mg daily.

Rifampicin is recommended for chemo-prophylaxis in close contacts of patients with *Haemophilus influenzae* type b and meningococcal infections. It is also given to the index case in order to eliminate asymptomatic nasopharyngeal carriage. The adult dose for *Haemophilus influenzae* type b infections is 600 mg daily for four days and for meningococcal infections it is 600 mg 12-hourly for two days.

Rifampicin in combination with erythromycin is recommended for the treatment of severe *Legionella* sp. infections. The drug is also used in combination with other anti-

staphylococcal agents in serious staphylococcal infections at a dose of 20 mg/kg daily.

ADVERSE DRUG REACTIONS

Gastrointestinal upset is common with rifampicin. Patients complain of heartburn, epigastric distress, nausea, vomiting, anorexia, flatulence, abdominal cramps and diarrhoea.

The drug may also cause central nervous system effects such as drowsiness, fatigue, headache, mental confusion and visual disturbances. Myalgia and arthralgia are often experienced during the first few weeks of rifampicin therapy.

Rifampicin may induce a flu-like illness, particularly when it is taken on an intermittent basis. The drug can cause a range of hypersensitivity reactions, such as urticaria, pruritus, eosinophilia, anaphylaxis, exfoliative dermatitis and Stevens-Johnson syndrome.

Rifampicin often causes transient elevations in liver function tests (aspartate aminotransferase, bilirubin, alkaline phosphatase). On occasion it may cause an acute hepatitis and liver failure. It is also reported to cause a range of blood dyscrasias.

DRUG INTERACTIONS

Rifampicin induces the metabolism of a large number of drugs including warfarin, verapamil, oral contraceptives, methadone, sulfonylurea oral hypoglycaemics, corticosteroids, anticonvulsants, cyclosporin, theophylline, β-blockers and quinidine, resulting in a diminishment of their effects. Careful monitoring is required during and on discontinuation of rifampicin therapy.

Concurrent use of rifampicin and ketoconazole may not only result in decreased levels of ketoconazole but also decreased levels of rifampicin.

PRECAUTIONS AND CONTRAINDICATIONS

Rifampicin is contraindicated in patients with jaundice or a previous hypersensitivity reaction to the drug. A full blood picture and liver function tests should be carried out before commencing rifampicin and these parameters should be monitored regularly whilst drug therapy continues.

Rifampicin may turn body secretions, including urine, sweat and tears, orange in colour and patients should be warned of this. Patients should not wear soft contact lenses whilst taking rifampicin as these may become permanently stained.

POLYMIXINS

Polymixin B, Colistin

The polymixin group of antibiotics (A, B, C, D and E) were first isolated from spore bearing *Bacillus* sp. in 1947. Only two of these, polymixin B and polymixin E (colistin), are used clinically. These drugs are used either as sulfates or sodium sulfomethonates.

TRADE NAMES

Colistin: *Coly-Mycin*.

MECHANISM OF ACTION

Polymixins are bactericidal in action. They appear to act on the bacterial cell membrane by a type of detergent action resulting in increased permeability, swelling and rupture of the bacterium.

PHARMACOKINETICS

Polymixin B and colistin are not absorbed orally. They are absorbed slowly following intramuscular administration.

Both drugs distribute widely into body tissues, binding reversibly to liver, kidneys, heart and muscle. Neither polymixin B nor colistin attain therapeutic levels in the cerebrospinal fluid.

Colistin and polymixin B are both eliminated in the urine by glomerular filtration. The half-life of polymixin B in patients with normal renal function is about 5.1 hours and of colistin 2.2 hours. Both drugs accumulate in patients with renal failure.

SPECTRUM OF ACTIVITY

Polymixin B and colistin are active against most Gram negative bacteria except *Proteus* sp. and Gram negative cocci. They are particularly active against *Klebsiella* and *Pseudo-monas* sp. Polymixins are inactive against Gram positive organisms. Cross-resistance between the two polymixins is complete.

USES

Once the drugs of choice for the management of pseudomonal infections, their role has been taken over by antipseudomonal penicillins and cephalosporins. The major use of polymixins is now topical. Polymixin B in combination with other antimicrobials active against Gram positive bacteria is used in the treatment of skin and eye infections. Colistin administered via a nebuliser is used to clear pseudomonal respiratory tract infections in patients with bronchiectasis and cystic fibrosis. It may also be combined with kanamycin or neomycin and used as a bladder irrigation. Oral colistin is used in some institutions as part of a gastrointestinal decontamination program in immunocompromised patients.

Parenteral colistin is now reserved for serious Gram negative infections, particularly pseudomonal infections, which are unresponsive to less toxic agents or when such agents are contraindicated. The usual intramuscular or intravenous dose is 2.5–5 mg/kg daily given in two to four divided doses.

ADVERSE DRUG REACTIONS

Topical use of polymixins is associated with a low incidence of adverse effects, with hypersensitivity reactions rarely occurring.

Both polymixin B and colistin may cause nephrotoxicity, neurotoxicity and hypersensitivity reactions when administered parenterally. Nephrotoxicity may be manifested by albuminuria, haematuria, pyuria, azotaemia and excessive electrolyte losses. Neurotoxicity ranges from facial flushing, dizziness and mental confusion to seizures and coma. These drugs possess neuromuscular blocking actions and may induce respiratory paralysis. Pain at the site of injection is also frequently reported.

DRUG INTERACTIONS

Polymixins may potentiate or prolong the

INFECTIOUS DISEASES

30

skeletal muscle relaxation produced by neuromuscular blocking drugs and/or general anaesthetics. Concurrent administration of potentially nephrotoxic or neurotoxic drugs with polymixins may potentiate their toxicity. Combined use of these agents should be avoided if possible.

PRECAUTIONS AND CONTRAINDICATIONS

Polymixin B and colistin are contraindicated in patients with a history of polymixin allergy.

The dosage of both drugs should be reduced in patients with renal impairment as accumulation of the drug may result in toxic levels. Patients require careful monitoring for signs of nephro- or neurotoxicity.

PEPTIDE ANTIBIOTICS

Bacitracin, Gramicidin

Bacitracin and gramicidin are polypeptide antibiotics produced by *Bacillus subtilis* and *Bacillus brevis* respectively. While they are considered too toxic for systemic use they continue to be used topically.

MECHANISM OF ACTION

Bacitracin appears to act by interfering with bacterial cell wall synthesis preventing the incorporation of amino acids and nucleotides. The antibiotic may also damage the cell membrane. Gramicidin acts by interfering with bacterial plasma membrane function.

PHARMACOKINETICS

Neither drug is absorbed when administered topically.

SPECTRUM OF ACTIVITY

Gramicidin and bacitracin are highly active against Gram positive bacteria such as staphylococci, streptococci, anaerobic cocci, *Corynebacteria* and *Clostridia* sp. Bacitracin is also active against gonococci, meningococci and fusobacteria. However, these drugs are generally inactive against Gram negative bacteria.

USES

Both gramicidin and bacitracin are used topically in combination with other antimicrobials (often neomycin and polymixin B) to treat minor skin infections and eye and ear infections. Bacitracin has also been used in solution for wound irrigation or bladder instillation. Recent studies suggest that oral bacitracin at a dose of 25 000 units 6-hourly for 7–14 days, may be a suitable alternative to vancomycin in the treatment of pseudomembraneous colitis.

ADVERSE DRUG REACTIONS

Topical use of bacitracin and gramicidin is associated with few side effects. Hypersensitivity reactions rarely occur.

Administered parenterally bacitracin is associated with significant nephrotoxicity. Gramicidin is highly toxic to the erythrocytes (causing haemolytic anaemia), kidneys and liver.

AMINOCYCLITOL ANTIBIOTICS

Spectinomycin

Spectinomycin is an antibiotic obtained from cultures of *Streptomyces spectabilis*.

TRADE NAMES

Spectinomycin: *Trobicin*.

MECHANISM OF ACTION

Spectinomycin is bacteriostatic and acts by inhibiting bacterial protein synthesis by binding to the 30S ribosomal subunit.

PHARMACOKINETICS

Spectinomycin is not absorbed when given orally. However, it is rapidly absorbed following intramuscular injection with peak concentrations attained after one hour. The drug has a half-life of 1.2–2.8 hours in adults. Spectinomycin undergoes metabolism to a biologically active metabolite. Both the parent drug and its metabolite are eliminated in the urine by glomerular filtration.

SPECTRUM OF ACTIVITY

Spectinomycin is active against a wide range of Gram positive and Gram negative organisms. Importantly, it is active against penicillinase producing strains of *Neisseria gonorrhoeae*, but it is inactive against *Treponema pallidum* (syphilis) and *Chlamydia trachomatis*.

USES

Spectinomycin is used to treat acute gonococcal urethritis and proctitis in men and acute gonococcal cervicitis and proctitis in women when the organism is resistant to penicillin or the patient is allergic to penicillins. The usual dose is 2 g as a single dose given by deep intramuscular injection.

ADVERSE DRUG REACTIONS

Single doses of spectinomycin are generally well tolerated. The most common side effects reported are pain at the injection site, dizziness, nausea, fever, rash and headache.

PRECAUTIONS AND CONTRAINDICATIONS

Spectinomycin is contraindicated in patients with a previous allergy to the drug.

Since spectinomycin may mask or delay symptoms of syphilis any patient treated with spectinomycin for gonorrhoea should have a serological test for syphilis at the time of diagnosis and three months later.

Mupirocin

Mupirocin is the major fermentation metabolite produced by *Pseudomonas fluorescens*. Although the antimicrobial activity of the fermentation products of this organism was first described in 1887 it was not until 1971 that its major active metabolite, pseudomonic acid A, was isolated. Pseudomonic acid A is now known as mupirocin.

TRADE NAMES

Mupirocin: *Bactroban*.

MECHANISM OF ACTION

Mupirocin is thought to act by inhibiting RNA and protein synthesis. DNA activity and cell wall formation are affected to a lesser extent.

PHARMACOKINETICS

Minimal systemic absorption occurs when mupirocin is applied topically. The drug is not suitable for systemic use as it has too short a half-life (approximately 30 minutes) when given intravenously.

SPECTRUM OF ACTIVITY

Mupirocin is active against many Gram positive bacteria such *as Staphylococcus aureus* (including methicillin resistant strains) and many other staphylococci and streptococci. Enterococci are far less sensitive. With the exception of *Haemophilus influenzae* and *Neisseria* and *Branhamella* sp. Gram negative organisms are resistant to mupirocin. The drug is inactive against fungi and yeasts.

USES

Mupirocin formulated as a 2% ointment (in a polyethylene glycol base) is used to treat primary and secondary skin infections such as impetigo, folliculitis, ecthyma, eczema and minor burns, wounds and ulcers caused by susceptible organisms.

Mupirocin is also formulated in a soft paraffin base for use in the nose to eliminate staphylococcal nasal carriage, including methicillin resistant strains.

ADVERSE DRUG REACTIONS

Mupirocin has shown little potential to cause systemic toxicity or hypersensitivity reactions. Local reactions such as pain, stinging, burning, pruritus or skin rashes may occur. These may in part be due to the polyethylene glycol base.

DRUG INTERACTIONS

No clinically significant interactions have been reported with mupirocin.

PRECAUTIONS AND CONTRAINDICATIONS

The only contraindication to mupirocin use is known hypersensitivity to the drug or the vehicle. Safety in pregnancy has not been established.

30 INFECTIOUS DISEASES

NURSING IMPLICATIONS

ASSESSMENT

Previous hypersensitivity reactions generally preclude the further use of the same or a related antibiotic in a particular patient. A careful history of previous antibiotic exposure and drug allergies must therefore be taken.

When the dose of antibiotic (e.g. aminoglycosides, chloramphenicol) to be given is dependent on weight the patient should be weighed. Renal function should be assessed in all patients before commencement of any of these antibiotics; renal failure may necessitate dosage reduction for a number of these agents (e.g. aminoglycosides, penicillins, cephalosporins, aztreonam, imipenem) or preclude their use (e.g. tetracyclines). Liver function should be assessed in patients receiving chloramphenicol, erythromycin and clindamycin. Tetracyclines should not be prescribed for pregnant women or children under the age of 8 years. Mothers with young babies should be warned against breast feeding whilst receiving tetracyclines.

ADMINISTRATION

Antibiotic doses should be spaced evenly throughout the day to ensure adequate serum concentrations and minimise the risk of emergence of resistance.

Most oral antibiotics are best given on an empty stomach (i.e. 1 hour before food or 3 hours after food) to maximise absorption. If gastrointestinal intolerance occurs, seek advice from a pharmacist or the manufacturer about co-administration with meals. Tetracyclines in general should not be given with milk, antacids or iron preparations.

Antibiotics prescribed intramuscularly should be administered into large muscles, by deep injection. Administration of many β-lactams intramuscularly requires co-administration of a local anaesthetic. Prevention of accidental intravenous administration by aspiration of the needle is essential. Slow injection is recommended to minimise the risk of tissue damage and pain secondary to intramuscular injections. Similarly, intravenous antibiotics should be given slowly or by infusion to reduce the risk of phlebitis. Antibiotics of different groups (e.g. penicillins and aminoglycosides) should not be mixed prior to administration.

EVALUATION

Evaluation of antimicrobial therapy consists of assessment of efficacy and detection of adverse effects and superinfection. Efficacy may be assessed on the basis of clinical improvement, especially reduction in body temperature, and objective measurements such as white cell count, culture results and radiological examinations.

All patients should be monitored for the development of hypersensitivity reactions. Other monitoring for adverse effects is dependent on the antibiotic being used (e.g. chloramphenicol — full blood picture; cephamandole — coagulation profile; aminoglycosides — renal function, hearing and vestibular function).

Peripheral cannulae sites should be inspected regularly for signs of phlebitis and extravasation. Monitoring of aminoglycoside and chloramphenicol levels is critical; blood samples should be drawn at specific times in relation to the dose for peak and trough estimates.

QUINOLONES

Nalidixic acid, introduced into clinical practice in 1962, is the prototype for this group of agents. There are two distinct classes of quinolones — non-fluorinated quinolones (e.g. nalidixic acid, cinoxacin, acrosoxacin) and fluoroquinolones (e.g. norfloxacin, ciprofloxacin, enoxacin, pefloxacin, ofloxacin).

The fluoroquinolones, by virture of their broad spectrum of activity and oral route of administration, represent a significant advance in antimicrobial therapy. Resistance, however, poses a major threat to their long-term effectiveness.

MECHANISM OF ACTION

All quinolones, non-fluorinated and fluorinated, act by inhibiting DNA gyrase, a bacterial enzyme essential for DNA replication. The quinolones are bactericidal in action.

Non-Fluorinated Quinolones: Nalidixic Acid

TRADE NAMES

Nalidixic acid: *Negram*.

PHARMACOKINETICS

Nalidixic acid is rapidly and completely absorbed from the gastrointestinal tract with peak concentrations occurring within 1–2 hours of administration. Following absorption the drug only achieves clinically significant concentrations in the urine; negligible amounts of the drug enter the cerebrospinal fluid.

The drug undergoes metabolism in the liver leading to the production of at least one active metabolite, hydroxynalidixic acid. Nalidixic acid is also partly metabolised in the kidney. The half-lives of the parent drug and active metabolite are about 6–7 hours. Both are excreted principally in the urine with about 4% excreted in the faeces.

SPECTRUM OF ACTIVITY

Nalidixic acid is highly active against the majority of Enterobacteriaceae (including *Klebsiella*, *Proteus* and *Enterobacter* sp. and *Escherichia coli*). It is also active against some strains of *Salmonella* and *Shigella* sp. The drug is inactive against *Pseudomonas aeruginosa*, Gram positive organisms and anaerobes. However, resistance may develop during nalidixic acid therapy in up to 25% of cases.

USES

Nalidixic acid is now considered a third-line agent for the treatment of acute and chronic urinary tract infections caused by susceptible Gram negative bacteria. The introduction of safer agents, notably amoxycillin–clavulanic acid and the fluorinated quinolones, and problems of resistance and adverse effects mitigate against its use. The usual dose of nalidixic acid is 1 g orally 6-hourly.

ADVERSE DRUG REACTIONS

The most common adverse effects of nalidixic acid involve the central nervous system and include headache, malaise, drowsiness, dizziness, vertigo, syncope, sensory changes, visual disturbances, excitation, depression, confusion, toxic psychosis and rarely, seizures. The drug should be used with caution in patients with central nervous system disorders. Gastrointestinal side effects include nausea and vomiting, with diarrhoea and abdominal pain occurring less frequently. Hypersensitivity reactions have been reported, the most common being urticaria and rash. Eosinophilia, pruritus and photosensitivity reactions may also occur.

Nalidixic acid may cause blood dyscrasias, in particular haemolytic anaemia in patients with glucose-6-phosphate dehydrogenase deficiency. Renal and hepatic damage may also occur during nalidixic acid treatment.

DRUG INTERACTIONS

Nalidixic acid, being highly protein bound, may displace warfarin from its binding sites on serum albumin and potentiate its anticoagulant effect. The combination should be used only with regular monitoring of prothrombin times.

PRECAUTIONS AND CONTRAINDICATIONS

Nalidixic acid is contraindicated in patients with a history of hypersensitivity to the drug. Patients receiving nalidixic acid should be warned of the risk of photosensitivity reactions and advised to limit their exposure to direct sunlight and to use a sunscreen whilst on the drug.

30 INFECTIOUS DISEASES

If severe central nervous system reactions such as seizures, raised intracranial pressure or toxic psychosis occur, the drug should be withdrawn immediately and appropriate treatment measures instituted. The use of nalidixic acid is contraindicated in patients with known seizure disorders.

Animal studies have demonstrated nalidixic acid and related compounds can cause cartilage erosion in weight-bearing joints and other signs of arthropathy in sexually immature individuals. Although similar effects have not been seen in humans, use in individuals under 16 years of age is not generally recommended.

Fluorinated Quinolones: Norfloxacin, Ciprofloxacin

Norfloxacin and ciprofloxacin are the only fluoroquinolones commercially available in Australia at this time. Many more are available overseas and undoubtedly some of these will be released onto the Australian market in the future.

TRADE NAMES

Norfloxacin: *Noroxin*.
Ciprofloxacin: *Ciproxin*.

PHARMACOKINETICS

The oral bioavailability of all fluoroquinolones exceeds 50% and is greatest (>95%) for ofloxacin and pefloxacin. Following absorption they are widely distributed into body tissues and fluids, often attaining concentrations in excess of those found in serum. Drug concentrations tend to be very high in urine, high in kidney and prostatic tissue, but lower in prostatic fluid. The drugs distribute well into lung tissue, although concentrations in saliva and bronchial secretions tend to be lower than serum levels. High levels are attained in the faeces.

In general these drugs show poor penetration into the cerebrospinal fluid, with the exception of pefloxacin (40% of serum levels) and ofloxacin (90% of serum levels). Fluoroquinolones are concentrated in macrophages and leucocytes. Their half-lives range from 4–10 hours.

Elimination of ciprofloxacin, norfloxacin, enoxacin and fleroxacin is both renal and non-renal. Ofloxacin is excreted primarily in the urine, whilst pefloxacin undergoes non-renal elimination. With the exception of perfloxacin the half-lives of all the fluoroquinolones discussed are increased in patients with renal failure.

SPECTRUM OF ACTIVITY

Fluoroquinolones show excellent in-vitro activity against most Enterobacteriaceae, fastidious Gram negative bacilli including *Haemophilus* sp., and Gram negative cocci, such as *Neisseria gonorrhoeae, Neisseria meningitidis* and *Moraxella (Branhamella) catarrhalis*. In general ciprofloxacin is the most active against these organisms. *Pseudomonas aeruginosa* is also sensitive to fluoroquinolones, however other *Pseudomonas* sp. tend to be resistant.

When introduced into clinical practice the fluoroquinolones demonstrated excellent activity against staphylococci including methicillin-resistant strains. However, resistance amongst these organisms is becoming a problem. The fluoroquinolones tend to be less active against streptococci and enterococci and exhibit poor activity against anaerobic organisms. Ofloxacin and ciprofloxacin are active against *Mycobacterium tuberculosis* and other *Mycobacterium* sp. and like other fluoroquinolones exhibit activity against *Chlamydia trachomatis, Mycoplasma, Legionella* and *Rickettsiae* sp., *Coxiella burnetti* and *Plasmodium falciparum*.

USES

In usual doses (400 mg orally 12-hourly) norfloxacin serum levels are insufficient to treat systemic infections. Therefore, its use is limited to the treatment of complicated and uncomplicated urinary tract infections and the management of prostatitis and gonococcal urethritis. The drug has also proven effective in the treatment of gastroenteritis, including shigellosis and salmonellosis. Norfloxacin also may be given to patients undergoing chemotherapy to reduce the risk of Gram negative infections.

Ciprofloxacin, unlike norfloxacin, achieves therapeutic concentrations in many body fluids and tissues. It may be used in the treatment of urinary tract infections; respiratory tract infections (including bronchiectasis, bronchitis, lung abscess and pneumonia); skin and skin structure infections; and bone and joint infections. Ciprofloxacin has proven effective in the treatment of gastroenteritis caused by a wide range of enteric pathogens. It is effective for treatment of typhoid fever and the typhoid carrier state.

Ciprofloxacin may be used to treat penicillin-resistant gonococcal infections and chancroid. Although ciprofloxacin is not indicated in the treatment of *Neisseria meningitidis* meningitis, it may be given as a single dose (500–750 mg) to eliminate nasopharyngeal carriage.

In most instances ciprofloxacin may be administered orally, however in serious infections it may be given intravenously by infusion. The usual adult oral dose ranges from 250 mg orally 12-hourly for urinary tract infections to 750 mg 12-hourly for more serious infections. The intravenous dose is 200–400 mg 12–hourly given as a 30–60 minute infusion, dependent on the severity of the infection. Dosage reduction is necessary in patients with renal dysfunction.

ADVERSE DRUG REACTIONS

The fluoroquinolones are generally well tolerated and exhibit a similar spectrum of adverse effects to nalidixic acid. Gastrointestinal adverse effects have been reported most often and include nausea, abdominal discomfort, vomiting and diarrhoea. *Clostridium difficile* associated colitis is an infrequent complication of fluoroquinolone therapy.

Central nervous system symptoms are the next most common adverse effects of fluoroquinolones. These include headache, dizziness, vertigo, ataxia and sleep disturbances. Rarer, but more serious adverse effects include seizures, delirium and hallucinations. Seizures have been associated with the use of the drugs in patients with underlying brain lesions and as a result of drug interactions (see Drug Interactions).

Arthropathy is a concern with the use of fluoroquinolones, as it is with nalidixic acid. Because of cartilage erosion in weight-bearing joints, the use of these agents in children and pregnant or breast-feeding women is not generally recommended. Reversible arthritis and tendonitis have been associated infrequently with the use of fluoroquinolones in adults.

Rare cases of haematuria, interstitial nephritis and acute renal failure have been reported. Crystalluria may occur in patients receiving high doses of fluoroquinolones, particularly in the presence of a raised urinary pH. However, precipitation of these drugs in the urine has not been associated with renal impairment.

DRUG INTERACTIONS

Fluoroquinolones should not be administered with antacids containing magnesium, calcium or aluminium as these compounds reduce absorption of the antibiotics by forming non-absorbable complexes. In the case of ciprofloxacin, serum concentrations may be reduced by as much as 90%. Sucralfate, which contains aluminium, also diminishes the absorption of norfloxacin and ciprofloxacin.

The clearance of theophylline is reduced by enoxacin and to a lesser extent by ciprofloxacin and pefloxacin. Norfloxacin, ofloxacin and lomefloxacin appear to have a minimal effect on theophylline elimination. Reports of theophylline toxicity following co-administration of ciprofloxacin and enoxacin highlight the need for careful monitoring of theophylline levels if these combinations are prescribed.

Ciprofloxacin has been reported to enhance the effects of warfarin resulting in prolongation of prothrombin times. Thus patients receiving anticoagulants should have their prothrombin times monitored regularly if ciprofloxacin is prescribed.

30 INFECTIOUS DISEASES

Probenecid has been shown to interfere with the tubular secretion of fluoroquinolones resulting in high serum concentrations and prolongation of half-lives. In the case of ciprofloxacin, levels may be increased by as much as 50%.

PRECAUTIONS AND CONTRAINDICATIONS

Fluoroquinolones are contraindicated in patients with a history of hypersensitivity to any fluoroquinolone.

Patients receiving fluoroquinolones must maintain an adequate fluid intake to prevent precipitation of the drug in the urine (crystalluria). As quinolones may cause central nervous system stimulation they should be used with caution in patients with a history of seizures or other central nervous system disorders. Particular caution should be exercised when ciprofloxacin is given in combination with a theophylline derivative because ciprofloxacin may inhibit theophylline metabolism leading to toxicity (see Drug Interactions).

Dosage adjustment is required in patients with renal impairment because of potential drug accumulation and toxicity.

NURSING IMPLICATIONS

ASSESSMENT

The patient's history should be reviewed for evidence of hypersensitivity to any of the quinolones, renal or hepatic impairment, a history of convulsive disorders, psychosis or raised intracranial pressure, or asthma being treated with theophylline or a derivative. Evidence of pregnancy or breast feeding should be ascertained as these are considered contraindications to treatment. The patient's state of hydration should be determined and, if necessary, the patient should be rehydrated prior to commencing therapy. If the patient has an alkaline or acidic urine this should be corrected to avoid crystalluria in the case of alkaline urine or decreased urinary activity in the case of acid urine. The patient's concurrent medication should be reviewed for any potential drug interactions. The patient's age should be checked. If the patient is a pre-pubertal child the potential problem of cartilage erosion of the weight-bearing joints must be addressed. The patient's neurological function should be assessed and recorded. Specimens should be obtained prior to commencement of therapy and forwarded to the microbiology laboratory for culture and sensitivity testing. Clinical manifestations of the infection should be recorded to establish a baseline for observations.

ADMINISTRATION

The orally administered quinolones should be given one hour before or two hours after meals to minimise the influence of food on the rate and extent of absorption. The patient should be given plenty of fluids to maintain an adequate state of hydration and to minimise the risk of crystalluria. If the patient requires therapy with aluminium or magnesium containing antacids, these should be administered at least two hours after the dose of the quinolone. If the patient is to receive an infusion of ciprofloxacin it should be administered slowly over 30–60 minutes.

EVALUATION

During the course of treatment the patient should be monitored for signs of clinical improvement. If no improvement is apparent or deterioration occurs, antibiotic therapy should be reviewed. Further samples should be taken for microbiological examinations. The patient should be examined for sites of other infection particularly those due to secondary infection. The question of adequate drug absorption should be addressed if the patient is receiving oral therapy.

The patient's neurological function should be assessed periodically, with monitoring for central nervous system toxicity. Other body systems should be observed for possible side effects. Renal and hepatic function and urine pH should be monitored if patients are receiving drugs which might alter these parameters.

Ciprofloxacin may interfere with the metabolism of certain drugs, notably warfarin and theophylline. Increased monitoring of patients receiving these drugs is required. Patients receiving parenteral ciprofloxacin should have the injection site regularly inspected for signs of irritation, extravasation and phlebitis.

PATIENT EDUCATION

The patient should be advised to take the quinolone one hour before or two hours after meals, maintain an adequate fluid intake and avoid taking antacid preparations. The patient should be advised of the signs of adverse reactions, including hypersensitivity reactions, and to report these if they occur. He or she should also be advised to avoid prolonged exposure to direct sunlight, and that the quinolones may cause light-headedness and dizziness which could prove hazardous if driving or operating machinery. The patient should be instructed to complete the full course of treatment.

FOLATE ANTAGONISTS

Sulfonamides: Sulfacetamide, Sulfadiazine, Sulfadimidine, Sulfamethizole, Phthalylsulfathiazole

In 1935 Prontosil rubrum was introduced into clinical practice and a new era in the treatment of infectious diseases began. Since that time many sulfonamides have been synthesised. Today the use of sulfonamides for infectious diseases has decreased significantly. In part this is due to increased resistance to these antimicrobials and the introduction of more effective, less toxic alternatives.

MECHANISM OF ACTION

Sulfonamides are bacteriostatic in action and exert their effect by inhibiting the formation of folic acid in bacteria and parasites. Unlike humans who may utilise preformed folic acid absorbed from their diet, microorganisms are unable to absorb folic acid and must synthesise it intracellularly from para-aminobenzoic acid. Sulfonamides act by competitively inhibiting dihydrofolate synthetase, the enzyme responsible for converting para-aminobenzoic acid to dihydrofolic acid. (See Figure 30.3.)

PHARMACOKINETICS

The sulfonamides may be divided into three groups according to their different pharmacokinetic properties:

1. Absorbable, rapidly excreted (short acting) sulfonamides (e.g. sulfadimidine, sulfafurazole, sulfamethizole and sulfacetamide).

2. Absorbable, more slowly excreted (intermediate acting) sulfonamides (e.g. sulfamethoxazole, sulfadiazine).

3. Non-absorbable or very poorly absorbed sulfonamides (e.g. phthalylsulfathiazole).

Absorbable sulfonamides are widely distributed in the body tissue and fluids. Cerebrospinal fluid concentrations of some sulfonamides (e.g. sulfadiazine) may reach 35%–80% of serum concentration. The drugs cross the placenta and may be detected in breast milk.

The sulfonamides undergo hepatic metabolism. The parent drugs and their metabolites are then excreted principally in the urine by glomerular filtration. Short acting sulfonamides have half-lives in the range 4–8 hours and intermediate acting agents have half-lives in the range 7–17 hours.

SPECTRUM OF ACTIVITY

Sulfonamides were originally active against a wide range of Gram positive and Gram negative organisms, however increasing

INFECTIOUS DISEASES

30

PARA-AMINOBENZOIC ACID

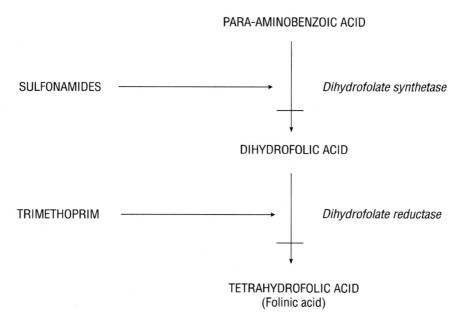

FIGURE 30.3 Mode of action of trimethoprim and sulfonamides

resistance has diminished the clinical use-fulness of these drugs. Apart from activity against bacteria, sulfonamides are active against Chlamydia trachomatis, Toxoplasma gondii and *Plasmodium* sp.

USES

The spectrum of use of sulfonamides has considerably diminished with the emergence of widespread resistance to these agents. Today, the most commonly used sulfonamide is sulfamethoxazole which is given in combination with trimethoprim.

Sulfonamides are occasionally used to treat non-obstructive urinary tract infections including pyelonephritis, pyelitis and cystitis caused by susceptible Enterobacteriaceae and *Staphylococcus aureus*. Urinary alkalinisation is carried out to enhance sulfonamide excretion into the urine and the drug's antibacterial activity.

Sulfonamides are considered the drugs of choice for the treatment of nocardiosis and toxoplasmosis. They may also be used as alternatives for the treatment of chancroid, chlamydial infections (except psittacosis) and elimination of meningococcal naso-pharyngeal carriage.

Sulfadoxine in combination with pyrimethamine may be used for the prevention of chloroquine resistant malaria, however co-existing antifolate resistance now exists in some areas of the world (e.g. Thailand). The combination has also been used in the treatment of falciparum malaria.

Silver sulfadiazine in combination with chlorhexidine is used topically in the management of burns.

ADVERSE DRUG REACTIONS

Side effects are common with sulfonamides. Hypersensitivity reactions contribute a large number of adverse effects and include dermatological reactions, drug fever, serum sickness, anaphylaxis, lupus erythematosus, vasculitis, fibrosing alveolitis, hepatitis and myocarditis. The incidence of such reactions appears to increase with increased dosage.

Sulfonamides have been reported to cause a number of blood dyscrasias such as haemolytic anaemia, agranulocytosis, thrombocytopenia and aplastic anaemia. Renal damage is also a problem with these drugs. They may precipitate in the kidney leading to renal colic, urolithiasis, oliguria, obstructive anuria, haematuria, proteinuria and elevations in serum urea concentration. These complications may be avoided by ensuring the patient has an adequate urine output (1500 mL/day) and by alkalinisation of the urine.

Hepatic complications resulting in jaundice have been reported with sulfonamides. Jaundice and kernicterus may occur in newborns or premature infants treated with sulfonamides. To avoid this these drugs should not be given to pregnant women near term, or newborn or premature infants.

Gastrointestinal upset occurs commonly with sulfonamides and it is generally recommended that these drugs be taken with food. Neurological side effects associated with sulfonamides range from headache and dizziness to acute psychosis and seizures.

DRUG INTERACTIONS

Sulfonamides have a synergistic action when given in combination with pyrimethamine or trimethoprim, which also act to inhibit folic acid synthesis (see Figure 30.3).

The combination of warfarin with certain sulfonamides (e.g. sulfamethoxazole) may result in potentiation of the anticoagulant effects of warfarin either due to displacement of warfarin from serum proteins or inhibition of warfarin metabolism.

The effects of certain sulfonylurea oral hypoglycaemic agents may be enhanced by sulfonamides due to displacement of these drugs from serum proteins. In addition, sulfamethizole is reported to inhibit the metabolism of tolbutamide.

Sulfonamides should be given with caution to patients receiving methotrexate as these drugs have the potential to displace methotrexate from protein binding sites or inhibit its renal excretion, thus enhancing its toxicity.

PRECAUTIONS AND CONTRAINDICATIONS

Sulfonamides are contraindicated in patients with a history of hypersensitivity to one of these agents.

The dose of these drugs should be reduced in patients with renal impairment or severe hepatic dysfunction. Excessive accumulation of the drug may occur putting these patients at greater risk of adverse effects.

Patients developing skin rashes, sore throats, arthralgia, jaundice, purpura, fever or pallor whilst receiving a sulfonamide should discontinue taking the drug immediately, as these may be early signs of more serious adverse reactions.

Trimethoprim

Trimethoprim is a synthetic antifolate antimicrobial. It is available alone or in combination with sulfamethoxazole.

TRADE NAMES

Trimethoprim: *Alprim*; *Triprim*.

MECHANISM OF ACTION

Trimethoprim acts by inhibiting dihydrofolate reductase, thus interfering with the production of tetrahydrofolic acid in bacterial cells (see Figure 30.3). Its action is slowly bactericidal.

PHARMACOKINETICS

Trimethoprim is well absorbed from the gastrointestinal tract with peak levels achieved 1–4 hours after administration. Following absorption the drug is widely distributed into the body tissues and fluids, including the cerebrospinal fluid. It crosses the placenta and is concentrated in breast milk.

Trimethoprim is excreted principally in the urine by glomerular filtration and tubular secretion. In patients with normal renal function it has a half-life of 8–11 hours.

SPECTRUM OF ACTIVITY

Trimethoprim is active against Gram positive aerobic cocci and most Gram negative organisms except *Pseudomonas aeruginosa*. It is active against common urinary pathogens including *Escherichia coli, Proteus mirabilis, Klebsiella pneumoniae* and *Enterobacter* sp.

30

INFECTIOUS DISEASES

USES

Trimethoprim may be used for the initial treatment of acute uncomplicated urinary tract infections caused by susceptible organisms. In females the drug may be given as a single 600 mg oral dose or as a 5-day course of 300 mg daily. In males a 5-day course is indicated. Patients with recurrent urinary tract infections may be given the drug prophylactically to prevent further episodes (the usual dose is 150 mg nightly).

Trimethoprim (20 mg/kg daily in divided doses) may also be used in combination with dapsone (100 mg daily) to treat *Pneumocystis carinii* infections in patients sensitive to sulfonamides.

ADVERSE DRUG REACTIONS

The most frequent adverse drug reactions reported with trimethoprim are rash (maculopapular or morbilliform) and pruritus. More serious dermatological reactions such as exfoliative dermatitis, Stevens-Johnson syndrome and toxic epidermal necrolysis have been reported rarely.

Gastrointestinal untoward effects include epigastric discomfort, nausea, vomiting and altered taste sensation. Thrombocytopenia, neutropenia, megaloblastic anaemia and leucopenia may occur as a result of trimethoprim's inhibition of dihydrofolate reductase. These effects are usually not seen with short courses of trimethoprim and when the dose is kept below 300 mg daily.

DRUG INTERACTIONS

Trimethoprim, when combined with sulfonamides or dapsone, produces a synergistic effect.

Trimethoprim may significantly reduce the hepatic metabolism of phenytoin. When the two drugs are administered together patients should be observed closely for signs of phenytoin toxicity.

PRECAUTIONS AND CONTRAINDICATIONS

Trimethoprim is contraindicated in patients with a history of allergy to the drug. It should not be administered to patients with severe renal impairment unless drug levels are monitored. The drug is also contraindicated in patients with severe haematological disorders or megaloblastic anaemia secondary to folate deficiency. It should be used with caution in the elderly or those with suspected folate deficiency. If folate supplementation is required, folinic acid should be given. Care should also be exercised when administering trimethoprim to patients with impaired hepatic function.

Trimethoprim–Sulfamethoxazole

The combination of trimethoprim with sulfamethoxazole (formerly named co-trimoxazole) in a weight to weight ratio of 1 to 5 is available for oral and parenteral administration. The combination makes use of two antimicrobials which inhibit sequential steps of bacterial metabolism (see Figure 30.3). In doing so, the drugs act synergistically. The combination also decreases the risk of emergence of resistance.

TRADE NAMES

Trimethoprim–sulfamethoxazole: *Bactrim*; *Resprim*; *Septrin*.

SPECTRUM OF ACTIVITY

The combination is bactericidal at concentrations at which its components are usually bacteriostatic. It is effective against a wide range of Gram positive and Gram negative bacteria including staphylococci, streptococci, pneumococci, *Escherichia coli, Neiserria, Klebsiella, Enterobacter, Proteus, Salmonella* and *Shigella* sp., *Haemophilus influenzae* and *Bordetella pertussis*. It is also active against *Pneumocystis carinii*.

USES

Concerns about the side effects profile of the trimethoprim–sulfamethoxazole combination (particularly in the elderly) and increasing bacterial resistance have reduced the product to a second line agent for most bacterial infections. Despite this, it is a very effective agent for the treatment of upper and lower respiratory tract infections, urinary tract infections, prostatitis, osteo-myelitis, skin and wound infections and sep-ticaemias caused by susceptible organisms. It is a useful alternative to third generation cephalosporins for the treatment of Gram negative enteric meningitis.

The combination is active against *Serratia marcesens, Pseudomonas cepacia, Xan-thamonas maltophilia* and *Acinetobacter* sp. which are common pathogens in superinfec-tions and often resistant to other antibiotics. It may be used in the treatment of infec-tions due to amoxycillin resistant strains of *Shigella* sp. It is an alternative to ciproflox-acin, the third generation cephalosporins, ampicillin and chloramphenicol in the treat-ment of enteric fever due to *Salmonella typhi* or *paratyphi*. In patients intolerant of erythro-mycin and tetracyclines, the combination may be used to treat chlamydial infections. The combination may also be used in the treat-ment of gonorrhoea.

Trimethoprim–sulfamethoxazole is the treatment of choice for *Pneumocystis carinii* pneumonia, a life threatening infection in immunocompromised patients. It is also of value in the treatment of nocardiosis, bru-cellosis and toxoplasmosis, and the preven-tion of Gram negative septicaemia in neutropenic patients.

The usual adult dose is trimethropim 160 mg plus sulfamethoxazole 800 mg 12-hourly. In pneumocystosis the dose is based on 20 mg/kg per day of trimethoprim, in four di-vided doses. The dose must be reduced in patients with renal impairment.

ADVERSE DRUG REACTIONS

Adverse effects reported with the combina-tion are similar to those reported with the individual components. An increased inci-dence of serious haematological and derma-tological reactions leading to death has been reported in patients over the age of 60 years.

DRUG INTERACTIONS

Drug interactions are similar to those of the individual components; importantly the combination may potentiate the effects of warfarin.

PRECAUTIONS AND CONTRAINDICATIONS

Trimethoprim–sulfamethoxazole is contrain-dicated in patients with a history of hy-persensitivity to the combination or either of its components.

Dosage reduction is required in patients with impaired renal and hepatic function. Use in patients over the age of 60 years is no longer recommended due to the in-creased number of deaths in this age group secondary to blood dyscrasias and severe skin reactions caused by the product.

NURSING IMPLICATIONS

ASSESSMENT

Before treatment with sulfonamides or trimethoprim, the patient's history should be reviewed for evidence of blood dys-crasias, renal impairment or liver disease. Evidence of any of these conditions could influence the decision to prescribe these drugs. They should not be used in preg-nant women near term or in women who are breast feeding. The nurse should also check for known hypersensitivity to any of the sulfonamides and related compounds such as the thiazide diuretics, chlorthali-done, acetazolamide and the sulfonylurea hypoglycaemic agents.

Obstetric and neonatal nursing staff should be aware that these drugs can pre-cipitate jaundice and kernicterus in the new-born or premature infant and they should not be given either to the mother prior to delivery or to the neonate.

The clinical manifestations of the infec-tion should also be recorded to establish a baseline for observations.

ADMINISTRATION

It is advisable to give these drugs with food or after meals to help eliminate nau-sea and gastrointestinal side effects. If the

INFECTIOUS DISEASES

30

more insoluble sulfonamides are being used, ensure that the patient drinks plenty of fluids during the day to minimise the risk of crystalluria.

EVALUATION

Once treatment has started, the nurse should evaluate the patient for clinical improvement and adverse effects. With respect to the latter, nurses must be alert for the development of blood dyscrasias. Signs and symptoms of these include sore throat, fever, prostration, ulceration of the mouth, rectum or vagina, bleeding gums, nose bleeds and unexplained bruising.

The skin should be observed for signs of hypersensitivity and photosensitivity reactions and the urine for signs of haematuria. The urine pH should be monitored and a urinary alkaliniser administered if ordered.

PATIENT EDUCATION

Patients should be advised to take the drug with food or after meals and to increase their fluid intake. Fair skinned patients should be told to avoid exposure to sunlight. They should be advised of the signs of adverse effects, including hypersensitivity reactions, and to report these if they occur. As with all anti-infective therapy, they should be advised of the importance of completing the prescribed course.

URINARY ANTISEPTICS

This group of drugs includes nitrofurantoin, hexamine mandelate and hexamine hippurate. These agents are used exclusively for the treatment of urinary tract infections.

Nitrofurantoin

Nitrofurantoin is a synthetic antibacterial nitrofuran compound.

TRADE NAMES

Nitrofurantoin: *Furadantin*; *Macrodantin*.

MECHANISM OF ACTION

Nitrofurantoin is thought to interfere with several bacterial enzyme systems involved in bacterial carbohydrate synthesis.

PHARMACOKINETICS

Nitrofurantoin is well absorbed from the gastrointestinal tract and rapidly excreted in the urine. It fails to achieve therapeutic levels in the serum or body tissues. It does however cross the placenta and is distributed into breast milk. The plasma half-life of nitrofurantoin is about 20 minutes in patients with normal renal function but is prolonged in patients with renal impairment.

SPECTRUM OF ACTIVITY

Nitrofurantoin is active against Gram negative and Gram positive urinary pathogens, particularly *Escherichia coli*. Some strains of *Klebsiella* and *Proteus* sp. are less sensitive, whilst *Pseudomonas aeruginosa* is resistant.

USES

Nitrofurantoin is indicated for the treatment of urinary tract infections such as cystitis, pyelitis and pyelonephritis due to susceptible pathogens. Because of its serious side effects it is not considered a first-line agent. The usual dose for such infections is 50–100 mg orally 6-hourly. The drug may also be given prophylactically to prevent recurrent urinary tract infections. In this case the dose is 50 mg nightly.

ADVERSE DRUG REACTIONS

Nausea with associated anorexia and vomiting are the most common adverse effects of nitrofurantoin therapy. Of more importance however, is the occurrence of pulmonary hypersensitivity reactions and peripheral neuropathy. Pulmonary reactions may be classified as acute, subacute or chronic. The acute form usually occurs during the first week of therapy and is characterised by fever, chills, cough, dyspnoea, chest pain and pulmonary infiltration. In general, it resolves on drug withdrawal. The subacute and chronic forms often have an insidious onset and may progress to irreversible pulmonary fibrosis.

Peripheral neuropathy occurs in about 1 in 5000 patients receiving nitrofurantoin and is more commonly seen in patients with renal dysfunction. Tingling or numbness occurring during nitrofurantoin treatment necessitates drug withdrawal. Blood dyscrasias (haemolytic anaemia, thrombocytopenia, agranulocytosis, eosinophilia, megaloblastic anaemia) and hepatotoxicity may also occur secondary to nitrofurantoin therapy.

DRUG INTERACTIONS

Probenecid may interfere with the renal excretion of nitrofurantoin, therefore diminishing its effectiveness and enhancing its potential toxicity. Nitrofurantoin antagonises the action of quinolone derivatives, hence co-administration of these agents is not recommended.

PRECAUTIONS AND CONTRAINDICATIONS

Nitrofurantoin is contraindicated in patients with a history of furan allergy, patients with moderate to severe renal impairment, pregnant women near term or infants under 1 month of age.

Haemolytic anaemia may occur in patients with glucose-6-phosphate dehydrogenase deficiency; any sign of haemolysis is an indication to withdraw the drug.

Hexamine Mandelate, Hexamine Hippurate

Hexamine (methenamine) was introduced as a urinary antibacterial agent in 1894. Today it is available in the form of hexamine mandelate and hexamine hippurate.

TRADE NAMES

Hexamine mandelate: *Mandelamine.*
Hexamine hippurate: *Hiprex.*

MECHANISM OF ACTION

The antibacterial action of hexamine and its salts is dependent on the release of formaldehyde in an acid medium. Formaldehyde is a non-specific antibacterial agent, which is generally bactericidal. Hippuric acid and mandelic acid also possess some antibacterial properties. Their presence also facilitates the liberation of formaldehyde.

PHARMACOKINETICS

Hexamine and its salts are readily absorbed from the gastrointestinal tract, although hexamine is partially hydrolysed in the stomach to formaldehyde and ammonia. Following absorption hexamine and its salts are excreted intact in the urine by glomerular filtration and tubular secretion. In the presence of an acidic urine, hexamine is hydrolysed to formaldehyde and ammonia. A urinary pH below 5.5 facilitates maximum hydrolysis. Peak urinary formaldehyde concentration are seen within 3–8 hours.

SPECTRUM OF ACTIVITY

Formaldehyde is active against essentially all Gram positive and Gram negative bacteria, including *Pseudomonas aeruginosa*, as long as the concentration is high enough. Resistance does not develop during hexamine therapy as bacteria do not become resistant to formaldehyde.

USES

Although hexamine and its salts have been used to treat uncomplicated urinary tract infections, they are now only used to suppress recurrent urinary tract infections in patients without indwelling catheters.

Hexamine mandelate is given in a dose of 1 g 6-hourly, whilst hexamine hippurate is given in a dose of 1 g 12-hourly. Evidence suggests that supplementary acidification of the urine is required less often in patients given hexamine hippurate. If the urinary pH is not less than 5.5 then ascorbic acid 1 g 6-hourly should be administered. Urinary acidification is particularly important when treating infections due to urea-splitting organisms such as *Proteus, Enterobacter* and *Pseudomonas* sp.

30 INFECTIOUS DISEASES

ADVERSE DRUG REACTIONS

Both hexamine salts are generally well tolerated, although some patients experience gastrointestinal side effects such as nausea, vomiting and diarrhoea. These effects are though to be due to local irritation caused by formaldehyde in the gut. Dermatological reactions, manifesting as skin rashes, urticaria and pruritus, may occur.

High levels of formaldehyde in the urinary tract can lead to bladder irritation, painful and frequent micturition, albuminuria and haematuria. Transient elevations in serum transaminases have also been reported during the use of hexamine hippurate.

DRUG INTERACTIONS

Hexamine salts should not be administered concurrently with sulfamethizole as formaldehyde and sulfamethizole form an insoluble complex in acid urine.

PRECAUTIONS AND CONTRAINDICATIONS

Hexamine and its salts are contraindicated in patients with a history of allergy to any of these drugs and in patients with renal insufficiency. In addition, hexamine hippurate should not be used in patients with known hepatic impairment or severe dehydration.

ANTIPROTOZOAL AND ANTIANAEROBIC AGENTS

Metronidazole

Metronidazole is one of a large group of synthetic compounds known as nitroimidazoles. Initially introduced to treat protozoal infections, it has more recently become the agent of choice for anaerobic infections.

TRADE NAMES

Metronidazole: *Flagyl; Metrogyl; Metrozine.*

MECHANISM OF ACTION

The exact mechanism of action of metronidazole is unknown. It has been postulated that within the cells of microorganisms possessing nitro-reductase enzymes, the nitro group of metronidazole is reduced and extremely active intermediate derivatives are produced. These intermediates then bind to the organism's DNA, inhibit its synthesis and cell death ensues. The lack of activity of metronidazole against aerobic bacteria has been rationalised on the basis that these organisms do not possess nitro-reductase activity.

Natural and acquired resistance to metronidazole is uncommon, and when it does occur is due to poor cell penetration and/or decreased nitro-reductase activity.

PHARMACOKINETICS

Metronidazole given orally is very well absorbed (>80%) from the gastrointestinal tract, with absorption not influenced by food. The drug is also well absorbed when administered rectally, however metabolism by bacteria in the rectum means higher doses must be given to achieve equivalent blood levels. Following absorption the drug is widely distributed into body tissues and fluids including vaginal, pleural and cerebrospinal fluids, and breast milk. The drug crosses the placenta.

The drug is metabolised in the liver and both unchanged drug (approximately 19%) and its metabolites are excreted in the urine. The half-life of metronidazole in patients with normal renal and hepatic function is around 6–8 hours.

SPECTRUM OF ACTIVITY

Metronidazole is active against a wide range of anaerobic bacteria including *Bacteroides fragilis* and other *Bacteroides* sp., *Clostridia*, *Fusobacterium* and *Eubacterium* sp. and anaerobic streptococci. The drug is not active against aerobic or facultative organisms.

Metronidazole is active against *Trichomonas vaginalis, Giardia lamblia, Entamoeba histolytica* and *Balantidium coli.*

USES

Metronidazole is now accepted as the agent of choice for the treatment and prevention of anaerobic infections due to susceptible organisms. The drug is used prophylactically to prevent postoperative anaerobic infections in procedures where contamination by anaerobes may occur, e.g., bowel surgery, vaginal hysterectomy and appendectomy. In these instances the drug is administered concurrently with other agents, commonly a cephalosporin, active against aerobic organisms.

When using metronidazole for these indications the drug may be given intravenously (500 mg 8–12-hourly by infusion over 20 minutes), orally (400 mg 8–12-hourly or rectally 1 g 8–12-hourly); wherever possible oral therapy should be used.

Vaginal trichomoniasis may be treated with a single oral dose of 2 g of metronidazole or alternatively with 400 mg 12-hourly for 5–7 days. *Gardnerella vaginalis* vaginosis may also be treated with the 5–7-day course. Giardiasis is best treated by giving a 2 g dose on three consecutive days. Amoebiasis is treated by giving 600–800 mg orally 8-hourly for 5–10 days. Acute ulcerative gingivitis usually responds to 200 mg orally 8-hourly for 5 days.

Metronidazole has been shown to be as effective as vancomycin for the treatment of *Clostridium difficile* induced pseudomembranous colitis at a dose of 200–400 mg orally 8-hourly for 5–10 days, although it has also been implicated in causing the condition. The drug also shows promise in the treatment of Crohn's disease. When administered orally the drug should be given after food.

ADVERSE DRUG REACTIONS

In general metronidazole is well tolerated when given in the standard doses. The most common adverse effects are gastrointestinal and include nausea (sometimes accompanied by headache), anorexia, furry tongue, dry mouth, abdominal discomfort and a metallic taste in the mouth. Metronidazole may also affect the central nervous system producing dizziness, ataxia, confusion, irritability, depression and, rarely, seizures. Peripheral neuropathy has been associated with large cumulative doses.

Hypersensitivity reactions and leucopenia have been reported. The drug may also discolour the urine (red-brown) and patients should be made aware of this.

DRUG INTERACTIONS

Metronidazole is a potent inhibitor of warfarin metabolism and concurrent use results in an enhanced anticoagulant effect. Dosage reduction of warfarin is usually necessary and prothrombin times must be monitored closely.

Patients taking metronidazole have experienced disulfiram-like reactions (e.g. flushing, vomiting, headache, abdominal cramps) after ingesting alcohol. Patients should avoid alcohol for 48 hours after completion of their course of therapy.

PRECAUTIONS AND CONTRAINDICATIONS

Metronidazole is contraindicated in patients with a history of allergy to the drug or other nitroimidazoles. The drug should be used with caution in patients with hepatic dysfunction, neurological disorders or blood dyscrasias. Dosage reduction is necessary in patients with liver disease.

Patients who develop neurological symptoms (particularly peripheral neuropathy) should be monitored closely and drug withdrawal considered. Nursing mothers should be advised against breast feeding for up to 24 hours after receiving metronidazole.

Tinidazole

Tinidazole, like metronidazole, is a synthetic nitroimidazole compound. The drug possesses a similar mechanism of action and spectrum of activity to metronidazole.

TRADE NAMES

Tinidazole: *Fasigyn.*

INFECTIOUS DISEASES

30

PHARMACOKINETICS

Tinidazole is rapidly absorbed from the gastrointestinal tract and widely distributed into body tissues and fluids. Concentrations in the cerebrospinal fluid exceed 80% of those in the serum. Unlike metronidazole, the drug is excreted mainly unchanged in the urine.

USES

Given as a single dose of 2 g tinidazole has been found to be effective in the treatment of vaginal and urogenital trichomoniasis, and giardiasis. The drug is also used in the treatment of amoebiasis. Tinidazole may be used as an alternative to metronidazole for surgical prophylaxis.

For information on adverse drug reactions, drug interactions, precautions and contraindications see metronidazole.

NURSING IMPLICATIONS

ASSESSMENT

Nursing assessment prior to administration of metronidazole or tinidazole should aim to identify current alcohol use and the presence of haematopoietic disorders. As the drugs are mutagenic, pregnancy should be excluded. Caution should be exercised if it is necessary to administer the drugs to nursing mothers. The mother should be advised to cease breast feeding during the course of treatment and for 24 hours after the last dose of metronidazole and 72 hours after the last dose of tinidazole.

ADMINISTRATION

The administration of metronidazole and tinidazole with food may minimise the risk of gastrointestinal upsets.

EVALUATION

When evaluating patients taking these drugs, watch for and report signs of allergy such as rash or pruritus. Numbness,

tremor, ataxia or paraesthesia may indicate central nervous system toxicity. Sore throat, fatigue and fever are indicative of leucopenia.

PATIENT EDUCATION

Avoidance of alcohol during a course of therapy with metronidazole or tinidazole should be stressed as these drugs exert a disulfiram-like effect which can cause distressing symptoms such as flushing, tachycardia, nausea, vomiting and even circulatory collapse. Patients should also be advised that these drugs may cause a metallic taste in the mouth and that the urine may become discoloured. All patients who are self-administering these drugs should be counselled regarding these adverse effects.

OTHER ANTIPROTOZOAL AGENTS

Pentamidine Isethionate

Pentamidine isethionate is an aromatic diamidine derivative antiprotozoal agent which has proven efficacy in the treatment and prevention of *Pneumocystis carinii* pneumonia. It may be used as an alternative to trimethoprim–sulfamethoxazole in the treatment of pneumocystosis in immunocompromised patients, including those with AIDS. The drug is also useful in a range of other parasitic diseases.

TRADE NAMES

Pentamidine isethionate: *Pentacarinat*.

MECHANISM OF ACTION

The exact mechanism of action of pentamidine has not been elucidated. The drug exhibits a 'cidal' action against *Pneumocystis carinii* possibly by inhibiting oxidative phosphorylation, nucleic acid and protein synthesis, glucose metabolism and/or dihydrofolate reductase activity.

PHARMACOKINETICS

Little information is available about the pharmacokinetics of pentamidine isethionate. Following intramuscular injection peak concentrations occur after about one hour. The drug is widely distributed in the body and accumulates in tissues particularly in the liver, lungs, spleen and adrenals. Pentamidine is eliminated slowly from the body, with around 6% excreted unchanged in the urine over a 15-day period.

SPECTRUM OF ACTIVITY

Pentamidine isethionate is active against *Pneumocystis carinii, Leishmania* sp. and some *Trypanosoma* sp.

USES

Pentamidine isethionate is used as an alternative to trimethoprim–sulfamethoxazole for the treatment and prevention of *Pneumocystis carinii* pneumonia. For treatment, the drug may be administered by intravenous infusion (over 1–2 hours) in a dose of 4 mg/kg daily for at least two weeks. Alternatively, it may be given by oral inhalation using a *Respirgard II* jet nebuliser. In this case, 600 mg is diluted in 6 mL of water and administered as an aerosol for 20 minutes daily. Administration of 150 mg of pentamidine twice monthly or 300 mg once a month as an oral inhalation has proven effective in preventing relapses.

Pentamidine is also used to prevent and treat African trypanosomiasis (sleeping sickness) and leishmaniasis (both kala-azar and the cutaneous form).

ADVERSE DRUG REACTIONS

Over 50% of patients given pentamidine experience side effects; some of which may be life threatening. The drug may produce sudden severe hypotension, cardiac arrhythmias, cardiac arrest and death. It is therefore recommended that the drug be administered slowly with the patient in the supine position.

Pentamidine has a toxic effect on the β-islet cells of the pancreas, which results in severe and prolonged hypoglycaemia in 5%–10% of patients. The drug demonstrates significant nephrotoxicity and it may produce acute renal failure. Its use has also been associated with the development of leucopenia, thrombocytopenia, abnormal liver function tests, gastrointestinal upset, acute pancreatitis, confusion, hallucinations, hyperkalaemia, hypocalcaemia, hyponatraemia and Stevens-Johnson syndrome.

Given intramuscularly the drug may cause sterile abscesses, pain, erythema, tenderness and induration at the site of injection. Intravenous use may cause phlebitis. The two most common adverse effects of inhaled pentamidine are cough and bronchospasm.

DRUG INTERACTIONS

As nephrotoxic effects may be additive, the concurrent or sequential use of pentamidine with other nephrotoxic agents should be avoided if possible.

PRECAUTIONS AND CONTRAINDICATIONS

Pentamidine isethionate is contraindicated in patients with a history of allergy to the drug. It should be used with caution in patients with hepatic and/or renal impairment, hypertension or hypotension, hyperglycaemia, leucopenia, thrombocytopenia or anaemia.

The drug should be administered with the patient lying down. The patient's blood pressure should be measured before the first dose and at regular intervals during and after administration until the course is completed. The following laboratory tests and monitoring should be carried out at regular intervals: serum electrolytes, creatinine levels, liver function tests, full blood picture, serum calcium, urinalysis (weekly) and electrocardiograms.

INFECTIOUS DISEASES

30

ANTITUBERCULAR AGENTS ▮▮▮▮▮▮

Tuberculosis remains an important disease and a subject of active research. The introduction of streptomycin (1945), para-aminosalicylic acid (1946) and isoniazid revolutionised the treatment of all forms of this disease. Today, antitubercular drugs can be divided into two groups:

  (i) First-line agents: isoniazid, rifampicin, ethambutol, pyrazinamide and streptomycin; and

  (ii) Second-line agents: ethionamide, prothionamide, para-aminosalicylic acid (PAS), kanamycin, capreomycin and cycloserine.

The initial treatment of tuberculosis includes the use of three or four first-line drugs, dependent on the treatment regimen selected. Multi-drug regimens are used to prevent the development of resistance or the selection of resistant subgroups of mycobacteria.

Traditionally, the treatment of tuberculosis has involved 18 months of therapy, initially with three drugs (1–3 months) then with two drugs. More recently, the emphasis has changed to the use of shorter courses of either nine months or six months. Also, in an effort to improve patient compliance intermittent (twice weekly) therapy is now used in some cases. The agents used for short course therapy are listed in Table 30.5.

FIRST-LINE AGENTS

Isoniazid

Isoniazid (isonicotinic acid hydrazide, INAH) is the most effective antitubercular drug available at this time. The drug is highly effective in virtually all types and stages of tuberculosis.

MECHANISM OF ACTION

The exact mechanism of action of isoniazid has not yet been established, although several mechanisms including interference with bacterial synthesis of proteins, nucleic acids, carbohydrates and lipids have been postulated. Recent evidence suggests that isoniazid inhibits the synthesis of mycolic acids (important constituents of the mycobacterial cell wall) by interfering with the enzyme mycolate synthetase (an enzyme unique to mycobacteria). Isoniazid is bactericidal at high concentrations and bacteriostatic at lower levels. Its bacteriostatic effects last for up to 72 hours after a single dose.

PHARMACOKINETICS

Isoniazid is readily and rapidly absorbed from the gastrointestinal tract. It diffuses into all body cavities, tissues and fluids (including the cerebrospinal fluid and breast

TABLE 30.5 Short course regimens for the treatment of tuberculosis

Regimen	Initial Phase (Months 1–2)	Maintenance Phase
6 months (4 drugs)	Rifampicin + isoniazid + pyrazinamide plus either ethambutol or streptomycin	Rifampicin + isoniazid
9 months (3 drugs)	Rifampicin + isoniazid plus either ethambutol or streptomycin	Rifampicin + isoniazid

milk) reaching concentrations comparable to those in the blood. The drug crosses the placenta.

Isoniazid is metabolised primarily in the liver, and the metabolites and unchanged drug are excreted in the urine. Isoniazid undergoes acetylation and the half-life of the drug is dependent on the acetylator status of the patient. In fast-acetylators its half-life is 1.2 hours and in slow acetylators 3.5 hours.

SPECTRUM OF ACTIVITY

Isoniazid is only active against mycobacteria, including *Mycobacterium tuberculosis, Mycobacterium bovis* and some strains of *Mycobacterium kansasii.*

USES

Isoniazid is a first-line antitubercular agent routinely used in both the initial and maintenance phases of tuberculosis therapy. The standard adult dose is 300–450 mg daily, preferably given one hour before breakfast. When given intermittently (twice weekly) for maintenance therapy the dose is 15 mg/kg (up to 750 mg). Pyridoxine is usually given with isoniazid to prevent development of isoniazid induced peripheral neuropathy.

Isoniazid is also used for the prevention of tuberculosis in certain high-risk groups of patients. In this instance the drug is given alone in a dose of 5–10 mg/kg daily (maximum 300 mg) for 6–12 months.

ADVERSE DRUG REACTIONS

Isoniazid is generally considered the safest of the first-line agents. The most important toxic effect of the drug is hepatic injury. About 10% of patients taking isoniazid develop abnormal liver function tests and a small number of these go on to develop hepatitis. Whilst the exact mechanism of this reaction has not been elucidated, it is thought that it may be due to the conversion of isoniazid to acetylhydrazine or related hepatotoxic metabolites which are capable of causing hepatic necrosis. The incidence of hepatotoxicity is higher in the elderly and those who consume alcohol. It

is also thought that isoniazid and rifampicin have additive hepatotoxicity.

Peripheral neuropathy is another adverse effect of concern. It results from pyridoxine deficiency secondary to isoniazid's ability to stimulate tryptophan metabolism. Common early signs are burning and tingling of hands and feet. Occasionally optic neuritis, seizures, ataxia and psychoses develop. The incidence of these neurotoxic effects is higher in slow acetylators and may be prevented by co-administration of pyridoxine.

Other side effects seen with isoniazid include hypersensitivity reactions (rashes, fever, lymphadenopathy and vasculitis), haematological reactions (agranulocytosis, haemolytic anaemia, thrombocytopenia), a rheumatic syndrome and a systemic lupus-like syndrome.

DRUG INTERACTIONS

Antacids containing aluminium hydroxide may decrease isoniazid absorption. Isoniazid may decrease the metabolism of phenytoin and carbamazepine, particularly in patients who are slow acetylators, resulting in potentiation of these drugs' toxicity.

PRECAUTIONS AND CONTRAINDICATIONS

Isoniazid is contraindicated in patients with acute liver disease or a history of isoniazid induced hepatitis. The drug should also not be used in patients with a history of serious adverse reactions to isoniazid such as drug fever, chills or arthritis.

All patients receiving isoniazid should have baseline liver function tests performed and repeated at regular intervals during therapy. Patients should be informed of the possibility of hepatotoxicity and instructed to cease the drug if symptoms of liver disease appear. Patients should be advised to abstain from alcohol whilst taking the drug.

Periodic ophthalmic checks are indicated during isoniazid therapy if visual symptoms occur.

Rifampicin

Rifampicin was introduced in 1970 and is now established as the first-ranking companion

INFECTIOUS DISEASES

30

drug to isoniazid. This drug is discussed in detail in the section on antibacterial agents.

SPECTRUM OF ACTIVITY

Rifampicin is active against *Mycobacterium tuberculosis* and other mycobacteria including *Mycobacterium avium-intracellulare* and *Mycobacterium leprae*.

USES

Rifampicin, like isoniazid, is used both in the initial and maintenance phases of tuberculosis treatment. The standard adult dose for patients weighing less than 50 kg is 450 mg daily and for those weighing more than 50 kg, 600 mg daily. The drug should be given one hour before breakfast.

Rifampicin exerts a prolonged bacteriostatic effect (up to three days) and therefore may be used in intermittent (twice weekly) maintenance regimens. In this case the adult dose is 10 mg/kg (up to 600 mg). Intermittent therapy is, however, associated with a higher incidence of flu-like and respiratory side effects.

For information on adverse drug reactions, drug interactions, precautions and contraindications and trade names see section on antibacterial agents.

Pyrazinamide

Pyrazinamide is a synthetic nicotinamide derivative.

TRADE NAMES

Pyrazinamide: *Zinamide*.

MECHANISM OF ACTION

The mechanism of action of pyrazinamide has not been fully elucidated. Its action is thought in part to be dependent on its conversion to pyrazinoic acid by mycobacterial pyrazinamidases. Pyrazinoic acid appears to have specific antimycobacterial activity. Pyrazinamide is bactericidal in an acid medium. Resistance to the drug, however, develops rapidly if it is used alone.

PHARMACOKINETICS

Pyrazinamide is well absorbed orally. Following absorption it distributes widely into body tissues and fluids including the lung, liver and cerebrospinal fluid. The drug is initially metabolised in the liver to pyrazinoic acid (major active metabolite), then further hydroxylated to 5-hydroxypyrazinoic acid before being excreted in the urine. The normal half-life of the drug is about 9–10 hours, but this may be prolonged in patients with renal or hepatic disease.

SPECTRUM OF ACTIVITY

Pyrazinamide is only active against *Mycobacterium tuberculosis*.

USES

Pyrazinamide is used in the initial phase of treatment for tuberculosis caused by *Mycobacterium tuberculosis*. The usual adult dose is 25 mg/kg daily (maximum 2 g daily) given in two or three divided doses. It may, however, be continued for the full duration of therapy dependent on the sensitivities of the infecting organisms. If used for maintenance therapy the drug may be given on an intermittent basis (twice weekly); the usual dose is 50 mg/kg (maximum 2.5 g).

ADVERSE DRUG REACTIONS

Pyrazinamide is relatively non-toxic when used at the recommended dosage of 25 mg/kg daily. However, at higher doses it is associated with a significant incidence of hepatotoxicity. The drug interferes with the excretion of uric acid leading to hyperuricaemia in most patients, although gout rarely occurs. Other side effects reported with pyrazinamide include nausea, vomiting, arthralgias, rashes, anaemia, drug fever and renal impairment.

PRECAUTIONS AND CONTRAINDICATIONS

Pyrazinamide is contraindicated in patients with a previous allergy to the drug or those with severe hepatic damage.

Patients receiving the drug should have regular monitoring of liver function tests (fortnightly) and the drug should be discontinued if signs of liver disease develop. The drug should be used with caution in patients with renal disease, a history of gout or diabetes mellitus (pyrazinamide may affect diabetic control).

Ethambutol

Ethambutol is a synthetic diamine derivative introduced into general use in 1966. It is bacteriostatic in action and has replaced para-aminosalicylic acid as a first line agent. In comparison to rifampicin and isoniazid it is a relatively weak antitubercular agent.

TRADE NAMES

Ethambutol: *Myambutol.*

MECHANISM OF ACTION

The mechanism of action of ethambutol is not fully understood. It is thought to act in part by inhibition of the synthesis of essential metabolites in susceptible bacteria, resulting in impaired cellular metabolism, arrest of cell division and cell death. The drug is only active against actively dividing bacteria.

PHARMACOKINETICS

Ethambutol is about 80% absorbed after oral administration. Following absorption the drug is distributed into most body fluids and tissues, with the highest concentrations found in erythrocytes, lungs, saliva and kidneys. The drug crosses the blood brain barrier when the meninges are inflamed.

The drug is excreted primarily unchanged (80%) in the urine by glomerular filtration. About 10% of the drug is metabolised to the inactive dicarboxylic acid derivative. In patients with normal renal function the half-life is 3–4 hours.

SPECTRUM OF ACTIVITY

Ethambutol is active against a wide range of mycobacteria, including some strains of *Mycobacterium avium-intracellulare.* Resistance to the drug develops rapidly when it is used alone, thus it is given in combination with other antitubercular agents.

Ethambutol is inactive against other bacteria, fungi and viruses.

USES

Ethambutol is used in the initial phase of treatment of tuberculosis in a dose of 20–25 mg/kg daily. If treatment is continued in the maintenance phase the daily dose should be reduced to 15 mg/kg. At these dosages the risk of damage to the optic nerve is markedly reduced.

The drug is also suitable for intermittent dosing. In this case the dose is 30–40 mg/kg (maximum 2 g). Dosage reduction is required in patients with renal impairment.

ADVERSE DRUG REACTIONS

Optic neuritis which produces a defect in visual acuity, especially red-green vision, is the most important adverse effect of ethambutol therapy. As mentioned this occurs more frequently when the daily dose exceeds 25 mg/kg. Discontinuation of the drug is usually associated with complete recovery. Other side effects include skin rashes, peripheral neuritis, hyperuricaemia and leucopenia.

PRECAUTIONS AND CONTRAINDICATIONS

Ethambutol is contraindicated in patients with a previous allergy to the drug or those with optic neuritis. All patients commenced on ethambutol should have baseline visual acuity testing carried out and this should be repeated periodically during therapy. Patients should be advised to contact their doctor if they notice any change in their vision.

Streptomycin

Streptomycin is rarely used these days. Its use is now restricted to those patients in whom other first-line agents cannot be used or who have infections due to multidrug resistant *Mycobacterium* sp.

The standard daily dose of streptomycin is 1 g for patients weighing more than 50 kg and 750 mg for patients weighing less than 50 kg. The dose should be reduced in the elderly and those with renal impairment. In all patients serum levels should be monitored; peak levels should be less than 20 mg/L and trough levels less than 3 mg/L. Streptomycin may also be used for intermittent therapy when, unlike other antitubercular drugs, the dose remains the same.

For information on mechanism of action, pharmacokinetics, adverse effects, precautions and contraindications see section on aminoglycosides.

SECOND-LINE AGENTS

Second-line drugs include such agents as para-aminosalicylic acid, prothionamide, ethionamide, kanamycin, cycloserine, clarithromycin and capreomycin. All are effective when used in appropriate circumstances, but are more toxic than first-line agents. Their use is now reserved for treatment of infection due to multidrug resistant *Mycobacterium tuberculosis* strains and some atypical mycobacterial infections. Recently, fluoroquinolones have been used to treat mycobacterial infections, however, their exact place in antitubercular therapy is yet to be established. The dosages and major toxicities of the second-line agents are shown in Table 30.6.

NURSING IMPLICATIONS

ASSESSMENT

The patient's general physical condition, history of drug hypersensitivity, liver or kidney disease or alcohol abuse, should be assessed before therapy is commenced. A history of liver damage contraindicates the use of isoniazid, pyrazinamide and rifampicin. Doses of ethambutol, streptomycin and capreomycin should be reduced in patients with poor renal function. Plasma concentrations of cycloserine and streptomycin should be monitored during therapy. Baseline visual function should be established before ethambutol therapy is commenced, and auditory function established prior to streptomycin therapy.

ADMINISTRATION

A daily dosage schedule is recommended for antitubercular agents. Gastrointestinal irritation caused by ethambutol can be reduced by giving the drug with food. Drug therapy may need to be closely supervised to ensure compliance.

EVALUATION

The patient's response to antitubercular drugs should be evaluated with close attention paid to adverse effects on the

TABLE 30.6 Second-line antitubercular agents

Drug	Dosage	Toxicity
Para-aminosalicylic acid	12 g orally daily in divided doses	Gastrointestinal, hepatic, renal, hypersensitivity
Prothionamide/ethionamide	500–750 mg orally daily in divided doses	Gastrointestinal
Capreomycin, kanamycin Clarithromycin	1 g IM daily 1 g orally daily	Renal, vestibular, auditory Gastrointestinal
Cycloserine	500–750 mg orally daily in divided doses	Neurological, haematological (rare)

liver, kidneys and central nervous system. Auditory and vestibular function should be monitored with streptomycin, haematological function with cycloserine and ethambutol, and ophthalmic function with ethambutol and isoniazid.

PATIENT EDUCATION

Patients should be made aware of the importance of compliance with the prescribed regimen. Patients prescribed rifampicin should be warned that it may interfere with the effectivenss of oral contraceptives and it will colour body secretions orange. The wearing of soft contact lenses is not advised during rifampicin treatment. Patients receiving ethambutol or isoniazid should be advised to immediately report any visual disturbances to their doctor.

ANTILEPROTIC AGENTS ■

The mainstay of the treatment of leprosy caused by *Mycobacterium leprae* is dapsone, which is effective in all forms and stages of the disease. In cases of dapsone intolerance (e.g. early polyneuritis, acute reaction or psychosis) or dapsone resistance, clofazimine may be substituted. Rifampicin is also a highly effective agent in the management of leprosy, however, rapid development of resistance to this agent precludes its use as a single agent.

COMBINATION THERAPY

Combination therapy is recommended for the treatment of all forms of leprosy:

a) *Paucibacillary leprosy* (intermediate, tuberculoid or borderline tuberculoid)
Dapsone 100 mg orally daily for 6 months
plus
Rifampicin 600 mg orally once monthly for 6 months

b) *Multibacillary leprosy* (borderline, borderline lepromatous or lepromatous)
Dapsone 100 mg orally daily
plus
Rifampicin 600 mg orally once monthly
plus
Clofazimine 50–100 mg daily
Prothionamide may be substituted for clofazimine if side effects are intolerable.

Dapsone

Dapsone is known as the 'parent sulfone' of a group of synthetic compounds, the sulfones, that have antileprotic activity.

MECHANISM OF ACTION

The exact mechanism of action of dapsone is unknown, however it may act in a similar manner to the sulfonamides as its activity is inhibited by para-aminobenzoic acid. Dapsone is generally bacteriostatic in action.

PHARMACOKINETICS

Dapsone is almost completely absorbed from the gastrointestinal tract following oral administration. It is distributed into most body tissues, including the skin, muscle, kidneys and liver. The drug crosses the placenta and is found in breast milk.

Dapsone is extensively metabolised in the liver, principally to acetyl derivatives. About 20% of the drug is excreted in the urine unchanged, the remainder is excreted as metabolites. The average half-life of the drug is 21 hours.

SPECTRUM OF ACTIVITY

Dapsone is active against *Mycobacterium leprae, Pneumocystis carinii* and *Plasmodium* sp.

INFECTIOUS DISEASES

30

USES

Dapsone is used in the initial phase of leprosy treatment (see above) and long-term maintenance therapy (which may be lifelong) of multibacillary leprosy.

Dapsone has been used in combination with pyrimethamine for the prevention of malaria (see Antimalarial Agents). This combination may also be used to prevent relapses of *Pneumocystis carinii* infections. Dapsone has been used in combination with trimethoprim (20 mg/kg/day) to treat pneumocystosis in AIDS patients. The drug is also used to treat a number of dermatological conditions including dermatitis herpetiformis and bullous pemphigoid.

ADVERSE DRUG REACTIONS

Dapsone therapy may be associated with considerable toxicity. Haemolytic anaemia and methaemoglobinaemia are common side effects. The drug may also cause the so called leprosy reaction states classified as reversal reactions and erythema nodosum leprosum. These occur as a result of activation of the body's defence mechanisms.

Dapsone may cause an acute hepatitis or a hypersensitivity cholestatic jaundice. It is potentially nephrotoxic causing nephrotic syndrome and/or acute renal failure in some patients. Gastrointestinal adverse effects include anorexia, abdominal pain, nausea and vomiting. The drug may also cause serious skin reactions (e.g. exfoliative dermatitis, erythema multiforme), peripheral neuropathy, phototoxicity, agranulocytosis, blurred vision, lupus erythematosus and an acute mononucleosis-type syndrome.

DRUG INTERACTIONS

The effectiveness of clofazimine may be reduced by concurrent administration of dapsone. The haematological toxicity of dapsone may be enhanced by the administration of other folate antagonists or other drugs associated with haemolytic anaemia (e.g. primaquine, nalidixic acid, nitrates).

PRECAUTIONS AND CONTRAINDICATIONS

Dapsone is contraindicated in patients with a history of allergy to the drug. It should not be given to patients with severe anaemia and should be used with extreme caution in patients with glucose-6-phosphate dehydrogenase deficiency.

All patients receiving dapsone should have regular monitoring of full blood picture and liver function tests. Patients should be instructed to report any pallor, sore throat, purpura, fever or jaundice to their doctor.

Clofazimine

Clofazimine has both antimycobacterial and anti-inflammatory activity. It is a phenazine dye.

MECHANISM OF ACTION

Clofazimine possibly acts by binding to mycobacterial DNA and inhibiting bacterial replication and growth. The drug appears to be slowly bactericidal.

PHARMACOKINETICS

Absorption of clofazimine from the gastrointestinal tract is variable, being dependent on the formulation administered and the presence of food which has an enhancing effect. Following absorption it is distributed principally into adipose tissue and cells of the reticuloendothelial system. The drug does not enter the cerebrospinal fluid, however it does cross the placenta and is distributed into breast milk. Clofazimine is excreted principally in the faeces, mainly as unchanged drug. The drug has a extremely long half-life of around 8 days.

SPECTRUM OF ACTIVITY

Clofazimine has a broad spectrum of activity against mycobacterium including *Mycobacterium leprae, Mycobacterium tuberculosis* and *Mycobacterium avium-intracellulare*.

USES

Clofazimine may be used in combination with dapsone in the treatment of multibacillary leprosy or instead of dapsone in dapsone resistance or intolerance. Clofazimine is also used to treat and prevent erythema nodosum leprosum and for the treatment of other mycobacterial infections, particularly those caused by *Mycobacterium avium-intracellulare*.

ADVERSE DRUG REACTIONS

Clofazimine is generally well tolerated in daily doses of 100 mg or less. The major adverse effects of the drug involve the skin (pink to brownish-black discolouration, ichthyosis and dryness), the eyes (reversible, dose related, red-brown discolouration of the conjunctiva, cornea and lacrimal fluid) and gastrointestinal tract (abdominal and epigastric pain, diarrhoea, nausea and vomiting). The gastrointestinal effects can be severe, particularly in patients on high doses, and include bowel obstruction, splenic infarction, haemorrhage and eosinophilic enteritis.

DRUG INTERACTIONS

See dapsone.

PRECAUTIONS AND CONTRAINDICATIONS

Clofazimine, because of its potential to cause gastrointestinal side effects, should be used with caution in patients with gastrointestinal symptoms such as diarrhoea or abdominal pain. Development of gastrointestinal symptoms may require a reduction in dosage or drug withdrawal.

Patients should be warned of the risk of skin discolouration (which is reversible but often persists for a long time) as well as discolouration of tears, urine, faeces, conjunctiva, breast milk, sebum and nasal secretions.

ANTIMALARIAL AGENTS ■■■■■

Malaria is one of the six most common infectious diseases of tropical and developing countries. Despite intensive programs to eradicate the disease, evidence suggests that in some areas it is on the increase. Although Australia is free from malaria, many cases of imported malaria are reported each year amongst visitors to endemic areas. Today the prevention and treatment of malaria is hindered by increasing resistance to antimalarial agents.

CHEMOPROPHYLACTIC AGENTS

The choice of antimalarial to prevent the development of malaria is determined by a number of factors including:

1. the risk of exposure to anopheline mosquitoes carrying malarial parasites;

2. patterns of antimalarial resistance;

3. duration of the person's stay in the malarious area;

4. the person's immune status;

5. the person's age and race; and

6. the person's history of adverse effects.

The agents that have been used for malaria prophylaxis include chloroquine, hydroxychloroquine, pyrimethamine–dapsone, pyrimethamine–sulfadoxine, mefloquine and doxycycline. The indications for currently recommended drugs are summarised in Table 30.7. Continuing and changing patterns of *Plasmodium falciparum* resistance have meant frequent revision of prophylactic recommendations.

Chloroquine

Chloroquine is a valuable antimalarial agent which has been used extensively over the last three to four decades for both the prevention and treatment of malaria. It is a synthetic 4-aminoquinolone derivative.

INFECTIOUS DISEASES

30

TABLE 30.7 Recommendations for malaria chemoprophylaxis

First Choice Agents	Alternative Agents
Areas without chloroquine resistant malaria Chloroquine	Doxycycline
Areas with chloroquine resistant malaria Doxycycline	Mefloquine Chloroquine plus doxycycline
Areas with multidrug resistant malaria (including mefloquine resistance) Mefloquine	Doxycycline Chloroquine plus doxycycline Chloroquine (plus treatment dose of mefloquine)*

*For long-term prophylaxis in low risk areas

TRADE NAMES

Chloroquine: *Chlorquin; Nivaquine.*

MECHANISM OF ACTION

Chloroquine is thought to act through a number of mechanisms including binding to nucleoproteins and inhibiting protein synthesis.

SPECTRUM OF ACTIVITY

Chloroquine is active against the asexual erythrocytic forms of most strains of *Plasmodium vivax, Plasmodium ovale* and *Plasmodium malariae*. Although the drug is active against *Plasmodium falciparum* resistance is becoming widespread. The drug is not active against the pre-erythrocytic or exo-erythrocytic forms of the plasmodia.

PHARMACOKINETICS

Chloroquine is rapidly and almost completely absorbed from the gastrointestinal tract. The drug is widely distributed in the body and is concentrated in many tissues and in erythrocytes. Chloroquine is partially metabolised and the parent drug and metabolites are excreted slowly in the urine. The drug has a half-life of 72–120 hours.

USES

Chloroquine may be used as a single agent for malaria chemoprophylaxis in persons travelling to areas where resistance to the drug is low or when the duration of possible exposure is short (less than eight weeks). However, it is more frequently used in combination with doxycycline because of problems with chloroquine resistant *Plasmodium falciparum*. In this setting it is used to prevent attacks of vivax, ovale and malariae malaria. The usual adult prophylactic dose is 300 mg of chloroquine base once weekly, commencing one week before entering the malarious area and continuing for four weeks after departing.

Chloroquine remains the drug of choice for the treatment of chloroquine sensitive *Plasmodium falciparum* infections and all other forms of malaria. The dose used is 600 mg of chloroquine base initially, followed by 300 mg 6–8 hours later, then 300 mg daily for two days. In patients with severe attacks, the drug may be given parenterally. In patients with vivax and ovale malaria, treatment with chloroquine should be followed by a course of primaquine to eradicate exo-erythrocytic forms of the parasites and prevent relapses.

ADVERSE DRUG REACTIONS

The side effects commonly seen with prophylactic doses of chloroquine are gastrointestinal disturbances, headache and skin eruptions. Following prolonged therapy, serious and sometimes irreversible toxicity can occur. This includes ocular changes (retinopathy being the most serious), gastrointestinal disturbances, dermatological reactions, neurological reactions and blood dyscrasias (including aplastic anaemia).

DRUG INTERACTIONS

Chloroquine may diminish the antibody response to rabies vaccine, hence coadministration is not recommended.

PRECAUTIONS AND CONTRAINDICATIONS

Chloroquine is contraindicated in patients with a history of allergy to the drug. The use of chloroquine in combination with pyrimethamine–sulfadoxine is no longer recommended. The combination has been associated with a higher incidence of serious and sometimes fatal skin reactions such as Stevens-Johnson syndrome.

Patients receiving long-term prophylactic therapy with chloroquine (more than three years) should have regular ophthalmological examinations (every 3–6 months). Patients should also be warned that the drug may affect visual accommodation. Haematological monitoring is also indicated in patients on long-term chloroquine therapy.

Chloroquine should be used with caution on patients with psoriasis as it may aggravate this condition.

Hydroxychloroquine

Hydroxychloroquine (*Plaquenil*) is a hydroxylated derivative of chloroquine and has a similar mode of action and spectrum of activity against *Plasmodium* sp. As with chloroquine resistance is a problem; *Plasmodium falciparum* resistant to chloroquine are also resistant to hydroxychloroquine.

Hydroxychloroquine has not been shown to have any therapeutic advantage over chloroquine. When used for malaria chemoprophylaxis the drug is given in a dose of 310 mg of base once weekly. It is only used when chloroquine is not available. Hydroxychloroquine is more commonly used in the treatment of systemic lupus erythematosus and rheumatoid arthritis.

Pyrimethamine Combinations: Pyrimethamine–Sulfadoxine, Pyrimethamine–Dapsone

Pyrimethamine, an antifolate drug which acts in a similar fashion to trimethoprim, is no longer used alone for malaria prophylaxis because of widespread resistance to the drug. Instead it is used in combination with a sulfonamide or sulfone, with which it acts synergistically.

TRADE NAMES

Pyrimethamine–Sulfadoxine: *Fansidar*.
Pyrimethamine–Dapsone: *Maloprim*.

MECHANISM OF ACTION

Pyrimethamine blocks the conversion of dihydrofolic acid to tetrahydrofolic acid by inhibiting dihydrofolate reductase. Sulfonamides, like sulfadoxine, inhibit the previous step of folate metabolism, the conversion of para-aminobenzoic acid to dihydrofolic acid. Thus, the combination has synergistic activity. Dapsone is also thought to exert an antifolate effect.

PHARMACOKINETICS

Pyrimethamine is well absorbed from the gastrointestinal tract following oral administration. It distributes mainly into the kidneys, lungs, liver and spleen. The drug is partially metabolised and the unchanged drug and metabolites are excreted in the urine. The average half-life of the drug is 100 hours. The average half-life of sulfadoxine is 200 hours and of dapsone 25 hours.

The pharmacokinetics of sulfonamides and dapsone have been discussed in detail previously in this chapter.

SPECTRUM OF ACTIVITY

Pyrimethamine alone and in combination with other folate antagonists inhibits the asexual erythrocytic forms of susceptible *Plasmodium* sp. Pyrimethamine–sulfadoxine and pyrimethamine–dapsone are active against many strains of *Plasmodium falci-*

INFECTIOUS DISEASES

30

parum, however, antifolate resistance is becoming a problem.

USES

Pyrimethamine–dapsone (25 mg/100 mg) given in a dose of one tablet weekly, has been used for malaria chemoprophylaxis and is preferred to pyrimethamine–sulfadoxine (25 mg/500 mg) once weekly because of serious side effects attributed to the latter (see below). Prophylaxis should commence two weeks before entering malarious areas and continue for four weeks after departing.

Pyrimethamine–sulfadoxine has also been used to treat acute attacks of chloroquine resistant *Plasmodium falciparum* malaria. In this case it is usually given as a single dose of three tablets (75 mg/1500 mg) in conjunction with quinine therapy.

ADVERSE DRUG REACTIONS

Pyrimethamine used alone or in low doses for malaria prophylaxis is associated with few side effects. Prolonged therapy with high doses (as used in toxoplasmosis) may result in folate deficiency and megaloblastic anaemia.

The combination of pyrimethamine and sulfadoxine has been reported to cause severe dermatological reactions including erythema multiforme, Stevens-Johnson syndrome and toxic epidermal necrolysis, some of which have resulted in fatalities. Aplastic anaemia and other blood dyscrasias, hypersensitivity reactions and hepatocellular necrosis have been attributed to the sulfonamide and sulfone components of the combinations. Pyrimethamine–dapsone should never be given in a dose greater than one tablet weekly, as a number of deaths have been reported with the use of higher doses.

PRECAUTIONS AND CONTRAINDICATIONS

The use of pyrimethamine–sulfadoxine or pyrimethamine–dapsone is contraindicated in patients with a known allergy to either component. These combinations should not be administered to pregnant women, nor should they be used in infants under the age of 4 weeks. They should be used with caution in patients with hepatic and/or renal impairment. Patients should be informed of the possible risk of adverse events and to discontinue the drug if they develop a rash, erythema, pruritus, urogenital lesions or a sore throat. Patients receiving long-term prophylaxis with these combinations should have regular haematological monitoring.

Mefloquine

Mefloquine is a quinolinemethanol derivative, structurally related to quinine. It is used both for the prevention and treatment of malaria, including chloroquine resistant *Plasmodium falciparum* infections.

TRADE NAMES

Mefloquine: *Lariam*.

MECHANISM OF ACTION

Like chloroquine, mefloquine is active against the asexual erythrocytic forms of plasmodia. Its mechanism of action is unknown.

PHARMACOKINETICS

Mefloquine is well absorbed from the gastrointestinal tract. Following absorption it is largely taken up in the liver, but also into erythrocytes, lungs, muscles, brain and retina. Mefloquine is extensively metabolised and only a small proportion of the drug is excreted unchanged in the urine. The average half-life of the drug is 21 days.

SPECTRUM OF ACTIVITY

Mefloquine is active against all species of malaria parasites including those resistant to chloroquine and/or antifolate drugs. Unfortunately, resistance to mefloquine is now becoming a problem, particularly in Asia.

USES

Mefloquine is indicated for short-term and long-term prophylaxis for patients travelling or living in areas where chloroquine resistance and antifolate resistance are common. In this situation the prophylactic dose is 250 mg weekly commencing one week before entering the malarious area and continuing for two weeks after departure. Mefloquine or doxycycline are now recommended in place of pyrimethamine combinations.

Mefloquine may also be used to treat acute attacks of malaria, including those due to chloroquine resistant *Plasmodium falciparum*. The dose for non-immune patients is 750 mg initially, followed by 500 mg 6–8 hours later. If the patient weighs more than 60 kg, then a further dose of 250 mg should be given in another 6–8 hours. If used to treat vivax malaria, follow-up therapy with primaquine will be required to clear the liver forms.

ADVERSE DRUG REACTIONS

The major concern associated with the use of mefloquine is central nervous system toxicity. Vertigo, confusion, psychosis and convulsions have been reported with both treatment and prophylactic doses. Use of the drug is therefore not advised in patients with a history of epilepsy or psychiatric illness, and those whose occupation requires fine coordination and spatial discrimination.

Mefloquine has also been reported to cause gastrointestinal disturbances, headache, nightmares, anaemia and bradycardia.

DRUG INTERACTIONS

Mefloquine may prolong cardiac conduction leading to bradycardia. When combined with β blockers, calcium antagonists and other agents which prolong cardiac conduction, severe bradycardia and cardiac arrest may occur. Mefloquine should not be used in combination with quinine or quinidine because of additive toxicity.

PRECAUTIONS AND CONTRAINDICATIONS

The safety of mefloquine in patients with renal impairment or severe liver disease has not yet been established, thus its use should be avoided in such patients. Because of its neurotoxicity the drug should be used with extreme caution in patients with a history of epilepsy or psychiatric disorder. Mefloquine is teratogenic in animals, and women of child-bearing age should take an effective contraceptive during, and for at least three months after their last dose of the drug. The drug should be used with caution in patients with cardiac disease.

Doxycycline

Doxycycline is used for the suppression or chemoprophylaxis of malaria caused by multidrug resistant (including chloroquine resistant) *Plasmodium falciparum*. The usual prophylactic dose is 100 mg orally daily, commencing two days prior to entering the malarious area and continuing for two weeks after departure. If used with chloroquine the dose is reduced to 50 mg daily. Once daily dosing poses problems of compliance, however taken correctly doxycycline is a highly effective agent.

For information on mechanism of action, pharmacokinetics, adverse effects, interactions, precautions and contraindications see the section on tetracyclines.

THERAPEUTIC AGENTS

Chloroquine remains the mainstay of treatment for all forms of malaria, except those caused by chloroquine resistant *Plasmodium falciparum*. For those infections quinine is the drug of choice. However, as already discussed mefloquine, pyrimethamine–sulfadoxine and doxycycline may be used as alternatives. Primaquine has a specific role in *Plasmodium vivax* and *Plasmodium ovale* infections.

Quinine

Quinine is a naturally occurring alkaloid obtained from the bark of the cinchona tree. Quinine was one of the first agents used to prevent and treat malarial infections. Today, its use is generally restricted

INFECTIOUS DISEASES

30

to the treatment of chloroquine resistant falciparum malaria.

MECHANISM OF ACTION

The exact mechanism of quinine's antimalarial activity has not been elucidated, but it appears to interfere with DNA function. Quinine also exerts a number of other effects on the body including skeletal muscle relaxation, local anaesthetic, analgesic, antipyretic and oxytoxic effects, and prolongation of cardiac conduction.

PHARMACOKINETICS

Quinine is rapidly and completely absorbed following oral administration. It is widely distributed into body tissues and fluids including the cerebrospinal fluid. The drug crosses the placenta and may be detected in breast milk. The drug is bound to serum proteins and the degree of binding is higher in patients with malaria (about 90%) compared with healthy volunteers. Quinine is extensively metabolised mainly in the liver, then excreted in the urine. The average half-life of the drug ranges between 7 and 12 hours in adults with malaria.

SPECTRUM OF ACTIVITY

Quinine is active against the asexual erythrocytic forms of all species of plasmodia, including chloroquine resistant *Plasmodium falciparum*. It does not act on pre-erythrocytic or exo-erythrocytic forms of the parasite.

USES

The primary indication for the use of quinine is the treatment of chloroquine resistant *Plasmodium falciparum* malaria. It is also indicated for the treatment of cerebral malaria, and for the treatment of vivax malaria when chloroquine cannot be given. In the latter case primaquine is required to effect a radical cure.

Wherever possible quinine should be given orally, the recommended dose being 600 mg (quinine sulfate) 8-hourly for three days, then 600 mg 12-hourly for seven days. If intravenous therapy is indicated (e.g. in comatose patients) quinine dihydrochloride injection is used. Quinine treatment is often supplemented with a course of tetracycline (250 mg 6-hourly for seven days) or pyrimethamine–sulfadoxine (75 mg/1500 mg) as a single dose.

ADVERSE DRUG REACTIONS

Oral quinine is generally well tolerated, however it may produce a syndrome known as cinchonism. Mild to moderate forms manifest as tinnitus, headache, nausea and mild visual disturbances. Severe cinchonism is associated with adverse gastrointestinal, central nervous system, cardiovascular and dermatological effects. Apart from cinchonism, quinine may cause hypersensitivity reactions, blood dyscrasias (including thrombocytopenia and haemolytic anaemia), hepatitis and cardiac conduction disturbances. Intravenous quinine may produce severe hypotension, arrhythmias and acute circulatory failure if given too rapidly. In cases of severe malaria, quinine therapy has been associated with pronounced hypoglycaemia.

DRUG INTERACTIONS

Quinine decreases digoxin clearance and concurrent use may result in digoxin toxicity. Mefloquine and quinine can have additive cardiac toxicity, thus concurrent use of the two drugs should be avoided. Extreme care should be exercised when initiating quinine therapy in patients who have received prophylactic mefloquine.

PRECAUTIONS AND CONTRAINDICATIONS

Quinine is contraindicated in patients with a known hypersensitivity to the drug. Such patients should be warned to avoid quinine containing products such as tonic water or *Bitter Lemon*. Quinine is also contraindicated in patients with glucose-6-phosphate dehydrogenase deficiency as it may cause haemolytic anaemia in this group of patients. The drug should be used with caution in patients with cardiac conduction defects.

Quinidine

Quinidine is a stereoisomer of quinine. The drug possesses similar antimalarial activity to quinine, but more potent antiarrhythmic activity. It may be used to treat malaria if quinine is unavailable.

Primaquine Phosphate

Primaquine is an 8-aminoquinoline derivative used specifically to eliminate liver forms of *Plasmodium vivax* and *Plasmodium ovale* and thus prevent recurrent attacks.

MECHANISM OF ACTION

Primaquine may act by interfering with DNA function.

PHARMACOKINETICS

Primaquine is well absorbed orally and appears to be widely distributed into body tissues and fluids. The drug is extensively metabolised in the liver and little is excreted unchanged in the urine. The average half-life of the drug is around 7 hours.

SPECTRUM OF ACTIVITY

Primaquine is active against the fixed tissue (liver) pre-erythrocytic and exo-erythrocytic stages of *Plasmodia* sp. and is gametocyticidal against *Plasmodium falciparum*.

USES

Primaquine is used to produce a radical cure of relapsing vivax and ovale malaria. In acute attacks of vivax malaria or mixed infections, patients should be treated first with a fast-acting blood schizonticide such as chloroquine. The usual dose of primaquine is 15 mg of base daily for 14 days. However, this may need to be increased for patients acquiring malarial infections in Papua New Guinea.

ADVERSE DRUG REACTIONS

The most common adverse effects of oral primaquine are nausea, vomiting, epigastric pain and abdominal cramps. These effects may be reduced by giving the drug with food. Acute haemolytic anaemia may occur in patients with glucose-6-phosphate dehydrogenase deficiency. The drug may also cause a number of other haematological problems.

PRECAUTIONS AND CONTRAINDICATIONS

Primaquine is contraindicated in patients with granulocytopenia and those receiving other agents which may cause haemolysis or which may suppress bone marrow function. Patients with proven glucose-6-phosphate dehydrogenase or NADH-methaemoglobin reductase deficiencies should receive the drug with careful haematological monitoring. In pregnant women, treatment with primaquine should be delayed until after delivery.

NURSING IMPLICATIONS

ASSESSMENT

When antimalarial drugs are administered, either prophylactically or to treat an acute attack, the nurse should be familiar with the type of drug to be used, its dosage regimen and adverse effects. Bearing in mind which drug has been ordered assessment should include such aspects as a history of cardiac, hepatic or renal impairment, haematological disorders, visual disturbances or convulsive disorders. Observation should include vital signs and the overall clinical appearance of the patient.

EVALUATION

If therapy is short term, evaluation should include observations for signs of gastrointestinal upsets (which can usually be remedied by giving the drug with meals) and allergic skin reactions.

During long-term therapy, the nurse should evaluate the patient for adverse effects such as visual impairment, blood dyscrasias, and cardiac, neurological, hepatic or renal problems, depending on the drug being used.

30 INFECTIOUS DISEASES

PATIENT EDUCATION

The nurse should advise patients of the importance of taking the medication strictly at the specified times and educate them concerning the signs of adverse effects and the importance of seeking medical advice if they occur.

Additional information on simple self-help measures to prevent mosquito bites and minimise the risk of malaria should be provided. These include the use of personal insect repellants containing diethyl toluamide; the use of mosquito nets, and sprays and coils to kill mosquitoes in non-airconditioned accommodation; and the wearing of light coloured clothing covering most of the body at and after dusk.

ANTIFUNGAL AGENTS ■■■■■■■■■

Most of the major antibiotics are produced by fungi and it is not surprising that fungi should be resistant to them. There are, however, some highly specialised antibiotics and synthetic compounds that are effective as antifungal agents and, in general, have little or no antibacterial activity. In this section the antifungals have been grouped according to those used predominantly to treat systemic infections and those used to treat superficial infections.

SYSTEMIC INFECTIONS

Amphotericin B

Amphotericin B is a member of the polyene group of antifungals. It is produced by the soil actinomycete *Streptomyces nodosus*. It was introduced into clinical practice in 1956 and remains the drug of choice for a number of systemic fungal infections despite its considerable toxicity.

TRADE NAMES

Amphotericin B: *Fungilin; Fungizone*.

MECHANISM OF ACTION

Amphotericin B binds to sterols in the cell membrane of susceptible fungi and yeasts leading to an increase in cell permeability and a resultant leakage of molecules out of the cell. The drug is fungistatic or fungicidal, dependent on the concentration of the drug and fungal susceptibility.

PHARMACOKINETICS

Amphotericin B is not absorbed to any significant degree following oral or topical administration. Information about distribution of amphotericin in the body following intravenous administration is limited. Concentrations attained in the cerebrospinal fluid are less than 5% of the serum concentration.

In patients with normal renal function the half-life of amphotericin B is about 24 hours. The drug undergoes metabolism in the body and only 5% is excreted unchanged in the urine.

SPECTRUM OF ACTIVITY

Amphotericin B exhibits a broad spectrum of antifungal activity. The drug is active against *Candida* sp. (except *Candida tropicalis*), *Cryptococcus neoformans*, some strains of *Aspergillus* sp., *Torulopsis glabrata*, *Coccidioides immitis*, *Histoplasma capsulatum*, *Rhodotorula* and *Blastomyces* sp. and *Sporotrichum schenckii*. It is not active against the dermatophytes or ring-worm fungi. Fungi resistant to amphotericin B are usually resistant to other polyene antifungals. Acquisition of resistance to the drug during therapy is not a problem.

USES

Parenteral amphotericin B is used to treat systemic fungal infections including aspergillosis, disseminated candidiasis, pulmonary or disseminated cryptococcosis, mucormycosis, coccidioidomycosis, and pulmonary or disseminated histoplasmosis. In these cases the drug is usually given by slow intravenous infusion in glucose 5% solution over 4–6 hours. In patients with meningitis who fail to respond to intravenous treatment, the drug may be given intrathecally or intraventricularly.

Amphotericin B is often given with flucytosine when treating cryptococcal infections, as the combination appears to have synergistic activity. Amphotericin B is often given empirically to febrile neutropenic patients who fail to respond to appropriate antibacterial therapy. Such patients may have primary fungal infections or have developed fungal superinfections whilst receiving antibiotics.

Given orally, in the form of suspension or lozenges, amphotericin B is used to treat superficial *Candida* sp. infections. The drug may be used topically to treat vaginal candidiasis and be instilled into the bladder to treat urinary tract infections.

The colloid amphotericin B should be reconstituted with water for injections, then added to a glucose 5% solution, which has been buffered to a pH above 5.5, before being administered by intravenous infusion. The drug will precipitate if mixed with electrolyte solutions containing sodium chloride or potassium chloride, and glucose solutions of low pH.

ADVERSE DRUG REACTIONS

Amphotericin B is considered the most toxic antimicrobial in use today. Adverse reactions during parenteral administration are common and include fever, chills, rigors, headache, anorexia, nausea and vomiting. These effects are considered to be dose related and are usually less severe when the drug is infused slowly and used on alternate days. Premedication with an antipyretic (e.g. aspirin, paracetamol), an antihistamine and an antiemetic may provide symptomatic relief. Pethidine given before the infusion may also help alleviate these symptoms.

Although uncommon, anaphylactoid reactions may occur. For this reason a test dose of amphotericin B (1 mg in 250 mL of glucose 5% solution, infused over 2–3 hours) should be given prior to commencing therapy. This initial dose should be followed by a 5–10 mg dose on the second day. Thereafter, the daily dose should be increased slowly until a maintenance dose of 0.5–1 mg/kg is achieved. If the patient is unable to tolerate the side effects, then the dose should be reduced. If azotaemia occurs dosage reduction or even drug withdrawal may be necessary for a few days until the serum creatinine returns to an acceptable level.

Nephrotoxicity occurs in almost all patients receiving intravenous amphotericin B. In general it is reversible, however permanent damage has been reported in some patients. Renal toxicity may be minimised by adequate alkalinisation of the urine, using a small initial dose of amphotericin B and increasing the dose slowly, and by sodium loading. Permanent damage is seen more commonly in patients receiving a cumulative dose of amphotericin greater than 4–5 g.

Hypokalaemia due to a renal tubular defect develops in 25% of patients and requires potassium supplementation. Hypomagnesaemia may also develop due to increased renal loss.

Amphotericin B causes bone marrow suppression and a normochromic normocytic anaemia may develop in up to 75% of patients. This generally does not require transfusion and is reversible on drug withdrawal. Phlebitis from intravenous administration is common, but it may be prevented or reduced by slow infusion or the addition of low dose heparin to the infusion. Rapid administration of amphotericin B may result in severe cardiovascular toxicity including cardiac arrest.

Intrathecal injections of amphotericin B may produce headache, urinary retention, paraesthesias, pain along lumbar nerves and palsies.

INFECTIOUS DISEASES

30

DRUG INTERACTIONS

The combination of amphotericin B and flucytosine is synergistic against *Cryptococcus neoformans, Candida albicans* and *Candida tropicalis*. It is thought that amphotericin B increases flucytosine penetration into fungal cells by increasing cytoplasmic membrane permeability.

Co-administration of amphotericin B with other potentially nephrotoxic drugs (e.g. aminoglycosides, cisplatin, vancomycin) should be avoided where possible as they may enhance renal toxicity due to amphotericin.

PRECAUTIONS AND CONTRAINDICATIONS

Amphotericin B is contraindicated in patients with a history of allergy to the drug, unless no other therapy is available.

Patients given amphotericin B should have the following parameters monitored prior to commencing therapy and at regular intervals during therapy: haemoglobin; serum potassium, magnesium, bicarbonate, urea and creatinine; leucocyte count, platelet count; and liver function. Monitoring of serum potassium concentrations are particularly important in patients receiving digoxin or skeletal muscle relaxants.

NURSING IMPLICATIONS

ASSESSMENT

Amphotericin B is a toxic drug and all patients should be carefully assessed prior to its administration. The patient's history should be reviewed for previously undisclosed allergy to the drug, and renal or haematopoietic disorders. Results of laboratory tests (e.g. blood urea nitrogen, creatinine and serum potassium levels) should be at hand before administration commences. Specimens should be taken for culture and sensitivity testing prior to commencement of therapy. When a systemic infection is to be treated with parenteral amphotericin B, the nurse should estab-lish baseline observations of vital signs before therapy is commenced.

ADMINISTRATION

Intravenous administration is by slow infusion over 4–6 hours in glucose 5% which has been buffered to the correct pH. Do not infuse amphotericin B in saline or ward stock glucose solutions. Administer premedications (e.g. aspirin, antihistamines, pethidine) and urinary alkaliniser as ordered.

EVALUATION

During intravenous administration, the patient's vital signs should be monitored regularly due to the high incidence of adverse reactions associated with this agent. Watch for signs of thrombophlebitis such as redness and pain along the vein. As this drug can cause severe skin irritation extravasation should be avoided during administration.

Patients should be evaluated for signs of nephrotoxicity and hypokalaemia. Monitor urine output, as oliguria or haematuria could indicate nephrotoxicity. Muscle weakness is a sign of hypokalaemia. Liver function tests and a full blood picture should be performed regularly.

Flucytosine

Flucytosine (5-fluorocytosine) was synthesised in 1957 for the treatment of leukaemia. It is related to the cytotoxic drugs fluorouracil and floxuridine but is ineffective as an anticancer agent. However, it does have selective antifungal activity.

TRADE NAMES

Flucytosine: *Ancotil.*

MECHANISM OF ACTION

Flucytosine appears to penetrate fungal cells where it is converted to fluorouracil, a known antimetabolite. This is then thought to act as a false substrate within fungal cells, interfering with nucleic acid and protein synthesis.

PHARMACOKINETICS

Flucytosine is well absorbed from the gastrointestinal tract and is widely distributed into body tissues and fluids including the cerebrospinal fluid.

In patients with normal renal function the half-life of flucytosine is in the range 2.5–6 hours, however this is increased in patients with renal impairment. The drug is excreted principally unchanged in the urine.

SPECTRUM OF ACTIVITY

Flucytosine is active against *Cryptococcus neoformans, Candida albicans* and other *Candida* sp. and *Torulopsis glabrata.*

USES

Flucytosine is used as a second-line agent only in the treatment of serious infections caused by susceptible strains of *Candida* and *Cryptococcus* sp. Fungaemia, endocarditis, and urinary tract infections caused by *Candida* sp. and meningitis and pulmonary infections caused by *Cryptococcus* and *Candida* sp. have been effectively treated with this agent. However, the drug should not be used alone for serious infections as drug resistance rapidly occurs.

Flucytosine is available as tablets and an intravenous infusion. The infusion must be stored at a temperature around 25°C as cooling may cause precipitation of the drug and heat may cause conversion to the cytotoxic drug fluorouracil.

ADVERSE DRUG REACTIONS

Although flucytosine appears to have a low order of toxicity compared with amphotericin B, its use is not without risk. The drug exerts its major toxicity on the rapidly proliferating cells of the bone marrow and lining of the gastrointestinal tract.

Moderate bone marrow hypoplasia may occur resulting in anaemia, leucopenia, pancytopenia, thrombocytopenia and agranulocytosis (rare). These effects occur more commonly in patients with high serum flucytosine levels (>100 mg/L) and/or those receiving concurrent amphotericin B. Gastrointestinal effects include nausea, vomiting, abdominal distension and diarrhoea.

Hepatic dysfunction has been reported in about 5% of patients receiving flucytosine and regular assessment of liver function should be performed.

DRUG INTERACTIONS

A synergistic action occurs when flucytosine is combined with amphotericin B in the treatment of infections due to *Cryptococcus neoformans, Candida albicans* and *Candida tropicalis.*

PRECAUTIONS AND CONTRAINDICATIONS

Flucytosine is contraindicated in patients with a history of allergy to the drug. It should be used with extreme caution in patients with bone marrow suppression or renal impairment. The dose must be reduced in renal failure and serum levels should be monitored routinely. All patients receiving flucytosine should have regular assessment of renal, hepatic and haematological function.

NURSING IMPLICATIONS

ASSESSMENT

Assessment of patients should aim to identify any previously undisclosed history of liver, renal or haematopoietic disorders. Patients who are especially at risk include those who have recently had (or are receiving) chemotherapy or radiotherapy for malignancies, as these therapies can cause bone marrow suppression.

ADMINISTRATION

To decrease the incidence of nausea which can occur with this drug, the administration of oral doses may be spread over 15 minutes.

INFECTIOUS DISEASES

30

EVALUATION

Blood counts should be done frequently during the course of therapy, and the nurse should evaluate the patient for signs of bone marrow depression such as bruising, bleeding, haematuria or sore throat. The nurse should observe for, and report, any adverse gastrointestinal effects (e.g. diarrhoea, jaundice) or signs of central nervous system toxicity such as confusion, headache and vertigo. Blood samples should be taken at appropriate times to determine flucytosine blood levels.

SYSTEMIC AND SUPERFICIAL INFECTIONS

A range of imidazoles and triazoles are now available which may be used to treat systemic and superficial fungal infections. These include the imidazoles, ketoconazole and miconazole, and the triazoles, fluconazole and itraconazole.

Ketoconazole

Ketoconazole is a synthetic imidazole derivative which may be administered topically and orally to treat a wide range of superficial and systemic fungal infections.

TRADE NAMES

Ketoconazole: *Nizoral.*

MECHANISM OF ACTION

The activity of ketoconazole is dependent on its ability to inhibit lipid biosynthesis in fungal cell membranes. The synthesis of ergesterol, the principal cellular sterol, is affected along with other cell membrane lipids. These changes result in increased cell membrane permeability. Ketoconazole may also inhibit uptake of nucleic acid precursors and synthesis of oxidative and peroxidative enzymes. The combination of these effects may result in cell death.

PHARMACOKINETICS

Ketoconazole is rapidly absorbed from the gastrointestinal tract in the presence of an acidic pH. In patients with achlorhydria or those receiving histamine$_2$ (H$_2$) antagonists, the bioavailability of ketoconazole is markedly reduced.

Following absorption, the drug is detected in the urine, bile, saliva, sebum, cerumen, synovial fluid and cerebrospinal fluid. Ketoconazole levels in the central nervous system are generally very low.

Ketoconazole is metabolised in the liver to inactive metabolites. It is excreted in the bile, with 20%–65% of the unchanged drug recovered in the faeces. Only 5%–10% of the drug is excreted in the urine. The normal half-life of the drug is about 8 hours.

SPECTRUM OF ACTIVITY

Ketoconazole is active against most dermatophytes (e.g. *Trichophyton rubrum, Microsporum canis), Candida* sp., *Malassezia furfur, Paracoccidioides brasiliensis, Histoplasma capsulatum, Coccidioides immitis* and *Cryptococcus neoformans.*

USES

Ketoconazole may be used in the treatment of chronic mucocutaneous candidiasis, oral thrush, oesophageal candidiasis, coccidioidomycosis, histoplasmosis, blastomycosis and paracoccidioidomycosis. It may be used to treat recalcitrant cases of superficial mycoses which fail to respond to conventional therapy such as tinea versicolor, tinea pedis, tinea corporis and tinea cruris.

The usual dose of ketoconazole is 200 mg orally, daily with food. Larger doses may be indicated for systemic infections. A 2% ketoconazole cream is also available for treatment of cutaneous infections.

It has also been used in the treatment of prostatic carcinoma as it inhibits testosterone production.

ADVERSE DRUG REACTIONS

Ketoconazole commonly causes anorexia,

nausea and vomiting. These adverse effects may be reduced by administering the drug with food or at bed-time. Abdominal pain, pruritus, headache, chills and fevers, dizziness and photophobia may also occur. Ketoconazole can suppress plasma testosterone levels and can cause gynaecomastia, decreased libido, and loss of potency in males and menstrual irregularities in women. High doses of ketoconazole may suppress cortisol production. The most serious adverse effect of the drug is hepatotoxicity which, although uncommon, may manifest as fatal hepatic necrosis.

DRUG INTERACTIONS

Ketoconazole is poorly absorbed in the absence of gastric acidity, hence H$_2$ antagonists and antacids decrease its absorption. They should be taken after the ketoconazole dose. When ketoconazole and rifampicin are administered concurrently the effects of both drugs are significantly reduced. Ketoconazole may inhibit the metabolism of warfarin, cyclosporin and corticosteroids, enhancing their effects. Patients on ketoconazole may experience a disulfiram-like reaction if they drink alcohol.

PRECAUTIONS AND CONTRAINDICATIONS

Ketoconazole is contraindicated in patients with a previous allergy to imidazole derivatives. It should not be given to pregnant women, patients with hepatic failure or those recovering from hepatitis.

Patients prescribed ketoconazole should have their liver function assessed prior to commencing the drug and periodically during therapy. Patients should be informed that the drug may affect their liver and that they should see their doctor if any signs or symptoms of liver disease (e.g. fatigue, dark urine, jaundice) develop whilst on the drug.

Miconazole

Miconazole is a synthetic imidazole derivative which is used topically and parenterally.

TRADE NAMES

Miconazole: *Daktarin*; *Monistat*.

MECHANISM OF ACTION

See ketoconazole.

PHARMACOKINETICS

Oral administration fails to produce clinically significant serum levels of miconazole. Given intravenously the drug is widely distributed in the body, penetrating inflamed joints, the vitreous humour of the eye and the peritoneal cavity. Entry into the cerebrospinal fluid is variable. If the drug is used to treat meningitis, intrathecal therapy must be used concurrently with intravenous therapy. Following intravenous administration the drug undergoes liver metabolism to inactive metabolites. These metabolites are excreted in the urine.

SPECTRUM OF ACTIVITY

Miconazole has a similar spectrum of activity to ketoconazole, however the drug does possess some additional activity against *Aspergillus* sp. Apart from its antifungal activity, miconazole also has some activity against Gram positive bacteria and *Acanthamoeba* sp.

USES

Topically, miconazole is used extensively to treat dermatophytosis and candidiasis. The drug is available as a 2% cream, vaginal cream, tincture, powder and an oral gel. The gel is used to treat oropharyngeal candidiasis.

Intravenous miconazole may be used to treat systemic fungal infection, however relapses after treatment are a problem. Treatment failures are also not uncommon. The introduction of fluconazole and itraconazole have significantly reduced the clinical role of parenteral miconazole. When used parenterally, miconazole is given in a dose of 200–1200 mg 8-hourly, as a 30–60-minute infusion.

ADVERSE DRUG REACTIONS

Miconazole applied topically may produce local irritation and burning at the site of application.

30 INFECTIOUS DISEASES

Parenteral miconazole use has been associated with the development of phlebitis, (rouleau formation appears on smears of peripheral blood), haemolytic anaemia, thrombocytopenia and thrombocytosis, skin rashes and hyponatraemia. Hyperlipidaemia may occur and appears to be vehicle rather than drug induced. Anaphylactoid reactions may also occur. Rapid administration of the drug may precipitate tachycardia and other cardiac arrhythmias.

DRUG INTERACTIONS

Miconazole has the potential to interact with hepatically metabolised drugs in a similar manner to ketoconazole. It has been reported to enhance the effects of warfarin and sulfonylurea oral hypoglycaemic agents.

PRECAUTIONS AND CONTRAINDICATIONS

Miconazole is contraindicated in patients with a history of allergy to imidazole derivatives or the intravenous infusion vehicle (*Cremophor EL*). Patients receiving parenteral miconazole should have the following parameters monitored periodically: haematocrit, haemaglobin, serum sodium and lipids.

NURSING IMPLICATIONS

ASSESSMENT

Patients who are to receive ketoconazole should be assessed for concurrent use of antacids or H2 antagonists, as the absorption of this drug is reduced when there is insufficient stomach acid. Their history should also be reviewed to exclude any previous allergy to the drug or related compounds or liver disease.

When patients are to receive parenteral miconazole, the nurse should establish baseline records of vital signs, ensure there is no history of allergy to this preparation or others known to contain *Cremophor EL*, and ensure that all laboratory results concerning the patient's haematopoietic function are at hand.

ADMINISTRATION

Ketoconazole should be administered at night or with food to minimise adverse effects. Intravenous infusions of miconazole should be given slowly over one hour. As the fluid can cause severe irritation to the skin, it is important to prevent extravasation during administration.

EVALUATION

Patients who are receiving oral ketoconazole should be observed for signs of adverse reactions such as allergy, gastrointestinal upset and hepatotoxicity. Nursing evaluation of patients receiving miconazole intravenously should include frequent recording of vital signs to detect early signs of cardiac arrhythmias or allergic reactions. Observation for signs of phlebitis and skin irritation at the infusion site is also necessary.

Fluconazole, Itraconazole

The triazoles are structurally similar to the imidazole antifungals but have a wider range of activity. Two triazoles, fluconazole and itraconazole, are now available for clinical use.

TRADE NAMES

Fluconazole: *Diflucan*.

MECHANISM OF ACTION

The triazoles block fungal cytochrome P-450 dependent enzymes, blocking synthesis of ergestrol, the principal sterol in the fungal cell membrane.

PHARMACOKINETICS

Fluconazole is readily absorbed orally (94% bioavailability), with absorption unaffected by food. Following absorption it is widely distributed in the body. Cerebrospinal fluid concentrations range between 57% and 93% of serum concentrations, and fungicidal levels are achieved in saliva, vaginal tissue and nails. Unlike ketoconazole it does not undergo metabolism, rather it is excreted unchanged in the urine. Fluconazole has a half-life of about 30 hours.

Itraconazole is also well absorbed from the gastrointestinal tract, however unlike fluconazole it does not enter the brain or cerebrospinal fluid in therapeutic concentrations and is extensively metabolised in the liver. Less than 5% is excreted in the urine unchanged. The normal half-life of itraconazole is about 17 hours.

SPECTRUM OF ACTIVITY

Fluconazole is active against many systemic fungal pathogens including *Candida albicans, Cryptococcus neoformans, Coccidioides immitis* and *Histoplasma capsulatum*. It is also active against many of the dermatophytes; however it has minimal activity against *Aspergillus* sp.

Itraconazole, unlike fluconazole, is active against *Aspergillus* sp.

USES

Fluconazole is used in the treatment of oropharyngeal and oesophageal candidiasis, and systemic *Candida* sp. infections (e.g. urinary tract infections, endocarditis, peritonitis, pneumonia). It is also indicated for the treatment and prevention of cryptococcal meningitis. Fluconazole is also highly effective in the treatment of superficial candidiasis and dermatophytosis, however the drug should be reserved for the treatment of infections refractory to conventional therapy. Fluconazole may be given orally or by intravenous infusion. The usual dose ranges from 100 mg to 400 mg daily.

Itraconazole in combination with flucytosine has been used to treat cryptococcal meningitis in AIDS patients, and appears effective in preventing relapses. The drug has been extensively used in the treatment of superficial mycoses, and is useful in the treatment of a number of systemic fungal infections, including those caused by *Aspergillus* sp. The usual dose of itraconazole is 100 mg daily for superficial infections and up to 400 mg daily for systemic mycoses.

ADVERSE DRUG REACTIONS

Fluconazole and itraconazole have both been well tolerated in clinical trials. Fluconazole has been reported to cause nausea, vomiting, headache, rash and modest elevations of serum aminotransferases. Rare cases of Stevens-Johnson syndrome, toxic epidermal necrolysis and acute hepatic necrosis have been reported in association with fluconazole use. The drug should be discontinued in patients with progressive liver dysfunction.

Itraconazole has been associated with a similar range of adverse effects, although overt liver disease has not been reported. The triazoles, unlike high-dose ketoconazole do not impair testicular and adrenal steroid production.

DRUG INTERACTIONS

Serum levels of fluconazole may be reduced by concurrent administration of rifampicin and increased by hydrochlorothiazide. Fluconazole may also increase the serum levels of phenytoin, warfarin, cyclosporin and sulfonylurea oral hypoglycaemic agents.

PRECAUTIONS AND CONTRAINDICATIONS

Fluconazole and itraconazole are contraindicated in patients with a history of allergy to triazoles. Itraconazole is contraindicated in pregnancy. The safety of fluconazole in pregnancy is yet to be established.

Patients receiving these drugs should have their liver function tests monitored, and the drugs should be withdrawn if signs or symptoms of liver disease appear. Patients on fluconazole who develop skin rashes should be monitored closely and the drug should be discontinued if the lesions worsen.

SUPERFICIAL INFECTIONS

Terbinafine

Terbinafine is an allylamine antifungal agent.

INFECTIOUS DISEASES

30

TRADE NAMES

Terbinafine: *Lamisil*.

MECHANISM OF ACTION

Terbinafine inhibits fungal squalene peroxidase thus preventing the conversion of squalene to ergesterol. This results in inhibition of cell wall synthesis and cell death.

PHARMACOKINETICS

Following oral ingestion, the drug is rapidly absorbed. It is widely distributed in the body and is concentrated in adipose tissue and skin where it may persist for days. Terbinafine is metabolised in the liver and its half-life is prolonged in patients with hepatic dysfunction. The drug has a half-life of about 4.6 hours in healthy adults.

SPECTRUM OF ACTIVITY

Terbinafine is active against dermatophytes (*Trichophyton, Microsporum* and *Epidermophyton* sp.), moulds (*Aspergillus* and *Scopulariopsis* sp.), dimorphic fungi and some yeasts.

USES

Topically, terbinafine is used to treat ringworm infections and cutaneous candidiasis.

Orally it is used to treat ringworm infections and onychomycosis (fungal infection of the nail) caused by dermatophytes. Terbinafine has been shown to clear such infection more quickly than griseofulvin. The usual oral dose is 250 mg daily. The duration of treatment for tinea pedis is 2–6 weeks, tinea cruris and corporis 2–4 weeks and onychomycosis 6–12 weeks.

ADVERSE DRUG REACTIONS

Side effects with oral therapy are generally mild and self-limiting. They include gastrointestinal upset (nausea, abdominal pain), cutaneous reactions (rash, pruritus) and central nervous system effects (headache, dizziness). Topical use may cause erythema, stinging and pruritus.

DRUG INTERACTIONS

The clearance of terbinafine is enhanced by the co-administration of enzyme inducing agents such as rifampicin. Conversely, its clearance is diminished by drugs such as cimetidine which inhibit cytochrome P-450.

PRECAUTIONS AND CONTRAINDICATIONS

Terbinafine should not be given to patients with a known allergy to the drug. In patients with hepatic dysfunction or who are receiving a drug which inhibits cytochrome P-450, drug accumulation may occur. Co-administration of enzyme inducing agents may diminish the effectiveness of the drug.

Clotrimazole, Econazole, Isoconazole, Ketoconazole, Miconazole, Bifonazole

MECHANISM OF ACTION

All these agents act by the same mechanisms as ketoconazole. When applied topically they exhibit minimal systemic absorption.

USES

The imidazoles are used topically to treat superficial dermatophyte infections and candidiasis. Econazole foaming lotion and ketoconazole cream are particularly effective for the treatment of pityriasis versicolor. They are used vaginally to treat vaginal candidiasis; evidence suggests that clotrimazole as a 500 mg pessary is the drug of choice. Clotrimazole is also effective for infections caused by *Trichomonas vaginalis*.

ADVERSE DRUG REACTIONS

Topically applied imidazoles appear to be well tolerated. Local burning or irritation may occur, blistering, erythema and pruritus have also been reported. Used in the vagina, these agents may cause rashes, irritation, itching, burning, lower abdominal cramps, bloating and slight urinary frequency.

Griseofulvin

Griseofulvin was isolated in 1939 from *Penicillium griseofulvum* but it was not until

1947 that its potential for the treatment of human fungal infections was realised.

TRADE NAMES

Griseofulvin: *Fulcin; Griseostatin; Grisovin.*

MECHANISM OF ACTION

Griseofulvin exerts its fungistatic action primarily by disrupting cell nuclear division. This results in abnormal DNA production which may arrest cellular division. The drug is deposited into keratin precursor cells rendering them an unfavourable environment for fungal invasion. Infected skin, hair or nails are then replaced with tissue not affected by the dermatophyte.

PHARMACOKINETICS

Absorption of griseofulvin from the gastrointestinal tract is variable and mainly occurs in the duodenum. The absorption of the microsized griseofulvin particles is enhanced by co-administration of a high fat meal or milk. Following absorption it concentrates in the skin, hair, nails, liver, fat and skeletal muscle. The drug is metabolised in the liver, then excreted in the urine as the inactive metabolites. Griseofulvin is also excreted in the faeces and perspiration. The elimination half-life of the drug is around 24 hours.

SPECTRUM OF ACTIVITY

Griseofulvin is highly active against the dermatophytes, *Trichophyton, Microsporum* and *Epidermophyton* sp. It is inactive against other fungi.

USES

Griseofulvin is used exclusively to treat tineas (ring worm infections) of the skin, hair and nails including tinea pedis, tinea cruris, tinea corporis, tinea capitis, tinea barbae and tinea unguium. Because the drug is not effective against other fungi, the infecting organism should be identified as a dermatophyte before treatment is commenced.

Response to griseofulvin therapy is dependent on the rate of keratinisation and the time necessary for desquamation of the infected keratinised tissues. Soles, palms and nails respond more slowly than less keratinised skin with the toe nails responding at the slowest rate. Consequently, the duration of griseofulvin treatment is dependent on the site of infection, e.g., tinea corporis 2–4 weeks, tinea capitis 4–6 weeks, tinea pedis 4–8 weeks and tinea unguium 4 months. The usual daily dose of griseofulvin is 330 mg (ultramicronised) or 500 mg (micronised).

ADVERSE DRUG REACTIONS

Griseofulvin is generally well tolerated with serious adverse effects occurring rarely. The most common adverse effects include central nervous system effects (e.g. headache, fatigue, lethargy, confusion) and alimentary tract disorders (e.g. nausea, vomiting, epigastric distress, thirst, glossitis). The drug may also induce hypersensitivity reactions ranging from urticaria and other rashes to lupus erythematosus and toxic epidermal necrolysis (rare). Photosensitivity may be a problem with griseofulvin therapy.

Griseofulvin has also been reported (rarely) to cause proteinuria, nephrosis, blood dyscrasias and hepatotoxicity.

DRUG INTERACTIONS

Griseofulvin induces liver microsomal enzymes and has been reported to reduce the efficacy of warfarin and oral contraceptive agents. Phenobarbitone may induce the metabolism of griseofulvin, thus diminishing its antifungal effect. Griseofulvin may potentiate the effect of alcohol, producing effects such as tachycardia and flushing.

PRECAUTIONS AND CONTRAINDICATIONS

Griseofulvin is contraindicated in patients with a history of allergy to the drug, porphyria or hepatocellular failure. Patients receiving the drug should have periodic monitoring of their liver and renal function, and full blood picture. They should also be warned to avoid excessive exposure to sunlight because of the possible risk of photosensitivity reactions.

30 INFECTIOUS DISEASES

NURSING IMPLICATIONS

ASSESSMENT

Patients who are to receive this drug should be assessed for any undisclosed history of hypersensitivity to the drug, hepatic disease or porphyria.

ADMINISTRATION

Griseofulvin is usually self-administered, and patients should be advised that taking it with a high fat meal will enhance its absorption. They should be told that completion of the whole course is required to avoid recurrence of the fungal infection.

PATIENT EDUCATION

As the drug can cause photosensitivity, patients should be advised to avoid excessive exposure to ultraviolet light.

Nystatin, Natamycin

Nystatin and natamycin are polyene antibiotics like amphotericin B, and were isolated from *Streptomyces* sp. in 1950 and 1955 respectively. Nystatin and natamycin have similar properties and are administered topically, mainly to treat *Candida* sp. infections.

TRADE NAMES

Nystatin: *Mycostatin*; *Nilstat*.
Natamycin: *Pimafucin*.

MECHANISM OF ACTION

Nystatin and natamycin act in the same manner as amphotericin B by binding to sterols on the fungal cell membrane and altering cell permeability.

PHARMACOKINETICS

Nystatin and natamycin are not absorbed orally or when applied to intact skin or mucous membranes.

SPECTRUM OF ACTIVITY

Nystatin and natamycin have a similar range of activity to amphotericin B, however, they are principally used to treat superficial *Candida* sp. infections.

USES

Nystatin is the most frequently prescribed topical polyene, although there is no evidence of its superiority compared to the other polyenes. It is used in the form of ointments and creams to treat *Candida* sp. infections of the skin. Oropharyngeal candidiasis may be treated with nystatin oral suspension or lozenges (100 000 units 6-hourly). Vaginal candidiasis responds well to nystatin administered either as a vaginal cream or pessaries over 14 days.

Otitis externa due to yeasts or fungi has been successfully treated with topical application of nystatin and natamycin. Nebulised nystatin suspension has also been used to treat pulmonary aspergillosis. Oral nystatin tablets are used to treat *Candida* sp. overgrowth in the lower gut.

ADVERSE DRUG REACTIONS

Oral and topical nystatin preparations are well tolerated, with mild gastrointestinal upset and local irritation occurring infrequently.

PRECAUTIONS AND CONTRAINDICATIONS

The only contraindication to nystatin or natamycin is a history of allergy to the drug.

Dosages for commonly used antifungal agents are listed in Table 30.8.

NURSING IMPLICATIONS

These substances are administered orally or applied locally. They are generally well tolerated. Patients should be instructed in the correct method of application and dosage regimen, and the importance of completing the entire course of therapy to ensure eradication of the infection.

TABLE 30.8   Dosages for antifungal agents

Drug	Strength(s)	Dose Range (Adults, Normal renal function)	Frequency of dosing
Amphotericin	50 mg, injection	0.25–0.6 mg/kg/day, or 0.5–1 mg/kg	Daily by slow IV infusion over 4–6 hours On alternate days
	10 mg, lozenge	10 mg	6-hourly
	100 mg, tablet	100–200 mg, oral	6-hourly
	100 mg/mL, suspension	100 mg (1 mL)	6-hourly
	Vaginal cream, topical cream and ointment		
Flucytosine	500 mg, tablet 2.5 g/250 mL injection	150 mg/kg/day, oral, IV	6-hourly, IV infusion over 20–40 minutes
Ketoconazole	200 mg, tablet Topical cream	200–400 mg, oral	Daily
Miconazole	200 mg/20 mL, injection	200–1200 mg IV	8-hourly infusion over 30–60 minutes
	100 mg, vaginal tablet, vaginal cream	Vaginally	Daily
	Topical cream, oral gel		12-hourly
Bifonazole	Topical cream		Daily
Clotrimazole	100 mg, 500 mg, vaginal tablet	Vaginally	Daily as single dose
	Vaginal cream		Daily
	Topical cream		12-hourly
Econazole	150 mg, vaginal ovules Vaginal cream, topical cream	Vaginally	Daily
Fluconazole	100 mg, injection, capsule	100–400 mg	Daily, IV infusion over 30–120 minutes
Itraconazole	100 mg, capsule	100–400 mg	Daily
Terbinafine	250 mg, tab	250 mg, oral	Daily
	Topical cream		12-hourly
Isoconazole	300 mg vaginal tablet Topical cream, solution	Vaginally	Single dose
Griseofulvin	125 mg, 330 mg, 500 mg, tablets	330–500 mg, oral	Daily
Nystatin	500 000 units, tablets, capsules	500 000–1 000 000 units, oral	6-hourly
	100 000 units, lozenge 100 000 units/mL, suspension	100 000 units (1 mL), oral	6-hourly
	100 000 units, vaginal tablets, vaginal cream	100 000 units, vaginally	Daily
	Topical cream, ointment, gel		

ANTIVIRAL AGENTS ▉▉▉▉▉▉▉▉

Viruses are too simple in structure to multiply by themselves. In order to multiply, a virus invades a cell, then uses the biochemical mechanisms of that cell to make new viral proteins and genetic material. This intimate relationship between virus and host cells makes it imperative that an effective antiviral agent can distinguish between the virus and the host. In the last two decades, the improved understanding of viral structures and multiplication has lead to the development of a large number of new antiviral agents.

The introduction of acyclovir marked a significant breakthrough in the treatment of herpes virus infections. The interest in antiviral research generated by the AIDS epidemic has led to a number of agents active against the human immunodeficiency virus and other viruses capable of causing secondary infections in AIDS patients.

There are seven steps in the viral infection of cells:

1. attachment to the cell membrane;

2. penetration into the cell;

3. uncoating of the viral nucleic acid (RNA or DNA) which then allows multiplication of the virus within the cell;

4. replication of the viral genome;

5. protein synthesis;

6. assembly of the virus; and

7. release of the new virus capable of infecting other cells.

Inhibition of any of these steps affords the opportunity to control viral infections. The possibilities for therapeutic intervention are summarised in Table 30.9.

TABLE 30.9 Mechanism of action of antiviral agents

Agents	Mode of Action
	Inhibition of:
Vaccines, immunoglobulin, interferons, inosiplex*	1. Attachment
Amantadine, rimantadine*	2. Penetration
Amantadine, rimantadine*	3. Uncoating
Foscarnet, ribavirin, amantadine	4. Replication RNA synthesis
Idoxuridine, acyclovir, ganciclovir, foscarnet, didanosine, zalcitabine, zidovudine	DNA synthesis
Interferons	5. Viral protein synthesis
Metasizon*	6. Assembly
Interferons	7. Release

*Not available in Australia

CYCLIC AMINE COMPOUNDS

Amantadine, Rimantadine

Amantadine is a cyclic amine compound first marketed in the 1960s for prophylactic use against influenza A virus. It was subsequently approved for use in the treatment of influenza A infections. Another cyclic amine compound, rimantadine, has been used extensively in Russia for the same indications.

MECHANISM OF ACTION

The exact mechanism of action of amantadine has not been fully elucidated. It is possible that it prevents penetration of the virus into the cell, but it is more likely that it inhibits the uncoating of the virus.

SPECTRUM OF ACTIVITY

Amantadine is only active against influenza A. It possesses minimal activity against influenza B and C. The drug is virostatic rather than virocidal, and spontaneous resistance can develop during therapy.

USES

Amantadine is used for prophylaxis against influenza infections in high risk patients (e.g. those with chronic airways limitation or diabetes mellitus) during influenza A epidemics. Prophylaxis should be commenced as soon as an influenza outbreak occurs or immediately after the patient comes in contact with the disease. The usual adult dose is 200 mg daily given in two divided doses for 10 days after a single exposure, or for four weeks or more if repeated exposure occurs during the epidemic. The dose should be reduced in patients with renal impairment and the elderly.

For information on pharmacokinetics, adverse drug reactions, drug interactions, precautions and contraindications see amantadine, Chapter 25 Neurological Disorders.

PURINE AND PYRIMIDINE NUCLEOSIDE ANALOGUES

This group of antiviral agents has been designed structurally to mimic the purine and pyrimidine nucleosides which are essential metabolites, and are required by viruses for normal growth and replication. The purine analogues include acyclovir, ganciclovir, vidarabine, didanosine (DDI) and zalcitabine (DDC) and the pyrimidine analogues idoxuridine, trifluorothymidine, zidovudine and ribavirin.

Acyclovir

Acyclovir is a cyclic analogue of guanine. Since its introduction in 1981 it has become the mainstay for the treatment of herpes simplex and varicella zoster infections.

TRADE NAMES

Acyclovir: *Zovirax*.

MECHANISM OF ACTION

After uptake into infected cells acyclovir is phosphorylated to its active form, acyclovir triphosphate, by viral thymidine kinase. Acyclovir triphosphate inhibits the viral DNA polymerase and/or acts as a chain terminator of viral DNA. Resistance to acyclovir occurs when a virus fails to produce the enzyme thymidine kinase.

PHARMACOKINETICS

Oral absorption of acyclovir is variable and poor; somewhere between 15%–20% of each dose being absorbed. Following absorption the drug is widely distributed in the body, including the cerebrospinal fluid. Approximately 70% of acyclovir is excreted unchanged in the urine by glomerular filtration and tubular secretion. In patients with normal renal function the average half-life of the drug is 2.9 hours.

INFECTIOUS DISEASES

30

SPECTRUM OF ACTIVITY

Acyclovir is clinically active against herpes simplex 1 and 2 viruses and the varicella zoster virus.

USES

Acyclovir may be used topically to treat cutaneous herpes simplex infections. It is used ophthalmically as a 3% ointment applied 4-hourly (five times daily) to treat herpes zoster keratitis. Systemically it is used for the treatment and prevention of herpes simplex infections in immunocompromised patients.

Acyclovir is also used in immunocompetent patients to treat severe mucocutaneous herpes simplex infections, genital herpes, herpes encephalitis and chickenpox. The drug is effective in reducing morbidity and preventing dissemination of shingles (herpes zoster) in patients with impaired immunity.

When treating herpes simplex 1 and 2 infections, the oral dose is 200 mg five times daily (4-hourly) and the intravenous dose 5 mg/kg 8-hourly. A dose of 10 mg/kg 8-hourly should be used for patients with varicella-zoster infections or herpes encephalitis. When given intravenously acyclovir should be well diluted (250 mg/50 mL of fluid) and infused over 60 minutes.

ADVERSE DRUG REACTIONS

Application of the eye ointment may be associated with burning or stinging; similar reactions occur when the drug is applied to the skin. Oral and intravenous acyclovir have been reported to cause gastrointestinal symptoms (e.g. nausea, vomiting, diarrhoea and abdominal pain), rashes and alterations in liver function tests. Headache and encephalopathic changes, including tremor, hallucinations, obtundation and coma, may occur. The latter are more likely in the presence of high serum levels of acyclovir. Acyclovir may precipitate in the renal tubules causing acute renal failure, particularly if the drug is given too rapidly intravenously. Adequate hydration of the patient will prevent this occurring.

DRUG INTERACTIONS

Probenecid inhibits the tubular secretion of acyclovir, resulting in higher and more prolonged serum levels of the drug. Acyclovir appears to enhance the neurotoxicity of zidovudine when given concurrently.

PRECAUTIONS AND CONTRAINDICATIONS

Acyclovir is contraindicated in patients with a history of allergy to the drug. The mutagenic and teratogenic potential of acyclovir remain to be fully evaluated; its use is therefore not recommended during pregnancy unless the benefits outweigh the risks.

Acyclovir should be used with caution in patients with renal impairment or dehydration or those receiving other nephrotoxic drugs. Serum urea and creatinine levels should be monitored regularly during therapy and adequate fluid intake maintained.

Patients with underlying neurological conditions, severe hepatic or renal impairment, or electrolyte abnormalities should be monitored closely for signs of neurotoxicity.

Ganciclovir

Ganciclovir, formerly known as DHPG (9-[(3-dihydroxy-2-propoxy)-methyl]guanine), is a synthetic guanine analogue structurally related to acyclovir.

TRADE NAMES

Ganciclovir: *Cymevene*.

MECHANISM OF ACTION

After entry into the infected cell, ganciclovir is phosphorylated to its active form ganciclovir triphosphate. Unlike acyclovir, this process is not dependent on viral thymidine kinase. The ganciclovir triphosphate acts by inhibiting viral DNA polymerase and/or limiting or ending DNA elongation.

PHARMACOKINETICS

Ganciclovir is poorly absorbed orally, and currently it is only administered intravenously. It is widely distributed into body tissues and fluids, including the cerebrospinal fluid. It is eliminated primarily in the urine by glomerular filtration. In patients with normal renal function the drug has a half-life of around 3.9 hours.

SPECTRUM OF ACTIVITY

Ganciclovir is active against all the herpes viruses including herpes simplex, varicella zoster, cytomegalovirus (CMV) and Epstein-Barr virus. Because of its toxicity however, its use has been restricted to severe cytomegalovirus infections.

USES

Approved indications for the use of ganciclovir are sight-threatening cytomegalovirus infections in AIDS and other immunocompromised patients, and for the treatment of cytomegalovirus pneumonitis in bone marrow transplant recipients. It has also been used to treat cytomegalovirus oesophagitis, colitis and central nervous system infections with varying success.

For cytomegalovirus retinitis the usual induction dose of ganciclovir is 5 mg/kg 12-hourly for 14–21 days, given as an intravenous infusion over one hour. The maintenance dose is 6 mg/kg daily five days a week or 5 mg/kg daily seven days a week. The dose should be reduced in patients with renal dysfunction or in patients with bone marrow suppression.

ADVERSE DRUG REACTIONS

The most important adverse effects of ganciclovir are neutropenia (25%–40%) and thrombocytopenia (20%); central nervous system effects, such as headache, psychosis, confusion and depersonalisation; and gastrointestinal problems, such as nausea, vomiting and diarrhoea. The severity of these side effects is dose-related and neutropenia appears to be the dose limiting untoward effect. Ganciclovir has been shown to be mutagenic, carcinogenic and teratogenic in animals.

DRUG INTERACTIONS

Ganciclovir myelosuppression is enhanced by the concurrent administration of zidovudine, and this may be the case with other myelosuppressive drugs. Seizures have been reported when ganciclovir is given in conjunction with imipenem–cilastatin, however, both drugs are capable of precipitating seizures when given alone.

PRECAUTIONS AND CONTRAINDICATIONS

Ganciclovir is contraindicated in pregnant women, nursing mothers and those patients with a previous allergy to ganciclovir or acyclovir. It should not be given to patients with a neutrophil count of less than 500 cell/mm^3 or platelet count below 2500 cell/mm^3. Regular monitoring of white cell and platelet counts must be carried out for all patients prescribed ganciclovir.

As ganciclovir has been shown to be carcinogenic it should be handled with the same precautions as cytotoxic drugs.

Vidarabine

Vidarabine was the first antiviral agent available for parenteral use. It is a purine nucleoside obtained from fermentation cultures of *Streptomyces antibioticus*.

TRADE NAMES

Vidarabine: *Vira-A*.

MECHANISM OF ACTION

Vidarabine and its major metabolite arabinoside hypoxanthine are phosphorylated intracellularly to mono-, di- and triphosphate derivatives. These competitively and selectively inhibit virus controlled DNA polymerase.

PHARMACOKINETICS

Vidarabine is poorly absorbed orally or when given by intramuscular or subcutaneous injection. Following intravenous injection it is rapidly metabolised to arabinoside hypoxanthine, which is 50 times less active than vidarabine. Both the parent drug and its major metabolite are widely distributed in the body, including the central nervous system. Most of the drug

INFECTIOUS DISEASES

30

is excreted in the urine as arabinoside hypoxanthine, with the unchanged drug accounting for only 2%. The half-life of vidarabine is 1–3 minutes, whilst that of arabinoside hypoxanthine is 5 hours. Accumulation of arabinoside hypoxanthine occurs in patients with renal insufficiency.

SPECTRUM OF ACTIVITY

Vidarabine is active against all herpes viruses — herpes simplex 1 and 2, varicella zoster, cytomegalovirus and Epstein-Barr virus. It is also active against other DNA viruses such as pox virus, rhabdovirus and vaccinia.

USES

Vidarabine has largely been replaced by acyclovir. It is still used ophthalmically to treat herpes simplex keratoconjunctivitis. Vidarabine may be used intravenously in cases of drug resistance to acyclovir. In this instance the dose is 15 mg/kg daily, given as a single infusion over 12–24 hours.

ADVERSE DRUG REACTIONS

The most common adverse effects of vidarabine are gastrointestinal (10%–15%) such as nausea, vomiting, diarrhoea and anorexia. At doses higher than 15 mg/kg vidarabine may cause bone marrow suppression (e.g. anaemia, thrombocytopenia and leucopenia) and neurotoxicity. The drug exhibits mutagenic, carcinogenic and teratogenic potential.

Didanosine

Didanosine (DDI) is an analogue of the naturally occurring purine inosine. It has recently been released for the management of human immunodeficiency virus (HIV) infections.

TRADE NAMES

Didanosine: *Videx*.

MECHANISM OF ACTION

Although the exact mechanism of action of didanosine is not fully understood, it is thought to inhibit viral reverse transcriptase after intracellular conversion to its active metabolite dideoxyadenosine-5- triphosphate. Didanosine exerts a virostatic effect.

PHARMACOKINETICS

Oral absorption of didanosine is variable and influenced by such factors as pH of the stomach, presence of food and the dosage form given. Didanosine is rapidly degraded by acidic pH, hence the commercially available tablets contain antacids to increase gastric pH. Food markedly reduces the rate and extent of didanosine absorption. Following absorption, the drug is widely distributed into body tissues and fluids, including the cerebrospinal fluid. It crosses the placenta and is found in amniotic fluid. The drug is minimally protein bound. The metabolic fate of didanosine is unclear, however in dogs it has been shown to be extensively metabolised. The drug is at least 50% excreted in the urine by both glomerular filtration and tubular secretion. The half-life of the drug is 1.3–1.6 hours in adults and 0.8 hours in children and adolescents.

SPECTRUM OF ACTIVITY

Didanosine is active against many human and animal retroviruses, including human immunodeficiency virus.

USES

Didanosine has been shown to increase CD4 counts, decrease p24 antigen levels and decrease symptoms in AIDS patients and those with severe AIDS related complex. Some patients unresponsive to zidovudine have shown clinical improvement on didanosine. It is indicated for use in patients intolerant of or unresponsive to zidovudine.

The adult daily dose is dependent on the patient's weight:
> 75 kg: 300 mg (2 × 150 mg tablets) 12-hourly
50–74 kg: 200 mg (2 × 100 mg tablets) 12-hourly
35–49 kg: 100 mg (2 × 50 mg tablets) 12-hourly

ADVERSE DRUG REACTIONS

The major dose limiting side effects are painful peripheral neuropathy (usually after 2–6 months) and potentially fatal pancreatitis. The drug should not be given with other drugs capable of causing pancreatitis such as pentamidine. Diarrhoea has been reported commonly, other side effects include nausea and vomiting, headache, insomnia, dry mouth, fever, rash, hyperuricaemia, hypokalaemia, increased aminotransaminase activity and thrombocytopenia.

DRUG INTERACTIONS

Antacids enhance the absorption of didanosine by increasing gastric pH, so may H_2 antagonists. The concurrent administration of didanosine with dapsone has been reported to reduce the effectiveness of dapsone in preventing relapses of *Pneumocystis carinii* infections. The absorption of ketoconazole and quinolones is reduced by the increase in gastric pH produced by the buffered didanosine tablets. The effects of didanosine and zidovudine appear to be synergistic in experimental studies. Clinical trials are now underway to determine the significance of this interaction. Tetracyclines should not be given with didanosine as they will chelate the antacid compounds and reduce didanosine absorption.

PRECAUTIONS AND CONTRAINDICATIONS

Didanosine is contraindicated in patients with a history of allergy to the drug. The drug is not a cure for HIV infections and patients given the drug may still develop opportunistic infections and other complications of AIDS and AIDS related complex. The drug should be used with extreme caution in patients with a history of pancreatitis, and the diagnosis of pancreatitis should be considered in any patient developing abdominal pain, nausea and vomiting whilst on the drug. Should pancreatitis develop the drug should be discontinued.

Patients should be monitored for clinical symptoms of peripheral neuropathy, their occurrence warrants drug withdrawal. If the peripheral neuropathy resolves, the drug may be restarted at a lower dose.

Dosage reduction is required in patients with renal impairment and/or hepatic dysfunction. The drug should be used with caution in patients with phenylketonuria as the tablets contain aspartame.

Zidovudine

Zidovudine (AZT, azidothymidine) is a thymidine analogue, and was the first commercially available agent for the treatment and prevention of human immunodeficiency virus infections.

TRADE NAMES

Zidovudine: *Retrovir*.

MECHANISM OF ACTION

Zidovudine, like other nucleoside analogues, is converted intracellularly to a triphosphate metabolite. Zidovudine triphosphate inhibits HIV multiplication by inhibiting viral reverse transcriptase and promoting termination of the viral DNA chain.

PHARMACOKINETICS

Zidovudine is well absorbed orally. It is widely distributed into body fluids and tissues, including the cerebrospinal fluid where concentrations reach 50%–60% of those in the plasma. The drug undergoes metabolism in the liver, and less than 25% of the drug is excreted unchanged in the urine. The drug has a short half-life of around 1–1.5 hours.

SPECTRUM OF ACTIVITY

Zidovudine is active against many human and animal retroviruses, including HIV.

USES

Oral zidovudine can decrease the frequency of opportunistic infections and prolong survival in patients with AIDS or AIDS related complex. The drug may also delay progression of disease in HIV-infected patients with CD4 lymphocyte counts of less than 500 cells/mm^3. However, the effectiveness of

INFECTIOUS DISEASES

30

zidovudine appears short lived, around six months. The drug is now given to patients with AIDS or AIDS related complex with opportunistic infections at a dosage of 100 mg 4-hourly (six times a day). A dose of 100 mg 4-hourly (five times a day) while the patient is awake is used in asymptomatic HIV-infected patients.

The drug is also given prophylactically to health-care workers following needle-stick injuries, however the effectiveness of zidovudine in this setting has yet to be confirmed.

ADVERSE DRUG REACTIONS

Severe anaemia and neutropenia are the usual dose-limiting toxicities of zidovudine therapy. The reduction in the recommended dose from 1200 mg daily to 500–600 mg, has been associated with a decreased incidence of neutropenia. Side effects commonly seen early in therapy include asthenia, headache, dizziness, insomnia, anorexia, nausea, vomiting, malaise and myalgia. Long-term zidovudine therapy has been associated with polymyositis on rare occasions.

DRUG INTERACTIONS

The concurrent administration of paracetamol and zidovudine has been associated with an increased incidence of neutropenia. The use of acyclovir or ganciclovir together with zidovudine may result in enhanced toxicity of either or both agents. Probenecid may increase and prolong serum zidovudine concentrations.

PRECAUTIONS AND CONTRAINDICATIONS

Zidovudine is contraindicated in patients with a previous history of life-threatening allergy to the drug. Because of its potential to produce anaemia and neutropenia, regular monitoring of the patient's full blood picture is required. As zidovudine may cause severe myopathy and myositis, patients should be advised to report any musculoskeletal symptoms to their doctor. Routine monitoring of creatine kinase and lactic acid dehydrogenase levels as early markers of muscle damage is advisable. The patient should be informed that zidovudine is not a cure and that opportunistic infections and progression of the disease may occur. Dosage adjustment is indicated in patients with renal and hepatic impairment, and those who develop myelosuppression.

Idoxuridine

Idoxuridine (IDU) is a halogenated thymidine analogue. It is only used topically as it is too toxic to use systemically.

TRADE NAMES

Idoxuridine: *Stoxil*; *Herplex, Herplex D.*

MECHANISM OF ACTION

Idoxuridine is phosphorylated by cellular enzymes to idoxuridine triphosphate. This is then incorporated into DNA in place of thymidine thus interrupting viral replication. The drug is however, non-selective, affecting both viral and host cells.

PHARMACOKINETICS

The drug is minimally absorbed when applied topically.

SPECTRUM OF ACTIVITY

Idoxuridine is active against herpes simplex 1 and 2 viruses, cytomegalovirus and varicella-zoster virus.

USES

Idoxuridine is used ophthalmically to treat herpetic keratoconjunctivitis and topically to treat cutaneous herpes simplex, vaccinia and varicella-zoster infections. It is also used dissolved in dimethylsulfoxide (DMSO) in concentrations up to 40% to treat skin infections, but the use of this solvent is controversial.

ADVERSE DRUG REACTIONS

Used topically in the eye, idoxuridine often causes irritation, redness, itching and mild oedema of the cornea or eyelid.

PRECAUTIONS AND CONTRAINDICATIONS

Topical skin preparations should not be

used in the eye. Use of idoxuridine during pregnancy is not advised.

Ribavirin

Ribavirin is a synthetic nucleoside that is structurally similar to pyrimidine. It is available for the treatment of respiratory syncytial virus bronchiolitis.

TRADE NAMES

Ribavirin: *Virazide*.

MECHANISM OF ACTION

Ribavirin undergoes intracellular phosphorylation to its active metabolites. These appear to act by interfering with RNA and DNA synthesis, and subsequently inhibiting viral protein synthesis and replication.

PHARMACOKINETICS

Ribavirin is rapidly absorbed when given orally or by aerosol. The drug appears to be concentrated in the lungs and liver. Ribavirin does not cross the blood-brain barrier. It is degraded in cells by deribosylation, amide hydrolysis and phosphorylation. The major route of elimination of the drug and its metabolites is in the urine, about 15% is excreted in the faeces. The average half-life of the drug in plasma is about 24 hours, however it is retained in red blood cells for many days.

SPECTRUM OF ACTIVITY

Ribavirin is virostatic against a wide range of DNA and RNA viruses, including respiratory syncytial virus, influenza A and B, measles, para-influenza, mumps, reoviruses, herpes simplex 1 and 2, Lassa fever, hepatitis A and HIV.

USES

Ribavirin aerosol is indicated for the treatment of severe lower respiratory tract infections due to respiratory syncytial virus in children under the age of 2 years. In this instance 6 g of the drug is administered daily via a small particle aerosol

generator (SPAG) as a 20 mg/mL solution over a period of 12–18 hours daily for 3–7 days.

Intravenous and oral ribavirin have been used experimentally to treat a wide variety of viral infections. The drug has been shown to reduce the mortality associated with Lassa fever.

ADVERSE DRUG REACTIONS

Ribavirin has been shown to be mutagenic, carcinogenic, teratogenic and toxic to the reproductive system in animal studies and therefore is contraindicated in pregnancy. Given by aerosol, ribavirin may induce acute deterioration in respiratory function in patients with bronchospastic lung disease (e.g. asthma). The drug may also cause rashes and conjunctivitis. Rare cases of anaemia, hypotension and cardiac arrest have also been reported.

Given intravenously the most important adverse effect is anaemia.

DRUG INTERACTIONS

Ribavirin may antagonise the antiviral effects of zidovudine by inhibiting its intracellular phosphorylation.

PRECAUTIONS AND CONTRAINDICATIONS

Ribavirin is contraindicated in pregnant women and women who are likely to become pregnant during exposure to the drug.

Patients receiving ribavirin should have their respiratory function closely monitored, as the drug may cause a sudden deterioration in function. Extreme caution should be exercised when administering the drug to patients with asthma or chronic obstructive lung disease.

Zalcitabine

Zalcitabine (dideoxycytidine, DDC) is a pyrimidine analogue derived from cytidine.

TRADE NAMES

Zalcitabine: *Hivid*.

30 INFECTIOUS DISEASES

MECHANISM OF ACTION

Zalcitabine is phosphorylated intracellularly to its active 5'-triphosphate form. It may then act by either incorporation of dideoxynucleoside triphosphates onto growing strands of viral DNA or competition with endogenous nucleoside triphosphates for reverse transcriptase.

PHARMACOKINETICS

Given orally, zalcitabine is about 80% absorbed, although absorption is diminished in the presence of food. It is widely distributed in the body with central nervous system levels of about 20% of those in the plasma. The drug is excreted primarily in the urine and has a half-life of about 1.2 hours.

SPECTRUM OF ACTIVITY

Zalcitabine is a potent, specific and relatively selective agent. It is equally active against HIV-1 and HIV-2 viruses and shows activity against zidovudine resistant strains. Apart from hepatitis B virus, it is not active against other viral pathogens.

USES

Zalcitabine is indicated for the treatment of HIV infection in patients either intolerant to zidovudine or with advanced disease (CD4 count < 300 cells/mm^3). In these patients, the usual daily dose is 750 micrograms 8-hourly.

The drug may also be used (in similar doses) with zidovudine in patients with advanced disease (CD4 count ≤ 200 cells/mm^3) who have received less than 12 months treatment with zidovudine.

ADVERSE DRUG REACTIONS

Of patients receiving zalcitabine, 20%–31% develop a peripheral neuropathy which may necessitate drug withdrawal. Patients at greatest risk are those with a pre-existing peripheral neuropathy or a CD4 count below 50 cells/mm^3. Zalcitabine may also produce myelosuppression (leucopenia, neutropenia, anaemia, thrombocytopenia) but is said to be less myelosuppressive than zidovudine.

Other adverse effects reported include pancreatitis (rarely fatal), oesophageal ulcers, cardiomyopathy, cardiac failure, alterations in liver function tests and anaphylactoid reactions.

DRUG INTERACTIONS

Concurrent use of drugs known to cause peripheral neuropathies (e.g. cisplatin, vincristine, gold, ribavirin) may potentiate the neurotoxicity of zalcitabine. Similarly, drugs which prolong the elimination of the drug (e.g. amphotericin B, foscarnet, aminoglycosides) may enhance its toxicity. The combination of didanosine and zalcitabine is not recommended because of the increased risk of pancreatitis.

PRECAUTIONS AND CONTRAINDICATIONS

Use is contraindicated in patients with a known allergy to the drug. It should be used with extreme caution in patients with peripheral neuropathy or pancreatitis or patients who are receiving drugs which may induce these conditions. Similar care is required with concurrent use of myelosuppressive agents.

OTHER ANTIVIRAL AGENTS

Foscarnet

Foscarnet (phosphonoformate) is a pyrophosphate analogue.

TRADE NAMES

Foscarnet: *Foscavir.*

MECHANISM OF ACTION

The exact mechanism of action of foscarnet is not known. It reversibly and competitively inhibits viral DNA polymerase of all herpes viruses and the RNA polymerase of influenza viruses probably by binding to the pyrophosphate binding site on the polymerases. Foscarnet also non-competitively inhibits the reverse transcriptase of retroviruses, including HIV.

PHARMACOKINETICS

Foscarnet is poorly absorbed orally, hence it is given intravenously. About 10%–28% of each dose is deposited in bone, where it may remain for months.

Foscarnet is mainly eliminated unchanged by the kidneys. The average half-life of the drug is 3–5 hours, but is extended in patients with renal impairment.

SPECTRUM OF ACTIVITY

Foscarnet is active against all human herpes viruses — herpes simplex 1 and 2, varicella-zoster, cytomegalovirus and Epstein-Barr and some retroviruses (e.g. HIV). The drug is virostatic thus it must be given on a continuous basis.

USES

Foscarnet has been used as an alternative to ganciclovir to treat cytomegalovirus infections, including retinitis. Usual dosage is 60 mg/kg intravenously 8-hourly for 14–21 days, followed by 90–120 mg/kg once daily as maintenance therapy. The drug is given as a 2-hour infusion. The dose should be reduced in patients with renal impairment.

ADVERSE DRUG REACTIONS

The major toxicity of foscarnet is renal damage, evident by increasing serum creatinine and proteinuria. Rare cases of nephrogenic diabetes insipidus have also been reported. Other side effects include nausea and vomiting, malaise, fatigue, headache, seizures, symptomatic hypocalaemia, hypercalcaemia, hypophosphataemia, hyperphosphataemia, hypomagnesaemia, penile ulcers, leucopenia and altered liver function.

PRECAUTIONS AND CONTRAINDICATIONS

Foscarnet is contraindicated in patients with a previous history of allergy to the drug. It should be used with caution in patients with renal or hepatic impairment, and regular monitoring of renal and hepatic function is required.

INTERFERONS

Interferons are glycoproteins produced by all species of animals and form part of the natural host defences. They may be divided into three classes: interferon alfa, interferon beta and interferon gamma. Whilst all interferons possess antiviral activity, it is interferon alfa which has been used most widely.

TRADE NAMES

Interferon alfa: *Roferon A; Intron A.*

MECHANISM OF ACTION

Interferons do not have direct antiviral activity. They act by inducing cellular enzymes which are capable of inhibiting many stages of viral growth. Thus causing breakdown of viral RNA and inhibition of viral protein synthesis. In the case of retroviruses, they may also inhibit viral assembly and release of viral particles.

SPECTRUM OF ACTIVITY

Interferons have a broad spectrum of activity against both DNA and RNA viruses.

USES

Interferon alfa is used for the treatment of genital warts which are caused by papillomavirus. In this case it is administered intralesionally in a dose of 1 million units three times weekly for three weeks. The drug is also effective in the treatment of hepatitis B and hepatitis C. Interferon has also been used intranasally to prevent rhinovirus colds and topically to treat herpes infections. Although interferon alfa has weak activity against HIV it appears to exhibit synergy when used with zidovudine, foscarnet and zalcitabine.

For information on pharmacokinetics, adverse drug reactions, drug interactions, precautions and contraindications see interferon alfa, Chapter 31 Cancer Chemotherapy.

INFECTIOUS DISEASES

30

NURSING IMPLICATIONS

See interferon alfa, Chapter 31 Cancer Chemotherapy.

FURTHER READING

Allan, J.D., Eliopoulos, G.M., and Moellering, R.C. Jr. (1986) 'The expanding spectrum of β-lactam antibiotics.' *Adv. Intern. Med.* 31: 116–46.

Breslin, T. (1991) 'Infections. Part VIII: Tuberculosis in Australia.' *Curr Ther,* 32: 49–59.

'Choice of cephalosporins.' (1990) *Med Lett Drugs Ther* 1990; 32: 107–10.

Davey, P.G. (1990) 'New antiviral and antifungal drugs.' *Br Med J*; 300: 793–8.

'Drugs for viral infections.' (1990) *Med Lett Drugs Ther,* 32: 73–8.

'Drugs for AIDS and associated infections.' (1991) *Med Lett Drugs Ther,* 33: 95–102.

Epstein, F.H. (1991) 'New mechanisms of bacterial resistance to antimicrobial agents.' *New Engl J Med*; 324: 601–12.

McEvoy, G.K. (ed.) (1992) *AHFS Drug Information 92*. Bethesda: American Society of Hospital Pharmacists, Inc.

Parenti, M.A., Hatfield, S.M., and Leydon, J.J. (1987) 'Mupirocin: A topical antibiotic with a unique structure and mechanism of action.' *Clin Pharm*; 6: 761–70.

Pedler, S.J., Edwards, C. *Pharm J* (1991) (1) Antibacterial agents; 246: 492–5.

Reese, R.E., Betts, R.F. (eds) (1991) *A practical approach to infectious diseases*, 3rd ed. Boston: Little, Brown and Company.

Rosenblatt, J.E. (1991) 'Laboratory tests used to guide antimicrobial therapy.' *Mayo Clin Proc*; 66: 942–8.

Scheife, R.T. (1991) 'Pharmacokinetic considerations in the choice of antimicrobials.' *Postgrad Med*; 114: 15–21.

Schneider, J., Hughes, J., and Henderson, A. (1990) 'Infectious diseases: prophylaxis and chemotherapy.' Sydney: Appleton & Lange.

Wilkowske, C.J. 'General principles of antimicrobial therapy.' (1991) *Mayo Clin Proc*; 66: 931–41.

Wiltink, E.H.H., Janknegt, R. (1991) 'Antiviral drugs.' *Pharm Weekblad Sci*; 13: 58–69.

Wolfson, J.S. (1991) 'New quinolone antimicrobial agents.' *Postgrad Med*; 114: 5–13.

Wood, M.J. (1991) 'More macrolides: Some may be improvements on erythromycin.' *Br Med J*; 303:594–5.

TEST YOUR KNOWLEDGE

1. Selection of an appropriate anti-infective agent should be based on a number of factors. What are those factors?

2. Combination therapy with anti-infective agents is indicated in certain circumstances. Which of the following statements is(are) specific justification(s) for combination therapy? (a) To delay the emergence of resistance to one drug through the use of a second drug. (b) To achieve prompt treatment of a desperately ill patient suspected of having a serious infection. (c) To allow for a reduction in the dosage of one or both drugs. (d) To achieve bactericidal synergism. (e) To cover a mixed infection.

3. Briefly describe three mechanisms whereby resistance can be transferred from one bacterium to another.

4. Which of the following statements correctly describe some of the properties of penicillins? (a) Patients who are allergic to benzylpenicillin will be allergic to the other penicillins. (b) The penicillins are bactericidal and act by disrupting the permeability of the cell membrane by binding to target enzymes (PBPs). (c) Oral penicillins should be administered 60 minutes before meals and at bedtime to achieve higher serum antibacterial activity. (d) Ampicillin is active against some Gram negative bacteria resistant to benzylpenicillin. (e) Semisynthetic penicillins can be administered in a mixed solution with gentamicin to treat serious staphylococcal infections.

5. List five indications for the use of each of the following agents.
(a) Benzylpenicillin (b) Ampicillin (c) Azlocillin (d) Flucloxacillin

6. Complete the following statements describing the administration and absorption of cephalosporins.
(a) .... and .... are well absorbed from the gastrointestinal tract. These cephalosporins are acid ....
(b) Cephalosporins administered by the intramuscular route cause .... and .... and occasionally sterile .... formation.
(c) The intravenous dose of cephamandole for an adult, in mild to moderate infections, is .... administered .... hourly.

7. Adverse effects to cephalosporins are similar to those encountered with the penicillins, nevertheless which of the following statements is correct: (a) patients with a history of delayed penicillin hypersensitivity can be treated with a cephalosporin; (b) diuretic agents or aminoglycosides may produce additive nephrotoxicity when used with a cephalosporin; (c) the cephalosporins appear to cause less immediate hypersensitivity reactions than the penicillins; (d) patients with hepatic dysfunction are at special risk of drug accumulation or toxic serum concentrations when receiving cephalosporins.

8. Which of the second generation cephalosporins are commonly prescribed for surgical prophylaxis?

9. List three β-lactams that may cause hypoprothrombinaemia, and a disulfiram-like reaction when alcohol is ingested?

10. What purpose does cilastatin serve in the combination product: imipenem–cilastatin?

11. (a) Clavulanic acid is a what? (b) When combined with amoxycillin it extends the spectrum of that drug to include *Proteus* sp. and *Pseudomonas aeruginosa*. True or false? (c) What adverse effects may occur after the discontinuation of amoxycillin/clavulanic acid?

12. Which of the following adverse effects may be experienced with tetracycline therapy:
(a) ototoxicity (b) thrombophlebitis (c) photosensitivity (d) nausea, heartburn and diarrhoea (e) hepatotoxicity

INFECTIOUS DISEASES

30 ■

13. (a) Parenteral gentamicin is used in the treatment of .... (b) Aminoglycosides are excreted almost entirely by the .... (c) High serum concentrations of the aminoglycosides may cause .... (d) In the presence of renal dysfunction the parenteral dose of the aminoglycoside should be .... or the dosage interval ....

14. (a) List some of the indications for the use of erythromycin (b) What erythromycin salt has been associated with hepatotoxicity?

15. (a) .... is a serious side effect associated with lincomycin and clindamycin therapy. (b) This side effect is due to the organism .... (c) .... in a dose of 125 mg orally 6-hourly is used to treat this side effect. (d) This drug (c) is generally administered intravenously to treat potentially life-threatening systemic .... infections. How should this IV dose be given?

16. Chloramphenicol is active against a wide variety of Gram positive and Gram negative organisms. Chloramphenicol is used infrequently, why?

17. How do the quinolones exert their antibacterial effect?

18. Are ciprofloxacin and norfloxacin both indicated for the treatment of bone and gastrointestinal tract infections? Explain your answer.

19. List three drug interactions that are known to occur with quinolones.

20. List three anti-infective agents that are known to colour the urine, and/or tears and other body fluid secretions. What advice would you give to a patient who wears soft contact lenses and is prescribed one of these agents?

21. Discuss the place of the combination product trimethoprim-sulfamethoxazole in the treatment of urinary tract infections or acute exacerbations of chronic bronchitis. What agents are preferred in these infections?

22. (a) Amphotericin B injection should be diluted in .... and administered over ..... hours. (b) .... and .... are triazole derivatives, ... is particularly active against *Aspergillus* sp. (c) Oral .... and .... may be used to treat tinea pedis. .... has been associated with fatal hepatic necrosis.

23. Doctor has prescribed ketoconazole 200 mg orally at 8 am daily, and cimetidine orally 400 mg bd. Can both these tablets be administered to the patient on the 8 am drug round? Explain your answer.

24. Explain how intravenous miconazole should be administered and what adverse effects the patient may experience.

25. (a) Metronidazole is one of the drugs of first choice for the treatment of ...., particularly those caused by *Bacteroides fragilis*. (b) The usual adult dose of metronidazole for intravenous infusion is .... mg administered .... hourly and infused over .... minutes. (c) Metronidazole in combination with .... may produce abdominal cramps, nausea, vomiting, headaches and flushing. (d) A patient who is breast feeding is ordered metronidazole as a single 2 g dose for trichomoniasis. What advice would you give the patient?

26. (a) Which antiviral agent(s) can be used to treat cytomegalovirus infections? (b) Which antivirals have activity against HIV? (c) What significant toxicity may accompany inhaled ribavirin therapy.

27. A patient is being treated for tuberculosis with a four drug regimen: isoniazid, rifampicin, pyrazinamide and ethambutol. How long would the four drugs continue and which two drugs would normally be continued for the entire 6 months?

28. What agents can be used by the traveller as prophylactic therapy against malaria when visiting a malaria-endemic region?

29. Your patient has been prescribed acyclovir 300mg IV 8 hourly. Discuss your approach to fulfilling this order safely and effectively.

30. A patient you are nursing has HIV infection and his treatment includes zidovudine 100 mg orally 4 hourly. He complains of fever and headache and asks you for some *Panadol*. What would be your response? Give reasons.

TABLE 30.10   Summary table — anti-infective therapy

DRUG GROUP Drug Name	Use	Action	Adverse Reactions	Nursing Implications
ANTIBACTERIAL AGENTS				
PENICILLINS Benzylpenicillin Phenoxymethylpenicillin Methicillin Cloxacillin Flucloxacillin Ampicillin Amoxycillin Amoxycillin–clavulanic acid Azlocillin Carbenicillin Mezlocillin Ticarcillin Ticarcillin–clavulanic acid Piperacillin	Wide variety of Gram positive and Gram negative aerobic and anaerobic infections	Bactericidal; inhibit bacterial cell wall synthesis	Relatively non-toxic; hypersensitivity reactions common; rarely: neurotoxicity, nephritis, haemolysis, hepatotoxicity	**Assess:** History of hypersensitivity, previous penicillin use, baseline temperature, signs of specific infection **Administer:** Around the clock; oral on an empty stomach; IM deep into large muscle, slowly, do not massage; IV slowly, at correct dilution, in compatible fluid **Evaluate:** Improvement in signs of infection; for hypersensitivity, drug toxicity and superinfection
CEPHALOSPORINS Cephazolin sodium Cephalothin sodium Cephamandole Cefoxitin Cephalexin Cefaclor Cefotaxime Ceftazidime Ceftriaxone Cefotetan Cefixime Latamoxef	Wide variety of Gram positive and Gram negative aerobic and anaerobic infections	Bactericidal; inhibit bacterial cell wall synthesis	Hypersensitivity reactions may occur; nephrotoxicity; haematological abnormalities: thrombophlebitis	**Assess:** As for penicillins; renal function; alcohol ingestion with some 2nd and 3rd generation agents **Administer:** As for penicillins **Evaluate:** As for penicillins; urine output

TABLE 30.10 continued

DRUG GROUP Drug Name	Use	Action	Adverse Reactions	Nursing Implications
MONOBACTAMS Aztreonam	Wide variety of Gram negative infections	Bactericidal; inhibits bacterial cell wall synthesis	Hypersensitivity reactions may occur; haematological abnormalities	**Assess:** As for penicillins **Administer:** Slow IV infusion around clock **Evaluate:** As for penicillins
CARBAPENEMS Imipenem	Wide variety of Gram positive and Gram negative aerobic and anaerobic infections	Bactericidal; inhibits bacterial cell wall synthesis	Hypersensitivity reactions may occur; CNS effects; haematological abnormalities: phlebitis; superinfections	**Assess:** As for penicillins **Administer:** Slow IV infusion around clock **Evaluate:** As for penicillins; CNS function
AMINOGLYCOSIDES Framycetin Gentamicin Tobramycin Amikacin Neomycin Netilmicin Kanamycin Streptomycin	Serious Gram negative infections and in combination with β lactams for Gram positive infections	Bactericidal; interfere with bacterial protein synthesis in ribosomes	Ototoxicity; nephrotoxicity; neuromuscular blockade; local irritation with IM and IV administration; hypersensitivity	**Assess:** As for penicillins; renal function; baseline hearing and balance **Administer:** As for IM/IV penicillins; reduce dose in renal impairment; high fluid intake **Evaluate:** As for penicillins; ototoxicity: hearing loss, dizziness, vertigo; nephrotoxicity: urine output, uraemia; neuromuscular blockade following surgery: respiratory depression, decreased pulse rate; monitor serum concentrations and auditory function

TABLE 30.10 continued

DRUG GROUP Drug Name	Use	Action	Adverse Reactions	Nursing Implications
TETRACYCLINES Chlortetracycline Tetracycline Doxycycline Methacycline Minocycline Roliltetracycline Oxytetracycline	Wide variety of Gram positive and Gram negative infections, particularly Gram negative infections not susceptible to penicillin; doxycycline: malaria prophylaxis and treatment	Bacteriostatic; inhibit protein synthesis by binding to bacterial ribosomes	Diarrhoea, nausea, heartburn, epigastric distress; superinfection with *Candida albicans*; hypersensitivity is uncommon; nephrotoxicity; hepatotoxicity; haematological abnormalities; thrombophlebitis with IV administration	**Assess:** As for penicillins; pregnancy; age: not to be given to children under 8 years or with growth impairment; liver disease, renal impairment **Administer:** As for penicillins; do not give with milk, iron or antacids **Evaluate:** As for penicillins; urine output, uraemia; jaundice
MACROLIDES Erythromycin Clarithromycin Roxithromycin Azithromycin	Wide variety of Gram positive infections and some Gram negative infections	Bacteriostatic in normal concentrations, bactericidal in high concentrations; inhibit protein synthesis in ribosomes	Least toxic of the antibiotics; abdominal cramps, nausea, vomiting, stomatitis, heartburn, anorexia, pruritus ani, occasional skin rash; thrombophlebitis with IV administration; occasional ototoxicity and hepatotoxicity	**Assess:** As for penicillins; liver function **Administer:** As for penicillins **Evaluate:** As for penicillins; liver impairment: jaundice, hepatomegaly, pale stools, dark urine; auditory function with IV administration

TABLE 30.10 continued

DRUG GROUP Drug Name	Use	Action	Adverse Reactions	Nursing Implications
MISCELLANEOUS AGENTS Lincomycin Clindamycin	Wide variety of Gram positive infections; Gram negative aerobic and anaerobic infections	Bacteriostatic in normal concentrations, bactericidal in high concentrations; inhibit protein synthesis in ribosomes	Nausea, vomiting, diarrhoea, cramping, pseudomembranous colitis; IV: transient flushing, syncope, cardiopulmonary arrest, thrombophlebitis; IM: pain	**Assess:** As for penicillins **Administer:** As for penicillins **Evaluate:** As for penicillins; diarrhoea containing blood or mucus; abdominal pain
Chloramphenicol	Wide variety of Gram negative and Gram positive infections including infections due to *Salmonella* sp., *Haemophilus influenzae*, *Vibrio cholera*, rickettsiae and *Mycoplasma* sp.; reserved for serious infections due to its toxicity	Bacteriostatic in low concentration, bactericidal in high concentration; inhibits bacterial protein synthesis	Aplastic anaemia, pancytopenia, haematopoietic toxicity; circulatory collapse in newborn (grey syndrome); optic neuritis; nausea, vomiting, glossitis, stomatitis; hypersensitivity reactions; anaphylaxis; angioedema; increased prothrombin time	**Assess:** As for penicillins; renal, hepatic and haemopoietic function **Administer:** As for penicillins **Evaluate:** As for penicillins, bone marrow suppression; grey syndrome in newborn; bleeding; optic neuritis
GLYCOPEPTIDE ANTIBIOTICS Vancomycin	Serious Gram positive infections, particularly those due to staphylococci resistant to other	Bactericidal; inhibits bacterial cell wall synthesis	Ototoxicity; nephrotoxicity; red-man syndrome with rapid IV infusion; pain, thrombophlebitis;	**Assess:** As for penicillins and aminoglycosides **Administer:** IV infusion over 60 minutes, 6 or

30 INFECTIOUS DISEASES

TABLE 30.10 continued

DRUG GROUP Drug Name	Use	Action	Adverse Reactions	Nursing Implications
	anti-infectives; antibiotic-associated colitis caused by *Clostridium difficile*		hypotension; rash; hypersensitivity reactions	12-hourly (reduce dose in renal impairment); oral, 6-hourly for 7–10 days (for antibiotic associated colitis) **Evaluate:** As for penicillins; ototoxicity: hearing loss, dizziness, vertigo; nephrotoxicity: urine output, uraemia; monitor serum concentrations
Teicoplanin	Serious Gram positive infections, particularly those due to staphylococci resistant to other anti-infectives	Bactericidal; inhibits bacterial cell wall synthesis	Ototoxicity; nephrotoxicity; pain, thrombophlebitis; hypotension; rash; hypersensitivity reactions	**Assess:** As for penicillins and aminoglycosides **Administer:** IM or IV bolus over 5 minutes, 24-hourly (reduce dose in renal impairment) **Evaluate:** As for penicillins; ototoxicity: hearing loss, dizziness, vertigo; nephrotoxicity: urine output, uraemia
CEPHALOSPORIN P ANTIBIOTICS Fusidic Acid	Severe Gram positive infections due to staphylococci	Bactericidal; inhibits protein synthesis	Mild GIT disturbance; rashes; jaundice, pain, thrombophlebitis and venospasm with IV use	**Assess:** As for penicillins; hepatic function **Administer:** Oral, 8-hourly; IV, over 2–4 hours **Evaluate:** As for penicillins; hepatic function

TABLE 30.10 continued

DRUG GROUP Drug Name	Use	Action	Adverse Reactions	Nursing Implications
RIFAMYCIN B ANTIBIOTICS Rifampicin	See section on antitubercular agents			
POLYMIXINS Polymixin B Colistin	Superficial and severe (colistin) Gram negative infections	Bactericidal, disrupt bacterial cell membrane	Topical use: hypersensitivity reactions; parenteral use: neurotoxicity, nephrotoxicity, hypersensitivity reactions	**Assess:** As for penicillins, renal function, neurological function **Administer:** Colistin: IM, IV, 6–12-hourly **Evaluate:** As for penicillins, renal function, serum albumin, serum electrolytes, mental status
PEPTIDE ANTIBIOTICS Bacitracin Gramicidin	Superficial Gram positive infections	Bactericidal, interfere with cell wall synthesis and/or cell membrane function	Topical use: hypersensitivity	**Assess:** Previous hypersensitivity **Administer:** Topically **Evaluate:** As for penicillins
AMINOCYCLITOL ANTIBIOTICS Spectinomycin	Penicillinase producing *Neisseria gonorrhoeae* infections	Bacteriostatic, inhibits protein synthesis	Pain at site of injection, dizziness, nausea, fever, rash, headache	**Assess:** As for penicillin, concomitant syphilis **Administer:** IM, single dose **Evaluate:** As for penicillins
Mupirocin	Superficial Gram positive infections	Bacteriostatic, inhibits RNA and protein synthesis	Local pain, stinging, burning, pruritus, skin rash	**Assess:** Previous allergy to drug or vehicle **Administer:** Topically **Evaluate:** As for penicillins

30 INFECTIOUS DISEASES

TABLE 30.10 continued

DRUG GROUP Drug Name	Use	Action	Adverse Reactions	Nursing Implications
NON-FLUORINATED QUINOLONES Nalidixic Acid	Gram negative infections of the urinary tract	Bactericidal; inhibits bacterial DNA synthesis	CNS: headache, malaise, drowsiness, dizziness, vertigo, syncope, sensory changes, visual disturbances, excitement, depression, confusion, seizures; GIT: nausea, vomiting, abdominal pain, diarrhoea; dermatological: rash, urticaria, photosensitivity reactions	**Assess:** History of hypersensitivity, convulsive disorder; weight, age, pregnancy, lactation; hepatic and renal function **Administer:** Orally, 6-hourly **Evaluate:** Reduction of clinical manifestations of infection; visual and CNS function; photosensitivity and hypersensitivity reactions **Educate:** Dosage regimen; signs of adverse reactions; photosensitivity
FLUORINATED QUINOLONES Ciprofloxacin Norfloxacin	Gram positive and Gram negative infections; systemic pseudomonal infection; gastrointestinal and urinary tract infections	Bactericidal; inhibit DNA-gyrase with disruption of DNA synthesis	CNS: dizziness, drowsiness, light-headedness, headache, confusion, convulsions; GIT: nausea, vomiting, diarrhoea dyspepsia, bitter taste; crystalluria; hypersensitivity; joint swelling; tendonitis; thrombophlebitis with IV use	**Assess:** History of hypersensitivity; possible interactions (e.g. with aminophylline, theophylline); renal, hepatic and CNS function; hydration status; pregnancy, lactation; should not be given to prepubertal children **Administer:** Orally on empty stomach, 12-hourly; IV over 30–60 minutes and maintain hydration

TABLE 30.10 continued

DRUG GROUP Drug Name	Use	Action	Adverse Reactions	Nursing Implications
				Evaluate: Reduction of clinical manifestations of infection; neurological and auditory function; fluid status and renal function; urine pH; photosensitivity reaction **Educate:** Dosage regimens; signs of adverse reactions; photosensitivity
FOLATE ANTAGONISTS Sulfacetamide Sulfadiazine Sulfadimidine Sulfadoxine Sulfamethizole Phthalylsulfathiazole	Chancroid; trachoma; nocardiosis; toxoplasmosis; malaria; Gram positive and Gram negative infections of urinary tract	Bacteriostatic; inhibits folic acid synthesis in bacteria and parasites	Hypersensitivity reactions; photosensitivity; agranulocytosis; thrombocytopenia; aplastic and haemolytic anaemia; jaundice; renal damage; CNS: headache, depression, malaise; GIT: nausea, vomiting; pain and thrombophlebitis with IV use	**Assess:** History of hypersensitivity to sulfonamide or related drugs; hepatic or renal disease; blood dyscrasias; pregnancy, lactation; concurrent use of anticoagulants, methotrexate, sulfonylurea hypoglycaemics, thiazides, uricosurics; baseline clinical signs of infection **Administer:** Oral, with food or after meals at equal intervals during day; IV, dilute according to directions, infuse over 20

30 INFECTIOUS DISEASES

TABLE 30.10 continued

DRUG GROUP Drug Name	Use	Action	Adverse Reactions	Nursing Implications
				minutes (sulfadiazine) or 60–90 minutes (trimethoprim–sulfamethoxazol) **Evaluate:** Abating signs of infection; hypersensitivity; blood dyscrasias (high fever, prostration, mucosal ulceration, lassitude, fatigue, dizziness, headache, unexplained bleeding, bruising); Stevens-Johnson syndrome (fever, headache, erythematous rash, rhinitis, conjunctivitis, stomatitis); renal dysfunction (decreased urinary output, blood in urine, renal colic); urinary pH (alkaliniser may be needed); maintain sufficient fluid intake to ensure at least 1500 mL output daily **Educate:** Importance of adequate fluid intake; report adverse effects; importance of completing course; photosensitivity

TABLE 30.10 continued

DRUG GROUP Drug Name	Use	Action	Adverse Reactions	Nursing Implications
Trimethoprim	Gram positive and Gram negative infections particularly of urinary tract; combined with sulfamethoxazole — urinary tract and other infections including *Pneumocystis carinii* pneumonia	Bactericidal; inhibits bacterial folic acid synthesis	Gastrointestinal upset; haematologic abnormalities (rare)	**Assess:** History of blood dyscrasias; renal impairment; liver disease; pregnancy, lactation; document clinical signs of infection **Administer:** Oral, with food **Evaluate:** Improvement in clinical manifestations of infection; blood dyscrasias (see sulfonamides above); observe skin for signs of hypersensitivity reactions **Educate:** Correct dosage regimen; report adverse effects
URINARY ANTISEPTICS Nitrofurantoin	Gram positive and Gram negative infections of urinary tract	Bacteriostatic in low concentrations, bactericidal in high concentrations; action enhanced in acidic urine; inhibits several bacterial enzyme systems	GIT disturbances; CNS: headache, dizziness, malaise, nystagmus, peripheral neuritis; acute allergic reactions; pulmonary toxicity; bone marrow depression; haemolytic and megaloblastic anaemias; brown colouration of urine; discolouration of infants' teeth	**Assess:** Impaired renal function; age; weight; pregnancy; blood dyscrasias; known hypersensitivity to drug **Administer:** Oral with food at equal intervals during 24 hours **Evaluate:** Reduction of clinical manifestations of infection; pH of urine; administer urinary acidifier if ordered where reabsorption

30 INFECTIOUS DISEASES

TABLE 30.10 continued

DRUG GROUP Drug Name	Use	Action	Adverse Reactions	Nursing Implications
				of drug is indicated in pyelonephritis; adverse effects **Educate:** Brown discolouration of urine
Hexamine Hippurate Hexamine Mandelate	Gram negative infections of the urinary tract	Releases the antibacterial formaldehyde in acid urine	GIT disturbances, rash, urticaria, pruritus; high doses and prolonged therapy lead to irritation of urinary tract	**Assess:** Hepatic and renal function; age; weight; fluid balance; pregnancy; pH of urine **Administer:** Oral with food at equal intervals during 24 hours **Evaluate:** pH of urine, maintain at or below 5.0; administer urinary acidifier as ordered; urinary output; if prolonged administration, test urine for protein and blood; rash, complaints of painful urination, gastric upsets

TABLE 30.10 continued

DRUG GROUP Drug Name	Use	Action	Adverse Reactions	Nursing Implications
ANTIPROTOZOAL AND ANTIANAEROBIC AGENTS Metronidazole	Protozoal infections; anaerobic bacterial infections, e.g. due to *Bacteroides fragilis* and *Clostridium* sp.	Uncertain; possibly inhibits DNA synthesis in susceptible microorganisms	Rash, pruritus, urticaria; GIT: nausea, anorexia, furry tongue, dry mouth, abdominal discomfort, metallic taste; CNS: headache, dizziness; leucopenia; darkening of urine, dysuria; interaction with alcohol; thrombophlebitis with IV administration of metronidazole	**Assess:** Pregnancy, lactation; current alcohol use, history of haematopoietic disorders **Administer:** Oral: with food to minimise GIT upset; IV metronidazole: infuse over 20 minutes **Evaluate:** Allergic reactions; GIT upsets; CNS toxicity; leucopenia; local irritation with IV use of metronidazole **Educate:** Self-evaluation for ADRs, e.g. metallic taste and discolouration of urine; avoid use of alcohol
Tinidazole	Protozoal infections; anaerobic bacterial infections, e.g. *Bacteroides fragilis*			

30 INFECTIOUS DISEASES

TABLE 30.10 continued

DRUG GROUP Drug Name	Use	Action	Adverse Reactions	Nursing Implications
Pentamidine isethionate	Protozoal infections including *Pneumocystis carinii* pneumonia	Uncertain; possibly antagonises folic acid metabolism in *Pneumocystis carinii*	Hypotension, cardiac arrhythmias; hypoglycaemia; nephrotoxicity; hypocalcaemia; leucopenia; anaemia; thrombocytopenia; GIT: nausea, vomiting, abdominal discomfort, anorexia, unpleasant taste; CNS: fever, confusion, hallucinations; bronchospasm; anaphylactic reactions; pruritus, urticaria, rash; abscess formation with IM use, phlebitis with IV use	**Assess:** Previous hypersensitivity; blood glucose; blood pressure; serum calcium; renal function; haematopoietic function; hydration status; hepatic function **Administer:** Deep IM injection; IV infusion over 60 minutes (minimises cardiac toxicity) **Evaluate:** Cardiac function and ECG; blood glucose, electrolytes; renal function; hydration status; complete blood picture; hepatic function

TABLE 30.10 continued

DRUG GROUP Drug Name	Use	Action	Adverse Reactions	Nursing Implications
ANTITUBERCULAR AGENTS				
Isoniazid	Tuberculosis; concomitant administration of pyridoxine advisable to prevent peripheral neuritis	Bactericidal or bacteriostatic; interferes with cellular synthesis and active only against rapidly growing tubercle bacilli	Resistance develops rapidly when used alone; vertigo, twitching of limbs; increased reflexes; urinary retention; psychoses, confusion, coma, convulsions if serum concentrations too high; peripheral neuritis; hepatitis; agranulocytosis, thrombocytopenia; anaemia	**Assess:** Physical condition; hepatic and renal function; full blood picture; alcohol use; CNS function; interacting drugs **Administer:** Oral, before breakfast **Evaluate:** Renal, hepatic and neurological function, haemopoietic parameters **Educate:** Need for compliance, multiple drugs and long-term therapy
Rifampicin	Tuberculosis; leprosy; some Gram positive and Gram negative infections	Bactericidal and bacteriostatic; interferes with RNA synthesis	Resistance develops when used alone; hepatocellular damage, jaundice; rare hypersensitivity reactions, flu-like syndrome; haematological changes; respiratory effects; reddish-orange colouration of urine, sweat, tears	**Assess:** Previous hypersensitivity; liver damage; interacting drugs; whether patient wears soft contact lenses **Administer:** Oral, before breakfast **Evaluate:** Liver function; haematological changes **Educate:** See isoniazid; interactions with oral contraceptives; colouration of urine, sweat, tears; staining of soft contact lenses

30 INFECTIOUS DISEASES

TABLE 30.10 continued

DRUG GROUP Drug Name	Use	Action	Adverse Reactions	Nursing Implications
Pyrazinamide	Tuberculosis due to *Mycobacterium tuberculosis*	Bacteriostatic and bactericidal	Resistance develops when used alone; hepatotoxicity, jaundice; gout; rash, arthralgia, fever, photosensitivity with reddish-brown skin discolouration; nausea, vomiting anorexia; thrombocytopenia; sideroblastic anaemia	**Assess:** Hepatic and renal function; porphyria; haematopoietic function; diabetes; gout **Administer:** Oral, 8–12-hourly **Evaluate:** Hepatic, renal and haematopoietic function **Educate:** See isoniazid; adverse effects; avoid excessive exposure to ultraviolet light
Ethambutol	Tuberculosis due to mycobacteria	Bacteriostatic; inhibits cellular metabolism	Resistance develops rapidly when used alone; ocular toxicity; peripheral neuritis (rare)	**Assess:** See isoniazid; visual function **Administer:** Oral, before breakfast **Evaluate:** Visual function **Educate:** See isoniazid; need for eye tests
ANTILEPROTIC AGENTS Dapsone	Leprosy; malaria prophylaxis	Bacteriostatic; interferes with cellular metabolism	Anaemia, leucopenia; reversal reaction (type I); erythema nodosum leprosum or lepromatous lepra reaction (type 2); cutaneous reactions; peripheral neuropathy; hepatitis; cholestatic jaundice;	**Assess:** Renal, hepatic and cardiovascular function; hypersensitivity to drug **Administer:** Oral, daily for some years in leprosy **Evaluate:** Adverse effects

TABLE 30.10 continued

DRUG GROUP Drug Name	Use	Action	Adverse Reactions	Nursing Implications
			albuminuria; nephrotic syndrome; anorexia, nausea, vomiting	**Educate:** To report sore throat, fever, pallor, purpura, jaundice, dark urine, skin rashes
Clofazimine	Leprosy; pyoderma gangrenosum	Active against various mycobacteria, inhibits DNA replication and growth	Pink-brownish discolouration of skin; ichthyosis, dry skin, pruritus, rash; reversible red-brown discolouration of eyes; dry, burning, itching, irritated, watery eyes; GIT: pain, diarrhoea, nausea, vomiting; CNS: dizziness, drowsiness, fatigue, headache, taste disorder; discolouration of urine and other body secretions	**Assess:** Baseline ocular and skin evaluations **Administer:** Oral, daily for some years **Evaluate:** Adverse effects particularly discolouration, severe abdominal colicky pain and persistent diarrhoea **Educate:** Warn about skin discolouration
ANTIMALARIAL AGENTS Chloroquine Hydroxychloroquine	Malaria due to *Plasmodium falciparum, P. vivax, P. ovale, P. malariae*	Blood schizonticide; complexes with DNA	Retinopathy; GIT disturbances; dermatological reactions; neurologic reactions; blood dyscrasias; chloroquine accumulates in the liver	**Assess:** Previous hypersensitivity; history of renal or hepatic disease, retinal or visual field defects; psoriasis; concurrent use of other drugs which are hepatotoxic, including alcohol; porphyria **Administer:** Prophylactic oral doses, same day each week with meals; in acute attacks, oral or parenteral doses as ordered

30 INFECTIOUS DISEASES

TABLE 30.10 continued

DRUG GROUP Drug Name	Use	Action	Adverse Reactions	Nursing Implications
				Evaluate: Ophthalmic examinations at regular intervals during long-term therapy, reports of blurred vision, blind spots, night blindness; GIT disturbances; skin reactions; neurological reactions; blood dyscrasias; hepatic function **Educate:** Correct dosage regimen; self-evaluation for adverse effects
Mefloquine	Chloroquine resistant malaria due to *Plasmodium falciparum*	Blood schizonticide; uncertain	GIT: diarrhoea, epigastric pain, nausea, vomiting; CNS: dizziness; muscle pain, tremor; seizures; bradycardia; haematological abnormalities	**Assess:** Previous hypersensitivity, history of seizures, renal, hepatic or cardiac disease **Administer:** Prophylaxis, same day each week; for acute attack, as ordered **Evaluate:** Haematological, neurological and cardiac function **Educate:** Compliance with regimen; self-evaluation for adverse effects

TABLE 30.10 continued

DRUG GROUP Drug Name	Use	Action	Adverse Reactions	Nursing Implications
Pyrimethamine	Malaria; toxoplasmosis	Blood schizonticide; antagonises folic acid, arresting sporogeny in mosquito	Dermatoses; folic acid deficiencies with bone marrow depression; GIT: anorexia, vomiting, nausea, glossitis; CNS with high dose: ataxia, tremor, seizures	**Assess:** If high doses to be used, history of hypersensitivity, convulsive disorders and folic acid deficiency **Administer:** Malaria prophylaxis: with meal same day each week; toxoplasmosis: same time each day **Evaluate:** Signs of folic acid deficiency (e.g. fever, sore tongue, rash, diarrhoea); renal and hepatic function; biweekly haematological studies during treatment of toxoplasmosis
Pyrimethamine–dapsone Pyrimethamine–sulfadoxine	Malaria due to chloroquine resistant *Plasmodium falciparum*	Blood schizonticide; antagonises folic acid, arresting sporogeny in mosquito	See pyrimethamine and dapsone See pyrimethamine and sulfonamides; fatalities have occurred due to erythema multiforme, Stevens–Johnson syndrome and toxic epidermal necrolysis	**Assess, Administer, Evaluate:** See pyrimethamine, dapsone and sulfonamides **Educate:** Importance of compliance with prophylactic regimen; cease therapy and consult doctor if adverse effects occur

30 INFECTIOUS DISEASES

TABLE 30.10 continued

DRUG GROUP Drug Name	Use	Action	Adverse Reactions	Nursing Implications
Primaquine	Malaria due to *Plasmodium vivax* and *Plasmodium ovale*	Tissue schizonticide; acts against fixed tissue (liver) stage of plasmodia	Abdominal cramps, epigastric distress; urticaria; haematological abnormalities	**Assess:** History of renal or haemopoietic disorders; document race of patient — some dark-skinned people demonstrate a primaquine sensitivity which can result in an acute anaemia **Administer:** With meals or antacids **Evaluate:** Gastrointestinal disturbances; evidence of haemolysis particularly in dark patients (decreased urinary output, dark or red urine, chills or fever) **Educate:** Self-evaluation for adverse effects, importance of regular blood tests
Quinine	Malaria due to chloroquine-resistant *Plasmodium falciparum*	Blood schizonticide; acts against erythrocytic phase of plasmodia	IV use: marked hypotension, hypoglycaemia; oral use: tinnitus, hearing impairment, dizziness, tremor, palpitations	**Assess:** Previous hypersensitivity; history of cardiac or renal disease; establish baseline blood pressure if being administered parenterally **Administer:** Oral doses — with meals as ordered; parenteral doses — in acute attacks, as ordered

TABLE 30.10 continued

DRUG GROUP Drug Name	Use	Action	Adverse Reactions	Nursing Implications
				Evaluate: Nausea, vomiting, diarrhoea, sweating, blurred vision, tinnitus, hearing deficiency; blood pressure and blood glucose during parenteral use **Educate:** Correct dosage regimen; self-evaluation for adverse effects
ANTIFUNGAL AGENTS Amphotericin B	Superficial and systemic fungal infections	Fungistatic; binds to sterols in fungal cell membrane and interferes with fungal cell permeability	Topical use: ADRs rare; parenteral use: high incidence of ADRs: fever, chills, anorexia, nausea, vomiting; thrombophlebitis; nephrotoxicity; hypokalaemia; hypomagnesaemia; reversible normochromic, normocytic anaemia; rarely liver function abnormalities, cardiac arrest after too rapid infusion	**Assess:** Previous allergy to drug; pregnancy, lactation; haematopoietic disorders; renal function; serum potassium; establish baseline observations of vital signs prior to parenteral administration **Administer:** IV, over 4 h by slow infusion in glucose buffered to correct pH **Evaluate:** Redness, swelling, pain at infusion site; muscle weakness (hypokalaemia), oliguria, haematuria; serum electrolytes and urea, complete blood picture, liver function tests; monitor vital

30 INFECTIOUS DISEASES

TABLE 30.10 continued

DRUG GROUP Drug Name	Use	Action	Adverse Reactions	Nursing Implications
			signs frequently during administration; monitor for signs of allergy and other adverse effects	
Flucytosine	Serious systemic infections caused by *Candida* and *Cryptococcus* sp.	Fungistatic; penetrates fungal cells where it is converted to fluorouracil which interferes with protein synthesis	Less toxic than amphotericin B; hypoplasia of bone marrow; nausea, vomiting, anorexia, abdominal bloating, diarrhoea; transient liver enlargement and alteration in liver function tests	**Assess:** Liver, renal and haematopoietic disorders; previous or concurrent radiotherapy or chemotherapy for malignancy **Administer:** Oral, each dose may be divided and given at 15-minute intervals to reduce nausea; IV, infuse over 20–40 minutes (do not heat or cool product) **Evaluate:** Complete blood picture; renal function; observe for confusion, headache, vertigo, bruising, bleeding, sore throat, GIT upsets; jaundice; report elevated blood urea, creatinine; serum concentrations
Fluconazole	Superficial and systemic fungal infections	Inhibition of fungal cytochrome P-450 dependent enzymes, interfering with ergesterol synthesis	GIT disturbance; rashes; hepatoxicity; dizziness, headache; haematological abnormalities; hypokalaemia	**Assess:** History for previous allergy, liver disease and haematological disorders **Administer:** Oral, 24-hourly; IV by slow infusion (200 mg/h)

TABLE 30.10 continued

DRUG GROUP Drug Name	Use	Action	Adverse Reactions	Nursing Implications
				Evaluate: GIT symptoms, skin rashes, muscle weakness (hypokalaemia), jaundice; interaction with other drugs, e.g. cyclosporin, warfarin
Itraconazole	Superficial and systemic fungal infections including aspergillosis	As for fluconazole	GIT disturbance; rashes; transient increase in liver function tests; hypokalaemia	**Assess:** History for previous allergy and liver disease **Administer:** Oral, 24-hourly with food **Evaluate:** As for fluconazole
Ketoconazole	Systemic and superficial fungal infections including dermatophytosis	Fungistatic; interacts with sterol or fatty acid metabolism in fungal cell altering membrane permeability; interferes with oxidative enzymes	Nausea, vomiting, diarrhoea, abdominal pain; rash; gynaecomastia; severe hepatotoxicity	**Assess:** Previous allergy to drug; liver disease; concurrent use of antacids, H2 antagonists or other interacting drugs **Administer:** Acidic solution to facilitate absorption in achlorhydria; drugs likely to decrease gastric acidity should be given 2 hours after the dose **Evaluate:** Hepatic function; interactions with other drugs, e.g. phenytoin, warfarin, cyclosporin

30 INFECTIOUS DISEASES

TABLE 30.10 continued

DRUG GROUP Drug Name	Use	Action	Adverse Reactions	Nursing Implications
				Educate: Report any signs of hepatotoxicity (abdominal pain, dark urine, pale stools, jaundice) to doctor
Miconazole	Topical and vaginal infections; IV for systemic candidiasis, histoplasmosis and other fungal infections	Fungistatic; interferes with sterol metabolism in fungal cell altering membrane permeability	Topical: ADRs rare; IV: phlebitis; pruritus; rash; nausea, vomiting; fever, chills; drowsiness; erythrocyte aggregation, anaemia, thrombocytosis; hyperlipidaemia; cardiac arrhythmias with rapid infusion	**Assess:** Previous allergy to drug or vehicle; haematopoietic disorders; establish baseline observations of vital signs prior to parenteral administration; ensure results of blood tests and/or electrolyte studies to hand **Administer:** IV by slow infusion over 30–60 minutes; prevent extravasation; topically or vaginally using correct procedure **Evaluate:** IV administration: vital signs, cardiac effects, allergic reactions, phlebitis and skin irritation at infusion site; topical and vaginal administration: oedema, pruritus, irritation at site of application **Educate:** Correct method for vaginal administration

TABLE 30.10 continued

DRUG GROUP Drug Name	Use	Action	Adverse Reactions	Nursing Implications
Clotrimazole Econazole Isoconazole	Topical and vaginal fungal infections	Fungistatic; interferes with sterol metabolism in fungal cell altering membrane permeability	Well tolerated. Topical: local blistering, burning, irritation; erythema; pruritus. Vaginal: rash, irritation, itching, burning; lower abdominal cramps, bloating; slight urinary frequency	**Assess:** History of previous allergy to imidazoles or sensitivity to antioxidants **Administer:** Using correct technique **Evaluate:** Signs of local irritation **Educate:** Correct method of vaginal administration
Griseofulvin	Mycoses of skin, hair and nails caused by dermatophytes, e.g. *Trictophyton*, *Microsporum* and *Epidermophyton* sp.	Fungistatic; disrupts division of cell nucleus	Relatively non-toxic; headache; epigastric pain, nausea, vomiting, diarrhoea, thirst, flatulence; oral thrush; hypersensitivity rashes; photosensitivity	**Assess:** History of hypersensitivity; hepatic disease or porphyria **Administer:** With high-fat foods **Evaluate:** Clinical response; adverse effects **Educate:** To take drug with high-fat food; to avoid excessive exposure to ultraviolet light; to complete prescribed course; self-evaluation for adverse effects

30 INFECTIOUS DISEASES

TABLE 30.10 continued

DRUG GROUP Drug Name	Use	Action	Adverse Reactions	Nursing Implications
Terbinafine	Tinea pedis, tinea cruris, tinea corporis, cutaneous candidiasis	Fungicidal, interferes with ergesterol synthesis by inhibiting squalene perioxidase	Topical use: erythema, pruritus, stinging; Oral use: nausea, abdominal pain, rash, pruritus, headache, dizziness	**Assess:** Previous hypersensitivity; possible interacting drugs **Administer:** Oral, daily; topical, 12-hourly **Evaluate:** Clinical response **Educate:** Need to complete full course of treatment
Nystatin	Topical and vaginal *Candida* sp. infections	Fungistatic; binds to sterols in fungal cell membranes and interferes with fungal cell permeability	Virtually no ADRs with topical application	**Assess:** Previous hypersensitivity **Administer:** Using correct technique **Evaluate:** Clinical response **Educate:** Importance of proper application and completion of prescribed course of therapy
ANTIVIRAL AGENTS Amantadine	Prophylaxis against influenza A infections, Parkinson's disease, see chapter 25	Uncertain; possibly interferes with viral penetration into susceptible cells	CNS: nervousness, lack of concentration, dizziness, light-headedness, slurred speech, ataxia, drowsiness, insomnia, blurred vision, dry mouth; palpitations; congestive heart failure, oedema, orthostatic hypotension; photosensitivity	**Assess:** History of psychiatric, cardiac, hepatic or renal disorders; hypertension; concurrent use of anticholinergic drugs, MAO inhibitors, tricyclic antidepressants and antipsychotic drugs; establish baseline BP and pulse rate

TABLE 30.10 continued

DRUG GROUP Drug Name	Use	Action	Adverse Reactions	Nursing Implications
				Administer: With food **Evaluate:** Signs of sympathomimetic and atropine-like side effects; BP (lying and standing), pulse rate, urinary output, changes in behaviour, slurred speech, drowsiness, insomnia, palpitations, blurred vision, dry mouth **Educate:** Drug for prophylactic use only (when used as antiviral agent); self-evaluation of adverse effects
Acyclovir	Herpes simplex and varicella-zoster infections (topical and systemic)	Virostatic; inhibits DNA polymerase in herpes virus	Ophthalmic: transient stinging; oral: nausea, vomiting, diarrhoea, arthralgia, fever, sore throat, muscle and leg pain; IV: phlebitis, rash, anaemia, leucopenia; neurotoxicity; raised liver enzymes; raised blood urea; renal tubular damage	**Assess:** Clinical signs of infection; weight; hepatic and renal function with systemic use **Administer:** Topical, as ordered using correct technique; oral, 4-hourly while awake; IV, over 60 minutes, maintain adequate hydration, prevent extravasation

30 INFECTIOUS DISEASES

TABLE 30.10 continued

DRUG GROUP Drug Name	Use	Action	Adverse Reactions	Nursing Implications
				Evaluate: Efficacy; topical: signs of local stinging or irritation; IV: behavioural changes, phlebitis; creatinine, BUN, urine output **Educate:** Topical: correct technique and importance of completing prescribed course; oral: 4-hourly while awake
Ganciclovir	Serious cytomegalovirus infections	Inhibition of DNA synthesis by competing with viral DNA polymerase and acting as a false nucleotide	Neutropenia, thrombocytopenia, retinal detachment, CNS toxicity (confusion, headache, delirium seizures), GIT disturbances, abnormal liver function tests, raised serum creatinine	**Assess:** History of previous allergy, renal disease, haematological disorders and concurrent use of bone marrow suppressing drugs **Administer:** IV, by slow infusion over 1 hour; avoid IM or SC; observe same administration precautions as cytotoxic drugs **Evaluate:** GIT upset, bleeding (thrombocytopenia), infection (neutropenia) CNS symptoms, extravasation
Vidarabine	Herpes simplex and Herpes zoster infections; varicella-zoster infections	Virostatic; inhibits host cell DNA polymerase preventing intracellular viral multiplication	IV: haematological changes; neurotoxicity; hypokalaemia, hypophosphataemia, hypoglycaemia; GIT: nausea,	**Assess:** Previous allergy to drug; pregnancy; weight; renal or hepatic disease; serum potassium levels;

TABLE 30.10 continued

DRUG GROUP Drug Name	Use	Action	Adverse Reactions	Nursing Implications
			vomiting, diarrhoea; CNS: malaise, weakness, tremor, hallucinations, confusion; pain, thrombophlebitis at infusion site	baseline clinical signs of infection **Administer:** Ophthalmic — as ordered using correct technique **Evaluate:** Ophthalmic — efficacy, local adverse effects (burning, irritation, pain, photophobia); IV — efficacy, adverse reactions (e.g. fluid overload, serum electrolytes, neurotoxicity, nausea, vomiting); liver function tests; complete blood picture **Educate:** Ophthalmic — correct technique and importance of completing prescribed course

TABLE 30.10 continued

DRUG GROUP Drug Name	Use	Action	Adverse Reactions	Nursing Implications
Idoxuridine	Ocular keratitis due to viral infections; herpes simplex skin lesions	Virostatic; inhibits growth and replication of viral DNA	Ophthalmic: allergy, pain and pruritus in eye or eyelids; corneal defects; topical: skin irritation, oedema; secondary bacterial infections	**Assess:** Previous allergy to drug **Administer:** Eye drops — use correct technique, avoid contact of dropper with eyelids or lashes, observe correct storage precautions **Evaluate:** Efficacy; adverse reactions (pain, pruritus in eye or lids) **Educate:** Ophthalmic — correct technique and importance of completing prescribed course
Ribavirin	Respiratory syncytial virus bronciolitis	Virostatic; inhibits viral protein synthesis and replication	Rashes; conjunctivitis; bronchospasm; anaemia; hypotension and cardiac arrest	**Assess:** Previous hypersensitivity, lung function, pregnancy **Administer:** Aerosol as ordered using correct technique **Evaluate:** Aerosol — efficacy, adverse effects (acute deterioration in respiratory function) **Educate:** Aerosol — correct technique and importance of compliance

TABLE 30.10 continued

DRUG GROUP Drug Name	Use	Action	Adverse Reactions	Nursing Implications
Zidovudine	Amelioration of symptoms of HIV infection	Virostatic; inhibits viral transcription by interfering with reverse transcriptase	Haematological: bone marrow toxicity with anaemia, granulocytopenia; CNS: headache, asthenia, malaise, somnolence, dizziness, paraesthesia, agitation, restlessness, insomnia; GIT: nausea, pain, diarrhoea, dyspepsia, anorexia, vomiting; other: myalgia, dyspnoea, fever, rash, taste perversion	**Assess:** Clinical signs of infection; neurological status; haematopoietic function; renal, hepatic function; concomitant drug therapy **Administer:** Oral, 4-hourly around clock **Evaluate:** Weekly or biweekly haematopoietic function, complete blood picture; efficacy; hepatic, renal function; neurological status **Educate:** Importance of compliance; not to share medication; not a cure for HIV infection; importance of monitoring for adverse effects (self and doctor); avoid use of paracetamol and paracetamol-containing products
Didanosine	Amelioration of symptoms of HIV infection	Virostatic; inhibits viral reverse transcriptase	Pancreatitis; peripheral neuropathy; GIT: diarrhoea, nausea, vomiting; dry mouth, insomnia, rash, fever hyperuricaemia,	**Assess:** Clinical signs of infection; history of pancreatitis or use of drugs capable of causing pancreatitis

30 INFECTIOUS DISEASES

TABLE 30.10 continued

DRUG GROUP Drug Name	Use	Action	Adverse Reactions	Nursing Implications
			hypokalaemia, altered liver function tests, thrombocytopenia	**Administer:** Oral, 2 tablets 12-hourly **Evaluate:** Symptoms of pancreatitis and peripheral neuropathy **Educate:** Importance of compliance; not a cure for HIV infection; importance of monitoring adverse effects
Zalcitabine	Amelioration of symptoms of HIV infection	Virostatic; inhibits viral reverse transcriptase	Peripheral neuropathy; myelosuppression; pancreatitis; cardiomyopathy; heart failure; oesophageal ulcers; hepatotoxicity; anaphylaxis	**Assess:** History of peripheral neuropathy, blood disorders and pancreatitis or use of drugs capable of causing these disorders **Administer:** Oral, 8-hourly **Evaluate:** Symptoms of peripheral neuropathy, blood disorders and pancreatitis; complete blood picture **Educate:** Importance of compliance; not a cure for HIV infection; self-evaluation of adverse effects

TABLE 30.10 continued

DRUG GROUP Drug Name	Use	Action	Adverse Reactions	Nursing Implications
Foscarnet	Cytomegalovirus infections	Virostatic; inhibition of DNA polymerase	Nephrotoxicity; haematological: anaemia, leucopenia; metabolic: hypo- and hypercalcaemia, hypo- and hyperphosphataemia, hypomagnesaemia; CNS disturbances including seizures; genital ulcers	**Assess:** Renal function, haematopoietic function, history of seizures **Administer:** IV by slow infusion **Evaluate:** Routine urinalysis and renal function tests; serum electrolytes; complete blood picture; observe for genital ulcerations. **Educate:** Inform patient of possibility of renal adverse effects and to report any polyuria/polydipsia

30 INFECTIOUS DISEASES

Cancer Chemotherapy

MICHAEL J. CAIN

O B J E C T I V E S

At the conclusion of this chapter the reader should be able to:

1. Discuss the aims of cancer chemotherapy;

2. Describe the general principles of antineoplastic drug therapy;

3. List the expected or common side effects of the anticancer agents in regular use;

4. Discuss cytotoxic drug administration and the procedures employed to limit the toxicity of individual agents; and

5. Prepare a nursing care plan that covers nursing assessment of the patient, potential problems related to drug administration and patient education.

CYTOTOXIC AGENTS ████████████████

The antineoplastic drugs are those agents which act with some degree of selectivity against the uncontrolled proliferation of cancerous cells. Most agents in use are cytotoxic, directly or indirectly affecting DNA or DNA function to cause cell death.

Cytotoxic agents are generally considered to have a particular affinity for cells that are in the process of dividing. Drugs described as 'cell cycle specific' act on specific parts of the cell division cycle and will only affect cells if they are present at the time that cells pass through that stage (see Figure 31.1). Importantly these drugs do not affect cells in the resting phase (G_0). Agents that are 'cell cycle non-specific' act on cells in any part of the cell cycle, although they often have a more profound effect on those cells actively dividing.

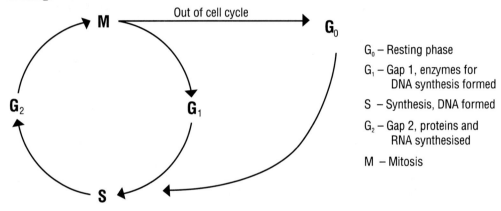

FIGURE 31.1   The cell division cycle

Increased susceptibility during active cell division is thought to explain two major observations in the treatment of malignant disease:

1. Malignancies that show the best response are, in general, those with a relatively rapid rate of growth and a large percentage of their cell population undergoing division (high growth fraction). These include testicular carcinoma, high grade lymphomas, acute leukemias and small cell carcinoma of the lung.

2. The principal adverse reactions of cytotoxic drugs develop in those non-malignant tissues which have a high growth fraction. These include bone marrow (causing myelosuppression), gastrointestinal mucosa (causing mucositis or diarrhoea), hair follicles (causing alopecia) and the gonads (causing menstrual irregularities, decreased spermatogenesis, sterility). See Figure 31.2.

Hormonal agents, biological response modifiers and steroids used in cancer treatment are significantly different in their modes of action when compared to cytotoxic drugs. In general these agents stimulate or block cellular receptors that play a part in the complex system of signals that control cellular proliferation and differentiation. For example, tamoxifen blocks the effect of oestrogen on breast tissue. The effect on breast cancer cells is to block one pathway that stimulates growth. Breast cancer cells may become dormant or may undergo programmed cell death (a normal cell process which removes damaged or excess cells). Hormones, steroids and biological response modifiers exhibit a very different range of toxicities.

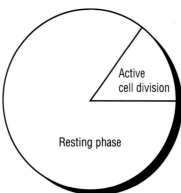

FIGURE 31.2   Generalised comparison of the growth fractions of malignant and non-malignant cell populations

DRUG COMBINATIONS AND DOSE SCHEDULES

Cytotoxic agents are used in combination for two reasons: firstly, to maximise response rate; and secondly, to prevent or delay the emergence of drug resistance.

In general only agents that produce a response rate of at least 15%–20% when used alone are included in combination treatments. The usual aim is to combine agents that have different 'dose limiting toxicities'. This allows each agent to be used at its highest tolerable dosage, thereby allowing maximal therapeutic effect. For example, the chemotherapy protocol BEP (comprising the drugs bleomycin, etoposide and cisplatin) used in the curative treatment of testicular cancer has little in the way of overlapping toxicity. Bleomycin dosage is limited by lung toxicity, etoposide by myelo-suppression and cisplatin by renal or neurological toxicity.

The schedule of drug administration (i.e. whether the drug is given as a single bolus, multiple small doses or an infusion over a period of hours or days) has largely been determined by the 'cell cycle specificity' of the agent and the premise that cycles or pulses of cytotoxic treatment have an improved therapeutic advantage. Drugs that are cell cycle specific, i.e. act primarily at one part of the cell cycle, are more active when given over an extended period. Prolonged exposure (over a number of days) allows more and more cells to enter the critical part of the cell cycle and hence be affected. Conversely, cell cycle non-specific drugs are, in theory, effective whether given as a single bolus or spread over a number of days. The cell cycle specific and non-specific cytotoxic agents are listed in Table 31.1.

CANCER CHEMOTHERAPY

31

TABLE 31.1 Cell cycle specific and non-specific cytotoxic agents

Cell cycle specific agents

Antimetabolites
Epipodophyllotoxins
Vinca alkaloids
Colaspase
Hydroxyurea
Bleomycin

Cell cycle non-specific agents

Alkylating agents
Anthracyclines
Anthracenediones
Platinum complexes
Dactinomycin
Mitomycin C

Malignant growths are considered to have a high percentage of cells in the process of dividing compared with normal cell populations. This, and the ability of normal cell populations to 'recruit' extra cells from the relatively protected resting phase, is thought to allow normal cell populations (e.g. white blood cells) to recover prior to the next treatment cycle while the tumour population does not. (See Figure 31.3.)

Resistance of cancer cells to cytotoxic drugs either from the start or developing during treatment is the most common cause of treatment failure. In theory the use of combinations of drugs that have differences in pharmacology (e.g. different mechanisms of action and ways in which the drug is handled by cells) reduces the chance of tumour resistance or delays its onset.

The philosophies and theories discussed in the simplest of terms above should be seen as generalisations only. There exists in current practice many recognised treatment protocols that do not fit entirely within these conventions.

AIMS OF CYTOTOXIC THERAPY

The way in which cancer chemotherapy is applied and the intensity of the doses used is determined by the balance between the expected outcome of treatment and the likely toxicity. Essentially, when the intended aim is cure, a high level of short-term toxicity is considered acceptable provided long-term effects are minimal. An example of agents with unacceptable long-

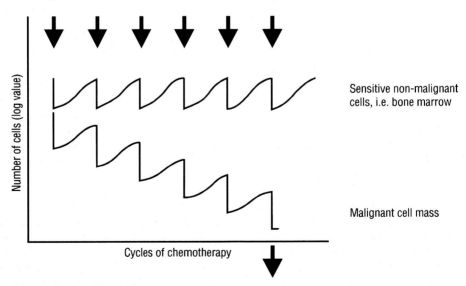

FIGURE 31.3 Basis for cycles of cytotoxic therapy

term toxicities are the alkylating agents, which may induce secondary malignancies and sterility. Where cure or long-term remission is expected alternative effective therapies, *if available*, are used.

Adjuvant chemotherapy is that used to treat patients who have undergone an apparently curative initial treatment, usually surgery. In this setting treatment is administered to reduce the rate of recurrence. Treatment is given with the knowledge that a percentage of patients will have achieved a true cure with the primary treatment and will consequently undergo chemotherapy unnecessarily. Unfortunately patients in this position cannot be identified at the time treatment needs to be given. Adjuvant therapy may improve the long-term disease free survival rate, e.g. from 55% to 75%, with 20% of patients in this example gaining obvious benefit. The toxicities of the treatment are closely assessed given that 55% of patients derive no benefit from treatment.

At the other end of the treatment spectrum is palliative therapy. This is used not with the intention of prolonging life but rather to relieve or prevent the symptoms of advanced malignancy. In this setting avoidance of short-term toxicity and hence maintenance of quality of life takes high priority, while long-term toxicities are largely irrelevant.

CYTOTOXIC SIDE EFFECTS

Cytotoxic agents are associated with a diverse range of side effects. A number of these are significant or typical of many cytotoxic agents and hence are discussed here rather than included in the individual monographs.

Myelosuppression, a reduction in the production of the different blood cell lines, is the most common limitation to increasing cytotoxic drug doses. The leucocytes (most importantly neutrophils) and platelets are more readily affected, while erythrocytes are usually reduced only after intense therapy or multiple cycles. Some cytotoxic agents are notable for their lack of bone marrow toxicity, these include bleomycin, cisplatin and vincristine.

The pattern of thrombocyte, leucocyte and erythrocyte depression varies in intensity and duration depending on the agent or combination of agents used, and the dosage. For example, cyclophosphamide and ifosfamide have a greater effect on leucocytes than platelets, while carboplatin treatment is often limited by significant thrombocytopenia, see Figure 31.4.

The duration of myelosuppression for leucocytes and platelets for many treatments is 21–28 days, however, if intensive high dose treatments are used this can be considerably longer. Other agents, e.g. lomustine and carmustine, have a delayed and prolonged effect with myelosuppression persisting for 6–8 weeks. Some agents, e.g. chlorambucil, have a cumulative effect on marrow function such that, without continued close monitoring and adjustment of dose, bone marrow function may be permanently reduced.

With the exception of bone marrow transplantation programs and the treatment of acute leukaemias, the intention with cytotoxic therapy is to avoid severe or life threatening myelosuppression and, more specifically, to avoid life threatening infection, haemorrhage and symptomatic anaemia.

Prior to the availability of the haematopoietic growth factors and autologous stem cell transfusions cytotoxic dosage was in most cases limited by myelosuppression. The primary exception to this being the treatment of acute leukaemia where severe myelosuppression is expected and the consequences of that myelosuppression form part of the accepted risk of treatment. The availability of granulocyte colony stimulating factors (filgrastim, lenograstim) and granulocyte-macrophage colony stimulating factor (molgramostim) and the greater availability of peripheral stem cell transfusions make it possible to further increase cytotoxic drug doses while avoiding significant or life threatening deficiencies in blood counts, most notably neutrophils.

CANCER CHEMOTHERAPY

31

The use of higher cytotoxic drug doses in most instances awaits proof of improved patient survival and hence has not been widely adopted. With myelosuppression ameliorated other dose limiting toxicities are encountered as doses are increased. Larger doses will in general increase the severity of many known but previously non-troublesome toxicities. Significant organ or tissue toxicities not associated with conventional doses may also emerge.

Nausea and vomiting have, to a large degree, become associated with anticancer treatment in general. Whilst symptoms can be severe with some therapies there are many agents which rarely induce significant nausea, vomiting or anorexia. Table 31.2 lists cytotoxic agents in relative order of emetic potential. In considering the relative potencies of these it is important to note that effects are usually related to dose, e.g. low dose oral cyclophosphamide is usually well tolerated but high dose intravenous therapy almost always requires prophylactic antiemetics. Nausea, vomiting and anorexia associated with cytotoxic drugs commonly last for 12–48 hours. The notable exception to this is cisplatin where effects can persist for seven or more days in susceptible patients.

Cytotoxic drugs damage or inhibit DNA function and are considered potentially mutagenic or carcinogenic. For this reason patients should take precautions to avoid pregnancy during treatment. When a patient who is already pregnant requires cytotoxic therapy the available options for treatment often pose an ethical and medical dilemma. Much is unknown about the effect of individual agents on the fetus. Judgements

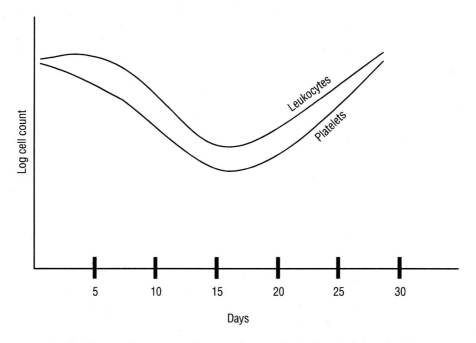

• Not all cytotoxics cause myelosuppression, e.g. bleomycin, vincristine, cisplatin

• Patterns of myelosuppression vary between agents in duration and selectivity

• Depth and duration of nadir both increase the risk of significant complications

FIGURE 31.4 Pattern of cytotoxic induced myelosuppression using carboplatin at standard dose as an example

TABLE 31.2 Incidence, onset and duration of cytotoxic induced vomiting

Agent	Incidence	Onset (hours)	Duration (hours)
Cisplatin	> 90%	1–6	7 days
Dacarbazine		1–3	1–12
Dactinomycin		2–6	12–24
Mustine hydrochloride		0.5–2.0	8–24
Cyclophosphamide >1 g		4–8	4–10
Carmustine		2–4	4–24
Lomustine		2–6	4–6
Doxorubicin		4–6	6
Daunorubicin		2–6	24
Cytarabine		6–12	3–5
Procarbazine		24–27	
Etoposide		3–8	
Mitomycin-C			
Methotrexate			
Fluorouracil		3–6	
Hydroxyurea		6–12	
Bleomycin		3–6	
Vinblastine	< 10%		
Vincristine			
Chlorambucil			
Busulphan			

are therefore made on a case by case basis. Breast feeding during treatment is poorly studied and not recommended for any cytotoxic drug.

Cytotoxic drugs, in particular the alkylating agents, have been associated with an increased risk of secondary malignancies in certain conditions. Alkylating agents are avoided where possible when treating malignancies for which a cure or long-term remission may be expected and an effective alternative exists.

Occupational exposure to cytotoxics may be hazardous and all agents are subject to the same stringent safeguards in handling. (See General Nursing Implications).

CANCER CHEMOTHERAPY

31

GENERAL NURSING IMPLICATIONS

In no other field of drug therapy are agents as uniformly toxic as those used to treat malignant disease. In general terms treatment is designed to allow maximal therapy while keeping toxicity within limits acceptable for the case being treated. With this as the aim there will still be a percentage of patients who experience unexpected and unacceptable toxicity. Awareness of the points salient to the prevention and management of side effects provides the opportunity to limit the incidence or severity of toxicity in many instances.

ASSESSMENT

Cytotoxic agents are given with the intent that likely benefits will outweigh the known or likely toxicities. A shift in this balance occurs if individual patients have characteristics that predispose them to toxicity and these characteristics are not given consideration prior to treatment.

Myelosuppression and poor marrow reserve are prime examples where administration of full doses of myelotoxic therapy is likely to result in serious toxicity. Before administering cytotoxic drugs the nurse should confirm that the patient has an adequate blood count or that the prescriber is aware and that the charted dose is fully intended.

In addition to adequate blood counts the presence of infection, mucositis or diarrhoea or any other significant toxicity due to prior treatment should be considered before administration of cytotoxic drugs. Supportive care measures, e.g. antiemetics, should be reviewed if prior outcomes were unacceptable. The nurse should ensure that the prescribing physician is aware of any such problems.

Treatment with the same therapy should not be given if there are obvious signs of disease progression whilst on therapy.

ADMINISTRATION

The majority of cytotoxic agents are given intravenously. The rate of administration, the dilution used, the order of administration, the selection of venous access and the avoidance of extravasation can all be significant to the efficacy and toxicity of therapy depending on the agents used. For protocols involving oral therapy correct administration usually involves the additional elements of patient education and compliance.

Many agents have side effects that can be avoided or minimised with appropriate measures. Examples of these include: adequate hydration to minimise renal damage with cisplatin; use of the protective agent mesna to prevent ifosfamide induced haemorrhagic cystitis; use of the specific antidote leucovorin to prevent the potentially life threatening toxicity of high dose methotrexate therapy; and use of effective antiemetics to prevent or minimise nausea and vomiting from highly nauseating therapies. In general these preventive measures are built into cytotoxic protocols or form part of standard practice within institutions.

Other preventive measures are more broadly applicable. These include the use of good administration techniques to prevent extravasation of agents with vesicant potential and initiation of appropriate mouthcare in patients at risk of cytotoxic induced mucositis. As with drug administration there are aspects requiring patient education and compliance.

In addition to causing side effects in patients cytotoxic drugs are also considered to be potentially toxic to healthworkers if handling precautions are not taken. Some cytotoxics are irritant to the skin, mucous membranes and eyes following accidental splashing. The major concern, however, is the theoretical risk of DNA damage leading to carcinogenesis and teratogenic effects. The basis for these concerns is the increased incidence of secondary cancers observed in some treated patients and animal studies and reports that healthworkers preparing cytotoxic agents for administration (dissolving, drawing up, diluting and administering) had small but detectable levels of cytotoxic drugs present in their urine and blood. Standards for handling cytotoxic drugs have since been dramatically improved. Drug preparation is considered the greatest source of exposure, primarily as a result of the drug being sprayed into the air. In all centres where cytotoxic drug therapy is used regularly drug preparation is carried out by specialised pharmacy services. Where the currently recommended guidelines have been implemented studies have been unable to detect contamination in healthworkers.

Nursing staff involved in the administration of cytotoxic drugs should be aware of the procedures for preventing exposure. Additionally procedures and facilities for dealing with cytotoxic spills and waste should be in place.

EVALUATION

Early recognition of adverse effects is important. Anaphylactic reactions and the inadvertent extravasation of vesicants into soft tissues are examples of immediate toxicities that may be significantly reduced in severity if appropriate action is taken early. Procedures and materials to deal with these problems must be readily available.

Although many side effects occur in the days or weeks following treatment myelosuppression is the most common and usually the most important. Most protocols are designed with the intention of avoiding significant myelosuppression, however, this will still occur in a percentage of patients. Patients who become febrile and unwell in the days following chemotherapy must be treated promptly. Any early signs of myelosuppression should be reported to the treating physician or clinic without delay.

PATIENT EDUCATION

Patient education, particularly for outpatient treatment, is of major importance. Nursing staff are well placed to provide or reinforce patient education.

Patients and their carers need to be made aware of the signs and symptoms of febrile neutropenia and thrombocytopenia and what action to take if such symptoms develop. Similarly, mucositis is a toxicity that requires recognition and response by the patient and carer. Other important but less generalised toxicities may be prevented or modified with appropriate patient education. Examples are listed under specific drugs.

The importance of taking oral chemotherapy strictly as prescribed and keeping appointments for regular blood tests needs to be stressed.

ALKYLATING AGENTS

As a class the alkylating agents make up the largest and most commonly used cytotoxic group. Although basically having the same mechanism of action, their considerable differences in reactivity, cellular uptake and pharmacokinetics mean that resistance to one alkylating agent does not necessarily result in resistance to others.

Alkylating agents derive their name from their ability to chemically add alkyl groups to the nucleophilic groups found on amino acids, proteins and, most importantly, the nucleic acids that make up DNA and RNA. Alkylation of nucleic acids disrupts and inhibits DNA and RNA function and is considered responsible for the significant cytotoxic, mutagenic and carcinogenic properties of these drugs. Some alkylating agents are highly reactive

CANCER CHEMOTHERAPY

31

when administered (e.g. nitrogen mustard), some require metabolism within the body to the known active agent (e.g. cyclophosphamide), while for others the active form of the drug remains unknown.

A significant component of cytotoxicity from this class of drugs is attributed to the cross linking of DNA strands by bifunctional alkylating agents. These agents which have, or are able to form, reactive sites at two locations on their structure, are considerably more potent than agents having only one reactive site.

Alkylating agents can be grouped according to chemical structure, see Table 31.3.

NITROGEN MUSTARDS

Chlorambucil

TRADE NAMES

Chlorambucil: *Leukeran.*

MECHANISM OF ACTION

Chlorambucil and its main metabolite are bifunctional alkylating agents. Chlorambucil is a derivative of mustine hydrochloride that is orally active and chemically less reactive.

PHARMACOKINETICS

Chlorambucil is absorbed orally reaching peak blood levels after 45–60 minutes. It has a half-life of approximately 60 minutes compared with 120 minutes for its active metabolite. Further metabolism to inactive compounds is the major means of elimination from the body. Less than 1% of each dose is excreted as unchanged drug in the urine.

USES

Chlorambucil is given orally according to a wide variety of protocols. Representative examples of the three main ways in which the drug is given are: intermittent single doses of 0.4 mg/kg every 2–4 weeks; cycles of 8–10 mg/m^2 daily for 10–14 days every 4–8 weeks; and continuous daily doses of 1–4 mg/m^2 or 0.03–0.1 mg/kg. Doses of 3–6 mg/m^2 daily for 3–6 weeks may be used as induction therapy prior to continuous daily dosing. Although absorption is probably better when the drug is taken on an empty stomach consistency of administration in relation to food is most important. Doses are usually adjusted on the basis of blood count responses to previous treatment.

Common indications for chlorambucil include chronic lymphocytic leukaemia, lymphomas, macroglobulinemia, polycythemia vera, trophoblastic neoplasms and advanced ovarian carcinoma. Chlorambucil is occasionally used to treat some non-malignant diseases.

ADVERSE DRUG REACTIONS

Myelosuppression is the usual dose limiting toxicity. Leucopenia and thrombocytopenia may occur depending on the dose used and

TABLE 31.3   Classification of alkylating agents

Group	Drugs
Nitrogen mustards	Chlorambucil, cyclophosphamide, ifosfamide, melphalan, mustine hydrochloride
Nitrosoureas	Carmustine, lomustine, streptozocin
Triazenes	Dacarbazine
Methane sulfonate esters	Busulfan
Ethylenimines	Thiotepa

duration of treatment. Inadvertent prolonged or excessive doses can result in pancytopenia and sustained bone marrow suppression.

Nausea, vomiting and anorexia are not normally significant with conventional dosage. Alopecia is usually not expected when chlorambucil is given alone in low doses. Infrequent or rare side effects include allergic skin reactions, interstitial pneumonitis and hepatotoxicity.

PRECAUTIONS AND CONTRAINDICATIONS

Marrow toxicity from previous treatment or other causes may preclude or delay the use of chlorambucil. Prior or concurrent radiotherapy to bone marrow will reduce tolerance to chlorambucil. Malignant infiltration of marrow also reduces tolerance to chlorambucil.

NURSING IMPLICATIONS

PATIENT EDUCATION

Patients should be made aware of the importance of taking chlorambucil strictly as prescribed. Additionally patients should know the signs of febrile neutropenia and what to do if such signs develop. The importance of keeping appointments for regular blood tests should be stressed. Chlorambucil tablets are heat sensitive and require refrigeration.

Cyclophosphamide

TRADE NAMES

Cyclophosphamide: *Cycloblastin; Cytoxan; Endoxan-Asta.*

MECHANISM OF ACTION

Cyclophosphamide is inactive and non-toxic, requiring two separate metabolic conversions to become active. The first step in activation occurs in the liver giving an in-

termediate form that is transported widely throughout the body. This intermediate form is taken up by cells and converted to the bifunctional alkylating agent phosphoramide mustard and a secondary metabolite, acrolein. Acrolein is considered responsible for the bladder toxicity of cyclophosphamide.

PHARMACOKINETICS

Absorption after oral administration is considered to be good. The effect of food on absorption is largely unknown. The elimination half-life of cyclosphosphamide is 3–10 hours with 10%–20% of unchanged drug excreted via the kidneys.

USES

Given orally, by slow intravenous injection or as a short intravenous infusion, cyclophosphamide is one of the most widely used antineoplastic agents. Dosages vary enormously depending on the disease treated, other drugs used and the treatment aim. Individual protocols should be consulted. As an indication, doses range from continuous daily treatment of 50 mg per day for some non-malignant diseases up to several grams by short intravenous infusion as part of bone marrow transplantation programs. Single intravenous doses of 350 mg– 1.2 g/m^2 and oral doses of 1.4–2.0 g/m^2 given over 5–14 days are indicative of cyclophosphamide doses used in conventional combination chemotherapy.

Some of the more common indications for cyclophosphamide include lymphomas, myeloma, leukaemias, neuroblastoma, retinoblastoma, ovarian carcinoma, breast carcinoma and a variety of sarcomas.

Oral cyclophosphamide is usually administered as a morning dose with instruction to the patient to take sufficient fluid to cause frequent emptying of the bladder (see Adverse Drug Reactions). If given in divided doses or as a night-time dose fluid intake should be sufficient to ensure middle of the night voiding.

Intravenous doses of cyclophosphamide may be given by slow intravenous injection,

CANCER CHEMOTHERAPY

31

although slow infusion in a volume of 100–1000 mL is more common. With high doses additional intravenous hydration may be required and possibly the specific uroprotectant, mesna.

ADVERSE DRUG REACTIONS

The usual dose limiting toxicity is myelosuppression, primarily leucopenia. Although cyclophosphamide is considered relatively 'platelet sparing', platelet levels will show a decline. Anaemia may occur with repeated therapy. The leucocytes reach their lowest level 8–15 days after a dose, with recovery occurring in 17–28 days.

Anorexia, nausea and vomiting are dose related. Symptoms are mild or absent with doses of 100 mg/m^2 but moderate to severe with doses greater than 1 g when prophylactic antiemetics are not given. Urological toxicity ranges from slight irritation on voiding to life threatening haemorrhagic cystitis. This toxicity is peculiar to cyclophosphamide and the related compound ifosfamide. Acrolein, a renally excreted metabolite of both drugs, causes acute damage to the bladder lining. Long-term damage, i.e. persistent haematuria and bladder fibrosis, can result. Toxicity is considered to be due to the concentration of acrolein in the bladder and the duration of contact.

Alopecia is common when cyclophosphamide is used to treat malignancies. Nail changes or banding corresponding to treatment cycles may be seen. Hypersensitivity reactions, skin rashes and lung toxicity are infrequent. Lung toxicity presents as a dry cough with dyspnoea on exertion.

Inappropriate water retention may occur 4–8 hours following doses of 50 mg/kg or more. This resolves within 24 hours. Cardiotoxicity only occurs with very large doses, e.g. 120–270 mg/kg over 1–4 days.

DRUG INTERACTIONS

Dapsone may inhibit cyclophosphamide's leucopenic effects. When given with suxamethonium, prolonged neuromuscular blockage may occur.

PRECAUTIONS AND CONTRAINDICATIONS

Marrow toxicity due to previous treatment or other causes may preclude or delay the use of cyclophosphamide. Hydration protocols for intravenous doses should be adhered to and the bladder emptied frequently. Concurrent urinary tract infection may exacerbate the risk of bladder toxicity. Prior or subsequent irradiation of the bladder may increase the risk of haemorrhagic cystitis. Doses should be reduced in the presence of severe renal dysfunction.

NURSING IMPLICATIONS

ASSESSMENT

The nurse should ensure that blood counts are acceptable. Cystitis or haematuria following previous cyclophosphamide treatment imply that the preventive hydration or other measures used may have been inadequate and may need to be reassessed. Urinary tract infection may increase the risk of bladder toxicity. Signs or symptoms of urinary tract infection prior to cyclophosphamide administration should be reported.

In those situations where urinalysis forms part of patient monitoring, pretreatment 'dip stick' urinalysis for blood provides a useful reference point. The presence of blood in the urine should be reported prior to administration of the drug.

EVALUATION

Patients receiving low to moderate doses should be encouraged to take sufficient fluid to allow frequent voiding. When doses are given other than in the morning, fluid intake should be sufficient to induce night voiding. High and very high dose treatments often involve vigorous hydration and use of the uroprotectant, mesna. Patients should be monitored for fluid retention when large intravenous doses are given.

Patients should be observed for signs and symptoms of cyclophosphamide induced bladder toxicity. Such symptoms should be reported with a view to reassessing hydration or other preventive measures.

PATIENT EDUCATION

Patients receiving oral treatment should be instructed that strict compliance with prescribed doses is highly important. The necessity for hydration and frequent voiding should be stressed. Patients should be made aware of the signs and symptoms of excessive myelosuppression and understand what action to take if these develop.

Ifosfamide

TRADE NAMES

Ifosfamide (iphosphamide): *Holoxan.*

MECHANISM OF ACTION

Ifosfamide is inactive and non-toxic, requiring two separate metabolic conversions to produce the active form. The first step in activation occurs in the liver giving an intermediate form that is transported widely throughout the body. This intermediate form is taken up by cells converted to a bifunctional alkylating agent and a secondary metabolite, acrolein. Acrolein is considered responsible for the bladder toxicity of ifosfamide.

PHARMACOKINETICS

Although ifosfamide is orally absorbed an oral form is not available. Its half-life at commonly used doses (1.2–2.0 g/m^2) is 3.5–7 hours with approximately 20% of the dose excreted unchanged in the urine. At higher doses (5–8 g/m^2) kinetics may be altered with the half-life increased and the fraction of unchanged drug excreted in the urine increased.

USES

Ifosfamide has been used in the treatment of a wide group of malignancies including small cell and non-small cell lung cancer, sarcomas, lymphomas, urogenital tumours including testicular carcinoma, cervical carcinoma and a variety of paediatric tumours.

The most common mode of administration for ifosfamide is by continuous infusion over 1–5 days or as daily short infusions for five days. Mesna is coadministered to prevent bladder toxicity. As with cyclophosphamide adequate hydration with a generous urine output plays an important role in preventing bladder toxicity.

ADVERSE DRUG REACTIONS

Myelosuppression is the usual dose limiting toxicity. Leucopenia is most significant, platelets are relatively spared. Anaemia may develop with intensive therapy or repeated cycles. Leucocytes reach their lowest level 7–14 days after treatment with recovery occurring 17 days after the last dose.

Serious bladder toxicity, which includes fatal haemorrhagic cystitis, initially prevented the use of ifosfamide except in restricted trials. Development of the effective uroprotectant, mesna, has allowed wide use with an acceptable level of safety. Bladder toxicity is qualitatively the same as that with cyclophosphamide.

Neurological toxicity ranging from drowsiness to a severe syndrome, including weakness, ataxia, seizures and coma, occurs depending on the dose used and patient risk factors such as renal dysfunction, advanced age and low albumin. Toxicity is less frequent and less severe when doses are divided over 4–5 days. Symptoms can appear after as little as two hours but are more commonly seen after 24–48 hours. Resolution of symptoms takes from three days to weeks.

Anorexia, nausea and vomiting are dose related. In 5-day fractionated treatments symptoms are mild to moderate. Cardiac arrhythmias have been observed during 3–5 day treatments. Alopecia is an expected side effect. In large doses ifosfamide frequently

CANCER CHEMOTHERAPY

31

induces fluid retention lasting less than 24 hours.

DRUG INTERACTIONS

Alcohol and chloral hydrate may increase the risk of neurotoxicity. Mesna uniformly causes a false positive reading for ketones with commonly used urine dipsticks.

PRECAUTIONS AND CONTRAINDICATIONS

Marrow toxicity from previous treatment or other causes may preclude or delay the use of ifosfamide. Protocols for hydration and mesna administration should be adhered to. Concurrent urinary tract infection may increase the risk of bladder toxicity. Prior or subsequent irradiation of the bladder may increase the risk of haemorrhagic cystitis.

Renal impairment and hypoalbuminemia increase the risk of neurotoxicity and are relative contraindications to ifosfamide use.

NURSING IMPLICATIONS

ASSESSMENT

The nurse should ensure that blood counts and renal function are acceptable. Urinary tract infection present at the time of administration may increase the risk of bladder toxicity. Signs or symptoms of urinary tract infection should be reported to the responsible medical officer. A pretreatment dip stick urinalysis for blood provides a useful reference point should results of tests after administration be positive.

ADMINISTRATION

Attention to hydration and the fluid balance is important. The nurse should ensure that mesna is administered correctly. The protocols for the requirements for each therapy should be consulted.

EVALUATION

During high dose treatments patients should be monitored for fluid retention. Diuretic therapy may be used to maintain fluid balance.

Patients should be observed for signs of ifosfamide induced bladder toxicity. In the event of frank haematuria ifosfamide infusion should be halted and the responsible medical officer contacted. The administration of mesna should not be interrupted. Mild symptoms or microscopic bleeding may not necessitate stopping ifosfamide but the protocol or medical officer should be consulted.

Patients should be observed for any signs of developing central nervous system toxicity. Such signs should be reported if they appear.

EDUCATION

Patients should be made aware of the signs and symptoms of excessive myelosuppression and understand what action to take if these occur.

Melphalan

TRADE NAMES

Melphalan: *Alkeran.*

MECHANISM OF ACTION

Melphalan is an orally active bifunctional alkylating agent derived from mustine hydrochloride.

PHARMACOKINETICS

Oral absorption of melphalan is highly variable and may be reduced by food. Melphalan has a half-life of 60–90 minutes. Only a small fraction is excreted unchanged by the kidney.

USES

Melphalan has been used in the management of multiple myeloma and ovarian carcinoma. Doses may be given in cycles of up to 1 mg/kg divided over 4–5 days and repeated every 4–6 weeks. Alternatively an induction course of 0.1–0.15 mg/kg day may be given for 7–14 days followed, after a break to allow blood counts to recover, by a daily maintenance dose of approximately 0.05 mg/kg per day.

High dose intravenous melphalan, up to 140 mg/m^2, or up to 220 mg/m^2 with stem cell transplantation, may be used in specialist centres. Oral melphalan is given on an empty stomach. Intravenous doses are given by slow injection or by infusion over 15–30 minutes.

ADVERSE DRUG REACTIONS

The dose limiting toxicity of melphalan is myelosuppression with equal suppression of leucocytes and platelets. The nadir occurs within 2–3 weeks and recovery in 4–6 weeks, depending on the dose used. Melphalan can cause cumulative bone marrow toxicity leading to marrow exhaustion if repeated or excessive doses are used.

When given in high doses, e.g. prior to bone marrow transplantation, mucositis becomes the dose limiting toxicity. Mucositis is not a feature of oral low dose therapy.

Anorexia, nausea and vomiting are mild and infrequent with conventional oral doses but moderate to severe with intravenous doses in excess of 70 mg/m^2. Similarly alopecia is uncommon at low doses but expected at high doses. Hypersensitivity reactions ranging from rashes to anaphylaxis are infrequent and mostly, but not entirely, restricted to intravenous treatment.

Melphalan injection is not considered to be vesicant but may cause some irritation if extravasation occurs.

PRECAUTIONS AND CONTRAINDICATIONS

Pre-existing marrow toxicity from previous treatment or other causes may preclude or delay the use of melphalan. Prior bone marrow irradiation, extensive prior chemotherapy and malignant infiltration of bone marrow can reduce bone marrow reserve and reduce tolerance to melphalan. Pancytopenia and

agranylocytosis can occur when dosages are not monitored closely. Melphalan should be given with caution to patients with renal failure, doses may need to be reduced.

NURSING IMPLICATIONS

PATIENT EDUCATION

Patients should be made aware of the importance of taking melphalan strictly as prescribed. In addition patients should be made aware of the signs and symptoms of excessive myelosuppression and what to do if such signs develop. The importance of keeping appointments for regular blood tests should be stressed.

Mustine Hydrochloride

TRADE NAMES

Mustine hydrochloride (nitrogen mustard, mechlorethamine): *Mustine.*

MECHANISM OF ACTION

Mustine hydrochloride was the first antineoplastic to be used widely in clinical practice. It is a highly reactive bifunctional alkylating agent.

PHARMACOKINETICS

Following injection mustine hydrochloride has a half-life of less than 10 minutes, primarily as the result of its highly reactive nature and rapid chemical breakdown in biological fluids. Less than 0.01% of a dose is excreted via the kidneys.

USES

The primary indication for mustine hydrochloride is the treatment of Hodgkin's lymphoma, most commonly at a dose of 6 mg/m^2 given on days 1 and 8 as part of the MOPP protocol (mustine, vincristine, procarbazine and prednisone or prednisolone).

CANCER CHEMOTHERAPY

31

As a single agent the dose per cycle rarely exceeds 0.4 mg/kg (approximately 16 mg/m^2) each 28 days.

Mustine hydrochloride instilled into the pleural space in doses of 10–30 mg can be used to treat malignant pleural effusions. Topical solutions and ointments have been used in the management of mycosis fungoides and some non-malignant skin diseases.

Intravenous mustine hydrochloride is administered by slow injection into the side arm of a fast flowing intravenous infusion of sodium chloride 0.9% or glucose 5%.

ADVERSE EFFECTS

The dose limiting toxicity of mustine hydrochloride is myelosuppression with leucopenia generally more pronounced than thrombocytopenia. The nadir occurs 7–14 days after administration with recovery usually within 28 days. Intrapleural administration of up to 20 mg is not usually associated with significant myelosuppression.

Nausea and vomiting commencing 1–8 hours after treatment and persisting for a few hours is common if prophylactic antiemetics are not given. Fever and chills occur 30–60 minutes after administration in a fraction of patients treated for Hodgkin's lymphoma.

Alopecia is an expected toxicity with repeated doses. Diarrhoea, taste changes and skin rashes are infrequent. Neurological toxicity is rare with doses of 0.4 mg/kg and less.

Mustine hydrochloride is a strong vesicant. Extravasation is usually (though not always) associated with pain at the site of injection. Inflammation and increasing pain follow taking 3–5 days to subside. Significant extravasations may cause tissue damage manifesting as skin induration and necrosis requiring up to six weeks to heal. Vein irritation and bluish-grey hyperpigmentation occurring progressively over several days is not due to extravasation.

Topical application of mustine hydrochloride is associated with a high incidence of contact dermatitis and hyperpigmentation.

PRECAUTIONS AND CONTRAINDICATIONS

Marrow toxicity due to prior treatment or other causes may preclude or delay the use of mustine hydrochloride.

Mustine hydrochloride is a strong vesicant, direct injection should be avoided. The access site should be repositioned if its integrity is in any way in doubt. In addition to the risk of extravasation, direct intravenous bolus injection via peripheral venous access has been associated with venous thrombosis.

NURSING IMPLICATIONS

ASSESSMENT

The nurse should ensure that blood counts are acceptable.

ADMINISTRATION

Reliable venous access and good technique are important in the administration of this vesicant agent. Administration should be performed by or under the direct supervision of those with considerable experience in giving vesicant agents. The integrity of the venous access should be monitored during delivery and the patient directed to report any significant pain at the site either during or after administration.

Procedures and requirements to deal with extravasation should be available.

PATIENT EDUCATION

Patients should be made aware of the signs and symptoms of excessive myelosuppression and understand what action to take if they occur.

NITROSOUREAS

Carmustine

TRADE NAMES

Carmustine (BCNU): *BiCNU.*

MECHANISM OF ACTION

Carmustine undergoes spontaneous degradation in the body to form a bifunctional alkylating agent. Carmustine may act in other ways although the clinical significance of this is unclear.

PHARMACOKINETICS

Carmustine disappears from the plasma rapidly as a result of chemical decomposition and hepatic metabolism to active compounds. The parent drug is undetectable in the blood 15 minutes after intravenous administration.

USES

Indications for carmustine include brain tumours, multiple myeloma, Hodgkin's lymphoma and malignant melanoma. When used alone doses of 150–200 mg/m^2 every six weeks can be given. In combination therapy dosages are reduced according to the myelosuppressive properties of the other agents used. Carmustine is administered over 1–2 hours as an infusion into the side arm of a fast flowing infusion of glucose 5% or sodium chloride 0.9%. Pain at the site of infusion often limits the rate of infusion when the drug is administered via peripheral venous access.

ADVERSE DRUG REACTIONS

The dose limiting toxicity of carmustine is myelosuppression with thrombocytopenia most prominent. The nadir is delayed compared with most agents, occurring after 4–6 weeks and persisting for a further 1–2 weeks. Carmustine has a cumulative effect on bone marrow. There is a greater or more persistent decline in the blood count with repeated cycles.

Anorexia, nausea and vomiting are dose related being moderately severe with doses of 150–200 mg/m^2 if prophylactic antiemetics are not used. Onset occurs within 2 hours and duration is 4–6 hours.

Dose related reversible elevations in liver function tests are common. High cumulative doses (1500 mg/m^2) have been linked with serious liver damage. Lung toxicity, occasionally occurring long after the completion of treatment, appears to be associated with high cumulative dose (1200–1500 mg/m^2). Carmustine is not a vesicant but often causes burning along the vein being perfused. Phlebitis may develop 7–10 days after infusion. Solutions of carmustine inadvertently spilt onto exposed skin may cause burning and local hyperpigmentation.

DRUG INTERACTIONS

Cimetidine, may increase carmustine induced myelosuppression. Serum levels of phenytoin may be reduced.

PRECAUTIONS AND CONTRAINDICATIONS

Marrow toxicity from previous treatment or other causes may preclude or delay the use of carmustine. Marrow suppression is delayed with carmustine therefore intervals between doses should be 6–8 weeks. Patients with reduced lung function, a history of smoking or prior chest irradiation are considered to be at an increased risk of lung toxicity.

NURSING IMPLICATIONS

ASSESSMENT

The nurse should ensure that blood counts are acceptable.

ADMINISTRATION

Carmustine should be administered according to established protocols. Burning along the venous tract proximal to peripheral venous access may necessitate slowing the rate of infusion.

CANCER CHEMOTHERAPY

31

EDUCATION

Patients should be made aware of the signs and symptoms of excessive myelosuppression and understand what action to take if they occur.

Lomustine

TRADE NAMES

Lomustine (CCNU): *CeeNu.*

MECHANISM OF ACTION

Lomustine undergoes spontaneous degradation in the body following oral absorption to form a bifunctional alkylating agent. Lomustine may act in other ways although the clinical significance of this is unclear.

PHARMACOKINETICS

Lomustine is rapidly absorbed from the gastrointestinal tract and has good penetration into the central nervous system. While lomustine has a short half-life of 90 minutes its active metabolites have elimination half-lives of 16–24 hours. The metabolites are eliminated primarily through the kidneys.

USES

Lomustine is used primarily in the treatment of brain tumours and Hodgkin's lymphoma. As a single agent oral doses of up to 130 mg/m^2 every 6–8 weeks can usually be given without causing clinically significant myelosuppression. When combined with other myelosuppressive agents lower doses are commonly used. Single doses of up to 200 mg/m^2 have been used in combination treatment of acute leukaemia. Lomustine is given orally, often in the early part of the evening to allow patients to sleep through the worst of any nausea.

ADVERSE DRUG REACTIONS

The dose limiting toxicity of lomustine is myelosuppression. The leucocyte and platelet nadir occurs at 4–6 weeks with recovery after a further 1–2 weeks. Low haemoglobin levels are common with repeated treatment and intensive therapies. A significant risk of nephrotoxicity has been reported with high cumulative doses of lomustine (greater than 1200 mg/m^2).

Anorexia, nausea and vomiting are common. Nausea and vomiting develop 2–6 hours after a dose and may persist for up to 36 hours. Anorexia may continue for an additional 2–3 days.

Rashes, stomatitis and hepatotoxicity are very infrequent. Lomustine may, in rare cases, induce pulmonary fibrosis.

PRECAUTIONS AND CONTRAINDICATIONS

Marrow toxicity from previous treatments or other causes may preclude or delay treatment with lomustine. Marrow suppression from lomustine is delayed, dosage intervals for treatment should be every 6–8 weeks.

Lomustine should be given with caution to patients with significant renal dysfunction.

Streptozocin

TRADE NAMES

Streptozocin (streptozotocin): *Zanosar.*

MECHANISM OF ACTION

Streptozocin and its methyl metabolite are classified as alkylating agents. They are weak alkylators and may have other more important actions.

PHARMACOKINETICS

Streptozocin has a half-life of 5–15 minutes, its metabolites have half-lives of up to 40 hours. Streptozocin and its metabolites are eliminated principally by the kidneys.

USES

Pancreatic islet cell carcinoma, Hodgkin's lymphoma and pancreatic adenocarcinoma are some of the indications for streptozocin. Intravenous doses of 500 mg/m^2 daily for five days every six weeks or 1000–1500 mg/m^2 given weekly for 4–6 weeks may be used. Administration is by slow intravenous injection over 3–5 minutes or by short intravenous infusion over 15–30 minutes in glucose 5% or sodium chloride 0.9%.

ADVERSE DRUG REACTIONS

The dose limiting toxicity of streptozocin is usually renal failure in the form of permanent tubular damage. Some degree of reversible dysfunction occurs in most patients. Nausea and vomiting can be severe if preventive measures are not taken. Hypoglycaemia occurring in the 24 hours after administration is the result of damage to pancreatic β cells.

Haematological toxicity is mild, diarrhoea and liver toxicity are rare. Rapid intravenous injection may cause pain or erythema at the injection site.

DRUG INTERACTIONS

Concurrent administration of streptozocin and other nephrotoxic drugs may increase renal toxicity.

PRECAUTIONS AND CONTRAINDICATIONS

Streptozocin should be used with caution in patients with renal or hepatic dysfunction.

NURSING IMPLICATIONS

ASSESSMENT

The nurse should ensure that blood counts are acceptable.

ADMINISTRATION

Pain at the site of administration may be reduced by slowing the rate of infusion when using peripheral venous access.

PATIENT EDUCATION

Patients should be made aware of the signs and symptoms of excessive myelosuppression and understand what action to take if they occur.

TRIAZENES

Dacarbazine

TRADE NAMES

Dacarbazine (DTIC): *DTIC-Dome*.

MECHANISM OF ACTION

The mechanism of action of dacarbazine is largely unknown. Its activity is due to unidentified active metabolites.

PHARMACOKINETICS

After intravenous administration the elimination half-life of dacarbazine is 30–50 minutes with approximately half the drug excreted unchanged via the kidneys. Dacarbazine has been detected in the urine for up to 12 hours following a dose.

USES

Doses of up to 1250 mg/m^2 per cycle (most commonly as 250 mg/m^2 on 5 consecutive days) may be used in the treatment of malignant melanoma. In the treatment of Hodgkin's lymphoma the drug is used in combination with other agents, e.g. the ABVD protocol (doxorubicin, bleomycin, vinblastine and dacarbazine), at a dose of 750 mg/m^2 per cycle (375 mg/m^2 on days 1 and 15).

Administration is by short infusion into the side arm of a fast flowing infusion of glucose 5% or sodium chloride 0.9%. When given via peripheral venous access to sensitive patients the rate of infusion may have to be slowed significantly to alleviate pain along the vein. Short intravenous injections over 2–4 minutes have also been used.

ADVERSE DRUG REACTIONS

Nausea and vomiting can be dose limiting if preventive measures are not taken. Dacarbazine causes myelosuppression although with standard doses (less than 1000 mg/m^2 per cycle) it is generally mild.

When given on consecutive days tolerance to the emetic effects of dacarbazine develops, such that with a 5-day course the incidence and severity of nausea and

CANCER CHEMOTHERAPY

31

vomiting is considerably reduced by the last day.

Fever, malaise and myalgias with or following administration affect a small percentage of patients. Photosensitivity, reported as burning in areas exposed to sunlight immediately after dacarbazine administration, is possible and more likely following high doses.

Dacarbazine is not a strong vesicant, however pain along the vein being infused, even in the absence of extravasation, is common and may complicate administration when peripheral venous access is used.

Mild and transient elevations in liver enzymes are common. Liver necrosis is very rare. Hypotension, transient watery diarrhoea and urine discolouration (brick red during or shortly after treatment) are associated only with high doses administered as a single brief infusion.

PRECAUTIONS AND CONTRAINDICATIONS

Marrow toxicity from previous treatment or other causes may preclude or delay the use of dacarbazine. Dacarbazine should be used with caution in patients with severe renal or hepatic dysfunction.

NURSING IMPLICATIONS

ASSESSMENT

The nurse should ensure that blood counts are acceptable.

ADMINISTRATION

Pain occurring along the vein being infused may necessitate a significant reduction in infusion rate. Extravasation of dacarbazine is painful but is not likely to cause soft tissue necrosis unless delivered in high concentration. Procedures to deal with inadvertant extravasation should be in place prior to administration.

Dacarbazine is rapidly degraded in the presence of sunlight. At room temperature

and under the less intense fluorescent lighting common in institutions dacarbazine is sufficiently stable to allow administration without extremes of light protection. Avoid administration in sunlit areas.

Rapid administration of high doses may cause hypotension.

PATIENT EDUCATION

Patients should be advised to avoid direct sunlight to the skin in the hours immediately following administration as this may result in a burning sensation in exposed areas. Patients given high doses may notice a brick-red discolouration of the urine within hours of administration. This is due to a metabolite and is without consequence but may cause distress in an uninformed patient.

Patients should be made aware of the signs and symptoms of excessive myelosuppression and should understand what action to take should they occur.

METHANE SULFONATE ESTERS

Busulfan

TRADE NAMES

Busulfan: *Myleran*.

MECHANISM OF ACTION

Busulfan is a bifunctional alkylating agent which is relatively specific for myeloid cells at low dose. Higher doses suppress the production of all blood cells.

PHARMACOKINETICS

Busulfan is rapidly absorbed from the gut reaching peak blood levels after 2–3 hours. Removal from the body is almost entirely by metabolism or as the result of chemical degradation. Only 1% of unchanged drug is eliminated via the kidneys.

USES

Doses of 2–6 mg per day are used in the treatment of chronic myelocytic leukaemia and polycythemia vera. High dose therapy, 1 mg/kg four times a day for four days, is used in conditioning regimens prior to stem cell transplantation.

Busulfan is given orally, there are no specific recommendations on administration with relation to food.

ADVERSE DRUG REACTIONS

Myelosuppression, which may be profound and prolonged, is the dose limiting side effect of busulfan. When used as part of stem cell transplantation protocols the dose limiting toxicities are mucositis and hepatotoxicity.

The nadir for myelosuppression is 11–30 days following a dose with recovery in 24–54 days. This delayed and prolonged myelosuppression complicates treatment when small daily doses are used. Relatively close monitoring of blood counts is required with prompt cessation of treatment with any early sign of pancytopenia.

Generalised skin darkening occurs in 5%–10% of patients. Weakness, anorexia, weight loss, gynaecomastia and dysmenorrhoea have been reported in some patients. Nausea and vomiting are rare at normal doses and infrequent and mild with high doses.

Busulfan induced cataracts develop only after years of continuous treatment. Lung toxicity is rare (although serious) and only reported with total doses in excess of 500 mg. Myoclonic epilepsy, severe liver toxicity, mucositis or diarrhoea are only associated with high dose treatments.

PRECAUTIONS AND CONTRAINDICATIONS

Excessive myelosuppression requires dose modification in patients receiving daily treatment. Prophylactic short-term anticonvulsant therapy may be considered with very high doses.

NURSING IMPLICATIONS

EVALUATION

Patients receiving high dose treatments should be observed for signs of seizure activity and jaundice. Protocols for the prevention and management of possible mucositis should be in place for high dose treatments.

PATIENT EDUCATION

Patients taking continous daily doses should be reminded of the importance of taking the correct dosage and of keeping appointments for regular blood tests. They should be made aware of the symptoms of excessive myelosuppression and the appropriate action to take in the event of this occurring.

ETHYLENIMINES

Thiotepa

MECHANISM OF ACTION

Thiotepa is an alkylating agent. Both thiotepa and its major metabolite, tepa, are active. It is likely that other metabolites also have activity.

PHARMACOKINETICS

After intravenous administration thiotepa is extensively metabolised, primarily by the liver. The drug's terminal elimination half-life is 80–125 minutes. Thiotepa, tepa and other metabolites are excreted in the urine in significant amounts.

USES

Athough used most commonly as a bladder instillation and to a lesser extent as ophthalmic drops in the treatment of pterygium, thiotepa used in high intravenous doses has come under renewed interest as a potentially useful drug in a number of areas.

CANCER CHEMOTHERAPY

31

Bladder instillations of 30–60 mg in 30–60 mL of water retained in the bladder for two hours are administered weekly for 4–6 weeks and then each 4–6 weeks as maintenance in the management of superficial tumours of the bladder. Patients are usually dehydrated prior to administration to prevent excess dilution of the solution in the bladder and are repositioned every 15 minutes after administration to ensure complete exposure of the bladder lining to the solution.

Intravenous doses of thiotepa are poorly defined. Areas of potential application include breast and ovarian cancers. Intravenous doses can be given over 3–5 minutes as a solution of 15 mg/10 mL, larger doses may be given by short infusion. Intramuscular administration in a suitable volume of procaine 2% has been used for small doses.

ADVERSE DRUG REACTIONS

The dose limiting toxicity for thiotepa is myelosuppression becoming significant with doses of 60–65 mg/m^2 per cycle. Stem cell transplantation is required with doses in excess of 180 mg/m^2. Bladder instillation is infrequently associated with significant myelosuppression.

Hypersensitivity, evident as rash, pruritus or urticarial reaction, is noted in 3% of patients given thiotepa bladder instillations. Hypersensitivity takes a number of cycles to develop. Once sensitised symptoms will manifest 1–24 hours after each administration.

Stomatitis, erythroderma, confusion, somnolence and liver toxicity are infrequent toxicities of very high dose treatment only.

DRUG INTERACTIONS

Suxamethonium activity may be prolonged following the administration of thiotepa.

PRECAUTIONS AND CONTRAINDICATIONS

Intravenous thiotepa should be given with caution to patients with significant renal or hepatic dysfunction or myelosuppression. Previous hypersensitivity to intravesical or intravenous thiotepa is usually a contraindication to further treatment.

NURSING IMPLICATIONS

ASSESSMENT

The patient's history should be reviewed for hypersensitivity to thiopeta. If the drug is to be given intravenously the nurse should ensure that blood counts are acceptable.

ADMINISTRATION

When used as a bladder instillation clear instructions or protocols for patient preparation (fluid restriction), patient positioning during administration and for the safe handling of waste should be established before administration.

ANTIMETABOLITES

In general antimetabolites can be considered inhibitors of DNA synthesis. They imitate substances involved in the normal process of forming DNA with the result that specific essential steps are blocked or faulty DNA is formed, or both. Antimetabolites are cell cycle specific for the S phase.

DEOXYCYTIDINE ANALOGUES

Cytarabine

TRADE NAMES

Cytarabine (cytosine arabinoside, ara-C): *Cytosar-U.*

MECHANISM OF ACTION

Cytarabine mimics the natural precursor of DNA, deoxycytidine. It inhibits the formation of DNA and when incorporated into DNA results in incomplete DNA formation and faulty function. Cytarabine is cell cycle specific for the S phase.

PHARMACOKINETICS

Following parenteral administration cytarabine is largely metabolised to the inactive renally excreted metabolite ara-U. The elimination half-life of cytarabine in conventional doses is 0.5–2.6 hours. It is considerably longer with high doses. Cytarabine penetrates into the central nervous system with cerebrospinal fluid levels approximately 40%–50% of plasma levels. Direct intrathecal injection produces high cerebrospinal fluid levels with low levels in the general circulation.

USES

Cytarabine is most commonly used in combination with other agents as treatment for acute leukaemias. It is less frequently used in the management of lymphomas. Given by direct intrathecal injection it is used for the prophylaxis and treatment of meningeal leukaemia and as treatment for meningeal carcinomatosis.

Dosages and administration vary widely depending on the protocol used. Continuous infusions of 100–200 mg/m^2 per day for 5–7 days are common. High dose therapies of 1–3 g/m^2 given over 1–3 hours twice daily for 4–6 days and low dose therapies using subcutaneous injections of 5–30 mg/m^2 twice daily for up to 21 days are used less commonly in selected cases. Bolus doses of up to 200 mg/m^2 by slow intravenous injection are less common.

Cytarabine can be prepared in sodium chloride 0.9% or glucose 5% in a suitable volume. Intrathecal doses of 50 mg/m^2 or 100 mg may be prepared in a volume of up to 10 mL and administered up to twice weekly in the active treatment of meningeal disease.

ADVERSE DRUG REACTIONS

The dose limiting toxicity of cytarabine is myelosuppression with both leucocytes and platelets affected. Haematological recovery occurs after 2–3 weeks with conventional doses but may be delayed following the high dose or extended treatments used in the treatment of leukaemia. Low haemoglobin values are common with intensive treatments for leukaemia.

Nausea and vomiting can be severe with high dose treatment but is generally mild with conventional doses and is well controlled with antiemetics. Stomatitis is common with conventional and high doses given over several days. Effects are seen after 4–7 days with recovery dependent on the dose and duration of treatment. Diarrhoea, diffuse abdominal pain and ileus are more common with more intensive treatment.

Neurological toxicity, evident as agitation, confusion and ataxia, occurs only with high dose treatment and then most commonly in the elderly and those with renal dysfunc-

CANCER CHEMOTHERAPY

31

tion. Other toxicities, almost entirely confined to high dose treatment, include a 5%–10% incidence of a painful palmar-plantar reaction, pulmonary oedema (which may be clinically significant in a few patients) and a chemical conjunctivitis which affects 38%–100% of patients. Cytarabine conjunctivitis can be prevented or lessened by the prophylactic use of steroid eye drops.

Alopecia is rare with low doses, common with standard doses and universal following high dose treatment. Maculopapular skin rash over the trunk is common with high doses but infrequent with conventional doses. Anaphylactic reactions are rare.

Intrathecal administration of cytarabine may cause nausea, fever and transient headache.

PRECAUTIONS AND CONTRAINDICATIONS

Marrow toxicity from previous treatment or other causes may preclude or delay the use of cytarabine. Cytarabine should be administered with caution to patients with significant renal or hepatic dysfunction. High dose cytarabine is contraindicated in the presence of renal failure or hepatic dysfunction. High dose treatment of patients over 50 years of age or those in a debilitated condition should be approached with particular caution.

Prophylactic steroid eye drops are useful for preventing or limiting ophthalmic toxicity with high dose treatments.

NURSING IMPLICATIONS

ASSESSMENT

If cytarabine is being used for treatment of cancers other than leukaemia the nurse should ensure that blood counts are acceptable.

ADMINISTRATION

The mode of administration is particularly important to the action of cytarabine. Con-fusion over administration times can result in under treatment or excessive toxicity depending on the circumstance. The protocol should be checked for the correct mode of administration.

Mucositis is common with standard and high dose cytarabine based antileukaemia treatments. Protocols for the prevention and management of mucositis should be established.

PATIENT EDUCATION

Appropriate mouth care plays a significant role in preventing secondary infection and subsequent delay in mucosal healing. Patients should be educated on the requirements for good mouth care to limit mucositis and encouraged to contact their physician or clinic if significant mucositis or diarrhoea occur. Patients should be made aware of the symptoms of severe myelosuppression and the appropriate action to take if they occur.

FLUOROPYRIMIDINES

Fluorouracil

TRADE NAMES

Fluorouracil (5-fluorouracil, 5-FU): *Fluroblastin.*

MECHANISM OF ACTION

Fluorouracil mimics uracil, a natural substrate required for the formation of DNA and RNA. Fluorouracil both inhibits the formation of DNA and, when incorporated into the nucleic acid structures, results in the formation of incomplete and faulty DNA and RNA. Fluorouracil is cell cycle phase specific for the S phase.

PHARMACOKINETICS

Oral fluorouracil absorption is highly variable and not considered a reliable means of administration in most situations. The plasma half-life of 8–23 minutes is the result of rapid metabolism to inactive compounds in the liver and other tissues. Only 10% of a dose is excreted in the urine unchanged.

USES

Fluorouracil has a wide range of indications including carcinoma of the colon, rectum, stomach, breast, pancreas and head and neck. Dosages used vary significantly and individual protocols should be consulted. Representative examples include: single doses of 30 mg/kg every 14–28 days; daily injections of 350–600 mg/m^2 for five days repeated every 21–35 days; boluses of 450–500 mg/m^2 weekly; and continuous infusions of 500–1000 mg/m^2 daily for 4–5 days repeated every 21–28 days.

Fluorouracil is administered as a 25–50 mg/mL solution by slow intravenous injection, higher doses may be given by short infusion. Continuous infusions are given in any suitable volume of glucose 5% or sodium chloride 0.9%.

ADVERSE DRUG REACTIONS

The dose limiting toxicity of fluorouracil is dependent on the mode of administration. For example, the dose for continuous infusions given over 4–5 days cannot be increased above 1 g/m^2 because of severe stomatitis; myelotoxicity is a dose limiting toxicity for standard bolus doses given daily for 5 days; and neurotoxicity limits the dose that can be given as a single bolus dose.

Myelosuppression, with leucocytes affected more than platelets, begins 4–7 days after a dose. Recovery usually occurs within 14 days of the last dose. Anaemia may develop with repeated cycles.

Stomatitis from fluorouracil can affect any site along the gastrointestinal tract. Symptoms may include dysphagia, retrosternal burning, diarrhoea and proctitis. Mucositis may be preceded by a dry sensation and erythema of the mucosa followed by formation of a white patchy membrane. In severe cases ulceration, necrosis and significant pain ensues.

Nausea, vomiting and anorexia are mild when they occur and are usually well managed by standard antiemetics. Partial alopecia is common.

A variety of skin rashes may occur with fluorouracil. Effects on nails include banding and more rarely discolouration. Hyperpigmentation of the tissue overlying vascular channels proximal to the infusion site can occur particularly with continuous infusions of fluorouracil given by peripheral veins. This peculiar side effect does not affect vein patency but may cause discomfort.

Chest pain mimicking Prinzmetal's angina occurs in up to 8% of patients receiving fluorouracil by continuous infusion. Myocardial infarction and cardiac related deaths have also been reported. The reported incidence of cardiotoxicity is lower with bolus doses of fluorouracil.

Blurred vision, excessive lacrimation and a chemical conjunctivitis may occur. Anaphylactic reactions to fluorouracil are rare but not unknown.

DRUG INTERACTIONS

Leucovorin when combined with fluorouracil gives an enhanced activity and toxicity. This interaction is used clinically to increase the activity of fluorouracil against some tumours.

PRECAUTIONS AND CONTRAINDICATIONS

Marrow toxicity from previous treatment or other causes may preclude or delay the use of fluorouracil.

Fluorouracil is contraindicated in patients in whom mucositis or diarrhoea resulting from prior fluorouracil treatments has not cleared. Such symptoms developing during a treatment course may warrant cessation of treatment. When combined with radiotherapy increased toxicity to the gastrointestinal epithelium contained within the radiation field can be expected. Dosages may be adjusted for this.

A history of cardiac disease is associated with an increased risk of fluorouracil induced cardiovascular toxicity.

CANCER CHEMOTHERAPY

31

NURSING IMPLICATIONS

ASSESSMENT

As re-treatment prior to resolution of fluorouracil induced mucositis or diarrhoea can result in severe toxicity such symptoms should be reported to the prescribing physician prior to further administration. The nurse should also ensure that blood counts are acceptable prior to starting a cycle of therapy.

EVALUATION

If chest pain of cardiac origin or myocardial infarction is suspected during a continuous infusion of fluorouracil the infusion should be stopped immediately and the responsible medical officer contacted. Similarly if symptoms occur during a course of bolus doses the responsible medical officer should be contacted before further doses are given.

PATIENT EDUCATION

Patients treated with fluorouracil should be warned of their increased susceptibility to solar radiation.

Fluorouracil is not a vesicant agent, however patients may notice some erythema and subsequent darkening along veins associated with peripheral venous administration. When evident this will occur over a number of days. Patients should be forewarned and advised that it is not of consequence in itself.

Appropriate mouth care plays a significant role in preventing secondary infection and subsequent delay in mucosal healing. Patients should be advised on appropriate mouth care and encouraged to contact their physician or clinic if significant mucositis or diarrhoea occur. Patients should be made aware of the signs and symptoms of excessive myelosuppression and understand what action to take should these occur.

Floxuridine

MECHANISM OF ACTION

Floxuridine (FUDR) is an antimetabolite with a mode of action very similar to that of fluorouracil. When given by rapid infusion a significant amount of the drug is converted to fluorouracil. Floxuridine is cell cycle specific for the S phase.

PHARMACOKINETICS

The liver is particularly efficient at removing floxuridine from the blood stream. This characteristic is exploited by use of hepatic artery infusions to treat hepatic tumours as little of the drug reaches the rest of the body.

USES

Intrahepatic artery infusion using doses of 0.1–0.2 mg/kg per day for 14 days in each 28-day cycle is used in the treatment of selected patients with carcinomas localised to the liver.

Floxuridine is diluted with glucose 5% or sodium chloride 0.9% to a suitable volume and administered usually as a continuous infusion.

ADVERSE DRUG REACTIONS

Intravenous doses of floxuridine have qualitatively the same toxicities as fluorouracil. When given by intrahepatic arterial infusion toxicity to the hepatobiliary system limits both the dose and duration of treatment.

Epigastric pain and/or vomiting associated with intra-arterial infusion may suggest slippage of the infusion catheter and misperfusion into the gastrointestinal arterial blood supply. Misperfusion can cause necrosis of the intestinal epithelium with haemorrhage, perforation and attendant symptoms.

Systemic toxicity associated with arterial doses of floxuridine is unusual.

DRUG INTERACTIONS

Leucovorin coadministered with floxuridine gives enhanced activity and toxicity.

PRECAUTIONS AND CONTRAINDICATIONS

Hepatic artery infusion should only be undertaken by those with experience in catheter placement and floxuridine usage.

When given intravenously floxuridine use has the same general nursing implications as fluorouracil.

Patients undergoing hepatic artery infusion should be advised to contact their physician if they develop significant epigastric pain and/or nausea and vomiting during the period of treatment.

PURINE ANTIMETABOLITES

Mercaptopurine

TRADE NAMES

Mercaptopurine (6-mercaptopurine, 6-MP): *Purinethol.*

MECHANISM OF ACTION

Mercaptopurine acts as a false purine. It inhibits the formation and intracellular conversion of purine bases essential to the synthesis of DNA and RNA and results in faulty DNA and RNA function. Mercaptopurine is cell cycle specific affecting cells in the S phase.

PHARMACOKINETICS

Oral mercaptopurine is rapidly although incompletely absorbed, with much of the drug metabolised by the liver before reaching the systemic circulation. Absorption is greater on an empty stomach. Elimination from the systemic circulation is mainly due to metabolism. Only a small percentage of drug is excreted unchanged in the urine. The elimination half-life of mercaptopurine is 1.5–7 hours.

USES

Mercaptopurine is used in combination with other agents in the treatment of acute lymphoblastic leukaemias, high grade lymphoblastic lymphoma and occasionally in acute non-lymphoblastic leukaemia. It has also been used as an immunosuppressant in the management of some non-malignant conditions.

Daily oral doses of 2.5 mg/kg, occasionally escalated to 5 mg/kg, are used during induction therapy for acute leukaemia. Maintenance doses are 1.5–2.5 mg/kg per day. Mercaptopurine is best administered on an empty stomach. It should not be given with cow's milk.

ADVERSE DRUG REACTIONS

The dose limiting toxicity of mercaptopurine is myelosuppression. A fall in leucocyte and platelet counts may occur within as little as five days with daily dosing but is commonly much slower in onset. Anaemia can occur with prolonged treatment.

Mild nausea, vomiting and anorexia are initially common but rarely persist with continued daily treatment. Mucositis, diarrhoea and reversible pancreatitis are infrequent. Reversible cholestatic jaundice may be a more common finding. Rash on stopping mercaptopurine, described as erythematous, often pruritic and appearing mainly on the face, neck and upper chest, is common in some patients.

DRUG INTERACTIONS

Allopurinol significantly inhibits the metabolism of mercaptopurine and can induce serious toxicity. A dosage reduction to 25%–33% of the intended dose of mercaptopurine is mandatory. Mercaptopurine may inhibit the anticoagulant effect of warfarin.

PRECAUTIONS AND CONTRAINDICATIONS

Treatment should be discontinued or suspended following an abnormally large fall in the leucocyte count and generally not restarted until the status of bone marrow function is established.

Mercaptopurine should be given with caution to patients with significant liver or renal dysfunction.

CANCER CHEMOTHERAPY

31

PATIENT EDUCATION

Patients treated with mercaptopurine on an outpatient basis should be aware of the importance of taking the correct dosage. Patients should be made aware of the signs and symptoms of excessive myelosuppression and be instructed to contact their physician or clinic should these occur.

Thioguanine

TRADE NAMES

Thioguanine (6-thioguanine): *Lanvis.*

MECHANISM OF ACTION

Thioguanine acts as a false purine inhibiting purine synthesis and, when incorporated into DNA, inhibiting DNA activity. Thioguanine is cell cycle specific affecting cells in the S phase.

PHARMACOKINETICS

Thioguanine is orally active but is subject to incomplete and variable absorption. The elimination half-life may be as long as 11 hours with metabolism almost entirely responsible for drug elimination.

USES

Thioguanine has been used in the treatment of acute non-lymphocytic leukaemia and acute lymphocytic leukaemia although it has been replaced by other drugs in many instances. It has also been used in the management of chronic myelogenous leukaemia.

As maintenance treatment doses of 75 mg/m^2 per day or 2 mg/kg per day are used initially with doses increased after four weeks if an inadequate response is seen. In combination with other agents as induction therapy doses of 75–200 mg/m^2 per day for 5–7 days have been used. Daily oral doses are given in one or two divided doses.

ADVERSE DRUG REACTIONS

Myelosuppression is the dose limiting side effect of thioguanine. Leucopenia is the initial manifestation, developing over 2–4 weeks with daily treatment. Significant thrombocytopenia and anaemia may also occur with continued therapy.

Nausea, vomiting and anorexia are infrequent and mild with usual doses. Significant diarrhoea, stomatitis and rash (urticarial or dermatitis-like) are infrequent side effects.

PRECAUTIONS AND CONTRAINDICATIONS

Thioguanine should be given with caution to patients with severe renal or hepatic dysfunction.

Occasional patients may show an early profound drop in leucocyte count. Therapy may be temporarily suspended at this time to ensure that significant unwanted marrow hypoplasia does not occur.

PATIENT EDUCATION

Strict adherence to planned doses must be stressed. The patient should be made aware of the signs and symptoms of febrile neutropenia and instructed on what action to take should these occur.

FOLATE ANTIMETABOLITES

Methotrexate

TRADE NAMES
Methotrexate (MTX): *Ledertrexate.*

MECHANISM OF ACTION

Methotrexate mimics intracellular folic acid competitively blocking dihydrofolate reductase to prevent the intracellular conversion of folates into their biologically active form. The drug also directly and indirectly inhibits thymidylate synthetase. Methotrexate is cell cycle specific for the S phase. Leuco-vorin (folinic acid) is a specific inhibitor of methotrexate. When given in appropriate dose it prevents further toxicity by any methotrexate remaining in the body.

PHARMACOKINETICS

Oral methotrexate absorption is considered unreliable with doses greater than 50 mg. Small doses of methotrexate can reliably be given by intramuscular injection.

Following intravenous administration methotrexate has an initial half-life in plasma of 2–3 hours. The final elimination half-life is 8–10 hours. With low doses up to 90% is excreted unchanged via the kidney. At higher dose a larger proportion is metabolised by the liver.

Penetration of methotrexate into the central nervous system (necessary to treat the central nervous system in some situations) is negligible with conventional doses, significant with moderate to high doses and uniformly high following direct intrathecal injection.

USES

Methotrexate is used in a very wide variety of doses to treat a diverse group of malignant and non-malignant diseases.

Psoriasis, rheumatoid arthritis and a variety of inflammatory or autoimmune conditions may be treated with weekly doses usually in the range of 5–15 mg.

Methotrexate has a significant role in the treatment of childhood acute lymphoblastic leukaemia, non-Hodgkin's lymphoma, choriocarcinoma and sarcoma. In combination with other agents it is useful against many cancers including those of the lung, breast and bladder. Administration is usually by slow intravenous injection although small doses may be given by intramuscular injection.

In combination with other cytotoxic drugs intravenous doses of methotrexate of 20–40 mg/m^2 are common. As a single agent doses of 50–100 mg/m^2 can be given up to weekly. Leucovorin rescue is not generally required for these doses.

Intermediate doses of 400–500 mg/m^2 are usually (although not always) given with 25%–33% of the dose as a bolus and the rest as an infusion over four or more hours depending on the protocol. Leucovorin rescue is mandatory. Although vigorous hydration is not usually employed patients should not be dehydrated at the time of infusion. In general, measurement of methotrexate levels and urine alkalinisation are not required unless specific risk factors exist.

High dose methotrexate protocols are employed in the treatment of acute lymphoblastic leukaemia and osteogenic sarcoma. Doses of 1–12 g/m^2 are administered by infusion over 4–42 hours (strict adherance to established protocols is essential for doses of this magnitude). Alternatively a loading or bolus dose, followed by an infusion may be given. Adequate hydration is essential during the first 48 hours. This ensures that the high levels of methotrexate passing through the kidney are diluted and not concentrated enough to form crystals. In addition, raising the urine pH to 7 or more increases the solubility of methotrexate and acts in concert with adequate hydration to prevent crystal formation. Blood samples are taken to monitor the elimination of methotrexate from the body and to guide the selection and duration of leucovorin rescue. The timing of assays and the adjustment of leucovorin doses varies with each protocol.

Intrathecal doses of 6–12 mg/m^2 to a maximum of 15 mg may be given every 2–5 days by lumbar puncture or omaya reservoir. Intrathecal treatment is indicated for prophylaxis or treatment of acute lymphoblastic leukaemia or high grade lymphoma and in the treatment of meningeal carcinomatosis.

ADVERSE DRUG REACTIONS

Without the use of the specific methotrexate inhibitor leucovorin, myelosuppression and mucositis are dose limiting. Methotrexate infrequently causes significant myelosuppression when given in low dose

CANCER CHEMOTHERAPY

31

or with leucovorin rescue. However, when myelosuppression does occur platelets and leucocytes are both affected. Anaemia may occur following repeated or prolonged courses.

Mucositis, beginning 3–7 days after treatment is the most common toxicity. Significant diarrhoea is uncommon.

High dose treatments (1–15 g/m^2) were initially associated with a high incidence of death due to severe renal toxicity. The use of adequate hydration, urine alkalinisation and the exclusion of high risk patients has largely eliminated this problem. Mild reversible renal toxicity not due to the formation of renal crystals occurs in many patients given high doses.

Alopecia is infrequent with low doses but significant with high dose treatment. Rashes are rare with low doses, however pruritic maculopapular rash with or without skin peeling occurs in approximately 7% of patients given doses of 400 mg to 10 g. Methotrexate enhances the effect of sun exposure, and can reactivate sun damage occurring 1–3 days prior to methotrexate administration.

Nausea and vomiting are infrequent and usually mild with conventional methotrexate doses. Without prophylactic antiemetics high dose therapy causes significant nausea and vomiting in most patients.

Following high dose treatment up to a quarter of patients experience dry eyes lasting 2–5 days.

Long-term daily low dose oral therapy has been associated with liver toxicity. When given in pulses, at intervals of a week or more, liver toxicity is less frequent. High dose treatment is not associated with long-term liver toxicity.

Reversible pneumonitis, characterised by cough, dyspnoea, fever or cyanosis, occurs in 3%–8% of patients. Symptoms develop hours to days after treatment. Pulmonary fibrosis is rare.

Intrathecal methotrexate rarely causes systemic effects, however 30% of patients experience meningeal irritation, characterised by headache, lethargy, fever or vomiting. Symptoms develop within a few hours and last commonly for 12 hours and infrequently for a few days. Encephalopathy manifested by confusion, irritability, ataxis, tremor or seizures, is infrequent when intrathecal methotrexate is used alone. Concurrent use of cranial irradiation and/or systemic methotrexate substantially increases risk.

High dose intravenous methotrexate (8–12 g/m^2) has been associated with behavioural changes, paraesthesias and less frequently seizures. Onset occurs on average 6 days after treatment with full recovery in minutes to days. Symptoms may not recur with treatment.

Reports of anaphylaxis with methotrexate are rare.

DRUG INTERACTIONS

Aspirin can significantly increase the toxicity of methotrexate and in general should be avoided at the time of methotrexate administration. NSAIDs and nephrotoxic drugs increase the likelihood of serious toxicity from high dose methotrexate.

Vaccines containing live attenuated organisms have caused serious infections in some patients treated with cytotoxic drugs including methotrexate.

PRECAUTIONS AND CONTRAINDICATIONS

Methotrexate should be used with considerable caution in patients with mild renal failure, liver dysfunction, pleural effusions or ascites. Significant renal failure is usually a contraindication to use.

Intravenous methotrexate should not be administered to patients who are dehydrated.

High dose and mid dose methotrexate should only be given to patients with good renal function. Hydration requirements, urine alkalinisation where applicable and rescue doses of leucovorin must be given in accordance with protocols. High dose methotrexate should only be carried out in centres with ready access to assay facilities that provide rapid reporting on methotrexate levels.

During high dose treatment NSAIDs, renally toxic drugs and non-essential medications should be avoided.

Methotrexate should be given with extreme caution if the patient is receiving concurrent irradiation. Pre-existing drug induced mucositis is a contraindication to treatment. Marrow toxicity from previous treatment or other causes may preclude or delay the use of methotrexate.

NURSING IMPLICATIONS

ASSESSMENT

Patients should be assessed for any indication of mucositis occurring as a result of previous similar doses of methotrexate. Where significant toxicity has occurred or is suspected and no change in therapy is made, the nurse should ensure that the prescribing physician is fully aware of this information.

The nurse should ensure that blood counts are acceptable.

ADMINISTRATION

Mid and high dose protocols vary considerably in terms of the need for, and application of, hydration, urine alkalinisation, drug administration, methotrexate assays and the use and modification of leucovorin rescue doses. Details pertaining to one protocol may not be relevant to another. The requirements for each protocol must be clear prior to starting therapy.

PATIENT EDUCATION

Patients should be advised to avoid the use of aspirin within 24 hours of methotrexate. Excessive sunlight exposure, particularly in the days leading up to treatment, should be avoided.

Where leucovorin rescue is utilised on an outpatient basis correct adherence to directions must be stressed.

ANTITUMOUR ANTIBIOTICS

The antitumour antibiotics are a diverse group of drugs having their origins in the natural products isolated from particular bacterial culture broths, most notably that of the species *Streptomyces*. Although labelled antibiotics and having antibiotic activity these agents are not clinically useful as such because they are cytotoxic at relatively low levels.

The toxicity of these agents varies with individual drugs or subgroups. In a number of cases toxicities are relatively unique. The actions of these agents are also varied with cell cycle phase specific and non-specific actions noted.

ANTHRACYCLINES

Daunorubicin

TRADE NAMES

Daunorubicin: *Cerubidin*.

MECHANISM OF ACTION

Daunorubicin binds tightly to DNA, intercalating part of its structure into the DNA helix, leading to DNA breaks and ultimately

inhibition of DNA synthesis and DNA related RNA synthesis. Although most toxic to cells in the S phase of the cell cycle daunorubicin is considered cell cycle non-specific.

PHARMACOKINETICS

Following intravenous administration daunorubicin has an elimination half-life of approximately 17 hours. Elimination is by metabolism, which includes the formation

CANCER CHEMOTHERAPY

31

of an active metabolite, as well as both hepatic and renal excretion. Forty per cent of the drug is removed by the liver with the remainder, much of it unchanged drug, excreted via the kidneys.

USES

The primary indication for daunorubicin is as part of combination induction and maintenance therapy for acute myelogenous leukaemia. Other uses are less certain.

While individual protocols should be consulted doses used include 25–45 mg/m^2 on three successive days combined with other agents as induction therapy or 30–60 mg/m^2 for 3–5 days as a single agent. Maintenance therapy utilises lower doses.

Administration is by slow intravenous injection over 3–5 minutes into the side arm of a fast flowing intravenous infusion of sodium chloride 0.9% or glucose 5%. Short infusions (over 30–45 minutes) can also be used. The drug is administered into a patent and ideally large vein with due respect for its vesicant nature. Central venous access, commonly available in leukaemic patients, is a preferable alternative to peripheral access.

ADVERSE DRUG REACTIONS

Myelosuppression with significant leucocyte and platelet decline is the dose limiting toxicity for individual doses of daunorubicin.

Severe haematological effects are usually the intention when treating leukaemia. With chronic treatment classic anthracycline cardiotoxicity limits treatment to an approximate total dose limit of 600 mg/m^2 (see doxorubicin).

Nausea and vomiting is dose related being moderate to severe with full doses and lasts for 24–48 hours after administration. Anorexia may persist for longer. Prophylactic antiemetics are usually effective.

Daunorubicin, like doxorubicin, may cause severe tissue damage if extravasated. Management measures for extravasation are unproven in value and in some cases may themselves be associated with significant toxicity. Prevention remains the most effective management. Extravasation is usually accompanied by an immediate burning sensation at the site involved (see doxorubicin).

Mucositis is infrequent with commonly used doses and generally not severe. High dose or repeated daily doses may cause significant mucositis. Alopecia is dose dependent being moderate to severe in doses commonly used. Pigmentation and/or banding of the finger or toe nails may occur in association with treatment cycles.

Reactivation of tissue damage incurred from radiation therapy in the days to weeks prior to daunorubicin administration is possible. A red discolouration of the urine may be seen in the 48 hours following a dose, depending on the dose given. This may alarm patients but is not of any consequence.

DRUG INTERACTIONS

Cyclophosphamide given in large doses may increase the cardiac toxicity of daunorubicin. Other cardiotoxic drugs, notably other anthracyclines, add to the cumulative cardiotoxicity of daunorubicin.

PRECAUTIONS AND CONTRAINDICATIONS

Daunorubicin should be given with caution and usually in reduced doses to patients with significant hepatic or renal failure.

Congestive cardiomyopathy may occur during or several months after cessation of therapy. Although considered irreversible appropriate management following early detection of cardiotoxicity may be important in limiting further toxicity and optimising cardiac output in some cases. The maximum cumulative dose tolerated may be less in patients who have pre-existing heart failure, have received cardiac irradiation, have been given other cardiotoxic drugs or who have significant hepatic impairment.

Daunorubicin is a strong vesicant agent, direct injection should be avoided. The venous access site should be changed if the integrity of the existing access is in any way in doubt.

Doxorubicin

TRADE NAMES

Doxorubicin (hydroxydaunorubicin): *Adriamycin.*

MECHANISM OF ACTION

See daunorubicin.

PHARMACOKINETICS

The elimination half-life of doxorubicin is 22–38 hours with most of the drug metabolised to active and non-active metabolites and excreted in the bile. Approximately 5% of a dose is excreted renally, most as unchanged drug.

USES

Doxorubicin is widely used against solid tumours, including carcinomas of the breast, ovary, bronchus, thyroid, stomach, sarcomas of soft tissue and bone, and both Hodgkin's and non-Hodgkin's lymphoma. It is also active against both acute lymphoblastic and myeloblastic leukaemia and multiple myeloma.

Doses totalling 60–75 mg/m^2 can be given by intravenous injection or infusion into the side arm of a fast flowing infusion of sodium chloride 0.9% or glucose 5% every 3–4 weeks as a single agent. The total dose may be given as a 5–10 minute injection on one day or divided and given over a number of sequential days. Alternatively the drug may be administered by short infusion. When given in combination with other myelosuppressive drugs in the treatment of solid malignancies dosage is usually reduced. Doses of 20 mg/m^2 can be given weekly as an alternative to full doses given every 3–4 weeks.

In the treatment of leukaemias individual protocols should be consulted, however doses of 30 mg/m^2 per day for three days may be given in combination with other agents. Doxorubicin as a continuous infusion of 9 mg/m^2 per day for four days in combination with vincristine and dexamethasone is used in the treatment of multiple myeloma. When administered by infusion particular attention should be paid to the risk of extravasation. The use of central venous access may be considered depending on patient variables, the duration of infusion and the relative risk of extravasation and possible tissue damage. (See Adverse Drug Reactions.)

ADVERSE DRUG REACTIONS

The dose limiting toxicity is myelosuppression affecting primarily leucocytes and platelets. The blood count nadir occurs 12–14 days after treatment.

Cumulative dosage is limited by cardiac toxicity. All anthracycline agents are cardiotoxic, capable of inducing cardiomyopathy with all the signs and symptoms of classical heart failure. Doxorubicin induced cardiomyopathy is the most extensively studied and is considered to typify the effects of this class of drug. The incidence of significant cardiomyopathy is less than 5% with total doses below 550 mg/m^2 but increases rapidly after this. Some subgroups of patients are considered to be at greater risk of cardiomyopathy, e.g. the elderly, those with pre-existing cardiomyopathy, those treated with mediastinal irradiation, high dose cyclophosphamide or other anthracyclines, and those with liver dysfunction.

Doxorubicin is strongly vesicant capable of causing serious and persistent tissue necrosis if extravasated. Extravasation is characterised by localised pain, usually immediate, with erythema and swelling occurring within hours. Darkening and demarcation of the area occur over 4–5 days. A central eschar may form with lesions which have the potential to deepen and expand over a number of weeks. The severity of extravasation injuries depends on the amount and concentration of solution extravasated.

Numerous management measures, ranging from extensive surgical excision to topical cooling, have been used to limit tissue damage. The most satisfactory management is prevention through the use of good administration technique and appropriate venous access.

CANCER CHEMOTHERAPY

31

Localised vein hypersensitivity or 'flare' should not be mistaken for extravasation. This transient reaction, described as erythematous streaking along the vein and local urticaria, is not a contraindication to further treatment and may not recur with subsequent administration.

Alopecia is dose related and common with doxorubicin. Mucositis beginning 5–13 days after therapy may be severe with high doses (more than 80 mg/m^2). Banding or pigmentation of the nails with each cycle is common but not significant. In occasional patients hyperpigmentation in the skin folds may occur. This skin change is not clinically significant and will fade after treatment stops. Patients may notice a red-orange discolouration of their urine due to the presence of the drug and its metabolites.

Doxorubicin can reactivate toxicity (skin, mucosa) in previously irradiated areas (radiation recall). This is most likely when radiotherapy is given in the seven days prior to doxorubicin administration but has occurred as late as 30 days after.

Nausea, vomiting and anorexia following doxorubicin administration can be moderately severe if not treated prophylactically. Symptoms may persist for a few days in some patients.

DRUG INTERACTIONS

Cyclophosphamide given in high doses may increase the risk of doxorubicin cardiotoxicity.

PRECAUTIONS AND CONTRAINDICATIONS

Doxorubicin should be given with caution and usually in reduced doses to patients with significant hepatic dysfunction or significant hepatic metastases. Doses may be adjusted on the basis of serum bilirubin, liver enzyme levels or significant tumour infiltration of the liver. Myelosuppression from previous treatment or other causes may preclude or delay the use of doxorubicin. See also daunorubicin.

Epirubicin

TRADE NAMES

Epirubicin: *Pharmorubicin.*

MECHANISM OF ACTION

See daunorubicin.

PHARMACOKINETICS

Following intravenous injection epirubicin is largely removed by metabolism and biliary excretion. At least one metabolite has significant cytotoxic function. The half-life of epirubicin is 15–38 hours. Approximately 11% of a dose is eliminated in the urine, primarily as metabolites.

USES

Epirubicin has been used in the treatment of a number of solid malignancies including breast, ovarian and gastric carcinoma, soft tissue sarcomas and non-Hodgkin's lymphoma. Additionally epirubicin has been used in the treatment of some acute leukaemias.

As a single agent doses of up to 120 mg/m^2 every three weeks have been used. Weekly doses of up to 45 mg/m^2 have also been used. When given in combination with other agents doses of up to 90 mg/m^2 are used.

Administration is by intravenous injection into the side arm of a fast flowing infusion of sodium chloride 0.9% or glucose 5%. Alternatively doses may be administered as a short infusion in a suitable diluent. The drug is administered into a patent and, ideally, large vein with due respect for its vesicant nature. Central venous access, where available, is preferable.

ADVERSE DRUG REACTIONS

Myelosuppression, most notably leucopenia, is the toxicity that limits individual doses. When used as a single agent doses of 90 mg/m^2 usually cause mild thrombocytopenia. Cumulative dosages are limited by cardiomyopathy. When compared to doxorubicin in equal doses epirubicin is less cardiotoxic. When compared in doses that cause the same degree of myelosuppression the difference is far less pronounced. The suggested cumulative dose limits for epirubicin is 900 mg/m^2.

Epirubicin extravasation is considered to carry the same risks as doxorubicin.

Alopecia is frequent. Nausea, vomiting and anorexia are dose related but amenable to antiemetic therapy. Mild to moderate mucositis is possible with higher dosage. Epirubicin may discolour the urine orange-red for 24 hours after treatment.

DRUG INTERACTIONS

Cyclophosphamide given at high dosage may increase the risk of epirubicin induced cardiotoxicity.

PRECAUTIONS AND CONTRAINDICATIONS

See doxorubicin.

Idarubicin

TRADE NAMES

Idarubicin: *Zavedos*.

MECHANISM OF ACTION

Idarubicin is a synthetic derivative of daunorubicin and has a similar action.

PHARMACOKINETICS

Idarubicin is subject to metabolism that includes the formation of an active metabolite. The elimination half-life of idarubicin is 13–19 hours compared with the 60-hour half-life of its active metabolite. Approximately 15% of a dose, measured as the drug and active metabolite, is excreted in the urine over 2–4 days. Idarubicin has been given orally in some clinical trials.

USES

Idarubicin in doses of 10–12 mg/m^2 daily for three days in combination with other agents is used to treat acute non-lymphoblastic leukaemia. It has also shown activity against acute lymphoblastic leukaemia and both Hodgkin's and non-Hodgkin's lymphoma.

Idarubicin is given by slow intravenous injection into the side arm of a fast flowing infusion of sodium chloride 0.9% or glucose 5%. The drug is administered into a patent and preferably large vein with due respect for its vesicant nature. Central venous access, commonly available in leukaemic patients, is a preferable alternative to peripheral access.

ADVERSE DRUG REACTIONS

The limiting toxicity for acute doses of idarubicin is myelosuppression. Although this is a desired effect in the treatment of leukaemia, the use of excessive doses may result in a prolonged myelosuppression and an associated higher risk of complications. Leucocytes are affected more than platelets although both may be severely suppressed. The nadir for both is 14–15 days with recovery after a period of 21 days. In leukaemic patients leucocyte counts may fall as early as three days after starting therapy.

Classical anthracycline cardiotoxicity limits the total cumulative dose of idarubicin that may be given. A total cumulative dose limit for idarubicin use has not been established but is likely to be 90 mg/m^2.

Nausea and vomiting following treatment occurs within 1–4 hours peaking at 2–4 hours. Symptoms may be moderate and are amenable to antiemetic treatment or prophylaxis. Mucositis may occur. Abdominal pain which may be associated with diarrhoea has occurred 1–10 days after treatment. A red-orange discolouration of the urine may occur in the 24 hours after treatment.

Alopecia from idarubicin based combination treatments for leukaemia is usually marked. Rash and dermatological toxicity is rare with the exception of a localised 'flare' reaction described as urticaria and streaking along the injection vein. This is not associated with drug extravasation.

Idarubicin is considered to be strongly vesicant when extravasated (see doxorubicin).

PRECAUTIONS AND CONTRAINDICATIONS

See daunorubicin.

CANCER CHEMOTHERAPY

31

NURSING IMPLICATIONS

ASSESSMENT

The nurse should ensure that blood counts are acceptable.

ADMINISTRATION

Reliable venous access and good technique are important when administering anthracycline drugs. Administration should be by or under the direct supervision of those with considerable experience in giving such agents. The integrity of the venous access should be monitored during delivery and the patient directed to report significant pain at the injection site, either during or shortly after administration. Procedures and provisions to deal with extravasation should be available.

Intensive treatment with anthracyclines may induce mucositis. Protocols for patients likely to be affected should be established at the time of administration.

PATIENT EDUCATION

Patients should be made aware of the signs and symptoms of severe myelosuppression and understand what action to take should these occur. Patients at risk of mucositis should be instructed on appropriate mouth care. Patients should be advised that a reddish-orange discolouration of the urine may occur in the 24 hours following administration and that this is of no consequence.

ANTHRACENEDIONES

Mitozantrone

TRADE NAMES

Mitozantrone (mitoxantrone): *Novantrone.*

MECHANISM OF ACTION

Mitozantrone is structurally similar to the anthracyclines and whilst its mode of action is unclear it is known to intercalate into DNA and inhibit DNA and RNA synthesis resulting in both single and double strand DNA breaks. Mitozantrone is considered to be cell cycle non-specific in action.

PHARMACOKINETICS

Mitozantrone is usually given intravenously. It has a highly variable half-life, reported to be 2–13 days. Significant hepatic metabolism is thought to occur with 25% elimination by the biliary system. Renal excretion accounts for 6%–11% of each dose.

USES

Mitozantrone is useful in the treatment of acute lymphocytic and non-lymphocytic leukaemia, non-Hodgkin's lymphoma, multiple myeloma, sarcomas and carcinomas of the bladder and breast. When used alone to treat solid tumours doses of up to 14 mg/m^2 can be given every three weeks. In combination with other agents doses of 10–12 mg/m^2 are more common. As part of induction therapy for acute leukaemia doses of 10–12 mg/m^2 given daily for 3–5 days may be used.

Mitozantrone is given by infusion over a minimum of 5 minutes into the side arm of a fast flowing infusion of sodium chloride 0.9% or glucose 5%.

ADVERSE DRUG REACTIONS

The dose limiting toxicity of mitozantrone in the treatment of solid tumours is myelosuppression. Leucopenia with a nadir at 10–14 days is the predominant haematological toxicity. Thrombocytopenia is less severe and mild anaemia may develop with repeated cycles. Blood counts generally recover within 21 days of a single 10–14 mg/m2 dose. Haematological recovery following larger doses occurs later.

Mitozantrone causes cardiotoxicity considered to be the same as that associated with the anthracyclines. The incidence is known to increase in association with the total cumulative dose although a definitive limit to total dose has not been clearly established.

Nausea, vomiting and anorexia following conventional doses of mitozantrone affects approximately 50% of patients although only 10% experience significant symptoms. Prophylactic antiemetics are effective for most patients.

With high doses, as given in the treatment of leukaemia, significant mucositis can occur. With lower dosage mucositis is infrequent and mild. Mitozantrone may cause a blue-green discolouration in the urine in the 24 hours following treatment.

The effect of extravasated mitozantrone on soft tissues has not been fully determined. While extravasation has not generally been associated with tissue necrosis, tissue damage has been reported. Local erythema, vein itching and venous streaking proximal to the administration site is unrelated to extravasation and may be a feature of overly rapid infusion.

PRECAUTIONS AND CONTRAINDICATIONS

Mitozantrone should be given with caution to patients with significant liver dysfunction or tumour infiltration into the liver. Myelosuppression from previous treatment or other causes may preclude or delay the use of mitozantrone. Mitozantrone in high total cumulative dose is associated with cardiomyopathy (see daunorubicin).

Although mitozantrone appears to be a mild vesicant it should be considered as potentially damaging if extravasated.

NURSING IMPLICATIONS

Although there are conflicting reports on the vesicant nature of mitozantrone reliable venous access and good technique are important. Mitozantrone may turn the urine blue-green in the hours after administration. See anthracyclines.

OTHER ANTITUMOUR ANTIBIOTICS

Bleomycin

TRADE NAMES

Bleomycin: *Blenoxane.*

MECHANISM OF ACTION

Bleomycin is a mixture of antibiotic substances noted to cause breaks in DNA and to bind to DNA. It is cell cycle specific for the G_2 phase. The cytotoxic action of bleomycin is measured in units of activity.

PHARMACOKINETICS

The drug is administered by intravenous, subcutaneous or intramuscular injection. Bleomycin has an elimination half-life of 120 minutes in patients with normal renal function.

Although intended for local effect only, intrapleural and intraperitoneal administration results in about 50% of the drug reaching the systemic circulation.

USES

Bleomycin is used in combination with other agents in the treatment of a wide group of solid tumours including Hodgkin's lymphoma, testicular carcinoma, squamous cell carcinomas of many sites, diffuse non-Hodgkin's lymphomas, some sarcomas and mycosis fungoides. Dosages range widely although 10–20 units/m^2 by intravenous, intramuscular or subcutaneous administration once or twice weekly is used in most protocols. Continuous infusions of 5–15 units/m^2 daily for a number of days have also been used.

Bleomycin is not a vesicant drug and may be injected in any suitable volume, usually 1–2 mL for subcutaneous or intramuscular injections or as a 2 units/mL solution when given by slow intravenous injection over 10 minutes.

Additionally, bleomycin has been instilled into the pleural cavity in the management of malignant pleural effusion, most commonly in doses of 30–60 units.

CANCER CHEMOTHERAPY

31

ADVERSE DRUG REACTIONS

In single doses bleomycin is well tolerated. Its most significant toxicity, pulmonary fibrosis, is related to the total cumulative dose given. The incidence of fibrosis with total doses of 300 units or less is approximately 1%. As doses increase above 400 units the risk rises significantly. Bleomycin lung toxicity presents as a dry, non-productive cough progressing to shortness of breath with basal rales. Lung toxicity is considered permanent.

Hair loss is common as are skin changes including hyperpigmentation, desquamation of pressure areas, hardening and tenderness in the fingertips, nail ridging and erythema. Mucositis is usually mild and more common with high doses or in the presence of renal dysfunction. Nausea and vomiting are infrequent. Significant haematological toxicity is rare.

Hypersensitivity to bleomycin can take a number of forms. Fever, chills and myalgias are most common, occurring 4–12 hours after treatment, and are self-limiting. In rare cases in sensitive individuals symptoms may be severe and fevers high. Urticaria, angioedema and hypotension are rare and may represent a severe form of the more common reaction rather than a true anaphylaxis.

DRUG INTERACTIONS

High concentration oxygen therapy given during anaesthesia has been associated with a significant increase in lung toxicity.

PRECAUTIONS AND CONTRAINDICATIONS

Bleomycin should be administered with caution to patients with chronic lung disease, renal impairment, previous or concurrent thoracic radiotherapy and advanced age. The use of high oxygen concentrations, notably during surgery, enhances the risk of lung toxicity in patients treated with bleomycin. Regular monitoring of lung function during treatment is recommended.

The suggested use of test doses of 2 units or less prior to initial bleomycin administration in lymphoma patients follows the observed higher incidence of severe hypersensitivity reactions in this group. This recommendation is not universally accepted as useful. Individual institutions will have their own practice.

NURSING IMPLICATIONS

EVALUATION

Signs of lung toxicity (non-productive cough, shortness of breath on exertion) in patients given bleomycin must be reported to the responsible medical officer prior to further treatment. During and immediately after administration the patient should be observed for symptoms of hypotension or other severe hypersensitivity reactions.

PATIENT EDUCATION

The patient should be warned of the likelihood of fever and chills in the 12 hours following treatment, the potential for darkening of the skin and the chance of mild skin changes over the hands, pressure areas and the nails. Reassurance should be given that these are not clinically significant and reversible over time. More severe skin rashes involving significant discomfort or the formation of bullae should be reported.

Patients receiving large doses of bleomycin should receive instruction on general mouthcare.

Dactinomycin

TRADE NAMES

Dactinomycin (actinomycin D, actinomycin): *Cosmegan.*

MECHANISM OF ACTION

The exact mechanism of action of dactinomycin is unclear. It is known to bind to DNA and to inhibit RNA synthesis. At higher doses DNA and protein synthesis are inhibited. Dactinomycin is cell cycle non-specific.

PHARMACOKINETICS

Dactinomycin is given by intravenous injection. It has an elimination half-life of approximately 36 hours with approximately 30% of the dose excreted renally. Biliary excretion accounts for up to 11%.

USES

Dactinomycin is used in the treatment of Wilms' tumour, some sarcomas and gestational choriocarcinomas, most commonly in combination with other agents. Representative doses are 300–500 micrograms/m^2 daily for five days, 2 mg/m^2 as a single dose in adults or doses of up to 15 micrograms/kg day for five days in children. Treatment cycles can be repeated every 3–6 weeks depending on blood counts.

Administration is by intravenous injection into the side arm of a fast flowing infusion of sodium chloride 0.9% or glucose 5% using reliable venous access and with due regard for its vesicant potential. Dactinomycin should not be administered through cellulose ester membrane filters.

ADVERSE DRUG REACTIONS

The dose limiting toxicity for dactinomycin is myelosuppression with the leucocyte and platelet nadir occurring 8–15 days following the start of a conventional five day treatment and 17–25 days after a single high dose.

Nausea, vomiting and anorexia are dose related and common in patients not treated with prophylactic antiemetics. Symptoms develop within a few hours of administration and last for up to 24 hours.

Mucositis, most commonly oral but also occurring elsewhere with associated pain or diarrhoea, may be evident in 30% of patients treated with a five day course. Onset of symptoms occurs after 1–4 days with resolution generally occurring in a further 3–5 days.

Alopecia following dactinomycin treatment is variable. An acne-like rash may

occur, most commonly in adolescents. Other rashes including reactivation of radiation effects (radiation recall), hyperpigmentation (most notably on the face), dry skin and maculopapular eruptions can occur.

Dactinomycin can cause phlebitis and when extravasated is a strong vesicant capable of significant tissue necrosis. Conservative management for dactinomycin extravasation includes the use of topical cooling. Heating is likely to increase toxicity.

Hepatic toxicity is rare and has been reported primarily in Wilms' tumour patients treated concurrently with vincristine. Lethargy, fever, fatigue and myalgia are frequently attributed to dactinomycin.

PRECAUTIONS AND CONTRAINDICATIONS

Pre-existing marrow toxicity from previous treatment or other causes may preclude or delay the use of dactinomycin. Dactinomycin should be given with caution to patients with significant hepatic dysfunction. Pre-existing drug induced stomatitis is a contraindication to dactinomycin administration.

Concurrent radiation and dactinomycin administration enhances radiation toxicity. Similarly dactinomycin given days to weeks after radiation therapy may result in the reactivation of radiation toxicity within the irradiated area.

Dactinomycin is considered a vesicant agent, direct intravenous injection is not recommended. The access site should be repositioned if the integrity of the venous access is in any way in doubt.

NURSING IMPLICATIONS

ASSESSMENT

The nurse should ensure that blood counts are acceptable.

ADMINISTRATION

Reliable venous access and good technique are important in administering this

CANCER CHEMOTHERAPY

31

vesicant drug. See mustine hydrochloride. Dactinomycin binds significantly to some cellulose ester membrane filters and generally should not be administered through these.

PATIENT EDUCATION

Patients should be advised on appropriate mouth care and encouraged to contact their physician or clinic if significant mucositis develops. Patients should be made aware of the signs and symptoms of severe myelosuppression and understand what action to take should these occur.

Mithramycin

TRADE NAMES

Mithramycin (plicamycin): *Mithracin.*

MECHANISM OF ACTION

The exact mechanism of action is unknown. Mithramycin is noted to bind to DNA and to inhibit RNA synthesis.

PHARMACOKINETICS

The kinetics and metabolism of mithramycin are very poorly characterised. The drug is not orally active. Approximately 40% of a dose is excreted renally as drug or metabolite within 15 hours.

USES

Clinical use of mithramycin is limited to the treatment of malignant hypercalcaemia, using low doses of 15–25 micrograms/kg every 2–10 days. Administration can be as a slow intravenous injection into the side arm of a fast flowing infusion of sodium chloride 0.9% or glucose 5%. The manufacturer's recommendation of administration over 4–6 hours in 1 L of glucose solution is intended to lessen the incidence of nausea associated with the larger doses of mithramycin no longer in clinical use. It is of doubtful advantage for the relatively low doses used to treat malignant hypercalcaemia.

ADVERSE DRUG REACTIONS

Repeated doses of mithramycin are limited by their potential for inducing a bleeding disorder. Mucocutaneous bleeding has occurred when mithramycin is administered on consecutive days. In doses used to treat hypercalcaemia haematological toxicity is rare.

Anorexia or nausea is frequent although normally mild. It should be noted that nausea and vomiting is a common symptom of hypercalcaemia and that effects due to mithramycin may be difficult to discern in this setting.

Mithramycin has been considered a vesicant drug although there is little evidence to support this. The manufacturers have suggested the use of local heat to minimise irritation or cellulitis following extravasation.

PRECAUTIONS AND CONTRAINDICATIONS

Mithramycin should be used with caution in the presence of myelosuppression, bleeding disorders, hepatic dysfunction, renal failure or drug induced stomatitis.

NURSING IMPLICATIONS

ADMINISTRATION

Mithramycin binds significantly to some membrane filters and in general should not be administered through these.

EVALUATION

Patients who have received multiple doses, particularly on consecutive days, should be observed for signs of mucocutaneous bleeding.

Mitomycin C

MECHANISM OF ACTION

Mitomycin C (mitomycin, MMC) binds to DNA causing cross linking and subsequent inhibition of DNA, RNA and protein synthesis. Mitomycin C is cell cycle phase non-specific but is more active against cells in the G_1 or early S phase.

PHARMACOKINETICS

Mitomycin C given by intravenous injection has an elimination half-life of 30–70 minutes. Most is metabolised with only 10% eliminated in the urine unchanged. When given as a bladder instillation less than 1% of the dose is absorbed into the systemic circulation.

USES

Mitomycin C is active against a wide variety of carcinomas including those of the stomach, rectum, anus, cervix, lung, breast and pancreas. The maximum single agent dose is 20 mg/m^2 which can be repeated every 6–8 weeks. Mitomycin C is often used in combination treatments at lesser doses and has been used in conjunction with radiotherapy.

Administration is by slow intravenous injection into the side arm of a fast flowing infusion of sodium chloride 0.9%. Alternatively the drug may be given as a short infusion in a suitable volume of sodium chloride 0.9%. Mitomycin C is a vesicant drug and should be administered via a reliable venous access with due regard for potential tissue toxicity.

Bladder instillations of 20–40 mg of mitomycin C as a 1 mg/mL solution may be used in the treatment of bladder carcinoma. Prior to treatment patients are usually dehydrated to prevent excessive dilution of the solution in the bladder by urine.

ADVERSE DRUG REACTIONS

Myelosuppression is the dose limiting toxicity of mitomycin C. The effects are delayed compared to most cytotoxic agents with the leucocyte nadir occurring after 3.5 weeks and platelets reaching their lowest point after approximately 4 weeks. Full recovery may take 6–8 weeks. Cumulative toxicity to the bone marrow is also a feature of mitomycin although this is rare with total doses less than 50 mg. Anaemia may occur with repeated cycles but is generally mild.

Mucositis and diarrhoea are infrequent and usually mild when they occur. Nausea and vomiting are dose related, but mild with doses commonly used. Symptoms develop 2–6 hours after administration and may last for 6–12 hours.

Mitomycin C is a strong vesicant capable of causing severe and prolonged soft tissue necrosis if extravasated. Extravasation commonly causes pain at the time of administration, erythema and oedema at the site may be evident within 24 hours. In serious cases tissue sloughing occurs in approximately 14 days.

Rash, primarily on the palms, soles and face, is common in patients who have received repeated bladder instillations of mitomycin C. Similar rashes have occurred following intravenous doses.

Other significant side effects include renal dysfunction associated with total cumulative dose and in rare cases a haemolytic-uraemic syndrome characterised by haemolytic anaemia, thrombocytopenia, renal failure and pulmonary oedema.

PRECAUTIONS AND CONTRAINDICATIONS

Intravenous mitomycin C should be administered with caution to patients with renal failure. Myelosuppression from previous treatment or other causes may preclude or delay the use of mitomycin C.

Mitomycin C is contraindicated in patients with prolonged bleeding times, coagulation disorders and hypersensitivity to the drug. Mitomycin C is a strong vesicant, direct injection should be avoided. The venous access should be changed if the integrity of the existing site is in any way in doubt.

NURSING IMPLICATIONS

ASSESSMENT

The patient's history should be checked for hypersensitivity related to

CANCER CHEMOTHERAPY

31

past mitomycin C exposure. The nurse should ensure that blood counts are acceptable (blood counts may not be taken prior to bladder instillations).

ADMINISTRATION

When used as a bladder instillation clear instructions or protocols for patient preparation (fluid restriction), patient positioning during administration and the safe handling of waste should be established prior to administration.

Intravenous administration requires reliable venous access and good technique to prevent soft tissue toxicity from extravasation. See mustine hydrochloride.

PATIENT EDUCATION

Patients receiving intravenous therapy should be made aware of the signs and symptoms of severe myelosuppression and understand what action to take if these should occur. Rash or other signs of hypersensitivity should be reported.

PLATINUM COMPLEXES ▬▬▬

Carboplatin

TRADE NAMES

Carboplatin: *Paraplatin.*

MECHANISM OF ACTION

Carboplatin becomes chemically reactive in the low chloride conditions found inside cells. Carboplatin is bifunctional, having two reactive sites on its molecule capable of binding to DNA to cause DNA cross linking with subsequent cell death. Toxicity is cell cycle nonspecific. The relative differences in toxicity between cisplatin and carboplatin are thought to be due to the lower chemical reactivity of the carboplatin molecule.

PHARMACOKINETICS

The reported pharmacokinetics of carboplatin vary widely depending on the assay used. The terminal elimination half-life when drug and metabolites are measured is 22–40 hours. Approximately 60%–80% of a dose is excreted renally in the first 24 hours, 30%–60% of the total as unchanged drug.

USES

The uses for carboplatin are still expanding but include carcinoma of the lung, head and neck, ovary and testis. Typical doses include 250–450 mg/m^2 as a single dose and 100 mg/m^2 daily for five days with both

repeated on a 4-weekly cycle. The usual mode of administration is infusion over 15–60 minutes in a suitable volume of glucose 5% or sodium chloride 0.9%. Continuous infusions have also been used.

ADVERSE DRUG REACTIONS

The dose limiting toxicity of carboplatin is myelosuppression, predominantly thrombocytopenia. Leucopenia occurs and can also be significant. The nadir for both is 14–21 days with recovery in 28–30 days. Anaemia is common with repeated courses.

Nausea and vomiting after high doses occur in up to 80% of patients not pretreated with antiemetics. Effects are dose related, evident after 6–12 hours and rarely persist for more than 24 hours.

Alopecia may be evident after three or more cycles. Serious renal toxicity does not occur with carboplatin in standard dose. Abnormal liver function tests, stomatitis, flu-like symptoms and hypersensitivity, manifesting as skin rash and pruritus, are infrequent.

Peripheral neuropathy, tinnitus, hearing loss and other neurological symptoms are reported in 2%–3% of patients.

DRUG INTERACTIONS

Phenytoin levels may be significantly decreased by carboplatin administration.

PRECAUTIONS AND CONTRAINDICATIONS

Myelosuppression from previous treatment or other causes may preclude or delay the use of carboplatin. Carboplatin is contraindicated in patients with severe renal failure. Treatment with reduced doses may be given to patients with mild to moderate renal impairment.

Peripheral neuropathy, especially due to prior cisplatin therapy, may be worsened by carboplatin. Hypersensitivity to carboplatin is usually, although not always, a contraindication to further treatment.

NURSING IMPLICATIONS

ASSESSMENT

The nurse should ensure blood counts are acceptable.

ADMINISTRATION

During infusion the patient should be observed for signs of hypersensitivity. If a hypersensitivity reaction is suspected the infusion should be halted and a medical assessment sought.

PATIENT EDUCATION

Patients should be made aware of the signs and symptoms of severe myelosuppression and understand what action to take should they occur.

Cisplatin

TRADE NAMES

Cisplatin (cisplatinum): *Platinol*.

MECHANISM OF ACTION

See carboplatin.

PHARMACOKINETICS

Renal filtration is the main means of elimination accounting for 20%–80% of drug

eliminated within 24 hours. The terminal elimination half-life of total cisplatin is 60–75 hours.

USES

Cisplatin is active against a wide variety of malignancies including but not limited to testicular cancer, ovarian carcinoma, squamous cell carcinoma of the head and neck, oesophagus, cervix and bladder, small cell carcinoma of the lung, osteogenic sarcoma, neuroblastoma, Hodgkin's and non-Hodgkin's lymphoma. Cisplatin can be used in conjunction with radiotherapy as a radiosensitiser.

The most commonly used doses are 60–120 mg/m^2 given as a 1–24 hour infusion on a 3–4-week cycle. Alternatively, doses may be given at a dose of 20–25 mg/m^2 per day for up to five days. Saline hydration, mannitol diuresis (with or without frusemide) and effective antiemetic therapy are necessary to prevent or limit the renal toxicity and severe emesis caused by cisplatin (see Adverse Drug Reactions). Doses of 60–120 mg/m^2 given over 1–6 hours have been administered with a variety of hydration protocols. Hydration at these doses has typically included 1–2 L of sodium chloride 0.9% prior to cisplatin with sufficient fluid to maintain an output of 150–400 mL/hour for the next 4–6 hours. Hydration recommendations for lesser doses and continuous infusions are not clearly defined.

ADVERSE DRUG REACTIONS

The dose limiting toxicity of cisplatin can be renal toxicity, nausea and vomiting or neurotoxicity. Adequate hydration and the use of effective antiemetics are significant in preventing renal and gastrointestinal toxicity from the dosages in regular clinical use.

Cisplatin can induce both acute and chronic renal damage. Although toxicity is minimised by appropriate hydration, cumulative renal impairment occurs in many patients.

Renal wasting of electrolytes is common leading to hypomagnesaemia and hypokalaemia after repeated cycles.

CANCER CHEMOTHERAPY

31

Severe acute nausea and vomiting occur with doses of cisplatin in excess of 50 mg if effective prophylactic antiemetics are not used. Symptoms begin 1–4 hours after administration and may persist for 24 hours. Less intense but persistent symptoms, commonly referred to as delayed nausea and vomiting, are frequent with larger doses and may last for up to a week in susceptible people. Treatment of acute nausea and vomiting with 5HT₃ antagonists (ondansetron, tropisetron, granisetron) in conjunction with steroids (e.g. dexamethasone) is successful for the majority of patients. Delayed nausea and vomiting can be difficult to control with the 5HT₃ antagonists being no more effective than metoclopramide in controlling vomiting and less effective in controlling nausea in most patients. This observation suggests that delayed nausea and vomiting are caused by a different mechanism than acute nausea and vomiting.

Cisplatin is ototoxic and capable of causing irreversible hearing loss starting with the high tones not used in conversation. With continued treatment cisplatin progressively affects lower tones causing profound deafness. The effects are often subclinical and detectable only with audiometry. Functional hearing loss is more likely with multiple high dose treatments. Tinnitus may occur in 10% of patients and unlike hearing loss usually abates. Vertigo is rare. Loss or alteration in taste is common.

Peripheral neuropathy, usually numbness and tingling in the extremities, may become evident with repeated cycles. In severe cases, associated with high cumulative doses, disturbance of gait has occurred. Other central nervous system toxicities noted have included autonomic neuropathy and, more rarely, slurred speech, transient blindness and convulsions.

Hypersensitivity reactions, evident as facial flushing, bronchospasm and hypotension in severe cases, are reported in 1%–5% of patients. Reactions are more common following multiple cycles.

Cisplatin has a mild effect on platelet and leucocyte counts. However anaemia, particularly after repeated cycles, can be significant with patients requiring transfusions in some instances. Phlebitis is infrequent. Cisplatin is not generally considered a vesicant drug although extravasation of concentrated solutions has, in rare instances, caused tissue necrosis. Alopecia is mild. Gynecomastia has been noted in males on rare occasions.

DRUG INTERACTIONS

Nephrotoxic drugs may enhance the renal toxicity of cisplatin. Phenytoin levels may be reduced by cisplatin administration. Probenecid may inhibit the excretion of cisplatin.

PRECAUTIONS AND CONTRAINDICATIONS

Cisplatin should be administered with caution to patients with pre-existing peripheral or autonomic neuropathy, renal dysfunction or hearing loss. Cisplatin is contraindicated in patients with severe renal dysfunction and those with a history of significant hypersensitivity to cisplatin or other platinum compounds.

Hydration and antiemetics should be administered. Intolerance to the required hydration may be a contraindication to the administration of cisplatin, e.g. patients with superior vena cava obstruction or significant heart failure.

Needles and administration sets containing aluminium are incompatible with cisplatin and should not be used.

NURSING IMPLICATIONS

ASSESSMENT

The nurse should ensure renal function and blood counts are acceptable.

ADMINISTRATION

Cisplatin should be administered along with hydration and antiemetics according to established protocols or institutional guidelines.

EVALUATION

During hydration the urine output should be monitored and the patient observed for signs of intolerance to the fluid given.

The patient should be observed for signs of hypersensitivity during administration. If hypersensitivity is suspected the infusion should be halted and medical assessment sought.

PATIENT EDUCATION

Patients should be provided with, or have ready access to, sufficient antiemetic therapy to last several days. Patients should be instructed to contact their physician or clinic if severe or debilitating symptoms occur.

EPIPODOPHYLLOTOXINS

Etoposide

TRADE NAMES

Etoposide (VP16, VP-16-213): *Vepesid.*

MECHANISM OF ACTION

Etoposide inhibits part of the function of the DNA unwinding topoisomerase II and induces DNA strand breaks. Etoposide is cell cycle phase specific for late S and early G$_2$ phases.

PHARMACOKINETICS

Oral etoposide has incomplete and variable absorption, approximately 50% with doses of 200 mg. Penetration into the cerebrospinal fluid is low, although levels attained in brain tumours may be significant. Disruption of the blood brain barrier with mannitol or glycerol has been used in some protocols to increase central nervous system penetration.

Approximately 50% of etoposide in the systemic circulation is excreted renally, either as unchanged drug or as metabolite. Another 16% is excreted via the bile. The terminal elimination half-life is 6–8 hours.

USES

Etoposide is active against a diverse group of malignancies including but not limited to testicular carcinoma, lung carcinomas, sarcomas, Hodgkin's and non-Hodgkin's lymphoma, acute myelogenous leukaemia, brain tumours and Kaposi's sarcoma.

Etoposide is given intravenously in combination with other agents in doses of 60–100 mg/m^2 for 3–5 days every 3–4 weeks or as a single agent in doses of 60–200 mg/m^2 for 5 days every 3–4 weeks. Oral etoposide may in some situations be substituted for intravenous doses. The oral dose is usually twice that of the intravenous dose. More recently oral doses of 50 mg/m^2 daily for 21 days repeated on a 28–35 day cycle have been used.

Oral doses, using either capsules or the injection liquid, should be given on an empty stomach. When the injection liquid is given orally it should be diluted in a suitable fluid, e.g. orange juice, to mask the sour taste. Intravenous doses are most commonly diluted in 500–1000 mL of sodium chloride 0.9% or glucose 5% and administered over 30–60 minutes.

ADVERSE DRUG REACTIONS

The usual dose limiting toxicity of etoposide is myelosuppression with leucopenia most significant. The leucocyte nadir occurs within 5–15 days, the platelet nadir by day 12. Recovery is usually complete by day 28.

Nausea, vomiting and anorexia are infrequent and usually mild. Mucositis is infrequent with all but very high doses. Alopecia is common, particularly when etoposide is administered over an extended period of days in each cycle. Properly diluted etoposide injection is not considered to be a vesicant

CANCER CHEMOTHERAPY

31

agent but may cause irritation if inadvertently extravasated.

Hypersensitivity to etoposide may take two forms. Hypotension related to the infusion rate and, less frequently, an anaphylactoid reaction manifesting as bronchospasm, dyspnoea, chest pain, hypotension, hypertension, flushing, lacrimation or tachycardia.

DRUG INTERACTIONS

Cyclosporin given with etoposide may increase myelosuppression. Inducers and suppressors of hepatic microsomal metabolism should be used with caution in patients treated with etoposide.

PRECAUTIONS AND CONTRAINDICATIONS

Etoposide should be administered with caution to patients with severe renal or hepatic failure. Myelosuppression from previous treatment or other causes may preclude or delay treatment.

Rapid intravenous administration should be avoided. Patients should be observed for signs of hypotension or hypersensitivity reaction during administration. In the event of hypotension the infusion should be stopped and may be tentatively restarted at a slower rate after correcting blood pressure. Other hypersensitivity reactions are managed on an individual basis.

Teniposide

TRADE NAMES

Teniposide (VM-26): *Vumon.*

MECHANISM OF ACTION

See etoposide.

PHARMACOKINETICS

Following intravenous administration teniposide is extensively metabolised, 10%–20% is excreted renally as unchanged drug, 30%–35% as metabolites. The elimination half-life is 20–48 hours.

USES

The role of teniposide in the treatment of malignancies is incompletely defined. Uses have included the treatment of paediatric tumours, acute lymphocytic leukaemia, lymphomas and small cell lung cancer. Doses used are highly variable ranging from 100–150 mg/m^2 per week to 400 mg/m^2 given in cycles every 3–4 weeks.

Teniposide is administered by infusion in 500 mL of sodium chloride 0.9% or glucose 5% over 30–60 minutes.

ADVERSE DRUG REACTIONS

Myelosuppression, principally leucopenia, is the dose limiting toxicity of teniposide. Leucocyte nadir occurs after approximately 7 days. Significant thrombocytopenia may also occur.

Nausea and vomiting from teniposide occurs in up to 20% of patients but is generally mild when it occurs and readily controlled. Symptoms develop after 3–6 hours and last for 6–12 hours. Mucositis, diarrhoea and skin rashes are infrequent. Partial alopecia occurs with repeated doses.

Hypersensitivity and hypotensive reactions to teniposide are similar to those seen with etoposide.

Teniposide in diluted solution may cause local irritation if extravasated into soft tissue.

DRUG INTERACTIONS

Inducers or suppressors of hepatic metabolism should be used with caution in patients receiving teniposide.

PRECAUTIONS AND CONTRAINDICATIONS

See etoposide.

NURSING IMPLICATIONS

ASSESSMENT

The nurse should ensure that blood counts are acceptable.

ADMINISTRATION

Intravenous etoposide and teniposide should be administered according to

protocol or institutional guidelines while observing for signs of hypersensitivity. If hypersensitivity is suspected the infusion should be stopped and a medical assessment sought.

PATIENT EDUCATION

Patients receiving treatment with oral etoposide should be instructed on the importance of strict adherance to the prescribed doses. Patients should be made aware of the signs and symptoms of severe myelosuppression and understand what action to take if they occur.

VINCA ALKALOIDS

Vinblastine

TRADE NAMES

Vinblastine: *Velbe*.

MECHANISM OF ACTION

Vinblastine binds to tubulin units within cells and blocks the formation of microtubules. Microtubules have a major role in the division of cells and in other processes essential to cell structure and function. Vinblastine is cell cycle phase specific for the M-phase of the cell cycle.

PHARMACOKINETICS

Vinblastine is given intravenously. It is rapidly taken up into tissues but does not penetrate into the cerebrospinal fluid. The elimination half-life is approximately 25 hours with most drug being metabolised, 5%–20% is eliminated unchanged by the kidneys.

USES

The primary indications for vinblastine are in the treatment of Hodgkin's lymphoma, as part of the ABVD (*Adriamycin*, bleomycin, vinblastine, dacarbazine) protocol, and testicular carcinoma as part of the PVB (platinum, vinblastine, bleomycin) protocol. (The latter protocol has largely been superseded.) Vinblastine has also been used in the treatment of breast carcinoma, choriocarcinoma, renal cell carcinoma, bladder carcinoma and Kaposi's sarcoma.

Intravenous doses of 3–6 mg/m^2 in combination with other agents are common. As a single agent or in tolerant patients doses may be escalated considerably. Direct intralesional injection of a 0.2 mg/mL solution has been used to treat individual Kaposi's sarcomas.

Vinblastine is a vesicant agent and should be administered over 1–5 minutes into the side arm of a fast flowing infusion of sodium chloride 0.9% or glucose 5%.

ADVERSE DRUG REACTIONS

Leucopenia is the dose limiting toxicity of vinblastine. The nadir occurs 4–9 days after treatment with recovery in 7–21 days. Thrombocytopenia is usually mild. Anaemia may occur with prolonged treatment.

Vinblastine induced peripheral neurotoxicity is uncommon except with high dose and prolonged therapy. Autonomic effects, primarily abdominal pain and constipation, are more frequent. The spectrum of effects is the same as that of vincristine, the incidence is less.

Nausea and vomiting due to vinblastine are mild and affect 10%–30% of patients. Mucositis is not common but may be significant at high doses. Alopecia is common. Dyspnoea, bronchospasm and hyponatraemia are significant but rare adverse reactions.

Vinblastine is a potential tissue vesicant. Inadvertent injection into tissues causes local pain that persists for 24–48 hours. Small extravasations are associated with cellulitis, larger amounts may induce necrosis.

CANCER CHEMOTHERAPY

31

Cold compresses are likely to worsen tissue damage and should not be used if extravasation is suspected.

PRECAUTIONS AND CONTRAINDICATIONS

Myelotoxicity from previous treatment or other causes may preclude or delay the use of vinblastine.

Vinblastine should be administered in reduced doses to patients with significant liver dysfunction. Concurrent administration of vinblastine with radiotherapy may heighten toxicity in irradiated areas, e.g. stomatitis, oesophagitis and radiation nephritis.

Vincristine

TRADE NAMES

Vincristine: *Oncovin.*

MECHANISM OF ACTION

See vinblastine.

PHARMACOKINETICS

Following intravenous administration vincristine is widely distributed into tissues, with the cerebrospinal fluid the notable exception. Elimination is largely by hepatic metabolism and biliary excretion. Renal elimination accounts for 10%–15% of each dose.

USES

Vincristine has wide therapeutic use including but not limited to acute lymphoblastic leukaemia, Hodgkin's and non-Hodgkin's lymphoma, Ewing's sarcoma, neuroblastoma, Wilms' tumour, multiple myeloma, breast carcinoma and small cell lung cancer. The most commonly employed dose is 1.4 mg/m^2 in adults and 2.0 mg/m^2 in children. Some physicians limit the dose to a maximum of 2.0 mg.

Vincristine is a vesicant agent. The drug is administered over as little as one minute into the side arm of a fast flowing infusion of sodium chloride 0.9% or glucose 5%. Alternatively vincristine may be given by infusion in a suitable volume of sodium chloride 0.9% or glucose 5% through a reliable venous access.

ADVERSE DRUG REACTIONS

The dose limiting toxicity of vincristine is neurotoxicity, which may be peripheral, autonomic or both.

Peripheral neuropathy is common with vincristine treatment. The initial signs are an asymptomatic reduction in achilles tendon reflex and sensory loss in a palmar-plantar distribution. With continued treatment peripheral paraesthesia and peripheral muscle weakness may develop, potentially leading to foot or wrist drop, ataxia and, in severe cases, gait abnormalities. Toxicity is dependent on the intensity of doses used. Symptoms are reversible although muscle weakness may be slow to resolve.

Autonomic neuropathy presents most commonly as abdominal pain or constipation 3–10 days after a dose with resolution over several days. In severe cases bowel obstruction can occur. Autonomic neuropathy can present as, or include, postural hypotension and bladder atony with urinary retention.

Cranial nerve palsies manifesting as bilateral ptosis, diplopia or hoarseness of the voice are uncommon and reversible. Jaw pain and headaches are infrequent.

Vincristine is a strong vesicant capable of causing cellulitis or frank tissue necrosis depending on the size of the extravasation. Cold compresses are likely to worsen necrosis and should not be used if extravasation is suspected.

Myelosuppression is rare with vincristine treatment. Nausea and vomiting may occur after 4–8 hours but are uncommon and mild. Alopecia is frequent with vincristine containing protocols. Rashes and hypersensitivity reactions are rare.

DRUG INTERACTIONS

Digoxin absorption may be inhibited by vincristine. Isoniazid may worsen vincristine induced neuropathy.

PRECAUTIONS AND CONTRAINDICATIONS

Vincristine should be given with caution and usually in reduced doses to patients with significant liver dysfunction. Caution should also be used in treating patients with neuromuscular disorders or those receiving other neurotoxic drugs.

Prophylactic use of laxatives is advisable in patients who have experienced vincristine induced constipation or who are considered at risk of doing so.

The neurotoxicity of vincristine is enhanced by radiotherapy. If the area treated includes the liver, serious liver toxicity can result.

Vincristine must never be used intrathecally, as such administration is always fatal.

Vindesine

TRADE NAMES

Vindesine: *Eldesine.*

MECHANISM OF ACTION

See vinblastine.

PHARMACOKINETICS

Vindesine has an elimination half-life of 24 hours. Metabolism has not been fully characterised although the majority of the drug is probably eliminated by the liver. Less than 15% of the drug is excreted intact in the urine.

USES

Vindesine has been used in the palliative treatment of leukaemias, non-small cell lung carcinoma, malignant melanoma, breast carcinoma and renal cell carcinoma.

Doses of 3 mg/m^2 in adults and 4 mg/m^2 in children repeated every 7–10 days are representative. Vindesine is a vesicant agent and is administered over 1–5 minutes into the side arm of a fast flowing infusion of sodium chloride 0.9% or glucose 5%.

ADVERSE DRUG REACTIONS

Vindesine has a toxicity profile that lies between that of vincristine and vinblastine.

Myelosuppression, particularly leucopenia, is the dose limiting toxicity. The leucocyte nadir occurs after 3–7 days with recovery generally within 14 days. Anaemia may develop with repeated doses.

Like vincristine, vindesine may cause peripheral and autonomic neuropathies although in general the effects are less intense.

Moderate nausea and vomiting may occur in a percentage of patients but is generally easily controlled. Stomatitis occurs in a fraction of patients but is usually mild. Alopecia of varying degrees and a flu-like syndrome are reported in up to 30% of patients.

Extravasation of vindesine may cause cellulitis or tissue necrosis depending on the amount involved. Cold compresses may worsen toxicity and are not recommended.

PRECAUTIONS AND CONTRAINDICATIONS

See vincristine.

NURSING IMPLICATIONS

ASSESSMENT

The nurse should ensure that blood counts are acceptable in patients receiving vinblastine and vindesine. Any signs of neurotoxicity noted with previous treatment with vinca alkaloids should be reported.

ADMINISTRATION

Reliable venous access and good techniques are important in the administration of the vinca alkaloids. See mustine hydrochloride.

PATIENT EDUCATION

Patients should be warned of the possibility of abdominal pain and constipation and provided with appropriate advice on how to manage these side effects.

CANCER CHEMOTHERAPY

31

MISCELLANEOUS AGENTS ▐███████████

Colaspase

TRADE NAMES

Colaspase (asparaginase, L-asparaginase): *Leunase.*

MECHANISM OF ACTION

Colaspase has a relatively unique mode of action. It acts by enzymatically degrading the body's circulating levels of the amino acid asparagine. In leukaemic cells that are unable to synthesise their own supply of asparagine (and hence rely on circulating asparagine) protein synthesis is inhibited. Asparaginase is specific for the G_1 phase of the cell cycle.

PHARMACOKINETICS

Colaspase cannot be given orally but may be given by intramuscular, subcutaneous or intravenous injection. The pharmacokinetics of the drug are poorly defined. Little unchanged drug is excreted renally. The elimination half-life has been quoted at 8–30 hours, however, detectable levels may persist for up to 3 weeks with associated suppression of plasma asparagine levels.

USES

The primary indications for colaspase are the treatment of acute lymphocytic leukaemia and certain high grade lymphomas.

Dosages vary considerably, however 6000–9000 units/m^2 day for 9–28 days is broadly representative of those in common use. Administration is by intravenous infusion in sodium chloride 0.9% or glucose 5% over a period of no less than 30 minutes, by subcutaneous injection or by intramuscular injection.

The common practice of using test doses prior to a course of treatment involves the administration of 1–10 units intradermally in a suitable volume. The site is examined after one hour for signs of hypersensitivity. Test doses are considered controversial by some physicians (see Adverse Drug Reactions).

ADVERSE DRUG REACTIONS

With the exception of hypersensitivity reactions there are no significant toxicities associated with single doses of up to 200 000 units. The duration of treatment, however, is limited as the removal of asparagine from the systemic circulation inhibits the synthesis of some biologically important proteins. With continued colaspase use deficiencies in clotting factors, albumin, insulin and thyroid binding globulin may result.

Hypersensitivity reactions most commonly involve urticarial rash, fever, chills or arthralgia. Other more severe reactions which occur in many affected patients include facial oedema, abdominal pain, hypotension or bronchospasm. Signs of significant hypersensitivity usually occur within 60 minutes. Deaths have been reported in rare instances.

Some degree of hypersensitivity develops at some time in 20%–40% of patients receiving repeated treatment. The risk of hypersensitivity increases with repeated doses, intermittent dosing and may be more common with intravenous administration. Risk is reduced with concurrent corticosteroid use. Test doses of 1–10 units may be given intradermally or subcutaneously prior to treatment or in situations where therapy is intermittent or has been interrupted for seven days or more. Erythema or a wheal appearing at the site should be assessed in terms of the risk of serious hypersensitivity. Test doses are not entirely reliable, false results do occur in a significant number of cases. For this reason the use of test doses has been abandoned by many physicians.

Reduced production of clotting factors by the liver is a common side effect of colaspase although this rarely causes clinical bleeding. Similarly there may be a reduction in pancreatic secretions including insulin. Clinically significant pancreatitis with overt hyperglycaemia may occur in up to 5% of patients. Mild alterations in liver function are very common. Serious and fatal hepatotoxicity is infrequent.

Nausea and vomiting are common but readily controlled. Depression, lethargy and disorientation are infrequent central nervous system side effects. Renal insufficiency and proteinuria are rare.

DRUG INTERACTIONS

Methotrexate's activity is reduced if given with or up to 10 days after colaspase.

PRECAUTIONS AND CONTRAINDICATIONS

Colaspase is contraindicated in patients with a history of true anaphylaxis with colaspase. Although test doses of colaspase are recommended prior to the first dose or when treatment is interrupted for more that seven days false negative results can occur. The drug should be initiated or restarted only in centres with facilities to deal with anaphylaxis.

Patients receiving hypoglycaemic therapy may have worsening of control. Hepatic, pancreatic and renal activity are usually monitored during therapy.

NURSING IMPLICATIONS

ASSESSMENT

Test doses of colaspase may be given depending on hospital policy or instruction from the physician.

Hydroxyurea

TRADE NAMES

Hydroxyurea: *Hydrea.*

MECHANISM OF ACTION

Hydroxyurea is considered to inhibit the formation of some of the essential components of DNA. It is cell cycle specific for the S phase.

PHARMACOKINETICS

Hydroxyurea is well absorbed from the gastrointestinal tract with peak levels occurring after 80–120 minutes. The plasma half-life is 2–4.5 hours with metabolism and elimination poorly understood.

USES

The primary indication for hydroxyurea is in the control of blood counts in patients with chronic myelogenous leukaemia. Doses may be given on a continuous basis at 0.5–3 g per day or as intermittent doses of up to 3 g/m^2 every three days. Powder filled capsules may be given as a single daily dose or divided over the day. Patients who experience difficulty in swallowing capsules may sprinkle the powder into water.

ADVERSE DRUG REACTIONS

The dose limiting toxicity of hydroxyurea is myelosuppression, primarily leucopenia. Leucocyte counts decline 3–7 days after a dose with recovery evident soon after stopping therapy. Significant thrombocytopenia is uncommon and anaemia less so.

Nausea and vomiting are mild to moderate when they occur. Symptoms are easily controlled and generally wane after a number of weeks of continued treatment. Stomatitis is rare.

Long term hydroxyurea use has been associated with skin atrophy, hyperpigmentation, erythema of the face and hands, partial alopecia and nail changes in a percentage of patients.

PRECAUTIONS AND CONTRAINDICATIONS

Hydroxyurea should be used with caution in patients with significant renal dysfunction.

NURSING IMPLICATIONS

PATIENT EDUCATION

Patients should be made aware of the importance of taking hydroxyurea only as instructed. Additionally patients should

CANCER CHEMOTHERAPY

31

be aware of the signs and symptoms of infection that may result from leucopenia and be instructed to contact their physician or clinic without delay should these develop.

Procarbazine

TRADE NAMES

Procarbazine: *Natulan*.

MECHANISM OF ACTION

Procarbazine was initially synthesised as a potential MAOI antidepressant. It was subsequently noted to have cytotoxic action via binding to DNA.

Procarbazine requires metabolism to as yet unidentified metabolites to exert its effects. Procarbazine inhibits DNA, RNA and protein synthesis and is cell cycle specific for cells in S and G_2 phase.

PHARMACOKINETICS

Oral absorption of procarbazine is rapid and complete. Procarbazine is extensively metabolised with more than 75% excreted as metabolites over 24 hours.

USES

Procarbazine use is largely restricted to the treatment of Hodgkin's lymphoma as part of the MOPP protocol (mustine, vincristine, procarbazine and prednisone or prednisolone). The usual dose is 100 mg/m^2 daily for days 1–14 of a 28-day cycle.

ADVERSE DRUG REACTIONS

Myelosuppression is the primary dose limiting toxicity of procarbazine. However, in doses commonly used myelosuppression is mild. Leucocyte and platelet decline begins after one week.

Anorexia, nausea and vomiting occur in relation to dose. Symptoms, usually mild but marked in some cases, are seen in 60%–90% of patients. Symptoms often fade or stop when daily administration is continued. Mucositis and diarrhoea are infrequent.

Postural hypotension with an insidious and progressive onset occurs in 10% of patients given doses of 150 mg/m^2 day. Hypertensive crisis resulting from MAOI type food interactions has been reported but may in fact be rare (see Drug Interactions).

Neurological symptoms including somnolence, confusion and peripheral neuropathy are infrequent with commonly used doses. In rare cases pneumonitis characterised by fever, dyspnoea and a dry cough may develop within hours or days of starting therapy.

DRUG INTERACTIONS

Alcohol ingestion during or two to three days after procarbazine administration may induce a disulfiram reaction. Symptoms include severe headache, facial flushing and sweating.

Metabolism of antihistamines and barbiturates may be inhibited by procarbazine with a resultant increase in effect.

Pethidine effects may be potentiated.

Procarbazine is a weak MAOI and if large amounts of foods rich in tyramine are ingested a hypertensive crisis manifesting as a severe headache could theoretically result. Actual reports of this are rare, however patients should be advised to avoid highly fermented products and those likely to be rich in tyramine.

PRECAUTIONS AND CONTRAINDICATIONS

Procarbazine should be used with caution in patients with moderate to severe renal or hepatic failure. Pre-existing marrow toxicity from previous treatment or other causes may preclude or delay treatment.

NURSING IMPLICATIONS

PATIENT EDUCATION

Patients should be educated on the importance of taking procarbazine strictly in accordance with instructions. The nurse should ensure that the patient is aware that alcohol and certain foods are to be avoided whilst taking procarbazine.

Patients should be made aware of the signs and symptoms of severe myelosuppression and understand what action to take if these occur.

Paclitaxel

TRADE NAMES

Paxlitaxel: *Taxol*; *Anzatax*

MECHANISM OF ACTION

Paclitaxel acts to promote and stabilise microtubule assembly. Normal dissociation of the tubulin units that make up the microtubular apparatus is inhibited leaving cells blocked in the G_2 and M phase of the cell cycle. Cell mitosis is inhibited with cell death following. Paclitaxel is cell cycle phase specific.

PHARMACOKINETICS

Paclitaxel has complex kinetics, its terminal elimination half-life varies between 3.3 and 8.4 hours. The major means of elimination is the liver with only 2.1–8.2% excreted via the kidney.

USES

Paclitaxel in doses of 135–175 mg/m^2 is used in the palliative control of relapsed epithelial ovarian cancer. Application as first-line therapy either alone or in combination is currently being studied. Other areas of investigational use include breast carcinoma, non-small cell lung cancer, leukaemia, and head and neck cancer. Doses of up to 200 mg/m^2 every 3 weeks as a single agent have been used without support from granulocyte colony stimulating factor or peripheral stem cell transfusions. Doses of 250–300 mg/m^2 have been administered with the support of granulocyte colony stimulating factor.

Paclitaxel is commonly diluted into 500 mL of glucose 5% and administered over 3–24 hours every 21 days. Because the paclitaxel formulation is capable of leaching plasticiser from PVC plastics non-PVC containers and giving sets (glass or polypropylene) are used. An in line 0.2 micron filter is required to remove the particulate matter that can form during storage of the commercial formulation.

ADVERSE DRUG REACTIONS

Without haematological support myelosuppression is the dose limiting toxicity of paclitaxel. Leucopenia is most significant. Neutrophil counts begin to fall after 8 days reaching a nadir at 8–11 days. Recovery occurs in 15–21 days with no cumulative effect resulting from repeated treatments. Platelet counts are only moderately reduced. Mild anaemia may occur. Doses above 200 mg/m^2 are capable of causing significant neutropenia. Heavily pretreated patients may be susceptible with lower doses.

Hypersensitivity reactions including dyspnoea, hypotension, bronchospasm, urticaria, angioedema and erythematous rash were initially reported in approximately 10% of patients. The subsequent introduction of dexamethasone, diphenhydramine and cimetidine (or similar agent) as prophylaxis has reduced this to 2% or less. With the exception of erythematous rash, symptoms most commonly occur during the first few minutes of infusion. If symptoms are to occur they are almost always with the first or second exposure to paclitaxel. In addition to stopping paclitaxel, plasma expanding fluids, bronchodilators and adrenaline may be used to manage severe hypersensitivity reactions.

Minor symptoms, such as mild hypotension, skin reactions, tachycardia, flushing and mild dyspnoea, may be managed without stopping treatment.

Myalgia and arthralgia beginning 2–3 days after paclitaxel is common and dose related. In a small number of patients effects are severe and debilitating. Symptoms resolve in 2–4 days and will usually recur with re-exposure to paclitaxel.

Peripheral neuropathy from paclitaxel is cumulative with repeated treatment and is dose related. Neuropathy may develop within 24–72 hours of a dose, characteristically as a burning sensation or sensory

CANCER CHEMOTHERAPY

31

loss in a classical glove and stocking distribution. Recognition of pressure, temperature, pain and vibration are commonly affected although symptoms are rarely severe. Neuropathy resolves slowly following discontinuation of therapy.

Benign sinus bradycardia is a common observation during paclitaxel administration. Infrequently, bradycardia has progressed to AV block. Life threatening ventricular arrhythmias are not associated with paclitaxel given as a single agent but are associated with the combination of paclitaxel and cisplatin.

Mucositis is rare with doses of less than 200 mg/m^2 . When mucositis does develop onset is 3–7 days after treatment with resolution generally in a further 5–7 days.

Paclitaxel has a profound but reversible effect on hair follicles. Hair loss is universally significant and rapid with commonly used doses. Both facial and body hair loss become evident 10–14 days after treatment. Repeated doses commonly result in total alopecia.

Nausea and vomiting due to paclitaxel are mild when they occur and generally easy to manage with antiemetics. Alterations in taste, headaches and diarrhoea are infrequent or mild. Paclitaxel is a mild vesicant.

DRUG INTERACTIONS

Experience with paclitaxel in combination with other drugs is still very limited hence it is good practice to avoid giving non-essential drugs during and around the time of paclitaxel administration.

The sequence of administration of cisplatin and paclitaxel has a profound effect on toxicity. The sequence of cisplatin followed by paclitaxel is associated with a 33% reduction in paclitaxel clearance and is more toxic than the converse sequence.

The clearance of paclitaxel may be reduced during ketoconazole administration.

PRECAUTIONS AND CONTRAINDICATIONS

Paclitaxel should be administered with caution to patients with pre-existing myelosuppression, prior intensive chemotherapy or radiotherapy to marrow sites, significant liver dysfunction, a history of cardiac conduction abnormality, or previous severe hypersensitivity reactions to paclitaxel or teniposide.

NURSING IMPLICATIONS

ASSESSMENT

Any obvious signs of current infection or any significant toxicity experienced as a result of previous paclitaxel treatment should be reported to the responsible medical officer. The nurse should ensure that directions or protocols for drug administration and patient monitoring during infusion have been specified or are available. Procedures and materials to deal with hypersensitivity reactions (including rapid access to medical advice) should be available.

ADMINISTRATION

Paclitaxel should be administered via non-PVC giving set and in line 0.2 micron filter according to protocol or specific directions. In line filters that contain only short sections of PVC lined tubing are considered safe to use (i.e. the *IVEX-2* filter). Reliable venous access should be used to minimise the risk of extravasation.

EVALUATION

During infusion, particularly the first 10 minutes, patients should be observed for respiratory or cardiovascular signs of hypersensitivity. Heart rate should be assessed regularly. Any significant symptoms should be reported to the responsible medical officer for assessment. Administration can be safely completed in many instances if symptoms are minor. If symptoms are clearly severe or if there is doubt the infusion should be stopped until a medical assessment can be made. The

patency of venous access should be assessed at regular intervals.

PATIENT EDUCATION

Patients should be advised to report any unusual symptoms occurring during infusion or any significant pain at the injection site. Patients should be advised of the risk of myalgias following treatment and to seek assistance if symptoms are severe. Patients should be aware of the signs and symptoms of myelosuppression and should know what to do if these should occur.

HORMONAL TREATMENTS

ANTIOESTROGENS

Tamoxifen

TRADE NAMES

Tamoxifen: *Genox; Kessar, Nolvadex, Nolvadex-D.*

MECHANISM OF ACTION

Tamoxifen is a non-steroidal antioestrogen. Its precise mechanism in controlling breast cancer is unknown although it has been noted that the drug and some of its metabolites retard cell proliferation and induce the death of oestrogen sensitive malignant cells.

PHARMACOKINETICS

Tamoxifen is adequately absorbed orally with significant metabolism in the liver to active and inactive metabolites. The terminal elimination half-life of the parent drug is long, in excess of seven days. Approximately 10% of a dose is eliminated in the urine unchanged. The majority of the drug is eliminated via the faeces.

USES

The primary indications for tamoxifen are the treatment of advanced breast cancer and adjuvant therapy following surgical excision of early breast cancer. Tamoxifen has some activity against epthelial ovarian carcinoma. Additionally tamoxifen has been used in combination with cytotoxic therapy for malignant melanoma and is being trialled as preventive therapy in premenopausal women considered at high risk of breast cancer. The most commonly employed doses are 10–40 mg per day.

ADVERSE DRUG REACTIONS

The most common adverse effects of tamoxifen are hormonally based. Hot flushes occur in 20%–27% of postmenopausal women treated with 20 mg per day. It should be noted that 8%–11% of such patients experience hot flushes whilst taking placebo. Similarly nausea, pain, headaches, fatigue and anorexia occur equally in treated and untreated patients. Vaginal bleeding and pruritus vulvae occur in a percentage of tamoxifen treated postmenopausal women. In premenopausal women hot flushes (33%), amenorrhoea (38%) or reduced menses (21%) have been reported.

Phlebitis and thrombosis have been associated with tamoxifen use although the incidence is not statistically different from that in control groups. When used with chemotherapy there is a significant increase in the risk of thrombosis.

Other toxicities of tamoxifen are rare or infrequent. Tumour 'flare', characterised by an initial worsening of tumour pain or hypercalcaemia, apparent within hours or days of starting treatment may occur in 3%–7% of patients with advanced breast cancer.

DRUG INTERACTIONS

Warfarin activity is enhanced by tamoxifen, caution is required when starting or stopping tamoxifen in warfarinised patients.

CANCER CHEMOTHERAPY

31

Aminoglutethimide

TRADE NAMES

Aminoglutethimide: *Cytadren*.

MECHANISM OF ACTION

Aminoglutethimide exerts an antioestrogenic action by inhibiting the synthesis of oestrogens and by enhancing the catabolism of oestrogen sulfate. Aminoglutethimide also inhibits the synthesis of glucocorticoids. Supplementation with replacement glucocorticoid (commonly cortisone acetate or hydrocortisone) is required for all but low doses of aminoglutethimide.

USES

The primary indication for aminoglutethimide is in the treatment of advanced breast cancer. The usual dose is 500–1000 mg per day in divided doses, normally in conjunction with replacement glucocorticoid. Such replacement may not be necessary with aminoglutethimide in doses of 125 mg twice daily.

For information on pharmacokinetics, adverse drug reactions, drug interactions, precautions, contraindications and nursing implications see Chapter 19 Endocrine Diseases.

PROGESTERONES

Medroxyprogesterone Acetate

TRADE NAMES

Medroxyprogesterone (MPA): *Provera*; *Farlutal*.

MECHANISM OF ACTION

Medroxyprogesterone is a synthetic progesterone with demonstrated activity against some malignancies and a poorly understood mechanism of action. In sensitive tumours there is a reduction in mitotic activity and atrophy of cells.

PHARMACOKINETICS

The oral bioavailability of medroxyprogesterone is low, approximately 10%. The unchanged drug has a terminal half-life of 59 hours with only 1% of absorbed drug excreted unchanged in the urine.

USES

Doses of up to 1000 mg per day have been used in the management of advanced breast cancer. Other possible indications for use in malignant disease include endometrial, ovarian, prostatic and renal cell carcinoma.

ADVERSE DRUG REACTIONS

High doses of medroxyprogesterone (greater than 400 mg per day) induce a significant non-fluid weight gain in up to 40% of patients. Weight gain can be useful in cachectic patients but may be worrisome and progressive in others. At doses of 1000 mg per day weight gain equivalent to 5% of body weight is evident in 50% of patients.

Medroxyprogesterone in high doses can induce cushingoid features, alter glucose tolerance in susceptible patients, and suppress levels of some reproductive hormones. Amenorrhoea, altered menstrual flow and hot flushes are noted in a percentage of women; impotence, hot flushes and headache in some men.

Nausea and vomiting, although generally mild, affect 4%–23% of patients at high doses. Hypertension may be induced in up to 40% of patients given high doses. Fluid retention (6%), heart failure (5%) and muscular cramp (up to 20%) have also been reported with high dose treatment.

Less frequent or uncommon reactions include tremor, nervousness, insomnia, depression, alopecia, acne, hirsutism, facial rash, pruritus or hypercalcaemia.

DRUG INTERACTIONS

The half-life of warfarin may be increased by high doses of medroxyprogesterone.

PRECAUTIONS AND CONTRAINDICATIONS

Medroxyprogesterone, particularly at high doses, can induce glucose intolerance in susceptible individuals. Patients with diabetes may need adjustment of their diabetic therapy. Hypertension, oedema and, in susceptible patients, congestive heart failure can develop insidiously with high dose therapy. Patients should be reassessed for these effects at regular intervals.

Megestrol Acetate

TRADE NAMES

Megestrol: *Megostat.*

MECHANISM OF ACTION

Megestrol is a synthetic progesterone with demonstrated activity against some malignancies. Its mechanism of action is poorly understood although in sensitive tumours there is a reduction in mitotic activity and atrophy of cells.

PHARMACOKINETICS

Oral megestrol is well absorbed with peak serum levels after 2–3 hours. The elimination half-life is 15–20 hours. Unchanged drug in the urine accounts for 12% of each dose, 20% is found in the faeces, the remainder is excreted as metabolites in the urine.

USES

Megestrol is used in the management of advanced breast or ovarian carcinoma, most commonly in doses of 160 mg per day. Doses of 80–800 mg per day have been used to treat malignant melanoma, endometrial carcinoma, prostate cancer and benign prostatic hypertrophy. It is also used in the management of anorexia, cachexia and weight loss in patients with malignancy or AIDS in doses of 160–320 mg per day.

ADVERSE DRUG REACTIONS

Although non-fluid weight gain is desirable in some patients it may be problematic in others. At doses of 160 mg per day an average increase in body weight of 10% may be seen (range, 0–24 kg), a third of patients having no increase. Weight gain tends to progress with continued treatment.

Increases in diastolic and systolic blood pressure (greater than 20 mmHg) are evident in 9% of patients. Oedema is reported in up to 20% of patients.

DRUG INTERACTIONS

The half-life of warfarin may be increased by megestrol in usual doses.

PRECAUTIONS AND CONTRAINDICATIONS

See medroxyprogesterone.

NURSING IMPLICATIONS

Patients with diabetes should be advised to monitor their diabetic therapy more closely during the initial weeks of therapy with medroxyprogesterone and megestrol.

BIOLOGICAL RESPONSE MODIFIERS ■

Interferon Alfa

TRADE NAMES

Interferon alfa-2a: *Roferon A.*
Interferon alfa-2b: *Intron A.*

MECHANISM OF ACTION

Two subtypes of interferon alfa are currently available in Australia. Although differing from each other by one amino acid the alfa-2a and alfa-2b subtypes are considered identical in action and toxicity. Other interferons, beta and gamma, have been commercially produced but are not in use in Australia. Interferon alfa binds to receptor sites on the surface of many cells resulting in a large number of cellular responses. These can be summarised as

CANCER CHEMOTHERAPY

31 ■

antiproliferative, antiviral and immune modulating. In receptive cells interferon alfa inhibits continued cell division preventing the entry of cells into the S phase of the cell cycle. Antiviral activity is not likely to have a significant role in the management of patients with malignancy. Modulation of immune response by increased macrophage and killer cell binding to tumour cells may play a major role.

PHARMACOKINETICS

Interferon alfa is not absorbed orally. Peak levels occur 2–4 hours following subcutaneous or intramuscular injection. The drug has a half-life of 4–8 hours. It is metabolised in the kidney.

USES

Interferon alfa has been used in the treatment of a diverse range of conditions. Some of the more recognised indications are hairy cell leukaemia, chronic myelogenous leukaemia, multiple myeloma, Kaposi's sarcoma, malignant melanoma and renal cell carcinoma. Dosages range from 3 million units three times weekly up to 18 million units daily.

Administration is by subcutaneous or intramuscular injection. For some patients flu-like side effects are lessened if the drug is given in the evening.

ADVERSE DRUG REACTIONS

Adverse effects with interferon alfa are common and diverse in nature. When commencing therapy up to 50% of patients experience flu-like symptoms (e.g. fever, chills, headache, nausea, vomiting, myalgias) within hours of the dose. These usually resolve with cessation of therapy. The most important dose limiting side effect is persistent fatigue. Although bone marrow suppression (e.g. anaemia, leucopenia and thrombocytopenia) occurs it is usually mild and reversible. Other side effects include confusion, depression, seizures and possibly cardiotoxicity.

DRUG INTERACTIONS

Interferon alfa may reduce the metabolism of theophylline, hence careful monitoring of theophylline levels is advised when the drugs are used in combination.

PRECAUTIONS AND CONTRAINDICATIONS

Interferon alfa should be used with caution in patients with debilitating cardiopulmonary conditions including congestive heart failure, unstable angina and obstructive airways disease. The flu-like symptoms associated with interferon may lead to an exacerbation of these conditions in some patients. Caution has also been advised for use in patients with significant hepatic impairment and seizure disorders.

NURSING IMPLICATIONS

PATIENT EDUCATION

Where interferon is to be self-administered or given by a care giver the nurse should ensure that adequate training in proper administration of the drug has been given. Advice on the disposal of associated needles and syringes should also be provided.

Patients should be informed of the likelihood of flu-like symptoms associated with interferon use. Paracetamol relieves these symptoms in many cases, patients should be advised to take 0.5–1 g of paracetamol either prophylactically or in response to symptoms. Patients should note the pattern of flu-like symptoms associated with treatment. A change in the pattern of fever may indicate that a secondary problem has developed, i.e. infection, disease progression.

Patients should be cautioned that fatigue associated with interferon may impair their ability to peform hazardous tasks, e.g. driving, and that a dulling of mental sharpness may also occur. If affected they should be advised not to drive a motor vehicle.

FURTHER READING

Baird, S.B., McCorkle, R., Grant, M. (1991) *Cancer Nursing*. Philadelphia: Saunders.

Cain, M., Tenni, P. (1992) *Drug Therapy in Cancer: A Practical Guide for Health Professionals.* Melbourne: Society of Hospital Pharmacists of Australia.

De Vita, V.T., Hellman, S., Rosenburg, S.A. (1989) *Cancer: Principles and Practice of Oncology.* Philadelphia: Lipincott.

Perry, M.C. (ed). (1992) *The Chemotherapy Source Book*. Baltimore: Williams and Wilkins.

TEST YOUR KNOWLEDGE

1. List four cytotoxic drugs that may cause tissue necrosis if inadvertently extravasated.

2. Rank the following drugs in order of their emetogenic potential from lowest to highest: doxorubicin, busulfan, fluorouracil, cisplatin.

3. Which cytotoxic drugs are considered cell cycle specific? Why are extended infusions of such drugs more effective against sensitive tumours?

4. Compare and contrast the aims of curative chemotherapy and palliative chemotherapy.

5. Why are cytotoxic drugs often used in combination and what are the desirable characteristics of those combinations?

6. Give examples of measures taken with cytotoxic drug administration to limit the toxicity of individual agents.

7. What agents used in cancer treatment do not have myelosuppression as their major or dose limiting toxicity?

8. What agents have been associated with cumulative and permanent toxicity to major organs?

9. What agents are commonly given by the intrathecal route?

CANCER CHEMOTHERAPY

31

Drugs Used in Critical Care

HEATHER J. LYALL

O B J E C T I V E S

At the conclusion of this chapter the reader should be able to:

1. Discuss the problems associated with drug therapy in the critical care patient;

2. Describe in general terms the resuscitative measures used in the management of cardiac arrest;

3. List the drugs commonly used in the treatment of hypertensive emergency, cardiac and/or circulatory disorders, stress induced gastritis and cerebral oedema;

4. Describe the mechanism of action of these drugs; and

5. List the nursing implications of the administration of these drugs.

DRUG THERAPY IN CRITICAL CARE

Critical care patients pose many challenges to effective drug therapy, e.g.:

- The presence of multiple medical problems hence the side effects of drugs are of greater significance;

- Patients who are intubated and/or unconscious can only be treated with drugs which can be administered parenterally or via a nasogastric or endotracheal tube;

- Renal and/or hepatic failure are not uncommon and can affect drug elimination;

- The pharmacokinetics of some drugs are altered in the seriously ill patient; and

- Multiple drug regimens increase the incidence of drug interactions, adverse drug reactions, drug incompatibility and fluid management problems.

Most intensive care units (ICUs) have developed protocols for the use of individual drugs. They may include guidelines for dosage, routes of administration, infusion strength, infusion rate, indications, contraindications, monitoring and adverse drug reactions. Such protocols differ from one unit to the next and should always be consulted prior to commencement of any drug therapy.

CARDIAC ARREST

Cardiac arrest is an abrupt cessation of cardiac pump function which progresses to death within minutes if active interventions are not undertaken promptly. Ventricular fibrillation is the most common electrical mechanism for cardiac arrest (65%–80%) followed by bradyarrhythmias or asystole (20%–30%).

The initial response to cardiac arrest is to institute cardiopulmonary resuscitation (CPR) until definitive interventions can be made by a trained resuscitation team. These interventions include:

1. defibrillation/cardioversion and/or pacing;
2. endotracheal intubation; and
3. insertion of an intravenous line for fluid and drug administration.

Electrocardiograph (ECG) monitoring should be instituted as soon as possible.

DRUGS USED IN CARDIAC ARREST

Adrenaline

MECHANISM OF ACTION

Adrenaline (epinephrine) is a naturally occurring catecholamine having potent stimulant effects on a adrenergic receptors resulting in vasoconstriction, and less potent effects on β adrenergic receptors resulting in increased chronotropy and contractility of the heart muscle and vasodilation. The beneficial effects of adrenaline during cardiac arrest are thought to be due primarily to α adrenergic receptor mediated increases in myocardial and cerebral blood flow and increased aortic pressure during ventilation and chest compression.

PHARMACOKINETICS

Adrenaline has a rapid onset of action, with a peak effect after 1–2 minutes and a duration of action of about five minutes. It is not effective orally due to rapid metabolism in the gut but is well absorbed if administered via an endotracheal tube. Elimination is via uptake and metabolism by sympathetic nerve endings and the circulating drug is metabolised in the liver.

USES

In the management of cardiac arrest, adrenaline is administered intravenously in doses of 0.5–1.0 mg (5–10 mL of a 1:10 000 solution) or via an endotracheal tube in doses of 1.0 mg (10 mL of a 1:10 000 solution). Doses are repeated at 5-minute intervals during resuscitation. Intracardiac administration carries the risks of coronary artery laceration, cardiac tamponade and pneumothorax and is used only where other routes of administration are persistently inaccessible.

Adrenaline is also administered by inhalation or subcutaneously for the treatment of acute bronchospasm or anaphylaxis in doses of 0.1–0.5 mg (0.1–0.5 mL of a 1:1000 solution), see Inotropic Agents.

Adrenaline is available as 1 mL ampoules and preloaded syringes of a 1:1000 solution (1 mg/mL) and 10 mL ampoules and preloaded syringes of a 1:10 000 solution (0.1 mg/mL).

ADVERSE DRUG REACTIONS

It has been suggested that adrenaline produces a β adrenergic mediated increase in myocardial oxygen consumption and reduction in perfusion which may be detrimental in cardiac arrest. Others believe β stimulation to be beneficial, increasing inotropy and coarsening ventricular fibrillation. The proven benefits of early adrenaline administration during resuscitation of cardiac arrest outweigh any concerns.

Continuous administration of adrenaline can produce adverse effects (see Inotropic Agents).

DRUG INTERACTIONS

Adrenaline should not be administered in the same intravenous line as alkaline solutions, e.g. sodium bicarbonate.

Comcomitant use of other sympathomimetic agents may produce additive effects and increase toxicity. α Adrenergic antagonists such as phentolamine and ergot alkaloids will antagonise the pressor response to adrenaline.

Adrenaline should be used with caution in patients receiving cyclopropane or halogenated hydrocarbon general anaesthetics as these agents increase cardiac irritability.

Lignocaine

TRADE NAMES

Lignocaine (lidocaine): *Xylocaine*; *Xylocard*.

MECHANISM OF ACTION

Lignocaine is a local anaesthetic and a class I (membrane stabilising) antiarrhythmic agent which acts by combining with fast sodium channels to inhibit recovery after repolarisation (phase 4 of the action potential). It shortens the action potential duration and, to a lesser extent, the effective refractory period of Purkinje and ventricular cells so that the ratio of effective refractory period to action potential duration is increased. Lignocaine controls ventricular arrhythmias without affecting automaticity in the sinoatrial (SA) node.

PHARMACOKINETICS

After an intravenous bolus it takes approximately two minutes for lignocaine to reach the central circulation. There is an early, rapid decline in plasma concentration due to distribution into tissue, followed by a slower elimination phase due to hepatic metabolism. The half life of lignocaine is prolonged in patients with myocardial infarction, and/or congestive cardiac failure and following continuous intravenous infusion for more than 24 hours.

DRUGS USED IN CRITICAL CARE

32

USES

Lignocaine is the drug of choice for the management of ventricular fibrillation during cardiac arrest and is given as an intravenous push of 1 mg/kg. Doses of 0.5 mg/kg are repeated every 8–10 minutes if necessary, to a total of 3 mg/kg. Following successful resuscitation a continuous intravenous infusion may be initiated at 2–4 mg/minute. With prolonged infusions the dose should be reduced after 24 hours or blood levels monitored. Plasma lignocaine concentrations of 1–5 micrograms/mL are therapeutic, with toxic symptoms occurring at concentrations greater than 5 micrograms/mL.

Lignocaine is available in many forms. The 100 mg/5 mL ampoules or 100 mg/10 mL preloaded syringes are used for bolus doses and 1000 mg/10 mL ampoules for preparation of infusions. Lignocaine solutions containing adrenaline are not used in this setting.

ADVERSE DRUG REACTIONS

Serious adverse reactions to lignocaine are uncommon and are dose related. High plasma concentrations may produce central nervous system effects including drowsiness, dizziness, disorientation, confusion, agitation, visual disturbances, nausea, paraesthesia and slurred speech, and cardiovascular effects including hypotension, arrhythmias, bradycardia and heart block.

Monitoring of blood levels during prolonged infusions will help to avoid adverse effects. If adverse effects occur the infusion rate should be immediately lowered or the infusion discontinued and re-instituted at a lower rate. Local thrombophlebitis may also occur in patients receiving prolonged intravenous infusions.

DRUG INTERACTIONS

Concurrent administration with other antiarrhythmic agents may produce additive cardiac effects and toxicity. Drugs which inhibit hepatic metabolism, e.g. cimetidine, or which reduce hepatic blood flow, e.g. propranolol, may result in increased plasma lignocaine concentrations and precipitate toxic symptoms.

PRECAUTIONS AND CONTRAINDICATIONS

Constant ECG monitoring is necessary during intravenous administration of lignocaine. Lignocaine infusions should be used with caution in patients with liver disease, congestive cardiac failure, marked hypoxia, severe respiratory depression, hypovolaemia or shock. Lignocaine is contraindicated in patients with known hypersensitivity to the amide local anaesthetics.

Bretylium

TRADE NAMES

Bretylium: *Critifib*.

MECHANISM OF ACTION

Bretylium is a class III antiarrhythmic agent. Its cardiovascular actions are complex and not completely understood. Initially bretylium releases noradrenaline from adrenergic neurones followed by adrenergic blockade. It facilitates electrical defibrillation and may also have a direct antifibrillatory effect on the myocardium. Bretylium prolongs the QT interval.

PHARMACOKINETICS

Antifibrillatory effects are seen about two minutes after intravenous injection. Bretylium is not metabolised, is renally excreted and has a half-life of 5–10 hours. It is removed by haemodialysis.

USES

Bretylium is a second-line agent used to control ventricular fibrillation which is resistant to lignocaine and defibrillation or which has recurred despite lignocaine. An intravenous bolus of 5 mg/kg is given followed by electrical defibrillation. If ventricular fibrillation persists the dose can be increased to 10 mg/kg and repeated at 15–30-minute intervals to a maximum of 30 mg/kg. Continuous intravenous infusions may be administered at a rate of 1–2 mg/minute. Bretylium is available as 100 mg/2 mL and 500 mg/10 mL ampoules.

ADVERSE DRUG REACTIONS

Transient hypertension may occur initially due to noradrenaline release. However, hypotension is the most frequent adverse effect of bretylium and often occurs within the first hour of therapy. Also, by increasing the QT interval the drug increases the risk of torsades de pointes, especially in hypokalaemic patients. Nasal stuffiness and diarrhoea have also been associated with bretylium use.

DRUG INTERACTIONS

Concurrent administration with other antiarrhythmic agents may produce additive cardiac effects and toxicity, including an increased risk of torsades de pointe.

PRECAUTIONS AND CONTRAINDICATIONS.

Constant ECG and blood pressure monitoring is necessary during bretylium administration. Dosage should be reduced in patients with significant renal impairment.

Atropine Sulfate

MECHANISM OF ACTION

Atropine is a parasympatholytic agent with peripheral and central anticholinergic activity. It reduces cardiac vagal tone, enhances the rate of discharge of the SA node and facilitates AV node conduction.

PHARMACOKINETICS

Atropine is given intravenously and is also well absorbed via the endotracheal route. It has its effect within minutes and is metabolised in the liver. Unchanged drug and metabolites are excreted in the urine.

USES

Atropine is used for asystole as a 1 mg intravenous push and repeated after five minutes if asystole persists. For bradycardia the dose is 0.5 mg intravenously every five minutes to a total dose of 2 mg. Atropine sulfate is available in 1 mL ampoules containing 0.6 mg or 1.2 mg and in 1 mg/10 mL preloaded syringes.

ADVERSE DRUG REACTIONS

Adverse reactions are dose related and reversible and include dry mouth, blurred vision, urinary retention, constipation and tachycardia.

PRECAUTIONS AND CONTRAINDICATIONS

Atropine should be used cautiously in the presence of myocardial ischaemia or infarction as excessive increases in heart rate may worsen the ischaemia or increase the zone of infarction.

Sodium Bicarbonate

MECHANISM OF ACTION

Sodium bicarbonate is an alkalinising agent.

USES

Sodium bicarbonate was previously used to correct the acidosis associated with cardiac arrest. It is now thought to be detrimental during resuscitation. Ensuring adequate ventilation is the mainstay of acid–base control.

Bicarbonate should only be used after defibrillation, cardiac compression, ventilatory support and pharmacological therapies such as adrenaline and antiarrhythmics have been employed, and at the discretion of the resuscitation team leader. When sodium bicarbonate is used an initial dose of 1 mmol/kg is given intravenously with subsequent doses of no more than half the original dose given at 10-minute intervals. Post-resuscitation administration is guided by measurements of arterial pH and partial pressure of carbon dioxide. Sodium bicarbonate is available as an 8.4% solution (1 mmol/ mL) in 100 mL vials and 50 mL preloaded syringes.

ADVERSE DRUG REACTIONS

Sodium bicarbonate may induce hyperosmolarity, hypernatraemia and hypokalaemia. It may also produce a paradoxical acidosis due to formation of carbon dioxide, which may then depress myocardial and cerebral cell function.

DRUGS USED IN CRITICAL CARE

32

DRUG INTERACTIONS

Sodium bicarbonate inactivates adrenaline and should not be given in the same line. Sodium bicarbonate forms a precipitate if mixed with calcium salts.

PRECAUTIONS AND CONTRAINDICATIONS

Sodium bicarbonate should be used with extreme caution in patients with congestive cardiac failure or other oedematous or sodium retaining conditions and in patients with severe renal impairment.

Calcium

MECHANISM OF ACTION

Calcium ions play a critical role in myocardial contraction and conduction. When released from the sarcoplasmic reticulum of cardiac muscle fibres calcium ions bind with troponin C (a contractile protein) to facilitate muscle contraction. The sarcoplasmic reticulum then reaccumulates calcium ions bringing about muscle relaxation. A slow inward movement of calcium ions also causes a slow depolarisation during the plateau of the action potential (phase 2).

USES

Calcium is contraindicated in the presence of ventricular fibrillation and should only be used when hyperkalaemia, hypocalcaemia or calcium channel antagonist toxicity is present. When necessary, 2 mL of a 10% solution of calcium chloride may be given intravenously over two minutes and repeated as necessary. Calcium chloride is available as a 10% solution in 10 mL ampoules and preloaded syringes.

ADVERSE DRUG REACTIONS

Rapid intravenous injection of calcium salts may cause vasodilation, hypotension, bradycardia and arrhythmias.

DRUG INTERACTIONS

Calcium enhances the inotropic and toxic effects of digoxin. Calcium salts form a precipitate if mixed with sodium bicarbonate.

PRECAUTIONS AND CONTRAINDICATIONS

Calcium salts are irritating to tissue and may cause necrosis or cellulitis if administered by intramuscular or subcutaneous injection.

An example of treatment sequences in the management of adult cardiac arrest is shown in Figure 32.1.

NURSING IMPLICATIONS

ASSESSMENT

Rapid assessment of the patient who collapses suddenly is vital and includes checking for carotid pulse, clear airway and breathing. Basic life support (CPR) and ECG monitoring should be instituted promptly and the resuscitation team summoned. CPR should be continued until the resuscitation team arrives.

ADMINISTRATION

Nurse members of the resuscitation team must be familiar with doses and methods of administration of all drugs used during resuscitation and with resuscitation protocols. A record of all measures taken, including the doses of drugs administered during resuscitation, should be kept. Many hospitals have a medical record form specifically for this purpose.

EVALUATION

ECG and monitoring of blood pressure, respiratory status and level of consciousness are used to evaluate the patient's response to resuscitation attempts, which should also be documented.

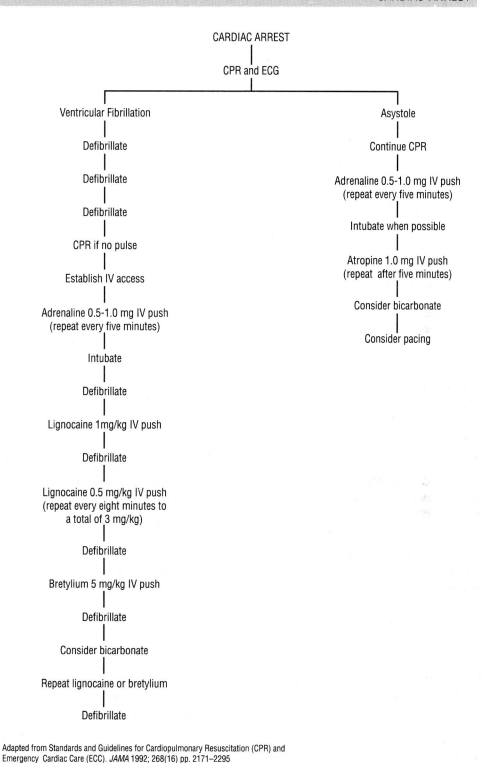

Adapted from Standards and Guidelines for Cardiopulmonary Resuscitation (CPR) and
Emergency Cardiac Care (ECC). *JAMA* 1992; 268(16) pp. 2171–2295

FIGURE 32.1   Example of treatment sequences in the management of adult cardiac arrest

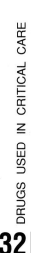

DRUGS USED IN CRITICAL CARE

32

HYPERTENSIVE EMERGENCY ████████

Hypertensive emergency (crisis) is a state of acute, severe hypertension and requires prompt control to avoid complications such as vascular damage, organ damage, cerebral haemorrhage and encephalopathy. Examples of hypertensive emergency include:

- Malignant hypertension of unknown pathogenesis;

- Accelerated hypertension as a result of uncontrolled essential or secondary hypertension (may deteriorate to malignant hypertension);

- Pregnancy induced hypertension (eclampsia and pre-eclampsia);

- Perioperative hypertension due to activation of the sympathetic nervous system and release of stress hormones;

- Drug related hypertension, e.g. during treatment with MAOIs or following abrupt withdrawal of antihypertensive agents; and

- Phaeochromocytoma (tumour of the adrenal medulla which produces excess catecholamines).

VASODILATORS

Direct vasodilators are effective in most forms of hypertensive emergency except that associated with phaeochromocytoma.

Sodium Nitroprusside

MECHANISM OF ACTION

Sodium nitroprusside has a direct action on vascular smooth muscle to produce peripheral arteriolar and venous vasodilation and a marked lowering of arterial blood pressure. Venous pressure is also lowered and some coronary vasodilation is seen. In hypertensive patients, a slight increase in heart rate and decrease in cardiac output normally occur.

PHARMACOKINETICS

Following intravenous administration reduction in blood pressure is almost immediate. Sodium nitroprusside is rapidly metabolised in the erythrocytes and tissues to cyanogen and further in the liver to thiocyanate. Continuous infusions are required to maintain its hypotensive effect which disappears within 10 minutes if the infusion is ceased.

USES

Sodium nitroprusside is effective in the management of hypertensive emergency, regardless of aetiology. Vials of sodium nitroprusside powder are reconstituted with either unpreserved water for injections or glucose 5% in water. *Sodium nitroprusside should not be administered by direct intravenous injection.* The concentrated solution is diluted with glucose 5% in water (no other diluent should be used). Infusion is initiated at a rate of 0.5 microgram/kg per minute and adjusted in 0.5 microgram/kg per minute increments every few minutes, until an adequate hypotensive response is achieved. The average rate required is 3 micrograms/kg per minute with a range of 0.5–10 micrograms/kg per minute. Sodium nitroprusside solutions are degraded by light and should be protected, generally by wrapping solution containers in aluminium foil.

Longer acting oral antihypertensive agents should be introduced as soon as possible and the sodium nitroprusside infusion slowed as they take effect. Infusions are generally ceased after 24–48 hours as adverse effects may occur if infusion is prolonged.

Sodium nitroprusside is also used in combination with β blocking agents to control blood pressure and left ventricular pressure in patients with acute aortic dissection.

ADVERSE DRUG REACTIONS

Nausea, vomiting, sweating, headache, restlessness, dizziness, muscle spasm and abdominal pain may occur and may be alleviated by a reduction in infusion rate. Prolonged infusion may lead to profound hypotension and accumulation of metabolites cyanogen and thiocyanate. Cyanogen produces methaemoglobinaemia and thiocyanate is neurotoxic.

PRECAUTIONS AND CONTRAINDICATIONS

Constant blood pressure monitoring is necessary during administration of sodium nitroprusside. Abrupt withdrawal will cause a rebound hypertensive effect and sodium nitroprusside is contraindicated in compensatory hypertension, e.g. arteriovenous shunt or coarctation of the aorta.

Infusions at the maximum recommended rate of 10 micrograms/kg per minute should never last longer than 10 minutes. Hydroxocobalamin binds cyanogen and may help prevent toxicity with prolonged infusions.

Hydralazine

TRADE NAMES

Hydralazine: *Apresoline*; *Alphapress*.

MECHANISM OF ACTION

Hydralazine reduces peripheral resistance and blood pressure via direct vasodilation, mostly in the arterioles. Increased heart rate and cardiac output occur, probably as a reflex response to decreased peripheral resistance, and may offset the hypotensive effect of the drug.

USES

Intravenous hydralazine is used in doses of 10–20 mg when rapid control of severe hypertension is required. Doses are repeated according to response. Hydralazine is a first-line agent in the treatment of eclampsia and pre-eclampsia. An initial intravenous dose of 5 mg is followed by doses of 5–20 mg every 20–30 minutes as necessary. Hydralazine is available in ampoules of 20 mg powder for reconstitution. Oral antihypertensive therapy should overlap and replace intravenous hydralazine once blood pressure is controlled.

ADVERSE DRUG REACTIONS

The most common reactions are headache, palpitation and tachycardia. Hydralazine induced tachycardia may exacerbate angina pectoris.

For further information see Chapter 12 Cardiovascular Diseases.

Diazoxide

MECHANISM OF ACTION

Diazoxide is a non-diuretic thiazide derivative which reduces blood pressure via direct vasodilation of peripheral arterioles. Its precise mechanism is not fully understood but may involve calcium antagonism. A reflex response to decreased peripheral resistance causes an increase in heart rate and cardiac output.

Diazoxide causes sodium and water retention and also reduces excretion of potassium, chloride, bicarbonate and uric acid. Renin secretion is increased and insulin secretion decreased.

PHARMACOKINETICS

Diazoxide has a hypotensive effect within 2–5 minutes of intravenous administration. The duration of effect varies, generally from 3–12 hours, but may be as long as 72 hours. Diazoxide is partially metabolised in the liver but mostly eliminated via urinary excretion.

USES

Intravenous diazoxide is used for emergency lowering of blood pressure in doses of 1–3 mg/kg (up to a maximum of 150 mg) every 5–15 minutes until an adequate blood pressure reduction is achieved. Subsequent dosing at intervals of 4–24 hours

DRUGS USED IN CRITICAL CARE

32

depends on individual patient response. *The use of 300 mg doses is no longer recommended.* Diazoxide is of particular value for malignant hypertension with renal impairment.

Slow intravenous administration of diazoxide produces a slow sustained fall in blood pressure but rapid intravenous injection is usually required for maximum effects in the emergency situation. Diazoxide is an alternative to hydralazine in the treatment of eclampsia and pre-eclampsia. Diazoxide is available in 300 mg/20 mL ampoules.

Oral antihypertensive therapy should overlap and replace intravenous diazoxide once blood pressure is controlled.

ADVERSE DRUG REACTIONS

Diazoxide may cause tachycardia, palpitations, headache, flushing, sweating, sensations of warmth, lightheadedness and transient weakness, all of which resolve on discontinuation of the drug.

Mild hyperglycaemia and sodium and fluid retention frequently occur. Insulin is rarely required except in the previously diabetic patient and a diuretic such as frusemide will overcome sodium and fluid retention. Diazoxide may aggravate gout.

Pain, or a feeling of warmth, frequently occurs along the injected vein, and cellulitis and phlebitis may result from extravasation.

DRUG INTERACTIONS

Excessive hypotension may result from concurrent administration of diazoxide with other hypotensive agents. Diazoxide may displace highly protein bound drugs (e.g. warfarin) from their protein binding sites. It can reduce the effect of insulin and oral hypoglycaemics.

PRECAUTIONS AND CONTRAINDICATIONS

Constant blood pressure monitoring is necessary during intravenous diazoxide administration. Diazoxide is contraindicated in patients with arteriovenous shunt or coarctation of the aorta. It should be used with extreme caution in patients with angina or myocardial infarction and those in whom sodium and fluid retention may be hazardous.

Diabetic patients and non-diabetic patients with renal impairment should be monitored for hyperglycaemia. Diazoxide injection is highly alkaline and extravasation should be avoided. Intramuscular and subcutaneous injections are contraindicated.

Nifedipine

TRADE NAMES

Nifedipine: *Adalat.*

MECHANISM OF ACTION

Nifedipine is a calcium channel antagonist which produces a reduction in peripheral resistance via arteriolar vasodilation.

USES

Liquid filled capsules of nifedipine 10 mg have been used, either bitten and swallowed or bitten and held under the tongue, for rapid reduction of less severe acute hypertension. There is no advantage in retaining the capsule and liquid under the tongue. The current recommendation is that the capsule should be bitten to release the contents and then swallowed immediately with water.

ADVERSE DRUG REACTIONS

Flushing, headache, dizziness and palpitations may occur following administration of nifedipine in this manner.

For further information on nifedipine see Chapter 12 Cardiovascular Diseases.

Phaeochromocytoma

Acute hypertensive crises associated with phaeochromocytoma are managed with 2–5 mg intravenous boluses of the α adrenergic antagonist phentolamine. β Adrenergic antagonists are introduced after sufficient α blockade is achieved.

Eclampsia and Pre-eclampsia

For information on the treatment of eclampsia see Chapter 20 Drug Therapy in Pregnancy and Labour.

ASSESSMENT

A knowledge of the patient's history is helpful in assessing the aetiology of a hypertensive crisis and hence its management. Baseline blood pressure levels prior to the crisis are helpful in setting goals for antihypertensive therapy.

MANAGEMENT

Continuous infusion of antihypertensive drugs must be by infusion pump. Constant blood pressure monitoring is required until blood pressure control is achieved. Knowledge of the characteristics of antihypertensive drugs used is essential. Patients should be observed for signs of hypotension, chest pain, arrhythmias and worsening hypertension, e.g. headache, visual disturbances, confusion.

DISORDERS OF CARDIAC AND/OR CIRCULATORY FUNCTION

INOTROPIC AGENTS

An inotrope is an agent which affects the contractility of cardiac muscle. Negative inotropic agents, e.g. β adrenergic antagonists, decrease cardiac contractility. Positive inotropes which increase cardiac contractility are used in the critical care setting to treat various problems involving disorders of cardiac and/or circulatory function.

Whilst all positive inotropes increase cardiac contractility their effects on the vasculature and heart rate vary. The choice of inotrope is based on analysis of all haemodynamic variables available. See Tables 32.1 and 32.2.

ADRENERGIC RECEPTOR AGONISTS

The cardiovascular responses to the adrenergic receptor agonists are shown in Table 32.2.

Noradrenaline

TRADE NAMES

Noradrenaline: *Levophed.*

MECHANISM OF ACTION

Noradrenaline is the endogenous transmitter at sympathetic nerve endings. At low doses it stimulates cardiac β receptors to produce increases in contractility and heart rate. As the dose is increased, stimulation of α receptors produces vasoconstriction and a marked increase in peripheral vascular resistance whilst effects on heart rate diminish.

PHARMACOKINETICS

Pressor response occurs rapidly after intravenous administration and disappears 1–2 minutes after infusion is discontinued. Noradrenaline is eliminated via uptake and metabolism by sympathetic nerve endings. Circulating drug is metabolised in the liver.

USES

Noradrenaline is used to correct hypotension and lowered systemic vascular resistance associated with shock, particularly septic shock, which persists after adequate fluid replacement. Noradrenaline may also be used to treat hypotension during spinal or general anaesthesia.

Intravenous infusion is begun at a rate of 0.05 microgram/kg per minute and titrated to response.

ADVERSE DRUG REACTIONS

Mesenteric vasoconstriction may lead to mucosal ischaemia and translocation of bacteria from the gut; renal vasoconstriction may lead to decreased urine output. These

DRUGS USED IN CRITICAL CARE

32

TABLE 32.1 Indications for inotropic agents in critical care

Indication	Inotropes used
Cardiac arrest	Adrenaline during resuscitation Dopamine and dobutamine for postresuscitation haemodynamic support
Anaphylactic shock	Adrenaline
Cardiogenic shock	Dopamine Dobutamine Adrenaline Milrinone
Acute congestive cardiac failure requiring inotropic support	Dopamine Dobutamine, especially with ischaemic heart disease Dobutamine + low dose dopamine
Septic shock	Dopamine ± dobutamine or noradrenaline
Artificial ventilation	Dopamine Dobutamine
Renal insufficiency	Dopamine
Acute pulmonary embolism requiring inotropic support	Dobutamine Dopamine or noradrenaline if hypotensive
Status asthmaticus	Adrenaline (inhaled)
Atrial Fibrillation	Digoxin

Adapted from: Lollgen, H. and Drexler, H. (1990) 'Use of inotropes in the critical care setting'. *Crit. Care Med.* 18, pp 556–560.

effects are most common in hypovolaemic patients. Noradrenaline increases myocardial oxygen consumption and cardiac work, which may be deleterious to the patient with myocardial ischaemia or infarction. Noradrenaline may produce cardiac arrhythmias, lactic acidosis or hyperglycaemia.

DRUG INTERACTIONS

The pressor response to noradrenaline is blocked by α receptor antagonists such as phentolamine and enhanced by atropine.

Noradrenaline should be administered with caution to patients receiving MAOIs as they inhibit its metabolism.

PRECAUTIONS AND CONTRAINDICATIONS

Extravasation causes local necrosis and noradrenaline should be administered via a central vein or a plastic catheter deep into a peripheral vein. Hypovolaemia should be corrected with fluid replacement prior to noradrenaline infusion.

Noradrenaline is contraindicated in hypertensive patients and is generally not used in patients with myocardial ischaemia or infarction, or decreased cerebral blood flow.

Adrenaline

MECHANISM OF ACTION

Adrenaline is the predominant circulating endogenous catecholamine released by the adrenal gland in response to sympathetic stimulation. It produces α receptor mediated vasoconstriction, β receptor mediated bronchodilation and increases in cardiac contractility and heart rate. It also inhibits

TABLE 32.2 Cardiovascular responses to adrenergic receptor agonists

Receptor Stimulated	Organ	Effect
α receptors	Vascular smooth muscle	Vasoconstriction
β1 receptors	Heart	Increased rate and contractility
β2 receptors	Vascular smooth muscle	Vasodilation

the release of mediators from stimulated mast cells during anaphylaxis.

PHARMACOKINETICS

Adrenaline has a rapid onset and short duration of action. It is taken up and metabolised by sympathetic nerve endings and circulating drug is metabolised by the liver.

USES

Adrenaline is inhaled or injected subcutaneously for the treatment of acute severe bronchospasm. It is also the drug of choice for the emergency treatment of anaphylactic shock when it is administered by subcutaneous or intravenous injection or intravenous infusion. Subcutaneous doses of 0.1–0.5 mg are given every 10–15 minutes as necessary and intravenous injections of 0.1 mg are given over 5–10 minutes. Intravenous infusions for cardiogenic shock are initiated at a rate of 5–10 micrograms/minute and titrated to response.

ADVERSE DRUG REACTIONS

Adrenaline may cause tachycardia, increased myocardial oxygen demand, arrhythmias, hypertension, fear, anxiety, headache, dizziness, excitability and weakness. The drug may increase tremor and rigidity in parkinsonian patients and may aggravate or induce psychomotor disturbances or psychosis in some patients. Nausea, sweating and pallor, respiratory weakness and apnoea have also been reported.

DRUG INTERACTIONS

See section on Cardiac Arrest.

Dopamine

TRADE NAMES
Dopamine: *Intropin*.

MECHANISM OF ACTION

The actions of dopamine are complex as it stimulates α, β and dopamine receptors. Its overall effect on cardiovascular function is dose dependent. Low doses stimulate dopamine receptors to increase renal blood flow and promote water and sodium excretion. As the dose increases β receptor stimulation produces an increase in cardiac contractility and heart rate. Further dose increases result in α receptor mediated vasoconstriction.

PHARMACOKINETICS

Dopamine has a fast onset (about five minutes) and short duration of action. It is metabolised in the liver, kidneys and plasma to inactive metabolites and about 25% is metabolised to noradrenaline within adrenergic nerve endings.

USES

Dopamine is used in the treatment of low cardiac output states. The dose is titrated according to required response, i.e. low doses are used for renal, afterload reduction and inotropic effects, higher doses are used if a pressor response is required in addition to renal preservation. However, due to the unpredictability of individual response at higher doses, dopamine is now often used in low doses in combination with other inotropes, e.g. with dobutamine for heart failure when a positive inotrope is indicated and with noradrenaline when inotropic effects,

DRUGS USED IN CRITICAL CARE

32

potent peripheral vasoconstriction and preservation of renal function are the therapeutic objectives. Low doses of dopamine are also used alone in patients with renal failure.

At infusion rates up to 2 micrograms/kg per minute, dopaminergic renal effects occur and higher rates (up to 5 micrograms/kg minute) produce β receptor mediated inotropic effects. α mediated vasoconstriction appears at about 5 micrograms/kg minute and dominates when the rate reaches about 10 micrograms/kg minute.

Dopamine is available in 200 mg/5 mL ampoules for preparation of infusions with either sodium chloride 0.9% or glucose 5% in water.

ADVERSE DRUG REACTIONS

Side effects are similar to other α and β adrenergic agonists. At inotropic doses it can worsen myocardial oxygen balance and thus aggravate or induce ischaemia and induce arrhythmias.

DRUG INTERACTIONS

As MAO is involved in dopamine metabolism, MAOIs prolong the effects of dopamine. α adrenergic effects are blocked by phentolamine, β effects by β blocking agents and dopaminergic effects may be reduced by haloperidol, phenothiazines and opiates.

PRECAUTIONS AND CONTRAINDICATIONS

Hypovolaemia should be corrected with fluid replacement before dopamine therapy is instituted. High doses of dopamine should be used with caution in patients with myocardial ischaemia or infarction. Extravasation should be avoided and dopamine administered via a central vein or a plastic catheter deep in a peripheral vein.

Dobutamine

TRADE NAMES

Dobutamine: *Dobutrex.*

MECHANISM OF ACTION

Dobutamine is a synthetic catecholamine with potent β_1 and weak α and β_2 agonist effects. It has little net effect on the vasculature but its positive inotropic effects increase cardiac output, stroke volume and, at higher doses, heart rate. In patients with congestive cardiac failure the rise in cardiac output usually leads to a fall in systemic vascular resistance so that blood pressure is not altered. Left ventricular filling pressure is also reduced, leading to improvements in coronary perfusion.

PHARMACOKINETICS

Dobutamine has a fast onset (about two minutes) and short duration of action and is metabolised in the liver.

USES

Dobutamine is used to increase cardiac output in patients with cardiac failure due to organic heart disease, cardiac surgical procedures, acute myocardial infarction or septic shock.

Intravenous infusion is initiated at a rate of 2.5–5 micrograms/kg per minute and titrated to response. Dobutamine is available as a powder in 250 mg vials which is reconstituted with water for injections and as a solution in 250 mg/20 mL vials which is diluted with glucose 5% for infusion.

ADVERSE DRUG REACTIONS

As with other adrenergic receptor agonists tachycardia and arrhythmias may occur. Precipitous falls in blood pressure occasionally occur but revert after reduction of the dose or discontinuation of the infusion.

DRUG INTERACTIONS

β adrenergic blockers antagonise the cardiac effects of dobutamine, resulting in dominance of α adrenergic effects (vasoconstriction).

PRECAUTIONS AND CONTRAINDICATIONS

Hypovolaemia should be corrected with fluid replacement prior to commencing dobutamine therapy.

PHOSPHODIESTERASE INHIBITORS

Amrinone, Milrinone

Phosphodiesterase inhibitors are a new group of inotropic agents which produce increased cardiac contractility and vasodilation by raising cyclic AMP levels. Amrinone and milrinone (*Primacor*) are the first in this group of drugs to undergo extensive clinical evaluation. They show promise in the treatment of acute and chronic congestive cardiac failure, milrinone in particular, as it is more potent than amrinone and better tolerated. Recent studies with these agents have demonstrated deleterious effects on mortality rate in patients with chronic cardiac failure. Further investigations will decide their role in critical care.

NURSING IMPLICATIONS

ASSESSMENT

Monitoring of the seriously ill patient requiring inotropic support is extensive: ECG, haemodynamic variables (e.g. blood pressure, central venous pressure, systemic vascular resistance index, cardiac output, pulmonary capillary wedge pressure and indices of ventricular function), urine output, fluid balance, arterial gases and pH, electrolytes, blood sugar and lactate, are all important parameters. The Swan-Ganz pulmonary artery catheter is used to monitor patients receiving inotropic therapy and a full knowledge of its function and uses is required. Rates of inotrope infusion are titrated to achieve preset haemodynamic goals.

ADMINISTRATION

Infusion control devices are used for all inotrope infusions. Most ICUs have protocols for the preparation of inotrope infusions in standard dilutions and these should always be followed unless otherwise stipulated. Inotropes should be administered via a central venous catheter and patients should be monitored for adverse effects.

STRESS INDUCED GASTRITIS

Critically ill patients are at risk of developing gastritis and bleeding due to gastric mucosal injury from ischaemia, hyperacidity, bacterial endotoxins and toxic agents such as alcohol, NSAIDs and bile salts. Mucosal injury also promotes the translocation of bacteria and endotoxins from the gut, a factor which is now thought to contribute to multiple organ system failure.

Factors which increase the risk of stress induced gastritis are a history of ulcer or gastrointestinal disease, coagulopathy, burns, multiple organ failure, shock, pancreatic disease, acute renal failure, head injury, multiple trauma, alcoholism, sepsis and certain drugs (heparin, corticosteroids, NSAIDs).

Improved critical care techniques and routine prophylactic therapy have greatly reduced the incidence of stress induced gastrointestinal haemorrhage over the past 20 years.

Prophylactic therapy is directed towards reducing gastric acidity and enhancing mucosal defences.

DRUGS USED IN CRITICAL CARE

32

ANTACIDS

Aluminium Hydroxide, Magnesium Hydroxide

MECHANISM OF ACTION

Antacids act by neutralising gastric acid. The antacids commonly used are combinations of aluminium hydroxide and magnesium hydroxide (e.g. *Mylanta*).

PHARMACOKINETICS

Antacids are minimally absorbed; the small amounts of aluminium and magnesium which are absorbed are excreted by the kidneys.

USES

In critically ill patients antacids are administered via a nasogastric tube in doses of 20–30 mL every 1–2 hours. For optimum treatment the pH of aspirated gastric secretions is measured prior to each dose. The dose is then titrated to maintain gastric pH at predetermined target levels (generally 3.5–5).

ADVERSE DRUG REACTIONS

Magnesium antacids cause diarrhoea and aluminium antacids cause constipation. Combining the two generally avoids these complications but either may still occur. As aluminium binds phosphate in the gut hypophosphataemia may occur unless patients are being fed parenterally. Hypermagnesaemia and hyperaluminaemia may occur, particularly with long-term administration or in patients with renal failure. See also complications of acid reducing therapy below.

DRUG INTERACTIONS

Antacids may affect the absorption of concomitantly administered oral drugs. However, in the critically ill patient, most drugs are administered parenterally.

PRECAUTIONS AND CONTRAINDICATIONS

Many antacids contain sodium as an impurity and should be used with caution in patients with congestive cardiac failure, renal failure or oedema.

H_2 RECEPTOR ANTAGONISTS

Cimetidine, Ranitidine, Famotidine

Cimetidine (*Tagamet*) is the most widely studied of the H_2 antagonists in the prevention of stress gastritis and has been found to be as effective as antacids. In studies to date, ranitidine (*Zantac*) and famotidine (*Amfamox, Pepcidine*) have been found to be as effective as cimetidine, possibly more effective. All three produce a more consistent increase in gastric pH if administered by continuous intravenous infusion as opposed to intermittent infusions. Recommended dosages are listed in Table 32.3.

Regular measurements of pH of gastric aspirate allow titration of dosage to achieve target pH levels of 3.5–5. If intermittent infusions are used, the frequency of dosage is altered, not the dose. All H_2 antagonists are compatible with parenteral nutrition solutions and may be administered in this manner.

For further information on the H_2 antagonists see Chapter 17 Gastrointestinal Disorders.

COMPLICATIONS OF ACID REDUCING THERAPY

Apart from the usual adverse reactions to these drugs a higher incidence of nosocomial pneumonia in critically ill patients treated with acid reducing regimens has been reported. It is thought that increased gastric pH promotes colonisation of gastrointestinal flora, creating a bacterial reservoir in the stomach from which the tracheobronchial tree may be contaminated.

Whilst acid reducing therapy is effective in preventing bleeding, endoscopic studies have shown that mucosal erosions still occur.

TABLE 32.3 Recommended dosage of H_2 antagonists for prophylaxis of stress gastritis

Drug	Dosage			Availability
	Intermittent infusion	Continuous infusion loading dose	Continuous infusion maintenance	
Cimetidine	300 mg every 4–6 h diluted to at least 20 mL and infused over at least 2 min, maximum 2 g/day	150 mg	Up to 100 mg/h	200 mg/2 mL ampoules
Ranitidine	50 mg every 6–8 h diluted to at least 20 mL and infused over at least 5 min, maximum 400 mg/day	25 mg	6.25 mg/h	50 mg/2 mL ampoules
Famotidine	10 mg every 6–12 h diluted to 5–10 mL, and infused over 1 min			20 mg powder vials

CYTOPROTECTIVE AGENTS

Sucralfate

Sucralfate (*Carafate, SCF, Ulcyte*) has been found to be as effective as antacids and H_2 antagonists in the prevention of bleeding from stress induced gastritis. It has no effect on gastric pH.

Sucralfate tablets are administered orally or dispersed in water via a nasogastric tube in doses of 1 g every six hours.

Sucralfate may adsorb other drugs in the gut and has been reported to reduce the bioavailability of cimetidine, digoxin, phenytoin, ranitidine, tetracycline and theophylline. Antacids bind to sucralfate and should not be administered within half an hour of sucralfate.

For further information on sucralfate see Chapter 17 Gastrointestinal Disorders.

PROSTAGLANDIN ANALOGUES

Misoprostol

Misoprostol (*Cytotec*) appears promising in the prophylaxis of stress induced gastritis, although few studies have been performed. Doses of 200 micrograms, given orally or via a nasogastric tube every four hours, have been found as effective as antacids in maintaining gastric pH above 4 and preventing bleeding.

For further information on misoprostol see Chapter 17 Gastrointestinal Disorders.

Choice of Prophylactic Therapy

All of the agents mentioned are effective in preventing stress induced bleeding from gastric erosions, however a uniform approach to prophylaxis has not been established. Antacid administration is labour

DRUGS USED IN CRITICAL CARE

32

intensive, requiring frequent dosing and gastric pH measurements for maximum efficacy. H_2 antagonists and prostaglandin analogues are expensive but more easily administered. Because of concerns over the increased incidence of nosocomial pneumonia associated with acid reducing therapy, sucralfate is the current drug of choice in many intensive care units.

However, recent studies suggest that translocation of bacteria and endotoxins from the gut into the systemic circulation is promoted by mucosal injury and acidic intramucosal pH. Agents, or combinations of agents, which prevent erosion and increase gastric pH may therefore become the therapy of choice.

NURSING IMPLICATIONS

ASSESSMENT

Gastric pH measurement is required for titration of acid reducing therapy to achieve target pH levels of 3.5–5. Patients should be assessed for any signs of bleeding, e.g. macroscopic blood in gastric aspirate, malaena or haematemesis.

ADMINISTRATION

Antacids require frequent administration and tablets of sucralfate or misoprostol must be well dispersed in water for administration via a nasogastric tube. Nasogastric tubes should be flushed with water following administration of any medication to avoid tube blockage. H_2 antagonists are more easily administered particularly if continuous infusions are used. They may also be added to parenteral nutrition solutions.

CEREBRAL OEDEMA

Cerebral oedema is an increase in water content of the brain. Vasogenic oedema occurs when a breakdown of the blood brain barrier allows protein and fluid to penetrate the brain. Non-vasogenic or cytotoxic oedema occurs when the blood brain barrier is intact but impaired metabolic processes in the neurones or a brain osmolarity higher than serum osmolarity draw fluid into cells.

Conditions associated with the development of cerebral oedema are head injuries, hydrocephalus, tumours and pseudotumours, osmolar imbalance, ischaemia and stroke, diabetic ketoacidosis, encephalopathy, toxins, infection and therapy with some cytotoxic drugs.

DIURETICS

Osmotic diuretics, particularly mannitol, and the loop diuretic frusemide are used to reduce cerebral oedema.

Mannitol

TRADE NAMES

Mannitol: *Osmitrol.*

MECHANISM OF ACTION

Mannitol is an inert molecule which is not metabolised and acts by raising serum osmolarity. This causes withdrawal of fluid from the normal brain across an intact blood brain barrier and diuresis.

PHARMACOKINETICS

Diuresis occurs within 1–3 hours of intravenous administration and lowering of intracranial pressure may occur within 15 minutes. Mannitol is not metabolised but excreted by the kidney. Effects on intracranial pressure may last for 3–8 hours after infusion is ceased.

USES

Mannitol is used to reduce non-vasogenic oedema when the blood brain barrier is intact, e.g. ischaemia, stroke, encephalopathy, head injury. It is used prior to and during neurosurgery. Initial doses of 1–2 g/kg may be used and doses of 0.25–0.5 g/kg repeated 6-hourly as required for 24–48 hours. Mannitol is available in 10% (50 g/500 mL) and 20% (100 g/500 mL) intravenous infusions. Doses are administered over 30–60 minutes. When used preoperatively, mannitol should be administered 1–2 hours prior to surgery.

ADVERSE DRUG REACTIONS

The most severe adverse effects of mannitol therapy are fluid and electrolyte imbalances including hypernatraemia, hypervolaemia and hypokalaemia. High doses (400–900 g daily) have caused reversible acute renal failure. Rebound rises in intracranial pressure occasionally occur about 12 hours after infusion is discontinued and can be minimised by mild fluid restriction.

PRECAUTIONS AND CONTRAINDICATIONS

Accumulation of mannitol due to renal failure or rapid administration of high doses may cause hypervolaemia and precipitate pulmonary oedema, particularly in patients with congestive cardiac failure. If mannitol does not produce a diuresis it should not be continued.

Mannitol should be used cautiously in patients with cerebral atrophy or vascular lesions as decompression may lead to intracranial bleeding.

Extravasation should be avoided as it may cause local oedema and necrosis.

Frusemide

Frusemide acts directly in the nephron to increase sodium and water excretion and may also reduce cerebrospinal fluid and oedema formation.

Frusemide is effective in acutely lowering intracranial pressure and is the diuretic of choice in patients with congestive cardiac failure. Frusemide can act synergistically with mannitol or dexamethasone. Frusemide has a wide therapeutic dosage range from 20 mg to as high as 400 mg. For cerebral oedema, intravenous doses of 20–40 mg are recommended but higher doses may be used. Doses are repeated as necessary. Frusemide should be infused slowly, up to 4 mg/minute.

For further information on frusemide see Chapter 12 Cardiovascular Diseases.

CORTICOSTEROIDS

Dexamethasone, Methylprednisolone

In cerebral oedema steroids may act through various mechanisms including blood brain barrier repair, decreased capillary permeability, stabilisation of membranes, increased cellular water and sodium excretion, prevention of release of lytic enzymes and changes in cerebral metabolism.

Dexamethasone is the steroid generally used but methylprednisolone has also been used. Efficacy in the treatment of cerebral oedema associated with tumours is well established. However, their value in head injury or stroke is not proven.

An initial intravenous dose of dexamethasone 10 mg is followed by doses of 4 mg every six hours until symptoms subside. Dosage may be reduced after 2–4 days and gradually discontinued over 5–7 days. In patients with recurrent or inoperable tumours, a maintenance dosage of 2 mg 2–3 times daily may be required. Oral dexamethasone should replace intravenous administration as soon as possible.

For further information on corticosteroids see Chapter 19 Endocrine Diseases.

BARBITURATES

Pentobarbitone, Thiopentone

Short acting parenteral barbiturates, such as pentobarbitone and thiopentone, have been used in the management of cerebral ischaemia and raised intracranial pressure associated with head injury, stroke and Reye's syndrome. They reportedly reduce cerebral blood flow and subsequently reduce cerebral oedema and intracranial pressure. Their use, however, is not widely established.

For further information on the use of these drugs see Chapter 24 Drugs Used in Anaesthesia.

SEDATION, ANALGESIA AND MUSCLE RELAXATION

Patients admitted to intensive care units frequently experience fear, anxiety, discomfort and pain. They are often disoriented and/or unable to communicate. Feelings of anxiety and fear may also be heightened by perception of their environment and awareness of the severity of their illness.

Anxiety and pain can lead to adverse haemodynamic effects and sedative and analgesic infusions are an important part of medical therapy in critical care.

ANALGESICS

Opioid analgesics are generally used and administered by intravenous or epidural infusion. Morphine is the drug most often used for intravenous infusion. Doses are titrated to response, but are generally in the range 1–10 mg/hour. As well as its analgesic properties morphine also causes a degree of sedation, however, a concomitant sedative infusion is often required. Morphine induced respiratory depression often improves ventilator compliance in the ventilated patient but should be monitored in the non-ventilated patient. Morphine may also cause reductions in blood pressure, heart rate and gastrointestinal motility.

Epidural infusions may contain a local anaesthetic (usually bupivacaine), an opioid analgesic (usually pethidine or fentanyl) or a combination of the two. They are used particularly following major surgery, especially abdominal or thoracic surgery. Most hospitals have protocols governing the use of epidural infusions and these should always be consulted. Morphine is generally not used in epidural infusions.

Analgesic infusions may be supplemented with oral, nasogastric or rectal administration of paracetamol or NSAIDs such as indomethacin or naproxen.

SEDATIVES

The short acting benzodiazepine, midazolam, has largely replaced the longer acting diazepam for sedation in critical care. It is safe and usually well tolerated. Doses used are generally in the range 1–10 mg/hour. Recovery time from sedation with midazolam is variable and increases with duration of infusion. Dosage is generally reduced over several hours to avoid withdrawal syndromes. Rapid reversal of midazolam sedation (e.g. for making neurological observations) can be achieved with the benzodiazepine antagonist flumazenil, but this agent is not used routinely to enhance awakening following cessation of benzodiazepine infusions. Morphine and midazolam are physically compatible and may be combined in the same infusion solution.

Alternatives to benzodiazepines are the short acting anaesthetic induction agents thiopentone and propofol. Propofol is gaining popularity due to its rapid reversibility but experience with continuous infusions beyond 3–4 days is not widely reported. Doses range from 1–4 mg/kg per hour. Propofol is formulated in a fat emulsion and should not be combined with any other drug infusion solutions. Propofol may cause hypotension. Convulsions following its administration have also been reported. Ketamine has also been used as an infusion of 0.5 mg/kg per hour, particularly in the presence of acute bronchospasm. See also Chapter 24 Drugs Used in Anaesthesia.

MUSCLE RELAXANTS

The neuromuscular blocking agents are used to induce skeletal muscle paralysis in patients who are poorly compliant with mechanical ventilation and during tracheal intubation or other procedures. Patients must be adequately sedated prior to administration of muscle relaxants.

Suxamethonium is the most potent of these agents. It is rapid in onset and short acting (3–5 minutes) and is the drug generally chosen for tracheal intubation or short procedures. The longer acting agents, pancuronium, atracurium and vecuronium, are used for longer procedures or to enhance ventilator compliance. They have a variable duration of action, generally about 45–60 minutes following a single dose and are often given intermittently as required.

Atracurium and vecuronium are relatively shorter acting and may be given by intravenous infusion. Again, infusion rates are titrated to response, but typical doses are 0.5–1.0 mg/kg per hour for atracurium and 0.01–0.1 mg/kg per hour for vecuronium. Atracurium is unaffected by renal failure but significant hepatic failure may lead to accumulation of a toxic metabolite. The effect of vecuronium is prolonged in renal failure and recovery of normal function may take hours to days. Both agents may cause hypotension.

NURSING IMPLICATIONS

Infusions of analgesics, sedatives and muscle relaxants must be administered by infusion pump. Doses of these drugs show a high degree of inter-individual variability and infusion rates are usually titrated to response. Patients should be observed for adverse effects and adequacy of response. Once an adequate response has been achieved, dose reduction should be attempted from time to time to avoid oversedation or drug accumulation. The opiate antagonist, naloxone, must be available for reversal of the effects of narcotics should this be required.

DRUGS USED IN CRITICAL CARE

32

FURTHER READING

Oh, T.E. ed. (1990) *Intensive care manual*, 3rd edn. Butterworths, Sydney.

Lollgen, H. and Drexler, H. (1990) 'Use of inotropes in the critical care setting' *Crit. Care Med.* 18, pp. 556–560.

'Standards and guidelines for cardiopulmonary resuscitation (CPR) and emergency cardiac care (ECC)'(1992) *JAMA* 268(16), pp. 2171–2295.

Weigelt, J.A. ed. (1991) 'Surgical Critical Care'. *Surgical Clinics of North America (August)*.

TEST YOUR KNOWLEDGE

1. List the problems encountered in the critical care patient which affect drug therapy.

2. List the drugs used in the management of cardiac arrest and their pharmacological action.

3. List the vasodilators used in the treatment of hypertensive emergency.

4. How is nifedipine administered for rapid lowering of blood pressure?

5. What is an inotrope?

6. What are the results of stimulation of: (a) dopamine receptors? (b) α receptors? (c) β receptors?

7. Which diuretics are used in the treatment of cerebral oedema and how do they work?

8. For which type of cerebral oedema are corticosteroids most useful?

CHAPTER 33

Parenteral Nutrition

MARIAN M. TOWNSEND

O B J E C T I V E S

At the conclusion of this chapter the reader should be able to:

1. Describe the value and appropriate use of parenteral nutrition;

2. List the nutritional requirements of individual patients and assess a formulation providing these requirements;

3. List the implications involved in nursing patients receiving parenteral nutrition;

4. Describe potential adverse effects of parenteral nutrition, including deficiency states.

PARENTERAL NUTRITION SERVICES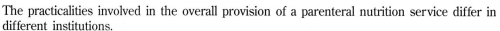

The practicalities involved in the overall provision of a parenteral nutrition service differ in different institutions.

In larger institutions, the service is the responsibility of a nutrition team which consists of a clinician, nurse, pharmacist and dietitian. The team defines local practice, coordinates the management of patients and advises and teaches other hospital personnel. It also may be involved in research.

An example of a request form and progress sheet used by a nutrition team is shown on the following page.

METABOLIC RESPONSES TO STARVATION AND INJURY

Any nutritional support aims to ensure the maximum chance of survival when appropriate amounts of food cannot be ingested. To assess and provide nutritional requirements the metabolic changes that occur in response to starvation and injury, which include trauma, surgery, sepsis and burns, need to be understood.

STARVATION

In the fasting state the metabolic changes which occur are geared to maintain glucose homeostatis and preserve body protein mass. Insulin levels fall and glucagon levels rise. Initially the glycogen stores in the liver and muscle are mobilised and converted to glucose. These reserves are sufficient for only 24–48 hours. After this, breakdown of muscle protein allows amino acids to act as a source of energy by means of conversion to glucose (gluconeogenesis) and to be used by the liver to synthesise albumin and other essential tissue proteins. Fat stores release triglycerides which allow fatty acids to act as an energy substrate (lipolysis). As time goes on up to 95% of energy production is derived from fat. This adaptation spares protein breakdown. A further important adaptation is a decrease in the basal metabolic requirement. Both these adaptations are responsible for the prolonged survival seen in starvation.

INJURY

The metabolic response to injury has three phases: the ebb phase; the flow phase; and the anabolic phase.

During the initial phase, the **ebb phase**, glycogen is mobilised to provide energy. This phase lasts for 6–18 hours.

The **flow phase** which follows is a time of increased energy requirements. Again, muscle and fat breakdown provide energy. However, as opposed to starvation, after injury only 80% of energy needs can be provided by fat, the rest is met by protein breakdown. This phase can last for 5–60 days depending on the severity of the injury, with marked weight and nitrogen loss (catabolic state). Nutritional support in this phase can only compensate for the breakdown of body tissue rather than rebuild it.

The third phase is the **anabolic phase** in which tissue lost in the previous phase can be replaced. It is now possible to place patients in an overall positive energy and nitrogen balance.

Patient Details

PARENTERAL NUTRITION REQUEST FORM

Procedure to request TPN

1. Complete this form and contact Director of Critical Care.
2. Submit the pink copy to the hospital Pharmacy Department.
3. Ensure adequate central venous access available.
4. Ensure appropriate pre-TPN investigations performed.

Clinical Details

Age . . . .   Sex . . . . . .   Attending Medical Officer: . . . .

Date fasting commenced: . . . .   Diabetes? ☐ Yes ☐ No

Liver Disease? ☐ Yes ☐ No   Renal Failure? ☐ Yes ☐ No

Relevant Clinical History

Nutritional Assessment

Height (cm): . . . .   Weight (kg): . . . .   Weight Loss: . . . .

Haemoglobin (g/L): . . . .   WCC: . . . .   Platelet count: . . . .

Albumin (g/L): . . . .   Creatinine: . . . .   Urea: . . . .

Recommended TPN Order

Nutrients	Commencement	Maintenance	Alterations
Amino acids (g)			
Glucose (g)			
Lipid (g)			
Energy (kJ)			
Volume (mL)			

TPN Team Information

Total Days on TPN: . . . .   Post-TPN albumin (g/L) . . . . . .   Discharge status: . . . .

Complications: Metabolic ☐   Infection ☐   Fluid Balance ☐

Comments: . . . .

. . . .

. . . .

. . . .

PARENTERAL NUTRITION

33

The needs of a starved patient therefore differ from those of an injured patient. However, many patients experience both states, e.g. starvation due to inability to eat before an operation for a gastric malignancy or lack of nutrition after gastrointestinal surgery. The particular circumstances of each patient must be recognised to ensure appropriate therapy.

INDICATIONS FOR PARENTERAL NUTRITION

Nutritional support is indicated for those patients who cannot eat, will not eat, should not eat or cannot eat enough. Parenteral nutrition is only indicated for nutritional support if the enteral route is not viable. Enteral support includes oral feeding, nasogastric feeding, nasoenteric feeding or liquid diets for the patient with a gastrostomy, duodenostomy or jejunostomy. Enteral feeding is less expensive and has fewer serious side effects than parenteral feeding. For further information on enteral nutrition see Chapter 34 Enteral Feeding.

Parenteral nutrition has been used in many diseases but, as a guide, is indicated if adequate enteral nutrition cannot be given for more than five days. It is used when it leads to an improved clinical outcome or helps recovery, not to prolong dying.

Indications for parenteral nutrition are:

- Enterocutaneous fistulae

- Preoperative preparation of cachetic patients

- Postoperative feeding of patients fed preoperatively or who develop surgical complications, e.g. prolonged ileus, intra-abdominal sepsis

- Inflammatory bowel disease, e.g. Crohn's disease, ulcerative colitis

- Pancreatitis, pancreatic absess, pseudocyst or fistulae

- Short bowel syndrome

- Hypermetabolic states, e.g. multiple trauma, severe burns

- Unconsciousness when tube feeding is contraindicated

- Liver failure, renal failure

- Radiation enteritis

- Necrotising enterocolitis, prematurity

Parenteral nutrition has also been used in cancer associated malnutrition, anorexia nervosa, chronic vomiting and chemotherapy induced diarrhoea. The question of definite clinical benefit remains unanswered in many situations.

NUTRITIONAL ASSESSMENT

The nutritional status of all patients should be assessed before beginning, and during treatment with parenteral nutrition. A careful evaluation of the patient's weight, recent weight loss, dietary intake, including recent changes, and a clinical examination is needed. Other indicators of nutritional status include:

- Anthropometric measurement, e.g. arm muscle circumference, triceps skin fold thickness (this assessment, ideally performed by a dietitian, assists in determining requirements);

- Measurement of protein stores, e.g. 24-hour urinary creatinine, creatinine height index;

- Indirect measurement of protein syn- thesis rates, e.g. serum albumin, serum transferrin, serum prealbumin; and

- Immune status determination, e.g. lymphocyte count, delayed hypersensitivity skin testing.

PARENTERAL NUTRITION FOR ADULTS

The basic adult nutritional requirements per kg per 24 hours are water 30 mL, amino acids 1.5 g, carbohydrate 5 g, fat 1 g, electrolytes, trace elements and vitamins. These are supplied in appropriate amounts to meet basal metabolic needs plus any additional requirements for stress.

Water

Water is the principal component of the human body, accounting for more than 50% of total body weight. Total body water varies depending on the body weight, fat content, age and sex of the patient. This water is divided into two main compartments, the intracellular fluid compartment (ICF) and the extracellular fluid compartment (ECF). The ICF accounts for 55% of total body water and the ECF for 35%. The ECF is subdivided into the intravascular component and the interstitial component. The remaining body water is located in connective tissue, bone and transcellular compartments.

The electrolyte content of the extracellular and intracellular compartments differ significantly. In the extracellular compartment, sodium, chloride and bicarbonate are the main electrolytes, whereas, in the intracellular compartment, potassium, mag-nesium and phosphate are the main electrolytes. These differences are maintained by pump systems on cell membranes. The osmolarity of all compartments is the same, with water moving freely to maintain osmotic equilibrium. Osmolarity is determined by the number of particles in solution, not the particle size or valence. The osmolarity of body fluid is maintained at 280–295 milliosmoles (mOsm) per L.

The amount of water required per day is approximately 30 mL per kg body weight. This will compensate for urine production, faecal loss and the replacement of insensible losses through respiration and sweating. The need is increased if there is fever, increased room temperature, increased metabolism or loss from the gastrointestinal tract, wounds, drains or fistulae. A patient who has compromised cardiac or renal function has reduced needs. The fluid balance of all patients is fundamental to allowing accurate assessment of fluid needs. Some fluid may be given as drug infusions and this must be taken into account. For further information on intravenous fluid therapy see Chapter 18 Fluid and Electrolyte Disorders.

Amino Acids

Amino acids contain nitrogen and are the building blocks of proteins. Proteins are found in all cell structures, all tissues especially muscle, enzymes and the blood. There are 20 amino acids in humans. Eight are regarded as essential, i.e., they cannot be synthesised in the body. These amino acids are leucine, isoleucine, lysine, methionine, phenylalanine, threonine, tryptophan and valine. The other amino acids are regarded as non-essential but are needed for optimal utilisation of the essential amino acids. The total daily requirement for a basal metabolic rate is 1 g of amino acid per kg body weight. For a moderate increase in metabolic rate, e.g. during sepsis, the requirement is 1.5–2 g per kg. Exact needs can be calculated from urea excretion using the following formula:

PARENTERAL NUTRITION

33

Nitrogen loss (g/24 hours) =
(0.028 × urinary urea in mmol/24 hours)
+ 2

where 2 represents non-urinary nitrogen excretion.

As each gram of nitrogen represents 6 g of amino acid, the amount of amino acid needed can be calculated.

Amino acids are available in various synthetic laevo-isomer amino acid solutions. They contain essential and non-essential amino acids and are hyperosmolar. The solutions differ in the amount and ratio of individual amino acids and the electrolyte content. The components of two commonly used amino acid solutions are listed in Table 33.1.

TABLE 33.1 Amino acid solutions

L-amino acids (% of total)	Synthamin 10%	Vamin N 7%
Isoleucine	6.07	5.56
Leucine	7.39	7.55
Lysine	5.87	5.56
Methionine	4.05	2.71
Phenylalanine	5.67	7.83
Threonine	4.25	4.27
Tryptophan	1.83	1.42
Valine	4.65	6.13
Cystine (Cysteine)	–	(1.99)
Tyrosine	0.40	0.71
Alanine	20.95	4.27
Arginine	11.64	4.70
Aspartic Acid	–	5.84
Glutamic acid	–	12.82
Glycine	10.42	2.99
Histidine	4.86	3.42
Proline	6.89	11.54
Serine	5.06	10.68
Essential amino acids	39.78%	41.03%
Aromatic amino acids	6.07%	8.54%
Branched chain amino acids	18.11%	19.24%
Nitrogen	16.69%	13.41%

The choice of formulation is determined by patient need and cost. Renal failure and liver failure patients have specific needs. For the effective utilisation of amino acids, i.e. synthesis of proteins, sufficient energy must be provided by glucose and/or fat to prevent the breakdown of amino acids to serve as an energy source. The optimal ratio of energy to nitrogen is approximately 630 kJ per 1 g of nitrogen.

Energy

The basal energy requirement is 125 kJ per kg of body weight per day. This is increased to 145–170 kJ per kg per day in stress, e.g. sepsis, surgery, burns. The more severe the stress, the higher the energy requirement. A patient with burns to more than 40% of the body will need more energy per kg of body weight than a patient with minor sepsis. Energy can be provided by glucose or fat.

GLUCOSE

Glucose yields approximately 16 kJ of energy per gram. Therefore 250 g glucose yields 4000 kJ. To obtain adequate amounts of glucose in a suitable volume, hyperosmolar concentrations of glucose must be used, e.g. 25%, 50%. Infusions of glucose at more than 7–8 g per kg of body weight per day is of little value due to an increase in carbon dioxide production and oxygen consumption. It may also lead to water retention and fatty infiltration of the liver. The amount of glucose given initially is less than the actual requirement of the patient. This is to optimise tolerance of the glucose and prevent hyperglycaemia.

Diabetic patients and others who do not tolerate the glucose need to have the amount decreased or have insulin administered, either as an addition to the parenteral nutrition solution or subcutaneously using a sliding scale.

FAT

Fat yields 38 kJ of energy per gram. It is a more concentrated source of energy than glucose. It also provides a balanced diet and supplies the essential fatty acids, linoleic acid and linolenic acid. Deficiency of essential fatty acids results in scaly dermatitis, alopecia, hepatomegaly, fatty liver, diminished skin pigmentation and, in infants, growth retardation. At least 100 g of fat per week is necessary to prevent this.

Fat is given in the form of soybean oil emulsified with egg yolk phospholipid, with the addition of glycerol to produce isotonicity. It is available as a 10% or 20% emulsion, *Intralipid*. Apart from providing the essential fatty acids, other advantages are its isotonicity, allowing it to be given peripherally, and its high energy density, supplying more energy in a smaller volume than glucose. Also, it does not lead to an increase in carbon dioxide production, as glucose does.

Fat is now commonly used not only to supply the essential fatty acids but also in combination with glucose as an energy source. In patients who have compromised respiratory function or glucose intolerance it is particularly beneficial. It is more expensive than glucose, and care must be taken to prevent cracking of the emulsion. It is contraindicated in patients with hyperlipidaemia and hepatocellular disease.

If too much fat is given (2 g/kg per day) the fat overload syndrome, with pyrexia, hyperlipidaemia, hepatosplenomegaly with impaired liver function, anaemia, thrombocytopenia, prolonged clotting time and spontaneous bleeding, may result. The deposition of lipid particles in pulmonary capillaries may also occur. The total energy provided, whether by glucose alone or glucose and fat, must be adequate for the utilisation of the amino acids.

Electrolytes

Initial electrolyte requirements may vary considerably as deficits or excesses are corrected. Table 33.2 is a guide to average daily requirements. The exact requirements are determined by an analysis of serum values and renal function, estimation of losses and consideration of electrolytes given concurrently, e.g. sodium contained in antibiotics such as piperacillin.

PARENTERAL NUTRITION

33

TABLE 33.2 Daily electrolyte requirements

Electrolyte	Chemical symbol	Dose (mmol/kg)	Deficiency	Toxicity
Sodium	Na	1–2	Weakness, confusion, convulsions, circulatory failure	CNS depression, muscle rigidity, tremor, convulsions
Potassium	K	1–2	Muscular weakness, cardiac conduction defects, arrhythmias	Muscular weakness, cardiac conduction defects, asystole
Calcium	Ca	0.1–0.15	Muscle cramps, tetany, rickets, seizures, cardiac conduction abnormalities	Abdominal pain, polyuria, cardiac arrhythmias, confusion, muscle weakness
Magnesium	Mg	0.1–0.2	Neuromuscular excitability, cramps, tetany, cardiac arrhythmias, mental changes	Impaired neuromuscular function, decreased cardiac function, respiratory depression
Chloride	Cl	1.3–1.9	Alkalosis	Acidosis
Phosphate	PO_4	0.5–0.7	Impaired cellular energy stores, paraesthesia, rickets	Effect on calcium homeostasis with ectopic calcification

Trace Elements

Trace elements (minerals) are required by numerous enzyme systems. Table 33.3 is a guide to daily requirements. Serum levels are, in general, not an accurate indication of need. As noted in the table some trace elements are only needed during long-term treatment.

TABLE 33.3 Daily requirements for trace elements

Trace element	Chemical Symbol	Dose (μmol)	Deficiency
Zinc	Zn	30–60	More common in gastrointestinal disease; rash progressing to pustular lesions, mental apathy, poor concentration, diarrhoea, alopecia
Copper	Cu	16	Neutropenia, anaemia, skeletal abnormalities
Chromium	Cr	0.4	Glucose intolerance, neuropathy
Iron	Fe	20	Anaemia
Iodine	I	0.4 May be obtained from topical use of povidone iodine	Hypothyroidism
Manganese	Mn	8	
Cobalt	Co	Give as vitamin B_{12}	As for vitamin B_{12}, i.e. anaemia, neuropathy
Selenium	Se	1.5	Long-term only; muscle pain, cardiomyopathy

Vitamins

Most vitamins are given on a daily basis, although vitamin K may be given once or twice weekly in appropriate doses. In general solutions should be protected from light to limit degradation. Table 33.4 is a guide to average daily doses. Certain disease states warrant the use of higher doses, e.g. an alcoholic patient will need more of the B group vitamins and folic acid.

PREPARATION OF SOLUTIONS

Traditionally, the amino acids, glucose, fat, electrolytes, trace elements and vitamins were administered separately. This involved the contents of multiple containers being infused simultaneously. This was cumbersome with a high potential for particulate and bacterial contamination and chemical instability or precipitation due to the complexity of the numerous ingredients. However, studies have documented the stability of some combined formulations.

The pharmaceutical industry now provides a range of glucose/amino acid mixtures with or without electrolytes. These have a shelf life of up to three months when stored at 4°C. Glucose/amino acid/fat mixtures available are stable for 30 days. This reasonably short shelf life limits their use. Additional electrolytes, trace elements, vitamins and other possible requirements, e.g. insulin, are added before administration.

The amount of each additive needed is calculated, either manually or with the aid of a computer program, according to the order of the clinician. The order of addition is very important to prevent precipitation of certain substances. This should be done by trained pharmacy staff in a laminar flow unit in a clean room using strict aseptic technique. This procedure is done according to the Code of Good Manufacturing Practice with strict standards for the clean room, equipment, clothing and technique being met. Quality control tests are performed on the environment and parenteral nutrition solutions produced. This minimises the risk of bacterial and particulate

TABLE 33.4 Average daily doses of vitamins

Vitamin	Dose	Deficiency	Toxicity
Retinol (A)	1 mg	Xerophthalmia, keratomalacia, night blindness	Exfoliative dermatitis, alopecia
Thiamine (B$_1$)	3 mg	Cardiomyopathy, neuropathy, encephalopathy	
Riboflavin (B$_2$)	3 mg	Stomatitis, cheilosis	
Niacin	40 mg	Pellagra	
Pyridoxine (B$_6$)	4 mg	Dermatitis, cheilosis, glossitis, neuropathy	Peripheral neuropathy
Folic Acid	2 mg	Anaemia	
Cyanocobalamin (B$_{12}$)	5 μg	Anaemia, neuropathy	
Ascorbic acid (C)	100 mg	Scurvy	
Ergocalciferol (D)	5 μg		Hypercalcaemia
E	10 mg		
K	100 μg	Haemorrhage	

PARENTERAL NUTRITION

33

contamination and, through a review of stability data, guarantees the provision of a safe, stable product. After it is checked by another person, it is appropriately labelled, including storage conditions and expiry date. If the needs of the patient are not met by one of these formulations or if the preparation is not part of the hospital's formulary, the individual ingredients are mixed in an empty sterile bag using the facilities mentioned above. If fat is part of the formulation the bag must not be made of polyvinyl chloride plastic, as fat can leach the phthalate plasticisers into the mixture. Ethylene vinyl acetate polymer bags are recommended. Further additions to the solution at ward level should not be made.

An example of a typical adult parenteral nutrition formulation is given in Table 33.5.

TABLE 33.5 A typical adult parenteral nutrition formulation

Amino acids	80 g
Glucose	350 g
Fat	50 g
Na	70 mmol
K	60 mmol
Mg	5 mmol
Phosphate	30 mmol
Vitamins (M.V.I.)	10 mL
Trace elements	
Total volume	2000 mL
Rate of infusion	84 mL per hour

M.V.I. = Multivitamin infusion

ADMINISTRATION

As previously mentioned the glucose and amino acids solutions used are hypertonic. The osmolarity of a 25% glucose solution is 1560 mOsm/L and that of a 10% amino acid solution with electrolytes is 1300 mOsm/L.

Hence they cannot be infused into a peripheral vein. Instead the product is administered into a large central vein which has a high blood flow for rapid dilution, most commonly the superior vena cava.

Some hospitals use peripheral parenteral nutrition using a formulation containing a lower concentration of glucose and a relatively high amount of fat which has a lower tonicity than conventional mixtures. This obviates the need of a central catheter. However, the central route is more common in most centres.

Catheter access to the administration site is generally via subcutaneous subclavican catheterisation after appropriate skin preparation. The cutaneous entry site of the silicone catheter is in the pectoral skin below the clavicle. The infraclavicular catheter entry site is separated from the exit site on the anterior chest wall by subcutaneous tunnelling.

This site is easy to keep clean and dress, usually with a transparent adhesive dressing, as it is flat, relatively immobile and does not collect perspiration or other secretions. The patient's arm and neck are free to move. Catheter placement should be performed by an experienced clinician under aseptic conditions. It is then checked radiologically before the parenteral nutrition begins. Complications of catheter insertion include central vein thrombosis, pneumothorax, haemothorax, air embolism, tracheal puncture, arterial puncture, haematoma, haemopericardium, hydropericardium and tamponade, arrhythmias (line touching tricuspid valve) and injury to the phrenic nerve, brachial plexus, or recurrent laryngeal nerve.

Administration of solutions is via a positive pressure volumatic infusion pump to ensure the correct administration rate. The line must not be used for giving other drugs, monitoring central venous pressure or obtaining blood. If a multilumen catheter is used, the distal port is used exclusively for parenteral nutrition, with the other lumens used for drug administration or central venous pressure monitoring.

COMPLICATIONS

The most frequent and potentially serious complication in patients receiving parenteral nutrition is catheter related sepsis, the source of which is most commonly the patient's own skin flora. The incidence of septicaemia can be reduced by using strict aseptic technique when changing lines and dressings. Protocols must be available and strictly adhered to. If the catheter is the source of the sepsis it must be removed.

Other complications are metabolic and include: hyperglycaemia, glycosuria, osmotic diuresis and dehydration; ketoacidosis in diabetes mellitus, refeeding syndrome; postinfusion (rebound) hypoglycaemia (minimised by a gradual reduction in the parenteral nutrition or ensuring oral intake is adequate before the parenteral nutrition is ceased); hyper or hyponatraemia; hyper or hypokalaemia; hyper or hypomagnesaemia; hyper or hypochloraemia; hypophosphataemia; hyper or hypocalcaemia; fluid overload, pulmonary oedema or congestive cardiac failure; trace elements and or vitamin deficiencies or toxicities; liver function abnormalities; and metabolic acidosis or alkalosis. These complications can be minimised by appropriate fluid and biochemical monitoring and adjustment of nutrients.

Air embolus can be prevented by correctly priming the giving set and carefully securing connections between the catheter and infusion line. Before and during disconnection the patient should perform the valsalva manoeuvre.

NURSING IMPLICATIONS

The role of the nurse is very important for the optimal use of parenteral nutrition and the prevention of complications. Responsibilities include:

- Maintaining an accurate fluid balance;

- Daily weighing;

- Checking the infusion device for function and that the infusion rate is constant. (If behind time, the rate must not be increased to catch up);

- Checking alarms and tubing for kinks or leaks;

- Regular blood glucose monitoring and urinalysis;

- Observing and documenting temperature, blood pressure, pulse and respiration;

- Adhering to the protocol for central line maintenance including inspection and line change;

- Checking the solution with the order before administration;

- Administering 5% or 10% glucose if the central line is removed suddenly to prevent hypoglycaemia;

- Oral hygiene of the patient due to a decrease in saliva production; and

- Informing the patient and family of the type of treatment being given and the reasons for the procedures and tests involved.

Communication of any abnormality detected to the appropriate medical personnel will help limit the extent of problems, e.g. an elevated temperature, increased blood glucose or inflammation at the catheter site may be the first signs of sepsis.

PARENTERAL NUTRITION

33

NEONATAL PARENTERAL NUTRITION

The requirements of the neonate are vastly different from those of the adult. For example, three amino acids, cysteine, tyrosine and histidine, are regarded as essential in the neonate but not in the adult.

Indications for parenteral nutrition in neonates include extreme prematurity, respiratory distress, gastrointestinal anomalies, abdominal wall defects and necrotising enterocolitis.

The average daily requirements for a neonate are listed in Table 33.6.

TABLE 33.6 Average daily requirements for a neonate per kg body weight per 24 hours

Fluid (premature infant)	150 mL
(term infant)	120 mL
Energy	440 kJ
Protein	up to 2.5 g
Glucose	10–15 g
Fat	up to 3 g
Sodium	3 mmol
Potassium	2 mmol
Calcium	0.9 mol
Chloride/Acetate	3 mol
Phosphate	0.9 mol
Zinc	1.4 µmol
Copper	0.6 µmol
Manganese	0.04 µmol
Vitamins	As ordered (see Further Reading)

Preparation of the solution is again done under aseptic conditions. Fat is not incorporated into the amino acid/glucose/electrolyte mixture, as the relatively high concentration of calcium, a divalent ion, would render the preparation unstable. Fat is given separately via a syringe pump. Administration is usually by a peripheral vein which limits the amount of glucose which can be given. In line bacterial filters and constant infusion pumps are used.

HOME PARENTERAL NUTRITION

There are certain patients who require long-term therapy. Developments have been made in this area to allow these patients to receive parenteral nutrition at home. It is given in a cyclic fashion over 12–14 hours, usually at night. Appropriate training and supervision of the patient, and an efficient mechanism for delivering solutions and supplies is essential. Medical, nursing, pharmacy and dietetic services must be available and coordinated. Nursing input may include training of the patient on catheter care, line changing and the aseptic addition of vitamins to the solution provided by the pharmaceutical industry or hospital pharmacy.

FURTHER READING

Phillips, G.D. and Odgers, C.L, (1986) *Parenteral and Enteral Nutrition, A Practical Guide*, 3rd edn, Churchill Livingston

Silk, D.B.A. (1983), *Nutritional Support in Hospital Practice*, Blackwell Scientific Publications.

'Adult Parenteral Nutrition', in L.Y. Young, M.A. Koda-Kimble (eds) (1992), *Applied Therapeutics - The clinical use of drugs*, 5th edn, Applied Therapeutics Inc., Vancouver, Wa. pp. 30.1-30.14

'Paediatric Parenteral Nutrition' in L.Y. Young, M.A. Koda-Kimble (eds) (1992), *Applied Therapeutics - the clinical use of drugs*, 5th edn, Applied Therapeutics Inc., Vancouver, Wa. pp. 32.1-32.17.

Understanding Parenteral Nutrition, A Nursing Perspective, Baxter Laboratories.

TEST YOUR KNOWLEDGE

1. Which of the following are indications for parenteral nutrition: (a) gastrointestinal sepsis; (b) pancreatic fistulae; (c) severe burns; (d) enterocutaneous fistulae in a patient with terminal metastatic disease receiving palliative care?

2. The total daily fluid needs of a 70 kg man with no excessive gastric loss or drainage from a wound is: (a) 500 mL; (b) 1000 mL; (c) 1750 mL; or (d) 2200 mL.

3. What are the essential ingredients of a total parenteral nutrition: (a) glucose; (b) thiamine; (c) insulin; (d) albumin; (e) a combination of amino acids?

4. 1 g of fat yields: (a) 9 kJ; (b) 9 kCal; (c) 4 kJ; or (d) 4 kCal.

5. 1 g of nitrogen is contained in: (a) 10 g glucose; (b) 1 g amino acid; (c) 6 g amino acid; or (d) 6 g fat.

6. Adequate utilisation of amino acid is most dependent on: (a) water; (b) energy; (c) heparin; or (d) zinc.

7. A suitable formulation for a 60 kg woman with intra-abdominal sepsis may include: (a) 20 g amino acid, 350 g glucose, 50 g fat; (b) 60 g amino acid, 350 g glucose, 50 g fat; (c) 60 g amino acid, 700 g glucose, 50 g fat; (d) 80 g amino acid, 700 g glucose, 100 g fat.

8. Potassium deficiency includes: (a) muscle weakness; (b) cardiac conduction defects; (c) tetany; (d) rickets.

9. The management of glucose intolerance could include: (a) reduction of glucose content; (b) substitution of fat for part of glucose content; (c) administration of insulin; (d) all of the above.

10. Possible signs of septicaemia include: (a) inflamed catheter site; (b) increased blood glucose; (c) rigors; (d) low white cell count.

PARENTERAL NUTRITION

33

TABLE 33.7 Summary table — parenteral nutrition

DRUG GROUP Drug Name	Use	Action	Adverse Reactions	Nursing Implications
PARENTERAL NUTRITION SOLUTIONS Composed of essential nutrients e.g. glucose, amino acids, electrolytes, trace elements, vitamins, fat	Metabolic support for patients who require gut rest or cannot use their enteral route	Nutrition	Catheter complications, sepsis, metabolic complications	**Assess:** Fluid balance/overload, weight; glucose and electrolyte levels; for sepsis; cardiovascular, respiratory and neurological status; anxiety **Administer:** Use infusion regulator, do not 'catch up' slow infusions; document discrepancies between orders and flow rates; taper off, rather than cease infusion abruptly; strict aseptic technique and care of catheter, handling solutions and lines; do not administer other medications, blood products through line, or take blood samples, or monitor central venous pressure; inform medical officer immediately if catheter obstructs, or is contaminated; refrigerate solutions if necessary **Evaluate:** Achievement of prescribed schedules, weight maintenance or gain, blood chemistry, anxiety reduction **Educate:** Purpose and expected results of therapy to patient and family

Enteral Feeding

HELEN A. KOHLHARDT

O B J E C T I V E S

At the conclusion of this chapter the reader should be able to discuss:

1. How to recognise the malnourished patient;

2. The role of enteral feeding in nutrition;

3. When to introduce enteral feeding as a nutritional support;

4. How to reduce the incidence of side effects due to enteral feeding;

5. Some of the products available for tube feeding; and

6. The relationship between 'normal feeding', enteral feeding and parenteral feeding.

NUTRITIONAL SUPPORT ▉▉▉▉▉▉▉▉▉▉▉▉

Parenteral feeding is nutritional support given intravenously. Enteral feeding is nutritional support given via the gastrointestinal tract. It may be supplementary to normal eating or provide the total nutritional needs of the patient by a special formula. The formula may be taken orally or administered by tube. If the gastrointestinal tract is functional, enteral feeding is the easiest, cheapest and safest way of administering nutritional support.

If it is necessary to supplement or substitute 'normal feeding' by enteral or parenteral feeding it is important to understand the psychological deprivation experienced by the patient. The importance of the regimen should be fully explained to the patient when possible and the patient should be encouraged to take an interest in the treatment and the monitoring of results.

All patients need the understanding and support of the health care team. A team effort involving the doctor, nurses, dietitian, pharmacist and biochemist is essential to achieve a satisfactory outcome. The nurse has a vital role in offering psychological support to the patient.

REQUIREMENTS FOR NUTRIENTS

The nutrient requirements of healthy individuals vary over a wide range and the requirements of any individual vary over time under different conditions. Tables of dietary allowances take this variation into account and the levels suggested are believed to meet the needs of 'practically all healthy persons'. It is recognised that a small number of healthy people may have needs in excess of the standard. For this reason dietary allowances are meant to be used as a guide for the feeding of groups of healthy people. When they are used as a guide for individuals, it is important to realise their limitations.

The Nutrition Committee of the National Health and Medical Research Council has established a guide for Australians, see Tables 34.1, 34.2, and 34.3. If the nutrients listed in the allowances are checked against the nutrients contained in various enteral and parenteral formulae it will be found that allowances are not suggested for many of the nutrients present in the formulae. The Nutrition Committee explains the reason for this as follows:

If the nutrients specified in daily allowances are provided by a mixed diet, it is unlikely that such a diet would be deficient in the other essential nutrients such as manganese, magnesium and copper. Some of these nutrients are referred to as trace elements or microtrace elements because they occur in our food and in our bodies in minute quantities. However, they are essential for normal body function.

It is when we consume a diet made up of a narrow range of foods that we are at risk of developing nutritional deficiencies. Some of the early attempts at enteral and parenteral feeding encountered problems relating to deficiencies of these elements and great care is now devoted to formulation and the monitoring of the patient's nutrient levels.

Recommendations for vitamin D are not considered necessary unless people are housebound or always indoors since the vitamin D status of Australians is determined by exposure to UV light from the sun.

NUTRITIONAL NEEDS OF PATIENTS

In recent years there have been a number of reports of iatrogenic (treatment induced) malnutrition or 'hospital' malnutrition, i.e. malnutrition which has developed while the

TABLE 34.1 Dietary allowances for use in Australia

Subject	Age (years)	Protein* (g)	Vitamin C (mg)	Vitamin A** retinol equivalents (μg)
Men	19–64	55	40	750
	64+	55	40	750
Women	19–54	45	30	750
	54+	45	30	750
Pregnant women 2nd and 3rd trimesters		+6	+30	+0
Lactating women		+30	+45	+450
Infants	0–0.5			
	breast fed	Not set	25	425
	bottle fed	2 g/kg body weight	25	425
	0.5–1	1.6 g/kg body weight	30	300
Children	1–3	14–18	30	300
	4–7	18–24	30	350
Boys	8–11	27–38	30	500
	12–15	42–60	30	725
	16–18	64–70	40	750
Girls	8–11	27–39	30	500
	12–15	44–55	30	725
	16–18	57	30	750

*Protein recommended dietary intake (RDI) figures based on: 0.75 g protein/kg ideal body weight/day for adults; 1.0 g protein/kg ideal body weight/day for children 4–18 years
**Vitamin A can also be supplied as β carotene

patient was undergoing hospital treatment. The nurse has a vital role in the early identification of such malnutrition.

Disease alters nutritional needs and it may alter the ability of patients to ingest, digest, absorb or metabolise nutrients or the mechanisms of excretion. Each patient should be monitored to provide appropriate nutritional assessment and to draw attention to the need for nutritional support as soon as possible. Symptoms associated with malnutrition are:

- loss of weight
- reduced muscle mass
- hypoproteinaemia
- oedema
- increased susceptibility to infection
- poor wound healing
- apathy

ENTERAL FEEDING

34

TABLE 34.2 Recommended dietary intakes (RDI) expressed as mean daily intake

Subject	Age (years)	Thiamine (mg)*	Riboflavine (mg)	Niacin, niacin equivalents (mg)**	Vitamin B$_6$ (mg)***	Total Folate (μg)§	Vitamin B$_{12}$ (μg)	Vitamin E α tocopherol equivalents (mg)
Infants	0–0.5							
	breast fed	0.15	0.4	4	0.25	50	0.3	2.5
	bottle fed	0.25	0.4	4	0.25	50	0.3	4.0
	0.5–1	0.35	0.6	7	0.45	75	0.7	4.0
Children	1–3	0.5	0.8	10	0.6–0.9	100	1.0	5.0
	4–7	0.7	1.1	12	0.8–1.3	100	1.5	6.0
Boys	8–11	0.9	1.4	15	1.1–1.6	150	1.5	8.0
	12–15	1.2	1.8	20	1.4–2.1	200	2.0	10.5
	16–18	1.2	1.9	21	1.5–2.2	200	2.0	11.0
Girls	8–11	0.8	1.3	15	1.0–1.5	150	1.5	8.0
	12–15	1.0	1.6	18	1.2–1.8	200	2.0	9.0
	16–18	0.9	1.4	16	1.1–1.6	200	2.0	8.0
Men	19–64	1.1	1.7	19	1.3–1.9	200	2.0	10.0
	64+	0.9	1.3	16	1.0–1.5	200	2.0	10.0
Women	19–54	0.8	1.2	13	0.9–1.4	200	2.0	7.0
	54+	0.7	1.0	11	0.8–1.1	200	2.0	7.0
Pregnant		+0.2	+0.3	+2	+0.1	+200	+1.0	+0
Lactating		+0.4	+0.5	+5	+0.7–0.8	+150	+0.5	+2.5

*   Thiamine recommendation based on 0.1 mg thiamine/1000 kJ
**   Niacin can also be supplied as tryptophan in dietary proteins
***   Vitamin B$_6$ RDI based on 0.02 mg/g dietary protein
§   Total folate is based on free plus conjugated folate

TABLE 34.3 Recommended dietary intakes (expressed as mean daily intake)

Subject	Age (years)	Calcium (mg)	Iron (mg)	Iodine (µg)	Zinc (mg)	Potassium mmol (mg)	Sodium mmol (mg)	Magnesium (mg)	Selenium* (µg)
Infants	0–0.5								
	breast fed	300	0.5	50	3.0	10–15 (390–580)	6–12 (140–280)	40	10
	bottle fed	500	3.0	50	3–6	10–15 (390–580)	6–12 (140–280)	40	10
	0.5–1	550	9	60	4.5	12–35 (470–1370)	14–25 (320–580)	60	15
Children	1–3	700	6–8	70	4.5	25–70 (980–2730)	14–50 (320–1150)	80	25
	4–7	800	6–8	90	6.0	40–100 (1560–3900)	20–75 (460–1730)	110	30
Boys	8–11	800	6–8	120	9	50–140 (1950–5460)	26–100 (600–2300)	180	50
	12–15	1200	10–13	150	12	50–140 (1950–5460)	40–100 (920–2300)	260	85
	16–18	1000	10–13	150	12	50–140 (1950–5460)	40–100 (920–2300)	320	85
Girls	8–11	900	6–8	120	9	50–140 (1950–5460)	26–100 (600–2300)	160	50
	12–15	1000	10–13	120	12	50–140 (1950–5460)	40–100 (920–2300)	240	70
	16–18	800	10–13	120	12	50–140 (1950–5460)	40–100 (920–2300)	270	70
Men	19–64	800	7	150	12	50–140 (1950–5460)	40–100 (920–2300)	320	85
	65+	800	7	150	12	50–140 (1950–5460)	40–100 (920–2300)	320	85
Women	19–54	800	12–16	120	12	50–140 (1950–5460)	40–100 (920–2300)	270	70
	55+	1000	5–7	120	12	50–140 (1950–5460)	40–100 (920–2300)	270	70
Pregnant		+300	+10–20 (2nd and 3rd trimesters)	+30	+4	+0	+0	+30	+10
Lactating		+400	+0	+50	+6	+0	+0	+70	+15

*Selenium intake should not exceed 600 µg/day.

34 ENTERAL FEEDING

Some patients are particularly at risk of developing malnutrition, e.g. the unconscious patient, patients with swallowing disorders or malabsorption, patients suffering severe shock or trauma (including severe burns), patients suffering from cancer, some postoperative patients, patients suffering from psychological disorders such as anorexia nervosa and severe depression or patients suffering from severe anorexia which may result from disease or from therapy. In these cases nutritional support should be given routinely and early.

The routine recording of height and weight on admission and the regular monitoring of weight are essential. Diminution in muscle mass, apathy and depression are indicators which should be heeded as symptoms often associated with malnutrition. Food intake should be monitored and patients who are consistently unable to consume an adequate diet should be given individual attention. Supplementary oral feeding introduced at this stage may give sufficient support.

Correct nourishment of the surgical patient is advantageous because postoperative recovery is enhanced, postoperative mortality is reduced, wound healing is accelerated and the patient is discharged from hospital earlier as a result.

More sophisticated physical measurements such as skinfold thickness, mid-arm circumference, total body nitrogen measurements and biochemical and haematological tests such as prothombin time, levels of vitamins in body tissues, serum albumin, serum calcium and phosphorus, haemoglobin levels and red cell counts may be used to assess nutritional status, but attention to weight and food intake are more likely to provide early warning.

FORMS OF NUTRITIONAL SUPPORT

The decision to introduce enteral or parenteral feeding will depend upon gastrointestinal function, the degree of malnutrition and the patient's willingness to take food. If gastrointestinal function is efficient, enteral feeding is indicated and is the preferred method.

The patient's normal diet may be supplemented with foods and fluids high in protein, calories and nutrients. If sufficient quantities of food and fluids cannot be taken orally, enteral nutrition via tube is the appropriate form of nutritional support. Such patients include those who are unconscious or have no gag reflex, upper gastrointestinal tract obstructions, elevated requirements and/or anorexia (when oral intake is insufficient to meet nutrient needs).

Enteral nutrition is contraindicated if the function of the patient's gastrointestinal tract is impaired. Such patients include those with paralytic ileus, extensive gastrointestinal tract pathology, organ failure exacerbated by gastrointestinal stimulus (e.g. acute pancreatitis), severe vomiting or diarrhoea and recent upper gastrointestinal tract surgery (when insertion of a nasoenteral tube may damage the wound site). In these cases parenteral nutrition should be instituted. Parenteral feeding may gradually be replaced by enteral feeding (as the situation resolves) which in turn is replaced by normal feeding.

ENTERAL FEEDING

When compared with parenteral feeding, enteral feeding is easier to administer, less likely to introduce infection, more physiologically acceptable, cheaper, more readily available and more flexible. Enteral feeding may be administered orally or by tube, see Table 34.4.

TABLE 34.4 Methods of enteral feeding

Oral feeding	Tube feeding
Normal diet	Nasogastric
Sip feeding supplementary to normal diet	Orogastric
Total nutritional requirements supplied by liquid formulae	Gastrostomy
	Fine needle jejunostomy

If patients are able to eat normal foods they should be encouraged to do so and detailed attention should be given to planning the meals and the food intake. The food consumed should be monitored and the intake of nutrients calculated and compared with estimated requirements. This should be done by the dietitian.

In sip feeding the liquid formula is taken in small quantities by the patient every 10–15 minutes over a prolonged period. This avoids gastric overload and is a simple method of administering a supplementary feeding. This method also reduces the likelihood of diarrhoea.

When the formula is taken by mouth special attention must be given to flavour, consistency, the frequency of administration and the amount given, as well as to the nutrients. It is important to watch for signs of 'taste fatigue', the change in attitude to a flavour after a period of time. It may be necessary to vary flavours to encourage patients to continue with the treatment.

Enteral feeding via tube is the administration of nutrient fluid to the gastointestinal tract through an indwelling tube. Nasogastric or orogastric tube feeding is the preferred method for short-term feeding. Gastrostomy feeding should be used for patients with severe oesophageal obstruction. It can be a temporary or permanent method of feeding. Jejunostomy feeding is indicated in the presence of pyloric obstruction, upper gastrointestinal entercutaneous fistulae and postoperatively after surgery involving the stomach and pylorus.

Even though complications following enteral tube therapy are few, there are several dangers which should be noted:

- **Dehydration** due to administration of hyperosmolar formulae.

- **Accidental intravenous administration** of a tube formula due to hooking up the tube containers to an intravenous giving set.

- **Microbial contamination** of the formula during preparation and setting up in the ward. Correct storage conditions must be maintained at ward level to minimise bacterial contamination.

- **Tissue perforation** in children.

- **Aspiration** of formula into the lungs.

NASOGASTRIC FEEDING

Factors to be considered with nasogastric feeding are: method of administration; nutritional adequacy and content of formula; water and electrolyte balance; osmolar load; possible complications; and selecting the formula.

Method of Administration

A thin, fine bore silastic tube with an internal diameter of 1 mm is the preferred method for nasogastric feeding. The position of the fine bore tube should be confirmed by X-ray. The formula is best administered by slow, continuous drip and should only be commenced after a successful

ENTERAL FEEDING

34

water trial to ensure gastric emptying. Many protocols are available from both hospitals and manufacturers to explain initiation of feeding and desired feeding procedures.

The formula should be started at a slow rate, e.g. 30–50 mL per hour at isotonic strength. If the formula is tolerated the rate may be increased to no more than 150 mL per hour or, if formulae are given intermittently and depending on the work load of nursing staff, not more than 300 mL per two hours. Most standard formulae are isotonic and do not require dilution when initially introduced. In rare cases when a hypertonic formula is used it should be introduced in diluted form and the strength increased as tolerated by the patient. Rate of adminstration and strength of formula should not be altered simultaneously. If necessary, the fine bore tube can be left in situ for several weeks. It is important to select a formula of a suitable consistency to flow through the tube. A pump is the preferred mode of delivery for all formulae especially the more viscous formulae.

Previously thick bore Ryle's tubes or double lumen tubes were used. These were uncomfortable for the patient and were frequently associated with nasopharyngeal ulceration, gastro-oesophageal reflux and sometimes stricture. The formula was usually administered by the bolus method when a given amount of formula was syringed into the tube at set intervals.

NUTRITIONAL ADEQUACY

It is of prime importance to calculate each patient's energy and protein requirements to prevent both undernutrition or the metabolic stress of overnutrition. Overnutrition can result in the development of a fatty liver, impaired glucose tolerance, renal stress and excessive carbon dioxide production.

Energy

To estimate energy requirements the various formulae available can be used. The Harris Benedict formula is given as an example.

Protein Requirements

Protein requirements vary with age, sex and medical condition. The requirements listed in Table 34.5 can be used as a guide.

TABLE 34.5 Estimating protein requirements

Medical condition	Protein requirement (g/kg body weight)
Medical patient, convalescing, mild trauma	1.0–1.5
Surgery, severe stress, trauma	1.5–2.0
Highly catabolic states	
Multiple trauma	2.0
Burns, acute phase	2.0–4.0
Liver disease	
No encephalopathy	1.0–1.5
With encephalopathy	0.5
Renal disease	
Predialysis	0.6
Haemodialysis	1.0–1.2
Continual peritoneal	
dialysis	1.2–1.5

Adapted from: Department of Nutrition and Dietetics 'Estimating protein requirements' in *Dieticians' pocket book*, May 1990. School of Community Health, Curtin University of Technology, Perth, pp. 39–40.

In addition, there is a need for vitamins, minerals, essential fatty acids, electrolytes and water.

The form in which nutrients are included in the formula (e.g. protein as casein, dipeptides, tripeptides or amino acids) will depend on the needs of the patient.

Most formulae are termed polymeric. In these formulae the protein, carbohydrate and fat is in a form that requires some digestion before absorption can occur.

Elemental formulae are sometimes used for enteral feeding. In these formulae the nutrients occur in simple forms which can

Harris Benedict formula for estimating energy requirements

Basal Energy Expenditure (BEE)

Male

66 + [13.7 × weight (kg)] + [5 × height (cm)] − [6.8 × age (years)] calories/day

278 + [57.5 × weight (kg)] + [20.9 × height (cm)] − [28.3 × age (years)] kJ/day

Female

655 + [9.6 × weight (kg)] + [1.7 × height (cm)] − [4.7 × age (years)] calories/day

2741 + [40 × weight (kg)] + [7.7 × height (cm)] − [19.6 × age (years)] kJ/day

Actual energy expended = BEE × activity factor × injury factor × thermal factor

Activity factor		Injury factor		Thermal factor	
Confined to bed	1.2	Uncomplicated	1.0		
		Postoperative/cancer	1.1	38°C	1.1
		Fracture	1.2	39°C	1.2
In bed but mobile	1.25	Sepsis	1.3	40°C	1.3
		Peritonitis	1.4	41°C	1.4
		Multitrauma	1.5		
Mobile	1.3	Multitrauma + Sepsis	1.6		
		Burns 30%–50%	1.7		
		50%–70%	1.8		
		70%–90%	2.0		

be absorbed without further digestion. They are absorbed in the upper gastrointestinal tract leaving minimal residue in the bowel. In these formulae, protein is supplied as amino acids or di- and tripeptides, carbohydrate as mono- and oligosaccharides and the fat content is low and supplied as medium chain triglycerides (MCT) which are relatively water soluble and can pass into the portal tract. Elemental formulae are expensive because of the processing involved. They should be reserved for patients with impaired digestion and absorption or inability to handle colonic residues (e.g. patients with intestinal fistulae).

Water and Electrolytes

Many patients are hypovolaemic when enteral feeding begins and require sufficient fluid to restore normal blood volume. Adults require 1500–2000 mL fluid/day or 35–45 mL/kg/day.

It is important that sufficient water is given to control the osmolarity of the formulae and to facilitate renal function. The more protein administered the more water required. Pyrexia increases water loss and each 1°C elevation in body temperature increases daily water requirements by 500–750 mL.

Allowance must be made for fluid losses from the gastrointestinal tract (e.g. due to vomiting, diarrhoea), surgical wounds, drains or fistulae and fevers.

Some conditions will reduce the water requirement, e.g. oedema, head injuries (cerebral oedema), oliguric or anuric renal failure, cardiac failure, respiratory distress syndrome and patients receiving humidified oxygen.

Potassium is concentrated in the intracellular fluids and as tissues are restored potassium needs increase. As protein requirements increase potassium requirements also increase.

ENTERAL FEEDING

34

Osmolar Load

The terms osmolarity and osmolality refer to the number of osmotically active particles in a given amount of solution.

Osmolarity is the number of osmotically active particles in 1 L of solution.

Osmolality is the number of osmotically active particles in 1 kg of solution.

The contents of the gut are rendered isotonic (the same osmolarity) with the body fluids in the duodenum and remain isotonic during the various stages of digestion and absorption. An osmolality of 300 mOsm/kg water is isotonic. If the gut contents have a higher osmolarity than the body fluids, water and electrolytes will be transferred across the mucosa of the gut until a balance is achieved. If nutrients such as glucose are unabsorbed and remain in the gut, water is absorbed into the colon and diarrhoea results.

The osmolality of a formula is important because it affects the amount of fluid drawn from the tissue into the gut and therefore the transit time of food through the gut and the absorption of nutrients. If large amounts of water are drawn into the gut and diarrhoea results, the food passes through the gastrointestinal tract more rapidly and there is insufficient time to absorb nutrients. Water and electrolytes as well as other nutrients will be depleted.

It is important to choose a formula of low osmolality. Problems with diarrhoea and absorption are lessened if an isotonic mixture is introduced and administered using a slow continuous drip and small hourly volume. The volume of feed per hour is increased slowly. Dilute (hypotonic) mixtures should be avoided as they do not provide sufficient nutrients.

Feeding carbohydrate as polymers of glucose and protein as dipeptides and tripeptides (rather than feeding glucose or sucrose and amino acids) reduces osmolarity by reducing the number of particles.

Selecting the Formula

Formulae should be selected with close attention to the individual needs of the patient. If the need for nutritional support is recognised early it may be possible to nourish the patient with small normal meals and milk based nutritional supplements, taken orally between meals. It is always desirable to maintain the patient's normal meals if possible.

There are a number of commercial formulae available which have been prepared with special attention to nutritional needs, electrolytes and consistency, see Table 34.6.

Details of these formulae are given in Tables 34.7 to 34.12. Tables 34.7 and 34.8 show comparisons of *Isocal, Osmolite, Ensure, Complan* and *Hospital Sustagen*. It can be seen from the tables that *Isocal, Osmolite, Ensure* and *Complan* may be used as complete nasogastric feeds as they supply all the nutrients required for life. *Hospital Sustagen* is more suitable for an oral supplement to an oral diet. Tables 34.9 and 34.10 give details of *Isocal High Calorie and Nitrogen (HCN), Ensure Plus, Traumacal, Two Cal High Nitrogen (HN)*, and *Ensure Plus High Nitrogen*. These are more concentrated formulae and may be used via a tube or orally for patients on restricted fluids or in need of concentrated nourishment, e.g. patients with burns. *Traumacal* with its high branch-chain amino acid content is especially produced for patients with major trauma.

Tables 34.11 and 34.12 give details of *Criticare High Nitrogen, Vital, Vivonex TEN, Elemental 0-28* and *Aminaid*. These are elemental formulae. They supply nutrients in a readily absorbable form and are useful for patients with digestion and absorption problems, so avoiding the use of the more expensive method of total parenteral nutrition. *Amin-Aid* with its very low protein and electrolyte content is especially produced for patients with renal failure.

Tables 34.13 and 34.14 give details of *Pulmocare* and *Glucerna*. These are formulae with a high fat content. They are useful for reducing carbon dioxide production (e.g. in respiratory patients) and assisting in glycaemic control. *Glucerna* also contains fibre.

Tables 34.15 and 34.16 give details of *Enrich*, *Jevity* and *Ultracal*. These formulae contain fibre. They are useful in patients with abnormal peristalsis (constipation or diarrhoea).

Formulae are available in powdered and liquid form. Particular attention should be given to the conditions under which formulae are prepared and stored to avoid bacterial contamination. Formulae should be stored under refrigeration but brought to room temperature before they are administered.

TABLE 34.6 Categories of enteral nutrition formulae

Formula	Indications
Polymeric Formulae Regular Isotonic, e.g. *Isocal, Osmolite, Ensure*	Used to establish and maintain feeding if there are no special requirements
Nutrient dense, higher protein and energy content than regular formula	
Hyperosmolar, e.g. *Ensure Plus, Isocal HCN, Traumacal* (high branch chain amino acids), *Ensure Plus HN, Two Cal HN*	Elevated nutrient requirements; fluid restriction
Fibre, e.g. *Enrich, Ultracal, Jevity*	Abnormal peristalsis, e.g. diarrhoea or constipation
High fat, low carbohydrate to reduce CO_2 production, e.g. *Pulmocare*	Respiratory insufficiency
High fat, fibre, low carbohydrate, to assist blood sugar level control, e.g. *Glucerna*	Hyperglycaemic patient
Elemental formulae (monomeric formulae) Hyperosmolar, absorbed in upper GIT with minimal or no digestion required, minimal stimulation of pancreatic, biliary and intestinal secretions, e.g. *Criticare HN, Vivonex TEN, Vital, Elemental 0-28, Traumaid* (high branch chain amino acids)	Impaired digestion and absorption, e.g. exocrine pancreatic dysfunction, small bowel mucosa pathology; inability to handle colonic residues, e.g. fistulae below jejunum
Low protein, minimal electrolytes, essential amino acids and histidine, high energy, e.g. *Amin-Aid*	Uraemic patient
High branch-chain amino acids and arginine, low aromatic amino acids and methione, minimal electrolytes e.g. *Hepatic-Aid*	Chronic liver failure

ENTERAL FEEDING

34

TABLE 34.7 Regular enteral formulae

Criterion	Isocal	Osmolite	Ensure	Complan	Hospital Sustagen
Protein source	Calcium caseinate Soy protein isolate	Sodium and calcium caseinate Soy protein isolate	Sodium and calcium caseinate Soy protein isolate	Dried whole milk/skim milk Sodium caseinate	Whole milk/skim milk Casein
g/L % total energy	34 g/L 13% energy	37.2 g/L 14% energy	37.2 g/L 14% energy	35 g/L 16% energy	61 g/L 24% energy
Fat source	Medium chain triglyceride (MCT) oil Soy oil	MCT oil. Corn oil. Soy oil	Corn oil	Corn oil. Milk fat	Milk fat
g/L % total energy	44 g/L 37% energy	38.5 g/L 31.4% energy	37.2 g/L 31.5% energy	32 g/L 32% energy	9.1 g/L 8% energy
Carbohydrate source	Glucose Oligosaccharides	Hydrolysed cornstarch (glucose polymers)	Corn syrup Sucrose	Lactose. Glucose Maltodextrins	Lactose Corn syrup solids
g/L % total energy	133 g/L 50% energy	145 g/L 54.6% energy	145 g/L 54.5% energy	116 g/L 52% energy	169 g/L 68% energy
Energy kJ/mL (cal/mL)	4.4 (1.05)	4.4 (1.06)	4.4 (1.06)	4.17 (0.9)	4.2 (1.0)
Osmolality (mOsm/kg water)	300	300	470	420	740–760
Lactose content	Nil	Nil	Nil	Yes	Yes
Flavour	Unflavoured	Unflavoured	Vanilla/Chocolate	Unflavoured	Vanilla/Chocolate
Presentation	Ready to use liquid: 355 mL per can, and 946 mL per can	Ready to use liquid: 237 mL per can, 946 mL per can, 237 mL bottle	Ready to use liquid: 237 mL per can, 946 mL per can; powder: 400 g can, 400 g + 1.4 L water to make 1.7 L	Powder: 500 g packet 225.8 g, add water to make 1 L	Powder: 1 kg powder, 260 g, add 820 mL water to make 1 L
Manufacturer	Mead Johnson	Ross Laboratories	Ross Laboratories	Boots	Mead Johnson
Indications for use	Tube feeding	Tube feeding	Tube feeding or oral	Tube feeding or oral	Oral supplement
Method of initiating tube feeding	30-50 mL, full strength, advance by 10-30 mL/h to a maximum rate of 100-125 mL/h, preferably by a 24-hour continuous method	30-50 mL, full strenth, advance by 10-30 mL/h to a maximum rate of 100-125 mL/h preferably by a 24-hour continuous method	30-50 mL, full strength, advance by 10-30 mL/h to a maximum rate of 100-125 mL h preferably by a 24-hour continuous method	Gradually introduce for long-term patients who are lactose tolerant after success with an Isocal feeding	Not recommended for tube feeding

TABLE 34.8 Biochemical analysis of regular enteral formulae

Constituents (per L)	Isocal	Osmolite	Ensure	Complan	Hospital Sustagen
Protein g	34	37.2	37.2	35	61.0
Fat g	44	38.5	37.2	32	9.0
Carbohydrate g	133	145	145	116	169.0
Kilocalories	1050	1060	1060	998	1000
Kilojoules	4400	4430	4430	4174	4186
Vitamin A µg (Retinol activity)	790	1450	1450	860	868
Vitamin B_1 mg (Thiamine)	2.0	1.6	1.6	1.4	5.7
Vitamin B_2 mg (Riboflavine)	2.3	1.8	1.8	1.7	5.7
Vitamin B_6 mg (Pyridoxine)	2.6	2.1	2.1	1.9	2.9
Vitamin B_{12} µg (Cyanocobalamine)	7.9	9.5	6.4	6.6	2.3
Niacin mg	31	27	27	17.4	67
Vitamin B_5 mg (Pantothenic acid)	13	10.5	5.6	2.2	21
Folic acid µg	211	422	210	340	57
Vitamin C mg (Ascorbic acid)	158	158	160	86	171
Vitamin E mg (α tocopherol)	26	17.5	17.5	10.4	3.9
Choline mg	264	317	316.5	170	69
Biotin µg	160	317	316.5	600	N/A
Vitamin D µg (Cholecalciferol)	5.2	5.3	5.3	4.4	5.7
Vitamin K_1 µg	130	38	38	92	N/A
Calcium mg	630	528	528	1120	2100
Phosphorus mg	520	530	530	940	1700
Copper mg	1.0	1.1	1.1	1.08	N/A
Iodine µg	79	79	79	122	N/A
Iron mg	9.5	9.5	9.5	16	8.6
Magnesium mg	210	211	214	152	N/A
Potassium mg (mmol)	1320 (33.8)	1014 (26)	1584 (40.6)	1370 (35)	2850 (73)
Sodium mg (mmol)	528 (22.9)	633 (27.5)	845 (36.7)	621 (27)	897 (39.0)
Chloride mg	1056	844	1443	1323	N/A
Manganese mg	1.6	2.6	2.1	1.74	N/A
Zinc mg	10.6	11.9	11.9	13	N/A
Osmolality (mOsm/kg water)	300	300	470	420	760 (chocolate) 740 (vanilla)

N/A: Not applicable

ENTERAL FEEDING

34

TABLE 34.9 Nutrient dense enteral formulae

Criterion	Isocal HCN	Ensure Plus	Traumacal	Two Cal HN	Ensure Plus HN
Protein source	Sodium and calcium caseinates	Sodium and calcium caseinates. Soy protein isolate	Sodium and calcium caseinates. Rich in branched chain amino acids leucine, isoleucine, and valine	Sodium and calcium caseinates	Sodium and calcium caseinates. Soy protein isolate
g/L % total energy	75 g/L 15% energy	55 g/L 14.7% energy	83 g/L 22% energy	83.7 g/L 16.7% energy	62.6 g/L 16.7% energy
Fat source	Soy oil. MCT oil	Corn oil	MCT oil. Soy oil	Corn oil MCT oil	Corn oil
g/L % total energy	102 g/L 45% energy	53.3 g/L 32% energy	68 g/L 40% energy	90.7 g/L 40.1% energy	49.9 g/L 30% energy
Carbohydrate source	Corn syrup solids	Corn syrup solids. Sucrose	Corn syrup solids. Sucrose	Hydrolysed corn starch. Sucrose	Hydrolysed corn starch Sucrose
g/L % total energy	200 g/L 40% energy	200 g/L 53.3% energy	143 g/L 38% energy	217.3 g/L 43.2% energy	199.9 g/L 53.3% energy
Energy kJ/mL (cal/mL)	8.4 (2)	6.3 (1.5)	6.3 (1.5)	8.4 (2)	6.3 (1.5)
Osmolality (mOsm/kg water)	640	690	490	690	650
Lactose content	Nil	Nil	Nil	Nil	Nil
Flavour	Unflavoured	Vanilla, chocolate, strawberry, egg nog, coffee	Vanilla	Vanilla	Vanilla
Presentation	Ready to use liquid: 237 mL per can	Ready to use liquid: 237 mL per can	Ready to use liquid: 237 mL per can	Ready to use liquid: 237 mL per can	Ready to use liquid: 237 mL per can
Manufacturer	Mead Johnson	Ross Laboratories	Mead Johnson	Ross Laboratories	Ross Laboratories
Indications for use	High energy and protein requirement. Tube feeding or oral. An infusion pump is recommended	High energy and protein requirement. Tube feeding or oral	High energy and protein requirement. Tube feeding or oral. An infusion pump is recommended	High energy and protein requirement. Tube feeding. An infusion pump is recommended	High energy and protein requirement. Tube feeding or oral. An infusion pump is recommended
Method of initiating tube feeding	Introduce gradually after establishing on an isotonic feeding	Introduce gradually after establishing on an isotonic feeding	Introduce gradually after establishing on an isotonic feeding	Introduce gradually after establishing on an isotonic feeding	Introduce gradually after establishing on an isotonic feeding

TABLE 34.10 Biochemical analysis of nutrient dense enteral formulae

Constituents (per L)	Isocal HCN	Ensure Plus	Traumacal	Two Cal HN	Ensure Plus HN
Protein g	75	55	83	83.7	62.6
Fat g	102	53	68	90.7	49.9
Carbohydrate g	200	200	143	217.3	199.9
Kilocalories	2000	1500	1500	2000	1500
Kilojoules	8400	6300	6300	8400	6300
Vitamin A µg (Retinol activity)	1500	1938	750	2901	2901
Vitamin B_1 mg (Thiamine)	3.8	2.1	1.9	2.5	3.2
Vitamin B_2 mg (Riboflavine)	4.3	2.4	2.2	2.9	3.6
Vitamin B_6 mg (Pyridoxine)	5	2.8	2.5	3.4	4.2
Vitamin B_{12} µg (Cyanocobalamin)	15	8.4	7.5	10.1	12.7
Niacin mg	62	28	38.3	33.8	42.2
Vitamin B_5 mg (Pantothenic acid)	25	14	12.5	16.9	21.1
Folic acid µg	400	565	200	675	844
Vitamin C mg (Ascorbic acid)	300	211	150	316	316
Vitamin E mg (α tocopherol)	50	23.3	25	35	35.1
Choline mg	500	420	250	630	625
Biotin µg	300	420	150	510	625
Vitamin D µg (Cholecalciferol)	10	7.1	5.0	10.5	10.6
Vitamin K_1 µg	250	51	125	76	76
Calcium mg	1000	705	750	1055	1055
Phosphorus mg	1000	705	750	1055	1055
Copper mg	2.0	1.4	1.5	2.1	2.1
Iodine µg	150	105	75	158	158
Iron mg	18	12.7	9.0	19.0	19.0
Magnesium mg	400	283	200	422	422
Potassium mg (mmol)	1700 (43)	2109 (53.9)	1400 (36)	2321 (62.8)	1814 (51.5)
Sodium mg (mmol)	800 (35)	1139 (46.6)	1200 (52)	1055 (57)	1181 (51.5)
Chloride mg	1200	1983	1600	1561	1603
Manganese mg	3.3	3.5	2.5	5.3	5.3
Zinc mg	19.8	15.8	15.0	23.8	23.8
Osmolality (mOsm/kg water)	640	690	490	690	650

ENTERAL FEEDING

34 ∎

TABLE 34.11 Elemental formulae

Criterion	Criticare HN	Vital	Vivonex TEN	Elemental 028	Amin-Aid
Protein source	60% free amino acids 40% small peptides	Hydrolysed whey, soy and meat protein 87% 13% free amino acids	Free amino acids	Crystalline synthetic amino acids in the proportions of human milk	Contents of each packet, when suspended in water (340 mL total), contains Rose's minimum daily requirements of eight essential amino acids plus 0.25 g histidine and provides 0.8 g nitrogen
g/L % total energy	38 g/L 14% energy	41.7 g/L 16.7% energy	38.2 g/L 15.3% energy	20 g/L 10.3% energy	19.4 g amino acids/L and 4% energy
Fat source g/L % total energy	Safflower oil 3 g/L 3% energy	Safflower oil. MCT oil 10.8 g/L 9.4% energy	Safflower oil 2.8 g/L 2.5% energy	Arachis oil (long chain fatty acids) 13.28 g/L 15.4% energy	Partially hydrogenated soy bean 46.2 g/L 21.2% energy
Carbohydrate source g/L % total energy	Hydrolysed corn starch Sucrose 222 g/L 83% energy	Hydrolysed corn starch Sucrose 185 g/L 73.9% energy	Maltodextrin. Modified starch 206 g/L 82.2% energy	Glucose polymer 144 g/L 74.3% energy	Maltodextrins Sucrose 365.6 g/L 74.8% energy
Energy kJ/mL (cal/mL)	4.2 (1.06)	4.2 (1.06)	4.2 (1.06)	3.1 (0.73)	8.4 (2.0)
Osmolality (mOsm/kg water)	650	500	630 (unflavoured)	317–684 depending on flavour and dilution	700
Lactose content	Nil	Trace	Nil	Nil	Nil
Flavour	Unflavoured. 'Chemical' taste due to amino acids and small peptides	Vanilla	Vanilla, orange/pine, lemon/lime	Unflavoured, orange	Berry, strawberry, lemon/lime, orange
Presentation	237 mL bottle. For tube feeding	79 g powder packet plus 225 mL water yields 300 mL. Tube or oral feeding	80 g powder packet Tube or oral feeding	100 g powder packet Tube or oral feeding	148 g (approx) per sachet 3 sachets plus 750 mL water yields 1020 mL
Manufacturer	Mead Johnson	Ross Laboratories	Norwich Eaton	Scientific Hospital Supplies	McGaw Laboratories, California
Indications for use	Impaired digestion and absorption. To reduce colonic residue	Impaired digestion and absorption. To reduce colonic residue	Impaired digestion and absorption. To reduce colonic residue	Impaired digestion and absorption. To reduce colonic residue. Tolerance should be assessed in patients with fat malabsorption	For acute renal failure or malnourished patient with chronic renal failure
Method of initiating tube feeding	Introduce at half strength, advance slowly to desired volume then increase to full strength	Introduce at half strength, advance slowly to desired volume then increase to full strength	Introduce at half strength, advance slowly to desired volume then increase to full strength	Introduce at dilution 1 in 7.5, then change to 1 in 5	Tube: introduce at isotonic strength (1/3 to 1/2 strength) advance slowly to desired volume then increase to full strength Oral: chilled and sipped slowly at full strength

TABLE 34.12 Biochemical analysis of elemental formulae

Constituent (per L)	Criticare HN	Vital	Vivonex TEN	Elemental 028 Unflavoured 1 in 5 dilution	Amin-Aid
Protein g	38	41.7	38.2	20	19.4
Fat g	3	10.8	2.8	13.28	46.2
Carbohydrate g	222	185	206	144	365.6
Kilocalories	1000	1000	1000	740	2000
Kilojoules	4200	4200	4200	3136	8400
Vitamin A μg (Retinol activity)	780	1833	750	650	nil
Vitamin B_1 mg (Thiamine)	2	2	1.5	1.2	nil
Vitamin B_2 mg (Riboflavine)	2.2	2.3	1.7	1.2	nil
Vitamin B_6 mg (Pyridoxine)	2.6	2.7	2	1.6	nil
Vitamin B_{12} μg (Cyanocobalamin)	7.9	8.0	6	3.6	nil
Niacin mg	32	26.7	20	8.4	nil
Vitamin B_5 mg (Pantothenic acid)	13	13.3	10	4	nil
Folic acid μg	210	533	400	166.6	nil
Vitamin C mg (Ascorbic acid)	159	200	60	56.6	nil
Vitamin E mg (α tocopherol)	27	22	10.5	16.6	nil
Choline mg	260	400	74	183.2	nil
Biotin μg	160	400	300	116.6	nil
Vitamin D μg (Cholecalciferol)	5.2	6.67	5	3.8	nil
Vitamin K_1 μg	132	47	22	50	nil
Calcium mg	530	667	500	375	nil
Phosphorus mg	530	667	500	400	nil
Copper mg	1	1.3	1	0.8	nil
Iodine μg	79	100	75	66.6	nil
Iron mg	9.5	12	9	8.4	nil
Magnesium mg	210	267	200	163.2	nil
Potassium mg (mmol)	1320 (33.8)	1333 (34)	782 (20)	932 (24)	neglible
Sodium mg (mmol)	630 (27.4)	467 (20.3)	460 (20)	600 (26)	338 (14.7)
Chloride mg	1060	900	819	666	nil
Manganese mg	2.6	3.3	0.9	1.2	nil
Zinc mg	10	15	10	8.4	nil
Osmolality (mOsm/kg water)	650	500	630 unflavoured	500 unflavoured	700

TABLE 34.13 High fat enteral formulae

Criterion	*Pulmocare*	*Glucerna*
Protein source g/L % total energy	Sodium and calcium caseinates 62.4 g/L 16.7% energy	Sodium and calcium caseinates 41.8 g/L 16.7% energy
Fat source g/L % total energy	Corn oil 92 g/L 55.2% energy	High oleic Safflower oil Soy oil 55.7 g/L 50% energy
Carbohydrate source g/L % total energy	Sucrose Hydrolysed corn starch 105.5 g/L 28.1% energy	Hydrolysed corn starch Fructose. Soy polysaccharide 93.7 g/L 33.3% energy
Dietary fibre	Nil	14.3 g/L
Energy kJ/mL (cal/mL)	6.3 (1.5)	4.2 (1.0)
Osmolality mOsm/kg water	490	375
Lactose content	Nil	Nil
Flavour	Vanilla	Vanilla
Presentation	Ready to use liquid 237 mL can	Ready to use liquid 237 mL can
Manufacturer	Ross Laboratories	Ross Laboratories
Indications for use	Respiratory insufficiency Chronic or acute retention of CO_2	Abnormal glucose tolerance
Method of initiating feeding	Tube or oral feeding Tube: introduce at 1/2 strength 30–50 mL/hour. Advance slowly to desired volume, full strength	Tube or oral feeding Tube: introduce slowly 30–50 mL/hour. Advance slowly to desired volume

TABLE 34.14 Biochemical analysis of high fat enteral formulae

Constituent (per L)	*Pulmocare*	*Glucerna*
Protein g	62.4	41.8
Fat g	92	55.7
Carbohydrate g	105.5	93.7
Fibre g	–	14.3
Kilocalories	1500	1000
Kilojoules	6300	4200
Vitamin A µg (Retinol activity)	2901	1935
Vitamin B_1 mg (Thiamine)	3.2	1.6
Vitamin B_2 mg (Riboflavine)	3.6	1.8
Vitamin B_6 mg (Pyridoxine)	4.2	2.1
Vitamin B_{12} µg (Cyanocobalamin)	12.7	6.3
Niacin mg	42.2	21.1
Vitamin B_5 mg (Pantothenic acid)	21.1	10.5
Folic acid µg	844	422
Vitamin C mg (Ascorbic acid)	316	211
Vitamin E mg (α tocopherol)	35	23.2
Choline mg	630	420
Biotin µg	630	320
Vitamin D µg (Cholecalciferol)	10.5	7
Vitamin K_1 µg	76	51
Calcium mg	1055	705
Phosphorus mg	1055	705
Copper mg	2.1	1.4
Iodine µg	158	105
Iron mg	19	12.7
Magnesium mg	422	283
Potassium mg (mmol)	1899 (48.6)	1561 (39.9)
Sodium mg (mmol)	1308 (56.9)	928 (40.4)
Chloride mg	1688	1435
Manganese mg	5.3	3.5
Zinc mg	23.8	15.8
Osmolality (mOsm/kg water)	490	375

ENTERAL FEEDING

34

TABLE 34.15 Fibre containing enteral formulae

Criterion	Enrich	Jevity	Ultracal
Protein source	Sodium and calcium caseinates. Soy protein isolate	Sodium and calcium caseinates	Sodium and calcium caseinates
g/L % total energy	39.7 g/L 14.5% energy	44.4 g/L 16.7% energy	44 g/L
Fat source	Corn oil	MCT oil Corn oil Soy oil	MCT oil Soy oil
g/L % total energy	37.1 g/L 30.5% energy	36.8 g/L 30% energy	45 g/L
Carbohydrate source	Hydrolysed corn starch. Sucrose	Hydrolysed corn starch	Maltodextrins
g/L % total energy	162 g/L 55% energy	151.7 g/L 53.3% energy	123 g/L
Fibre g/L	Soy polysaccharide 14.3 g/L	Soy polysaccharide 13.6 g/L	Oat Soy 14.4 g/L
Energy kJ/mL (cal/mL)	4.6 (1.1)	4.4 (1.06)	4.4 (1.06)
Osmolality (mOsm/kg water)	480	310	310
Lactose	Nil	Nil	Nil
Flavour	Vanilla, chocolate	Unflavoured	Unflavoured
Presentation	Ready to use 237 mL can	Ready to use 237 mL can	Ready to use 237 mL can
Manufacturer	Ross Laboratories	Ross Laboratories	Mead Johnson
Indications for use	To moderate transit time in colon (i.e. constipation or diarrhoea) secondary to gastric motility disorders	To moderate transit time in colon (i.e. constipation or diarrhoea) secondary to gastric motility disorders	To moderate transit time in colon (i.e. constipation or diarrhoea) secondary to gastric motility disorders
Method of initiating feeding	Tube or oral. Tube: preferably introduced after establishing on an isotonic feed. Infusion pump recommended	Tube or oral. Tube: introduced gradually at full strength. Infusion pump recommended	Tube or oral. Tube: introduced gradually at full strength. Infusion pump recommended

TABLE 34.16 Biochemical analysis of fibre containing enteral formulae

Constituent (per L)	*Enrich*	*Jevity*	*Ultracal*
Protein g	39.7	44.4	44
Fat g	37	36.8	45
Carbohydrate g	162	151.7	123
Fibre g	14.3	13.6	14.4
Kilocalories	1100	1060	1060
Kilojoules	4600	4400	4400
Vitamin A µg (Retinol activity)	1973	2072	1260
Vitamin B_1 mg (Thiamine)	1.6	1.7	3.2
Vitamin B_2 mg (Riboflavine)	1.9	1.9	3.6
Vitamin B_6 mg (Pyridoxine)	2.2	2.3	4.2
Vitamin B_{12} µg (Cyanocobalamin)	6.8	7.2	12.7
Niacin mg	21.5	22.6	49
Vitamin B_5 mg (Pantothenic acid)	10.8	11.3	21
Folic acid µg	430	456	340
Vitamin C mg (Ascorbic acid)	215	226	250
Vitamin E mg (α tocopherol)	24	25.1	42
Choline mg	431	449	420
Biotin µg	325	337.5	250
Vitamin D µg (Cholecalciferol)	7.2	7.6	8.5
Vitamin K_1 µg	50.7	54.8	106
Calcium mg	717	907	850
Phosphorus mg	717	755	850
Copper mg	1.4	1.5	1.7
Iodine µg	108	113	127
Iron mg	12.9	13.6	15.2
Magnesium mg	287	302	340
Potassium mg (mmol)	1688 (43.3)	1561 (40)	1610 (41)
Sodium mg (mmol)	846 (36.8)	928 (40.4)	930 (40)
Chloride mg	1435	1435	1440
Manganese mg	3.6	3.8	2.5
Zinc mg	16.2	17	17
Osmolality (mOsm/kg water)	480	310	310

ENTERAL FEEDING

34

POSSIBLE COMPLICATIONS

A list of possible complications associated with enteral feeding and recommendations to alleviate them are listed in Table 34.17.

Diarrhoea is the most common complication. It can be largely avoided by attention to the components of the formula and its administration.

It should be remembered that digestion and absorption are impaired in malnourished patients. Deficiencies of enzymes in the gastric mucosa are common. For example, lactose (sugar of milk) intolerance is common because of the deficiency of the enzyme lactase. Milk based foods and feedings are unsuitable for lactase deficient patients. The possible causes of diarrhoea with recommendations are listed in Table 34.18.

MONITORING

The aim of the treatment should always be to restore the nutritional status of the patient and to return the patient to normal eating as speedily as possible. The following measures are useful in monitoring the efficacy of treatment:

- daily weight
- mid arm circumference
- skin fold thicknesses
- urine volume and osmolarity
- stool frequency, consistency and volume
- serum osmolarity
- blood glucose
- haemoglobin and packed cell volume
- serum electrolytes and blood urea
- serum albumin
- serum prealbumin
- serum transferrin
- total lymphocyte count

TABLE 34.17 Possible complications with enteral feeding

Possible Complications	Recommendations
Delayed gastric emptying (symptoms include abdominal distension, cramping, vomiting, increased gastric residual)	• Reduce flow rate • Elevate bed head, lie patient on right side • Give metoclopramid • Pass tube through pylorus • Check bowel sounds to exclude paralytic ileus
Aspiration	• Check bowel sounds to exclude paralytic ileus • Check gastric emptying • Ensure nasogastric tube in stomach • Consider tracheo-oesophageal fistula if patient has had nasogastric and ET tubes in long term
Paralytic ileus	• Cease feed; repeat water trial when bowel sounds are present
Hyperglycaemia, glycosuria	• Give fluid replacement and insulin/oral hypoglycaemic drugs
Hypernatraemia	• Give additional water
Dehydration	• Review formula

TABLE 34.18   Possible causes of diarrhoea

Possible Causes	Recommendations
High flow rate Hyperosmolar formula	• Check introduction of feed
Contaminated formula	• Check protocol and asceptic technique • Formula bags must not be left at room temperature in excess of 12 hours
Prolonged broad spectrum antibiotic use	• Cease unnecessary antibiotics • Introduce *Lactobacillus acidophilus* yoghurt via side port
Drug induced: e.g. antacids, digoxin, potassium supplements, quinidine, chemotherapeutic agents	• Review drug therapy
Impaired digestion and/or absorption	• Consider elemental formula
Impacted bowel	• Enema
Bacterial contamination of gut High gastric pH	• Stool culture • Discontinue gastric pH control • *Lomotil* is not recommended for infective diarrhoea
Clostridium difficile	• Give oral vancomycin or metronidazole
Abnormal peristalsis, e.g. neurological disorders, diabetic autonomic neuropathy	• Give *Lomotil* or loperamide • Fibre enriched formula or add *Metamucil* via side port

NURSING IMPLICATIONS

ASSESSMENT

Before the patient commences an enteral feeding program the nurse should establish baseline documentation of height and weight, current nutritional state and fluid and electrolyte status. Before preparing to administer the formula the nurse should check the type and amount of formula to be given and the rate and frequency of administration.

ADMINISTRATION

Enteral feeding formulae are usually administered by a slow continuous drip using a fine bore intragastric tube. The position of the tube should be confirmed by X-ray. When preparing and setting up, contamination of the formula should be avoided and care taken to avoid accidentally connecting the formula to an intravenous line. The nurse should check that the formula is administered via the correct enteral administration set and that the container is not left suspended for long periods as bacterial contamination of the line could occur. The use of enteral feeding pumps permit well regulated delivery of formulae.

EVALUATION

A careful record of fluid intake and output should be kept. Weight should be monitored three times a week. The rate of

ENTERAL FEEDING

34

administration should be checked during feeding. The patient should be observed for signs of delayed gastric emptying, e.g. nausea, vomiting, regurgitation and distension, and monitored carefully for signs of hyperglycaemia, glucosuria, dehydration and diarrhoea, which should be reported if they occur.

PATIENT EDUCATION

The feeding regimen should be explained and, where possible, patients encouraged to take an active interest in their treatment and progress.

FURTHER READING

Department of Nutrition and Dietetics. (1990) *Dieticians' Pocket Book.* School of Community Health, Curtin University of Technology, Perth.

Kaminski, M.V. (ed) (1985) *Hyperalimentation. A guide for clinicians.* Jr Marcel Dekkes Inc, New York.

National Health and Medical Research Council. (1991) *Recommended dietary intakes for use in Australia.* AGPS, Canberra.

Parenteral and enteral nutrition. A practical guide. 3rd edn. Churchill Livingstone (1986).

Rombeau, J., Caldwell, M. (1984) *Enteral and tube feeding clinical nutrition*, Volume 1. W.B. Saunders, Philadelphia.

TEST YOUR KNOWLEDGE

1. List three features (symptoms) that may become evident in a patient suffering from malnutrition.

2. Discuss reasons for introducing enteral nutrition via tube, giving patient groups as examples.

3. When is enteral feeding contraindicated? Give examples.

4. Explain the reason for emphasis on the osmolality of enteral formulae.

5. Give two reasons for using a nutrient dense formula instead of a regular formula.

6. Define an elemental formula.

7. List three possible causes of diarrhoea in patients receiving enteral feeding.

8. Explain the difference between bolus feeding and continuous drip feeding.

Antiseptics, Disinfectants and Infection Control

ANNE E. McFARLANE

O B J E C T I V E S

At the conclusion of this chapter the reader should be able to:

1. Define the terms disinfectant and antiseptic;

2. Define the terms bactericidal and bacteriostatic;

3. List the main groups of disinfectants and antiseptics and describe their uses;

4. List the uses of disinfectants and antiseptics;

5. List examples of possible misuses of disinfectants and antiseptics;

6. List the limitations to the use of disinfectants;

7. Discuss the nursing implications of the selection and use of an antiseptic solution; and

8. List the principles of hand hygiene.

ANTISEPSIS

HISTORY

Antony van Leeuwenhoek first described the 'little animals' he saw under his self-made microscopes in 1677. Nearly 200 years elapsed before some practical application was seen in controlling microorganisms. Louis Pasteur, in the second half of the nineteenth century, demonstrated that microbes contaminated sterile culture media and was able to control unwanted fermentations in beer and wine by gentle heating (pasteurisation). In the 1860s Joseph Lister applied Pasteur's theory of airborne microbes to surgery and reasoned that infections in wounds were the result of airborne contamination. By using dressings soaked in phenol for application to surgical wounds, especially amputations, he found a marked reduction in the incidence of serious infections. This process became known as antiseptic surgery, later to be replaced by aseptic surgery.

CLASSES OF ANTISEPTICS AND DISINFECTANTS

ALCOHOLS

Ethanol, Isopropyl Alcohol

Alcohols are bactericidal in combination with water. Ethanol is most effective at 70%–80% v/v dilution and isopropyl alcohol at 50%–60% v/v. Alcohols may be used as bactericidal agents but are more commonly used as solvents for other disinfectants, e.g. iodine or chlorhexidine, and to potentiate their antibacterial activity. They should not be used in the theatre when diathermy is being used due to the risk of fire, on humidicribs or in confined spaces where toxic amounts of vapour may be inhaled. Alcohols have poor penetration of organic matter so are unsuitable for dirty surfaces.

DIGUANIDES

Chlorhexidine

Chlorhexidine (*Hibitane*) is bactericidal although bacteriostatic in high dilutions. Bacterial spores are resistant to it. Chlorhexidine is inactivated by many materials and is incompatible with soap. Dilutions (as final concentrations of chlorhexidine gluconate) for various uses are given in Table 35.1.

TABLE 35.1 Dilutions and uses of chlorhexidine gluconate

Dilutions	Uses
0.02% (1 in 5000) in aqueous solution	Bladder and vaginal irrigation (solution must be sterile)
0.05% (1 in 2000) in aqueous solution	Swabbing of genitourinary area prior to collection of midstream urine (MSU) samples
0.5% in 70% ethanol	Preoperative skin preparation; emergency disinfection of clean instruments and glass thermometers
1%	Cream: burns; aqueous solutions: preoperative skin preparation near sensitive tissues
4% in lotion (e.g. *Hibiclens*)	Hand disinfection

QUATERNARY AMMONIUM COMPOUNDS (QACs)

Cetrimide, Benzalkonium Chloride, Cetylpyridium Chloride

Cetrimide (*Cetavlon*), benzalkonium chloride (*Zephrin*), cetylpyridium chloride (*Cepacol*) are bactericidal and bacteriostatic at high dilution. They have the advantage of being surface active so concentrate on all types of surfaces giving rapid bactericidal action. They are at least partially inactivated by serum proteins, gauze, soap and phospholipids. An alcoholic solution of 0.5% cetrimide in 70% alcohol may be used for preoperative skin disinfection after ensuring the area is free of soap.

DIGUANIDE–QAC COMBINATIONS

Chlorhexidine–Cetrimide

Both chlorhexidine and cetrimide have limitations as antiseptics, however, when used together (*Savlon Hospital Concentrate*) these limitations are overcome to some extent. Combining antiseptics is uncommon and, as a general rule, most should not be mixed.

A 1 in 100 aqueous dilution of *Savlon Hospital Concentrate* is used for routine skin and wound disinfection ('clean' wound) and 1 in 30 for wounds which are 'dirty', i.e. contain grease or tar and require greater detergency.

A 1 in 30 alcoholic solution is also available but it is irritant to mucous membranes and open wounds. It may be used for preparing a surface as a 'sterile field' or for emergency instrument sterilisation (usually with antirust). Precleaning to remove debris is essential for the disinfectant to work.

Sachets of *Savlon Hospital Concentrate* may be mixed with warm water for use in the delivery ward. The addition of this product to baths has also been advocated but, due to its detergency, it makes the bath extremely slippery. Therefore, care should be exercised when adding it to a bath particularly if patients are unsteady on their feet.

PHENOLICS

Chlorinated Phenols, Bisphenols

The chlorinated phenols (*Dettol, Medol, Clearsol 50, Printol, Prephen, Sudol*) and the bisphenols (e.g. hexachlorophane) are bactericidal. They are incompatible with some plastics and natural materials such as rubber and *Pseudomonas* sp. grow readily in phenolics if contaminated. *Dettol* was used for skin disinfection at a 5% dilution for clean situations but more effective antiseptics have superseded it.

Medol, Clearsol 50, Printol, Prephen and *Sudol* are suitable for environmental disinfection. The usual dilution of *Medol* is 1% for a clean area and 1.5%–2% for dirty areas or theatres. A 2% dilution with 0.5% sodium nitrite (antirust) can be used for instrument disinfection. The problem in using it for inanimate objects is its blanching effect on perspex, e.g. in humidicribs. Prolonged immersion of endoscopic instruments may damage lens cement.

Hexachlorophane has been used in hand soap (2%–3%) and in a detergent emulsion for skin antisepsis where its value depends on a cumulative effect by repeated application. This effect is removed by alcohol.

CHLORINE COMPOUNDS

Chlorine Gas, Sodium Hypochlorite, Calcium Hypochlorite, Chlorinated Lime, Inorganic and Organic Chloramines

Chlorine gas, hypochlorites (e.g. sodium hypochlorite — household bleach, *Milton* 1%, *Absol* 5%, and calcium hypochlorite —

35

Virusorb), chlorinated lime (*Dakin's solution, Eusol*), inorganic and organic chloramines (*Chloramine-T Tablets* for colostomy or ileostomy bags) are bactericidal although organic matter and alkaline pH reduce activity. Due to a relatively low toxicity they are useful for the disinfection of clean, impervious surfaces such as babies' feeding bottles, baths, wash basins and food equipment.

Containers of sodium hypochlorite should be covered to avoid the escape of chlorine, thereby reducing potency, and changed at least every 24 hours. It must be remembered that the article must be in contact with the solution for antimicrobial activity, so upturned dummies and teats are unlikely to be sanitised. Hypochlorite is corrosive to metallic surfaces and instruments. Sodium hypochlorite is available as a 1% stabilised solution (*Milton*), a 1.5% solution (*Johnson & Johnson's Antibacterial Solution*) and a 5% solution with detergent (*Absol*). In the past a 1 in 20 dilution of *Milton* was used in removing slough from granulation tissue, e.g. in leg ulcers, but is now believed to be toxic to fibroblasts. There are no indications for the use of chlorine solutions in wound care. It is also used for blood spills from patients. (See Table 35.2.)

TABLE 35.2 Dilutions and uses of hypochlorites

Dilutions	Uses
125 ppm (e.g. 1 in 80 dilution of *Milton*)	Baby feeding bottles and teats, food utensils, face masks
10 000 ppm (1% sodium hypochlorite)	Surfaces contaminated with blood.

ppm = parts per million

IODINE COMPOUNDS

Iodine, Iodophors

Iodine (tincture of iodine, weak iodine solution) has been used as an antiseptic for intact skin but has been superseded by iodophors, which are complexes of iodine held in loose chemical combination with detergent surfactants. Iodophors (povidone iodine) are less staining than iodine and do not elicit the same degree of hypersensitivity so patients who are allergic to iodine may tolerate iodophors. The other major difference is their method of application. Tincture of iodine is applied and cleaned off with alcohol, whereas iodophors should be allowed to dry on the skin for maximum activity. Iodophors are bactericidal. Activity is reduced in alkaline pH and in the presence of organic matter.

Povidone iodine (*Betadine, Viodine*) is a solubilised form of iodine. It is a complex of iodine containing 9%–12% available iodine. Povidone iodine 7.5%–10% (equivalent to 0.75%–1% w/v iodine) is used for disinfection in surgical scrubs, preoperative skin preparations, ointments, throat gargles and cold sore paints.

ALDEHYDES

Formaldehyde, Glutaraldehyde

Formaldehyde is biocidal (being sporicidal above 40°C) as a 4% aqueous solution. Formalin is an aqueous solution of formaldehyde 34% to 38% and is used diluted 2–20 times with water. Formalin 10% in buffered solution is the usual strength for specimen preservation. It is too irritant for use on living tissue. Formalin in sodium chloride 0.9% should never be labelled or referred to as 'formal saline' as the confusion with normal saline has proven disastrous.

Glutaraldehyde (*Aldecyde 28, Cidex, Sonacide, 3M Instrument Disinfectant, Wavicide*) has a wide range of activity, being tuberculocidal and slowly sporicidal. The biocidal activity is greatest at pH 7.5 to 8.5. It is used as a 2% solution, requiring a supplement activator before use, or as a 1% stabilised solution. It is particularly useful for disinfection of endoscopy equipment.

MISCELLANEOUS PRODUCTS

Mercury Compounds

These are still occasionally used as antiseptics, although their use for antiseptic purposes is not recommended. Nitromersol is used as a 1 in 200 tincture (*Metaphen*). Mercurochrome has been used as a 2% solution. They are often allergenic, are poor antiseptics and are potentially dangerous due to their mercury content. Mercurochrome 10%–20% may be used as an adjunct to skin grafts in stomal therapy but not for its antiseptic properties.

Triphenylmethane Dyes

The triphenylmethane dyes, crystal violet (Gentian Violet), brilliant green and malachite green (*Triple Dye, Bonney's Blue*) are mainly used for their staining properties including as a skin marking dye for radiotherapy. Crystal violet (0.5% aqueous solution or 1% solution with 20% alcohol) has been used topically for staphylococcal, *Candida albicans* and mycotic skin infections but is now considered a potential carcinogen and is a Schedule 4 drug.

The activity of antiseptics and disinfectants under optimal conditions is shown in Table 35.3.

TABLE 35.3 Activity of antiseptics and disinfectants under optimal conditions

Group	Gram positive bacteria (e.g. *Staphylococcus* sp.)	Gram negative bacteria (e.g. *Pseudomonas* sp.)	Acid fast bacteria (e.g. tubercle)	Spores (e.g. *Clostridia* sp.)
Alcohols	+	+	+	−
Chlorhexidine	+	+	+	−
QACs	+	+	−	−
QAC-Chlorhexidine	+	+	−	−
Phenolics	+	+	+	−
Chlorine compounds	++	++	++	++
Iodophors	+	+	+	+
Aldehydes				
Formaldehyde	++	++	++	+
Glutaraldehyde	++	++	+	++

ANTISEPTICS, DISINFECTANTS AND INFECTION CONTROL

35

USES, LIMITATIONS AND MISUSE OF DISINFECTANTS AND ANTISEPTICS ▬

USES

The definite uses of disinfectants and antiseptics may be categorised as:

- Disinfection of the hospital environment with an agent effective in clean or dirty conditions;

- Disinfection of clean articles or surfaces; and

- Skin antisepsis.

A range of different products is required as no one disinfectant can provide the complete antimicrobial range and properties.

The efficiency of disinfectants and antiseptics depends on:

1. contact time allowed (no product causes instant disinfection);

2. range of antimicrobial activity of the individual product;

3. concentration used (if dilutions are used exact portions of disinfectant and water must be measured before mixing);

4. temperature;

5. initial load of microorganisms (the act of cleaning is itself a disinfection process);

6. presence of a protective film (e.g. blood, pus, milk, excreta, oil) preventing contact of the disinfectant with the microorganisms;

7. texture of the surface (a porous surface may also prevent contact);

8. inactivation of the product (e.g. by contaminants, detergents, containers, fibres, textiles);

9. pH of the medium; and

10. type of diluent (e.g. alcohol, water, hard water).

LIMITATIONS

Disinfectants should not be recommended under the following circumstances:

- When sterilisation is necessary other than in an emergency;

- When disinfection can be better accomplished by pasteurisation, e.g. anaesthetic equipment;

- When it is unnecessary, e.g. in routine cleaning of hospitals (in these cases, regular strict cleaning procedures using simple detergents is more important than disinfection and is also more cost effective); and

- When diathermy is being performed alcoholic solutions should never be used, either in the theatre or preoperatively in the ward where garments may absorb excess flammable liquid.

A general limitation to the use of all disinfectants and antiseptics is the life of diluted solutions at ward level. Antiseptics used on living tissue ideally should be packaged in sterile disposable containers and used once only then discarded. Disinfectants, once opened or diluted, should be replaced every 24 hours or more frequently if particularly prone to contamination or recommended by the manufacturer.

Antiseptics should not be mixed, poured from one bottle to another or topped up.

MISUSE

Not only can some microorganisms survive and thrive in disinfectants and antiseptics, cases have been reported where particular organisms may come to depend on the product for their survival. It is very important for all personnel to realise that these solutions are not self-sterilising.

Some causes of contamination are: contamination of QACs and clear soluble phenolics with *Pseudomonas aeruginosa* from bark stoppers; inactivation of chlorhexidine by cork and soap; and absorption of QACs by gauze swabs or mophead material.

SPECIFIC USES OF ANTISEPTICS

Wounds, Burns, Skin Infections

For these conditions a general cleansing action is required together with antisepsis. A suitable product is chlorhexidine 0.015% with cetrimide 0.150% in aqueous solution (*Savlon Hospital Concentrate* 1–100).

Preoperative Skin Preparation

It is desirable to initially remove organisms by washing, taking care to remove all soap. An alcohol swab may then be used to 'defat' the skin. Antisepsis is then performed using povidone iodine, aqueous or, more commonly, alcoholic chlorhexidine, or chlorhexidine and cetrimide. This should be coloured to demarcate the area of application and be applied twice to ensure mechanical removal of surface contaminants, aid penetration and allow ample time (approximately two minutes) for bactericidal action.

Insertion of Subclavian Catheters

This should be regarded as an operative procedure and similar steps to those outlined above should be taken, i.e. removal of hair, initial cleaning including defatting with alcohol, then application of povidone iodine 10% solution (available in impregnated swabsticks), allowing the area to dry. After insertion of the catheter the entry site is covered with a dressing. There is increasing evidence that the insertion of peripheral catheters should follow the same procedure as that for central lines.

Mucous Membrane Antisepsis

As these areas are sensitive care must be used in selecting the appropriate product. For cleansing sites adjacent to sensitive tissues, aqueous chlorhexidine 1% may be used. Iodophors tend to be irritant to conjunctival and urethral tissues due to their acidity.

In urinary tract procedures aqueous chlorhexidine is suitable. Swabbing of the genitourinary area prior to catheterisation should be carried out with aqueous chlorhexidine 1%. Prior to collection of urine specimens it may be useful to swab with aqueous chlorhexidine 0.05% to reduce contamination of the sample. Bladder and vaginal irrigation is carried out using *sterile* aqueous chlorhexidine 0.02%.

Infants' Skin

Hexachlorophane emulsion 3% has been used. The cumulative effect reduces staphylococcal infections but may increase the risk of Gram negative colonisation. However, there have been conflicting reports on neurological toxicity from dermal absorption of the product. As a result, guidelines have been issued to suggest that hexachlorophane emulsion could continue to be used in maternity hospitals on newborn babies but that extended use should be avoided and the practice not continued at home. In addition, the emulsion should be washed off with water, and newborn infants' clothing be changed immediately after application of hexachlorophane emulsion.

Umbilical cords are commonly treated with alcoholic chlorhexidine or special methylated spirits, although there is a trend to not treat them at all. Other products used for washing newborn babies include triclosan 2% (*Phisohex*) and chlorhexidine 1%–2%.

Handscrubbing

For surgical or invasive procedures, hand disinfection with a long acting bactericidal agent prior to gloving is necessary. The most commonly used antiseptics are povidone iodine 7.5% handscrub (e.g. *Betadine Surgical Scrub*) and chlorhexidine 4% in detergent solution (e.g. *Hibiclens*). Chlorhexidine has a rapid action but povidone iodine has a long lasting and cumulative effect as well as a broader spectrum of activity. It is possible to purchase scrub brushes already impregnated with antiseptic. Less irritation and chafing of hands and forearms occurs if the area is wet with water before applying the solution. The use of a barrier cream, especially at night, may also be necessary.

Handwashing

For routine tasks and non-invasive procedures as well as when leaving work scrubbing is not necessary. Handwashing is, however, required. Chlorhexidine 2% (*Hibiclens G, Novaclens 2*) has been advocated for non-critical hand cleansing and chlorhexidine in alcohol (*Hibicol, Hexol*) is available for emergency cleansing where a sink is unavailable. This product is allowed to dry on the skin.

NURSING IMPLICATIONS

Disinfection means the destruction of bacteria but not necessarily of fungi, viruses or spores. Sterilisation means 100% destruction of all types of microorganisms. Thus '99% sterilised' or 'partially sterilised' are contradictory terms. Select the correct term when referring to either disinfection or sterilisation.

Bacteria may grow in solutions of disinfectants and antiseptics, particularly those of weaker strength. These solutions must be carefully handled to avoid contamination and should not be stored in a moist, warm area which might promote the growth of organisms.

The disinfectant or antiseptic should only be used in the recommended dilutions and be available at ward level as ready to use solutions. These must not be diluted further. If dilutions have to be prepared, exact quantities of the disinfectant and water must be measured before mixing. Antiseptics are ideally a once only use item in disposable containers. Disinfectants and antiseptics must never be 'topped up'. Instruments wherever possible should be sterilised. Disinfection by 'pasteurisation' is the next best process. The presence of dried organic matter, such as blood, pus, excreta, oil or milk, on instruments will form a protective layer which will negate the effect of a disinfectant. Make sure all instruments for disinfection have been thoroughly cleaned mechanically before immersion.

All soap must be removed from instruments and skin before disinfectants and antiseptics are used. The effect of some antiseptics on the skin is destroyed by alcohol. Care must be taken when applying one product after another.

Alcoholic solutions of antiseptics should not be used near sensitive tissues such as the conjunctiva and urethra.

INFECTION CONTROL ▬▬▬▬▬

INFECTION CONTROL COMMITTEES

While hospitals may have monitored levels of infections in wards for many years, this was normally a function of the Department of Microbiology alone. However, in the mid 1970s, with the increasing presence in hos-

pital wards of methicillin resistant *Staphylococcus aureus* (MRSA), infection control committees started to appear in hospitals to set policies and procedures to control nosocomial or hospital acquired infections.

These committees had multidisciplinary representation with the key figure the infection control nurse. The value of having a full-time registered nurse in this role soon became apparent with more precise information on the type, location and incidence of infections obtained through regular infection surveys. Summaries of these information gathering exercises were then disseminated to key personnel in the hospital. This led to better preventive methods being established with the cooperation of medical, surgical, nursing, microbiology, pharmacy and cleaning staff meeting to combat a problem of mutual interest and concern. Policies on antibiotic usage, disinfectants and antiseptics, waste disposal and isolation techniques were strengthened and integrated. Possible vectors for the transmission of organisms about the hospital were identified and measures taken to prevent the spread of any infection from its source.

New guidelines were laid down for staff and patient hygiene, handling of staff and patient infections and the duties of infection control personnel. State departments of health began issuing recommendations for infection control policies and hospitals started to produce infection control procedure manuals. Various personnel from different hospitals and different disciplines began to meet to discuss items of common interest and formed infection control groups within the States.

Terms of Reference for an Infection Control Committee

1. To develop and periodically review written standards for hospital infection control.

2. To develop a practical system for monitoring, reporting, evaluating and record keeping of hospital associated infections amongst patients and personnel.

3. To develop, review and coordinate the hospital antiseptic and disinfectant policy.

4. To develop and coordinate procedures for isolation of patients.

5. To facilitate the teaching of information pertinent to infection control and isolation policies to employees on all levels, including medical staff and students, and provide advice on infection control matters.

6. To assist in educational and research programs related to infection control and epidemiology.

7. To provide assistance in the development of an employee health program.

Structure of the Committee

The committee may comprise the following personnel: the director of medical services, a microbiologist or infectious diseases physician, the infection control nurse, the director of nursing or designate, the director of pharmacy or deputy, the general services manager representing domestic, laundry and catering staff, a representative of the central sterilising department and the theatre supervisor. Other people may need to be coopted from time to time, e.g. the charge nurse of a particular ward.

The Infection Control Nurse

The person appointed would ideally be a registered nurse with at least three years postbasic experience and would be responsible to the director of nursing with a functional responsibility to the chairman of the infection control committee.

A working knowledge of microbiology and an understanding of statistical analysis and research methods would be required. The person would need to be able to act as a consultant and advisor on all matters of infection control, e.g. be able to demonstrate methods of aseptic and isolation techniques as applied to nursing and other disciplines and to evaluate equipment, furniture and fittings in relation to the prevention of cross infection and adequate infection control.

Besides enthusiasm and dedication, other important qualities necessary are tact and diplomacy.

ANTISEPTICS, DISINFECTANTS AND INFECTION CONTROL

35

FURTHER READING

Australian National Council on AIDS. (1993) *Infection control guidelines, AIDS and related conditions.* AGPS, Canberra.

Bennet, J.V., Brachman, P.S. (1992) *Hospital Infections.* 3rd edn. Little Brown, Boston.

Brennan, S.S., Leaper, D.J. (1985) 'The effect of antiseptics on the healing wound'. *British Journal of Surgery,* 72, pp. 780–782.

Brennan, S.S., Foster, M.E., Leaper, D.J. (1986) 'Antiseptic toxicity in wounds healing by secondary intention'. *Journal of Hospital Infection,* 8, pp. 263–267.

Cruse, P.J.E., Foord, R. (1980) 'The epidemiology of wound infection: a 10-year prospective study of 62 939 wounds'. *Surgical Clinics of North America,* 60(1), pp. 27–40.

Ferguson, A. (1988) 'Best performer'. *Nursing Times,* 84(14), pp. 52–55.

Gardner, J.F., Peel, M.A.A. (1991) *Introduction to sterilisation, disinfection and infection control.* 2nd edn. Churchill Livingstone, Melbourne.

Nichols, R.L. (1991) 'Surgical wound infection'. *American Journal of Medicine,* 91(suppl 3B), pp. 545–645.

Rutala, W.A. (1990). 'APIC guidelines for selection and use of disinfectants'. *American Journal of Infection Control,* 18(2), pp. 99–117.

Spanswick, A., Gibbs, S., Ekelund, P. (1990) 'Eusol—the final word'. *Professional Nurse,* pp. 211–214.

TEST YOUR KNOWLEDGE

1. Define the terms disinfectants and antiseptics.

2. Disinfectants are normally used: (a) when sterilisation is required; (b) on instruments that cannot be autoclaved or heated; (c) in detergent solutions to clean ordinary floors; or (d) after the original container has been opened for more than one week.

3. The definite uses of disinfectants and/or antiseptics are: (a) general disinfection of the hospital environment; (b) disinfection of clean articles or surfaces; (c) skin antisepsis; (d) sterilisation of surgeons' hands and arms.

4. Write down the class or classes of the following chemicals and their most common dilution in use (e.g. *Milton* chlorine compound, 1 in 80): (a) ethanol; (b) *Savlon Hospital Concentrate*; (c) *Medol*; (d) chlorhexidine; (e) povidone-iodine (use dilution expressed as percentage of available iodine).

5. (a) Sterilisation means at least 95% destruction of microorganisms (true/false); (b) bacteria may grow in ward solutions of disinfectants and antiseptics (true/false); (c) instruments wherever possible should be sterilised (true/false); (d) the efficacy of disinfectants is decreased by dried films of pus and excreta but not of blood or milk (true/false); (e) instruments for chemical disinfection should be thoroughly cleaned and free from soap (true/false).

6. Describe a desirable procedure to prevent cross-contamination during ward dressings.

TEST YOUR KNOWLEDGE — ANSWERS ▬▬▬▬

CHAPTER 1 PHARMACODYNAMICS

1. List three different mechanisms by which drugs may produce pharmacological effects.

A. Drugs may act at receptors, either by producing an effect similar to that observed when a naturally occurring compound binds to the receptor (i.e. a receptor agonist) or by producing an effect opposite to this (i.e. a receptor antagonist). Many drug products are identical to a naturally occurring compound, e.g. insulin or growth hormone. These drugs are produced using genetic engineering techniques. Drugs may produce their effects by inhibiting the actions of an enzyme, e.g. angiotensin converting enzyme inhibitors such as enalapril and captopril. Antimetabolites act by interfering with normal chemical reactions within the body, e.g. cytotoxic drugs used in cancer chemotherapy.

2. Describe two examples of the ways in which the pharmacodynamic response produced by a drug may vary in relation to the disease state being treated.

A. Patients with HIV infection may be more likely to develop a skin rash during treatment with some antibiotics. Immediately after a stroke, patients are often more susceptible to the hypotensive effects of drugs. Elderly or very young patients may have altered sensitivity to a variety of drug treatments.

3. Describe two different types of adverse drug reaction.

A. An adverse drug reaction may be related to an exaggerated therapeutic response to a drug (e.g. insulin induced hypoglycaemia). Other adverse drug reactions may be predictable on the basis of the drug's known effects (e.g. cytotoxic induced hair loss). Drugs may produce effects because of their similarity to other active compounds (e.g. spironolactone induced breast enlargement), or simply through idiosyncratic effects which are not predictable.

4. Outline at least one situation in which a relatively minor adverse drug reaction may assume a greater clinical significance.

A. Examples include drug induced anaemia in the patient with congestive cardiac failure or chronic obstructive airways disease, and drug induced hypokalaemia in the patient treated with digoxin.

5. Name three different drugs which may produce hepatic enzyme inhibition.

A. Cimetidine, erythromycin, ciprofloxacin.

6. Define the term low therapeutic index.

A. Drugs of low therapeutic index may be defined as those for which the dose or serum level producing the desired therapeutic effect is similar to that which produces serious adverse effects.

7. Outline three serious medical complications associated with intravenous drug abuse.

A. Examples include a range of psychiatric problems, complications related to 'fillers' such as talcum powder, risk of infection with HIV or hepatitis, bacteraemia associated with poor injection technique, and the risk of overdose.

8. Name five drugs or drug groups which may produce drug dependence.

A. Examples include alcohol, nicotine, opioids, cocaine, amphetamines, barbiturates and benzodiazepines.

9. Describe the common symptoms of an acute drug withdrawal reaction.

A. Features of varying severity may include psychological syndromes (e.g. dysphoria, anxiety); autonomic instability (e.g. wide variations in heart rate, blood pressure, body temperature); and seizures.

CHAPTER 2 PHARMACOKINETICS

1. Describe two different practical applications for the use of pharmacokinetics in the formulation of individual drug treatment regimens.

A. Enteric coating may be used to allow the oral administration of drugs which are not stable when exposed to the acidic environment of the stomach. When a drug has a very short half-life, formulation as a sustained release dose form may prolong clinical effects. Depot injection formulations are another example of this type of product.

2. Outline the ways in which the gastrointestinal transit time may influence the oral absorption of drugs.

A. Dissolution of the drug within the gastrointestinal tract may be the slowest step in the absorption process; circumstances which lead to a slower transit through the gastrointestinal tract may lead to enhanced absorption; increased exposure of acid-labile drugs to gastric acid arising from delayed stomach emptying may reduce the extent of absorption.

3. Define the term significant first pass effect.

A. A drug is said to undergo a significant first pass effect when a substantial proportion of the dose administered by mouth is metabolised in the liver before reaching the systemic circulation.

4. Calculate the oral bioavailability (as a percentage) for a drug for which 90% of the administered dose is not absorbed after oral administration.

A. The oral bioavailability of the drug described would be 10% (i.e. if 90% is not absorbed only 10% is).

5. Define the term enterohepatic cycling.

A. Enterohepatic cycling occurs when a drug is metabolised to a compound which is excreted into the lumen of the gastrointestinal tract via the bile and is subsequently reabsorbed into the general circulation after further modification by bacterial flora in the bowel.

6. Calculate the volume of distribution for a drug when the administered IV dose is 150 mg and the observed peak plasma concentration is 3 mg/L (assume that the process of distribution is complete).

A. The volume of distribution is calculated by dividing the known amount of drug in the body by the observed serum concentration, in this case 150 ÷ 3 mg/L. The volume of distribution is 50 L.

7. What is the term used for that proportion of drug in the plasma which is not bound to plasma proteins. List three clinical situations in which the concentration of proteins in the plasma may change.

A. The proportion of drug not bound to plasma proteins is the free fraction. Plasma protein concentrations change during pregnancy, cirrhosis of the liver, nephrotic syndrome and malnutrition.

8. Define the term pro-drug.

A. A pro-drug is a compound which is converted by metabolism to an active form after the drug has been administered.

9. List at least four drugs which may cause severe toxicity in patients with altered kidney function.

A. Examples include amikacin, tobramycin, gentamicin, vancomycin, lithium, flucytosine, cisplatin, digoxin and acyclovir.

10. Define the term elimination half-life.

A. The elimination half-life of a drug is that period of time required for the serum concentration of a drug to decline by 50%, e.g. if the drug concentration decreases from 10 mg/L to 5 mg/L in 4 hours, the elimination half-life of that drug is 4 hours.

CHAPTER 3 DRUG ADMINISTRATION

1. Describe the responsibilities of the nurse in drug therapy.

A. The nurse is responsible for the administration of medication to the patient and should have a thorough knowledge of drug therapy and administration techniques.

2. What is the function of the State Poisons Acts?

A. The State Poisons Acts are designed to control the packaging, labelling, distribution, storage, sale and use of the many potent drugs available.

3. What schedules of the poisons list are of particular importance to the nurse?

A. Schedules 4 and 8.

4. Name two drugs which are listed in Schedule 8 of the poisons list.

A. Morphine, pethidine, papaveretum.

5. Five factors are involved in ensuring that drug administration procedures are designed correctly. What are these factors?

A. That the **right patient** receives the **right drug**, in the **right dose**, by the **right route**, at the **right time**.

6. Describe the correct procedure for using a metered dose aerosol.

A. The usual procedure for using a metered dose aerosol is: shake the aerosol; breathe out in a relaxed fashion to the end of a normal breath; place the open end of the mouthpiece between the lips; breathe in slowly through the mouth, at the same time pressing the cannister firmly down into the plastic mouthpiece with the index finger; breathe in slowly and completely then remove the aerosol from the mouth and hold the breath for 5–10 seconds before breathing out; if a second inhalation is necessary wait for 2 minutes before repeating the inhalation.

7. An IV injection of methylprednisolone has been prescribed. Two injectable preparations are available. What are they and which is the appropriate preparation for IV use?

A. Depo-Medrol and Solu-Medrol. Solu-Medrol is the appropriate preparation for IV use.

CHAPTER 4 DOSE CALCULATIONS

1. Convert the following percentages into quantitative terms: (a) hydrocortisone eye ointment 0.5%; (b) timolol 0.25% eye drops; (c) betamethasone dipropionate cream 0.05%; (d) pilocarpine 6% eye drops.

A. *(a). 5 mg/g; (b) 2.5 mg/mL; (c) 500 micrograms/g; (d) 60 mg/mL.*

2. Convert the following quantitative terms into percentages: (a) betamethasone 0.2 mg/g; (b) clotrimazole 10 mg/g;

A. *(a) 0.02%; (b) 1%.*

3. How many frusemide 40 mg tablets must be given for a 10 mg dose?

A. $\frac{1}{4}$ *tablet.*

4. How many digoxin 0.25 mg tablets must be given for a dose of 125 micrograms?

A. $\frac{1}{2}$ *tablet.*

5. How many haloperidol 500 microgram tablets must be given for a 1 mg dose?

A. *2 tablets.*

6. A dose of 350 mg of potassium chloride has been ordered. A solution containing 1 g in 4 mL is available. What volume must be given?

A. *1.4 mL.*

7. A 100 mg dose of erythromycin has been ordered. Erythromycin suspension containing 125 mg/5 mL is available. How much must be given?

A. *4 mL.*

8. From ampoules containing atropine 0.6 mg/mL what volume must be given to give a dose of 900 micrograms?

A. *1.5 mL.*

9. A dose of 160 mg of frusemide is ordered. Each ampoule contains 250 mg/25 mL. How much should you give?

A. *16 mL.*

10. Cefotaxime 1.5 g IV is ordered. 2 g vials are available. What volume of reconstituted solution would you administer?

A. *Reconstitute with 9.0 mL (see Table 4.1) giving 200 mg/mL. Administer 7.5 mL.*

11. What flow rate in drops per minute must be maintained using an administration set delivering 20 drops/mL to give 1 L of normal saline by IV infusion over 12 hours?

A. *28 drops/min.*

12. How many drops per minute must be maintained to administer 50 mL of dextrose glucose 10% over 1 hour using a set delivering 60 drops per mL?

A. *50 drops/min.*

13. How long will it take 1 L of Hartmann's solution to run through at 50 drops per minute using a set that delivers 60 drops per mL?

A. *20 hours.*

14. How long will 500 mL of glucose 5% take to run through a 20 drop per mL giving set which is set at 40 drops per minute?

A. 4.2 hours.

15. A patient is ordered 1000 mL of sodium chloride 0.9% containing 20 mmol of potassium to be given over 8 hours using an infusion pump. Calculate at what rate the pump should be set (mL/h)?

A. 125 mL/h.

16. An infusion of morphine is prepared with 50 mg morphine diluted to 50 mL with normal saline in a 50 mL syringe. A dose of 0.03 mg/kg per hour is ordered. At what rate should the syringe pump be set to deliver this dose for a 60 kg patient?

A. 1.8 mL/h.

17. A 70 kg patient is ordered glyceryl trinitrate infusion to commence at a rate of 0.2 microgram/kg/min. The concentration of the prepared infusion solution is 100 micrograms/mL. At what rate (mL/h) should the infusion be set?

A. 8.4 mL/h.

18. How much sodium hypochlorite concentrate (100%) is required to make 100 mL of 1:20 solution?

A. 5 mL.

CHAPTER 5 PAEDIATRIC THERAPEUTICS

1. Name two factors which affect drug absorption in the neonate.

A. Decreased gastric acid and delayed gastric emptying.

2. Why does excretion of drugs alter with age?

A. Increasing renal maturity leads to greater excretion of renally excreted drugs such as gentamicin.

3. Name two drugs used particularly in neonates.

A. Alprostadil and exogenous surfactant.

4. If amoxycillin mixture is available as a 250 mg/5 mL mixture how much is needed for a dose of 350 mg?

A. 7 mL.

5. Name two tablets which should not be crushed or chewed.

A. Nuelin SR and Theo-Dur.

CHAPTER 6 GERIATRIC THERAPEUTICS

1. List five physiological changes that are known to occur with ageing that may impact on drug therapy. Discuss the three ways that these changes may impact on drug therapy causing an adverse drug reaction.

A. The physiological changes that are known to occur with ageing and may impact on drug therapy are: changes in homeostatic capacity, altered tissue responsiveness, reduced glomerular filtration rate, changes in hepatic function, reduction in organ mass, reduction *in coronary and organ blood flow and specific alterations in body composition. A drug may cause an adverse drug reaction through an increase in drug plasma concentration, an increase in the duration of drug action (i.e. the half-life) or an increase in the sensitivity of the body or specific organ to the drug.*

2. Why is serum creatinine unsuitable as an indicator of renal function in the aged. List five drugs which should be used with care in the aged with known or suspected reduced renal function.

A. Serum creatinine is not a good indicator of renal function in the aged because the older person is likely to have an altered body composition which may allow the creatinine to appear normal even in quite poor renal function. The creatinine clearance is a more accurate determinant of renal function. Drugs which should be used with care in the aged with known or suspected poor renal function are angiotensin converting enzyme inhibitors, allopurinol, aminoglycosides, acyclovir, cephalosporins, cimetidine, ciprofloxacin, digoxin, ethacrynic acid, lithium, metformin, methyldopa, nitrofurantoin, non-steroidal anti-inflammatory agents, norfloxacin, penicillins, quinidine, sulfonamides, tetracyclines, thiazide diuretics, triamterene, trimethoprim.

3. Why should the anticoagulant warfarin be administered with care in the aged?

A. Warfarin is highly protein bound which may make it more likely to be involved in drug interactions with other highly protein bound drugs; altered serum composition may change warfarin's disposition hence increasing its blood levels; the haemopoietic system may be more sensitive to warfarin and the incidence of bleeding increased.

4. Name the three mechanisms by which a drug may cause confusion as an adverse drug reaction.

A. A drug may cause confusion by crossing the blood brain barrier directly, by disturbing the extracellular environment, or through anticholinergic activity.

5. Mrs A is a 71-year old widow who has recently been exhibiting quite unusual behaviour. Her daughter is concerned about her mother's ability to remain independent and wishes to pursue nursing home admission arrangements. She fears the development of a dementing illness. Over the last two to three months Mrs A has become confused, easily fatigued and very irritable. She developed a disturbing obsessive/compulsive behaviour constantly complaining that her lace window curtains were dirty and required frequent washing. Detailed questioning revealed that she thought they were yellow-green and possibly mouldy. Her prescribed medications are: frusemide 40 mg daily in the morning; digoxin 250 micrograms daily; paracetamol 500 mg, 1–2 tablets 4-hourly when required; piroxicam 20 mg at night; *Mylanta* suspension, 20 mL when required; and *Coloxyl* 120 mg, 1–2 tablets at night.

(a) Consider how appropriate each drug and drug combination is for this patient. List five drug interactions, drug–disease interactions or administration factors to be considered in the review of Mrs A's medication.

(b) Which drug could be suspected of precipitating the confusion, fatigue and irritability? What other symptom could also be caused by this drug?

(c) What measures could be taken to improve Mrs A's compliance and maintain her independence?

A. (a) In the review of Mrs A's medication regimen the following points could be considered for further evaluation. It would appear that the dose of digoxin may be too high for a woman of this age. Digoxin is renally cleared. Digoxin can upset the stomach and should be administed after food. Piroxicam is a non-steroidal anti-inflammatory agent with a particularly long half-life. An agent with shorter action may be more appropriate. A drug interaction could potentially exist between Mylanta and digoxin if they are administered together. The combination of digoxin and frusemide may indicate the need for additional potassium supplementation. Low potassium levels in the body can cause fatigue. Piroxicam can cause fluid retention which may aggravate cardiac failure and increase the need for frusemide and digoxin. Mylanta is used to treat the upper gastrointestinal tract disorder of heartburn and acidity. Its use may be required due to this disorder being caused by piroxicam and/or digoxin. Both can irritate the stomach particularly if taken on an empty stomach.

(b) The sudden onset of confusion, fatigue and irritability could be linked to digoxin toxicity. Digoxin has a low therapeutic index and toxicity readily occurs if doses are too high or are not being cleared effectively. In the aged the normal symptoms of toxicity, such as nausea and vomiting, may be absent and replaced by symptoms occurring in the most vulnerable organ system, the central nervous system. The vision disturbance of yellow-green haze is characteristic of digoxin toxicity.

(c) To optimise Mrs A's quality of life and independence it is important, first to ensure that each medication and its dosage is appropriate and, second that she is able to comply with the regimen. To assist Mrs A we could provide education on the use and importance of each drug; enlist the aid of Mrs A's daughter; establish a medication card; establish compliance aids, e.g. Webster packing; ensure that other health professionals involved in Mrs A's care are aware of the identified problems and intervention plan; regularly review Mrs A's progress.

CHAPTER 7 DRUG SAFETY IN PREGNANCY AND LACTATION

1. Describe the mechanisms involved in drug transfer to the fetus. Which drugs will be more likely to accumulate in the fetal bloodstream?

A. While some substances are actively transported across the placenta by enzymatic reaction and pinocytosis, the majority are transferred by passive transport, some by facilitated diffusion where the size and shape of the molecule makes a contribution but for the most part by simple diffusion from an area of high concentration to that of low concentration. Drugs likely to accumulate in the fetal blood stream include alcohol, barbiturates, anaesthetic agents and phenothiazines.

2. List some of the drugs which should be avoided during early pregnancy.

A. Diethylstilboestrol, warfarin, isotretinoin, etretinate, tetracyclines, alcohol, iodides.

3. List those drugs which are contraindicated whilst breast feeding.

A. Phenindione anticoagulant, iodides and carbimazole, benzodiazepines (in low birthweight babies), chloramphenicol, ergot preparations, lithium compounds, oestrogens, radioactive preparations, sulfonamides.

CHAPTER 8 IMMUNISATION

1. Define immunity.

A. Immunity is a state of resistance or lessened susceptibility to infection. It may be innate or acquired.

2. What is an antigen?

A. *An antigen is a substance which induces the production of antibodies. It may be a protein, a polypeptide or a polysaccharide.*

3. What are antibodies?

A. *Antibodies are immunoglobulin molecules which react specifically with an antigen. They are produced by hosts in response to antigenic stimulation, usually from an infection.*

4. Describe (a) active immunity; (b) passive immunity.

A. *(a) Active immunity is induced by infection or immunisation. (b) Passive immunity is conferred by exogenous antibodies in the form of human immunoglobulin or heterologous antisera such as antitoxin or antivenom. Infants derive passive immunity by transplacental passage of maternal antibodies.*

5. Which is the drug of choice for the treatment of anaphylactic shock: adrenaline; an antihistamine; a corticosteroid?

A. *Adrenaline.*

CHAPTER 9 POISONINGS AND THEIR TREATMENT

1. List nine common groups of substances causing poisoning.

A. *The answer to this question could include a huge number of substances. Examples of common groups are analgesic drugs, respiratory system drugs, sedatives, antidepressants, opiates, cardiovascular drugs, pesticides, corrosives, cleaners, handyman products, venomous insects and animals.*

2. (a) List three initial steps in management of a poisoned patient. (b) Note exceptions to generalisations in 2(a).

A. *(a) Maintain vital functions; remove contact between poison and patient; treat symptomatically, administer specific antidote if available for specific toxin. (b) There are three important situations where gastric emptying and charcoal should NOT be used: following ingestion of corrosive substances or petroleum distillates or if the patient is convulsing.*

3. List two substances likely to cause serious delayed poisoning effects.

A. *Some substances causing delayed effects are paracetamol, sustained release preparations of theophylline and larger doses of carbamazepine and tricyclic antidepressants.*

4. For which of the following would you contact a Poisons Information Centre:

(a) advice on ingredients of a substance swallowed by an infant; (b) advice on how to manage a particular poisoning; (c) advice about a plant poisoning; (d) advice on where to send a redback spider.

A. *(a), (b), (c), (d). All enquiries listed could be answered by a Poisons Information Centre.*

5. List four poisons which have antidotes. Name the antidotes.

A. *See Table 9.5.*

6. The LD_{50} of a drug 'X' is said to be 700 mg/kg (oral, rats). The potential fatal dose in humans will be: (a) 700 mg/kg; (b) 1 g/kg; (c) 100 mg/kg; (d) cannot tell from data.

A. (d)

7. If a patient presents having ingested 700 mg/kg of drug 'X' referred to in the previous question they should be: (a) observed closely and are likely to have significant toxic effects; (b) sent home at once, 700 mg/kg in rats doesn't mean it will harm humans.

A. (a)

8. You are asked to prepare activated charcoal slurry for administration to a poisoned patient. The ratio of activated charcoal:water you should use is: (a) 1:1 (equal parts); (b) 1:5; (c) 1:8 to 1:10 (within this range); (d) 1:15 to 1:20 (within this range).

A. (c)

CHAPTER 10 DRUGS AND THE AUTONOMIC NERVOUS SYSTEM

1. Describe briefly: (a) the structure of the autonomic nervous system (ANS); (b) the role of cholinergic receptors and which transmitters are present; (c) the role of adrenergic receptors and which transmitters are present.

A. (a) The ANS consists of two sets of fibres, afferent and efferent, which integrate in the CNS. Afferent fibres bring information into the ANS. Efferent autonomic signals are transmitted to the body through two major subdivisions, the sympathetic and parasympathetic nervous systems. Stimulation of the sympathetic nervous system produces the 'fear, fright and flight' response; stimulation of the parasympathetic system generally produces opposite effects to sympathetic stimulation. The sympathetic system has long postganglionic fibres with many branches from the ganglia whereas the parasympathetic system has short postganglionic fibres with no branching after the ganglia. (b) Cholinergic receptors are of two types: nicotinic and muscarinic. Nicotinic receptors are mainly involved at ganglia and skeletal muscle junctions. Muscarinic receptors are mainly found in all effector cells stimulated by the postganglionic neurons of the parasympathetic nervous system. Acetylcholine is the transmitter. (c) Adrenergic receptors are involved in the postganglionic neurons of the sympathetic nervous system, either presynaptically or postsynaptically. There are two types of receptors: α and β. The transmitter is noradrenaline.

2. Define the following terms: (a) agonist; (b) antagonist; (c) parasympathomimetic; (d) anticholinergic.

A. (a) An agonist is an agent which acts on the receptor in a similar way to the transmitter present. (b) An antagonist is an agent which prevents the action of the transmitter at the receptor. (c) A parasympathomimetic stimulates muscarinic receptors or mimics the effect of postganglionic parasympathetic nerve stimulation. (d) An anticholinergic (or parasympatholytic) antagonises the effect of postganglionic parasympathetic nerve stimulation.

3. What is the response to sympathetic stimulation of the following organs: (a) heart; (b) lungs; (c) uterus?

(a) Sinus tachycardia, increased force of contraction of atria and ventricles. (b) Relaxation of tracheal and bronchial muscle. (c) Variable; stimulation of β_2 receptors will cause relaxation of the uterus.

4. What is the response to parasympathetic stimulation of the following organs: (a) intestine; (b) blood vessels; (c) heart?

A. *(a) Increased tone and motility, relaxation of sphincters and stimulation of secretions. (b) No effect on veins; dilation of arterioles except coronary arterioles which are constricted. (c) Decrease in heart rate, decreased AV conduction and decreased atrial contractility.*

5. Give two examples of drugs that have the following actions: (a) parasympathomimetic; (b) anticholinesterase; (c) sympathomimetic; (d) β adrenergic blocker; (e) α adrenergic blocker.

A. *(a) Pilocarpine, bethanechol, carbachol. (b) Neostigmine, pyridostigmine, edrophonium, distigmine, ecothiopate iodide, physostigmine salicylate. (c) Adrenaline, dobutamine, dopamine, ephedrine, fenoterol, isoprenaline, methoxamine, noradrenaline, orciprenaline, phenylephrine, ritodrine, salbutamol, terbutaline, tetrahydrazoline, tramazoline. (d) Propranolol, pindolol, timolol, alprenolol, sotalol, atenolol, metoprolol. (e) Tolazoline, phenoxybenzamine, phentolamine, prazosin.*

CHAPTER 11 RESPIRATORY DISEASES

1. Define the term bronchodilator and describe how drugs of this type are thought to produce their therapeutic effects.

A. *Bronchodilators are drugs used to increase the diameter of the small airways, primarily through the relaxation of bronchial smooth muscle.*

2. Provide examples of three separate types of bronchodilator drugs and briefly outline the various routes by which they may be administered.

A. *β agonists such as salbutamol, terbutaline and fenoterol work by stimulating β2 adrenoreceptors. These drugs may be given orally or intravenously, but are usually administered by inhalation (either by nebuliser or metered dose inhaler). Ipratropium bromide is an anticholinergic bronchodilator which is always administered by inhalation. Theophylline and its derivatives may be given intravenously, rectally or orally.*

3. Give three examples of drugs which are β2 agonists and describe the common adverse reactions observed with this class of drugs.

A. *Salbutamol, fenoterol, terbutaline, salmeterol and formoterol are all β2 agonists. Common adverse reactions include tremor, tachycardia, insomnia, anxiety and hypokalaemia.*

4. Outline the correct chronological order for the administration by inhalation of the following drugs: terbutaline, budesonide and ipratropium bromide.

A. *Terbutaline should be given first, followed by ipratropium and lastly budesonide.*

5. Provide examples of three drugs which may result in theophylline toxicity if administered concurrently with this agent.

A. *Cimetidine, erythromycin and ciprofloxacin are all capable of decreasing theophylline clearance and causing drug toxicity.*

6. Describe at least two situations in which the systemic administration of corticosteroid drugs may exert an important influence on the course of other intercurrent disease states.

A. *Steroids may destabilise blood glucose control in diabetes, exacerbate heart failure because of salt and water retention, prolong the healing of skin ulcers or cause weight gain which will negatively impact on a variety of disease states.*

7. Outline a range of adverse effects which might be expected to occur in patients treated with long-term oral corticosteroid therapy.

A. *Adverse effects include osteoporosis, peptic ulceration, anaemia, susceptibility to infection, depression, hirsutism, cataracts, proximal myopathy, friable skin, suppression of adrenal cortex.*

8. Give two examples of corticosteroid drugs which can be administered by inhalation.

A. *Beclomethasone and budenoside.*

9. List at least four factors which should be taken into account when selecting antibiotic therapy for the treatment of respiratory tract infections.

A. *Likely pathogen, local sensitivity patterns, site of acquisition (e.g. community or hospital), sputum penetration, drug interactions, history of allergy.*

10. Provide four examples of drug therapy which can produce adverse drug reactions which affect the respiratory tract.

A. *β blockers (e.g. propranolol) may cause asthma; aspirin and NSAIDs are known to cause bronchospasm in some patients; ACE inhibitors (e.g. lisinopril, enalapril) may cause cough or even anaphylaxis; allergies to drugs (e.g. penicillins, sulfonamides, contrast dye) may result in life threatening bronchospasm; other drugs (e.g. amiodarone, methotrexate) may produce adverse pulmonary effects which are not related to bronchospasm.*

CHAPTER 12 CARDIOVASCULAR DISEASES

1. Define the terms: (a) cardiac arrhythmia; (b) diuretic; (c) congestive cardiac failure.

A. *(a) Cardiac arrhythmia is a disturbance of the normal rhythm of the heart. There are a number of causes including abnormal SA node rhythm conduction blocks and ectopic foci generating premature beats.*
(b) Diuretics block the reabsorption of sodium within the kidney. This leads to decreased reabsorption of water resulting in increased formation of urine and reduction in oedema.
(c) Congestive cardiac failure is the inability of the heart to maintain adequate cardiac output when the body is at rest or undergoing normal activity.

2. Match the following drugs to the disease state in which they are used.

Drugs: Digoxin, sotalol, clofibrate, isosorbide dinitrate, frusemide.

Disease state: Oedema, angina pectoris, congestive cardiac failure, hyperlipidaemia, cardiac arrhythmias.

A. *Digoxin — congestive cardiac failure; sotalol — cardiac arrhythmias; clofibrate — hyperlipidaemia; isosorbide dinitrate — angina pectoris; frusemide — oedema.*

3. Match each of the following drugs to the side effect which may result from its use.

Drugs: Nicotinic acid, captopril, verapamil, procainamide, disopyramide.

Side effect: SLE syndrome, urinary retention, cough, flushing, constipation.

A. *Nicotinic acid — flushing; captopril — cough; verapamil — constipation; procainamide — SLE syndrome; disopyramide — urinary retention.*

4. Match each of the following drugs to its pharmacological class.

Drugs: Atenolol, chlorothiazide, diltiazem, enalapril, bumetanide, colestipol.

A. *Atenolol — β blocking drug; chlorothiazide — diuretic (thiazide); diltiazem — calcium channel blocker; enalapril — ACE inhibitor; bumetanide — diuretic (loop); colestipol — bile acid sequestrant.*

CHAPTER 13 BLOOD DISORDERS

1. List two examples of each of the following: (a) anticoagulants; (b) clotting agents; (c) fibrinolytic agents; (d) drugs affecting platelet function; (e) drugs affecting red cell growth.

A. *(a) Heparin, low molecular weight heparin, phenindione, warfarin, orgaron; (b) oxidised cellulose, thrombin; (c) streptokinase, urokinase, tissue plasminogen activator (tPA, alteplase), anistreplase; (d) aspirin, dipyridamole, sulfinpyrazone, ticlopidine; (e) erythropoietin, iron, folic acid, vitamin B_{12}.*

2. Name the antidotes for: (a) heparin; (b) warfarin.

A. *(a) protamine; (b) vitamin K.*

3. Describe the pharmacological actions of: (a) streptokinase; (b) thrombin; (c) low dose aspirin.

A. *(a) Streptokinase converts plasminogen to plasmin which then acts to degrade fibrin, fibrinogen and other proteins involved with clot formation; (b) thrombin activates the conversion of fibrinogen to fibrin which enhances clot formation; (c) in low doses aspirin inhibits the formation of thromboxane A_2 by inhibiting the enzyme prostaglandin cyclo-oxygenase.*

4. List the disease states in which the following drugs are used: (a) intravenous immunoglobulin; (b) vitamin B_{12}; (c) warfarin; (d) tranexamic acid; (e) G-CSF.

A. *(a) Primary and secondary hypogammaglobulinaemia, HITTS, ITP, other thrombocytopenias, prevention of specific infections; (b) pernicious anaemia, vitamin B_{12} deficiency; (c) treatment of DVTs and PE, prevention of clot formation after myocardial infarction, transient ischaemic attacks (TIAs), artificial heart valve and other prosthesis implantation, bacterial endocarditis; (d) tranexamic acid is used to decrease bleeding from extravascular sites following trauma or surgery (e.g. prostate or urinary tract surgery), to decrease excessive menstrual losses, to decrease gastrointestinal bleeding when the site cannot be identified, for prophylaxis before surgery in haemophiliacs; (e) G-CSF is used to decrease neutropenia associated with chemotherapy, bone marrow transplantation and other chronic neutropenias.*

5. What are the common adverse effects of (a) oral iron preparations; (b) heparin; (c) GM-CSF.

A. *(a) Nausea, black and 'tarry' stools, constipation, stained teeth (with liquid preparations); (b) bleeding, haematuria, epistaxis, petecchiae, internal haemorrhage, melaena, bruising etc, pruritus, fever, HITTS; (c) fever, headache, fluid retention, myalgias.*

6. List some of the drugs which interact with (a) warfarin; (b) iron.

A. *(a) Drugs which may increase the action of warfarin are: allopurinol, amiodarone, chloral hydrate, cimetidine, diflunisal, erythromycin, ibuprofen, indomethacin, ketoprofen, mefenamic acid, metronidazole, nalidixic acid, streptokinase, sulfonamides, sulindac, tetracyclines, thyroxine, tricyclic antidepressants. Drugs which may decrease the action of warfarin are: barbiturates, griseofulvin, rifampicin, oestrogens in oral contraceptives, sucralfate, vitamin K. (b) Tetracycline antibiotics, quinolone antibiotics (e.g. ciprofloxacin, norfloxacin).*

7. List the nursing implications in the use of: (a) dextran; (b) aminocaproic acid; (c) parenteral iron preparations.

A. (a) As an allergic reaction to dextran may occur soon after administration starts the patient should be observed closely at the commencement of the infusion. If a reaction develops the infusion should be stopped immediately. Resuscitation equipment, adrenaline, corticosteroids and antihistamines should be readily available. If dextran 1 is used it should be given 15 minutes before commencing the dextran 40 or 70 infusion. The two infusions should not be given at the same time. The patient should be monitored for signs of volume expansion and overload, e.g. increased pulse and respiratory rates, wheezing, shortness of breath. Renal function should be checked before infusions are commenced. If impairment is found, therapy may have to be decreased or discontinued. (b) Renal function should be measured and the dose altered accordingly. Patients are often very worried and anxious about blood loss. Accurate assessment of any blood loss is essential. Doses can be high and the patient may find it easier to take a liquid rather than a large number of tablets. If an oral formulation of aminocaproic acid is not available the IV form can be substituted in an emergency. The reverse does not apply. Infusions of aminocaproic acid must be given slowly to minimise the risk of bradycardia or cardiac arrhythmias. Continuous assessment of blood loss and checking for signs of hypercoagulation is necessary. Renal function should be monitored as renal impairment is an indication for reduction in dose. (c) Intramuscular injection of iron can be very painful. To avoid staining the skin a 'Z' track injection technique should be used. The dose should be split between the two buttocks. Once the haemoglobin level has returned to normal, patients feel much better and may be tempted to stop therapy. They should be reminded of the need to continue therapy to replace body stores of iron. Organ damage from excess iron levels should be evaluated and appropriate therapy given.

CHAPTER 14 DRUGS USED IN RENAL FAILURE

1. Name one drug which is commonly used to treat hypocalcaemia in patients with renal osteodystrophy.

A. Calcitriol.

2. What are the indications for use of aluminium hydroxide and/or calcium carbonate, and what is their main side effect?

A. To reduce serum phosphate concentration. Calcium carbonate can also be used as a calcium supplement and to reduce metabolic acidosis. Constipation is the main side effect of both agents.

3. Name two drugs which may be used to treat hyperkalaemia.

A. Sodium bicarbonate; glucose (and insulin); polystyrene resins; salbutamol.

4. Are diuretics of any value in the treatment of hypertension in patients with renal failure?

A. Diuretics are of limited value.

5. Should potassium sparing diuretics be administered to patients with renal failure?

A. No, they can cause fatal hyperkalaemia.

6. What is the most common adverse reaction of erythropoietin. List two other reported adverse reactions.

A. Hypertension. Hyperkalaemia; flu-like symptoms, seizures; skin reactions; clotting of arteriovenous fistulae and shunts.

7. Name three commonly used immunosuppressive agents and list their main side effects.

A. *Prednisolone: infections, Cushingoid appearance (high dose), peptic ulceration, sodium and fluid retention, hypertension, osteoporosis, poor wound healing, cataracts.*

Azathioprine: leucopenia, red cell aplasia, thrombocytopenia, megaloblastic anaemia.

Cyclosporin: nephrotoxicity, hypertension, hyperkalaemia, hepatotoxicity.

8. Name two drugs which require modification of dosage regimen when administered to patients with renal failure.

A. *Allopurinol; amikacin; amphotericin B; antacids containing magnesium; cefotaxime; cefoxitin; ceftazidime; cimetidine; digoxin; flucytosine; gentamicin; methotrexate; netilmicin; potassium salts; procainamide; tobramycin; trimethoprim–sulfamethoxazole; vancomycin.*

CHAPTER 15 DRUGS USED IN BLADDER DYSFUNCTION

1. List: (a) the types of drugs which can be used to relax the bladder; (b) the indications for the use of such agents; (c) what precautions need to be taken?

A. *(a) Anticholinergic agents, tricyclic antidepressants, β adrenergic sympathomimetic agents, calcium channel blockers, smooth muscle relaxants. (b) Detrusor instability, neurogenic bladder dysfunction, leakage around an indwelling catheter, to improve bladder capacity and compliance in intermittent catheterisation and neurogenic bladder.*
(c) Overdosage causing retention, bladder outlet obstruction, myasthenia gravis and glaucoma, elderly patients.

2. How may the detrusor be stimulated? Under what circumstances are such agents: (a) indicated; (b) dangerous; (c) unhelpful?

A. *With cholinergic agents. (a) Ineffective or inadequate bladder contractions causing voiding problems. (b) Bladder outlet obstruction. (c) When the bladder is incapable of contraction (i.e. acontractile).*

3. What types of drugs can cause urinary retention?

A. *Anticholinergic agents, tricyclic antidepressants (but not tetracyclic antidepressants), calcium channel blockers, ganglion blockers, anaesthetic agents, opioids, α adrenergic agents.*

4. List: (a) the drugs which can be used to lower bladder outlet resistance; (b) their indications; (c) their side effects.

A. *(a) α adrenergic blockers, striated muscle relaxants. (b) Temporary relief of obstruction whilst awaiting surgery; mild bladder neck obstruction in younger male patients who wish to retain fertility; mild sphincter dyssynergia in neuropathic bladder. (c) Incontinence, hypotension, loss of seminal emission and ejaculation.*

CHAPTER 16 LIVER DISEASES

1. What is the most commonly expected adverse effect on commencing interferon treatment and how can it be managed?

A. *Flu-like illness occurs in most patients. The symptoms may be relieved with paracetamol or aspirin.*

2. What is the treatment of choice for hepatitis A infection?

A. *There is no treatment, only supportive measures until the episode spontaneously resolves.*

3. (a) Into which muscle should hepatitis B vaccine be given for adults? (b) At what interval should the doses be given?

A. *(a) Deltoid muscle. (b) Initial, 1 month later and 6 months later.*

4. What is the theory behind the use of lactulose in hepatic encephalopathy?

A. *To help decrease the blood ammonia levels by promoting excretion from the bowel and inhibiting ammonia producing bacteria in the colon.*

5. What dose of spironolactone is used to treat ascites?

A. *100–400 mg daily. Doses greater than 100 mg should be given as divided doses.*

CHAPTER 17 GASTROINTESTINAL DISORDERS

1. Name three drugs from different chemical classes which can be used to heal peptic ulcers.

A. *i. Mylanta, Aludrox, Gastrogel, Gaviscon, Mucaine; ii. cimetidine, ranitidine, famotidine, nizatidine; iii. misoprostol; iv. omeprazole; v. sucralfate, bismuth.*

2. By which route should vancomycin be given when used to treat *Clostridium difficile* associated diarrhoea?

A. *Oral route.*

3. Name two drugs, the clearance of which can be reduced by the concomitant administration of cimetidine.

A. *Theophylline, warfarin, phenytoin.*

4. What ongoing monitoring should be instituted for patients taking sulfasalazine or azathioprine.

A. *Complete blood picture.*

5. Metoclopramide, domperidone and cisapride are all referred to as prokinetic agents. Explain the meaning of the term prokinetic.

A. *Drugs which increase gastric motility.*

6. Describe the mechanism whereby non-steroidal anti-inflammatory drugs damage gastric mucosa.

A. *Systemic inhibition of prostaglandins I_2 and E_2.*

7. Which of the three currently available 5-aminosalicylic acid derivatives used to treat inflammatory bowel disease should not be given to patients sensitive to sulfonamide drugs?

A. *Sulfasalazine.*

8. What effect does the administration of metronidazole have on anticoagulation status of patients taking warfarin?

A. *It increases the anticoagulant effect.*

9. Do tricyclic antidepressants cause diarrhoea or constipation?

A. Constipation.

10. Describe the mechanism of action of omeprazole. Does it suppress acid output to a greater or lesser extent than that achieved with the H_2 receptor antagonists?

A. Omeprazole inhibits hydrogen ion release from the proton pump within the parietal cell. Greater acid suppression can be achieved with omeprazole compared with that obtained with the H_2 receptor antagonists.

CHAPTER 18 FLUID AND ELECTROLYTE DISORDERS

1. The water content of a 70-kg 25-year old male is approximately: (a) 7 L; (b) 28 L; (c) 42 L; (d) 63 L.

A. (c)

2. The most abundant electrolytes of the extracellular space are: (a) sodium and chloride; (b) sodium and potassium; (c) sodium and calcium; (d) chloride and potassium.

A. (a)

3. The most abundant electrolyte of the intracellular space is: (a) sodium; (b) potassium; (c) calcium; (d) phosphate.

A. (b)

4. An isotonic solution has: (a) the same osmolality as plasma; (b) the same concentration of potassium as plasma; (c) the same concentration of sodium as plasma; (d) an osmolality of approximately 290 mosmol per kg.

A. (a) and (d)

5. The electrolyte sodium is: (a) a cation; (b) primarily involved with regulation of the water balance of the ICF; (c) primarily involved with bone formation; (d) primarily involved with blood clotting.

A. (a)

6. A patient who is volume depleted may have: (a) increased pulse, decreased urine output and thirst; (b) increased pulse, normal urine output and hypertension; (c) decreased pulse, normal urine output and hypertension; (d) decreased pulse, decreased urine output and hypertension.

A. (a)

7. The following solutions are all crystalloids: (a) 0.9% NaCl in water, Hartmann's solution, 5% albumin; (b) 0.9% NaCl in water, Hartmann's solution, 'Haemaccel'; (c) fresh frozen plasma, dextran 40 in 0.9% NaCl, 5% glucose; (d) 0.9% NaCl in water, 0.9% NaCl + 30 mmol KCl in water, Hartmann's solution.

A. (d)

8. A 70-kg 40-year old healthy male has had an uncomplicated hiatus hernia repair. A suitable IV regimen for use in the 24-hour nil by mouth period after operation might be: (a) 1 L Hartmann's over 24 hours; (b) 3 L 5% glucose, each litre over 8 hours; (c) 1 L Hartmann's over 8 hours, 1 L 0.9% NaCl + 30 mmol KCl over 8 hours, 1 L 5% glucose + 30 mmol KCl over 8 hours; (d) 500 mL dextran 40 in 0.9% NaCl over 1 hour, then 1 L 0.9% NaCl and 10 mmol KCl over 23 hours.

A. (c)

9. A 50-kg 70-year old female with chronic renal failure and congestive cardiac failure has had an uncomplicated hysterectomy. A suitable IV regimen for use in the 24-hour nil by mouth period after operation might be: (a) 1 L Hartmann's over 6 hours, then 3 L 5% glucose each litre over 6 hours; (b) 1 L 4% glucose + 0.18% NaCl with 60 mmol KCl over 24 hours; (c) 1 L Hartmann's over 12 hours then 1 L 5% glucose over 12 hours; (d) 500 mL 0.9% NaCl + 60 mmol KCl over 24 hours.

A. (c)

10. Part of the treatment of metabolic alkalosis might include: (a) infusion of 500 mL 8.4% sodium bicarbonate over 1 hour; (b) infusion of 1 L 0.9% NaCl + KCl over 8 hours; (c) rebreathing into a bag; (d) infusion of 30 mL neutral insulin in 1 L 5% glucose over 24 hours.

A. (b)

CHAPTER 19 ENDOCRINE DISEASES

1. Which of the following drugs are used in the treatment of acromegaly: octreotide, somatrem, norethisterone, bromocriptine, desmopressin?

A. Octreotide, bromocriptine.

2. Tetracosactrin is an analogue of which of the following hormones: oestrogen, testosterone, corticotropin, triiodothyronine, glucagon?

A. Corticotropin.

3. Which of the following statements are true: (a) Thyroxine is the active thyroid hormone in the body. (b) Intolerance to cold is a symptom of thyroxine overdose. (c) Propylthiouracil is used in the treatment of myxoedema coma. (d) Triiodothyronine can be given parenterally. (e) Thyroxine administration may enhance the action of warfarin.

A. (d) and (e).

4. Which of the following drugs are sulfonylurea oral hypoglycaemics: tolbutamide, oestriol, glipizide, metformin, glucagon?

A. Tolbutamide, glipizide.

5. Which of the following statements is true: (a) Insulin is effective if given by mouth. (b) Insulin should be stored under refrigeration. (c) Metformin is given by subcutaneous injection. (d) Metformin is used to treat NIDDM (type 2 diabetes). (e) Glibenclamide is a biguanide oral hypoglycaemic.

A. (b) and (d).

6. Which of the following drugs are used in the treatment of androgen deficiency: methyltestosterone, medroxyprogesterone acetate, bromocriptine, cyproterone acetate, mesterolone?

A. Methyltestosterone, mesterolone.

7. Sodium and water retention is a side effect of which of the following drugs: oestriol, fludrocortisone: mesterolone, insulin, chlorpropamide?

A. Oestriol, fludrocortisone, mesterolone.

8. Which of the following drugs are corticosteroids: hydrocortisone, aminoglutethimide, oxymetholone, betamethasone, prednisolone?

A. Hydrocortisone, betamethasone, prednisolone.

9. Which of the following are adverse effects of corticosteroid therapy: (a) Salt and water retention. (b) Hypoglycaemia. (c) Intolerance to heat. (d) Muscle weakness. (e) Skin atrophy.

A. (a), (d) and (e).

10. Which of the following drugs are used in the treatment of hyperadrenalism: aminoglutethimide, oestradiol, carbimazole, mitotane, mefenamic acid?

A. Aminoglutethimide, mitotane.

CHAPTER 20 DRUG THERAPY IN PREGNANCY AND LABOUR

1. List the drugs used prophylactically to prevent pre-eclampsia.

A. Low dose heparin, low dose aspirin.

2. What drugs should be avoided in the treatment of pre-eclamptic hypertension?

A. Diuretics and ACE inhibitors such as captopril, enalapril.

3. What are the two important side effects of continuous heparin therapy during pregnancy?

A. Continuous use of heparin during pregnancy may increase the risk of heparin induced thrombocytopenia and bone demineralisation resulting in osteoporosis.

4. What are the vitamin preparations that may be used during pregnancy in women taking antiepileptic drugs?

A. Folic acid and vitamin K in those women taking phenytoin, primidone and phenobarbitone.

5. Why is human insulin usually chosen for use in pregnant diabetic women who require insulin?

A. Exposure to insulin derived from animal sources, especially beef insulin, may lead to the development of anti-insulin antibodies.

6. Which drugs when used for treatment of pregnancy associated conditions may interfere with control of asthma?

A. β blocking agents. The non-selective β blockers, e.g. propranolol and pindolol, are more likely to induce bronchospasm than the cardioselective β blockers, e.g. atenolol and metoprolol.

7. Discuss the use of drugs in premature labour at 30 weeks gestation.

A. Drugs used in premature labour include drugs used to inhibit uterine contractions and corticosteroids to mature the fetal lung. The β sympathomimetic agents, salbutamol, terbutaline and ritodrine, are the drugs most commonly used to inhibit uterine contractions. Initial administration is by intravenous infusion and the rate of infusion is slowly increased until contractions have ceased. Side effects include increased maternal and fetal heart rate, hyper- or hypotension. Maternal blood pressure and heart rate and fetal heart rate need to be monitored. Other drugs that may be used to inhibit labour when β sympathomimetic agents cannot be used are indomethacin and nifedipine.

Corticosteroids administered to the mother have been shown to mature the fetal lung. Two doses of betamethasone are given at 12-hour intervals by intramuscular injection.

8. Which drugs can be used to induce uterine contractions in normal labour?

A. For controlled induction of labour, synthetic oxytocin and prostaglandins may be administered. At the completion of labour the oxytocic drugs oxytocin and ergometrine are used routinely to prevent postpartum haemorrhage.

9. What other drugs are commonly used at the time of delivery and why?

A. Phenothiazines such as chlorpromazine, promethazine and prochlorperazine are used as adjuncts to pain relief in labour, as well as for sedation and treatment of nausea. Metoclopramide is used as an antiemetic, and recently, to assist in the promotion of lactation. Lignocaine is used for local anaesthesia prior to episiotomy. Lignocaine, bupivacaine and mepivacaine are used for epidural anaesthesia. Narcotics, especially pethidine, are used for pain relief during labour and following caesarean section.

CHAPTER 21 CONTRACEPTION AND INFERTILITY

1. List the main female hormones and describe the role of these hormones in the normal ovarian cycle.

A. The two principal female sex hormones are oestrogen and progesterone. Oestrogen is produced throughout the entire menstrual cycle and is responsible for the regrowth of the lining of the uterus after each menstruation (the proliferative phase). Oestrogen is necessary to stimulate the endometrium just prior to its conversion to a secretory state. Progesterone is produced from the ruptured egg follicle (the corpus luteum) after ovulation, and is therefore present only in the latter half of the menstrual cycle. It is responsible for maintaining pregnancy and is mainly involved in the secretory phase of the menstrual cycle.

2. What types of contraceptive 'pill' are available, and what factors would determine the type of pill chosen for a particular patient?

A. There are basically two types of contraceptive pills, the combined oestrogen/ progestagen pill and the 'mini-pill' or progestagen-only pill. The combined pill is available in fixed strength and variable strength (biphasic and triphasic) combinations. Factors to consider in choosing a pill for a particular woman are age, length of menses, length of cycle, breast size, fat and hair distribution, history of acne, lactation, and any history of thrombosis or smoking. The logical starting point is a low-dose balanced triphasic formulation. If there is history of acne or hirsutism a more oestrogenic biphasic preparation may be appropriate. If irregular bleeding is a problem, then a low-dose fixed formulation may be appropriate. The mini-pill is used in the immediate postpartum period for lactating mothers and in oestrogen intolerance (e.g. smokers over 35 years, hypertensive patients and patients with a history of thrombosis).

3. Which of the following are adverse effects of oestrogen? Acne, depression, weight gain, leucorrhoea, hypertension, water retention, migraine, leg cramps, thrombosis, breakthrough bleeding.

A. Leucorrhoea, hypertension, water retention, migraine, leg cramps, thrombosis.

4. What are some of the possible causes of 'pill failure'?

A. Malabsorption (e.g. due to diarrhoea, vomiting); induction of hepatic microsomal enzymes (e.g. by anticonvulsant drugs or rifampicin); interruption of normal enterohepatic cycling of oestrogens (e.g. by broad spectrum antibiotics).

5. List the main drugs available for treatment of female infertility .

A. Oestrogen and/or progesterone; clomiphene; bromocriptine; danazol; gonadotrophins (HCG, menotrophin, urofollitrophin).

CHAPTER 22 MUSCULOSKELETAL DISORDERS

1. Which of the following drugs are used in musculoskeletal diseases: pheniramine, aspirin, ibuprofen, chlorthalidone, indomethacin, penicillamine, phenmetrazine?

A. Aspirin, ibuprofen, indomethacin, penicillamine.

2. List one disease state for which the following drugs are used: (a) sodium aurothiomalate, (b) lignocaine, (c) methyl salicylate, (d) baclofen, (e) probenecid, (f) naproxen.

A. (a) Rheumatoid arthritis; (b) haemorrhoids, anal or genital pruritus; (c) chronic inflammation, fibrositis, neuralgia; (d) multiple sclerosis, spinal cord lesions; (e) gout; (f) rheumatoid arthritis, osteoarthritis.

3. List two adverse effects often seen with the following drugs: (a) indomethacin, (b) baclofen, (c) colchicine, (d) sulindac.

A. (a) Gastrointestinal symptoms, blood dyscrasias, CNS effects (headache, vertigo, lightheadedness, confusion, hallucinations, depression, psychosis); (b) gastrointestinal symptoms, musculoskeletal system effects (asthenia, muscle weakness, hypotonia, muscle incoordination, tremors), CNS effects (daytime sedation, lethargy, vertigo, headache, dizziness); (c) nausea, abdominal discomfort, vomiting, diarrhoea; (d) constipation, diarrhoea, nausea, epigastric pain.

4. Write brief notes on the nursing implications for the use of: (a) non-steroidal anti-inflammatory drugs (NSAIDs), (b) drugs used for the treatment of gout, (c) topical enzyme preparations.

(a) Most NSAIDs are better tolerated if given with or after food. Assess patient's history for peptic disease and for other medications to determine any potential interactions. A history of renal or hepatic impairment and blood dyscrasias should be noted. Patients taking high doses of aspirin should be monitored closely for toxicity.
(b) Most drugs used in the treatment of gout should be given with food to reduce gastric irritation. Observe patients for changes in joint pain, swelling and frequency of attacks. A history of renal or liver impairment should be noted.
(c) Clean and debride area to be treated as necessary. Avoid healthy skin when applying and apply at least once daily. Document progress and note allergic reactions.

5. List four drugs or drug groups with actions that may be altered by concomitant administration of aspirin.

A. Anticoagulants (e.g. warfarin), antidiabetic agents, methotrexate, valproic acid, uricosuric agents, corticosteroids, antacids, alcohol.

CHAPTER 23 PAIN RELIEF

1. Define the terms analgesic and antipyretic.

A. An analgesic is a drug which alleviates pain. An antipyretic is a drug which prevents or allays fever.

2. What are the major contraindications to paracetamol?

A. Impaired kidney and liver function.

3. List the uses of codeine.

A. Pain relief (especially pain of visceral origin); somatic pain (usually combined with aspirin or paracetamol); severe diarrhoea (due to its constipating effect); and cough suppression (however, pholcodine is now mainly used).

4. What advice would you give to a patient who has been prescribed dextropropoxyphene?

A. That the drug should not be taken with alcohol as the CNS effects of both may be potentiated and that constipation may be a problem.

5. List the naturally occurring opium derivatives commonly used and the synthetic opioids.

A. The opium derivatives include morphine, codeine and papaveratum; the synthetic narcotics include pethidine, methadone, dextromoramide, oxycodone and pentazocine.

6. State the nursing implications of giving narcotic drugs.

A. The type and frequency of pain should be documented as an aid in assessing the pain; the patient should be observed for signs of pain (e.g. increased pulse and respiration rate, facial expression, posture, guarding muscular action, restlessness, sweating, pallor); legal requirements for administration of narcotics (e.g. entry of dose in drug register) should be adhered to.

7. To which class of drug does ketorolac belong? Where and how does this class of drug exert its effect?

A. Ketoralac is a non-steroidal anti-inflammatory (NSAID) which is more effective as a pain reliever than as an anti-inflammatory agent. It acts peripherally by inhibiting prostaglandins.

8. State the most important principles for the use of analgesia in the patient requiring palliative care.

A. i. Analgesia should be continuous and sufficient to keep the patient as pain free as possible (therapy for breakthrough pain should also be available). ii. Laxatives should be commenced at the beginning of opioid therapy to avoid the discomfort of constipation. iii. As the disease progresses other symptoms (e.g. nausea, dry or painful mouth, dysphasia, anorexia, insomnia) should be treated to keep the patient as comfortable as possible.

CHAPTER 24 DRUGS USED IN ANAESTHESIA

I. Isoflurane and enflurane are examples of commonly used volatile anaesthetic agents. True or false?

A. True.

2. Most volatile agents are extremely inflammable. True or false?

A. False.

3. Giving a patient 100% nitrous oxide is a common way to give the drug. True or false?

A. False.

4. Halothane is known to occasionally have an adverse effect on the liver and cause a form of hepatitis. True or false?

A. True.

5. The duration of action of suxamethonium is about 30 minutes. True or false?

A. False.

6. Muscle twitching (fasciculations) is usually observed after the administration of atracurium. True or false?

A. True.

7. Most skeletal muscle relaxant drugs used today are of the depolarising type. True or false?

A. False.

8. The duration of action of thiopentone injection is short. This is because it is rapidly metabolised by the liver. True or false?

A. False.

9. Accidental injection of thiopentone into an artery can result in major complications such as gangrene and limb loss. True or false?

A. True.

10. Peripheral nerve stimulators are a useful way of monitoring the effectivness of skeletal muscle relaxants. True or false?

A. True.

11. Local anaesthetics can be divided into two chemical groups, the esters and amides. True or false?

A. True.

12. Pain, light touch, pressure and movement are all equally affected by injection of local anaesthetic agents. True or false?

A. False.

13. Adrenaline is added to some local anaesthetic preparations to increase their duration of action. True or false?

A. True.

14. Preparations containing lignocaine and adrenaline should not be used to anaesthetise fingers and toes. True or false?

A. True.

15. Large doses of local anaesthetic agents if accidentally given intravenously can cause cardiac arrhythmias and convulsions. True or false?

A. True.

16. Muscle aches and pains are common after using vecuronium. True or false?

A. False.

17. Papaveretum and hyoscine are sometimes used together as a premedication. True or false?

A. True.

18. Isoflurane can be safely administered from a halothane vapouriser. True or false?

A. False.

19. Ether is (a) no longer used in Australia; (b) highly flammable; (c) a volatile anaesthetic; (d) still used in some overseas countries; or (e) all of the above.

A. (e).

20. Propofol (a) is dissolved in water in the ampoule; (b) causes unconsciousness for about 1 hour after a single injection; (c) sometimes causes pain on injection; (d) has the trade name *Hypnovel*; or (e) all of the above.

A. (c).

21. Flumazenil reverses action of drugs such as (a) diazepam (benzodiazepines); (b) morphine (opiates); (c) thiopentone (barbiturates); or (d) general anaesthetic agents.

A. (a).

22. Local anaesthetics act by (a) increasing the movement of sodium into the neurone; (b) decreasing the movement of sodium into the neurone; (c) increasing the movement of potassium into the neurone; (d) decreasing the movement of potassium into the neurone; or (e) primarily affecting calcium movement.

A. (b).

23. The transmitter chemical at the neuromuscular junction is (a) noradrenaline; (b) adrenaline; (c) nicotine; (d) muscarine; or (e) acetylcholine.

A. (e).

24. Which of the following side effects is not associated with morphine use (a) histamine release; (b) sedation; (c) nausea; (d) hypertension; or (e) vomiting.

A. (d).

25. Neostigmine acts by (a) increasing the amount of acetylcholine at the neuromuscular junction; (b) increasing the amount of noradrenaline at the neuromuscular junction; (c) decreasing the amount of acetylcholine at the neuromuscular junction; (d) decreasing the amount of noradrenaline at the neuromuscular junction; or (e) increasing the concentrations of both noradrenaline and acetylcholine at the neuromuscular junction.

A. (a).

CHAPTER 25 NEUROLOGICAL DISORDERS

1. Define the term 'epilepsy'.

A. Epilepsy is a disorder of the central nervous system in which an uncontrolled discharge from brain cells results in transient episodes of unconsciousness or psychic function with or without convulsive movements.

2. List extracranial factors which may lead to secondary epilepsy.

A. Extracranial factors include anoxia; poisons (e.g. alcohol, ethyl chloride, lead, cocaine); metabolic disturbances (e.g. uraemia, alkalosis, liver failure, hypoglycaemia); withdrawal of medications (e.g. hypnotics, opiates).

3. List three drugs used in the treatment of major seizures and complex partial seizures.

A. *Phenytoin, carbamazepine, sodium valproate, clonazepam, phenobarbitone, clobazam, methylphenobarbitone, primidone, vigabatrin, lamotrigine.*

4. State the nursing implications of giving phenytoin by IV injection.

A. *It is extremely important that IV injection be given slowly at a constant rate of not more than 50 mg per minute. Deaths have occurred from too rapid injection of phenytoin.*

5. What is the new terminology for classical and common migraine?

A. *Migraine with aura, and migraine without aura.*

6. Describe three classes of drugs used in the long-term management of migraine and list the drugs in each class.

A. *Drugs which alter catecholamine action: clonidine, β blockers (e.g. propranolol, pindolol), tricyclic antidepressants (e.g. amitriptyline), MAOIs (only used when other therapy has failed because of potential problems); antiserotonin drugs: cyproheptadine, methdilazine, pizotifen, methysergide; miscellaneous: phenytoin, anxiolytics (e.g. benzodiazepines).*

7. List the drugs used in an acute attack of migraine.

A. *Soluble aspirin or soluble paracetamol; antiemetic (e.g. metoclopramide); ergotamine; sumatriptan.*

8. What is the new drug used in the treatment of migraine?

A. *Sumatriptan.*

9. State any nursing implications of drugs used in migraine.

A. *The use of most of the drugs (excluding the analgesics) causes vasoconstriction. It is important to notice and report any non-transient claudication, coldness of extremities (gangrene is a danger from prolonged peripheral vasoconstriction), nausea, vomiting, anorexia, backache, chest pain or depression. Ensure the patient learns to rise slowly from the lying position to avoid postural hypotension.*

10. Why may it be of benefit to give IM metoclopramide 10 minutes before other medication in the acute migraine attack?

A. *To overcome gut stasis occurring during migraine, i.e. to restore peristalsis and so overcome the dumping effect of any other recently taken drugs such as analgesics.*

11. What adverse effect does prolonged use of ergotamine have?

A. *Prolonged use may give rise to gangrene.*

12. Describe Parkinson's disease.

A. *Parkinson's disease is a chronic, slowly progressive nervous disorder characterised by muscular rigidity, tremors, drooling, restlessness, shuffling gait and other neurological symptoms.*

13. Describe how a decarboxylase inhibitor added to levodopa benefits the patient.

A. *The decarboxylase inhibitor prevents the peripheral breakdown of levodopa by the enzyme decarboxylase. A much smaller dose of levodopa is required than when levodopa is given alone resulting in less dose related side effects for the patient.*

14. List other drugs used in Parkinsonism.

A. *Selegiline hydrochloride, amantadine, bromocriptine, anticholinergics (benzhexol, biperidine, benztropine, orphenadrine, procyclidine).*

CHAPTER 26 PSYCHIATRIC DISORDERS

1. It is advisable to recommend the use of a sunscreen agent to patients taking which one of the following drugs: methaqualone, chlorpromazine, benztropine, droperidol, temazepam, lithium carbonate?

A. Chlorpromazine.

2. Tardive dyskinesia is an adverse reaction brought about by which two of the following drugs: lithium carbonate, oxazepam, chlorpromazine, perphenazine, chlordiazepoxide, trimipramine, doxepin, amitriptyline?

A. Chlorpromazine, perphenezine.

3. With which of the following drugs should tyramine rich foods be avoided: amitriptyline, tranylcypromine, phenelzine, haloperidol, thioridazine?

A. Tranylcypromine, phenelzine.

4. A 52-year-old process worker presents with a 6-month history of insomnia. There is no history of anxiety or depressive illness. The physician decides to prescribe a hypnotic drug. Which of the following would be the most suitable drug: nitrazepam, oxazepam, temazepam, chlorpromazine, chloral hydrate? Give the reasons for your choice.

A. Temazepam as it is a short acting hypnotic which is safe in overdose.

5. Why is the antiparkinsonian agent L-dopa unsuitable for counteracting extrapyramidal side effects caused by chlorpromazine?

A. Because L-dopa may antagonise the antipsychotic action of chlorpromazine (it increases the available dopamine). Also, L-dopa can produce hallucinations and lowered blood pressure even in patients with Parkinson's disease and these effects would not be desirable in psychotic patients.

6. A 45-year-old manic depressive patient who has had uneventful lithium carbonate therapy for seven years develops the following symptoms: lethargy, confusion and a slight tremor of the hands. On taking a history the psychiatrist discovers that in recent months the patient has been placed on the following therapy: glibenclamide 5 mg in the morning for mild diabetes and methyldopa 250 mg three times daily and chlorothiazide 500 mg in the morning for hypertension. Which of the newly prescribed drugs may have caused the patient's symptoms and by what mechanism?

A. Chlorthiazide, a thiazide diuretic, reduces the renal clearance of lithium. In this case the increased plasma lithium concentration is revealed by lethargy, confusion and the slight hand tremor; all are signs of lithium toxicity.

7. Antipsychotic agents are useful in the treatment of insomnia and anxiety states. Is this statement true or false?

A. False.

8. Methylphenidate is used for the treatment of which two of the following conditions: manic depressive illness, narcolepsy, childhood hyperkinetic states, tardive dyskinesia?

A. Narcolepsy, childhood hyperkinetic states.

9. Tricyclic antidepressants are most useful in the treatment of which one of the following types of depression: depression associated with manic depressive illness, major depressive illness, depression secondary to organic brain disease, depression secondary to personal loss?

A. Major depressive illness.

10. Describe the nursing procedure you would follow after the administration of an intravenous dose of diazepam.

A. Monitor vital signs, noting any hypotension, tachycardia, respiratory depression or muscle weakness.

CHAPTER 27 EYE DISORDERS

1. What is the action of homatropine on the eye?

A. Mydriatic (dilates the pupil) and cycloplegic (paralyses accommodation).

2. Name two ocular and two systemic side effects of atropine.

A. (a) Photophobia, increased intraocular pressure, redness, swelling; (b) dry mouth, hallucinations, nausea, tachycardia, restlessness, confusion.

3. What are the main contraindications for timolol?

A. Asthma and severe heart disease.

4. What are the side effects of *Diamox*?

A. Nausea, diarrhoea, hypokalaemia, tingling of the extremities.

5. Which drop should be instilled first: (a) adrenaline or pilocarpine; (b) adrenaline or timolol?

A. (a) Pilocarpine; (b) adrenaline.

6. How long should you keep eye drops (a) with preservative and (b) without preservative, once opened?

A. (a) 28 days for an outpatient, 7 days for an inpatient; (b) 3 days under refrigeration.

7. When is fluorouracil used as a subconjunctival injection?

A. To stop formation of scar tissue after a filtering operation for glaucoma.

8. Give the name of an antifungal eye drop and its dosage.

A. Natamycin 5% eye drops every 1–2 hours.

9. What are the storage requirements for cephalothin eye drops?

A. Refrigeration.

10. What is the dosage of acyclovir tablets in herpes zoster ophthalmicus?

A. 800 mg five times a day.

CHAPTER 28 SKIN DISEASES

1. A cream consists of: (a) an oily substance dispersed in water; (b) an aqueous substance dispersed in oil; (c) a white powder evenly suspended in an aqueous vehicle; (d) (a) and (b); (e) (a), (b), and (c).

A. (d) A cream is an emulsion and may consist of oil globules dispersed in water (an oil in water emulsion) or water globules dispersed in an oily medium (a water in oil emulsion).

2. Photosensitivity is: (a) an abnormal fear of being photographed; (b) a burn caused by contact with photographic chemicals; (c) damage to the skin as a result of exposure to sunlight or artificial light.

A. (c).

3. The doctor has ordered betamethasone cream to be applied to a small weeping lesion on the patient's arm. You are unable to obtain cream but can obtain betamethasone ointment. What is likely to be the effect on the lesion if you use it?

A. Ointments do not absorb secretions and form a protective coating over the skin. Drying (and therefore healing) of the lesion is prevented and the skin may become soft and 'mushy'.

4. A friend asks for advice about the 'tinea' lesion between her toes. The lesion is red and weeping and the skin is cracked. Would it be better to apply an antifungal powder or cream? Why?

A. Cream. Powder in contact with secretions may absorb moisture and form coarse granules which will cause further irritation to an already painful lesion. A cream will absorb moisture but remain soft. When the lesion has healed an antifungal powder may be used to prevent reinfection.

5. The doctor has ordered salicylic acid 20% paint for a young woman with several warts on her hand. What instructions would you give the patient for its use?

A. The patient must be instructed to prevent spread of the paint onto the surrounding skin. The simplest way to do this is to carefully smear soft paraffin on the skin around and up to the edge of the wart. When the salicylic paint has dried the soft paraffin can be removed with a tissue. Another method is to cut a hole the size of the wart in zinc oxide plaster and position this over the wart but this is more cumbersome and requires some skill to cut the hole to the right size.

6. You have been applying neomycin soaks to a large infected area on the back. The lesion is healing rapidly, then for no apparent reason it again becomes inflamed and this inflammation persists in spite of continuing treatment. What would you suspect has happened?

A. The inflammation is probably due to the development of sensitivity to neomycin which, when applied topically, can cause allergic contact dermatitis.

7. An extensive infected leg ulcer has been irrigated with a solution of neomycin 0.5% for 10 days and, while the infection seems to be clearing, there is as yet little evidence of healing. The appropriate action is to: (a) continue the treatment; (b) change to another treatment to speed up the healing process; (c) draw to the attention of the attending medical officer that prolonged treatment with neomycin may have serious side effects.

A. (c) Application of neomycin solution to an extensive denuded area can result in significant systemic absorption of neomycin. If this continues for a prolonged period vestibular damage and hearing impairment may occur.

CHAPTER 29 ANTIHISTAMINES

1. Describe how antihistamines are thought to act.

A. Antihistamines appear to occupy H_1 receptor sites to the exclusion of histamine.

2. Which of the following drugs are antihistamines: (a) phenylbutazone (*Butazolidin*); (b) diphenhydramine (*Benadryl*); (c) promethazine (*Phenergan*); (d) phenytoin (*Dilantin*); (e) dexchlorpheniramine (*Polaramine*); (f) dextropropoxyphene (*Doloxene*)?

A. (b), (c) and (e).

3. List four conditions for which antihistamines may be used.

A. Allergic reactions such as itching from urticaria and pruritus, insect bites and stings and allergic rhinitis.

4. (a) What are the two most prominent adverse reactions to antihistamines? (b) List two others.

A. (a) Sedation and dry mouth. (b) Dizziness, blurred vision, loss of appetite, muscle weakness, hypotension (if given IV) and, paradoxically, wakefulness and hyperexcitability.

5. Name two non-sedating antihistamines.

A. Terfenadine, azatadine, loratadine.

6. Which of the following antihistamines are long acting: (a) terfenadine; (b) dexchlorpheniramine; (c) astemizole; (d) azatadine; (e) mebhydrolin.

A. (a), (c) and (d).

CHAPTER 30 INFECTIOUS DISEASES

1. Selection of an appropriate anti-infective agent should be based on a number of factors. What are those factors?

A. The likely infecting organism, known or proven antimicrobial sensitivities, ability of the anti-infective to reach the site of infection at the necessary concentration. The route of administration will be determined by the severity of the infection, as will the dose and frequency of drug administration. The ability of the patient to excrete the drug is important, as is a history of hypersensitivity or adverse effects to the anti-infective agent. The patient's immune status is important — 'cidal' rather than 'static' drugs should be used in the immunocompromised host.

2. Combination therapy with anti-infective agents is indicated in certain circumstances. Which of the following statements is(are) specific justification(s) for combination therapy? (a) To delay the emergence of resistance to one drug through the use of a second drug. (b) To achieve prompt treatment of a desperately ill patient suspected of having a serious infection. (c) To allow for a reduction in the dosage of one or both drugs. (d) To achieve bactericidal synergism. (e) To cover a mixed infection.

A. (a), (b), (c), (d), (e)

3. Briefly describe three mechanisms whereby resistance can be transferred from one bacteria to another.

A. (i) Conjugation involves the transfer of extranuclear particles of genetic material (DNA), known as plasmids, while the bacteria are in direct contact with another. (ii) Transduction involves the transfer of genetic material through the infection of bacteria by a virus (bacteriophage). (iii) Transformation involves the uptake of genetic material by one bacteria after lysis of another.

4. Which of the following statements correctly describe some of the properties of penicillins? (a) Patients who are allergic to benzylpenicillin will be allergic to the other penicillins. (b) The penicillins are bactericidal and act by disrupting the permeability of the cell membrane by binding to target enzymes (PBPs). (c) Oral penicillins should be administered 60 minutes before meals and at bedtime to achieve higher serum antibacterial activity. (d) Ampicillin is active against some Gram negative bacteria resistant to benzylpenicillin. (e) Semisynthetic penicillins can be administered in a mixed solution with gentamicin to treat serious staphylococcal infections.

A. (a), (c), (d)

5. List five indications for the use of each of the following agents: (a) Benzylpenicillin. (b) Ampicillin. (c) Azlocillin. (d) Flucloxacillin.

A. (a) Benzylpenicillin: pneumococcal meningitis; meningococcal meningitis; pneumococcal pneumonia; cellulitis; streptococcal endocarditis; gas gangrene; Lyme disease.
(b) Ampicillin: shigellosis; bronchitis; urinary tract infections; listeriosis; enterococcal infections; salmonellosis; pneumonia; bacterial meningitis; otitis media; acute sinusitis.
(c) Azlocillin: pseudomonal infections including urinary tract infections, pneumonia, septicaemia and osteomyelitis; febrile episodes in neutropenic patients in combination with an aminoglycoside; amoxycillin resistant Proteus sp. infections. (d) Flucloxacillin: staphylococcal infections including osteomyelitis, septicaemia, septic arthritis, urinary tract infections, pneumonias, meningitis, toxic shock syndrome, abscesses, mastitis and skin infections.

6. Complete the following statements describing the administration and absorption of cephalosporins.

(a) .... and .... are well absorbed from the gastrointestinal tract. These cephalosporins are acid .... (b) Cephalosporins administered by the intramuscular route cause .... and .... and occasionally sterile .... formation. (c) The intravenous dose of cephamandole for an adult, in mild to moderate infections, is .... administered .... hourly.

A. (a) Cephalexin, cefaclor, stable. (b) Pain, redness, abscess. (c) 1 g, 8-hourly.

7. Adverse effects to cephalosporins are similar to those encountered with the penicillins; nevertheless, which of the following statements is correct? (a) patients with a history of delayed penicillin hypersensitivity can be treated with a cephalosporin; (b) diuretic agents or aminoglycosides may produce additive nephrotoxicity when used with a cephalosporin; (c) the cephalosporins appear to cause less immediate hypersensitivity reactions than the penicillins; (d) patients with hepatic dysfunction are at special risk of drug accumulation or toxic serum concentrations when receiving cephalosporins.

A. (a), (b), (c)

8. Which of the second generation cephalosporins are commonly prescribed for surgical prophylaxis.

A. Cefoxitin, cefotetan, cephamandole.

9. List three β-lactams that may cause hypoprothrombinaemia, and a disulfiram-like reaction when alcohol is ingested?

A. Cephamandole, cefotetan, latamoxef.

10. What purpose does cilastatin serve in the combination product imipenem–cilastatin?

A. Cilastatin prevents the breakdown of imipenem in the kidney. This results in higher imipenem levels and a reduced risk of nephrotoxicity.

11. (a) Clavulanic acid is a what? (b) When combined with amoxycillin it extends the spectrum of that drug to include *Proteus* sp and *Pseudomonas aeruginosa*. True or false? (c) What adverse effects may occur after the discontinuation of amoxycillin–clavulanic acid?

A. *(a) β-lactamase inhibitor. (b) False. (c) Cholestatic jaundice, rash, diarrhoea.*

12. Which of the following adverse effects may be experienced with tetracycline therapy: ototoxicity, thrombophlebitis, photosensitivity, nausea, heartburn and diarrhoea, hepatotoxicity?

A. *All except ototoxicity.*

13. (a) Parenteral gentamicin is used in the treatment of .... (b) Aminoglycosides are excreted almost entirely by the .... (c) High serum concentrations of the aminoglycosides may cause .... (d) In the presence of renal dysfunction the parenteral dose of the aminoglycoside should be .... or the dosage interval ....

A *(a) Gram negative bacterial infections. (b) Kidneys. (c) Ototoxicity, nephrotoxicity. (d) Decreased, increased.*

14. (a) List some of the indications for the use of erythromycin. (b) What erythromycin salt has been associated with hepatotoxicity?

A. *(a) Cellulitis, pneumonia, acne, psitticosis, Q fever, Legionnaires disease, gonorrhoea, Rocky Mountain spotted fever. (b) All salts and the base although the incidence is highest with the estolate salt.*

15. (a) .... is a serious side effect associated with lincomycin and clindamycin therapy. (b) This side effect is due to the organism .... (c) .... in a dose of 125 mg orally 6-hourly is used to treat this side effect. (d) This drug (c) is generally administered intravenously to treat potentially life-threatening systemic .... infections. How should this IV dose be given?

A. *(a) Pseudomembraneous colitis. (b)* Clostridium difficile. *(c) Vancomycin. (d) Staphylococcal. As an infusion over 60 minutes.*

16. Chloramphenicol is active against a wide variety of Gram positive and Gram negative organisms. Chloramphenicol is used infrequently; why?

A. *Chloramphenicol may cause serious adverse effects, notably blood marrow suppression including irreversible aplastic anaemia, and the grey baby syndrome.*

17. How do the quinolones exert their antibacterial effect?

A. *Inhibition of DNA gyrase.*

18. Are ciprofloxacin and norfloxacin both indicated for the treatment of bone and gastrointestinal tract infections? Explain your answer.

A. *Only ciprofloxacin may be used to treat systemic infections as norfloxacin does not achieve clinically significant concentrations except in the urogenital tract.*

19. List three drug interactions that are known to occur with quinolones.

A. *(i) Antacids cause a decrease in fluoroquinolone absorption. (ii) Ciprofloxacin causes a decrease in theophylline metabolism and an increase in theophylline toxicity. (iii) Ciprofloxacin potentiates warfarin's anticoagulant effect. (iv) Sucralfate decreases fluoroquinolone absorption. (v) Probenecid increases serum concentrations of fluoroquinolones.*

20. List three anti-infective agents that are known to colour the urine, and/or tears and other body fluid secretions. What advice would you give to a patient who wears soft contact lenses and is prescribed one of these agents?

A. Metronidazole, rifampicin, nitrofurantoin, tinidazole. Patients receiving rifampicin should be advised not to wear soft contact lenses as they may become permanently discoloured.

21. Discuss the place of the combination product trimethoprim–sulfamethoxazole in the treatment of urinary tract infections or acute exacerbations of chronic bronchitis. What agents are preferred in these infections?

A. Trimethroprim–sulfamethoxazole is a useful agent for the treatment of both urinary tract infections and acute exacerbations of chronic bronchitis. Resistance, however, is becoming a problem particularly with Escherichia coli *and* Haemophilus influenzae. *The product is associated with a higher incidence of adverse effects, particularly in the elderly, than other commonly prescribed agents for these conditions, namely amoxycillin, amoxycillin–clavulanic acid, trimethoprim and cephalexin.*

22. (a) Amphotericin B injection should be diluted in .... and administered over ..... hours. (b) .... and .... are triazole derivatives. .... is particularly active against *Aspergillus* sp. (c) Oral .... and .... may be used to treat tinea pedis. .... has been associated with fatal hepatic necrosis.

A. (a) Glucose 5% (buffered), 4–6 hours. (b) Fluconazole, itraconazole, itraconazole. (c) Ketoconazole, griseofulvin; ketoconazole.

23. Doctor has prescribed ketoconazole 200 mg orally at 8 am daily, and cimetidine orally 400 mg bd. Can both these tablets be administered to the patient on the 8 am drug round? Explain your answer.

A. No, ketoconazole requires an acid stomach for absorption. The dose of cimetidine should be delayed for two hours.

24. Explain how intravenous miconazole should be administered and what adverse effects the patient may experience.

A. Miconazole should be given as a slow IV infusion over 30–60 minutes. IV miconazole can cause phlebitis and anaphylactoid reactions. Too rapid administration can cause tachycardia and other cardiac arrhythmias.

25. (a) Metronidazole is one of the drugs of first choice for the treatment of ...., particularly those caused by *Bacteroides fragilis*. (b) The usual adult dose of metronidazole for intravenous infusion is .... mg administered .... hourly infused over .... minutes. (c) Metronidazole in combination with .... may produce abdominal cramps, nausea, vomiting, headaches and flushing. (d) A patient who is breast feeding is ordered metronidazole as a single 2 g dose for trichomoniasis. What advice would you give the patient?

A. (a) Anaerobic infections. (b) 500 mg, 8–12-hourly, 20 minutes. (c) Alcohol. (d) Cease breast feeding for 24 hours after the dose as the drug is excreted in the breast milk giving it a bitter taste.

26. (a) Which antiviral agent(s) can be used to treat cytomegalovirus infections? (b) Which antivirals have activity against HIV? (c) What significant toxicity may accompany inhaled ribavirin therapy.

A. (a) Ganciclovir, foscarnet. (b) Zidovudine, didanosine, ribavirin, zalcitabine. (c) Acute deterioration in respiratory function, particularly in patients with underlying lung disease (e.g. asthma).

27. A patient is being treated for tuberculosis with a four drug regimen: isoniazid, rifampicin, pyrazinamide and ethambutol. How long would the four drugs continue and which two drugs would normally be continued for the entire 6 months?

A. 1–2 months, then continue with rifampicin plus isoniazid as maintenance therapy.

28. What agents can be used by the traveller as prophylactic therapy against malaria when visiting a malaria endemic region?

A. Chloroquine, mefloquine, pyrimethamine–dapsone, pyrimethamine–sulfadoxine, doxycycline.

29. Your patient has been prescribed acyclovir 300 mg IV 8-hourly. Discuss your approach to fulfilling this order safely and effectively.

A. Check the patient's weight, renal function and the indication for acyclovir use. These will indicate whether or not the dose is appropriate. Calculate the volume of reconstituted solution required to give a dose of 300 mg (250 mg/10 mL; 300 mg = 12 mL). Dilute the acyclovir in 100 mL of sodium chloride 0.9% solution before administering. Check that the patient is adequately hydrated before commencing the infusion. Infuse the drug over one hour. Monitor the patient for clinical improvement and signs of drug toxicity, particularly nephrotoxicity and neurotoxicity.

30. A patient you are nursing has HIV infection and his treatment includes zidovudine 100 mg orally 4-hourly. He complains of fever and headache and asks you for some *Panadol*. What would be your response —- give reasons.

A. The patient should not have paracetamol as an analgesic as it may potentiate the bone marrow toxicity of zidovudine.

CHAPTER 31 CANCER CHEMOTHERAPY

1. List four cytotoxic drugs that may cause tissue necrosis if inadvertently extravasated.

A. Mustine hydrochloride, daunorubicin, doxorubicin, epirubicin, idarubicin, dactinomycin, mitomycin C, vinblastine, vincristine and vindesine are all considered potent vesicants.

2. Rank the following drugs in order of their emetogenic potential from lowest to highest: doxorubicin, busulfan, fluorouracil, cisplatin.

A. Busulfan, fluorouracil, doxorubicin and cisplatin.

3. Which cytotoxic drugs are considered cell cycle specific? Why are extended infusions of such drugs more effective against sensitive tumours?

A. Cytarabine, floxuridine, fluorouracil, mercaptopurine, thioguanine, methotrexate, bleomycin, etoposide, tenopiside, colaspase, hydroxyurea, vincristine, vinblastine and vindesine are all considered cell cycle specific. Extended exposure to cell cycle specific drugs results in greater cell kill as more and more tumour cells move from the resting phase to the part of the cell cycle where the drug causes cell damage.

4. Compare and contrast the aims of curative chemotherapy and palliative chemotherapy.

A. With curative treatment or where long-term remission is expected, short-term toxicities are usually accepted if they are unavoidable in achieving the aims of the treatment. Avoidance of long-term toxicities, e.g. permanent organ damage, secondary malignancies and sterility, will be of greater concern and are avoided wherever possible. Conversely, with palliative treatment where symptom control is the aim, avoidance of the short-term toxicities that reduce quality of life will take higher precedence. Long-term toxicities such as sterility and secondary malignancies will have little or no bearing on the selection of chemotherapy for these patients.

5. Why are cytotoxic drugs often used in combination and what are the desirable characteristics of those combinations?

A. *In general, combinations of drugs are used to increase the effectiveness of chemotherapy and to prevent or delay the onset of drug resistance. When used in combination, cytotoxic drugs should ideally be active against the malignancy being treated, and have little overlapping toxicity and different pharmacological actions.*

6. Give examples of measures taken with cytotoxic drug administration to limit the toxicity of individual agents.

A. *(a) Adequate or suprahydration to prevent toxicity in patients receiving cyclophosphamide, ifosfamide, mid to high dose methotrexate and cisplatin; (b) attention to venous access and administration technique to reduce likelihood of drug extravasation; (c) slow administration of etoposide and tenopiside to limit incidence of hypotension and other 'hypersensitivity' reactions; (d) use of the protective agent mesna to prevent ifosfamide induced haemorrhagic cystitis; (e) use of leucovorin to prevent toxicity of high dose methotrexate; (f) use of effective antiemetics to prevent or minimise nausea and vomiting; (g) other examples exist.*

7. What agents used in cancer treatment do not have myelosuppression as their major or dose limiting toxicity?

A. *Bleomycin, cisplatin, vincristine, colaspase, hormonal agents and interferon.*

8. What agents have been associated with cumulative and permanent toxicity to major organs?

A. *Anthracyclines (doxorubicin, daunorubicin, epirubicin, idarubicin) and mitozantrone induce cumulative cardiotoxicity; bleomycin causes lung fibrosis; cisplatin induces renal dysfunction; other examples exist.*

9. What agents are commonly given by the intrathecal route?

A. *Methotrexate and cytarabine are the only agents regularly injected directly into the CSF.*

CHAPTER 32 DRUGS USED IN CRITICAL CARE

1. List the problems encountered in the critical care patient which affect drug therapy.

A. *Multiple medical problems; unconsciousness and/or intubation; renal and hepatic failure; altered pharmacokinetics; multiple drug regimens.*

2. List the drugs used in the management of cardiac arrest and their pharmacological action.

A. *Adrenaline (increased myocardial and cerebral blood flow); lignocaine (management of ventricular fibrillation); bretylium (alternative to lignocaine in management of ventricular fibrillation); atropine (for asystole or bradycardia); sodium bicarbonate (correction of acidosis); calcium chloride (for calcium channel antagonist toxicity, hyperkalaemia or hypocalcaemia).*

3. List the vasodilators used in the treatment of hypertensive emergency.

A. *Sodium nitroprusside; diazoxide; hydralazine.*

4. How is nifedipine administered for rapid lowering of blood pressure?

A. *A nifedipine 10 mg capsule should be bitten and swallowed with water.*

5. What is an inotrope?

A. An inotrope is an agent which affects contractility of cardiac muscle.

6. What are the results of stimulation of: (a) dopamine receptors? (b) α receptors? (c) β receptors?

A. (a) Renal vasodilation and increased water and sodium excretion; (b) vasoconstriction; (c) vasodilation, increased contractility of heart muscle and increased heart rate.

7. Which diuretics are used in the treatment of cerebral oedema and how do they work?

A. Mannitol (acts by osmosis) and frusemide (direct effect on nephrons to promote diuresis, decreased cerebrospinal fluid and oedema formation).

8. For which type of cerebral oedema are corticosteroids most useful?

A. Cerebral oedema associated with tumours.

CHAPTER 33 PARENTERAL NUTRITION

1. Which of the following are indications for parenteral nutrition: (a) gastrointestinal sepsis; (b) pancreatic fistulae; (c) severe burns; (d) enterocutaneous fistulae in a patient with terminal metastatic disease receiving palliative care?

A: (a), (b), (c).

2. The total daily fluid needs of a 70 kg man with no excessive gastric loss or drainage from a wound is: (a) 500 mL; (b) 1000 mL; (c) 1750 mL; or (d) 2200 mL.

A: (d).

3. What are the essential ingredients of a total parenteral nutrition: (a) glucose; (b) thiamine; (c) insulin; (d) albumin; (e) a combination of amino acids?

A: (a), (b), (e).

4. 1 g of fat yields: (a) 9 kJ; (b) 9 kCal; (c) 4 kJ; or (d) 4 kCal.

A: (a).

5. 1 g of nitrogen is contained in: (a) 10 g glucose; (b) 1 g amino acid; (c) 6 g amino acid; or (d) 6 g fat.

A: (c).

6. Adequate utilisation of amino acid is most dependent on: (a) water; (b) energy; (c) heparin; or (d) zinc.

A: (b).

7. A suitable formulation for a 60 kg woman with intra-abdominal sepsis may include: (a) 20 g amino acid, 350 g glucose, 50 g fat; (b) 60 g amino acid, 350 g glucose, 50 g fat; (c) 60 g amino acid, 700 g glucose, 50 g fat; (d) 80 g amino acid, 700 g glucose, 100 g fat.

A: (b).

8. Potassium deficiency includes: (a) muscle weakness; (b) cardiac conduction defects; (c) tetany; (d) rickets.

A: (a), (b).

9. The management of glucose intolerance could include: (a) reduction of glucose content; (b) substitution of fat for part of glucose content; (c) administration of insulin; (d) all of the above.

A: (d).

10. Possible signs of septicaemia include: (a) inflamed catheter site; (b) increased blood glucose; (c) rigors; (d) low white cell count.

A: (a), (b), (c).

CHAPTER 34 ENTERAL FEEDING

1. List three features (symptoms) that may become evident in a patient suffering from malnutrition.

A. Loss of weight, reduced muscle mass, hypoproteinaemia, oedema, apathy, poor wound healing, increased susceptibility to infection.

2. Discuss reasons for introducing enteral nutrition via tube, giving patient groups as examples.

A. Patients unable to ingest any nutrition, e.g. those who are unconscious or have absent/poor gag reflex or upper GIT obstructions; and patients who are unable to ingest sufficient quantities of food and fluids, e.g. those with increased nutrient requirements (severe trauma, burns, postoperative patients) or with psychological disorders (anorexia nervosa, severe depression).

3. When is enteral feeding contraindicated? Give examples.

A. Enteral feeding is contraindicated if the gastrointestinal tract is non-functional (e.g. due to paralytic ileus, extensive GIT pathology, severe vomiting or diarrhoea, acute pancreatitis).

4. Explain the reason for emphasis on the osmolality of enteral formulae.

A. If the formula has a higher osmolality than the body fluids, water and electrolytes will be transferred across the mucosa into the gut. Rapid passage of food through the GIT, reduced nutrient absorption and diarrhoea can result. When introducing a formula it is important to choose a formula of low osmolality (300 mOsm/kg water).

5. Give two reasons for using a nutrient dense formula instead of a regular formula.

A. Elevated nutrient requirements and fluid restriction.

6. Define an elemental formula.

A. An elemental formula has its nutrients supplied in a readily absorbable form. Protein is supplied in the form of amino acids or di- and tripeptides, carbohydrate as mono- and oligosaccharides. The fat content is low and generally in the form of medium chain triglycerides.

7. List three possible causes of diarrhoea in patients receiving enteral feeding.

A. Formula has been introduced too quickly or is hyperosmolar; formula is contaminated; the patient is receiving antibiotics; the patient has impaired digestion and/or absorption, a compacted bowel, Clostridium difficile in the bowel, a bacterial overgrowth in the GIT, abnormal peristalsis.

8. Explain the difference between bolus feeding and continuous drip feeding.

A. For bolus feeding the formula is syringed into the enteral tube at set intervals. For continuous drip feeding the formula is delivered at a set flow rate continuously, i.e. 24 hours per day.

CHAPTER 35 ANTISEPTICS, DISINFECTANTS AND INFECTION CONTROL

1. Define the terms disinfectants and antiseptics.

A. Disinfectants are bactericidal agents usually used on inaminate objects. Antiseptics are bacteriostatic or slowly bactericidal agents usually used on living tissue.

2. Disinfectants are normally used: (a) when sterilisation is required; (b) on instruments that cannot be autoclaved or heated; (c) in detergent solutions to clean ordinary floors; or (d) after the original container has been opened for more than one week.

A. (b).

3. The definite uses of disinfectants and/or antiseptics are: (a) general disinfection of the hospital environment; (b) disinfection of clean articles or surfaces; (c) skin antisepsis; (d) sterilisation of surgeons' hands and arms.

A. (a), (b), (c).

4. Write down the class or classes of the following chemicals and their most common dilution in use (e.g. *Milton* chlorine compound, 1 in 80): (a) ethanol; (b) *Savlon Hospital Concentrate*; (c) *Medol*; (d) chlorhexidine; (e) povidone iodine (use dilution expressed as percentage of available iodine).

A. (a) Alcohol, 70%; (b) QAC–diguanide combination, 1 in 100; (c) phenolic, 1%; (d) diguanide 0.02%; (e) iodophor, 1% available iodine.

5. (a) Sterilisation means at least 95% destruction of microorganisms (true/false); (b) bacteria may grow in ward solutions of disinfectants and antiseptics (true/false); (c) Instruments wherever possible should be sterilised (true/false); (d) the efficacy of disinfectants is decreased by dried films of pus and excreta but not of blood or milk (true/false); (e) instruments for chemical disinfection should be thoroughly cleaned and free from soap (true/false).

A. (a) False; (b) true; (c) true; (d) false; (e) true.

6. Describe a desirable procedure to prevent cross-contamination during ward dressings.

A. Wash hands before procedure. Complete dressing according to procedure manual in an aseptic manner, avoiding interruptions. Use gloves and other protective garments as per hospital policy. Wash hands after procedure.

APPENDIX — COMMON PRESCRIPTION AND MEDICAL ABBREVIATIONS ■

Common Prescription Abbreviations

Weight, measure and strength

mL (ml, cc) millilitre
L (l) litre
μg (mcg, microg) microgram
mg milligram
g gram
kg kilogram
iu, IU international units
mEq milliequivalent
mmol millimole
μmol (micromol) micromole

Dose form

cap, caps capsules
gtt, guttae drops
inj injection
mist, mixt mixture
neb solution for inhalation
pess pessary
pulv powder
sol, soln solution
supp suppository
susp suspension
tab, tabs tablets
tinct, tr tincture

Route of administration

po by mouth
pr by rectum
pv by vagina
IM intramuscular
IV intravenous
SC, sc subcutaneous
LE left eye
RE right eye

Time of administration

ac before meals
cc with meals
pc after meals
m, mane morning
n, nocte night
bd, bid twice daily
tds, tid three times daily
qds, qid four times daily
q4h, qqh every 4 hours
q6h every 6 hours
stat immediately, at once
sos if necessary
prn when necessary

Miscellaneous

et and
aq water
ex aq with water
c with

Common Medical Abbreviations

ADR adverse drug reaction
ANS autonomic nervous system
AV atrioventricular

BEE basal energy expenditure
BP blood pressure

CCF congestive cardiac failure
CHF congestive heart failure
CNS central nervous system
CPR cardiopulmonary resuscitation
CSF cerebrospinal fluid
CVP central venous pressure

DNA deoxyribonucleic acid
DVT deep vein thrombosis
ECG electrocardiogram
EEG electroencephalogram
ENT ear, nose and throat
ESR erythrocyte sedimentation rate

GI gastrointestinal
GIT gastrointestinal tract

5-HT 5-hydroxytryptamine

kJ kilojoules

MAO monoamine oxidase
MAOI monoamine oxidase inhibitor
MRSA methicillin resistant
Staphylococcus aureus

NS normal saline
NSAID non-steroidal anti-inflammatory drug

PN parenteral nutrition

REM rapid eyeball movement
RDS respiratory distress syndrome
RNA ribonucleic acid

SLE systemic lupus erythematosus

TPN total parenteral nutrition

UV ultraviolet

GLOSSARY

Absorption The process by which a drug enters the systemic circulation. The term absorption is used when the drug is administered orally, topically, intramuscularly or by other routes.

Adverse Drug Reaction A response to a drug that is noxious and unintended and which occurs in humans at doses used for prophylaxis, diagnosis or treatment of disease.

Ageing Ageing changes can be defined as those time related alterations not due to disease, occuring in individuals after maturity. These changes are more or less common to all members of the species and increase the probability of death. They are universal, progressive, irreversible and deleterious.

Agonist A compound which binds to a receptor and produces a similar effect to that of a naturally occurring (endogenous) compound within a body system. The result is usually an increase in the rate, intensity or extent of a physiological process.

Allergen A substance capable of inducing an allergy.

Anaesthetic, general A drug used to produce and/or maintain unconsciousness.

Anaesthetic, local A drug used to produce a loss of pain sensation in a specific localised area of the body.

Analgesic A drug which alleviates pain.

Antagonist A drug which binds to a receptor and produces a physiological effect which is different in nature or less intense than that which occurs with the naturally occurring compound. The result is that the rate, extent or intensity of the function of the cell or body system is decreased.

Anthropometric measurements Objective measurements of weight, height, skinfold thickness and arm muscle circumference used in nutritional assessment.

Antibacterial A drug used to combat an infection caused by bacteria.

Antibiotics Substances produced by microorganisms that, in high dilution, are antagonistic to the growth of other microorganisms. Some antibiotics are made synthetically.

Antibody An immunoglobulin which responds specifically to an antigen. It is produced by plasma cells of a host in response to antigenic stimulation, after infection or immunisation.

Antiemetic A drug used to reduce nausea and vomiting.

Antiepileptic (anticonvulsant) A drug which works on the central nervous system to prevent epileptic seizures.

Antifungal A drug used to combat an infection caused by fungi.

Antigen A substance which induces the production of families of sensitised lymphocytes and subsequently of antibodies. An antigen may be a protein, a polypeptide or a polysaccharide.

Antileprotic A drug used to combat an infection caused by *Mycobacterium leprae*.

Antimalarial A drug used to combat an infection caused by malarial (*Plasmodium*) parasites.

Antimetabolite A substance bearing a close resemblance to one required for normal physiological functioning and exerting its effect by interfering with the utilisation of the essential metabolite.

Antimicrobial A drug used to combat an infection caused by a microorganism, e.g. bacteria, fungi, protozoa, virus.

Antiprotozoal A drug used to combat an infection caused by protozoa.

Antipyretic A drug which prevents or allays fever.

Antiseptic Bacteriostatic or slowly bactericidal agent usually used on living tissue.

Antisialogogue A drug used to reduce the secretion of saliva.

Antitubercular A drug used to combat an infection caused by tubercle bacilli.

Antiviral A drug used to combat an infection caused by a virus.

Bacterial spores Thick-walled resting cells produced by certain bacteria (from soil) including those causing tetanus and gas gangrene.

Bactericidal agent An agent which causes death by destroying the bacterium. By combining with proteins and other cell protoplasm components they destroy or remove pathogenic microorganisms in the non-sporing or vegetative state.

Bacteriostatic agent An agent which stops growth division and multiplication of a bacterial cell without necessarily causing its death.

Basal metabolic rate (BMR) The energy consumed in performing necessary physiologicol work at rest. It is measured in kilojoules (or kilocalories. 1 kCal = 4.18 kJ).

Bioavailability The fraction or percentage of the total administered dose of a drug which reaches the systemic circulation. The oral bioavailability of a drug is that fraction of the total dose administered orally which reaches the systemic circulation.

Broad spectrum This term denotes a wide range of antimicrobial activity, e.g. activity against Gram positive and Gram negative organisms.

Catabolism The breaking down of tissues so that the constituents of living matter are reduced to waste material and are eliminated from the body (applies to catabolic diseases which cause wasting).

Catecholamines A group of sympatho-mimetic drugs including adrenaline.

Chemotherapy The drug treatment of disease in which the causative organism is destroyed or removed with minimal harm to the host.

Children Older than 2 years and less than 12 years of age.

Colonisation The presence of bacteria that are not causing infection and/or disease.

Cough Suppressants, antitussives Drugs used to decrease the cough reflex and provide relief from the symptoms of cough.

Counter-irritation Superficial irritation intended to relieve some other irritation.

Counter-irritant An agent which produces counter-irritation.

Cracking An oily layer developing in a lipid emulsion or in a formulation containing a lipid emulsion. A cracked emulsion is unsuitable for use.

Disinfectant Bactericidal agent usually used on inanimate objects.

Disposition Loss of drug from the systemic circulation due to distribution and/or elimination.

Distribution The movement of drugs and metabolites between different compartments within the body.

Drug formulation The process by which a drug product is designed, usually governed by knowledge of the compound's pharmacokinetic profile, e.g. a drug which is rapidly eliminated from the body may be formulated as a sustained release preparation.

Dysmorphogen A substance which, when given to a pregnant woman, causes minor or less obvious congenital abnormalities.

Elimination The means by which a compound is removed from the body.

Elimination half-life The time taken for the plasma concentration of a drug to decline by 50%, given that the processes of absorption and distribution are complete.

Enteral By the intestinal route.

Enteral feeding Nutritional support via the gastrointestinal tract.

Enterohepatic cycling The process by which a drug is first converted to a metabolite which is excreted into the bowel in the bile, the bacteria in the gut then convert the metabolite back to the parent drug which is reabsorbed into the systemic circulation.

Enzyme inhibitor A compound which decreases the activity of enzymes, producing an alteration in the production or breakdown of a chemical compound within the body and changing the nature of the physiological process caused by that compound.

Excretion The process by which a drug or metabolite is irreversibly removed from the internal environment of the body.

Exotoxin A toxin excreted by intact organisms, e.g. tetanus or diphtheria toxins.

Expectorant A drug which promotes the evacuation of the secretions of the bronchial tree (mucus or sputum).

Fungicidal agent An agent which kills fungi.

Gastrostomy The establishment of a communication between the interior of the stomach and the skin surface for tube feeding in patients who are unable to swallow.

Gonadotrophin A substance having a stimulating effect on the gonads. In the female the pituitary hormones follicle stimulating hormone (FSH) and leutinising hormone (LH) are said to have a gonadotrophic effect on the ovaries.

Gram positive organisms Those organisms that retain the primary dye complex of the Gram's staining technique (methyl violet) and appear dark purple on microscopic examination, e.g. *Streptococcus viridans* and *Staphylococcus aureus*.

Gram negative organisms Those organisms that are decolourised by acetone applied to the smear after methyl violet in the Gram's staining test. These organisms take up the counterstain, e.g. basic fuchsin, and appear pink on microscopic examination. Some examples are *Haemophilus influenzae, Escherichia coli, Klebsiella pneumoniae* and *Proteus mirabilis.*

Heterologous antiserum A preparation of antibodies obtained from mammalian species such as horses, sheep, dogs and rabbits. It is available for prophylaxis or treatment of disease or envenomation.

Hyperosmolar Solutions which have a higher osmolarity than body fluids.

Hypoproteinaemia A condition in which there is an abnormally reduced quantity of protein in the plasma, such as occurs in nephrosis, hepatic dysfunction or as the result of too little protein in the diet.

Hypovolaemia A condition in which the blood volume in the body is diminished.

Jejunostomy The establishment of an opening into the jejunum through the wall of the abdomen.

Immunity A state of resistance or lessened susceptibility to infection. It may be innate or acquired.

Immunity, active Immunity induced by infection or immunisation.

Immunity, passive Immunity conferred by exogenous antibodies in the form of human immunoglobulin or heterologous antisera such as antitoxin or antivenom. Infants derive passive immunity by transplacental passage of maternal antibodies.

Immunisation, vaccination These terms are often used interchangeably to describe the same process. Vaccination is a term formerly restricted to the administration of vaccines to induce active immunity. Immunisation includes the two concepts of inducing active immunity by the administration of vaccines and providing passive immunity by giving immunoglobulins or antisera.

Immunoglobulin, normal immunoglobulin A solution of antibodies prepared by plasma fractionation from pooled human blood donations. The antibody spectrum would be representative of the combined experience of the blood donor population.

Metabolite A new chemical substance produced within the body as a result of chemical reactions in the liver, kidneys, lungs, gut wall and other sites. The outcome of this process is that the drug undergoes a chemical reaction such as oxidation or demethylation with the end result, the metabolite, having greater water solubilty than the parent drug. In this way, the elimination of the drug from the body via the kidneys is facilitated.

Metered dose inhaler (MDI) A term used to described a drug delivery system which enables the drug to be delivered directly into the respiratory tract. These systems work by using a chemical propellant (i.e. metered dose *aerosol*) or can be driven by the patient's own inspiration of air through the device. These devices are commonly referred to as 'puffers'.

Mucolytic A drug used in an attempt to alter the characteristics of the sputum, making it less sticky and viscous and therefore easier to expectorate.

Muscarinic antagonists Drugs which reverse the muscarinic effects of acetylcholine, e.g. decrease in heart rate, bronchoconstriction, increase in gastric motility and intestinal secretions, stimulation of the salivary glands.

Muscle relaxant A drug used to paralyse the skeletal muscles.

Neuroleptanalgesia A deep trance-like state with a reduced appreciation of pain, produced by the administration of a combination of an opioid (narcotic) analgesic and a neuroleptic agent.

Narrow spectrum This term denotes a restricted range of antimicrobial activity, e.g. erythromycin has a range of activity restricted to Gram positive organisms and the polymyxins are active solely against Gram negative organisms.

Nebuliser A device which enables a solution of drug to be converted into a fine mist or spray which is then usually driven into the respiratory tract using a current of air or oxygen.

Nitrogen balance The input of nitrogen minus the loss of nitrogen.

Nitrogen balance, positive (anabolic state) The input of nitrogen is greater than the loss. This implies that protein is being synthesised by the body.

Nitrogen balance, negative (catabolic state) The loss of nitrogen is greater than the input. This implies muscle is being broken down to produce glucose.

Nystagmus Oscillatory movements of the eyeballs.

Oxytocic A drug that stimulates uterine contraction, i.e. a drug that mimics the effects of natural oxytocin.

Progestagen A synthetic steroid with progesterone-like activity which can be given orally, parenterally or vaginally to promote effects in the endometrium, ovary, breast and hypothalamic/pituitary area. These progestational effects can also be seen during pregnancy.

Premedication Drugs ordered by the anaesthetist for administration in the ward before the patient leaves for the operating theatre.

Organisms, non-pathogenic (commensals) Organisms that co-exist harmlessly with host cells.

Organisms, pathogenic Organisms capable of causing infection thereby harming the host.

Osmolarity A description of the number of particles in a solution. It is measured in milliosmoles (mOsm) per L.

Parenteral feeding Nutritional support given intravenously.

Parenteral nutrition, total The intravenous administration of utilisable forms of nutrition in sufficient amounts to meet energy requirements and promote tissue anabolism. These nutrients included water, amino acids, carbohydrate, fat, electrolytes, trace elements and vitamins.

Parenteral nutrition, partial The provision of a portion of these nutrients, the remainder being provided by another source.

Pharmacodynamics The study of effects of drugs within the body including mechanisms of drug action and physiological and biochemical effects of drugs upon the patient.

Pharmacokinetics The study of the movement of drugs and their breakdown products, *metabolites*, in the body, including absorption, distribution and elimination.

Pseudomembranous colitis An acute inflammatory response in the colon associated with antibiotic use. Characteristic exudative mucosal plaques are visible on colonic examination.

Pro-drug A drug administered in an inactive precursor form which is subsequently converted by metabolism to the active drug moiety.

Receptor A location or chemical structure within a cell or organ system where a drug, hormone or other chemical binds, usually producing a change in the function of the cell or body system. Drugs may bind to receptors and produce a beneficial (therapeutic) effect or an adverse side effect.

Refeeding syndrome The metabolic and physiological consequences of too rapid repletion of fluid, electrolytes, glucose and vitamins in a depleted patient. Compartmental shifts result in severe biochemical abnormalities and can lead to cardiac failure.

Rubefacient An agent that reddens the skin.

Serotonin (more commonly referred to as 5-HT (5-hydroxytryptamine) A neurotransmitter in the central nervous system. It also acts as a potent vasoconstrictor.

Spectrum The range of activity of a drug against microorganisms.

Teratogen A substance which, when given to a pregnant woman, causes serious malformations in the infant.

Therapeutic drug monitoring The practice of measuring the concentration of a drug in the blood or plasma, the aim being to adjust the individual dosage schedule so that the blood level falls within a range of concentrations likely to produce the desired therapeutic response without toxicity.

Tocolytic A drug that causes relaxation of the uterus or cessation of contractions.

Tuberculocidal agent An agent which kills cells of *Mycobacterium tuberculosis*. (35)

Vaccine A suspension of attenuated live or killed microorganisms (bacteria, viruses or rickettsiae) or fractions thereof, administered to induce immunity and prevent infectious disease.

Vaccine, attenuated A preparation of live microorganisms treated and cultured in a way that loss of virulence is achieved but a capacity to stimulate immunity is retained.

Valsalva manoeuvre Expiration against an expired glottis.

Virucidal agent An agent which kills viruses.

Volume of distribution The theoretical volume of blood or plasma which would be consistent with a known amount of drug in the body and the observed blood or plasma concentration when measured.

INDEX

This index contains entries for drugs, drug groups, diseases, disease groups and subjects. Drug therapy is assumed in all headings, so 'infectious diseases' includes (and is slightly broader than) 'anti-infective therapy'. Tables and figures (indicated by a **t** or **f** after the page number) have been indexed selectively, often only with a heading for the main topic.

All discussion of a drug is indexed under its **generic name**, which is shown in bold. *Trade names* are shown in italic type, with a reference to the generic name.

Alpha and beta have been spelt out in the index (e.g. 'beta blocking agents'). Numbers have been ignored in listing. Word-by-word listing has been used, so 'anti-infective' is listed before 'antiadrenal'. Prepositions have been ignored when listing subdivisions.

A

Abbocillin V, VK see phenoxymethylpenicillin
absence seizures 512, 524-525
Absol see sodium hypochlorite
absorption 11-12, 21-25
    geriatric 82
    paediatric 66-67
ABVD protocol 797, 825
ACE inhibitors 5
    adverse respiratory effects 174
    in cardiovascular disease 189-193, 193t, 249
    in pregnancy 391
acetazolamide 596
Acetopt see sulfacetamide
acetylcholine 145-146
acetylcysteine
    in eye disorders 602
    mucolytic 172
    in poisoning 130-131, 136t
acetylsalicylic acid *see* aspirin
Achromycin see tetracycline
acid-base imbalance 346
acid pepsin disease 302-310
acidosis 346
    predialysis therapy 251
Aclin see sulindac
acne 619, 621, 623, 626
    and oral contraceptives 410
acontractile bladder 277, 279
acromegaly 356-357
Acthargel see corticotropin
Actilyse see tissue plasminogen activator
actinomycin D *see* dactinomycin
activated charcoal in poisoning 127-129, 127t
active immunisation 110-115
Actrapid see insulin
acyclovir 733-734
    in eye infections 599
    in skin infections 627
Adalat see nifedipine

adjuvant chemotherapy 783
administration of drugs 12, 21-25, 36-50, 66-67
    anti-infectives 658-659
    chemotherapy 32-33, 91, 659, 781, 786-787
    record keeping 39-40, 119
    rectal 24, 43-44, 67
administration sets 58-59, 61t
adrenal hormones 375-383
adrenaline 151, 152t, 153
    in anaesthesia 505
    bronchodilator 159
    in cardiac arrest 840-841
    in cardiac disorders 850-851
    in eye disorders 594
adrenergic blockers *see* alpha blocking agents;
    beta blocking agents
adrenergic drugs *see* sympathomimetic
    (adrenergic) agents
adrenergic receptor agonists *see* sympathomimetic
    (adrenergic) agents
Adriamycin see doxorubicin
Adroyd see oxymetholone
adsorbents in diarrhoeal disease 319
adverse drug reactions 9-10 *see also* drug induced
    illness
    cytotoxic drugs 780, 783-787, 784f-785f
    geriatric 85-90, 85t, 87f
    immunisation 119-120
    ocular 603
    psychiatric 554
    respiratory 173-175, 173t
aerosol administration 47-48, 176
Agarol see liquid paraffin
age *see also* geriatric therapeutics; paediatric
    therapeutics
    and drug response 8
    and immunisation 117
Agon see felodipine
agonists 5
AIDS *see* immunisation; viral infections
Airol see tretinoin

P

paclitaxel 831-833
paediatric therapeutics 66-77 *see also* neonates
    antiseptics 905
    aspirin 462
    dexamphetamine 577
    epilepsy 512, 516-525
    immunisation 111, 115t
    naloxone 134-135
    poisoning by 125-128, 131, 133, 647
pain relief *see* analgesia
Palfium see dextromoramide
palliative care 480-482 *see also* terminal pain
    chemotherapy 783
Panadeine see paracetamol and codeine
Panadol see paracetamol
Panafcort see prednisone
Panafcortelone see prednisolone
Pancrease see pancreatic enzymes
pancreatic enzymes 312
Pancrex see pancreatic enzymes
pancuronium
    in anaesthesia 500-501
    in critical care 859
papaveretum 475
paracetamol 464-466, 465t
  and codeine
    for immunisation reactions 119
    in labour 403
    in migraine 537-538
    poisoning by 130-131, 297, 298t
    in pregnancy 388
Paradex see dextropropoxyphene
paraffin 619
paraldehyde 525
Paraplatin see carboplatin
parasitic infections
    liver 295-296
    skin 629-631
parasympathetic nervous system 144-151, 147t
    ocular control 592
parasympatholytics *see* anticholinergic agents
parasympathomimetics *see* cholinergic agents
parenteral administration 24-25, 32, 42-43
parenteral nutrition 862-873, 863t, 874t
    administration 870, 872
    adult 865-869, 866t, 868t, 870t
    indications for 864
    neonatal 872, 872t
    solution preparation 869-870, 872
parkinsonism 85, 527-534
    and antipsychotic drugs 558
Parlodel see bromocriptine
Parnate see tranylcypromine
paroxetine 572
Parvolex see acetylcysteine
pastes 617
patent ductus arteriosus 69, 72
patient education 49
patients' rights 48-49
    long-term care centres 89
    to refuse medication 49, 560

Pavulon see pancuronium
Paxyl see lignocaine
pediatric *see* paediatric
D-Penamine see penicillamine
Penbritin see ampicillin
penicillamine
    in musculoskeletal disorders 435-436
    in poisoning 135, 138t
    in Wilson's disease 299
penicillins 6, 660-667, 665t
    adverse allergic reaction 10, 598
    penicillin G *see* benzylpenicillin
    penicillin V *see* phenoxymethylpenicillin
    in skin infections 625-626
Pentacarinat see pentamidine
pentamidine 704-705
pentazocine 477
penthienate 270-271
Penthrane see methoxyflurane
pentobarbitone 578-580
    in cerebral oedema 857-858
pentosanpolysulfate 274
Pentothal see thiopentone
Pepcidine see famotidine
peppermint oil 312
peptic ulcer 302-303
Percodan see oxycodone
Pergalen see heparinoids
Pergonal see menotrophin
Periactin see cyproheptadine
pericyazine 555-559
perindopril 192-193
permethrin 630
perphenazine 555-559
Persantin see dipyridamole
Pertofran see desipramine
pethidine 474-475
    in critical care 858
    in labour 403, 475
petit mal seizures *see* absence seizures
petroleum jelly *see* soft paraffin
phaeochromocytoma 848
pharmacodynamics 4-17
    drug interactions 11
    geriatric 84
pharmacokinetics 20-33, 20f
    drug interactions 11-13
    geriatric 82-84
    paediatric 66
Pharmorubicin see epirubicin
phenelzine 153-154, 154t
    antidepressant 573-574
    in migraine 535-536
Phenergan see promethazine
phenindione 225-226
    in lactation 106t
pheniramine 313, 644-646
phenobarbitone 518-520
    in pregnancy 395-396
phenol 618, 634
phenolic disinfectants 901, 905

TO THE OWNER OF THIS BOOK

We are interested in your reaction to *Pharmacology and drug information for nurses*, fourth edition, by the Society of Hospital Pharmacists of Australia.

1. What was your reason for using this book?

    _____ university course _____ continuing education course
    _____ college course   _____ personal interest
    _____ TAFE course   _____ other (specify)

2. In which school are you enrolled? _____

3. Approximately how much of the book did you use?
    _____ 1/4   _____ 1/2   _____ 3/4   _____ all

4. What is the best aspect of the book?

5. Have you any suggestions for improvement?

6. Would more diagrams / illustrations help?

7. Is there any topic that should be added?

Fold here

- -

(Tape shut)

- -

REPLY PAID 5
The Acquisitions Editor
Harcourt Brace & Company, Australia
Locked Bag 16
MARRICKVILLE, NSW 2204